CATARACT SURGERY TODAY

The Best Cataract and Refractive IOL Articles
from *Cataract & Refractive Surgery Today*

Editor
David F. Chang, MD

BMC
BRYN MAWR COMMUNICATIONS LLC

ISBN: 978-0-615-29703-3

All articles published in this book were previously printed in *Cataract & Refractive Surgery Today* and are being reprinted with the express permission of the authors and Bryn Mawr Communications LLC, the publisher of *Cataract & Refractive Surgery Today* (hereafter, collectively "Bryn Mawr Communications LLC"). This publication is intended for health care professionals and providers only. All information contained in this publication, including but not limited to text, graphics, and images, is for informational purposes only, and is not intended to be a substitute for professional medical advice.

Although great care is taken by the Publisher and Editors to ensure that all information is accurate, it is recommended that readers seek independent verification of advice on drug or other product usage, surgical techniques, and clinical processes prior to their use. The opinions expressed in this publication are solely those of the authors and are not attributable to Bryn Mawr Communications LLC, the sponsors, the publication, or the Editorial Board. References made in articles may indicate uses of medical equipment or drugs at dosages, for periods of time, and in combinations not included in the current prescribing information.

Bryn Mawr Communications LLC makes no warranties or representations, express or implied, as to the accuracy or completeness, timeliness, or usefulness of any opinions, advice, services, or other information contained in this book.

Bryn Mawr Communications LLC shall not be liable for any direct, indirect, incidental, special, consequential, or exemplary damages, including without limitation, damages for any injury, loss of profits, goodwill, or other losses resulting from any use of the information contained in this book or any decision or action or non-action taken by you in reliance upon the information contained in this book.

Published by: Bryn Mawr Communications LLC
1008 Upper Gulph Road
Suite 200
Wayne, PA 19087 USA
Telephone: 484-581-1800
Fax: 484-581-1818
www.bmctoday.com
www.crstoday.com

Printed in Canada.

TABLE OF CONTENTS

TABLE OF CONTENTS

CAPSULORHEXIS AND HYDRODISSECTION

PHACO TECHNIQUE AND TECHNOLOGY

SECTION II: STRATEGIES FOR COMPLICATED CASES

MATURE CATARACTS

IFIS AND SMALL PUPILS

TRAUMA AND WEAK ZONULES

COMPLICATED CATARACTS AND COMORBIDITIES

SECTION III: COMPLICATIONS

OPERATIVE COMPLICATIONS

ENDOPHTHALMITIS PROPHYLAXIS

SECTION IV: INTRAOCULAR LENSES

Aspheric IOLs

COMPLICATIONS OF IOLs

ASTIGMATISM MANAGEMENT

REFRACTIVE IOLs

COMPLICATIONS OF PREMIUM IOLs

ACKNOWLEDGEMENTS & DEDICATION

This textbook is a compilation of 200 of the best cataract and IOL articles published in *Cataract & Refractive Surgery Today* during my 5-year tenure as co-chief medical editor. Together, they span a period of remarkable progress and change in our field. When *CRSToday* was launched in 2001, cataract and refractive surgeons occupied seemingly separate worlds with different types of practices and concerns. Back then, corneal topography and wavefront analysis were of as much interest to cataract surgeons as biometry and IOL formulas were to keratorefractive surgeons—which is to say very little. *CRSToday* was among the first publications to recognize the importance of integrating the education of cataract and refractive surgeons, and it was the vision of publisher David Cox to pair and focus on these two subspecialties in a single trade journal. The first annual *CRSToday* Refractive IOL Symposium in 2004, planned a year before the 2005 ruling by the Centers for Medicare & Medicaid Services (CMS), mirrored the journal by mixing cataract and refractive topics, faculty, and panel discussions. The seismic paradigm shift in our practices brought about by new refractive IOLs and the CMS ruling has validated *CRSToday*'s vision and mission. Now, more than ever, cataract and refractive surgeons need to learn from each other.

In an early editorial,[1] I outlined our desire at *CRSToday* to complement rather than replace the role of peer-reviewed journals. Our goal was to provide what I called the four C's of content: information that was current (timely), concise (summarizing), credible (evidence-based), and clinically relevant (practical). Although challenging for the editorial staff to manage, every other month we have devoted the issue to a special cover series focusing on an important topic in IOLs or cataract surgery. TASS, IFIS, CTRs, MICS—whatever the hot topic or acronym was—we assembled at least 10 different articles to cover it with unparalleled depth and balance in a single issue. This would not have been possible without the generous voluntary efforts of the several hundred authors who accepted our invitation to write original articles on all varieties of cataract-related topics. My job was easy—simply to select the topics and the individuals whose opinions I most wanted to read.

The editorial process has been akin to compiling a modular cataract textbook, which was published and updated in monthly installments. Indeed, in 2005 we created the first *Virtual Textbook of Cataract Surgery* on our Web site, www.crstoday.com, to provide international ophthalmologists with free online access to our cataract articles. This newly printed textbook is the result of my belief that this exceptional educational content merited publication as a stand-alone reference. My favorite cover focus was on the history of modern cataract surgery, which featured articles written by many of the key pioneers themselves. Published in March 2004, that issue included the last ophthalmology article written by Charles Kelman, MD,[2] along with numerous tributes to him[3] that he was able to read just months before he passed away. We have combined several of these historical articles together to provide the introduction to this textbook.

It has been an honor and a privilege to share the medical editorship of *CRSToday* with my friends and refractive counterparts, John F. Doane, MD, and Stephen G. Slade, MD. Their insight, imagination, and personalities have made this collaboration fun, and they have taught me a lot. All along, David Cox has been the charismatic leader who continues to inspire the innovation and creativity that so characterize *CRSToday* and its three sister publications. Vice President Adam Krafczek, Jr, and the rest of BMC Group work long hours but always manage to have fun in the process. Whether it is *CRSToday*'s Web site, Eyetube.net, a CME event or meeting, or a social reception, their trademark is a quality and first-class product. Finally, as mentioned, *CRSToday* publishes original articles written by ophthalmologists rather than by staff reporters conducting physician interviews. Although this greatly multiplies the amount of editing and deadlines to manage, Gillian McDermott and her editorial team are true professionals, and Gillian is the best editor with whom I have worked. Kudos and my personal thanks go to Sara Smith, Alicia Fagan, Julia T. Lewandowski, and, on *CRSToday Europe*, Laura Suarez. Finally, my thanks go to Jennifer Kreatsoulas for an exceptional job overseeing the layout and publication of this textbook.

In closing, I want to thank all of my friends in the cataract and refractive surgical teaching community for their support and their dedication to clinical research and education. Your voluntary contributions to *CRSToday* have been but one more example of your commitment to sharing your experience, wisdom, and enthusiasm with your colleagues. It is to those of you who regularly donate that most precious of assets—your time—toward educating others, that I dedicate this textbook. ■

Editor's Note: *Parts of this acknowledgement are excerpted from my November 2008 editorial in* CRSToday.[4]

David F. Chang, MD

1. Chang DF. My four cherished Cs of content. *Cataract & Refractive Surgery Today.* 2005;5(2):7. Available at: http://www.crstoday.com/PDF%20Articles/0205/Medpg.html. Accessed January 5, 2009.
2. Kelman CD. The genesis of phacoemulsification. *Cataract & Refractive Surgery Today.* 2004;4(3):57-59. Available at: http://www.crstoday.com/Old%20Archives/0304/crst0304%20art/crst0304_f3_kelman.pdf. Accessed January 5, 2009.
3. Dodick JM, Bechert CH, Gimbel HV, et al. Reflections on Charles Kelman and the early days of phaco. *Cataract & Refractive Surgery Today.* 2004;4(3):62-64. Available at: http://www.crstoday.com/Old%20Archives/0304/crst0304%20art/crst0304_f4_reflections.pdf. Accessed January 5, 2009.
4. Chang DF. Getting by with a little help from my friends. *Cataract & Refractive Surgery Today.* 2008;8(11):7. Available at: http://www.bmctoday.net/crstoday/2008/11/article.asp?f=CRST1108_Medpage.php. Accessed January 5, 2009.

ABOUT THE EDITOR

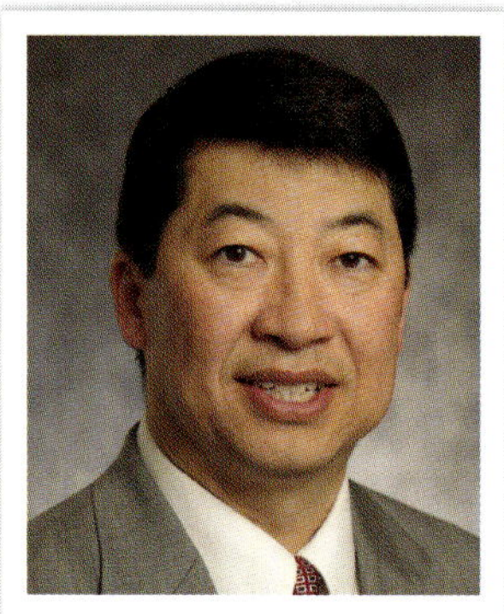

David F. Chang, MD, is a summa cum laude graduate of Harvard College and earned his medical degree at Harvard Medical School. He completed his ophthalmology residency at the University of California, San Francisco (UCSF), where he is now a Clinical Professor. He is also an Adjunct Professor of Ophthalmology at the Chinese University in Hong Kong. Dr. Chang is serving a 5-year term as chair of the American Academy of Ophthalmology (AAO) Annual Meeting Program Committee, having previously chaired the Cataract Program Subcommittee. He organized and was the program co-chair for the first eight AAO "Spotlight on Cataracts" symposia. He is also on the program committees for the American Society of Cataract and Refractive Surgery (ASCRS) Annual Meeting and the *Ocular Surgery News* (*OSN*)/Vindico Hawaiian Eye Meeting.

Having chaired the ASCRS Cataract Clinical Committee, Dr. Chang joined the ASCRS Executive Committee in 2009 and will eventually serve as president. He chairs the AAO Cataract Preferred Practice Pattern Panel, and is the immediate past Chair of the AAO Practicing Ophthalmologists' Curriculum Panel for Cataract and Anterior Segment, which developed the American Board of Ophthalmology (ABO) knowledge base for the Maintenance of Certification (MOC) examination. Dr. Chang serves on the medical advisory board of two global humanitarian organizations, Himalayan Cataract Project and Project Vision. He is also on the Board of Directors for the Pan American Association of Ophthalmology and is the current president of the Cordes Society (UCSF ophthalmology alumni society).

In addition to the AAO Achievement and Senior Achievement awards, Dr. Chang is a four-time AAO Secretariat Award recipient (2003, 2006, 2007, and 2009). He was the inaugural recipient of the UCSF Department of Ophthalmology's Distinguished Alumni Award (2005). In 2006 he became only the third ophthalmologist to ever receive the Charlotte Baer Award honoring the outstanding clinical faculty member at the UCSF Medical School. Dr. Chang was the third recipient of the Strampelli Medal from the Italian Ophthalmological Society (2007). He is the 2009 Binkhorst Medal Lecturer (ASCRS) and 2009 Lim Lecturer at the Asia Pacific Association of Cataract & Refractive Surgery (APACRS) Meeting.

Dr. Chang has been selected to deliver the following named lectures: Transamerica Lecture (UCSF), Williams Lecture (UCSF), Wolfe Lecture (University of Iowa), DeVoe Lecture (Columbia-Harkness), Gettes Lecture (Wills Eye Hospital), Helen Keller Lecture (University of Alabama), Kayes Lecture (University of Washington, St. Louis), Thorpe Lecture (Pittsburgh Ophthalmology Society), Schutz Lecture (New York University Medical Center), Wallace-Evan Lecture (Casey Eye, Oregon), Kambara Lecture (Loma Linda), Jules Stein Lecture (UCLA-Jules Stein), Proctor Lecture (UCSF/Proctor Foundation), and keynote lectures at the Indian Intraocular Implant & Refractive Society Annual Meeting, Argentinean Society of Ophthalmology Annual Meeting, and the Chinese American Ophthalmological Society's 20th anniversary meeting. He is on the scientific advisory board for the UCSF Collaborative Vision Research Group, American Medical Optics, Allergan ATLAS, Calhoun Vision, Medennium, Peak Surgical, and Visiogen, and is the medical monitor for the Visiogen Synchrony accommodating IOL FDA monitored trial.

Dr. Chang served for 5 years as co-chief Medical Editor for *Cataract & Refractive Surgery Today* and was the Cataract Editor for two online educational sites: the AAO's "Specialty Clinical Updates" and the *OSN* "Ophthalmic Hyperguides." He is the editor of *Mastering Refractive IOLs — the Art and Science* (Slack 2008) and *Curbside Consultation in Cataract Surgery* (Slack 2007), the series editor for all seven *Slack Curbside Consultation Ophthalmology* textbooks, and the principal author of *Phaco Chop* (Slack 2004). His co-authored 2005 study on intraoperative floppy iris syndrome (IFIS) and tamsulosin is one of the five most cited papers from the *Journal of Cataract and Refractive Surgery* (Source: *Editorial, JCRS 1/08*).

CONTRIBUTING AUTHORS

Iqbal Ike K. Ahmed, MD, FRCSC
Assistant Professor
University of Toronto, Ontario
Clinical Assistant Professor
University of Utah
Salt Lake City, UT

Everett Ai, MD
Director
California Pacific Medical Center
San Francisco, CA

Leonardo Akaishi, MD
Hospital Opthalmologic of Brasilia
Brasilia, Brazil

Ricardo Alarcon, MD
Servioftalmos
Bogotá, Colombia

David Allen, BSc, FRCS, FRCOphth
Consultant Ophthalmologist
Sunderland Eye Infirmary
Sunderland, England

Omar Almallah, MD
Susskind & Almallah Eye Associates
Toms River, NJ

David J. Apple, MD
Professor
John Moran Eye Center
Salt Lake City, UT

Lisa Brothers Arbisser, MD
Eye Surgeons Associates, PC
Iowa and Illinois Quad Cities
Adjunct Associate Clinical Professor
John Moran Eye Center
Salt Lake City, UT

Priscilla Perry Arnold, MD
Chair, Government Relations
ASCRS

Steve A. Arshinoff, MD, FRCSC
Lecturer, University of Toronto
Toronto, Ontario, Canada
Clinical Adjunct Assistant Professor
McMaster University
Hamilton, Ontario, Canada

Pablo Artal, PhD
Laboratorio de Optica
Centro de Investigacion
en Optica y Nanofisica (CiOyN)
Universidad de Murica
Campus de Espinardo
Murcia, Spain

Ehud I. Assia, MD
Associate Professor
Sackler Faculty of Medicine
Tel Aviv University
Tel Aviv, Isreal
Director, Department of Ophthalmology
Meir Medical Center
Kfar Saba, Israel

Kerry Assil, MD
CEO and Medical Director
Assil Eye Institute
Beverly Hills, CA

Brock K. Bakewell, MD, FACS
Clinical Assistant Professor
University of Utah
Salt Lake City, UT
Codirector
Fishkind, Bakewell, Maltzman Eye Care
and Surgery Center
Tucson, AZ

Peter Barry, FRCS
Consultant Ophthalmic Surgeon
Royal Victoria Eye and Ear
St. Vincent's University Hospitals
Dublin, Ireland

Thomas L. Beardsley, MD
Asheville Eye Associates
Asheville, NC

Ashley Behrens, MD
Assistant Professor
Wilmer Eye Institute
Baltimore, MD

George Beiko, BM, BCh, FRCSC
Lecturer, University of Toronto
Toronto, Ontario, Canada
Assistant Professor
McMaster University, Ontario
Hamilton, Ontario, Canada

Robert Bellucci, MD
Chief of the Hospital Ophthalmic Unit
Hospital and University of Verona
Verona, Italy

Stanley J. Berke, MD
Associate Clinical Professor
Albert Einstein College of Medicine
New York, NY
Chief, Glaucoma Service
Nassau University Medical Center
East Meadow, NY
Founding Partner
Ophthalmic Consultants of Long Island
Lynbrook, NY

Victor Bohórquez, MD
Servioftalmos
Bogotá, Colombia

Rosa Braga-Mele, MEd, MD, FRCSC
Associate Professor
University of Toronto
Director of Cataract Unit and Surgical Teaching
Mount Sinai Hospital
Toronto, Ontario, Canada

Richard E. Braunstein, MD
Associate Professor
Edward S. Harkness Eye Institute of
Columbia University Medical Center
New York, NY

Frank A. Bucci Jr, MD
Medical Director
Bucci Laser Vision Institute
and Ambulatory Surgery Center
Wilkes Barre, PA

Scott E. Burk, MD, PhD
Clinical Ophthalmologist
Cincinnati Eye Institute and
Volunteer Faculty
University of Cincinnati
Cincinnati, OH

Carlos Buznego, MD
President and Anterior Segment Surgeon
Center for Excellence in Eye Care
Voluntary Assistant Professor
Bascom Palmer Eye Institute
Miami, FL

Stephen Bylsma, MD
Assistant Clinical Instructor
University of California Los Angeles
Los Angeles, CA
Private Practice
Santa Maria, CA

Herve M. Byron, MD
Clinical Professor
New York University Medical Center
New York, NY

Jennifer Calafati, MD
University of Toronto
Toronto, Ontario, Canada

Louis Catania, OD
Senior Refractive Consultant
Nicolitz Eye Consultants
Jacksonville, FL

Lenka Champion, MD
Nicolitz Eye Consultants
Jacksonville, FL

Jonathan D. Christenbury, MD
Medical Director
Christenbury Eye Center
Charlotte, NC

Y. Ralph Chu, MD
Founder and Medical Director
Chu Vision Institute
Edina, MN
Adjunct Associate Professor
University of Minnesota
Minneapolis, MN
Clinical Professor
John Moran Eye Center
Salt Lake City, UT

Robert J. Cionni, MD
Medical Director
The Eye Institute
Salt Lake City, UT

Susan Clouser, RN, MSN, CRNO
Staff Nurse
Healthsouth Surgery Center of Dallas
Dallas, TX

Christopher S. Connor, MD
Associate Clinical Professor
Dartmouth Medical School
Hanover, NH

D. Michael Colvard, MD
Assistant Clinical Professor
Keck School of Medicine
University of Southern California Los Angeles
Los Angeles, CA
Director, Colvard Eye Center
Encino, CA

Garry P. Condon, MD
Associate Professor
Drexel University College of Medicine
Pittsburgh, PA

Minas Coroneo, MD, MS, MSc, FRACS, FRANZCO
Director, Ophthalmic Surgeons
Sydney Biotech
Sydney, Australia

Alan S. Crandall, MD
Professor and Senior Vice Chair of Ophthalmology and Visual Sciences
Director of Glaucoma and Cataract
John A. Moran Eye Center
Salt Lake City, UT

Daniel G. Dawson, MD
Bascom Palmer Eye Institute
University of Miami Miller School of Medicine
Miami, FL

Elizabeth A. Davis, MD
Adjunct Clinical Assistant Professor
University of Minnesota
Minneapolis, MN
Director, Minnesota Eye Laser and Surgery Center
Minnesota Eye Consultants
Bloomington, MN

James A. Davison, MD, FACS
President, Wolfe Eye Clinic
Marshalltown, IA

Andrea P. DaMata, MD
Cincinnati Eye Institute
Cincinnati, OH

Steven J. Dell, MD
Director of Refractive and Corneal Surgery
Texan Eye and Dell Laser Consultants
Austin, TX

Uday Devgan, MD
Maloney Vision Institute
Associate Clinical Professor
University of California Los Angeles
Los Angeles, CA

Terence M. Devine, MD
Chief of Ophthalmology
The Guthrie Clinic
Sayre, PA

Steven Dewey, MD
Colorado Springs Health Partners
Colorado Springs, CO

Deepinder K. Dhaliwal, MD
Associate Professor
University of Pittsburgh School of Medicine (UPMC)
Director, Cornea and Refractive Surgery Services
Director and Founder, Center for Integrative Eye Care
Director, UPMC Laser/Aesthetic Center
UPMC Eye Center
Pittsburgh, PA

H. Burkhard Dick, MD
Professor, Chairman, and Director
Center for Vision Science
Ruhr University Eye Hospital
Bochum, Germany

David M. Dillman, MD
Medical Director
Dillman Eye Care Associates
Danville, IL

John F. Doane, MD
Discover Vision Centers
Kansas City, MO
Clinical Assistant Professor
Kansas University Medical Center
Lawrence, KS

Eric D. Donnenfeld, MD
Ophthalmic Consultants of Long Island
Long Island, NY
Clinical Professor
New York University
New York, NY
Trustee, Dartmouth Medical School
Hanover, NH

Paul J. Dougherty, MD
Clinical Instructor
Jules Stein Eye Institute
University of California Los Angeles
Los Angeles, CA
Medical Director
Dougherty Laser Vision Institute
Camarillo, CA

Henry F. Edelhauser, PhD
Professor and Director of Ophthalmic Research
Emory University School of Medicine
Atlanta, GA

Paul H. Ernest, MD
Associate Clinical Professor
Kresge Eye Institute
Detroit, MI

I. Howard Fine, MD
Clinical Professor
Oregon Health & Science University
Portland, OR
Drs. Fine, Hoffman & Packer, LLC
Eugene, OR

William J. Fishkind, MD, FACS
Clinical Professor
University of Utah
Co-Director of Fishkind, Bakewell, Maltzman Eye Care and Surgery Center
Tucson, AZ

Luther L. Fry, MD
Fry Eye Associates, PA
Garden City, KS
Clinical Assistant Professor
University of Kansas Medical Center
Kansas City, MO

Devarshi U. Gajjar, PhD
Iladevi Cataract & IOL Research Centre
Raghudeep Eye Clinic
Memnagar, Ahmedabad, India

Johnny L. Gayton, MD, MD, FSEE
Founder and CEO, Eyesight Associates
Warner Robins, GA
Adjunct Clinical Professor
Mercer Medical School
Macon, GA

Adrian Glasser, PhD
Associate Professor
University of Houston
Houston, TX

James P. Gills, MD
Founder and Director
St. Luke's Cataract & Laser Institute
Tarpon Springs, FL

Howard V. Gimbel, MD
Professor and Chairman
Loma Linda University
Loma Linda, CA
Medical Director and Senior Surgeon
Gimbel Eye Center
Calgary, Alberta, Canada

Todd Gothard, MD
Wolfe Eye Clinic
Cedar Rapids, IA

D. Rex Hamilton, MD, MS
Assistant Professor
Jules Stein Eye Institute
Medical Director
University of California Los Angeles Laser Refractive Center
Los Angeles, CA

Dennis P. Han, MD
Professor
Medical College of Wisconsin
Milwaukee, WI

Jeffrey S. Heier, MD
Clinical Instructor
Harvard Medical School
Ophthalmic Consultants of Boston
Boston, MA

Bonnie Henderson, MD
Ophthalmic Consultants of Boston
Assistant Clinical Professor
Harvard Medical School
Boston, MA

Warren E. Hill, MD
Private practice
Mesa, AZ

Richard S. Hoffmann, MD
Clinical Associate Professor
Oregon Health & Science University
Portland, OR
Drs. Fine, Hoffmann, and Packer, LLC
Eugene, OR

Jack T. Holladay, MD, MSEE, FACS
Clinical Professor
Baylor College of Medicine
Houston, TX
President, Holladay LASIK Institute
Bellaire, TX

Simon Holland, MB, FRCSC
University of British Columbia
Pacific Laser Eye Centre
Vancouver, British Columbia, Canada

Suber S. Huang, MD, MBA
Professor and Vice Chairman
Case Western Reserve University
Director, Vitreoretinal Diseases and Surgery
University Hospitals of Cleveland
Cleveland, OH

John D. Hunkeler, MD
Founder and Medical Director
Hunkeler Eye Institute
Overland Park, KS
Chairman, Department of Ophthalmology
University of Kansas School of Medicine
Kansas City, KS

David G. Hwang, MD
Professor
Director, Cornea Service
University of California San Francisco
San Francisco, CA

J. Michael Jumper, MD
Retina Service Chief
California Pacific Medical Center
West Coast Retina Medical Group
San Francisco, CA

Thomas Kasper, MD
Johann Wolfgang Goethe-University
Frankfurt, Germany

Charles D. Kelman, MD (Deceased)
Clinical Professor
New York Medical College
New York Eye and Ear Infirmary
Manhattan Eye, Ear and Throat Hospital
New York, NY

Bhairavi V. Kharod, MD
Duke University Eye Center
Durham, NC

Terry Kim, MD
Associate Professor
Duke University Eye Center
Durham, NC

Thomas Kohnen, MD
Professor and Deputy Chairman
Johann Wolfgang Goethe-University Clinic
Frankfurt, Germany
Visiting Professor
Baylor College of Medicine
Houston, TX

Gregg T. Kokame, MD
Associate Clinical Professor
University of Hawaii
Honolulu, HI

Manus C. Kraff, MD
Kraff Eye Institute
Chicago, IL

Robert Kaufer, MD
Medical Director
Kaufer Clinica de Ojos
Buenos Aires, Argentina

Judy E. Kim, MD
Associate Professor
Medical College of Wisconsin
Milwaukee, WI

Michael C. Knorz, MD
Professor
University of Heidelberg
Medical Faculty Mannheim
Medical Director
FreeVis LASIK Centre
Mannheim, Germany

Douglas D. Koch, MD
Professor
Allen, Mosbacher, and Law Chair in Ophthalmology
Baylor College of Medicine
Houston, TX

Richard P. Kratz, MD, DSci
Clinical Professor
University of California
Irvine, CA

Baruch D. Kuppermann, MD, PhD
Chief of Retina Service
University of California
Irvine, CA

Stephen S. Lane, MD
Adjunct Clinical Professor
University of Minnesota
Stillwater, MN

Richard A. Lewis, MD
Consultant, Glaucoma
Sacramento, CA

Brian Little, FRCS, FRCOphth, FHEA
Consultant Ophthalmologist
Honorary Senior Lecturer
Royal Free Hospital NHS Trust
London, United Kingdom

Christopher Liu, FRCOphth
Consultant Ophthalmic Surgeon
Sussex Eye Hospital
Honorary Clinical Senior Lecturer
Brighton and Sussex Medical School
Brighton, United Kingdom
Director, Tongdean Eye Clinic
Hove, United Kingdom

Richard L. Lindstrom, MD
Founder and Attending Surgeon
Minnesota Eye Consultants
Adjunct Professor Emeritus
University of Minnesota
Minneapolis, MN

Dwayne K. Logan, MD
CEO, Atlantis Eyecare
Anaheim, CA

Boris Malyugin, MD, PhD
Chief of the Department of
Cataract and Implant Surgery
Deputy Director General
S. Fyodorov Eye Microsurgery Complex
Moscow, Russia

Francis S. Mah, MD
Assistant Professor, Medical Director
The Charles T. Campbell Ophthalmic
Microbiology Laboratory
University of Pittsburgh
School of Medicine
Pittsburgh, PA

William F. Maloney, MD
Director
Maloney Eye Center
Vista, CA
Associate Clinical Professor
University of California Irvine
Irvine, CA

Nick Mamalis, MD
Professor of Ophthalmology
John Moran Eye Center
Salt Lake City, UT

Lisa Martén, MD
South Texas Eye Institute
San Antonio, TX

Samuel Masket, MD
Private practice
Century City, CA
Clinical Professor
David Geffen School of Medicine
University of California Los Angeles
Jules Stein Eye Institute
Los Angeles, CA

Daniela M. Marques, MD
Medical Director
Marques Eye Institute
São Paulo, Brazil

Frederico F. Marques, MD
Medical Director
Marques Eye Institute
São Paulo, Brazil

Thomas R. Mazzocco, MD (Retired)
Valley Eye Center
Van Nuys, CA
Professor
University of California San Francisco
San Francisco, CA

J.E. "Jay" McDonald II, MD
McDonald Eye Associates
Fayetteville, AR

H. Richard McDonald, MD
California Pacific Medical Center
Associate Clinical Professor
University of California San Francisco
San Francisco, CA

Erik L. Mertens, MD, FEBOphth
Medical Director
Antwerp Eye Center
Antwerp, Belgium

Marc Michelson, MD
Clinical Professor
University of Alabama at Birmingham
Medical Center
Birmingham, AL

David Mills, MD
Nicolitz Eye Consultants
Jacksonville, FL

Daniel M. Miller, MD, PhD
Voluntary Assistant Professor
University of Cincinnati
Cincinnati, OH

Kevin M. Miller, MD
Kolokotrones Professor of Clinical
Ophthalmology
Jules Stein Eye Institute
David Geffen School of Medicine
University of California Los Angeles
Los Angeles, CA

Kensaku Miyake, MD
Director and Head
Shohzankai Medical Foundation
Miyake Eye Hospital
Nagoya, Japan

Satish Modi, MD, FRCSC
Assistant Clinical Professor
Albert Einstein College of Medicine
Bronx, NY
Seeta Eye Centers
Poughkeepsie and Fishkill, NY

Douglas Morck, DVM, PhD
University of Calgary
Alberta, Canada

Raja Narayanan, MD
Clinical Instructor
University of California Irvine
Irvine, CA

Ayman Naseri, MD
Assistant Professor
University of California San Francisco
Chief of the Department of Ophthalmology
San Francisco VA Medical Center
San Francisco, CA

Robert B. Nelson, PA-C
Executive Director
Island Eye Surgicenter
Carle Place, NY

Nastasia Nianiaris

Louis D. "Skip" Nichamin, MD
Medical Director
Laurel Eye Clinic
Brookville, PA

Ernst Nicolitz, MD
Nicolitz Eye Consultants
Jacksonville, FL

Terrence P. O'Brien, MD
Professor
Bascom Palmer Eye Institute
University of Miami Miller School of Medicine
Palm Beach Gardens, FL

Randall J. Olson, MD
The John A. Moran Presidential Professor and
Chair of Ophthalmology
CEO, John A. Moran Eye Center
Salt Lake City, UT

James M. Osher, MS
University of Cincinnati College of Medicine
Cincinnati, OH

Robert H. Osher, MD
Medical Director Emeritus
Cincinnati Eye Institute
Professor
University of Cincinnati College of Medicine
Cincinnati, OH

Richard Packard, MD, FRCS, FRCOphth
Consultant Ophthalmic Surgeon
Prince Charles Eye Unit
Windsor, United Kingdom

Mark Packer, MD
Clinical Associate Professor
Casey Eye Institute
Portland, OR
Drs. Fine, Hoffman, & Packer
Eugene, OR

Deepak Pandita, MS
Iladevi Cataract & IOL Research Center
Raghudeep Eye Clinic
Memnagar, Ahmedabad, India

Rahul Patel, MD
Dean A. McGee Eye Institute
Oklahoma City, OK

Adolfo Pena, MD
Ruhr University Eye Hospital
Bochum, Germany

Jay S. Pepose, MD, PhD
Professor of Clinical Ophthalmology and Visual
Sciences
Washington University School of Medicine
Director, Pepose Vision Institute
St. Louis, MO

Lillian Roth Pontacolone, RN, CNOR
Director of Nursing, Quality Assurance
Island Eye Surgicenter
Carle Place, NY

John W. Potter, OD, FAAO
Vice President, Patient Services
TLC Laser Eye Centers
Dallas, TX

Mamidipudi R. Praveen, DOMS
Iladevi Cataract & IOL Research Center
Raghudeep Eye Clinic
Memnagar, Ahmedabad, India

Michael Raizman, MD
Associate Professor
Tufts University School of Medicine
Boston, MA

Shetal M. Raj, MBBS, MS
Iladevi Cataract & IOL Research Center
Raghudeep Eye Clinic
Memnagar, Ahmedabad, India

Tal Raviv, MD, FACS
Assistant Professor, New York Medical College
Valhalla, NY
New York Eye and Ear Infirmary
New York, NY

El-Karim Rhemtulla, MD, FRCSC
Private practice
St. Catherines, Ontario, Canada

Gerald J. Roper, MD
Roper Advanced Eye Care
Batesville, IN

Kenneth J. Rosenthal, MD, FACS
Surgical Director, Rosenthal Eye
and Facial Plastic Surgery
Great Neck, NY
Associate Professor
John A. Moran Eye Center
Salt Lake City, UT

Thomas W. Samuelson, MD
Minnesota Eye Consultants, PA
Clinical Associate Professor
University of Minnesota
Minneapolis, MN

Edwin J. Sarver, PhD
President, Sarver and Associates, Inc.
Carbondale, IL

Paul Sanghera, MD
Lecturer, University of Toronto
Toronto, Ontario, Canada

Tina A. Scheufele, MD
New England Eye Center
Tufts-New England Medical Center
Boston, MA

Daniel M. Schwartz, MD
Shirley Reich Chair of Ophthalmology
Director Retina Service
University of California San Francisco
San Francisco, CA

Gary S. Schwartz, MD
Associated Eye Care
St. Paul, MN

Barry Seibel, MD
Clinical Assistant Professor
University of California Los Angeles
Los Angeles, CA

Donald N. Serafano, MD
Clinical Associate Professor
University of Southern California Los Angeles
Los Angeles, CA

Steven P. Shearing, MD (Retired)
Shearing Eye Institute
Las Vegas, NV

Bradford J. Shingleton, MD
Ophthalmic Consultants of Boston
Assistant Clinical Professor
Harvard Medical School
Boston, MA

Anurag Shrivastava, MD
Stanford University
Stanford, CA

Jack A. Singer, MD
Singer Eye Center
Randolph, VT

Kuldev Singh, MD, MPH
Professor
Director, Glaucoma Service
Stanford University
Stanford, CA

Joel K. Shugar, MD, MSEE (Deceased)
Medical Director
Nature Coast EyeCare Institute
Perry, FL

Robert M. Sinskey, MD
Clinical Professor
Jules Stein Eye Institute
Los Angeles, CA
Medical Director Emeritus
Southern California Lions Eye Institute
Costa Mesa, CA

Roger F. Steinert, MD
Vice Chair of Clinical Ophthalmology
Director of Cataract, Refractive,
and Corneal Surgery
University of California Irvine
Irvine, CA

Michael E. Snyder, MD
Voluntary Assistant Clinical Professor
Cincinnati Eye Institute
Cincinnati, OH

Tracy Swartz, OD, MS
Adjunct Faculty
Indiana University School of Optometry
Bloomington, IN

Christopher N. Ta, MD
Associate Professor and
Director of Residency Program
Stanford University School of Medicine
Stanford, CA

Mehran Taban, MD
Cole Eye Institute
Cleveland Clinic Foundation
Cleveland, OH

Juan Tabernero, MSc
Laboratorio de Óptica
Universidad de Murcia
Murcia, Spain

Diamond Y. Tam, MD
University of Toronto
Toronto, Ontario, Canada

Audrey Talley-Rostov, MD
Northwest Eye Surgeons
Seattle, WA

Manfred R. Tetz, MD
Professor and Director
Eye-Center-Spreebogen
Berlin, Germany

William B. Trattler, MD
Director of Cornea
Center for Excellence in Eye Care
Voluntary Assistant Professor
Bascom Palmer Eye Institute
Miami, FL

Abhay R. Vasavada, MS, FRCS
Director, Iladevi Cataract & IOL Research Centre
Raghudeep Eye Clinic
Memnagar, Ahmedabad, India

Li Wang, MD, PhD
Cullen Eye Institute
Houston, TX

Ming Wang, MD, PhD
Medical Director of Refractive Surgery
Aier Eye Hospital System
Shanghai, China
Clinical Associate Professor
University of Tennessee
Memphis, TN
Director, Wang Vision Institute
Saint Thomas Hospital
Nashville, TN

Bruce Wallace III, MD
Medical Director
Wallace Eye Surgery
Alexandria, LA
Clinical Professor
Louisiana State University School of Medicine
New Orleans, LA
Assistant Clinical Professor
Tulane School of Medicine
Tulane, LA

Liliana Werner, MD, PhD
Research Associate Professor
John A. Moran Eye Center
Salt Lake City, UT
Director of Preclinical Research
Berlin Eye Research Institute
Berlin, Germany

John R. Wittpenn, Jr, MD
Associate Clinical Professor
State University of New York at Stony Brook
Ophthalmic Consultants of Long Island
Stony Brook, NY

Michael Y. Wong, MD
Clinical Instructor
Robert Wood Johnson Medical School
New Brunswick, NJ
Medical Director
Wills Eye Laser
Princeton, NJ

J. Trevor Woodhams, MD
Surgical Director
Woodhams Eye Clinic
Atlanta, GA

Sam S. Yang, MD
California Pacific Medical Center
San Francisco, CA

Peter A. Zakrzewski, MD
University of British Columbia
Vancouver, British Columbia, Canada

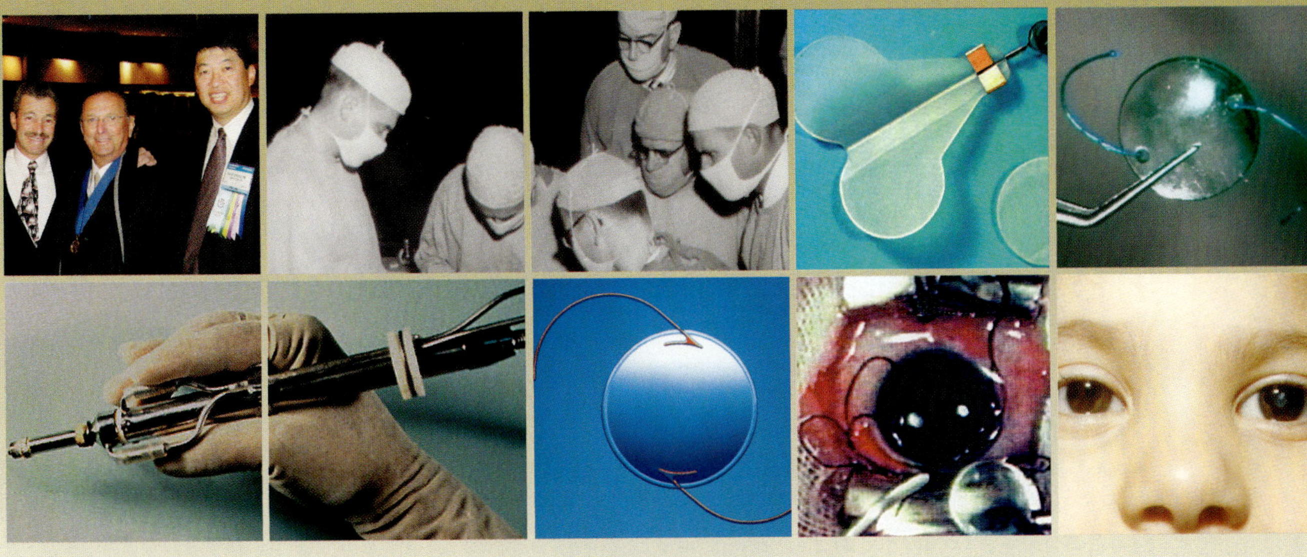

THE HISTORY OF MODERN CATARACT SURGERY

A Historical Look Back: Honoring Those With the "Right Stuff"

DAVID F. CHANG, MD

At its 2003 annual meeting held in Anaheim, California, the AAO hosted a special spotlight session to honor Charles Kelman, MD, one of three inaugural recipients of the newly established AAO Laureate Award. There was palpable excitement for this special first-time event, and Dr. Kelman's address captivated an overcapacity crowd. Afterward, past and present-day innovators followed Dr. Kelman's speech with thoughtful presentations on the history and future of phacoemulsification. As I sat in the audience, I could not help but feel some regret that so many other ophthalmologists were missing a unique and moving tribute to a figure who is arguably ophthalmology's most important living legend. For those present that evening, it was an unforgettable opportunity to pause and reflect upon what an extraordinary success story we are all blessed to be a part of. It was these sentiments that inspired this month's cover focus.

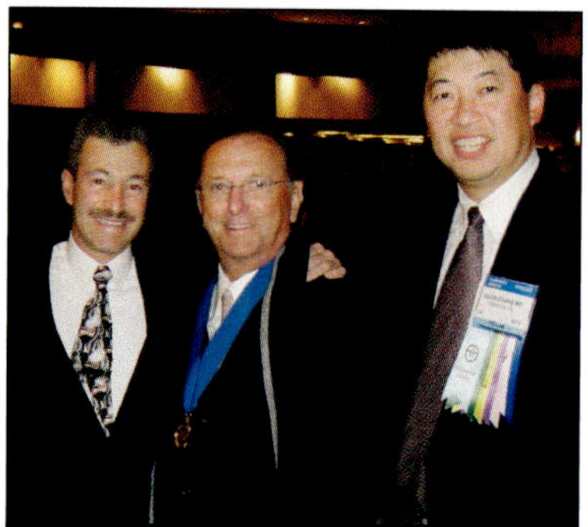

Charles Kelman, MD, (center) with Dr. Chang and *CRSToday* editorial board member Robert Osher, MD, (left) at the AAO tribute.

Modern cataract surgery has restored vision to more people than any other single operation. However, beyond just volume, it has been our collective progress in the technology and techniques initially conceived of by Sir Harold Ridley and Dr. Kelman that has made this one of the most important achievements in the history of medicine. Today, we are privileged not only to perform this miraculous operation on a routine basis, but also to be able to hear firsthand accounts of the origins of phacoemulsification and IOLs from so many of the pioneers themselves—a list that includes Dr. Kelman; Steven Shearing, MD; Thomas Mazzocco, MD; Richard Kratz, MD; Robert Sinskey, MD; and (until recently) Sir Harold. Like our first astronauts, these individuals had the curiosity and courage to test the accepted limits of and explore the uncharted territory in their field. Through their stories, we can appreciate their accomplishments and perhaps better understand what gave these individuals such determination to innovate and succeed—in other words, "the right stuff."

Like so many surgeons, I have been inspired by several of these ophthalmic giants on a personal level. Dr. Kelman was indirectly responsible for my career choice. I was first drawn to ophthalmology when I saw a 35-mm film of phacoemulsification as a medical student in 1978. Ironically, I am now on the faculty of Dr. Kelman's AAO and ASCRS phacoemulsification courses. I fulfilled my residency at the University of California San Francisco, which counted Dr. Shearing among its former residents and Dr. Mazzocco among its clinical faculty. By studying a videotape of Dr. Mazzocco performing phacoemulsification, I learned the Kratz iris-plane phaco technique as a second-year resident in 1983. Finally, it is a tribute to the humility of each of these individuals that it took some serious arm-twisting to coax them to write pieces for this issue.

At *Cataract & Refractive Surgery Today*, we would like to salute the pioneers of cataract surgery with this minifocus. In presenting their firsthand accounts, we hope that their spirit and commitment to innovation will further inspire all who have the privilege of following in their footsteps. Continually striving to improve lens replacement surgery—whether by pursuing newer techniques and technology or by simply improving our individual surgical skills—is the most fitting way for us to honor the vision, courage, and determination of these early leaders. ■

This editorial originally appeared in the March 2004 issue of CRSToday.

Flashback

HERVE M. BYRON, MD

In August 1960, I performed my first cataract extraction on a private patient at the New York Eye and Ear Infirmary. He had been admitted the previous night for the trimming of his eyelashes and irrigation of the nasolacrimal sac on his cataractous eye. That morning, the patient was brought into the OR on a stretcher and moved to the operating table.

After performing a sterile prep and drape, a modified Atkinson akinesia, and a retrobulbar injection of anesthesia, I started the procedure while standing and wearing a 3X loupe. I entered the anterior chamber with a keratome. After placing a 6–0 black silk suture at the superior limbus, I enlarged the incision to 160° with Castroviejo corneal-scleral scissors and made a small peripheral iridectomy at the base of the iris. The cataract was then tumbled out of the globe intracapsularly with a Castroviejo crossaction lens forceps. I injected Miochol-E (Novartis Ophthalmics, Inc., Duluth, GA) into the anterior chamber to constrict the pupil and maintain the integrity of the vitreous behind the iris. I used several 6–0 black silk sutures on Grieshaber needles to close the incision. Next, I placed an antibiotic ointment in the inferior cul de sac, closed the eyelids, and placed a slightly moist eye pad and metal shield over the patient's eye to protect it.

The patient was then carefully moved back to a stretcher and returned to the hospital room, which was already darkened for his visual comfort. He was kept on absolute bed rest for 72 hours before being allowed bathroom privileges with the assistance of a nurse. No bending, lifting, or walking was permitted for the first 5 to 7 postoperative days. I visited the patient in the hospital each day to examine his operated eye and change the dressing.

If no operative complications occurred, patients were discharged between the 8th and 10th postoperative days with their operated eye still covered and instructions to come to my office on the following day. Thereafter, postoperative visits were scheduled weekly for 4 to 6 weeks, during which time the operated eye remained covered with a pad and shield. Sometime between the fourth and sixth visits, if the eye were healing satisfactorily, the patient was fitted with temporary, unsightly aphakic spectacles. He was still prohibited from bending, lifting, or performing any strenuous exercise, including sex.

Finally, by the eighth postoperative week, the eye was usually completely healed. The patient would undergo a final refraction and receive a prescription for aphakic spectacles. No further eye drops or cover was necessary, and the patient could return to work and resume all normal activities. Many patients complained that they had little peripheral vision and that they had difficulty with depth perception and fusion using their aphakic spectacles.

Some of you younger ophthalmologists will think this scenario bogus, because you cannot believe that, only 45 years ago, cataract surgery was so primitive. That was the reality, however.

This ongoing column will celebrate the principal characters in the most dynamic and glorious journey in the history of eye surgery. As a former flight surgeon in the Air Force, I can compare our mission with the one to conquer outer space. The evolution of contemporary cataract surgery involved overcoming many professional and governmental obstacles through the creative genius and tenacity of many true pioneers. Consider how cataract patients are treated today in your OR, and you will appreciate what we have accomplished in the past 45 years. We are now space-walking in the OR. All of your comments and feedback are deeply appreciated. ■

This article originally appeared in the August 2005 issue of CRSToday.

A History of Modern Cataract Surgery

ROBERT M. SINSKEY, MD

Cataract surgery began around 800 BC, when couching was the procedure of choice. In the 1700s, Jacques Daviel published the first account of a cataract extraction through a limbal incision. Anesthesia for cataract surgery did not exist until the late 1800s when topical cocaine was introduced. Walter Atkinson, MD, made the procedure for local anesthesia easier with the invention of his retrobulbar needle. Aspects of these surgical practices remained when I was a fellow, but great changes were on the horizon.

THE 1950s

In 1951, I traveled to Japan to examine the survivors of the atomic bomb for radiation effects on the eyes. I visited the Red Cross hospital in Hiroshima where ophthalmologists were performing extracapsular cataract extraction on mature cataracts under topical anesthesia (cocaine drops). Surgeons created a 180° corneal section, stripped off the anterior capsule with a toothed forceps, expressed the nucleus, washed out the cortex, and then replaced the cornea. No sutures were used. Both of the patient's eyes were covered (Figure 1), and he had to lie flat on his back, without bathroom privileges, for 10 days. The complication rates were horrendous.

In 1954, I was chief resident at Duke University in Durham, North Carolina. I performed intracapsular cataract extraction with retrobulbar anesthesia and three corneal-scleral, 6–0, black, silk track sutures (Figure 2). Only the operated eye was patched, and the sutures, which felt like rope in the eye, remained in place for 4 to 6 weeks. After recovering from surgery, patients had to wear thick glasses. Although the surgery itself was relatively painless, the postoperative course was onerous. Patients were bedridden for 5 days and were not permitted to bend over or lift anything for an additional 6 weeks. In addition, they wore Coke-bottle cataract glasses. As a result, people postponed surgery until they could no longer see well enough to get around.

THE EARLY IOLs

In 1949, Sir Harold Ridley had introduced the IOL. High complication rates resulted from the insertion of these crudely made lenses, which came loose in time when the nylon loops dissolved (Figure 3). Consequently, two kinds of surgeons evolved in England in the 1950s and 1960s: (1) those who put IOLs in and (2) those who took them out.

In the late 1960s, Cornelius Binkhorst, MD, developed four- and two-loop, iris- and capsule-supported IOLs that had a much improved complication rate. His innovation renewed the interest of intraocular surgeons in the US and Europe. Turgot Hamdi, MD; Norman Jaffe, MD; Herve Byron, MD; and Henry Hirschman, MD, were the earliest American pioneers of intraocular implants.

In 1974, I attended the International Congress of Ophthalmology in Paris. After the conference, I joined a busload of American doctors who spent a week with Dr. Binkhorst in Terneuzen, the Netherlands, and with Jan Worst, MD, in Groningen, the Netherlands. We wanted to learn about IOLs and to begin implanting them when we returned to our home towns. Richard Kratz, MD, a couple of other surgeons on the bus, and I combined phacoemulsification with the implantation of a two-loop Binkhorst lens or a Worst Medallion lens. We felt that these designs were superior to the purely iris-supported lenses or the anterior angle-supported lenses of Peter Choyce, MD, after intracapsular cataract extraction.

In 1977, Steven Shearing, MD, of Las Vegas reported[1] on the first flexible, J-loop PCIOL (the design of Joaquin Barraquer, MD). This lens stimulated the practice of extracapsular cataract extraction, but it did not increase interest in phacoemulsification, which was still frowned upon by 90% of American eye surgeons and 98% of eye surgeons worldwide, according to my estimates.

LIMITING PHACOEMULSIFICATION

In the mid-1970s, the US government decided that Medicare

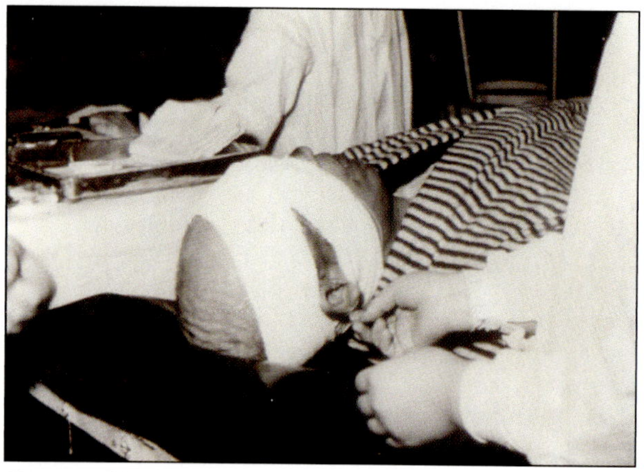

Figure 1. This photograph was taken in Japan in 1951. Cataract surgery required bilateral eye coverings and demanded that patients remain supine for 10 days.

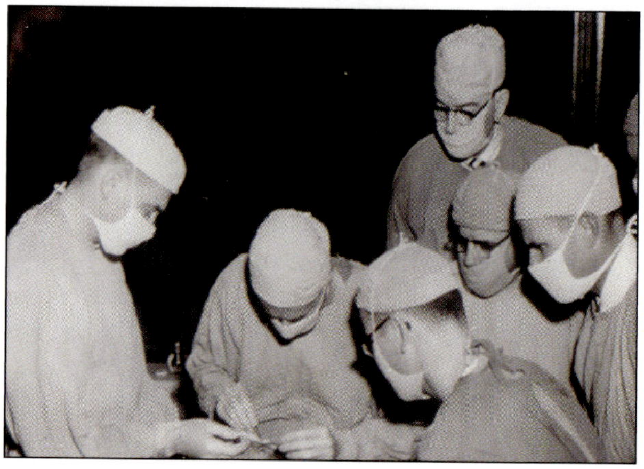

Figure 2. Townley Payton, MD, observes Dr. Sinskey in this photograph, taken in 1954. Dr. Payton was a famous corneal surgeon and the father of David Payton, organizer of Orbis International.

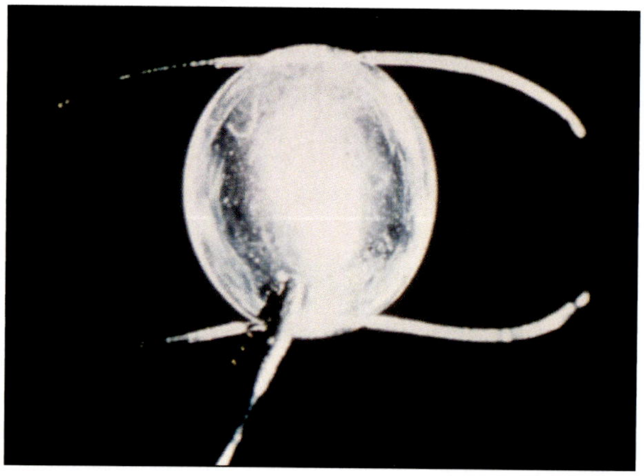

Figure 3. The nylon loops of the explanted lens designed by Joaquin Barraquer, MD, had dissolved.

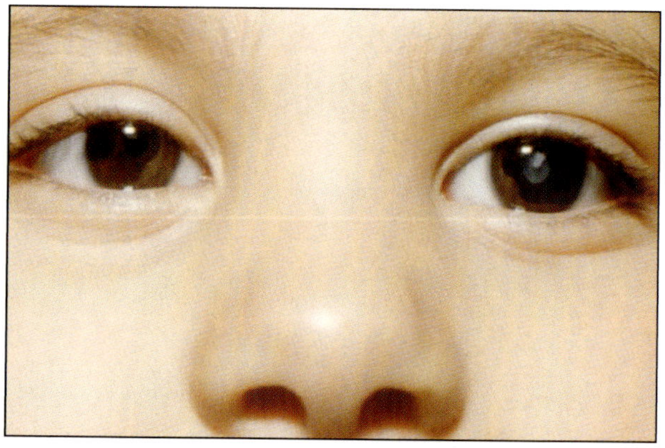

Figure 4. After performing cataract surgery, the author implanted an IOL into the right eye of a 3-year-old child. Surgery on the patient's left eye followed in 1980.

would not reimburse ophthalmologists for cataracts removed via phacoemulsification, and it designated the procedure experimental. Dr. Kratz and a number of other physicians, including myself, convinced the government that phacoemulsification was simply another way to perform cataract surgery. We explained that, if Medicare did not pay for the surgery, insurance companies would follow suit, thereby stifling the development of innovative and different ways of performing any type of surgery. We subsequently went through the same process with IOLs.

Phacoemulsification involved expensive equipment, including the phaco machine (invented in 1979 by Charles Kelman, MD, in conjunction with Cavitron, $40,000) and a microscope (preferably a coaxial-type microscope [Carl Zeiss Meditec Inc., Dublin, CA] with an assistant microscope attachment, $20,000). The combination of the equipment's price and the procedure's level of difficulty limited the number of surgeons performing phacoemulsification.

THE 1980s

In 1980, Danièle Aron Rosa, MD, introduced the Nd:YAG laser, which opened the cloudy posterior capsule noninvasively. That same year, David Miller, MD, and Robert Stegmann, MD, introduced Healon (now manufactured by Advanced Medical Optics, Inc., Santa Ana, CA), a viscoelastic that made cataract surgery dramatically easier and safer. Also in 1980, I modified the J-loop lens to make it easier to implant. Then, because the complication rate from acrylic PCIOLs with polypropylene loops was so low, I decided to start implanting these lenses in children. It took years before I was able to convince pediatric ophthalmologists to perform the procedure (Figure 4).

Phacoemulsification finally underwent a surge of popularity in 1984, when Thomas Mazzocco, MD, introduced the first flexible, silicone-plate IOL that could be introduced through a 3-mm incision. The lens caused complications because of its plate design, and the silicone caused increased tissue reaction. Only when the foldable optic was changed to an acrylic three-piece design with polypropylene loops or an acrylic single-piece with loops did the complication rate drop precipitously. Later, the silicone used in the lenses was modified to be as inert as acrylic.

THE BENEFITS OF PHACOEMULSIFICATION

In the early days of phacoemulsification, we surgeons did not realize all the advantages of the small incision and of leaving the posterior capsule intact. The benefits included lower occurrences of retinal detachment, iritis, and corneal complications from vitreous contact; lower amounts of postoperative astigmatism; early mobilization of the patient; and the ophthalmologist's total control of the eye during surgery (despite interruptions such as from the patient coughing or an elevated IOP). We thought that by eliminating hospitalization for cataract surger, we would reduce insurance costs and save Medicare a lot of money. Instead, because patients could have a relatively painless procedure that immediately achieved superb postoperative results, they chose to undergo the surgery as soon as their golf score dropped or the moment they were unhappy with their vision for any reason.

CATARACT SURGERY TODAY

Advances such as topical anesthesia, sutureless incisions, ultraviolet protection in IOLs, and accommodating technologies are leading surgeons to remove the crystalline lens whether it is cloudy or not (refractive lens exchange). Because the litigious US public is so intent on a perfect result, the stress level of the ophthalmic surgeon has increased dramatically. At the same time, insurance payments for cataract surgery have dropped dramatically. Future research in ophthalmology seems to be shifting toward correcting retinal problems such as senile macular degeneration and retinitis pigmentosa as well as toward artificial corneal implants. ■

This article originally appeared in the July 2006 issue of CRSToday.

1. Metcalfe JS, James A. Emergent innovation systems and the delivery of clinical services: the case of intra-ocular lenses. Centre for Research on Innovation and Competition and School of Economic Studies, University of Manchester. Available at: http://www.mot.chalmers.se/dept/idy/home/stanmetcalfe.pdf. Accessed June 7, 2006.

The Genesis of Phacoemulsification

CHARLES D. KELMAN, MD

Four years after my residency, I drafted a grant proposal to study the effects of freezing on the ciliary body, retina, and choroid. I went to bed concerned that the Hartford Foundation would not find the topic of interest, awoke in the middle of the night, and, almost in a trance, added an addendum to my application that would affect the rest of my life and the lives of 100 million patients: "in addition to the freezing studies, this investigator will develop a method for removing a cataract through an incision small enough so that no hospitalization will be required."

Mr. E. Pierre Roy, the head of the John A. Hartford Foundation, could easily have rejected my application and put an end to this matter. Instead, he had confidence in my abilities and gave me a 3-year grant, although I did not have the vaguest idea of how to realize my idea.

INITIAL STRUGGLES

Mr. Roy's confidence was misplaced for 2 years and 8 months, while I tried everything I could imagine. I first attempted to capture the cataract within a folding lens bag (Figure 1), crush it inside the bag with manual disintegrators, and then remove the device containing the fragmented lens material from the eye. The rotating devices I tried simply spun the cataract around inside the anterior chamber. High-speed cutting needles, a miniature blender, drills, tiny meat grinders, engraving tools—nothing worked. All the devices yielded opaque corneas in animal eyes.

I had meanwhile allowed my hair to grow down to my shoulders, and my teeth badly needed a cleaning. Sitting in my dentist's chair, I became interested in the ultrasonic tool he was using to clean my teeth. He explained that its high-frequency vibration removed tartar without disturbing the tooth itself. I raced out of his office with the bib still hanging around my neck and returned 1 hour later with a cataractous lens. Because I was able to engrave lines on the lens without its jumping off my finger, I believed that I could break up a cataract inside the eye without its spinning or vibrating against the corneal endothelium.

Cavitron Corporation ultimately made a prototype with a handpiece that incorporated I/A (Figure 2), rather than only irrigation, as with the original dental instrument. My first efforts with this device resulted in opaque corneas until I began using a physiologic solution, imported from the Barraquer Institute in Barcelona, Spain, in place of the simple saline solution. I also realized that the high temperatures that the procedure created inside the eye would denature the corneal proteins.

After several months of successful animal testing, I operated on my first human subject, a man suffering from a painful blind eye due to burned-out glaucoma. The strong surge of suction caused the cornea to collapse 30 to 40 times during the 70-minute phacoemulsification. The next day, his eye was a bag of pus that had to be removed.

I spent 2 years seeking a way to prevent corneal collapse and finally found a company in North Carolina that manufactured a device that sensed arterial flow. Cavitron Corporation incorporated this feature into the phacoemulsification device's aspiration line with an air-relieved valve. If the speed of the current in the aspiration line exceeded the speed of the irrigation, then a valve opened to halt suction immediately.

One year later, I worked up the nerve to operate on the eye of a patient with central retinal artery occlusion and no light perception. If I had failed that time, I probably would have abandoned the project. A specially designed, three-dimensional micromanipulator supported the weight of the cumbersome phaco handpiece and steadied the phaco tip inside the eye for long periods of time. I deemed the operation a success when the patient achieved light perception postoperatively. The severe striate keratitis present on the first postoperative day subsided after 6 weeks.

HURDLES

The Hospital

At that time, there were no rules against performing new procedures. Nonetheless, after I had successfully completed a few more cases, the chief surgeon at Manhattan Eye and Ear Hospital tried to convince the board to rescind my operating privileges. Ultimately, they established a committee to oversee the results of every patient. Fortunately, by this time, my results were quite good.

The Profession

Although I began teaching phacoemulsification in 1970 with the first commercially available machine, the profession vehemently

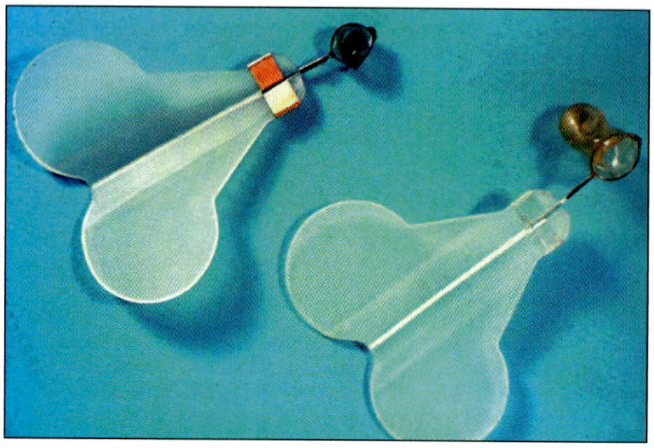

Figure 1. One of the many unsuccessful devices created by the author for small-incision cataract surgery involved folding lens bags and manual disintegrators.

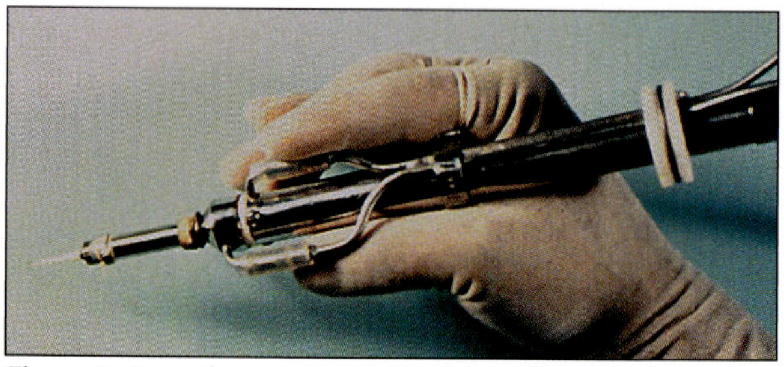

Figure 2. An early prototype of the phaco handpiece.

protested the adoption of the technique. Most if not all surgeons at that time used only loupes for magnification. As a result, they had to learn to use an operating microscope as well as to perform phacoemulsification. Many politically important ophthalmologists were older and either unwilling or unable to learn these new modalities. The fact that I, the technique's main proponent, was playing the saxophone and singing in the casinos of Atlantic City and appearing on the *Johnny Carson Show* did not help the cause (Figure 3).

The Companies

The lead engineer at Cavitron Corporation had encoded and threatened to withhold all the critical information about the new phacoemulsification machine in a play for a promotion to vice president around 1971. Cavitron Corporation fired him, but the company was then ready to abandon the project. Fortunately, Alan McMillan, an entrepreneur from California, took over the project and developed a new model, which he eventually sold to Cooper Vision (Fairport, NY) and, finally, Alcon Laboratories, Inc. (Fort Worth, TX).

The Study

The AAO initiated a major comparative study of phacoemulsification and intracapsular cataract extraction (ICCE). At my insistence, the chairman of the Department of Mathematics and Statistics at Columbia University in New York monitored the study's results. The investigators' reluctant conclusion was that phacoemulsification delivered the same quality of results as ICCE, but the report's conclusion stated that ICCE was the preferred and only method to use in many instances.

The Classification

The next major attack on phacoemulsification occurred when opponents got the FDA to classify the procedure as experimental and, therefore, nonreimbursable. Reversing this decision required thousands of letters from patients and an appearance before the FDA by the renowned television doctor, Marcus Welby, MD.

The IOL

As IOLs became more popular in the late 1970s, many surgeons gave up on phacoemulsification, because implanting the lenses required larger incisions. The advent of lenses that could fit through a smaller incision, such as the Omnifit (Precision-Cosmet Company, Inc., and Heyer Schulte) and foldable IOLs, revived the procedure.

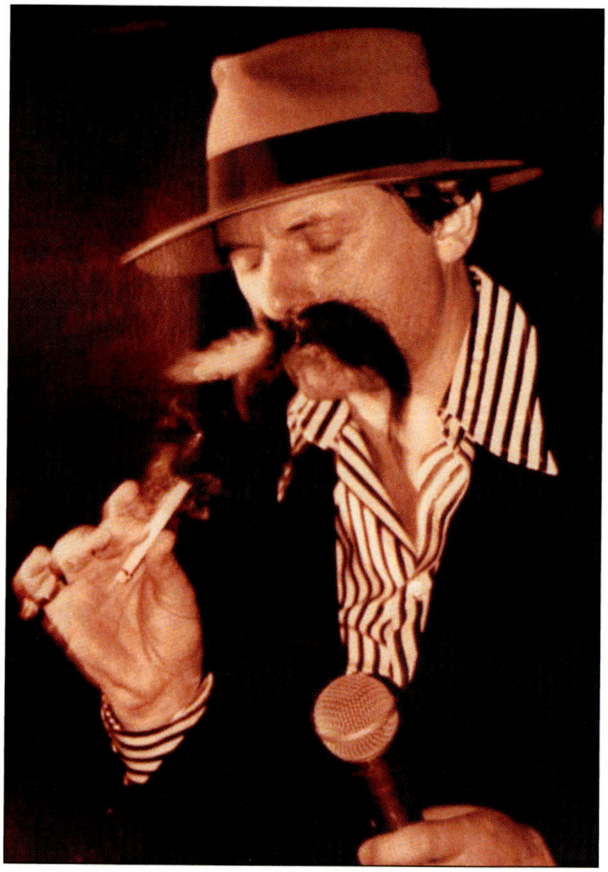

Figure 3. The author was well known for his musical and comedic performances.

CONCLUSION

When I began performing phacoemulsification, no accurate way for measuring an eye's endothelial cell count existed. Although patients' corneas recovered, I am certain that the endothelial cell loss was unacceptable in very early cases. If I had not been in the right place at the right time and had an obsessive motivation, I believe we would still be performing ICCE.

I thank my colleagues, supporters, and collaborators. I also thank my opposition for inspiring me to try harder. ■

This article originally appeared in the March 2004 issue of CRSToday.

Sir Harold Ridley

DAVID J. APPLE, MD

The story of Sir Harold Ridley, born in 1906, and his groundbreaking invention of the IOL is well known and one of the high points of ophthalmology in the 20th century.[1-4] In the mid-1980s, many physicians (including members of the academic medical establishment) still did not accept much of his work.[5-8] Even his lens implant,[9-11] inarguably one of the most important innovations in the history of ophthalmology and a blessing to society, was widely criticized. Sir Harold's presentations regarding his invention were often met with skepticism, invective, and scorn. Scientific research on his implant that my colleagues (The Apple Korps) and I had performed in our laboratory between 1982 and 1985 strongly supported and, indeed, verified much of his work.[1,2] He was pleased to learn of our publications and, in 1985, summoned me to his retirement cottage (Figures 1 and 2) in Stapleford, England, near Salisbury, where we first met.[4,6] We developed a close personal and professional relationship that lasted until his death on May 25, 2001.

After our initial meeting, I began visiting Sir Harold and his wife, Elisabeth, three times per year, and I was able to observe his important accomplishments personally.[3,4] I soon became convinced of the injustice under which he labored[5-8] and felt compelled to help secure the recognition and high honors that he and his family deserved.

POLITICS IN OPHTHALMOLOGY

Overview

Contributing to the lack of recognition for Sir Harold was the fact that some clinical complications occurred early on, many due to variations in the surgical techniques of other surgeons. These complications made some ophthalmologists hesitant to implant an IOL. Also, Sir Harold was not an aggressive advocate of lens implantation. My research then and as late as 2 years after his death[3,4] (involving the close study of his papers and other items provided to me by his sons, Nicholas and David) has clearly demonstrated that numerous vagaries of ophthalmic politics (including jealousy and a lack of foresight) were the major causes of our specialty's long-delayed acceptance of IOLs.[5-8]

Ridley Versus Duke-Elder

It is no secret that Sir Harold had major differences with one of the most prominent ophthalmologists of the 20th century, Sir Stewart Duke-Elder. They had various disagreements as early as the 1930s, at which time Sir Harold was the youngest ophthalmologist to receive a full consultant appointment at Moorfield's Eye Hospital in London. Their differences increased as World War II began.

Sir Harold had a special and sincere interest in the field of tropical ophthalmology. His father was an ophthalmologist in the British Royal Navy of the early 20th century, a position providing his family with a worldwide outlook. Also, Elisabeth Ridley had been raised in India. Even more important to Sir Harold's affinity for the field of tropical ophthalmology were the actions of Sir Stewart, the Director of the Institute of Ophthalmology in London. Sir Stewart was a prominent author of some of the most important, comprehensive volumes on the field of ophthalmology of his time (1940s through the 1960s). Almost all ophthalmologists of my generation read these volumes as their bible. He was also well known as the Queen's Ophthalmologist.

By 1943, Sir Stewart was in charge of almost all ophthalmology assignments for the British military. He sent Sir Harold to an apparently obscure assignment in Ghana, Africa, where he found his way into the rural bush to study various endemic diseases. Rather than hibernate in obscurity, Sir Harold assessed the opportunities there and immersed himself in clinical studies on what was and still is one of the most important blinding diseases afflicting that underprivileged region: onchocerciasis (river blindness). The rest is history.

His work in Africa ranks among the most important of his non-IOL contributions. During his wartime service in Ghana, Sir Harold managed not only to perform clinical examinations on affected patients, but he also completed histopathological analyses of the microorganisms causing this disease. This work resulted in the publication of his classic 1945 monograph.[12] He himself painted a figure showing this disease's fundus (ophthalmoscopic) changes, now universally termed the *Ridley Fundus.*

Even after the war, following Sir Harold's invention of the IOL[9-11,13,14] (Figure 3), he and Sir Stewart could not communicate. The latter was never able to accept the IOL.

RESISTANCE TO THE IOL

The huge backlash against Sir Harold's invention and surgical procedure by many of his peers occurred within the academic establishment in both England and the US. Derrick Vail, MD, of Chicago, for example, was very critical.[7,8]

Based on numerous interviews with his contemporaries who observed the evolution of the IOL firsthand, the emergence of this device necessitated a radical paradigm shift. Prior to that time, eye surgeons routinely learned to take things out of the eye (ie, foreign bodies, inflammatory material, tumors). The implementation of the IOL required a new thought pattern, namely, the concept of putting something into the eye. This new idea was difficult for many to accept. Sir Harold's IOL[9-11,13,14] was a new and important adjunct to cataract surgery (in his own words, a "cure of aphakia"), but it also represented a much broader and more significant innovation. Without realizing it, Sir Harold effectively helped to pioneer the modern field of biomedical engineering, specifically, the field of artificial device implantation. His IOL long preceded the introduction of all major devices designed for tissue/organ replacement and implantation into the body's various delicate and vital tissues and organs (eg, heart pacemakers, artificial kidneys, artificial hearts).

ENTERING THE MODERN ERA

During the latter half of the past century, the field of ophthalmology sufficiently recovered from the wreckage of World War II to progress into the era that we now term a *Golden Age of Ophthalmology and the Visual Sciences.* Sir Harold's inventions represented both an actual and symbolic beginning of this modern period, which was characterized by (1) extensive closures of institutes and sanitaria for the blind, (2) the substantial decrease in the number of blinded eyes submitted to anatomic-pathology laboratories such as the one directed by myself since the 1970s, and (3) surgeons' markedly increased ability to treat and manage eyes injured by various types of disease or trauma—eyes almost assuredly lost in former times.

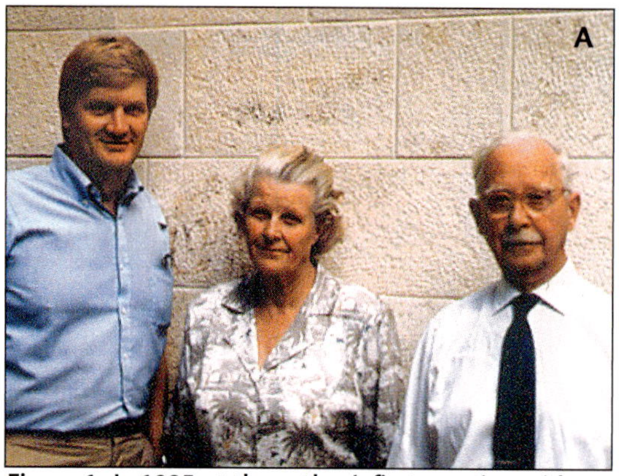

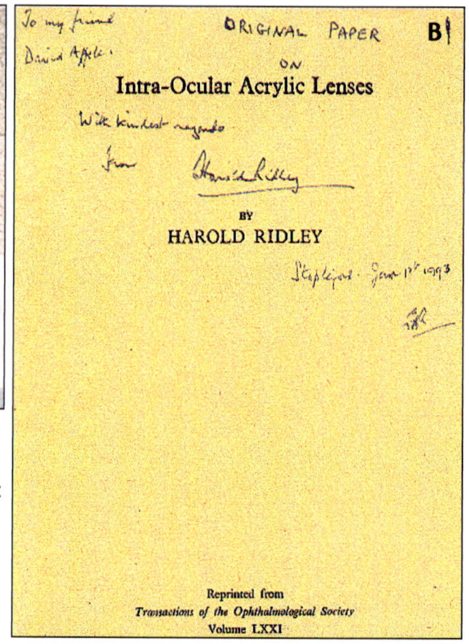

To my friend David Apple.

ORIGINAL PAPER ON

Intra-Ocular Acrylic Lenses

With kindest regards from Harold Ridley

BY

HAROLD RIDLEY

Stapleford. June 1st 1993

Reprinted from
Transactions of the Ophthalmological Society
Volume LXXI

Figure 1. In 1985, at the author's first meeting with Elisabeth and Harold Ridley in Stapleford, England. Sir Harold was despondent about the ophthalmologic establishment's lack of acceptance of his invention (From left: David J. Apple, MD, Mrs. Ridley, Sir Harold) (A). Sir Harold gave his first clinical/scientific publication on his invention to Dr. Apple (B).

ACCEPTANCE

One pivotal event that helped remedy Sir Harold's lack of acceptance occurred in 1986, when he was elected a fellow of the highly prestigious Royal Society. Further, in 1989, I presented his credentials and a list of his accomplishments to my former university, the Medical University of South Carolina. I was dumbfounded that some members of the administration and even my department were loathe to honor Sir Harold because they were unaware of his scientific and clinical accomplishments and of his gift to humanity. Fortunately, the president of the university at that time, Dr. James B. Edwards, rapidly grasped my intentions, and the university did agree to confer an honorary doctor's degree on Sir Harold that year (Figure 4). A torrent of honors for him followed, and he was belatedly knighted in London by Queen Elizabeth II on February 9, 2000, less than 1 year before his death (Figure 5).

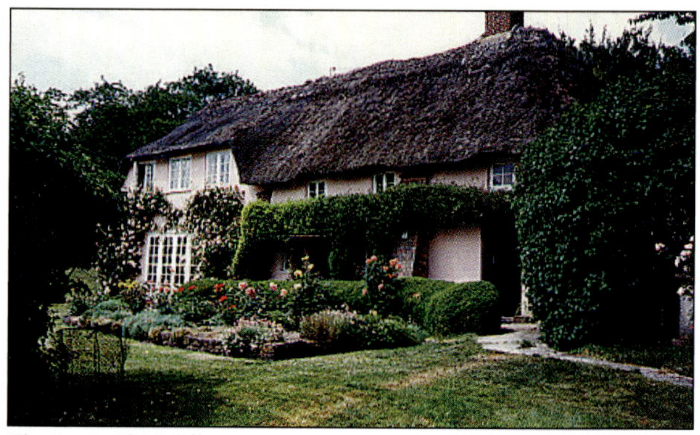

Figure 2. The Ridleys' retirement home, Keeper's Cottage, is a magnificent cottage in an idyllic region of south central England.

THE IMPACT OF THE IOL

Since its inception, the IOL has benefited well over 60 million cataract patients worldwide. Surgeons annually

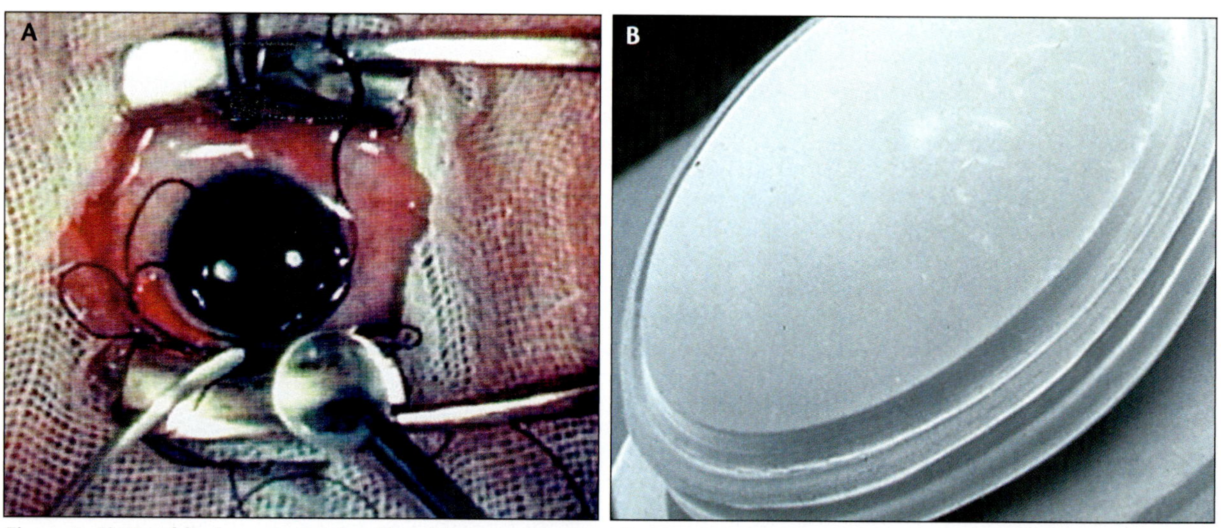

Figure 3. Sir Harold's cinematographer filmed IOL operation No. 7 in May 1951 (A). Sir Harold has grasped the IOL (Rayner Intraocular Lenses Ltd., East Sussex, UK) for insertion into the open wound, immediately after removing the cataractous, opaque crystalline lens. The operation was performed with minimal draping. Most surgeons of that era, including Sir Harold, wore no gloves, and lighting was provided by the simple flashlight held by the nurse. The IOL was a round, plastic disc (B).

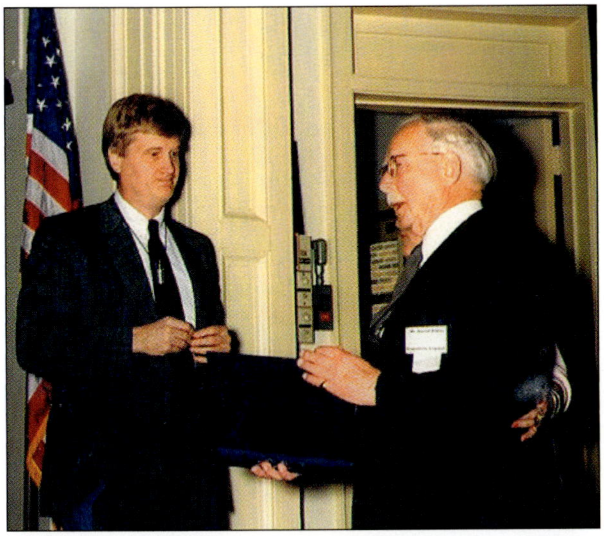

Figure 4. The author had the privilege of presenting the first university/academic award, an honorary doctor's degree, to Sir Harold in 1989.

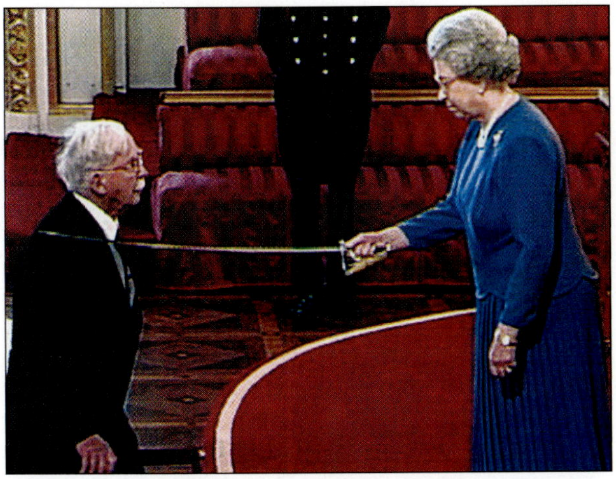

Figure 5. Queen Elizabeth II conferred a belated Knighthood upon Sir Harold in 2000.

implant more than 6 million IOLs today. Unfortunately, the IOL's market penetration into the underprivileged world has been slow, delayed largely by financial and logistical matters, as well as a lingering lack of acceptance in the 1990s by some of our specialty's leaders. An important turning point was a 1990 World Health Organization meeting in Geneva, Switzerland, that I had the privilege of attending and advising. The attendees established minimal required criteria for IOL quality, discussed various cost issues, and provided the support from the World Health Organization that was necessary to enhance the acceptance of implants worldwide.

As lens implantation gradually becomes widespread, the demand for the procedure increases, and the number of implantations should more than double by the year 2020. This development is a positive one, because, as the underprivileged world population grows and populations age, the incidence of disabling cataracts will rise rapidly. Almost all of us will develop cataracts if we live long enough. Thus ends a great story.

CONCLUSION

During the final decade of his life, Sir Harold and I worked together in accumulating and cataloging his writings, photographs, films, and other memorabilia. I have completed several short biographies of him and am currently writing a brief overview of his professional life for the *Biographical Memoirs of the Royal Society*. With the support of Sir Harold's wife and three children, I am also acting as his designated, official biographer and writing a full-length biography—an effort that I hope will establish forever his incredible legacy.

As I was working on that biography and sorting through some of his papers in January 2004, I found one of his writings from 1989 that is appropriate to this discussion and, indeed, is a quotation from him that I will always treasure:

"I had 25 years in the wilderness and would have been spared much suffering if David Apple, the one who at last took the trouble to read and analyze the early implant papers, had appeared in the 1950s—had that happened a whole generation of cataract patients might then have enjoyed full visual rehabilitation instead of suffering the abnormalities of aphakia." ■

This article originally appeared in the March 2004 issue of CRSToday.

1. Apple DJ, Kincaid MC, Mamalis N, et al. *Intraocular Lenses: Evolution, Designs, Complications, and Pathology*. Baltimore, MD: Williams and Wilkins; 1989.
2. Apple DJ, Mamalis N, Googe JM, et al. Complications of intraocular lenses. A histopathological review. *Surv Ophthalmol*. 1984;29:11-54.
3. Apple DJ, Ram J, Foster A, Peng Q. Elimination of cataract blindness. A global perspective entering the new millennium. *Surv Ophthalmol*. 2000;45(special delivery suppl):1-196.
4. Apple DJ. Auffarth GU, Peng Q, Visessook N. *Foldable Intraocular Lenses. Evolution, Clinicopathologic Correlation, and Complications*. Thorofare, NJ: Slack, Inc.; 2000.
5. Theobald GD. In regard to the Ridley implant. *Arch Ophthalmol*. 1953:36:1471.
6. Duke-Elder S. *System of Ophthalmology: Diseases of the Lens and Vitreous, Glaucoma and Hypotony*. Vol. XI. St. Louis, MO: CV Mosby; 1969:1-291.
7. Vail D. Discussion of Ridley, H. Further observations on intraocular acrylic lenses. *Trans Am Acad Ophthalmol Otolaryngol*. 1953;57:104:99.
8. Vail D. A dream cometh through a multitude of business. *Am J Ophthalmol*. 1952;35:1701-1703.
9. Ridley NHL. Intraocular acrylic lenses. *Trans Ophthalmol Soc UK & Oxford Ophthalmol Congress*. 1951:LXXI:617-621.
10. Ridley NHL. Intraocular acrylic lenses after cataract extraction. *Lancet*. 1952;1:118-119.
11. Ridley NHL. Further observations on intraocular acrylic lenses in cataract surgery. *Trans Am Acad Ophthalmol Otolaryngol*. 1953;57:98-106.
12. Ridley NHL. Ocular onchocerciasis: including an investigation in the Gold Coast. *Br J Ophthalmol*. 1945;(suppl):1-58.
13. Choyce DD. *Intra-Ocular Lenses and Implants*. London, England: H. K. Lewis & Co. Ltd.; 1964.
14. Apple DJ, Sims J. Harold Ridley and the invention of the intraocular lens. *Surv Ophthalmol*. 1996;40:279-292.

Recreating the Posterior Chamber Lens

STEVEN P. SHEARING, MD

The history of IOLs began in 1949 with Sir Harold Ridley's insertion of an artificial lens into the posterior chamber. Although placing an IOL within the space from which the cataract had been removed seemed (and seems still) a natural, almost obvious choice, ophthalmologists abandoned posterior chamber lens implantation within a few years. I reawakened surgeons' interest in posterior chamber IOLs by integrating the concept of compressibility into posterior chamber lens design. An open-looped, compressible, posterior chamber IOL became the first commercially successful, FDA-approved, posterior chamber lens (the Shearing 101 lens; IOLAB Corporation). To this day, the open-looped configuration is a mainstay of posterior chamber lens design. This article describes the genesis of my idea.

THE ORIGIN OF AN IDEA

I consider the creation of my lens design in terms of an experiment in thought. I underwent my training in the late 1960s when IOLs were so out of favor that they were never even discussed. Ophthalmologists' attitudes changed dramatically in the 1970s.

In late 1973, I attended a phacoemulsification course taught by Richard Kratz, MD, and Robert Sinskey, MD. The following year, I traveled to the Netherlands to observe the work of Cornelius Binkhorst, MD, and Jan Worst, MD. During the next 18 months, I implanted IOLs at my practice in Las Vegas. In a way, I was an ideal person to reevaluate IOL design, because I had enough experience to question the pronouncements of those who promoted themselves as authorities. Yet, I was uncommitted to any particular lens or technology.

In contrast to phacoemulsification (invented by Charles Kelman, MD) and the YAG laser (developed by Danièle Aron Rosa, MD), IOLs were relatively low-tech. Unfortunately, the assistance of skilled engineers and physicists was unavailable to me, and a research grant was out of the question. They proved unnecessary, however. My real task was to rethink what others had already done.

EARLIER LENSES

To me, IOLs were clearly the future of cataract surgery. When Ridley replaced a cataractous lens with an artificial IOL, he had taken the most important step in cataract surgery since Dr. Jacques Daviel invented the operation. He was vilified for his innovation and then ignored, but progress could not be stalled forever. First, Dr. Binkhorst and then Peter Choyce were being widely hailed in the ophthalmic community for their contributions to IOL design. Yet, the number of IOL-related complications with these lenses was disturbingly high. Too many eyes sustained serious damage. I found that the incidence of IOL dislocation increased as the quality of my extracapsular surgery improved. I theorized that there was less inflammatory glue to lock the lens in place, and I did not want to be dependent on inflammation for fixation.

Dr. Binkhorst's solution to the problems associated with IOLs in the 1950s was to invent an iris-supported lens, but the iris was proving to be too flimsy a structure on which to hang a lens. Too often, the IOL failed to fixate, even with extracapsular surgery. Rising interest in Choyce's anterior chamber lens showed that I was not the only surgeon having difficulty with iris-supported lenses. Although anterior chamber lenses seemed to solve the problem of fixation (except for "propellering"), their implantation could damage delicate tissue as they were jammed into a limited space. This very problem had been the initial inspiration for Dr. Binkhorst's invention of the iris-supported lens.

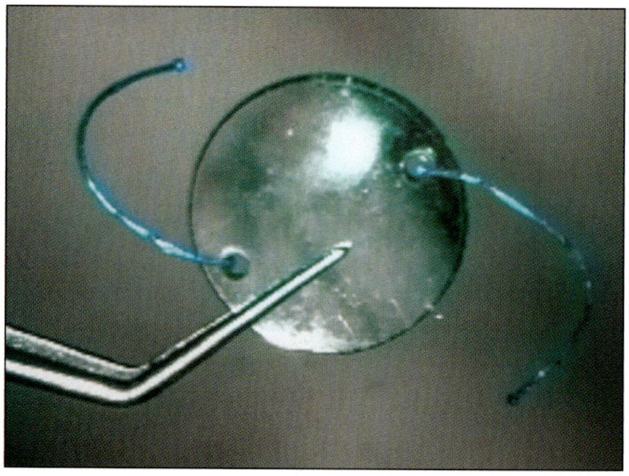

Figure 1. Note the primitive lens-haptic juncture and hand-shaped loops of this early prototype of the Shearing 101 lens.

NEW THINKING

If Choyce's anterior chamber lens (the Mark VIII lens), which had been denigrated for more than a decade, was worth the reconsideration suggested by multiple well-known surgeons, did not the same hold true of Ridley's posterior chamber lens? Considering the problems with existing lenses, I concluded it did. Removing a patient's natural lens certainly created adequate space in the posterior chamber for an IOL, but Ridley's lens—despite its large and heavy optic—was too small to fill the space. The lens inevitably shifted, damaged tissue, and often failed to fixate. Why had Ridley not simply filled the available space as the anterior chamber lens surgeons later did?

A careful review of the early literature suggested that Ridley's operation had been technically difficult. He had been caught on the horns of a dilemma. The shorter or smaller his posterior chamber lens, the easier it was to insert atraumatically through the pupil and into the posterior chamber. The longer the lens, the closer it came to achieving centration and then fixation (but at the price of increased trauma). By compromising, Ridley failed to achieve either goal; the surgery was difficult, and the lens did not fixate.

A SOLUTION

The posterior chamber lens needed to be short for the purposes of insertion but long for centration and fixation. These seemingly incompatible goals led to the concept of compressibility. I theorized that, if a lens could be compressed for insertion but had the memory to expand to its original shape once safely inside the posterior chamber, it would fill the space left by the extracted natural lens. Because the lens would be stable, capsular fixation would also be likely. In the mid-1970s, all lens optics were made of rigid PMMA. Softer, more flexible haptic materials were newly available, however, and I believed that compressible or flexible lens haptics could facilitate atraumatic IOL insertion and fixation.

At the annual AAO meeting in 1976, I approached executives from IOLAB Corporation about creating a compressible posterior chamber lens, because that manufacturer was the first to use haptics of polypropylene (PROLENE; Ethicon Inc., Somerville, NJ). Because polypropylene was both flexible and nonbiodegradable, it was the most suitable haptic material for a compressible IOL at the time. I believed it would be possible to make a three-piece lens with open-looped, polypropylene haptics and an overall diameter slightly greater than that of the posterior chamber.

To avoid manufacturing problems, I decided to mimic manufacturing techniques already shown to work with older, known IOLs. I requested that the company manufacture an IOL resembling the long-abandoned anterior chamber lens of Dr. Joaquin Barraquer, but with polypropylene haptics incorporating my recommended dimensions (Figure 1). The company's executives were reluctant to proceed. I indicated my willingness to pay, not only for the lenses I used, but also for any additional startup costs. The company, therefore, was guaranteed a profit from the outset. Moreover, I agreed to work with them exclusively to develop a commercial lens. They accepted this proposal.

Within a few weeks, I was testing IOL prototypes in cadaver eyes. In March 1977, with great trepidation and hesitation, I implanted the first compressible posterior chamber IOL in the eye of a living patient. Insertion proved relatively easy, and the lens immediately achieved fixation. Postoperatively, the eye was quiet, and the patient saw well. During a routine slit-lamp examination, it was easy not to notice the presence of the IOL. My idea had become reality. ■

This article originally appeared in the March 2004 issue of CRSToday.

Creating a Foldable Lens

THOMAS R. MAZZOCCO, MD

Although by the 1970s the technique of Kelman Phaco Emulsification had been perfected to allow the removal of a cataract through a 3-mm incision, most surgeons still performed extracapsular cataract extraction, because IOL insertion required the enlargement of the phaco wound to between 6 and 8 mm. Even so, a small cadre of ophthalmologists, including myself, continued to perform phacoemulsification in the belief that the procedure was a superior method of cataract extraction and that smaller incisions were beneficial.

Charles Kelman, MD, deserves credit for the idea of inserting an IOL through a 3-mm incision. During his frequently held phaco courses in the early 1970s, he showed a model of an anterior chamber lens with a 3-mm optic that he had designed and used. Unfortunately, because this IOL was angle-fixated, its centration over the pupil could not be ensured, and Dr. Kelman abandoned the design due to the excessive amount of glare it caused.

Every day, I observed the beautiful 3-mm incision I produced during phacoemulsification and longed for a method of IOL insertion that would not require me to enlarge the wound. I realized that patients needed an IOL with an optic of between 5.5 and 6.0 mm in order to achieve good visual acuity without glare.

BRAINSTORMING

My first idea was to cut a lens in half, possibly with a laser, and then glue it back together inside the anterior chamber after insertion. I decided that the adhesive posed an insurmountable problem: toxic chemicals might leach into the anterior chamber, and there was a likelihood of postoperative monocular diplopia.

I next considered the possibility of a 3-mm optic to which a surgeon could attach a collar of dark plastic by posts or a groove in order to produce a 6-mm zone of opacity with a 3-mm, clear, central optical zone (Figure 1). This assembly would occur within the anterior chamber after lens insertion. I felt that gaining FDA approval of the dye within the plastic would be problematic. Dr. Kelman later produced an elegant, small optic with opaque wings; regrettably, unexpectedly strong fibrosis of the capsular bag moved the wings back over the optic.

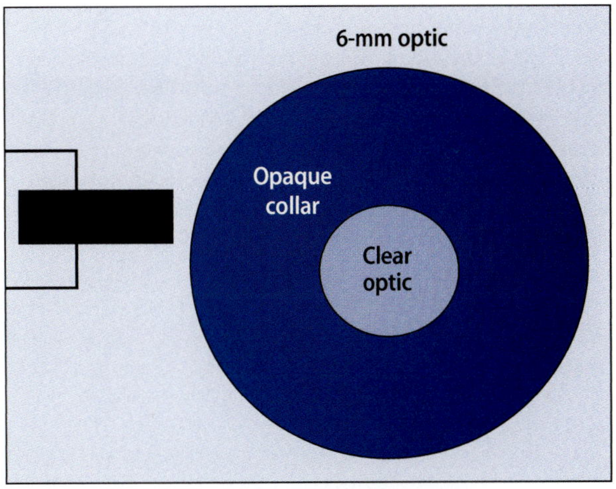

Figure 1. One of the author's design ideas was a 3-mm optic to which the surgeon could attach a dark plastic collar after inserting the pieces into the anterior chamber.

Finally, I began to consider using a soft material that could be folded and inserted through the 3-mm phaco incision. Other soft implants existed in 1980, but they were used primarily to lessen the degree of trauma to the delicate ocular structures. Edward Epstein, MD, of Johannesburg, South Africa, had considerable experience with soft implants. When we at STAAR Surgical Company (Monrovia, CA) settled on silicone as a suitable starting lens material, Dr. Epstein offered to assist us with the early insertions. He himself had unsuccessfully requested silicone material from Dow Corning Corporation (Midland, MI) during the late 1960s with the hope that he could construct IOLs from the material. His aim had been to create an atraumatic lens, but not for folding, because 3-mm incisions were not made in the 1960s.

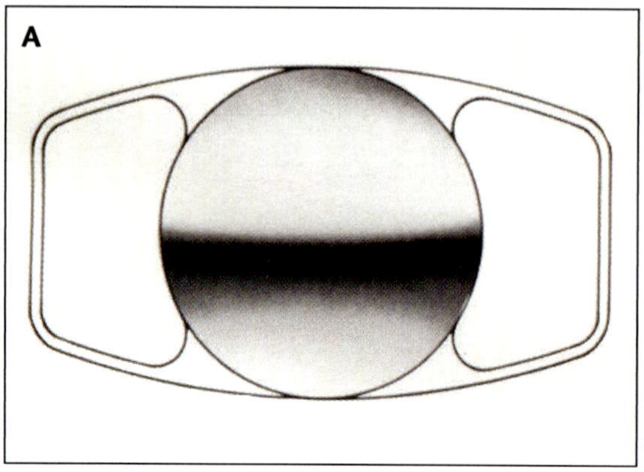

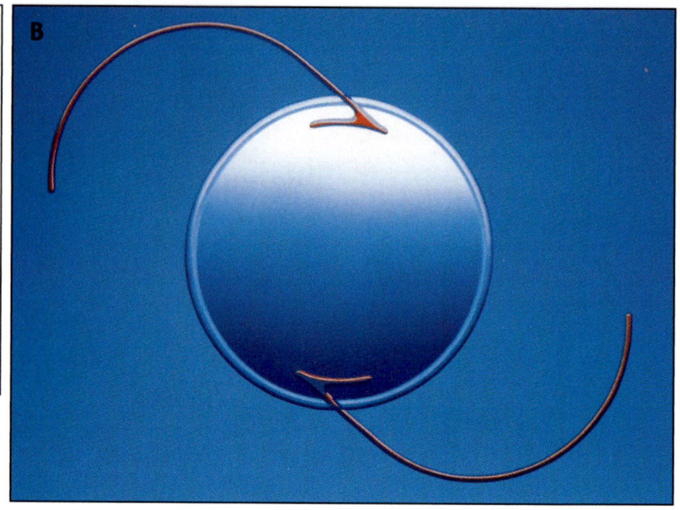

Figure 2. Early lenses by STAAR Surgical Company included the first foldable posterior chamber IOL, model AA 4004 (A), and the AQ 2010V (B).

LENS DESIGN

From the start, when the FDA approved the lenses for insertion in 1984, STAAR Surgical Company produced both one- and three-piece IOLs (Figure 2). I personally favored the three-piece design (polyimide haptics, silicone optic) because of its familiarity, but the simplicity and ease of manufacture led us to focus on the one-piece, molded lens. The early one-piece lenses were very pliable in the haptic area, a design that worked for sulcus fixation. The popularization of in-the-bag fixation led many surgeons to implant the soft haptics within the capsular bag. This technique resulted in the deformation of the soft haptics, owing to fibrosis of the bag, and led to IOL decentration. The surgeon then had to reposition the lens haptics in the sulcus. A thicker, stronger haptic solved this problem; some surgeons still use this lens model with strong haptics today. The sobriquet *Mazzocco Taco*, coined by Tom Waggoner, Cofounder of STAAR Surgical Company, to describe our earliest lenses has stuck and refers to all of our folding lens designs.

The development of a foldable IOL for insertion through a small incision was slow at first. Now, 20 years after the first insertion of a foldable lens, more than 80% of IOLs are foldable or deformable. My dream of inserting a large optic through a small incision is now a reality that has resulted in "come and go" cataract surgery with early ambulation, physical healing, and visual recovery. Only patients and surgeons who have experienced the old, large-incision surgery can really appreciate how far the field has come. ■

This article originally appeared in the March 2004 issue of CRSToday.

Cataract Surgery and IOLs

RICHARD P. KRATZ, MD, DSci

For those of you who only know phacoemulsification and IOLs, it is difficult to understand what a crude procedure cataract extraction used to be or the restrictive and disfiguring nature of aphakic spectacles. I performed my first extracapsular cataract extraction (ECCE) in 1945. Since then, the field of cataract surgery has changed profoundly to intracapsular cataract extraction (ICCE) and then phacoemulsification with the implantation of an IOL.

ECCE

In the 1940s, the indication for cataract extraction was a visual acuity of 20/100 or worse in the patient's better eye. The surgeon washed his hands briefly, then rinsed them with alcohol. Gloves were not used, operating microscopes were unknown, and most ophthalmologists did not use loupes. Assistants held the lighting and directed it at any angle the surgeon requested. Ophthalmologists created the 180° corneal incision just anterior to the superior limbus with the von Graefe knife. A toothed forceps removed the anterior capsule, and the surgeon squeezed the nucleus from the eye via the pressure of a squint hook dragged across the cornea. There was no cortical cleanup, because cortex could not be seen without magnification and a red reflex. Most surgeons either placed no sutures or maybe one or two 6–0 black silk sutures, which were considered to be very small.

In 1948, I took the basic science course at Moorfields Eye Hospital in London and saw the same technique used by Harold Ridley. Actually, the subsequent fibrosis from not performing cortical cleanup was the only reason that most of his lenses fixed in the posterior chamber. Years later, some of my Binkhorst two-loop IOLs subluxated, and Cornelius Binkhorst, MD, revealed that he always left a little cortex at the 12-o'clock position to initiate fibrosis.

ICCE

From the 1950s to the 1980s, ICCE became the dominant cataract extraction technique, primarily because it avoided a return to the OR for 25% of ECCE patients to remove flocculated cortex that filled the anterior chamber. The moment of truth was when the surgeon had removed the crystalline lens without rupturing the capsule or disrupting the vitreous face. Treating vitreous loss involved multiple cellulose sponges and excisions. There were no vitrectors, and, without magnification, the vitreous strands could not be well visualized. The development of new capsular forceps, suction cups, and, later, Alpha Chymar trypsin and cryoextractors added to ICCE's popularity. Manufacturers also introduced improved needles and thinner suture materials during this period.

PHACOEMULSIFICATION

In 1971, I took the first phaco course offered by Charles Kelman, MD. Attendance was limited to six students, and the class was held once a month. By September 1972, Robert Sinskey, MD, and I were teaching phacoemulsification to 25 ophthalmologists each month. We simplified the procedure by moving the emulsification from the anterior chamber to the iris plane in order to protect the cornea. We modified the machine and added hydrodissection, two-handed surgery, and the scleral tunnel incision.

Many ophthalmologists were opposed to phacoemulsification. They said that the learning curve was too great and the complications too many. In 1973, some prominent ophthalmologists found that they were losing their cataract patients to surgeons who practiced the newer technique. They convinced Medicare to declare phacoemulsification experimental and not payable. Continuing to perform phacoemulsification exposed the surgeon to malpractice and a loss of license. This situation lasted until 1974, when an AAO committee found that ICCE and phacoemulsification had an equal number of complications. Medicare then reinstated its approval and payment.

IOLs

Design

In the 1970s, IOLs were angle or iris supported. The rigid angle-supported IOLs were either too large and painful or so small that they rotated in the anterior chamber. Some lenses abraded the iris stroma and caused UGH syndrome. ACIOLs with compressible loops often caused angle-closure glaucoma. Iris-supported IOLs resulted in irregular pupils, and they often subluxated into the anterior or posterior chamber.

In 1977, Steven Shearing, MD, showed his capsular-bag–fixated J-loop IOL to me when he had implanted it in only four eyes. It was the first IOL design since those of Harold Ridley and John Pearce to be completely in the posterior chamber. The IOL immediately became my lens of choice, and I invited Dr. Shearing to join the Sinskey/Kratz phaco/IOL course. William Simcoe, MD, also introduced a PCIOL with C loops. Thomas Mazzocco, MD, taught at our phaco/IOL course and invented the first foldable IOL in 1982. Today, most of the IOLs used in the world are based on Drs. Shearing's, Simcoe's, and Mazzocco's inventions.

California

Because the early IOLs had a relatively high complication rate, many ophthalmologists strongly opposed their use. Gradually, the successes of Norman Jaffe, MD; Henry Clayman, MD; Henry Hirschman, MD; Miles Galin, MD; Dennis Shepherd, MD; Ralph Anderson, MD; and Herve Byron, MD, gained recognition, and more ophthalmologists and their patients began to prefer IOLs to aphakic spectacles.

In 1975, the California State FDA (with the cooperation of the US FDA) declared that IOLs were drugs rather than devices and were thus under the FDA's jurisdiction. My colleagues and I were shocked when the California State FDA suddenly declared IOLs experimental and banned them from use in California but not in the other 49 states. Two-thirds of the world's supply of IOLs were made in California, and the companies were prohibited from manufacturing them.

The companies obtained a legal opinion that a lens implant had to be manufactured, packaged, and sterilized before it could be called an *IOL*. They continued making the lenses and sent them to nearby Las Vegas for sterilization and shipment. Dr. Hirschman, Mary Kay Michaelis, MD, and the American Implant Society obtained a restraining order that allowed California ophthalmologists to resume using IOLs.

FDA Hearing

In 1980, the US FDA held a hearing in Washington, DC, in an effort to ban IOLs. The most vocal opponent of the IOL was Sidney Wolfe, MD, of Ralph Nader's Health Research Group. He misleadingly stated that the complication rate was 50% and requested that IOLs be outlawed. He achieved this statistic by including even the most minor adverse reactions in his total and then dividing by the number of patients instead of merely stating the number of patients who had one or more problems.

Testifying on behalf of IOLs were a doctor and a pilot, both of whom had received lens implants. They stated that they would not have been able to continue their work if they had had to depend on aphakic glasses. Actor Robert Young, who played the part of Dr. Marcus Welby on a popular television series, was the third and most effective speaker. He stated that he had nearly been blind from cataracts when I implanted his IOLs in 1976. When he left the hearing, he was greeted by reporters from all of the major TV channels. One reporter asked, "Dr. Welby, what do you think of IOLs?" He replied, "First of all I am not a doctor. I am an actor who plays the part of Dr. Welby." At that point, he grabbed the reporter by the tie and said, "But let me tell you that implants saved my career and should be available to all Americans." That statement was on all of the news channels, and even the FDA could not go against the advice of America's favorite doctor.

CONCLUSION

Sir Harold Ridley proved that the eye could tolerate an artificial lens. Dr. Kelman demonstrated how to remove the nucleus and cortex through a small incision. Drs. Shearing and Simcoe showed where to place the lens. Dr. Mazzocco proved that the IOL could be folded and inserted through a small incision. Now, we surgeons should turn our attention to preventing cataracts. ■

This article originally appeared in the January 2006 issue of CRSToday.

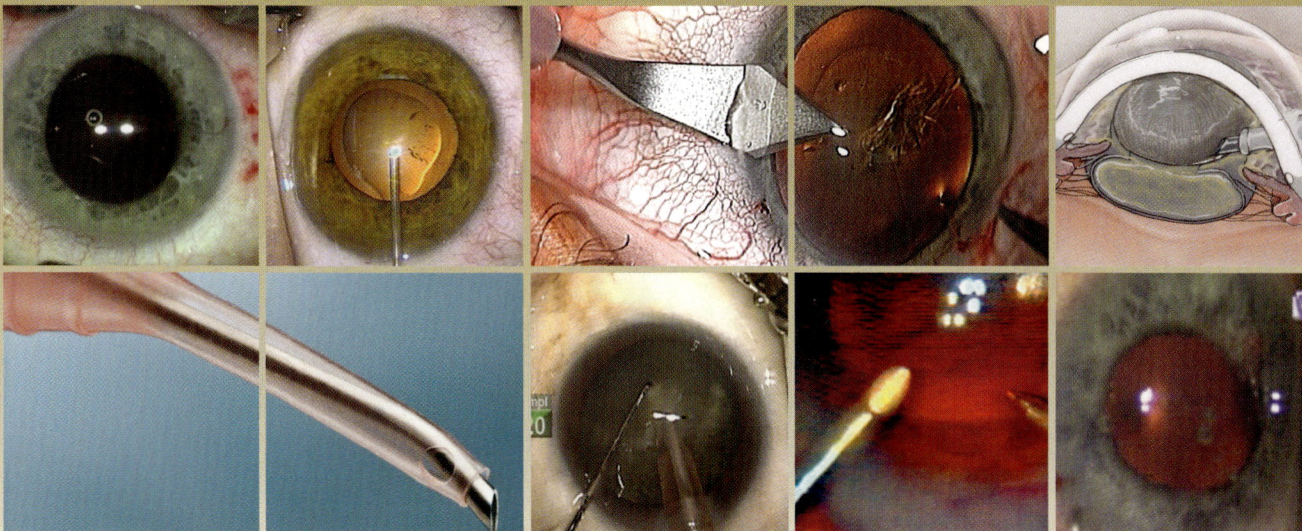

CATARACT SURGICAL TECHNIQUE

ANESTHESIA AND INCISION

CAPSULORHEXIS AND HYDRODISSECTION

PHACO TECHNIQUE AND TECHNOLOGY

CHAPTER 1

Tips on Topical Anesthesia for Cataract Surgery

TERRENCE P. O'BRIEN, MD

The goals of anesthesia in outpatient cataract surgery are to maintain the patient's safety and comfort, anesthetize the ocular tissues properly, and, in more complicated cases, achieve akinesia while maintaining normal intraocular and orbital pressures. Over the past several years, the trend in cataract surgery has been to transition from anesthesia delivered by needle injection to topical anesthesia. Following are some tips from my experience on using Xylocaine 2% Jelly (AstraZeneca LP, Wilmington, DE) during cataract surgery.

THE MOVE TO TOPICAL

The main impetus for cataract surgeons' transition to topical anesthesia is the risk associated with needle injections. Injury to the ocular or periocular structures can result in complications ranging in severity from posterior positive pressure to iris prolapse, and even to choroidal hemorrhage and retinal detachment. An injury to the ocular muscles, either from the needle itself or owing to a toxic effect of the anesthetic, can result in postoperative diplopia, which can be permanent and require the patient to wear prisms or undergo strabismus surgery. Other potential complications include retrobulbar hemorrhage, optic nerve injury, and the misdirection of anesthesia into the subarachnoid space or even an artery.

Although peribulbar blocks evolved as a method to reduce the risk of retrobulbar hemorrhage, they can still result in orbital hemorrhage, globe perforation, and retinal detachment. A subTenon's injection generally lowers the risk of retrobulbar hemorrhage and retinal detachment, but it often yields incomplete akinesia, as can a peribulbar block. Retrobulbar blocks still have a place, however, especially in more complicated surgeries for which we desire excellent anesthesia and akinesia, as well as a rapid onset of action.

Another factor in the switch to topical anesthesia is the increasingly high expectations of patients. They frequently want immediate results without pain, without downtime, and often without sutures—all at an affordable cost. Fortunately, advances in surgical technique and technology (such as smaller incisions, foldable IOLs, and newer phacoemulsification software) lend themselves to the use of topical anesthesia.

This method of anesthesia allows cataract surgeons to eliminate the risks associated with needle injection. It offers the additional advantage of keeping the cornea well lubricated. From a patient's perspective, visual recovery is rapid with topical anesthesia. This modality augments patients' postoperative comfort by eliminating the need for a patch after surgery. More importantly, topical anesthesia permits the early application of eye drops postoperatively, including anti-infectives and anti-inflammatory agents that help prevent complications and improve surgical outcomes. At The Wilmer Eye Institute, we use lidocaine 2% gel formulation for approximately 90% of routine cataract cases.

TOPICAL AGENTS

The most widely used topical agents are proparacaine, tetracaine, cocaine, lidocaine, and bupivacaine. Ophthalmologists use proparacaine daily. Both proparacaine 0.5% and tetracaine 0.5% have a rapid onset of action (within 1 minute) and a duration of 15 minutes. Tetracaine may be slightly more toxic to the ocular surface. Cocaine, used at a concentration of 0.5% to 2%, also acts rapidly, but its duration of action is slightly shorter. In addition, cocaine may loosen the corneal epithelium and cause recurrent erosion or a corneal abrasion intraoperatively. The drug also acts as a vasoconstrictor and may dilate the pupil, so its use has been limited. Bupivacaine 0.75% has a slow onset of action but is a potent amide anesthetic. The drug is rarely used in a topical application but mainly as an injectable anesthetic.

Lidocaine has many favorable properties, such as rapid diffusion and penetration. This potent, long-acting agent may be administered topically, via needle injection, or even intraocularly with the preservative-free preparation used by cardiologists and other practitioners intravenously. The 2% gel formulation I favor has a lidocaine concentration of 20 mg/mL and comes in a small 5-mL tube.

A randomized study in which I participated compared 2% lidocaine gel with topical tetracaine drops in terms of corneal anesthesia, patient comfort, and patients' need for additional anesthesia.[1] All patients underwent uncomplicated cataract surgery via phacoemulsification through a clear corneal incision and received an IOL implant. Quantitative and subjective data revealed no significant difference in the level of patient comfort between the groups of subjects, and both sets of eyes achieved the desired anesthetic effect.

TIPS FOR USAGE

Topical anesthesia works best with limbal and clear corneal incisions. Additionally, the projected operating time should be short, due to the briefer duration of action of topical versus needle-injection anesthesia. Challenging or difficult cases requiring a longer duration of operating time should therefore be avoided.

Patient Selection

When choosing the method of anesthesia, it is wise to assess the patient's demeanor preoperatively. If the patient is less than cooperative in the clinical examination area, this behavior may be worse in the operating room. Such a person is not suited to topical anesthesia, nor is an individual who received retro- or peribulbar anesthesia when undergoing cataract surgery in the fellow eye, because the experience will be markedly different and may provoke anxiety.

It is also important to avoid this method in "office squeezers," patients who display a marked squeezing or muscular spasm during tonometry or indirect ophthalmoscopy. Young, anxious patients tend to fare worse with topical anesthesia as well. This method is also inappropriate in those who are markedly hard of hearing, are suffering from significant dementia, or are otherwise incommunicative.

Timing and Supplementation of Anesthesia

In cases using retrobulbar or peribulbar anesthesia, the nurse anesthetist or anesthesiologist renders the patient nearly unconscious for the period of time surrounding the injection. For topical anesthesia, it is better not to deeply sedate the patient. Otherwise, he may wake up in the middle of surgery and be disoriented.

In cases that will require extensive iris manipulation, use supplemental intracameral, nonpreserved lidocaine 1%. Also, track operating time and supplement with topical anesthesia if the duration of the procedure is longer than usual. Additional gel may be applied.

Treat Both Eyes

I have found it helpful to place a single drop of topical proparacaine 0.5% in the fellow eye, because it keeps the patient comfortable. Otherwise, contact with the fellow eye during the draping process can cause the patient to blink or move and become less compliant.

The adjunctive use of a topical NSAID in the operative eye both pre- and postoperatively, meanwhile, offers the advantages of reducing inflammation, providing additional analgesia, and preventing CME.[2,3]

Dim the Illumination

I have also found it helpful to dim the illumination of the operating microscope initially so that the patient is not startled by the bright light. You can then gradually increase the illumination as needed for visualization intraoperatively. Interestingly, you may find that you require less microscope brightness than you have routinely used.

Employ Verbal Anesthesia

Of enormous benefit to the patient is calmly and continuously providing information during surgery. In exit survey polls that we have conducted, cataract surgery patients have stated that they have been very comforted by the surgeon's or the surgical team's telling them what to anticipate intraoperatively. Remarks can range from "Now you hear the sound of the phaco machine" to "We're going to place the lens inside the eye, so you may feel a little pressure."

Also bear in mind the adage, "It ain't over till it's over." Warn the patient when you will be removing the lid speculum, because a reflexive squeeze could cause the anterior chamber to flatten or the iris to prolapse. ■

This article originally appeared in the September 2002 issue of CRSToday.

1. Barequet IS, Soriano ES, Green WR, O'Brien TP. Provision of ocular anesthesia with single application of lidocaine 2% gel. *J Cataract Refract Surg.* 1999;25:626-631.
2. Roberts CW. Pretreatment with topical diclofenac sodium to decrease postoperative inflammation. *Ophthalmology.* 1996;103:636-639.
3. Brown RM, Roberts CW. Preoperative and postoperative use of nonsteroidal antiinflammatory drugs in cataract surgery. *Insight.* 1996;21:1:13-16.

CHAPTER 2

Should I Change My Incision?

RANDALL J. OLSON, MD

The introduction of clear corneal incisions made a dramatic impression on ophthalmologists across the United States in the mid-1990s. Attracted by the elimination of conjunctival manipulation and sutures, many surgeons, including myself, adopted this approach. Twelve years later, it is interesting to assess how ophthalmologists' views of these incisions have evolved. Clearly, all of their pluses remain, but an increased incidence of endophthalmitis continues to raise concern. The question becomes whether surgeons should abandon the clear corneal incision.

CLEAR CORNEAL INCISIONS AND ENDOPHTHALMITIS

My colleagues and I at the John A. Moran Eye Center in Salt Lake City had a quality care program to prospectively look at endophthalmitis. Unfortunately, it takes time to differentiate a trend from a cluster of cases when the incidence of disease is low. By 1999, however, my colleagues and I could detect a problem.[1] In a prospective, randomized study, Nagaki et al[2] found the incidence of endophthalmitis to be 4.6 times higher than with corneoscleral incisions and confirmed our findings.[3] Our own series of 15,000 cases[4] showed an incidence of endophthalmitis of approximately one in 400 for clear corneal incisions versus none for more than 1,200 corneoscleral tunnels performed during the same time period.

The confusing factor is that many ophthalmologists did not have a problem with clear corneal incisions.[5] For example, I have not had a case of endophthalmitis with clear corneal surgery. Clear corneal incisions are therefore not responsible for the increased overall incidence of endophthalmitis in the US. Why, however, do they potentially increase the risk of this complication?

Some important clues suggest a rational approach for cataract surgeons. Work by my colleagues and me[6] showed a 44-fold increase in the rate of endophthalmitis when clear corneal incisions leaked. Studying such a case reveals the problem. With each blink, the tear film moves in and out of the eye with gross contamination that is dramatically different from a leak between sutures in which fluid always flows out of the eye. We also found a 14-fold higher risk of endophthalmitis if there were complications at the time of surgery such as zonular rupture or a broken capsule—a figure that is many times greater than in a previous study looking at endophthalmitis in association with vitrectomy after cataract surgery.[6]

Clear corneal incisions have been associated with a high incidence of hypotony soon after surgery.[7] Is this hypotony related to a shutdown ciliary body, or does it represent leakage of the wound? In their excellent study,[8] Masket and Belari showed that scrupulous attention to details of the incision resulted in no eyes with an IOP below 10 mm Hg among the patients they analyzed soon after surgery. Hypotony, as reported,[7] therefore probably represents incisions that are leaking, a major concern in the early postoperative period.

The key is careful scrutiny at the end of the cataract case to identify a marginal wound. Any unstable incisions deserve a suture, and such a careful approach can minimize the risk of endophthalmitis.

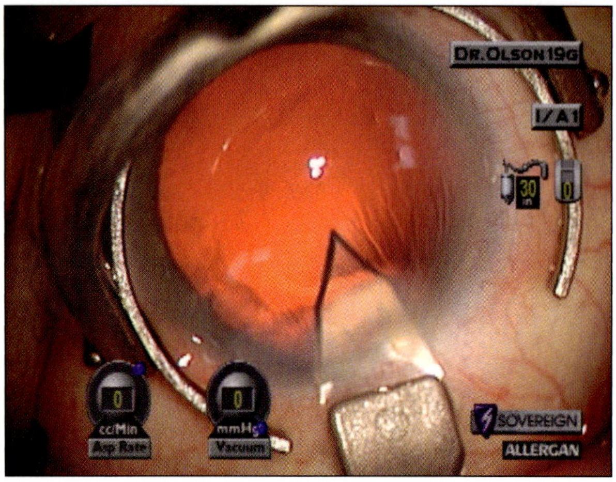

Figure 1. Because the entry to the wound was not parallel to the corneal plane, one side is shorter (concern about leakage), and one side is into the conjunctiva (concern about conjunctival ballooning).

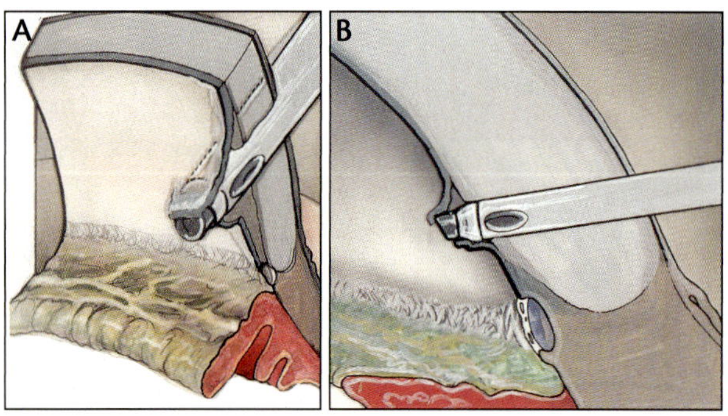

Figure 2. Small single tears of Descemet's membrane are easily created (A and B) and missed. Without the endothelial pump to seal the wound, there is a greater risk of leakage.

MARGINAL WOUNDS

Length

If marginal wounds are the cause of infection, then defining that term is important. To me, if any point across the wound is shorter than 2 mm, the incision is marginal. The shortened region often is at one edge of the wound or the other, either due to tearing of the periphery during the surgeon's manipulation of instruments or the entry of the keratome (particularly a diamond blade) not parallel to the corneal plane (Figure 1). A wound is only as strong as its weakest point.

My selection of 2 mm is based on a presentation by Masket.[9] He showed, in human eye-banked eyes, that any wound shorter than 2 mm could leak, whereas clear corneal incisions that were 2 mm or longer at all points were very resistant to leakage. His findings certainly jibe with my clinical experience.

Descemet's Detachment

Any area of Descemet's detachment (Figure 2) will result in a marginal incision. An intact Descemet's membrane is necessary for the endothelial pump to close the wound and produce a watertight incision. Small, single tears of Descemet's membrane are not uncommon and can escape the surgeon's notice. The easiest way to see them is to watch for the membrane to "flap in the breeze" during irrigation through the stab incision.

Tears

A torn wound is a marginal one. Although tears are not always easy to detect, the key for me is to look at the incision at the end of the case to see how well it lines up. If it has a tendency to pout or looks distorted, particularly with obvious damage to either edge, I consider it a torn wound. This problem usually results when the surgeon tries to force instrumentation through too small an incision. Such wounds may appear to be closed after stromal hydration, but, again, I become concerned about potential leakage if their edges do not line up perfectly.

Fishmouthing

"Fishmouthing" is an obvious change at the end of the case in which the incision gapes. The occurrence often relates to low scleral rigidity (eg, due to high myopia or keratoconus). I have also seen gaping wounds in cases of corneal transplantation, old lacerations near the incision, and scleral buckles.

Approach

To me, all marginal wounds deserve a single 10–0 nylon suture. Any doubt about the incision's integrity on my part prompts me to place a suture. Although only necessary in a small percentage of my cases, suturing reassures me that I am addressing the risk of a leaky wound. I remove these sutures at 1 week. One pearl is not to bury the knot but to cut the sutures close to the knot, because trying to dislodge a knot from inside the incision may reopen it. It is easy to cut the knot with the edge of a hypodermic needle and remove it without placing stress on the wound.

CONCLUSION

Clear corneal incisions are safe if appropriately cared for, but they are exceedingly unforgiving. It is essential to be scrupulous in the creation of the wound and to recognize and suture marginal incisions. I think that cataract surgeons need not abandon clear corneal incisions if they use this cautious approach. When reviewing videotapes of my surgeries, I find that I often spend more time checking the wound than I do removing the nucleus. ■

Supported in part by a grant from Research to Prevent Blindness, Inc., to the Department of Ophthalmology and Visual Sciences, University of Utah.

This article originally appeared in the June 2007 issue of CRSToday.

1. Jensen MK, Fiscella RG, Crandall AS, et al. A retrospective study of endophthalmitis rates comparing quinolone antibiotics. *Am J Ophthalmol.* 2005;139:141-148.
2. Nagaki Y, Hayasaka S, Kadoi C, et al. Bacterial endophthalmitis after small-incision cataract surgery. Effect of incision placement and intraocular lens type. *J Cataract Refract Surg.* 2003;29:20-26.
3. Sarayba MA, Taban M, Ignacio TS, et al. Inflow of ocular surface fluid through clear corneal cataract incisions: a laboratory model. *Am J Ophthalmol.* 2004;138:206-210.
4. Wallin T, Parker J, Jin Y, et al. Cohort study of 27 cases of endophthalmitis at a single institution. *J Cataract Refract Surg.* 2005;31:735-741.
5. Monica ML, Long DA. Nine-year safety with self-sealing corneal tunnel incision in clear cornea cataract surgery. *Ophthalmology.* 2005;112:985-986.
6. Javitt JC, Street DA, Tilsch JM, et al. Cataract Patient Outcomes Research Team. National outcomes of cataract extraction. Retinal detachment and endophthalmitis after outpatient cataract surgery. *Ophthalmology.* 1994;101:100-105.
7. Shingleton BJ, Wadhwani RA, O'Donoghue MW, et al. Evaluation of intraocular pressure in the immediate period after phacoemulsification. *J Cataract Refract Surg.* 2001;27:524-527.
8. Masket S, Belari S. Proper wound construction to prevent short-term ocular hypotony after clear corneal incision cataract surgery. *J Cataract Refract Surg.* 2007;33:383-386.
9. Masket S. What is the relationship between clear corneal incisions and endophthalmitis? Paper presented at: The New Orleans Academy of Ophthalmology Meeting; February 9, 2007; New Orleans, LA.

CHAPTER 3

Clear Cornea Versus Scleral Pocket

ASHLEY BEHRENS, MD

During the past few years, the popularity of clear corneal incisions for cataract surgery has increased dramatically. The most recent surveys estimate that more than 72% of ophthalmic surgeons in the United States favor this approach and more than 90% of them prefer unsutured cataract incisions,[1] originally introduced by I. Howard Fine, MD, in 1992.[2] Clear corneal incisions are widely accepted for their obvious benefits over other approaches. Some recent reports, however, have shown an increase in the rate of endophthalmitis,[3] and this rise has been temporally related to the introduction of the clear corneal approach. Case series comparing the incidence of endophthalmitis with clear corneal versus scleral tunnel incisions have favored the latter, which are associated with lower rates of infection.[4]

In an effort to explain this discrepancy, since 2002, Peter McDonnell, MD, has been leading a group effort of which I am a part at the Wilmer Eye Institute in Baltimore. We have developed several experimental designs to evaluate the watertightness of sutureless clear corneal incisions in ex vivo and in vivo models. This article summarizes the results of our research to date and shares potential methods for optimizing the cataract incision.

OUR RESEARCH

Using conventional clear corneal incisions in human donor globes, we observed the ingress of extraocular fluid using a dye (India ink) placed on the surface of the globe by means of an ink-soaked sponge in the vicinity of the wound. The most interesting finding was that the ink tended to flow into the eye through clear corneal wounds only during hypotony. Shingleton et al have shown that more than 20% of patients develop IOPs of 5 mm Hg or below during the first 30 minutes after cataract surgery using clear corneal incisions.[5] Cataract surgeons usually check the wound's integrity by increasing the IOP to detect outflow (Seidel method) but rarely check for extraocular fluid inflow, which could be more dangerous.

The donor globe model has been criticized, because it disregards the function of the endothelial cell pump, which ultimately may enhance the adherence of the wound's edges. We therefore attempted to reproduce the effects of ocular rubbing or blinking in patients during cataract surgery by applying slight pressure in the vicinity of the wound after mild limbal bleeding. Doing so allowed the validation of the endothelial cell pump's effects in the closure of the wound during the early postoperative period. We observed in these cases that the blood-tinged fluid reached the anterior chamber, signaling the wound's permeability to extraocular fluid (Figure 1), even after the hydrosealing of the wound.[6]

More recently, we analyzed the corneal wound's architecture in postoperative patients using anterior segment optical coherence tomography (Visante; Carl Zeiss Meditec, Inc., Dublin, CA).[7] This technology allows the evaluation of clear corneal wounds in the early postoperative period while preserving their actual shape, due to the noncontact nature of the procedure. In a short series, we detected evident gaping of the incisions in some patients at the 24-hour postoperative visit; these eyes thus may be at increased risk of bacterial invasion into the anterior chamber. Another interesting finding of this study was that most clear corneal incisions were associated with a localized Descemet's membrane detachment in the area of the incision (Figure 2). The complication may be associated with stretching of the wound during phacoemulsification or the insertion of the IOL.

All of these findings may contribute to the possible inflow of extraocular fluid into the anterior chamber through clear corneal incisions and would increase the risk of bacterial contamination.

POSSIBLE SOLUTIONS DERIVED FROM CORNEAL BIOMECHANICS

The clear corneal approach is currently the most common type

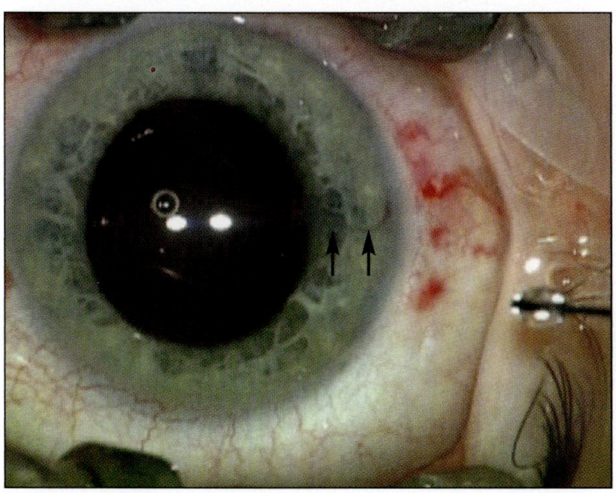

Figure 1. Blood-tinged fluid (arrows) flows into the anterior chamber after the investigators release slight pressure in the vicinity of the wound.

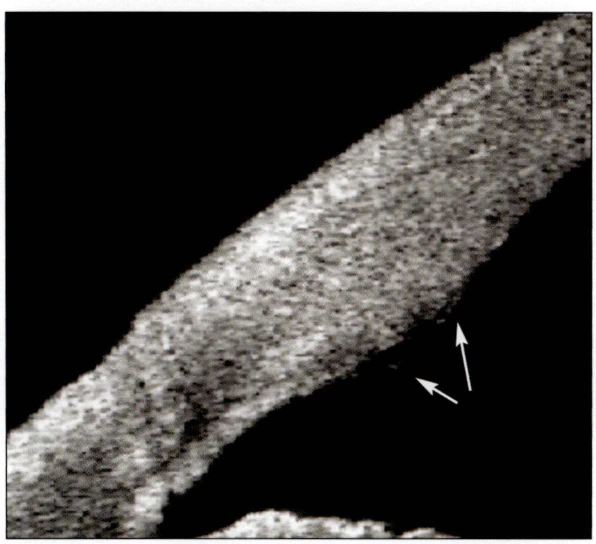

Figure 2. A localized, subclinical Descemet's membrane detachment (arrows) in the area of the incision may contribute to gaping of the wound.

of incision used for cataract surgery. It facilitates the procedure itself and contributes to the rapid postoperative recovery of the patient. Although we have not identified an indisputable cause-effect relationship between the use of sutureless clear corneal incisions and the development of postoperative endophthalmitis after cataract surgery, we believe that there is a strong association that deserves closer attention. Any method that promotes a complete sealing of these wounds is advantageous, because it will prevent the leakage of aqueous and the inflow of extraocular fluid and bacteria into the eye.

One common method for inducing the apposition of the wound's edges is hydrosealing. The surgeon injects the wound's edges with balanced salt solution in order to produce a localized corneal edema on both lips of the incision. In one of our published case series, the routine hydrosealing of the wound's edges did not appear to be as effective at preventing the inflow of extraocular fluid as it was at averting leakage.[6] Perhaps a new design in incisional architecture or other forms of hydrosealing the wound would more securely seal these wounds.

The use of sutures has repeatedly proven to prevent the inflow of India ink in our experimental models. One or two sutures placed on the incision may secure those wounds during the critical period of healing. The use of reabsorbable sutures instead of nylon has also been proposed. Many surgeons at the Wilmer Eye Institute are adopting this practice, especially for cases in which the clear corneal wounds do not appear to be watertight. Unfortunately, we do not have evidence that this strategy prevents the development of endophthalmitis, but it may—at least hypothetically—avoid postoperative inflow.

In the near future, another approach could be the use of novel methods for closing the wound such as corneal adhesives. At least one group of investigators has published the use of a commercially available cyanoacrylate derivative to seal cataract wounds in patients.[8] At our laboratory, we are testing three different, reabsorbable components of sealants for closing the cataract incision.[9,10] It seems that the sealing capacity of these adhesives is superior to standard nylon 10–0 sutures in ex vivo models, and they may add stability to the eye immediately after surgery. More studies are necessary, however, to evaluate the adhesives' biocompatibility in animal models before their clinical use.

CONCLUSION

Clear corneal incisions have been instrumental to the advancement of cataract surgery, but some adjustments to this approach may be required. The quest for a perfectly configured wound and/or improved materials for closing the corneal wound are still an important area of clinical research. ■

This article originally appeared in the June 2007 issue of CRSToday.

1. Learning DV. Practice styles and preferences of ASCRS members—2003 survey. *J Cataract Refract Surg.* 2004;30:892-900.
2. Fine IH. Clear corneal incisions. *Int Ophthalmol Clin.* 1994;34:59-72.
3. West ES, Behrens A, McDonnell PJ, et al. The incidence of endophthalmitis after cataract surgery among the U.S. Medicare population increased between 1994 and 2000. *Ophthalmology.* 2005;112:1388-1394.
4. Cooper BA, Holekamp NM, Bohigian G, Thompson PA. Case-control study of endophthalmitis after cataract surgery comparing scleral tunnel and clear corneal wounds. *Am J Ophthalmol.* 2003;136:300-305.
5. Shingleton BJ, Wadhwani RA, O'Donoghue MW, et al. Evaluation of intraocular pressure in the immediate period after phacoemulsification. *J Cataract Refract Surg.* 2001;27:524-527.
6. Herretes S, Stark WJ, Pirouzmanesh A, et al. Inflow of ocular surface fluid into the anterior chamber after phacoemulsification through sutureless corneal cataract wounds. *Am J Ophthalmol.* 2005;140:737-740.
7. Behrens A, Stark WJ, Pratzer KA, McDonnell PJ. Dynamics of small incision clear cornea wounds after phacoemulsification surgery in the early postoperative period using optical coherence tomography. *J Refract Surg.* In press.
8. Meskin SW, Ritterband DC, Shapiro DE, et al. Liquid bandage (2-octyl cyanoacrylate) as a temporary wound barrier in clear corneal cataract surgery. *Ophthalmology.* 2005;112:2015-2021.
9. Reyes JM, Herretes S, Pirouzmanesh A, et al. A modified chondroitin sulfate aldehyde adhesive for sealing corneal incisions. *Invest Ophthalmol Vis Sci.* 2005;46:1247-1250.
10. Noguera G, Lee WS, Castro-Combs J, et al. Novel laser-activated solder for sealing corneal wounds. *Invest Ophthalmol Vis Sci.* 2007;48:1038-1042.

CHAPTER 4

Why I Do Not Use Clear Corneal Incisions

JOHN R. WITTPENN, JR, MD

Clear corneal incisions allow for quick, sutureless surgery and rapid visual rehabilitation after phacoemulsification. I do not feel, however, that slightly faster surgery counterbalances the potentially higher risk of endophthalmitis.

RISK OF ENDOPHTHALMITIS

The pathogens responsible for endophthalmitis can only enter the eye through the incision in the ocular surface. Recent reports on an increased incidence of endophthalmitis with clear corneal incisions, however, reveal that, despite the use of newer antibiotic prophylaxis, a significant percentage (25% to 33%) of cases occur later than 1 week postoperatively.[1,2]

McDonnell and others have demonstrated that a reduction in the IOP after surgery can result in poor apposition of the edges of the clear corneal incision, with the potential for fluid to flow across the cornea and into the anterior chamber, thus increasing the risk of endophthalmitis.[3,4] Surgeons can decrease this risk by rapidly closing the external wound with a suture or covering it with conjunctiva. Until the incision has sealed completely, the instillation of a rapidly active, broad-spectrum antibiotic is essential to maintaining the surface's sterility.

An issue, however, is that the majority of today's cataract surgeons prefer a uniplanar or straight stab incision. More than 10 years ago, Langerman demonstrated that a uniplanar incision will readily leak with focused pressure on its posterior lip.[5] The egress of fluid will not necessarily occur at the end of the procedure, when significant corneal edema can make the wound appear to be well sealed. Testing the incision on the next day by pressing a cotton-tipped applicator on the posterior aspect of the wound will produce a leak. For a temporally placed incision, the exact same pressure can be achieved when the patient rubs a knuckle over the lateral aspect of his eye. In other words, temporal clear corneal incisions pose the highest risk of patient-induced brief leakage with subsequent hypotony.

Until the eye pressurizes, fluid and any pathogens present on the ocular surface can be drawn into the anterior chamber. This mechanism probably accounts for the appearance of virulent endophthalmitis beyond 1 week after cataract surgery with a clear corneal incision.[1,2]

THE TRIPLANAR INCISION

Langerman showed that a properly executed triplanar or Langerman hinge is extremely stable and does not leak when pressure is applied to its posterior lip.[5] I routinely place this incision at the superior limbus and cover it with conjunctiva when performing cataract surgery. I begin by turning down the conjunctiva superiorly or superotemporally while taking care to leave the Tenon's insertion intact. I generally incise the conjunctiva 1 to 2 mm anterior to the Tenon's insertion to create access to the surgical limbus without opening Tenon's capsule. At the surgical limbus or the blue line, I use a crescent knife to make a deep vertical incision with an aim of 80% to 90% of full thickness. I then come up off the base and tunnel horizontally into clear cornea for approximately 1.5 mm. I make the final part of the incision with a 2.6-mm slit blade that enters along the same plane and then plunges as straight as possible into the anterior chamber to create a triplanar incision.

After completing the procedure, I pull the conjunctiva back over the external incision and pinch it closed with light cautery. The slight foreign body sensation my patients feel from the pinched closing of the conjunctiva is no worse than what they experience with the clear corneal incision.

In a significant majority of my patients, the conjunctiva will remain over the cataract incision. In a few cases, there is some conjunctival retraction, and the edge of the wound is exposed. Most will be fully covered by conjunctiva, however, within the first 5 to 8 days postoperatively. If conjunctiva has fully sealed the incision at this point, I will stop the topical antibiotic. If there has been any retraction or I can still see the external opening of the wound, I will prescribe antibiotics for an additional week.

Because of their location and the presence of blood vessels, I believe that my preferred cataract incisions heal much more quickly than those made in clear cornea. I therefore prefer to place my cataract incisions at the surgical limbus using a triplanar configuration and cover them with conjunctiva. In glaucoma patients who have filtering blebs or may need filtering surgery, however, I perform clear corneal incisions but always place a suture.

CONCLUSION

I have not observed any real benefit to patients from the uniplanar, clear corneal incision compared with the more stable, triplanar incision described by Langerman[5] and placed beneath the conjunctiva at the surgical limbus. I can even use my incision with a temporal approach when circumstances (eg, ocular anatomy) warrant such an approach. Any time saved by the clear corneal incision cannot justify the increased risk to patients of potentially devastating endophthalmitis. ■

This article originally appeared in the June 2007 issue of CRSToday.

1. Deramo VA, Lai JC, Fastenberg GM, et al. Acute endophthalmitis in eyes treated prophylactically with gatifloxacin and moxifloxacin. *Am J Ophthalmol.* 2006;142:721-725.
2. Moshirfar M. Endophthalmitis following use of fourth generation fluoroquinolones after uncomplicated cataract surgery: a retrospective, observational case series. *Ophthalmology.* In press.
3. McDonnell PJ, Taban M, Sarayba M, et al. Dynamic morphology of clear corneal cataract incisions. *Ophthalmology.* 2003;110:2342-2348.
4. Taban M, Rao B, Reznik J, et al. Dynamic morphology of clear corneal cataract wounds–effect of incision angle and location. *Surv Ophthalmol.* 2004;49(suppl 2):S62-S72.
5. Langerman D. Architectural design of a self-sealing corneal tunnel, single-hinge incision. *J Cataract Refract Surg.* 1994;20:84-88.

CHAPTER 5

The Architecture of Clear Corneal Incisions

I. HOWARD FINE, MD; RICHARD S. HOFFMAN, MD; AND MARK PACKER, MD

The role of unsutured clear corneal incisions for cataract surgery in the apparently increased incidence of postoperative endophthalmitis is under intense scrutiny, and the literature on this subject is not conclusive.[1-10] Making a definitive determination requires, in part, understanding these incisions' architecture better. We therefore studied their anatomy with optical coherence tomography (OCT).

BACKGROUND

Clear corneal incisions, which involve an incision in the plane of the cornea with a length equal to 2.0 mm, were first described in 1992,[11] and we continue to construct them in essentially the same manner in our practice. In 1992, our incisions were as wide as 4.0 mm, but, more recently, the maximum width has ranged from 3.5 to 3.8 mm, if not sutured.

In an artist's view of the profile of clear corneal incisions, Figure 1A shows the single-plane incision and its apparently inherent lack of stability, as one surface can easily slide over another. Charles Williamson, MD, of Baton Rouge, Louisiana, innovated an alteration of that incision that involves a shallow, perpendicular groove prior to the incision of the cornea into the anterior chamber (Figure 1B). David Langerman, MD, of Orangeburg, New York, deepened the perpendicular groove in the belief that doing so led to greater stability (Figure 1C).

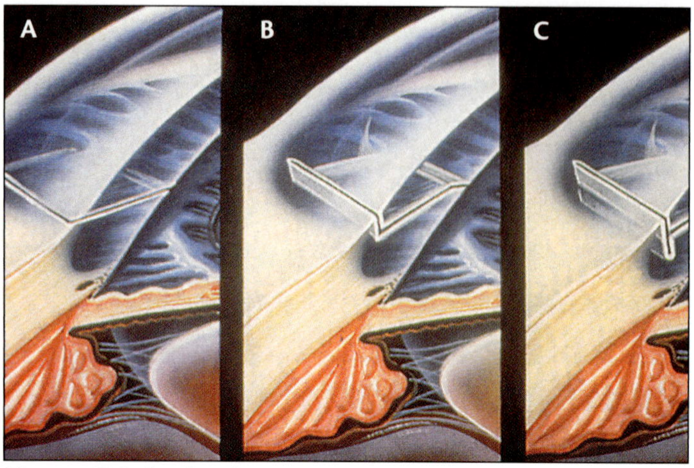

Figure 1. This drawing shows a cross-section of clear corneal incisions circa 1992 (A to C).

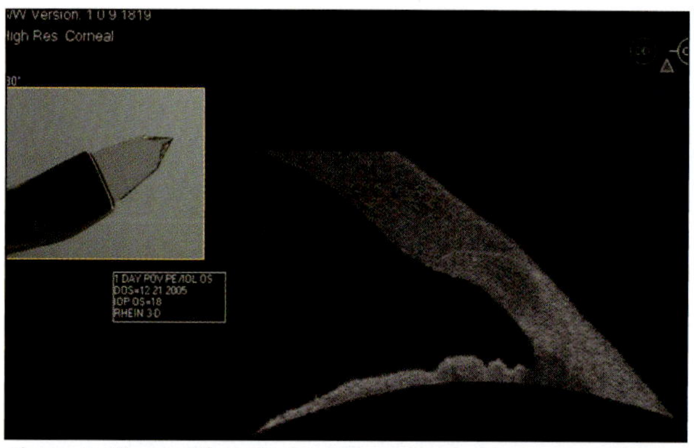

Figure 2. Seen with OCT, this 2.5-mm wide, clear corneal incision was made with the 3D Trapezoidal 2.5- to 3.5-mm blade. An image of the blade is inset.

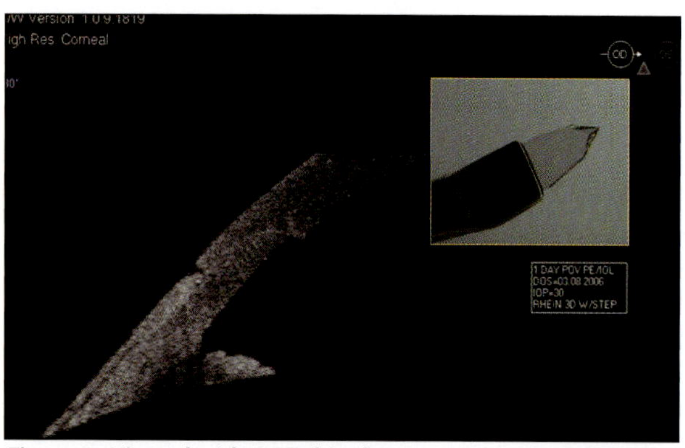

Figure 3. Viewed with OCT, this clear corneal incision has a 300-µm groove at its external edge. Gaping of both the external and internal lips of the incision is evident. An image of the 3D blade (Rhein Medical Inc.) is inset.

We have abandoned these grooved incisions in favor of a paracentesis-style incision due to gaping of the groove and the difficulties associated with persistent foreign body sensation and the pooling of mucus and debris in the groove. More importantly, the grooved incisions represent a disruption in the fluid barrier created by an intact epithelium that allows for a vacuum seal as a result of endothelial pumping.

The construction of the cataract incision begins with the blade flattened against the surface of the globe with the point of the knife at the edge of the clear cornea; the blade advances for 2 mm into the cornea in the plane of the cornea before incising Descemet's membrane. Early on, incisions were made with knives that had straight sides. These blades were subsequently replaced by trapezoidal knives that allowed surgeons to enlarge the incision without violating its architecture by cutting sideways. Since 1992, we have recommended stromal hydration, which thickens the cornea, forces the incision's roof onto its floor, and facilitates endothelial pumping to the upper reaches of the cornea. We also have strongly recommended testing the seal of the incision with a Seidel test using fluorescein.[12] These practices have not changed since 1992, except for eliminating the depression of the posterior lip of the incision.

OUR STUDY: CLEAR CORNEAL INCISIONS

Methodology

The Visante OCT anterior segment imaging system (Carl Zeiss Meditec, Inc., Dublin, CA) allowed us to obtain the first view of the clear corneal incision in a living eye during the early postoperative period. The details of the corneal periphery and the anterior chamber angle, including the regularity with which the corneal epithelium blends into the conjunctiva and the clear corneal stroma blends into the sclera, are clearly visible.

For the study, Dr. Fine created all of the clear corneal incisions. The OCT images of each operative eye were taken on the first postoperative day, within 24 to 30 hours of cataract surgery, and they are representative of multiple images from several patients. The incision's width is defined as the measurement parallel to the limbus. Its length is the distance, in a straight line, between the external incision and the entrance through Descemet's membrane. Dr. Fine used several types of knives to create the clear corneal incisions: the 3D Trapezoidal Blade (Rhein Medical Inc., Tampa, FL); the Simplicity and Black Metal Blades (Accutome, Inc., Malvern, PA); the Clear Cornea Fixed Angle Blade (ASICO, Westmont, IL); the Superstealth Blade (Mastel Precision, Inc., Rapid City, SD); the Kojo Slit and Atomic Edge Metal Blades (BD Ophthalmic Systems, Franklin Lakes, NJ); and the 2.2-mm Metal Blade (Alcon Laboratories, Inc., Fort Worth, TX).

Actual Shape of the Incision

Figure 2, which was taken on the first postoperative day, shows that clear corneal incisions constructed in the way we described are curvilinear, not a straight line as shown in Figure 1. The arcuate incisions have an arc that is considerably longer than the chord length originally estimated for the length of the incision. It is important to note that the architecture of the incision allows for a fit not unlike tongue-and-groove paneling, which adds a measure of stability and makes the sliding of one surface over the other considerably less likely.

The construction of the incision shown in Figure 3 was preceded by the creation of a 300-µm groove at the incision's external edge. The incision itself has a curved or arcuate configuration, but the gaping of the external groove—visible on the first postoperative day—is accompanied by a similar offset of the internal lips of

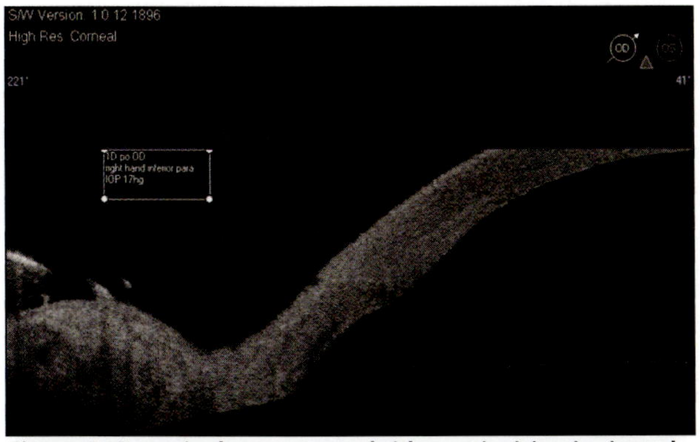

Figure 4. A routinely constructed sideport incision is viewed with the Visante OCT.

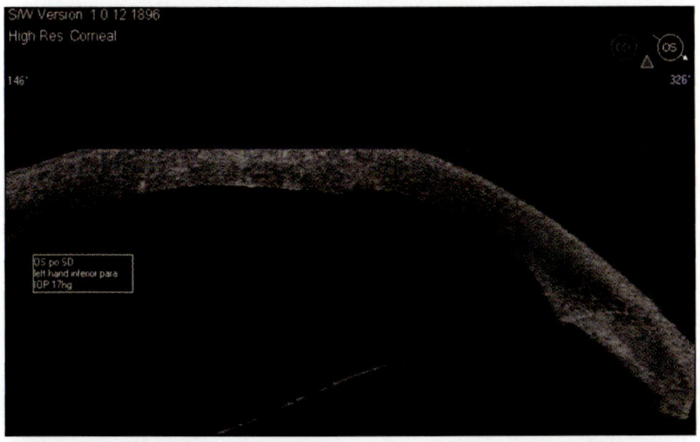

Figure 5. An appropriately constructed sideport incision is viewed with the Visante OCT.

the incision, which appears to be somewhat less stable than a paracentesis-style incision.

Conclusions Drawn

All of the OCT images demonstrate the persistence on the first postoperative day (meaning at least 24 hours after surgery) of stromal swelling from stromal hydration, which many critics of clear corneal incisions believed disappeared within 1 to 2 hours. To confirm that the swelling was due to stromal hydration rather than surgical trauma, we took OCT images of cases in which there was no stromal hydration of the incision. In these incisions, there is less thickening around the incision and some gaping of its internal lip.

Some of the eyes were hypotonous, but the incisions were still perfectly well sealed, a finding that contradicts current thinking regarding hypotony and self-sealability.[13] In addition, proper construction surprisingly resulted in a longer incision in the arc length rather than the measured chord length and in greater stability (like tongue-in-groove paneling).

Our findings demonstrate some of the characteristics that we believe have contributed to the safety of clear corneal incisions and that, in conjunction with other prophylactic measures, can result in the absence of endophthalmitis. We have not had a single case of infectious endophthalmitis in more than 10 years and 10,000 cases. Endophthalmitis prophylaxis involves many factors, including a proper preoperative antibiotic regimen; the preparation of the surgical field, including Betadine (The Purdue Frederick Company, Stamford, CT) and draping over the lashes and meibomian orifices; the incision's construction; surgical technique, including atraumatic surgery; phaco power modulations to avoid heating the incision; not grasping the roof of the incision with a toothed forceps, which would abrade the epithelium and disrupt the fluid barrier for endothelial pumping; the incision's closure utilizing stromal hydration; testing for leakage; and the use of postoperative antibiotics.

Although an attention to all of the details for endophthalmitis prophylaxis is essential, the construction of the incision leading to proper architecture is of primary importance in preventing endophthalmitis, as concluded in a recent white paper from the ASCRS.[14] All clear corneal incisions are not the same. An incision in the plane of the cornea with a chord length of at least 2 mm appears to produce uniquely advantageous architecture for adequate self-sealability.

OUR STUDY: SIDEPORT INCISIONS

We have performed bimanual microincisional phacoemulsification for more than 6 years. In our experience, sideport incisions, through which we use irrigating choppers in one hand and an unsleeved phaco needle in the other, are a little more difficult to seal than our coaxial sideport incisions were. Researchers' attention has recently focused on possible damage to sideport incisions from an unsleeved phaco tip.[15-18] It is important to note that, by their own admission, these investigators have not completed a learning curve in bimanual microincisional phacoemulsification, so some of what they demonstrated may be the result of their novice status with respect to this technique. Nonetheless, we decided to look at our sideport incisions with OCT (Figure 4), and we were surprised to find that many of them more closely resembled the clear corneal incisions seen in Figure 1 than they did our preferred architecture.

We therefore began to use the same amount of time and care in constructing sideport incisions as we do with our larger incisions. We were thus able to achieve exactly the same architecture (Figure 5).

Examining our sideport incisions with OCT forced us to recognize that their proper architecture requires the same appropriate construction as for temporal clear corneal incisions. The blade must be advanced in the plane of the cornea for an adequate length (approximately 1.5 mm) before it incises Descemet's membrane.

CONCLUSION

Proper architecture can be achieved, independent of the knife used, through the incision's appropriate construction. An unfailing attention to detail for both temporal clear corneal and sideport incisions is required. ■

This article is an extension of Fine IH, Hoffman RS, Packer M. Profile of clear corneal cataract incisions demonstrated by ocular coherence tomography. J Cataract Refract Surg. *2007;33:94-97.*

This article originally appeared in the June 2007 issue of CRSToday.

1. Cooper BA, Holekamp NM, Bohigian G, Thompson PA. Case-control study of endophthalmitis after cataract surgery comparing scleral tunnel and clear corneal wounds. *Am J Ophthalmol.* 2003;136:300-305.
2. Nakagi Y, Hayasaka S, Kadoi C, et al. Bacterial endophthalmitis after small-incision cataract surgery: effect of incision placement and intraocular lens type. *J Cataract Refract Surg.* 2003;29:20-26.
3. Eifrig CW, Flynn HW, Scott IU, Newton J. Acute-onset postoperative endophthalmitis: review of incidence and visual outcomes (1995-2001). *Ophthalmic Surg Lasers.* 2002;33:373-378.
4. Miller JJ, Scott IU, Flynn HW Jr, et al. Acute-onset endophthalmitis after cataract surgery (2000-2004): incidence, clinical settings and visual acuity outcomes after treatment.

Am J Ophthalmol. 2005;139:983-987.
5. Monica ML, Long DA. Nine-year safety with self-sealing corneal tunnel incision in clear cornea cataract surgery. *Ophthalmology*. 2005;112:985-986.
6. Masket S. Is there a relationship between clear corneal cataract incisions and endophthalmitis? *J Cataract Refract Surg*. 2005;31:735-741.
7. Mollan SP, Gao A, Lockwood A, et al. Postcataract endophthalmitis: incidence and microbial isolates in a United Kingdom region from 1996 through 2004. *J Cataract Refract Surg*. 2007;33:265-268.
8. Ng JQ, Morlet N, Bulsara MK, Semmens JB. Reducing the risk for endophthalmitis after cataract surgery: population-based nested case-control study. Endophthalmitis population study of western Australia sixth report. *J Cataract Refract Surg*. 2007;33:269-280.
9. Moshirfar M, Feiz V, Vitale AT, et al. Endophthalmitis after uncomplicated cataract surgery with the use of fourth-generation fluoroquinolones: a retrospective observational case series. *Ophthalmology*. 2007;114;686:691.
10. Lundstrom M, Wejde G, Stenevi U, et al. Endophthalmitis after cataract surgery: a nationwide prospective study evaluating incidence in relation to incision type and location. *Ophthalmology*. 2007;114:866-870.
11. Fine IH. Self-sealing corneal tunnel incision for small-incision cataract surgery. *Ocular Surgery News*. May 1992;10:9:38-39.
12. Fine IH. Clear corneal incisions. *Int Ophthalmol Clin*. 1994;34:59-72.
13. Realini T. Wound construction key to avoiding endophthalmitis. *EyeWorld*. February 2007;12:2:64-66.
14. ASCRS Cataract Clinical Committee. Special report: association between CCI and endophthalmitis [white paper]. *EyeWorld*. January 2007 (suppl). Available at: http://www.eyeworld.org/ewweeksupplementarticle.php?id=187&strict=&morphologic=&query=association%20between%20CCI%20and%20endophthalmitis. Accessed May 16, 2007.
15. Vasavada AR. Phaco tips and corneal tissue. *Cataract & Refractive Surgery Today*. June 2005;5(suppl):6:9-10.
16. Weikert M, Koch D. Phaco wounds study. *Cataract & Refractive Surgery Today*. June 2005;5(suppl):6:11-13.
17. Berdahl JP, DeStafano JJ, Kim T. Corneal wound architecture and integrity after phacoemulsification: evaluation of coaxial, microincision coaxial, and microincision bimanual techniques. *J Cataract Refract Surg*. 2007;33:510-515.
18. Osher RH, Injev VP. Microcoaxial phacoemulsification: part 1: laboratory studies. *J Cataract Refract Surg*. 2007;33:401-407.

CHAPTER 6

Are All Corneal Incisions the Same?

AYMAN NASERI, MD

Ophthalmic surgeons are concerned about the risk factors for the development of endophthalmitis. Although much of the focus on prevention has traditionally related to antibiotic prophylaxis, some investigators argue that sutureless clear corneal incisions may contribute to the development of this uncommon, yet devastating, complication of routine cataract surgery.[1] They argue that there is a temporal correlation between an observed rise in the rate of endophthalmitis and the widespread use of sutureless clear corneal incisions.[2]

Other researchers report that there is no statistically significant increase in the rate of endophthalmitis during the same time period at their institutions as those of the aforementioned investigators. These reports fail to identify a statistical link between clear corneal incisions and endophthalmitis.[3,4] Instead, these examiners suggest that the route of antibiotic administration may be one of the most important factors in preventing endophthalmitis.[5,6]

This article discusses the risk of endophthalmitis relative to types of incisions.

NO TWO INCISIONS ARE ALIKE

Differences in a Cut's Characteristics

One implied yet important assumption underlying the debate regarding clear corneal incisions is that they are all equal. Surgeons know, however, that there can be great variation in certain aspects of cataract incisions. Incisions can vary in length, location, angle, anterior and posterior thicknesses, shape, etc. There is also a considerable difference in the types of blades used, with many surgeons deferring to what works best for them.

Disparity in Wound Handling

Even if surgeons could consistently produce identical incisions, cataract surgery requires manipulation of the wound. This fact is obvious to a beginning surgeon, who is often uncomfortably surprised at the steep angle required for a phaco probe to reach the cataract in a highly myopic patient. Most of the studies that have implicated clear corneal incisions as a risk factor for endophthalmitis have not commented on these incisions' architecture at the end of each case.

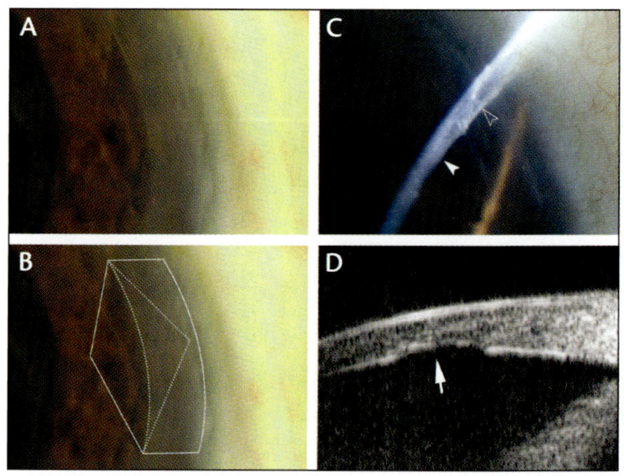

Figure 1. A clear corneal wound following uncomplicated phacoemulsification is pictured. The wound is characteristic of an everted corneal tongue (A). The same wound is shown with a schematic overlay of the everted clear corneal tongue (B). A slit beam shows thinning of the internal aspect of the wound (solid arrow) and thickening of the peripheral cornea (open arrow) from the everted tissue (C). Ultrasound biomicroscopy demonstrates a disruption in the acoustic reflectivity of Descemet's membrane and associated thinning corresponding to the folded tongue (arrow) (D).

Link Between Variability and Endophthalmitis?

Because there is heterogeneity in surgeons' clear corneal incisions, there may be a subgroup of wounds that increase the risk of endophthalmitis. If one could identify such a subgroup, one might better understand the variation in the rates of endophthalmitis across institutions and countries.

IDENTIFYING INCISIONS AT RISK

Inferotemporal

Increased scrutiny of clear corneal incisions has already allowed some surgeons to identify features that may influence the risk of

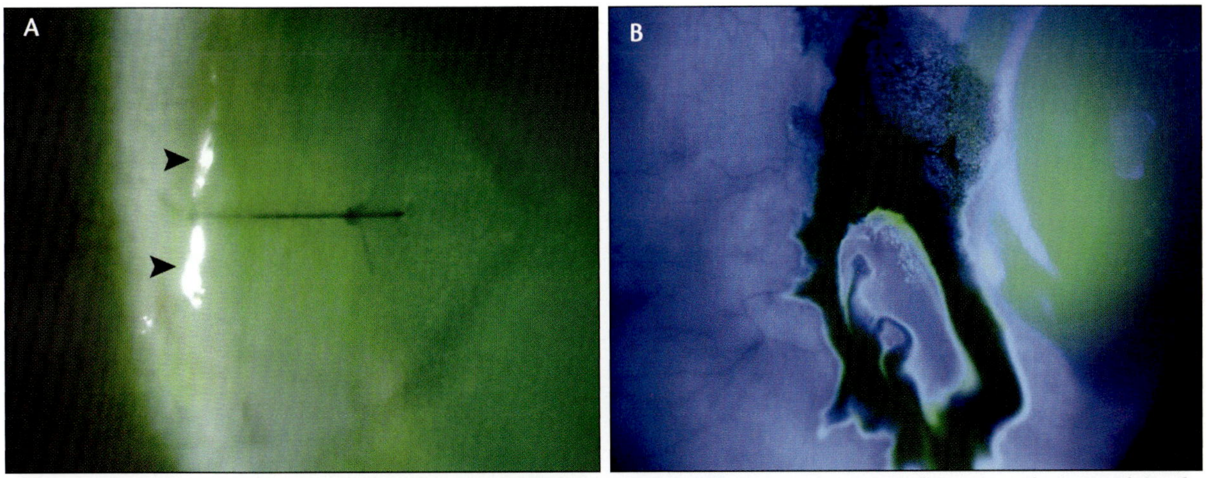

Figure 2. Pictured is a clear corneal wound after uncomplicated phacoemulsification with a 10–0 nylon suture. The internal tip of the corneal tongue is seen protruding from the wound (arrows) (A). A positive Seidel of the same wound resulted (B).

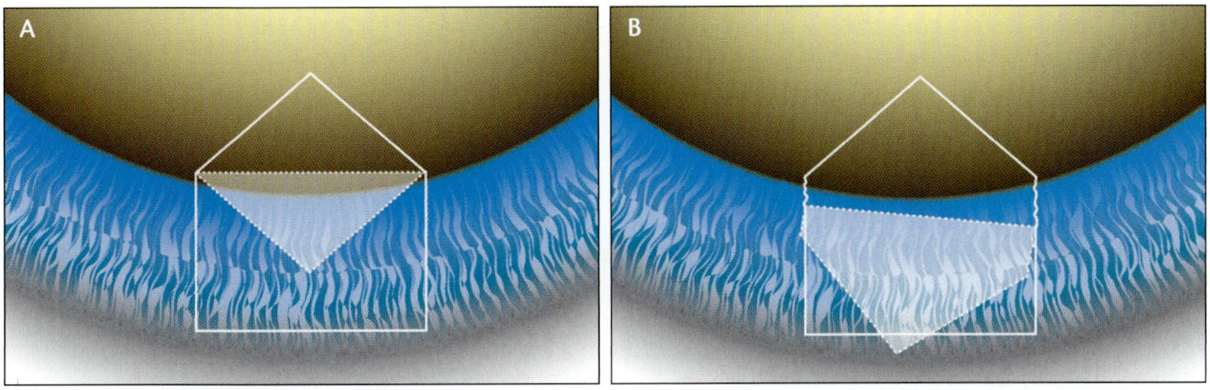

Figure 3. Two types of corneal tongues can be created during construction of the clear corneal wound for phacoemulsification. A type-one corneal tongue is observed when the internal hinge of the corneal flap is preserved; the tissue usually remains within the length of the incision as pictured in Figure 1 (A). With a type-two corneal tongue, a tear along the lateral aspect of the tunneled wound allows for a longer piece of tissue (B), which may even protrude at the ocular surface, especially with short incisions such as that shown in Figure 2.

endophthalmitis. Investigators from the Bascom Palmer Eye Institute in Miami observed that 86% of cases of endophthalmitis at their institution occurred in right eyes with incisions located inferotemporally.[3] Perhaps this observation should encourage right-handed surgeons to avoid inferiorly located incisions by sitting superotemporally when operating on a right eye. Ophthalmologists performing glaucoma filtering procedures often take this step already.

Rectangular

Investigators suggest that the shape of the incision is key to its self-sealing.[7] They argue that square incisions are superior to rectangular ones, because the former are more stable and therefore resistant to early postoperative hypotony and leakage. Perhaps surgeons should create square incisions.

Leaky

Although an incision prone to leakage is clearly undesirable in itself, a relationship between a leaking wound and endophthalmitis was highlighted in a 2005 cohort study from the University of Utah in Salt Lake City.[8] Researchers found that a wound leak on the first postoperative day was associated with a 44-fold increased risk of endophthalmitis. Although the timing of the causative bacterial inoculum is not known in most cases of endophthalmitis, this correlation with a postoperative wound leak suggests that the bacteria gain entry during the early postoperative period in at least some cases.

NEW RISK

Clear Corneal Tongue

My colleagues and I recently described a flaw in the construction of clear corneal wounds that could be a cause of postoperative wound leak.[9] We identified three patients who had undergone uncomplicated cataract procedures by two different surgeons. All three had leaking wounds in the postoperative period. A careful examination of the clear corneal incisions in each case revealed a common feature: the posterior lip of corneal tissue consisting of posterior stroma, Descemet's membrane, and endothelium was folded outward into the lumen of the incision. We described this everted tissue as a clear corneal tongue, and its presence could be confirmed by a slit-lamp examination and ultrasound biomicroscopy (Figure 1).

Although none of the patients in our study developed endophthalmitis, one patient had a positive Seidel sign 16 days postoperatively despite the placement of a suture at the time of surgery. This patient's clear corneal tongue was not only folded back into the wound, but the posterior tissue actually extruded from the eye and required a return to the OR to revise the wound (Figure 2). Another patient had a positive Seidel sign on postoperative day 9, suggesting that this mechanism of destabilizing the wound may lead to late leakage.

Two Categories

My colleagues and I described two types of clear corneal tongues. Type one consists of a simple folding of the free triangular flap frequently created by modern keratomes. Type two represents a lateral tear of the interior portion of the incision (Figure 3). The type-two tongue allows a larger piece of posterior tissue to evert toward the external eye, as occurred in our patient who had a wound leak despite the presence of a well-placed radial suture. We hypothesized that the type-two corneal tongue is created either by the side-cutting elements characteristic of some diamond keratomes or by the surgeon's manipulation of the wound when removing the cataract.

The folding of posterior tissue into the wound undermines the self-sealing properties of a clear corneal incision, because the tissue barrier prevents wound apposition at the internal entry site. Fluid can therefore enter rather than seal the wound via a valve-like mechanism. If endothelial pumping is a component in the closure of clear corneal incisions, it also would be compromised, because Descemet's membrane and the endothelium are inverted and folded into the wound itself. Repositioning the corneal tongue restores the normal anatomy that supports a valve-like, self-sealing wound.

CONCLUSION

I have observed clear corneal tongues intraoperatively for several years now. I stumbled upon the observation when I decided to stop performing stromal hydration of cataract incisions at the end of surgery. At that time, I began to notice that some wounds leaked at the end of surgery, whereas others did not. I realized that the clear corneal tongue was a key difference between wounds that leaked and those that did not. I then developed a technique for closing the wound that involves repositioning the corneal tongue and avoiding stromal hydration. Although this process adds some time to the end of the case, I feel more comfortable with a wound that I know is self-sealing without the temporary assistance of stromal hydration.

As investigators pay more attention to the issue of clear corneal incisions' architecture, I am hopeful that surgeons can continue to improve the incisions' creation and closure. If one can combine a sensible clear corneal incision with evidence-based antibiotic prophylaxis, I am confident that efficient, safe, high-quality cataract surgery will be ensured for patients now and in the future. ■

This article originally appeared in the June 2007 issue of CRSToday.

1. Cooper BA, Holekamp NM, Bohigian G, Thompson PA. Case-control study of endophthalmitis after cataract surgery comparing scleral tunnel and clear corneal wounds. *Am J Ophthalmol.* 2003;136:300-305.
2. Taban M, Behrens A, Newcomb RL, et al. Acute endophthalmitis following cataract surgery: a systematic review of the literature. *Arch Ophthalmol.* 2005;123:613-620.
3. Miller JJ, Scott IU, Flynn HW, et al. Acute-onset endophthalmitis after cataract surgery (2000-2004): incidence, clinical settings, and visual acuity outcomes after treatment. *Am J Ophthalmol.* 2005;139:983-987.
4. Mollan SP, Gao A, Lockwood A, et al. Postcataract endophthalmitis: incidence and microbial isolates in a United Kingdom region from 1996 through 2004. *J Cataract Refract Surg.* 2007;33:265-268.
5. Ng JQ, Morlet N, Bulsara MK, Semmens JB. Reducing the risk for endophthalmitis after cataract surgery: population-based nested case-control study. *J Cataract Refract Surg.* 2007;33:269-280.
6. Lundstrom M, Wejde G, Stenevi U, et al. Endophthalmitis after cataract surgery: a nationwide prospective study evaluating incidence in relation to incision type and location. *Ophthalmology.* 2007;114:866-870.
7. Masket S, Belani S. Proper wound construction to prevent short-term ocular hypotony after clear corneal incision cataract surgery. *J Cataract Refract Surg.* 2007;33:383-386.
8. Wallin T, Parker J, Jin Y, et al. Cohort study of 27 cases of endophthalmitis at a single institution. *J Cataract Refract Surg.* 2005;31:735-741.
9. Tam DY, Vagefi MR, Naseri A. The clear corneal tongue: a mechanism for wound incompetence after phacoemulsification. *Am J Ophthalmol.* 2007;143:526-528.

CHAPTER 7

The Stromal Hydration of Clear Corneal Incisions

ABHAY R. VASAVADA, MS, FRCS; MAMIDIPUDI R. PRAVEEN, DOMS; DEVARSHI U. GAJJAR, PhD; AND DEEPAK PANDITA, MS

Dr. Vasavada regularly performs stromal hydration, at both the clear corneal temporal incision and paracentesis, as part of his strategy for sealing the wound after cataract surgery. Further, he has found stromal hydration to be a useful adjunct in clear corneal cataract surgery, because it allows the adequate approximation of the anterior and posterior aspects of the corneal tunnel.

Today, surgeons perform stromal hydration to enhance the sealing of the wound and thus preclude the need for sutures. The stromal hydration of the incisions was advocated and popularized by Fine.[1] In a recent study, he and his colleagues used anterior segment optical coherence tomography to evaluate the profiles of the clear corneal incision's construction and architecture. They found persistent stromal swelling from stromal hydration, even on the first postoperative day.[2] Furthermore, Wong found that stromal hydration assists in securing clear corneal incisions, thereby helping to prevent endophthalmitis.[3]

Some critics of clear corneal incisions maintain that stromal hydration is detrimental to structural integrity. This assertion presumes that the endothelial pump has no effect on stromal hydration.

We decided to investigate whether hydrating the corneal stromal incision has any impact on the ingress of fluid from the ocular surface into the anterior chamber. This article summarizes our findings.

METHODOLOGY

We prospectively randomized 80 consecutive patients undergoing phacoemulsification to an evaluation of the self-sealing

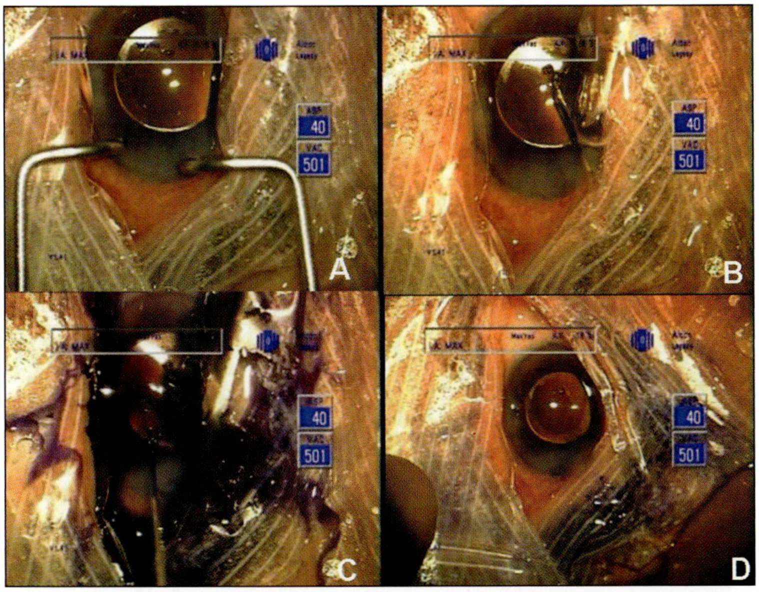

Figure 1. The surgeon removes the speculum from the eye (A) and instills trypan blue (B, C). Two minutes later, he performs gentle irrigation with BSS Plus (D).

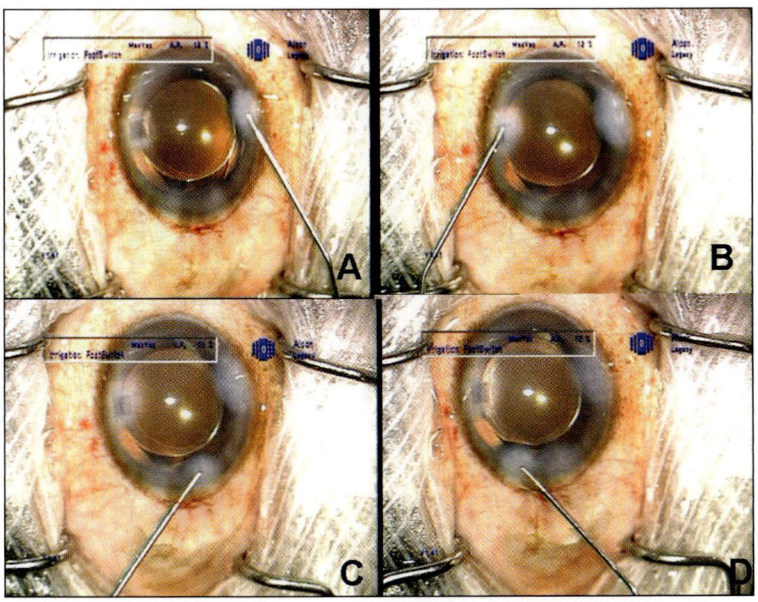

Figure 2. The surgeon performs stromal hydration with BSS Plus of the side walls of the main incision to help appose the roof and floor of the incision (A, B). He seals the two paracentesis incisions by hydrating the stroma (C, D).

property of the corneal incision in response to stromal hydration. For this trial, we used 0.0125% trypan blue solution as a tracer for quantifying the ingress of fluid from the ocular surface into the anterior chamber, and we measured the optical density of the dye in the fluid aspirated from the anterior chamber. We performed microcoaxial phacoemulsification by creating two clear corneal paracentesis incisions of 1 mm and a single-plane temporal clear corneal tunnel of 2.2 mm with an internal entry of at least 1.5 mm. We measured the internal entry with specially designed calipers. If it were less than 1.5 mm, we excluded the eye from the study. We used standardized surgical techniques with the Infiniti Vision System (Alcon Laboratories, Forth Worth, TX). Immediately after completing the cataract procedure, we randomly assigned the eyes to group 1 or 2. For group 1, we gently irrigated the main incision, including the stroma of the sidewalls, with BSS Plus (Alcon Laboratories, Inc.) to facilitate the apposition of the roof and floor of the incision. We continued injecting BSS Plus at the internal ends of the lateral walls to seal the internal entry completely. In both the groups, we removed the speculum from the eye to facilitate the application of trypan blue (0.0125%, pH = 7.39, osmotic pressure = 1.22; Shah & Shah, Calcutta, India) over the conjunctival surface with a micropipette. Patients were advised to blink voluntarily.

After 2 minutes, we gently irrigated the eyes with BSS Plus to wash the excess trypan blue from the ocular surface. Subsequently, we collected 0.1 mL of anterior chamber aspirate by means of a 27-gauge needle mounted on a tuberculin syringe and calculated the amount of dye present (Figure 1). At the end of the trial, in both groups, we sealed the paracentesis incisions along with the main incision by hydrating the stroma with BSS Plus (Figure 2).

We estimated the amount of trypan blue in the aspirate from the anterior chamber by measuring the optical density with a UV-Visible spectrophotometer (Lambda 25; PerkinElmer, Inc., Waltham, MA). We created a standard curve at 595 nm where the maximum absorbance was found when undiluted trypan blue solution was scanned from 190 to 1,100 nm. Simultaneously, using normal saline, we created another standard curve from serial dilutions of undiluted trypan blue (0.012%) down to diluted trypan blue (1:100,000), and we measured absorbance levels at 595 nm. The samples of aspirated aqueous containing trypan blue were measured for optical density by adding 0.9 mL of normal saline to the cuvette. The optical-density values were converted into dilution factors using the standard graph mentioned earlier. The quantitative difference in the ingress between the two groups was determined by comparing the dilution factors. The dilution factor of trypan blue was converted into log values, because the values were increasing and to simplify our calculations. The results were expressed as mean and median values.

OBSERVATIONS

We studied the ingress of trypan blue into the anterior chamber in both groups (Table 1). We found that it was several times lower in the eyes of group 1 (stromal hydration) versus group 2 (not hydrated). The mean log value was significantly higher for group 1, a finding indicating less penetration of trypan blue into the anterior chamber compared with that for group 2 (3.12 ±0.48 vs 2.14 ±0.60, $P<.001$). Similarly, there was a statistically significant difference in the mean dilution of trypan blue in the aqueous aspirate.

TABLE 1. A COMPARISON OF LOGS OF DILUTION AND DILUTION FACTORS OF TRYPAN BLUE'S INGRESS INTO THE ANTERIOR CHAMBER BETWEEN THE TWO GROUPS

	Log of Dilution			Dilution Factor	
Group	N	Mean	Median	Mean	Median
Stromal hydration	40	3.125 ±0.47	3.2	1:11337±30341.45	1:1585
No stromal hydration	40	2.145 ±0.60	2.2	1:220 ±154.15	1:170
	P<.001			P<.001	

Note: Mann-Whitney U test.

The higher the dilution, the lower the penetration of trypan blue into the anterior chamber (1:11,337 ±30,341.46 [group 1] vs 1:220 ±154.15 [group 2], P<.001).

CONCLUSION

Our clinical trial is the first of its kind to demonstrate the impact of hydrating corneal incisions on the ingress of extraocular fluid into the anterior chamber during microcoaxial phacoemulsification.[4] We believe that hydrating these incisions may help to prevent aqueous leakage and also, to some extent, the inflow of fluid from the ocular surface into the anterior chamber, because it restricts the ingress of small particles. In our experience, a corneal incision coupled with stromal hydration is consistently self-sealing and resistant to collapse. In some situations, when Dr. Vasavada notices any distortion or stretching of the incision or even a short internal entry (which raises questions about the integrity of the incision), he does not hesitate to place a single 10–0 Vicryl suture (Ethicon Inc., Somerville, NJ). The situations in which he has found stromal hydration most helpful are cases involving large incisions during standard coaxial phacoemulsification.

Our clinical findings provide evidence in favor of the hydration of corneal incisions after phacoemulsification. The benefits of stromal hydration are far from imaginary. ■

This article originally appeared in the June 2007 issue of CRSToday.

1. Fine IH. Corneal tunnel incision with a temporal approach. In: Fine IH, Fichman RA, Grabow HB, eds. *Clear Corneal Cataract Surgery and Topical Anesthesia.* Thorofare, NJ: Slack, Inc.; 1993:25.
2. Fine IH, Hoffman RS, Packer M. Profile of clear corneal cataract incisions demonstrated by ocular coherence tomography. *J Cataract Refract Surg.* 2007;33:94-97.
3. Wong MY. Securing clear corneal incisions. *Cataract & Refractive Surgery Today.* 2003 March. Available at: http://www.crstodayarchive.com/03_archive/0303/051.html. Accessed April 20, 2007.
4. Vasavada AR, Praveen MR, Pandita D, et al. Effect of stromal hydration of clear corneal incisions: quantifying ingress of trypan blue into the anterior chamber after phacoemulsification. *J Cataract Refract Surg.* 2007;33:623-627.

CHAPTER 8

Achieving a Watertight Incision

FRANK A. BUCCI JR, MD; PAUL H. ERNEST, MD; EHUD I. ASSIA, MD; AND BROCK K. BAKEWELL, MD

FRANK A. BUCCI JR, MD

Constructing a watertight, clear corneal cataract incision is mandatory to ensuring a stable anterior chamber without hypotony. In addition, it has recently been suggested that clear corneal incisions have contributed to the rising incidence of endophthalmitis over the past decade. Some clinicians have proposed "retreating" to using scleral tunnels with sutures exclusively instead of clear corneal incisions with a suture when indicated on occasion. In the mid-1990s, when the complication rate related to phacoemulsification was higher than acceptable, the ophthalmic community's response was to better educate the beginning phaco surgeon instead of retreating to the extracapsular technique. I suggest we take a similar approach now, because clear corneal incisions do not cause endophthalmitis; rather, poorly constructed clear corneal incisions that leak contribute to the complication.

My preferred technique for achieving a watertight seal at the time of phacoemulsification is to construct a clear corneal incision with three planes. After placing viscoelastic in the anterior chamber through the paracentesis site, I use a diamond blade with its footplates set at a depth of 370µm to create the first plane. This straight corneal groove is approximately 3 mm in length and is located just inside the clear cornea.

I create the second plane with a trapezoid diamond blade, which contains a progressive width of 2.6 to 2.9 mm. I place the tip of the trapezoid blade in the bottom of the groove and tip it upward so the path of the blade is parallel to the curvature of the peripheral cornea. The blade progresses through the clear cornea for a length of approximately 1.50 to 1.75 mm. Performing this step requires excellent visualization of the diamond blade's tip.

The final step begins with my changing the angulation of the trapezoid diamond. I point the tip of the trapezoid diamond to the theoretical center of the lens, and the keratome fully penetrates the clear cornea into the anterior chamber. My opposite hand provides countertraction by placing the second instrument in the paracentesis site, which is 3 clock hours clockwise to the temporal wound. At the completion of the procedure, all clear corneal incisions receive stromal hydration. A flat, 27-gauge cannula fits nicely into an appropriately constructed incision. I challenge the watertight seal of the wound with a dry Weck-Cel sponge (Medtronic Xomed Ophthalmics, Inc., Minneapolis, MN) and/or the 27-gauge cannula. I prefer to leave the eye somewhat firm, which I believe enhances the self-sealing–valve nature of the three-planed incision.

PAUL H. ERNEST, MD

A secure cataract incision is based on three components: (1) geometry; (2) the incision's location; and (3) the instrument's distortion of ocular tissue during microincisional cataract surgery.

A square wound with an adequate corneal component is the most secure incision that one can create, as demonstrated by laboratory studies in cadaveric models and living animal models.[1-7] Studies in both models have shown that the endothelial pump plays no role in the wound's stability.[4] The fact that there have been so many reports of endophthalmitis with nonsquare incisions but not with square incisions is further confirmation. Using contemporary lens technology and cartridge delivery systems, one can construct a cataract incision that is 2.50 to 2.75 mm wide. Started at the proper location (as described later), it can have a tunnel at least 2.50 mm long.

There is an area of the limbus that is approximately 0.50 to 0.75 mm where there is no sub-Tenon's space. By starting one's incision in this area and carrying the cut anteriorly 2.00 mm into the cornea, one can achieve a square geometry and avoid the potential for conjunctival ballooning during surgery.

I create a horizontal groove using a crescent blade. With the same keratome, I construct a tunnel into the cornea. I enter the anterior chamber with a blade that is 2.50 to 2.75 mm in width. It is important to avoid dragging posterior conjunctiva into the incision when using the keratome. Otherwise, the outermost edge of the blade will create a small hole in the conjunctiva—the source of conjunctival ballooning.

A second advantage of starting the incision in the limbal area is that resultant fibroblastic activity seals the incision within 7 days. In contrast, clear corneal incisions take 30 to 60 days to seal with fibroblastic activity.[4]

In microincisional cataract surgery, incisions are 1.0 to 1.5 mm wide. Placing instruments through these incisions will cause ovalization of the tissue. This distortion will destabilize the incision independent of its geometry and location. To avoid this problem, one should create a slightly larger and longer incision. Stromal hydration can help re-approximate the tissue after surgery. If leakage persists, the surgeon should close the incision with a suture.

EHUD I. ASSIA, MD

Several factors may affect the wound's stability. First, making a long corneal incision (minitunnel) is more significant than making a bi- or triplanar incision. Second, one should avoid corneal burn. The surgeon should direct the handpiece parallel to the incision. Tilting of the probe (for example, in deep-set eyes) may strangle the sleeve and decrease flow, which is required to cool the tip. One should also avoid prolonged continuous activation of ultrasonic energy—a simple precaution to take with new phaco machines that may be thus programmed.

The third issue is the incision's location. A superior incision is inconvenient, and a lateral incision tends to gape. I favor an oblique incision, which I can comfortably create and which will cause the least amount of astigmatism.

Fourth, using an anterior chamber maintainer throughout surgery maintains a steady chamber and prevents distortion of the corneal dome. A leaking incision is readily visible upon irrigation through a sideport.

Finally, the smaller the incision, the more watertight. Microincisional cataract surgery usually involves the bimanual technique (ie, an irrigating chopper or cannula in the surgeon's second hand). I prefer using an anterior chamber maintainer specifically designed for microincisional cataract surgery. I insert a new model of thinly walled, large-pored tube through a 1.2-mm inferior incision, where it provides more fluid than any available irrigating chopper. I find that irrigating instruments often flush nuclear pieces during surgical manipulations, whereas the modified anterior chamber maintainer allows me to use whichever instrument I like in my second hand. The chamber's stability does not depend on instruments inserted and withdrawn several times during surgery.

BROCK K. BAKEWELL, MD

When attempting to create a watertight wound during phaco surgery, it is important to keep three things in mind: (1) the entrance into the cornea should be parallel to the limbus and should not "fishmouth"; (2) the corneal tunnel should be at least 1.5 mm in length, as originally described by I. Howard Fine, MD,[8] but preferably closer to 2.0 mm; and (3) the surgeon should not stretch the wound to any significant degree during phacoemulsification or the insertion of the IOL.

A watertight, uniplanar incision is best achieved by applanating or applying posterior pressure while the blade remains parallel to the iris as it advances toward the anterior chamber. The resultant entrance wound is parallel to the limbus rather than curved away from it (fishmouthing), which shortens the corneal tunnel at its sides.

It is easier to make the incision watertight by lengthening it, closer to 2.00 or 2.25 mm, but elongation may cause striae during phacoemulsification that will worsen visualization. If the entrance of the incision begins in the far peripheral cornea where the conjunctival vessels are reflective, then a 2.00- or 2.25-mm incision will not cause striae.

When introducing the IOL, it is important not to stretch the wound, or corneal hydration will be required for a tight seal. While inserting the IOL, I enlarge the incision to 3 mm if I am using an Unfolder (Advanced Medical Optics, Inc.; Santa Ana, CA). With an SA60 lens (Alcon Laboratories, Inc., Fort Worth, TX), I insert the Monarch injector (Alcon Laboratories, Inc.) only into the initial aspect of the incision rather than entirely into the anterior chamber. I can then inject the IOL with a B cartridge without stretching a 2.8-mm incision.

These steps and an attention to detail usually produce a watertight incision and eliminate the need for corneal hydration. ■

This article originally appeared in the January 2006 issue of CRSToday.

1. Ernest PH, Rhem M, McDermott M, et al. Phacoemulsification conditions resulting in thermal wound injury. *J Cataract Refract Surg.* 2001;27:1829-1839.
2. Ernest PH, Kiessling LA, Lavery KT. Relative strength of cataract incisions in cadaver eyes. *J Cataract Refract Surg.* 1991;17:668-671.
3. Ernest PH, Lavery KT, Kiessling LA. Relative strength of scleral tunnel incisions with internal corneal lips constructed in cadaver eyes. *J Cataract Refract Surg.* 1993;19:457-461.
4. Ernest PH, Tipperman R, Eagle F, et al. Is there a difference in incision healing based on location? *J Cataract Refract Surg.* 1998;24:482-486.
5. Ernest PH, Lavery KT, Kiessling LA. Relative strength of scleral corneal and clear corneal incisions constructed in cadaver eyes. *J Cataract Refract Surg.* 1994;20:626-629.
6. Ernest PH, Fenzl R, Lavery KT, Sensoli A. Relative stability of clear corneal incisions in a cadaver eye model. *J Cataract Refract Surg.* 1995;21:39-42.
7. Ernest PH, Neuhann T. Scientific studies and their clinical relevance. The implications for cataract incisions. *J Cataract Refract Surg.* 2005;5:22-25.
8. Maloney W. Advanced phacoemulsification: recent advances. Course presented at: The ASCRS/ASOA Symposium on Cataract, IOL and Refractive Surgery; April 12, 1992; San Diego, CA.

CHAPTER 9

Improving the Seal of a Clear Corneal Incision

MICHAEL Y. WONG, MD

The increasing popularity of clear corneal incisions in cataract surgery has been accompanied by a worrisome suggestion that the incidence of bacterial endophthalmitis[1] and toxic anterior segment syndrome[2] is also on the rise. This article describes a simple, quick, inexpensive technique to tightly appose both lips of the incision and thus secure and prolong the seal.

TECHNIQUE

Prior to creating the clear corneal incision, I make a supraincisional stromal pocket 0.5 mm anterior to the intended entrance. With a simple stab of a diamond or metal keratome, I create a 2-mm pocket that resembles an equilateral triangle, its base toward the limbus. The pocket's depth can be anywhere from one-third to two-thirds stromal thickness.

I hydrate the stroma through this pocket with balanced salt solution at the end of the case, thus creating a bulge that exerts an inward pressure on the external lip of the clear corneal incision. The internal lip is pressed outward by the IOP. The combined pressure makes for a tight apposition of both lips of the incision and thus prevents the egress or ingress of fluid through the wound for a period of 24 hours. By that time, the ciliary body is producing aqueous, and the endothelial pump has brought the lamellae of the stroma tightly together. The seal is firm enough to withstand fluctuations in IOP, whether high or low.

One may create two pockets instead of one if desired, and I have found that there is tremendous latitude in the dimensions of the pocket(s) without impairing the effect (Figures 1 and 2). There are no significant complications of this technique. Formally described as *stromal hydration of a supraincisional pocket*, the technique is colloquially called the *Wong Way*.

INCREASED MARGIN OF SAFETY

A perfectly constructed, square or nearly square clear corneal incision created with a diamond knife is safe and secure.[3,4] The outward forces of the IOP press up on the internal aspect of the corneal lip to provide a sufficient seal until the endothelial pump dries the internal channel of the incision. In practice, however, conditions are less than perfect. Many surgeons employ a metal knife, the incision's edges are not as clean or long as desired, its lips shrink because of heat from the phaco tip or become stretched by the IOL's insertion, or the limbal structures are weakened by a limbal relaxing incision. The Wong Way can provide a margin of safety in these instances.

EFFECTIVE SEAL THROUGH VULNERABLE PERIOD OF HYPOTONY

The structural weakness of a standard clear corneal incision can be exposed in the postoperative period when additional biomechanical stress occurs with blinking, rubbing of the eye, ocular movement, and hypotony from a relative shutdown of the ciliary body. In vitro, hypotony in a cadaveric eye results in an inflow of India ink placed on the ocular surface.[5] In vivo, the release of aqueous through a clear corneal incision to manage a postoperative pressure spike can result in temporary hypotony with a subsequent superficial inflow of fluorescein placed in the tear film.[6] The resilience of the sclera causes the globe to expand from a relatively collapsed state in hypotony to produce a vacuum action. This situation may be one of the causes of toxic anterior segment syndrome.

In contrast, the Wong Way incision remains watertight in the presence of hypotony, as evident upon hydrating the pocket at the end of a cataract operation without reforming the anterior chamber and exerting external pressure with a cellulose sponge. The IOP is low, and the incision does not leak. In the estimated 20% of patients who experience postoperative hypotony,[7] the eye would thus be protected from a superficial influx of fluid that might contain bacteria or other toxic substances.

MORE EFFECTIVE LOCATION OF STROMAL HYDRATION

The stromal hydration of the sides and superior roof of the clear corneal incision can create the impression that the wound is watertight while the patient is on the operating table. This fluid, however, is often resorbed during the first few hours after surgery, because it is relatively close to the endothelial pump. Further, my experience with LASIK surgery has shown that apposing stromal

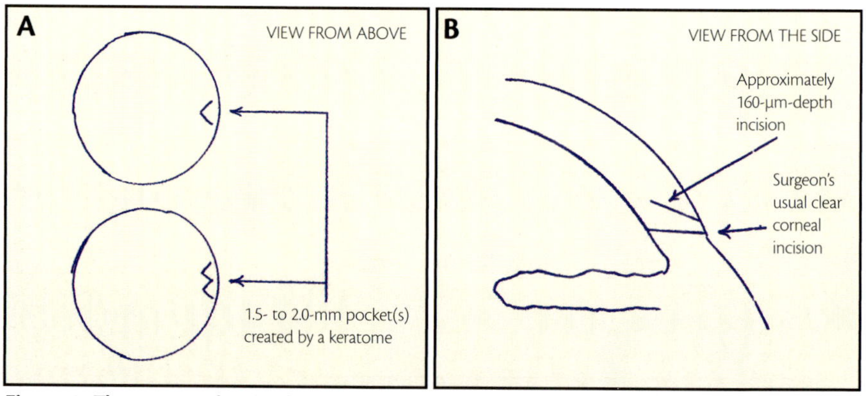

Figure 1. The surgeon begins by creating a stromal pocket that is 1.5 to 2.0 mm wide. If using two stab incisions, he places them side by side so that the incision resembles an upside down W (A). A side view shows the pocket to be just anterior to and above the usual entry into the anterior chamber (B).

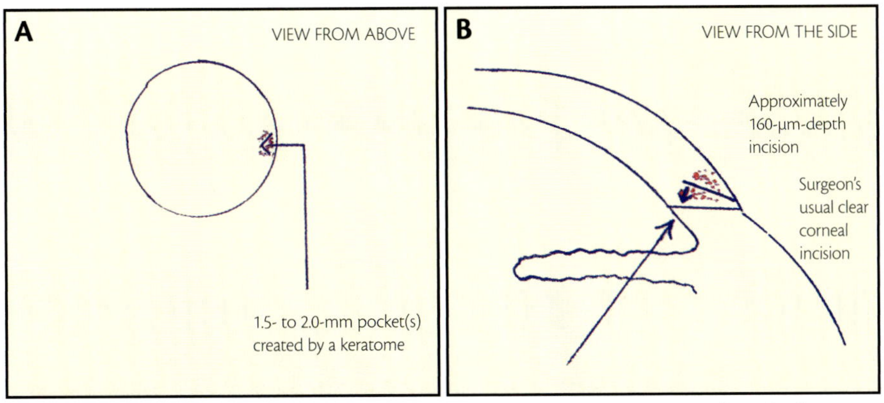

Figure 2. At the conclusion of the case, the surgeon uses a 30-gauge cannula to hydrate the tip and edges of the supraincisional stromal pocket with balanced salt solution (A). The reformed anterior chamber pushes upward on the internal aspect of the corneal lip, while the stromal hydration pushes downward on the wound (B).

lamellae are more adherent when desiccated. Stromal hydration within the channel of the clear corneal incision works in opposition to this concept.

On the other hand, stromal hydration in a separate and distinct stromal pocket that is external and anterior to the clear corneal incision typically lasts for 24 to 36 hours. The inward pressure remains beyond the time period of ciliary shutdown and hypotony. Further, because this supraincisional pocket of fluid is distal to the clear corneal incision with regard to the endothelium, the stromal lamellae within the channel of the clear corneal incision are desiccated and secure before the endothelium resorbs the supraincisional fluid.

ALTERNATIVES

Concern over a possible association between clear corneal incisions and the risk of endophthalmitis[1] has prompted some surgeons to switch back to scleral tunnels. Relying on a thin layer of conjunctiva that often retracts with blinking, however, is an unreliable defense. Other surgeons suggest sealing the clear corneal incision with a fibrin adhesive, but doing so adds time, expense, and potential toxicity,[8] and it may interfere with the desiccation of the stromal lamellae within the channel.

USES

I prefer to hydrate a supraincisional pocket with every clear corneal incision for cataract surgery. Other surgeons use the technique only when the seal of the wound is tenuous at the end of a case. I also find that the technique is useful for a paracentesis of questionable competence, when the corneal structure is less rigid than usual (eg, when the clear corneal incision is within a limbal relaxing incision or with a young patient), and in situations when anterior chamber stability is of the utmost importance during the early postoperative period (eg, after the insertion of a Crystalens accommodating IOL [Eyeonics, Inc., Aliso Viejo, CA]).

CONCLUSION

The Wong Way aids in sealing a clear corneal incision quickly, easily, and intuitively, and it entails no additional expense. Practically speaking, this technique is complication free. The best thing I can say about the Wong Way is that the worst thing that can happen is nothing. ■

This article originally appeared in the June 2007 issue of CRSToday.

1. Taban M, Behrens A, Newcomb RL, et al. Acute endophthalmitis following cataract surgery. *Arch Ophthalmol.* 2005;123:613-620.
2. Mamalis N, Edelhauser H, Dawson D, et al. Toxic anterior segment syndrome. *J Cataract Refract Surg.* 2006;32:324-333.
3. Ernest P, Kiessling LA, Lavery KT. Relative strength of cataract incisions in cadaver eyes. *J Cataract Refract Surg.* 1991;17:668-671.
4. Masket S, Belani S. Proper wound construction to prevent short-term ocular hypotony after clear corneal incision cataract surgery. *J Cataract Refract Surg.* 2007;33:383-386.
5. McDonnell PJ, Taban M, Sarayba M, et al. Dynamic morphology of clear corneal cataract incisions. *Ophthalmology.* 2003;110:2342-2348.
6. Chawdhary S, Anand A. Early post-phacoemulsification hypotony as a risk factor for intraocular contamination: in vivo model. *J Cataract Refract Surg.* 2006;32:609-613.
7. Shingleton B, Wadhwani R, O'Donoghue M, et al. Evaluation of intraocular pressure in the immediate period after phacoemulsification. *J Cataract Refract Surg.* 2001;27:524-527.
8. Realini T. Wound construction key to avoiding endophthalmitis. *EyeWorld.* February 2007. Available at: http://www.eyeworld.org/article.php?sid=3635&strict=&morphologic=&query=realini%20AND%20construction. Accessed May 15, 2007.

CHAPTER 10

Tissue Adhesives for Wound Closure in Cataract Surgery

BHAIRAVI V. KHAROD, MD, AND TERRY KIM, MD

Clear corneal incisions have marked a breakthrough in phacoemulsification, because they reduce surgical time, speed patients' postoperative recovery, and reduce the rate of induced astigmatism. They also significantly decrease the incidence of the complications associated with scleral tunnels such as conjunctival manipulation and hyphema. Studies, however, have suggested a potentially increased risk of postoperative endophthalmitis with clear corneal incisions.[1,2] For that reason, many ophthalmologists have become interested in strengthening the seal of these wounds. This article focuses on one such method, tissue adhesive.

CLEAR CORNEAL INCISIONS AND ENDOPHTHALMITIS

Recently, a multinational prospective study conducted by the ESCRS demonstrated that the risk of endophthalmitis following phacoemulsification was 0.38%.[1] Many peer-reviewed studies have compared the incidence of postoperative endophthalmitis with clear corneal versus scleral tunnel incisions. For example, a large, retrospective, comparative, case-controlled study evaluated the incidence of postoperative endophthalmitis in clear corneal incisions with or without sutures versus scleral tunnel incisions. The investigators compared 38 patients with culture-positive, acute, postcataract surgery endophthalmitis and 371 randomly selected control patients who underwent uncomplicated cataract surgery. They also compared the type of incision and use of a suture during cataract surgery between patients with endophthalmitis and controls. The researchers reported a threefold greater risk of endophthalmitis with clear corneal incisions than scleral tunnel incisions. The placement of a suture did not affect the incidence of endophthalmitis.[2]

In other studies, investigators have noted that self-sealing wounds were associated with the ingress of fluid into the anterior chamber in cases involving hypotony, minimal manipulation of the wound, and a postoperative fluctuation in IOP.[3,4] Several other studies have demonstrated foreign bodies (including retained cotton fiber, cilia, and ointment) in the anterior chamber following clear corneal incisions.[5-11] This research demonstrated the fragility of a clear corneal incision in the early postoperative period and the possible contamination of the anterior chamber by extraocular fluid entering through these wounds.

Nonetheless, a prospective case series involving 3,500 consecutive cataract surgeries performed by one surgeon using local anesthesia found different results. A 3- X 2-mm beveled clear corneal incision was employed in each procedure, and no cases of endophthalmitis were reported.[12]

TISSUE ADHESIVES AND CLEAR CORNEAL INCISIONS

Tissue adhesives have been utilized for various purposes in ophthalmology, including corneal perforations, wound repair, and amniotic membrane transplantation. They have also been used as sealants for glaucoma and plastics procedures. Traditionally, ophthalmologists choose cyanoacrylate-based glues, but fibrin-based glues are gaining popularity as substitutes for sutures.[13,14] Other new adhesives on the horizon include polyethyelene glycols, modified chondroitin sulfates, acrylic copolymers, and biodendrimers.

Many studies have demonstrated the efficacy of cyanoacrylate-based glue as a suture substitute in clear corneal incisions. In a prospective interventional case series, Meskin et al used 2-octyl cyanoacrylate with parabens (Liquid Bandage; Johnson & Johnson, Skillman, NJ) to seal the wound after clear corneal cataract surgery. In this series, a single surgeon created a 2.75-mm, triplanar, clear corneal incision in 51 patients. At the conclusion of each case, he sealed the wound with 2-octyl cyanoacrylate with parabens. All 51 eyes were found to have watertight wounds immediately after the application of the glue and at all postoperative visits. The most frequent complaint was a transient foreign-body sensation, which was reported by 31 patients (61%). Other side effects included bulbar conjunctival hyperemia and the retention of glue on the second postoperative visit.[15]

Hermel et al conducted a similar study in bovine and rabbit eyes and demonstrated that the wounds in eyes with cyanoacrylic adhesives showed greater resistance in the early postoperative period than sutures. Seven days after the operation, however, the resistance of the incisions was similar among the groups.[16]

Shigemitsu et al compared the tensile strength of wounds that were not sutured, sutured using various techniques, or treated with various biotissue adhesives. They demonstrated that both cyanoacrylate and fibrin glue had tensile strength comparable to the sutures used in cataract surgery.[17]

Ritterband et al evaluated the effect of fluctuations in IOP on wounds that were sealed with cyanoacrylate glue. They made 3-mm clear corneal incisions in human donor globes. They used a transscleral cannula to alter the IOP while placing droplets of India ink on the wound. The eyes without glue were noted to leak with manual pressure at the wound's edge. None of the eyes with tissue adhesive showed an ingress of India ink with varying IOP or manual manipulation of the wound.[18]

Researchers have also evaluated the histological inflammatory activity with bioadhesives such as fibrin and cyanoacrylate versus unsutured valved closure and suturing. Alvarado et al demonstrated that fibrin bioadhesive induced a greater inflammatory response than other techniques at 1 week postoperatively, whereas cyanoacrylate adhesive caused less inflammatory activity than the suturing material. On day 30, both fibrin and cyanoacrylate adhesives had generated a slightly greater inflammatory response than sutured and unsutured techniques for closure. The study also showed that healing may be better with fibrin than cyanoacrylate glue in both the early and late postoperative period.[19]

Similarly, Henrick et al found that wounds sealed with organic tissue glue (Tisseel; Baxter Healthcare Corporation, Glendale, CA) had a higher incidence of inflammation than those closed with sutures. They found no difference in the wounds' integrity between these two methods of closure.[20]

Fibrin-based adhesives have been shown to have equal efficacy as cyanoacrylate glue with the added advantages of biocompatibility, the ability to be applied over larger surface areas, and an enhanced ability to secure amniotic membrane or conjunctival grafts. The potential disadvantages of human fibrin glue are the theoretical risk of viral transmission and the complexity of their preparation and application.[21]

Other glue materials such as Dermabond (2-octyl cyanoacrylate; Ethicon Inc., Somerville, NJ) have been shown to seal clear corneal incisions effectively such that their tensile strength is comparable to wounds closed by sutures.[22]

NOVEL TISSUE ADHESIVES

Many new adhesives are under investigation as alternate modalities to seal corneal wounds. In various studies, modified chondroitin sulfate aldehyde adhesive[23] and acrylic copolymer tissue adhesive[24] have proven successful.

Dendrimers are another promising class of tissue adhesives. Velazquez et al showed that, for both linear and stellate corneal wounds, biodendrimer adhesives provided a higher mean leakage pressure than closure with sutures.[25]

Dendritic macromers are also under investigation. Some macromers cross-link to form macroscopic gels, including hydrogels. Wathier et al evaluated several macromolecules. Their studies showed that hydrogel sealants produced from various macromolecules were effective in sealing corneal incisions (Figure 1). Their results also demonstrated that hydrogel sealants withstand higher pressures and stress placed on a wound than conventional self-sealed or sutured wounds. The hydrogel sealants offered the added advantages of easy preparation, reduced (four to six times) surgical time compared with conventional suturing, and minimized trauma to tissue[26,27] (Figure 2).

CONCLUSION

Although no conclusive evidence exists to demonstrate a definitive relationship between clear corneal incisions and an increased risk of endophthalmitis, many ophthalmologists are investigating

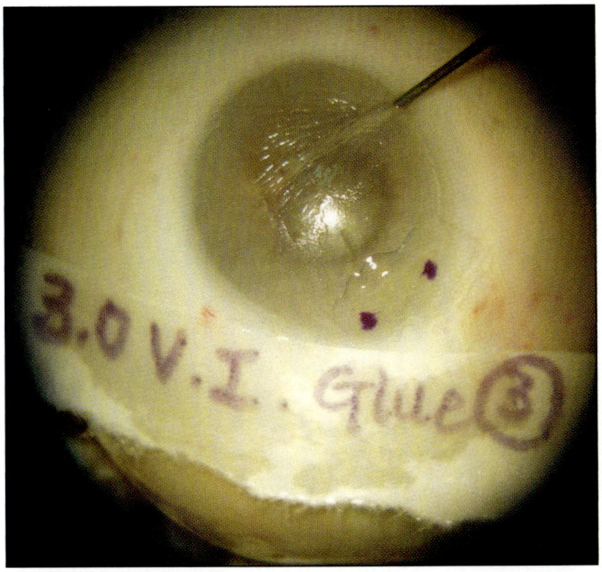

Figure 1. A clear, dendritic polymer has been used to seal this 3-mm clear corneal incision in a human eyebanked eye.

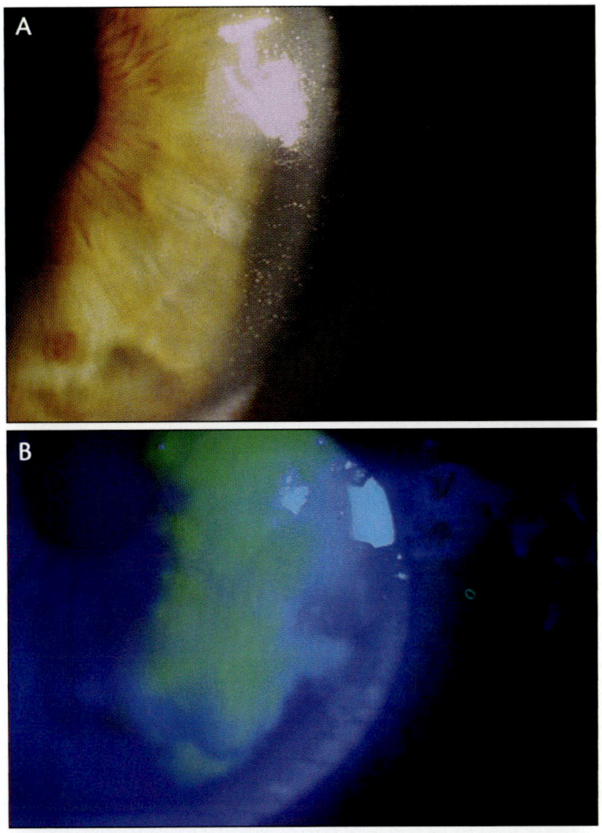

(Courtesy of Hyperbranch Medical Technology, Inc.)

Figure 2. Preliminary testing of a synthetic, dendritic sealant has demonstrated successful results on human patients (A; stained with fluorescein, B).

methods of sealing cataract incisions prophylactically. Traditionally, nylon sutures have been the most widely employed method of closing the wound. Tissue adhesives, however, have been quickly gaining in popularity as substitutes for sutures. Cyanoacrylate glue has been used most frequently, but other tissue adhesives, including human fibrin glue, are also employed. The disadvantages of cyanoacrylate and fibrin glues include a complex preparation process, foreign-body sensation, conjunctival hyperemia, and a possibly increased inflammatory reaction. Fibrin glue has the added theoretical risk of viral transmission. Other investigational bioadhesives may provide a safer, more biocompatible, and more effective alternative for closing corneal incisions after cataract surgery. ■

This article originally appeared in the June 2007 issue of CRSToday.

1. Seal DV, Barry P, Gettinby G, et al. ESCRS study of prophylaxis of postoperative endophthalmitis after cataract surgery: case for a European multicenter study. *J Cataract Refract Surg.* 2006;32:396-406.
2. Cooper MA, Holekamp NM, Bohigian G, Thompson PA. Case-control study of endophthalmitis after cataract surgery comparing scleral tunnel and clear corneal wounds. *Am J Ophthalmol.* 2003;136:300–305.
3. Chawdhary S, Anand A. Early post-phacoemulsification hypotony as a risk factor for intraocular contamination: in vivo model. *J Cataract Refract Surg.* 2006;32:609-613.
4. Taban M, Sarayba MA, Ignacio TS, et al. Ingress of India ink into the anterior chamber through sutureless clear corneal cataract wounds. *Arch Ophthalmol.* 2005;123:643-648.
5. Yuen HK, Lam RF, Kwong YY, et al. Retained presumed intraocular cotton fiber after cataract operation: long-term follow-up with in vivo confocal microscopy. *J Cataract Refract Surg.* 2005;31:1582-1587.
6. Rofail M, Briner AM, Lee GA. Migratory intraocular cilium following phacoemulsification. *Clin Experiment Ophthalmol.* 2006;34:78-80.
7. Galloway GD, Ang GS, Shenoy R, Beigi B. Retained anterior chamber cilium causing endophthalmitis after phacoemulsification. *J Cataract Refract Surg.* 2004;30:521-522.
8. Kargi SH, Oz O, Erdinc E, et al. Tolerated cilium in the anterior chamber. *Ocul Immunol Inflamm.* 2003;11:73-78.
9. Werner L, Sher JH, Taylor JR, et al. Toxic anterior segment syndrome and possible association with ointment in the anterior chamber following cataract surgery. *J Cataract Refract Surg.* 2006;32:227-235.
10. Aralikatti AK, Needham AD, Lee MW, Prasad S. Entry of antibiotic ointment into the anterior chamber after uneventful phacoemulsification. *J Cataract Refract Surg.* 2003;29:595-597.
11. Chen KH, Lin SY, Li MJ, Cheng WT. Retained antibiotic ophthalmic ointment on an intraocular lens 34 months after sutureless cataract surgery. *Am J Ophthalmol.* 2005;139:743-745.
12. Monica ML, Long DA. Nine-year safety with self-sealing corneal tunnel incision in clear cornea cataract surgery. *Ophthalmology.* 2005;112:985–986.
13. Marticorena J, Rodriguez-Ares MT, Tourino R, et al. Pterygium surgery: conjunctival autograft using a fibrin adhesive. *Cornea.* 2006;25:34-36.
14. Szurman P, Warga M, Grisanti S, et al. Sutureless amniotic membrane fixation using fibrin glue for ocular surface reconstruction in a rabbit model. *Cornea.* 2006;25:460-466.
15. Meskin SW, Ritterband DC, Shapiro DE, et al. Liquid bandage (2-octyl cyanoacrylate) as a temporary wound barrier in clear corneal cataract surgery. *Ophthalmology.* 2005;112:2015-2021.
16. Hermel B. Studies on the use of tissue adhesives in cataract microsurgery [in Polish]. *Polim Med.* 1980;10:3-18.
17. Shigemitsu T, Majima Y. The utilization of a biological adhesive for wound treatment: comparison of suture, self-sealing sutureless and cyanoacrylate closure in the tensile strength test. *Int Ophthalmol.* 1996-1997;20:323-328.
18. Ritterband DC, Meskin SW, Shapiro DE, et al. Laboratory model of tissue adhesive (2-octyl cyanoacrylate) in sealing clear corneal cataract wounds. *Am J Ophthalmol.* 2005;140:1039-1043.
19. Alvarado Valero MC, Mulets Homs E, Alio Y Sanz JL. Bioadhesives in ocular surgery [in Spanish]. *Arch Soc Esp Oftalmol.* 2001;76:559-566.
20. Henrick A, Kalpakian B, Gaster RN, Vanley C. Organic tissue glue in the closure of cataract incisions in rabbit eyes. *J Cataract Refract Surg.* 1991;17:551-555.
21. Bhatia SS. Ocular surface sealants and adhesives. *Ocul Surf.* 2006;4:146-154.
22. Leung GY, Peponis V, Varnell ED, et al. Preliminary in vitro evaluation of 2-octyl cyanoacrylate (Dermabond) to seal corneal incisions. *Cornea.* 2005;24:998-999.
23. Reyes JM, Herretes S, Pirouzmanesh A, et al. A modified chondroitin sulfate aldehyde adhesive for sealing corneal incisions. *Invest Ophthalmol Vis Sci.* 2005;46:1247-1250.
24. Alio JL, Mulet ME, Cotlear D, et al. Evaluation of a new bioadhesive copolymer (ADAL) to seal corneal incisions. *Cornea.* 2004;23:180-189.
25. Velazquez AJ, Carnahan MA, Kristinsson J, et al. New dendritic adhesives for sutureless ophthalmic surgical procedures: in vitro studies of corneal laceration repair. *Arch Ophthalmol.* 2004;122:867-870.
26. Wathier M, Johnson MS, Carnahan MA, et al. In situ polymerized hydrogels for repairing scleral incisions used in pars plana vitrectomy procedures. *ChemMedChem.* 2006;1:821-825.
27. Wathier M, Jung PJ, Carnahan MA, et al. Dendritic macromers as in situ polymerizing biomaterials for securing cataract incisions. *J Am Chem Soc.* 2004;126:12744-12745.

CHAPTER 11

The History of the Capsulorhexis Technique

HOWARD V. GIMBEL, MD

With the development of the in-the-bag single-plane posterior chamber IOLs in the early 1980s, it became obvious to me, and others, that a capsular opening without any extending tears would facilitate placement of both loops into the capsular bag. These tears always originated at a "V" of can-opener capsulotomies.

CONTINUOUS CURVILINEAR CAPSULORHEXIS

My first thoughts on how to avoid these V-shaped notches in the capsulotomy occurred in 1983 while watching James Gills, MD, of Tarpon Springs, Florida, tear a short arc using the scissors as a forceps after a cut in the capsule. I reasoned that tears with a cystatome could be directed in a curvilinear fashion. Because I was not using viscoelastics routinely at that time, at first, I tore the capsule in arc-like sections leaving small bridges to stabilize the flap in the turbulence of the irrigation fluid until the circle was mostly complete. After performing more than 1,000 of these procedures in my Canadian practice, I made my first public presentation of the concept with a video titled, "The Continuous Tear Capsulotomy" at the American Intraocular Implant Society film festival in Boston in April 1985.[1] My development and some of its advantages were also reported on in an ophthalmic trade publication.[2] In the fall of 1985, this video was shown at the IOLAB intraocular lens company booth at the AAO meeting in San Francisco. An illustrated information sheet on the new technique was distributed by IOLAB. The video was shown again in 1986 at the AAO film festival. When viscoelastics became routine, the technique changed to a full circle tear, which capsular forceps designed by Peter Utrata of Columbus, Ohio, facilitated. The new technique was appreciated and adopted with enthusiasm by those surgeons implanting the STAAR Surgical silicone plate-haptic IOL (STAAR Surgical, Monrovia, CA).

Thomas Neuhann, MD, from Munich, Germany, developed a technique that started a smooth, circular capsular opening with a subincisional needle puncture and then completed it with arcs taken both ways from this puncture. He coined the term *capsulorhexis*, which appropriately uses the Greek suffix rhexis meaning "to tear." He presented his capsulorhexis technique at the German Society of Ophthalmology meeting in the fall of 1985 and published a description of the technique in a German medical journal in 1987.[3]

Calvin Fercho, MD, of Fargo, North Dakota, presented a circular capsular opening technique at the Welsh Cataract Congress, in Houston in September 1986 titled "Continuous Circular Tear Anterior Capsulotomy."

Kimiya Shimizu, MD, in Kanagawa, Japan, reported on a method of opening the capsule in a smooth, round fashion at the Japanese ophthalmic surgeons' meeting in January 1987.

The name *continuous curvilinear capsulorhexis* (CCC) was selected as the most appropriate for the technique, because the opening it created did not have to be exactly circular to have all of the desired qualities.[4,5]

A number of modalities other than tearing have been evaluated to open the capsule. The Fugo plasma blade (Medisurg Research & Management Corporation, Norristown, PA) has proven very efficacious, especially when tearing is prevented by fibrosis in the capsule such as in late traumatic cataract cases.[6,7]

The intact CCC has made the nucleus' removal more efficient and safe.[8] In addition, cortex removal can be more complete, lens epithelial cell removal can be made possible, and the IOL's implantation can be easier, safer, and more secure. If in-the-bag fixation is not possible because of a posterior capsular tear, the intact CCC may be used for optic capture fixation described as Anterior Rhexis Fixation by Tobias Neuhann, MD, of Munich, Germany at the 1991 ASCRS Film Festival.[9]

TWO-STAGE CAPSULORHEXIS

I developed two-stage capsulorhexis in June 1988, and it has extended the possibilities for achieving a CCC in challenging and

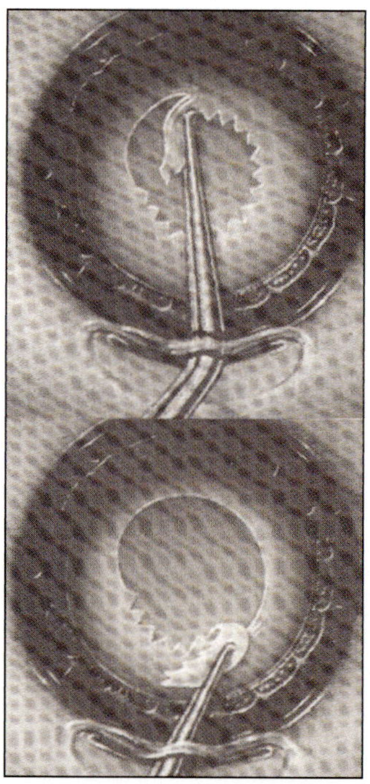

Figure 1. Following a tangential snip at the can-opener margin, an additional ribbon of capsule is removed in the process of converting to a smooth-edged CCC.

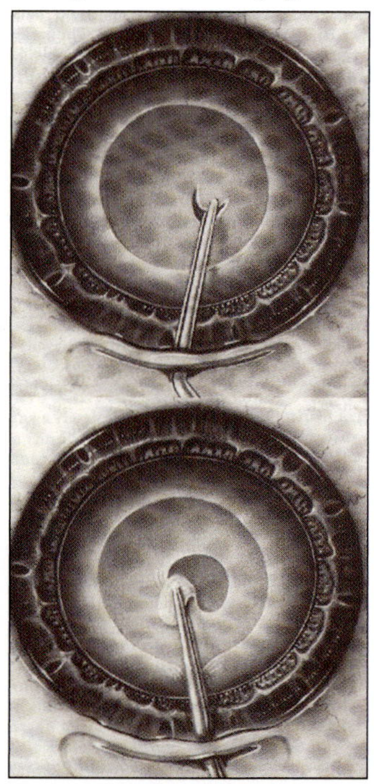

Figure 2. Using principles of CCC, PCCC is used to convert a posterior capsular tear into a continuous tear opening resistant to extension.

complicated cases.[10] This technique was first employed before capsular stains were used when the original capsulectomy was purposefully made small or can opener-like for safety reasons in white cataracts. The initial anterior capsular opening was converted to a CCC of the desired diameter by making a tangential snip on one side of the opening with a Vannas scissors (Katena Products, Inc., Denville, NJ). The second tear was then extended with forceps to remove a strip or ribbon of additional capsule (Figure 1). Short radial tears were turned back using a forceps, and for large radial tears, a snip and tear in the opposite direction was used to complete the opening.

POSTERIOR CCC

It was soon recognized that the intra- and postoperative advantages of the CCC could also be applied to make a smooth continuous curvilinear tear in the posterior capsule, a technique I first utilized on November 26, 1987, for removing a dense plaque on the posterior capsule. Naming it *posterior continuous curvilinear capsulorhexis* (PCCC), I presented this technique on April 30, 1989, at the Storm Eye Institute Ophthalmology Update Meeting in Charleston, South Carolina.

The PCCC technique was used in the making of a primary opening or used to advantage in cases where small, linear or triangular tears in the posterior capsule occurred during cataract surgery without extending too far toward the capsule's equator.[11] I first used a PCCC on September 27, 1988, after a tear inadvertently developed in the posterior capsule as I was polishing it with a stainless steel irrigation/aspiration tip. The posterior capsular tear was completed into a continuous smooth circular opening (Figure 2). The IOL was placed in the bag with no extension of the posterior capsular opening. No vitreous presented.

I then started to intentionally make 4.0- to 4.5-mm PCCCs in pediatric cataract surgery, and, without vitrectomy, capture the optic with the PCCC.[12] As expected, the secondary cataract "pearls" have all spilled into the anterior chamber without obstructing the visual axis.

CONCLUSION

Although the impetus to develop a CCC opening was the propensity of multiple adjoining tears in the can-opener technique to extend to the equator and even to the posterior capsule during lens removal and IOL placement, the strength of the CCC opening not only made phacoemulsification safer but also has lead to many other techniques. These techniques include in-the-bag lens disassembly, optic capture, lens epithelial cell removal, and safe strategies for managing small posterior capsular tears, posterior capsular plaques and with posterior CCC, optic capture for IOL fixation, and for maintaining a clear visual axis without vitrectomy. ■

This article originally appeared in the October 2007 issue of CRSToday.

1. Gimbel HV. Continuous tear capsulotomy. Film presented at: The American Intraocular Implant Society; April 1985; Boston, MA.
2. Gimbel HV. Capsulotomy method eases in-the-bag PCL. *Ocular Surgery News.* July 1, 1985;3:13:2-3.
3. Neuhann T. Theorie und operationstechnik der kapsulorhexis. *Klin Monatsbl Augenheilkd.* 1987;190:542-545.
4. Gimbel HV, Neuhann T. Development, advantages, and methods of the continuous circular capsulorhexis technique. *J Cataract Refract Surg.* 1990;16:31-37.
5. Gimbel HV, Neuhann T. Continuous curvilinear capsulorhexis. *J Cataract Refract Surg.* 1991;17:110-111.
6. Fugo RJ. Fugo blade to enlarge phimotic capsulorhexis [letter]. *J Cataract Refract Surg.* 2006;32:1900.
7. Sing D. Use of the Fugo blade in complicated cases [letter]. *Cataract Refract Surg.* 2002;28;573-574.
8. Gimbel HV. Evolving techniques of cataract surgery: continuous curvilinear capsulorhexis, down-slope sculpting, and nucleofractis. *Semin Ophthalmol.* 1992;7:193-207.
9. Neuhann T, Neuhann TH. The rhexis-fixation lens [film]. Film presented at: The ASCRS Symposium on Cataract, IOL and Refractive Surgery; April 1991; Boston, MA.
10. Gimbel HV. Two-stage capsulorhexis for endocapsular phacoemulsification. *J Cataract Refract Surg.* 1990;16:246-249.
11. Gimbel HV. Posterior capsule tears using phacoemulsification: causes, prevention and management (PCCC). *Eur J Implant Ref Surg.* 1990;2:63-69.
12. Gimbel HV, DeBroff BM. Posterior capsulorhexis with optic capture: maintaining a clear visual axis after pediatric cataract surgery. *J Cataract Refract Surg.* 1994;20:658-664.

CHAPTER 12

Why Did We Abandon the Can-Opener Capsulotomy?

DAVID J. APPLE, MD

In 1754, Jacques Daviel, MD, originated the extracapsular cataract extraction procedure and provided, for the first time, a cataract removal technique that spared surgeons and patients from the perils and complications of the ancient couching technique.[1] The latter technique was, of course, laden with complications such as hemorrhage, inflammation, and infection. Dr. Daviel's procedure permitted for the first time an extraction of the crystalline lens as opposed to pushing the lens into the interior of the eye.

A BRIEF HISTORY

Residual Peripheral Tears

From Daviel's time until the mid-20th century, the anterior capsular opening (anterior capsulotomy) maneuvers, including the can-opener procedure, consisted of procedures where one or more jagged residual peripheral tears were left. Whenever such a tear exists there is a high likelihood that the tear(s) would extend to the periphery toward and even around the equator. Therefore, the diameter and shape of the capsular opening are not well controlled.

Lack of Equatorial Support

In the 1940s, when Sir Harold Ridley invented the IOL he used an extracapsular cataract extraction procedure pioneered by the Austrian ophthalmologist, Anton Elschnig, MD.[1] This technique was not unlike the can-opener procedure, but the diameter of the capsulotomy orifice was much greater. Elschnig's procedure was characterized by a very large opening, and it also left numerous tears extending into the equator, so that not only was the entire anterior capsule removed, but some of the equatorial capsule was torn away. Ridley intended his lenses to be inserted into the capsular bag. In many instances, however, this was not possible because little or no equatorial support was left that could tightly sequester the lens periphery into the bag. His implants were actually most commonly on-the-bag, rather than in-the-bag as we know it. It is well known that the most common complication Ridley had to handle was an inferior decentration (sunset syndrome). Most authorities have attributed this dilemma to the excess weight of the implant, which was only partially true. The lack of capsular support at the equator was equally or even more important than the IOL's weight in the pathogenesis of this problem.

Attempts to Securely Fixate the IOL

By the 1970s and 1980s, surgeons were still searching for a better way to achieve high-quality symmetrical fixation of the IOLs' haptics, initially attempting ciliary sulcus fixation. Many soon realized the disadvantages of this type of fixation as compared with fully sequestering the pseudophacos in the capsular bag.[2-4] They therefore began to change to a goal of achieving in-the-bag fixation. Although the trend towards in-the-bag fixation was a step in the right direction, most surgeons still continued with the can-opener capsulotomy technique.

It soon became clear that most in-the-bag lenses did not end up in the capsule as planned. Rather most were situated with one haptic in and one haptic out of the bag, almost invariably causing an unwanted IOL decentration.[4] This was noted clinically by many surgeons at that time and we confirmed this in our pathological studies. By the mid-1980s, only 30% of IOLs were actually situated in the bag, 10% were in the cilary sulcus, and 60% were situated asymmetrically although most surgeons attempted a more accurate surgical result. Usually, the lens would be centered upward (sunrise syndrome) because the superior hapatic would generally end up in the soft tissues of the ciliary sulcus, whereas the inferior (ie, trailing) haptic would end up in the inferior capsular fornix.

At first, many surgeons feared that the quality of their surgery was poor, leading to the high incidence of such unwanted asymmetric fixations. I recall that many were genuinely distressed, believing that they could not successfully localize the haptics of the lens where they intended. Their distress was compounded by their need to deal with subsequent decentrations that followed. Young residents in training today cannot imagine what a problem this was, especially during the nascent years of flexible PC-IOLs between 1977 to 1985.

Scientific analysis gradually made it clear that the problem was not surgeons' "miss-aiming" of the haptics, but rather the so-called "pea-podding" effect in which, in many cases, a lens haptic initially implanted correctly within the bag would spring out via a capsular rent at the peripheral jagged edge characteristic of the can-opener.

THE INVENTION OF THE CAPSULORHEXIS

The invention of the continuous curvilinear capsulorhexis (CCC) by Thomas Neuhann, MD, of Munich, Germany, and Howard Gimbel, MD, of Alberta, Canada, (there were early possible mentions of this technique by two surgeons, Drs. Stein and Fercho) provided for the first time a means of avoiding capsular tears, which is the main reason that the CCC became the procedure of choice. As the CCC was adopted throughout the 1980s and 1990s, this in turn, decreased the incidence of many cases of tear-induced decentration that presented as a result of pea-podding that was so common in the era of the can-opener.

I was involved in running wet labs for surgeons in the early years when CCC was being introduced around 1984. One not only had to teach the technique but also justify it. In these labs and lectures, I discerned that it was sometimes difficult for surgeons to perceive its advantages by simply providing a didactic presentation without an accompanying demonstration. I found one means of demonstrating its safety and efficacy using what I have termed the "story of the peanut bag."

All of us have sometimes noted the difficulty in opening an airline-provided sealed peanut bag in the absence of a precut tear in the bag's periphery. In sharp contrast, when such preformed tears are present, it is easy to extend the tear and open the bag. This extension of the tear in the peanut bag is analogous to the extension of a radial tear.

During this period a major American airline went out of business. I remember vividly that their peanut bags had no preformed tears. Thus, it was easy to joke that their lack of an appropriate preformed tear with subsequent difficulty in opening peanut bags might have been one reason for the company's demise. Of course, there was no relationship to the airline's financial misfortunes and the peanut bags, but this fable helped me demonstrate to surgeons during the early years of the CCC the pathophysiology and potential negative implications of having or not having a preformed tear. Some of the best scientific studies on the pathophysiology of the CCC were performed by Assia et al.[5] In clinical surgery, of course, any radial tear is analogous to the preformed tear of the peanut bag, whereas the smooth edge of the CCC is analogous to the peanut bag that is difficult to open in the absence of the preformed tear.

Why mention this nonsensical story of the peanut bag? This tale is by no means just a historical vignette. We still use it today to help explain this technique to patients or lay individuals—especially to preoperative patients who are interested but have difficulty in understanding the intricacies of this stage of the procedure.

How can we be sure that the CCC technique works so well? One has to simply ask our young residents-in-training today if they have ever seen or heard of the pea-podding phenomenon. The CCC has almost made this complication an issue of the past!

CONCLUSION

In summary, the reason that surgeons transitioned away from the can-opener capsulotomy was to solve a problem, difficult to comprehend and solve in those early years, but very simple as viewed now in retrospect with 20/20 hindsight. The almost total eradication of the complication of pea-podding by the introduction of the CCC represented one more critical step in our move to today's modern cataract/IOL operation. The capsulorhexis is one of several techniques and devices such as hydrodissection and phacoemulsification that have made modern small-incision cataract/IOL surgery the wonderful procedure that benefits our patients today. ■

This article originally appeared in the October 2007 issue of CRSToday.

1. Apple, DJ. *Harold Ridley and the Fight for Sight.* Thorofare, NJ: Slack, Inc.; 2006.
2. Apple DJ, Reidy J, Googe J, et al. A comparison of ciliary and capsular bag chamber intraocular lenses. *J Am Intraocular Implant Soc.* 1985;11:44-63.
3. Apple DJ, Aufferth G, Peng Q, Visessook N. *Foldable Intraocular Lenses.* Thorofare, NJ: Slack, Inc.; 2000.
4. Ram J, Apple DJ, Peng Q, et al. Update on fixation of rigid and foldable posterior chamber lenses (IOLs). Part I. Elimination of decentration to achieve precise optical correction and centration. *Ophthalmolgy.* 1999;106:883-890.
5. Assia EI, Apple DJ, Barden A, et al. An experimental study comparing various anterior capsulotomy techniques. *Arch Ophthalmol.* 1991;109:642-647.

CHAPTER 13

Strategies for Managing the Difficult Capsulorhexis

DAVID F. CHANG, MD

There are four general conditions that increase the risk of a radial capsulorhexis tear: poor visibility, eye movement, chamber shallowing, and increased capsular elasticity. These situations may arise either because of the ocular anatomy or due to poor surgical technique.

POOR VISIBILITY

A good red reflex and visibility are important in order to manipulate the flap and monitor the direction of the tear as it develops. A surgeon's delayed recognition of a peripherally escaping tear may preclude any chance to redirect it in time.

Ocular causes of a poor red reflex include tear film debris, decreased corneal clarity, small pupils, anterior cortical opacity (anterior spokes or white cataract), nuclear opacity (brunescence), and vitreous opacities such as asteroid hyalosis or hemorrhage. Errors in surgical technique may also compromise visibility. Excessive drying can cloud the corneal epithelium. Poor irrigation fluid runoff may submerge the cornea. Clumsy instrument maneuvers might create corneal striae or displace the globe out of optimal microscope alignment. Finally, excessive downward pressure from the capsulotomy needle's tip will penetrate and stir up the epinucleus. This can cause focal loss of the red reflex right at the area where the flap inserts.

With challenging cases, surgeons must pay greater attention than usual to sharp focus, a clear corneal tear film, and positioning the eye so as to optimize the red reflex. The surgeon should increase the microscope zoom if necessary. Furthermore, a surgeon should consider trypan blue dye whenever he anticipates difficulty with visualizing the anterior capsule. He can apply dye even after he initiates the capsulotomy, because trypan blue preferentially stains the capsule but not the cortex.

EYE MOVEMENT

The potential for eye movement is characteristic of topical anesthesia or an unintentional consequence of a poor regional block. A sudden unanticipated head or eye movement may cause a peripheral radial tear. Patients must be cooperative enough to have surgery under topical anesthesia, and using appropriate levels of sedation and communication should enhance their cooperation. Fixation is improved by avoiding excessive microscope light intensity, which can induce squeezing. During the capsulotomy, the cornea should be moistened in a way so as to avoid startling the patient or surgeon. One way to eliminate the need for an assistant to manually wet the cornea during surgery is to lubricate it in the following manner. The surgeon first smears a few streaks of a dispersive ophthalmic viscosurgical device (OVD) such as Viscoat (Alcon Laboratories, Inc., Fort Worth, TX), Amvisc Plus (Bausch & Lomb, Rochester, NY), or Occucoat (Bausch & Lomb) onto the corneal surface. Adding several drops of balanced salt solution will create an even, but viscous wetting layer that will resist evaporation and provide superb clarity.

ANTERIOR CHAMBER SHALLOWING

The natural anterior convexity of the equatorial lens tends to steer any capsular tear toward the periphery. The shallower the chamber is, the more convex the anterior capsule becomes, and the more the tear tends to run radially "downhill." The direction of the tear is most easily controlled if the anterior capsular surface is flattened.

A shallow anterior chamber may be the natural result of a small globe, narrow angles, or an intumescent lens. Severe zonular laxity may result in an unexpectedly shallow chamber despite a normal axial length. A common cause of anterior capsular convexity is intraoperative shallowing of the anterior chamber due to escape of fluid or OVD through the wound. Excessive instrument pressure on the posterior incision lip will "burp" the chamber through a momentary wound gape, and the surgeon should interrupt the capsulotomy step to inject more OVD.

Because it creates more of a mass effect, a maximally cohesive OVD is better able to flatten the anterior capsular convexity when compared with a dispersive OVD. The latter better resists being burped out through the incision however. The soft-shell technique originated by Steve A. Arshinoff, MD, FRCSC, from the University of Toronto combines the complementary advantages of each OVD by placing the cohesive agent directly over the anterior capsule and blocking the incision with the dispersive OVD[1] (Figure 1). Healon5 (Advanced Medical Optics, Inc., Santa Ana, CA) is a maximally cohesive and viscoadaptive OVD that combines both of these desirable characteristics in a single agent.[2]

CAPSULAR ELASTICITY AND PSEUDOELASTICITY

The more elastic a material is, the more difficult it is to control how it tears. As an example, latex is more difficult to tear accurately than paper. As one attempts to tear an elastic material, it first stretches before abruptly splitting. Because of the rebound energy, the resulting tear is overly rapid and tends to slingshot away from, rather than toward, the grasping instrument. Because pediatric anterior capsules are very thin and elastic, the flap tends to spiral outward and is very difficult to control.[3] Similarly, the adult posterior capsule has less tensile strength, and it is thinner and more elastic than the anterior capsule. It behaves more like the pediatric anterior capsule, and accomplishing a posterior capsulorhexis is more challenging for this reason.

Lacking sufficient circumferential tension, a capsule that is not taut will also exhibit elastic behavior. As the surgeon pulls on the anterior capsular flap, the peripheral capsule should be immobile if he is to control the precise direction of the tear. This situation occurs if the zonules are intact, but weak zonules give rise to a condition that I call *capsular pseudoelasticity*,[4,5] where the anterior capsule is of normal adult thickness but behaves as though it is more lax and pliant due to insufficient zonular traction. Because the peripheral capsule will move along with, and in the same direction the flap is being pulled, the tear is difficult to control and will tend to slingshot radially. Poor surgical technique whereby the capsular flap is allowed to become too long can also create pseudoelasticity. The farther the grasping point of the capsular forceps is from the tearing point, the more pliant the flap becomes, and the more difficult it is to direct the tear. If the tear tends to spiral radially outward, the surgeon must regrasp the flap closer to the leading edge of the tear.

In higher-risk cases, I consider the capsulorhexis to be a "zonular stress test," because the first indication of how weak the zonules are becomes evident during this step. If the anterior capsule is very lax, the capsulotomy needle's tip will tend to dimple and indent it, rather than immediately puncture it. Next, as the surgeon tugs the capsular flap, the peripheral lens capsule is likely to stretch and move along with the flap toward the forceps. With extreme zonular weakness, the entire lens may start to move with the capsular forceps. The surgeon needs to take great care to avoid outward spiraling of the tear. In addition to using capsular forceps to regrasp the flap more frequently, employing the tear recovery technique originated by Brian Little, MD, from the Royal Free Hospital NHS Trust, in London, United Kingdom, is invaluable in these situations.

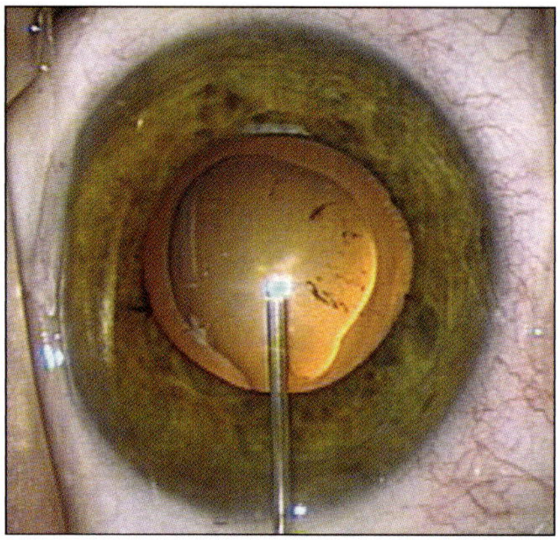

Figure 1. Soft-shell technique. After first injecting the dispersive OVD (Viscoat), the cohesive OVD (Provisc), is injected over the convex anterior capsule. This step pushes the dispersive OVD into the cornea and against the inner incision wall.

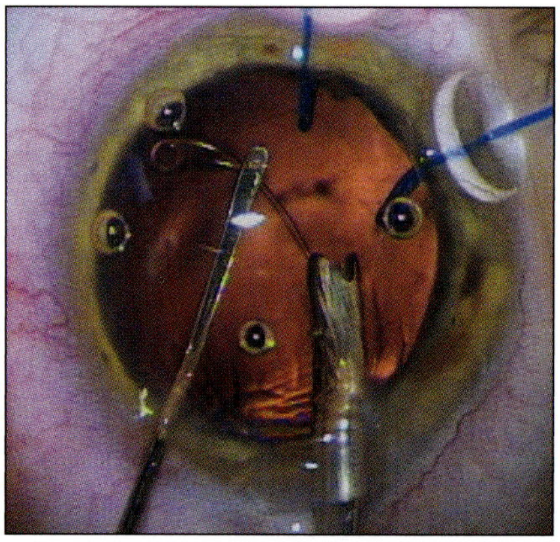

Figure 2. Mackool capsular retractors (Impex Surgical, Staten Island, NY) are long enough to be able to hook the capsulorhexis edge and yet support the equatorial capsule.

If pseudoelasticity is severe, the surgeon can use iris hooks or specially designed capsular retractors to help anchor the bag during the capsulorhexis step.[6] Richard Mackool, MD, Director of The Mackool Eye Institute and Laser Center in Astoria, New York, has designed self-retaining retractors that are elongated enough to hook a small-diameter capsulorhexis from the limbus[7] (Figure 2). After completing several clock hours of the capsulorhexis, one or more capsular retractors can be placed. These retractors stabilize the bag and provide helpful countertraction against the tugging flap. Care must be taken to avoid placing too much tension on the capsular edge with the retractors, as this force alone can extend the tear uncontrollably. A surgeon can use the capsular tension segments created by Ike Ahmed MD, FRCSC, from the University of Toronto and the University of Utah in Salt Lake City, in a similar manner. A surgeon should never insert a capsular tension ring before completing the capsulorhexis, however, because the expansive force of the ring will extend the tear. If the pupil is of borderline size, enlarge its diameter with iris retractors. Optimal visualization of the peripheral capsular region is of far greater importance here than with a routine case.

Opinions differ regarding the target diameter of the capsulorhexis in eyes with loose zonules. A larger-diameter capsulorhexis will make nuclear and cortical removal much easier, but it is much harder to complete in eyes with capsular pseudoelasticity. With weakened zonules, the more peripherally the tear advances, the more it wants to veer radially outward, and the more difficult it is to rescue the flap. In comparison, a smaller-diameter capsulorhexis is easier to control. It increases the margin for error by allowing more time to recognize and rescue a peripherally escaping tear. Although a small-diameter capsulotomy may somewhat hinder the subsequent surgical steps, it is far preferable to having a torn capsular edge, particularly when other risk factors are present.

For this reason, I believe that one should always aim for a smaller-diameter capsulorhexis in the presence of significant zonular laxity. Successful completion of a continuous circumlinear edge is more important than attaining the optimal size. The surgeon must mentally visualize its diameter during nuclear emulsification, however, so as not to tear it with the chopper shaft or phaco tip. Bimanual instrumentation is superior for cortical cleanup in loose capsular bags and greatly improves subincisional access through a small capsulorhexis. Modern injectors facilitate implantation of foldable IOLs through a small capsular opening. Finally, the surgeon should secondarily enlarge the capsulorhexis after the IOL and capsular tension ring are safely implanted.

CONCLUSION

In summary, achieving an intact capsulorhexis is crucial to the safety of the cataract procedure. To maximize the odds of success, the surgeon needs to make the diameter smaller when he encounters difficulty. Given the long-term importance of having a properly sized capsular opening, the surgeon should secondarily enlarge a small capsulorhexis following IOL insertion when the surgical conditions are more favorable. ■

This article originally appeared in the October 2007 issue of CRSToday.

1. Arshinoff SA. Dispersive-cohesive viscoelastic soft shell technique. *J Cataract Refract Surg.* 1999;25:167-173.
2. Arshinoff SA. Using BSS with viscoadaptives in the ultimate soft-shell technique. *J Cataract Refract Surg.* 2002;28:1509-1514.
3. Saini JS, Jain AK, Sukhija F, et al. Anterior and posterior capsulorhexis in pediatric cataract surgery with or without trypan blue dye. Randomized prospective clinical study. *J Cataract Refract Surg.* 2003;29:1733-1737.
4. Chang DF. Phacoemulsification in high-risk cases. In: Wallace RB, ed. *Multifocal IOLs and Refractive Cataract Surgery.* Chapter 11. Thorofare, NJ: Slack; 2001.
5. Chang DF. Strategies for the difficult capsulorrhexis. In: Chang DF, ed. *Phaco Chop.* Chapter 12. Thorofare, NJ: Slack; 2004.
6. Lee V, Bloom P. Microhook capsule stabilization for phacoemulsification in eyes with pseudoexfoliation-syndrome-induced lens instability. *J Cataract Refract Surg.* 1999; 25:1567-1570.
7. Mackool RJ. Capsule stabilization for phacoemulsification (letter). *J Cataract Refract Surg* 2000;26:629.

CHAPTER 14

Mastering the Complicated Capsulorhexis

MICHAEL E. SNYDER, MD

An intact capsulorhexis is a vital component in any cataract surgery. In complex cases, the capsulorhexis is even more critical and, sometimes, it can determine either the success or failure of the planned case. There are several instances in which the capsulorhexis can be particularly challenging. These technical challenges tend to occur most commonly in cases in which an intact capsulorhexis is so vitally important. In this article, I review various principles of performing a capsulorhexis and discuss some of the procedure's related challenges and techniques.

ACCESSING THE CATARACT

As surgeons, when we create a capsulorhexis, our goal is to create a continuous opening in the anterior capsular membrane. This opening allows adequate access to the cataractous lens material while maintaining adequate membrane structure for the safe implantation and long-term centered fixation of an IOL and, perhaps, a capsular tension ring and/or iris prosthetic device.

THE HYPERMATURE OR INTUMESCENT LENS

In cases in which the cataract has become either hypermature or intumescent, the cortical material has broken down, and, in the process, created an osmotic flow gradient, bringing additional fluid into the capsular bag. This situation causes a commensurate increase in the intracapsular hydrostatic pressure. Sudden release of this pressure gradient into the anterior chamber with the initiation of the capsular opening can create a forceful and rapid efflux of fluid, potentially causing a complete splitting of the capsular bag (Argentinean blue flag syndrome). This incident obviously markedly endangers the safe completion of the case and could lead to a dislocation of the nucleus into the posterior segment.

There are few maneuvers that will prevent this occurrence. First, staining the capsule with either trypan blue or indocyanine green will aid in visualization. Before attempting to open the anterior capsule, ensure that the anterior chamber is overpressurized, such that the anterior chamber pressure exceeds the endolenticular pressure. Typically, this step will require the generous use of an ophthalmic viscosurgical device (OVD) that has good cohesive properties. Under the operative microscope, the surgeon should see (at least) a slight flattening of the convexity of the anterior capsular surface. Next, a 25-gauge short needle (5/8") is placed on a 3-mL syringe, filled only halfway with balanced salt solution. The needle's tip is placed through the paracentesis, taking care not to allow any OVD to escape. With the needle's tip oriented with the bevel down, the needle pierces the capsular bag axially, and the syringe's plunger is immediately withdrawn to evacuate liquid contents from the confines of the bag (Figure 1). This process will effectively decompress the bag and neutralize the pressure gradient between the anterior chamber and intralenticular space. The remainder of the capsulorhexis can now be safely completed with the surgeon's preferred technique.

CAPSULORHEXIS IN THE PRESENCE OF ZONULAR COMPROMISE

Routine capsulorhexis requires a balance between the centripetal forces applied to the anterior capsule by the surgeon against the centrifugal countertraction force from the zonular apparatus and the force of the lens material against the forniceal equator of the bag. In cases of zonular compromise, the "normal"

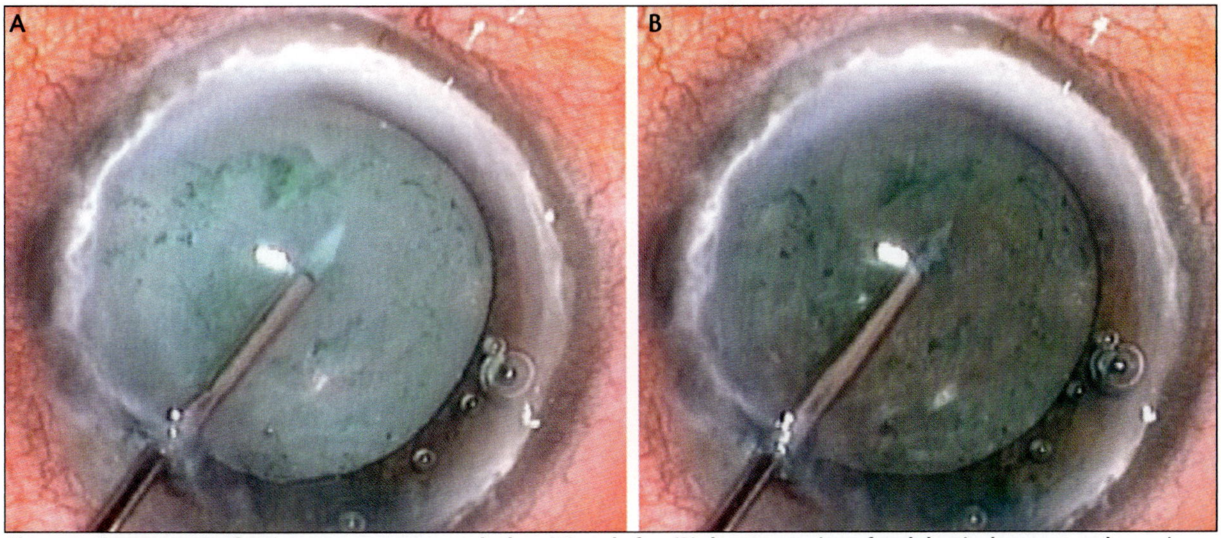

Figure 1. Appearance of an intumescent cataract before (A) and after (B) decompression of endolenticular pressure by aspiration of liquefied cortex.

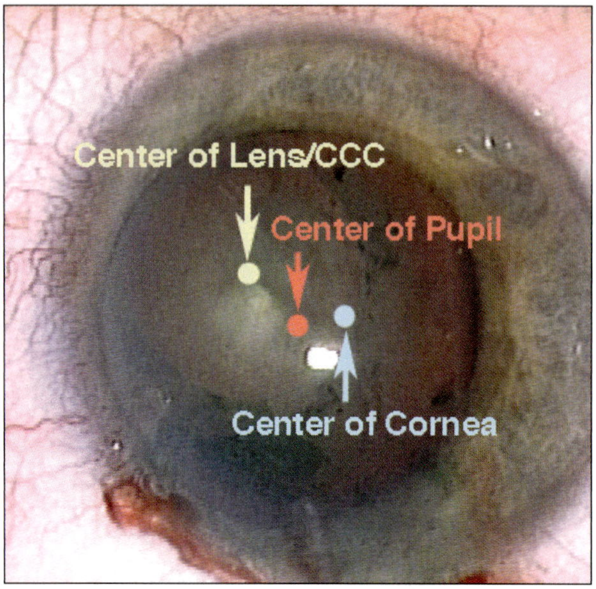

Figure 2. The geometric center of the lens does not always correspond to the visual axis or the corneal center.

balance of forces does not exist, and creating a continuous curvilinear capsulorhexis (CCC) becomes challenging. In some cases, the zonular compromise is not suspected until the initiation of the anterior capsular tear, in which a "pincushion" effect is noted as an attempt to puncture the anterior capsule is initiated and the capsule indents significantly before the needle will penetrate. This sign indicates diffuse zonular laxity and should alert the surgeon that he must be extremely attentive at this point. In cases where the zonular abnormality is well known, and, perhaps, the lens is subluxated, we need to determine where the CCC should be centered. There may be a temptation to make the CCC centered on the pupil center or the geometric center of the cornea, as we do in a routine case. This temptation should be avoided. If the crystalline lens is decentered, we must actively concentrate on keeping the CCC centered on the axis of the cataractous lens (Figure 2). An overly eccentric CCC can sometimes make capsular tension ring placement difficult, because during insertion, the ring tends to migrate out of the bag if the peripheral portion of the CCC is too near the equator.

Often, in cases of severe zonular compromise, the crystalline lens must be stabilized by either supporting the already torn portion of the capsulorhexis' margin with a hook similar to the Kuglen hook (Katena Products, Inc., Denville, NJ), flexible iris, or capsule retractor. Alternatively, one can stabilize the capsule with a forceps. Placement of an Ahmed segment (Morcher GmbH, Stuttgart, Germany) focally can stabilize the bag for completion of the capsulorhexis as well, provided that the portion that has already been opened is of sufficient size to place the segment without excessive manipulation. Although it has not yet been reported, focal placement of an Assia Anchor (Hanita Lenses, Kibbutz Hanita, Israel) could theoretically be used to stabilize the lens-bag complex to complete the capsulorhexis.

Regardless of the stabilization method selected, one should not attempt to recenter the lens-bag complex at least until the capsulorhexis has been completed.

With regard to CCC size, a larger capsulorhexis will facilitate the lens' removal from the bag, yet, if the CCC does not overlap the margin of the IOL, the surgeon should be aware that the lens will sit slightly anterior relative to the zonular plane, thus altering the IOL's refractive effectiveness. Accordingly, an IOL with less power may be appropriate compared to what might have been selected for cases in which the CCC margin covers the IOL edge.

CAPSULAR PLAQUE

In some cases, an anterior capsular plaque may exist along the planned path of the continuous tear capsulorhexis. In such cases, three effective techniques will allow the completion of a continuous capsulotomy. First, if the plaque is small in size, the planned path of the CCC can be altered to come either central or peripheral to the location of the plaque. If the plaque is too large to circumnavigate, the portion of the pathway that goes through the path of the intended capsulotomy can be extended with microscissors. If this technique is selected, it is critical that the surgeon begin the scissors portion of the cut slightly outside the point at which the continuous tear meets the plaque. This method will ensure maintained structural integrity of the capsular opening. In contradistinction, if the surgeon were to initiate the scissors cut just inside the point at which the tear meets the plaque, the weakest point of the capsular opening will be located exactly where the tear meets the plaque. In such an instance, further manipulations or expansion of the capsular bag may be much more likely to result in a peripheral, radial extension of the capsular opening with compromised integrity.

Once the plaque has been completely cut, the continuous tear can be completed.

ERRANT PERIPHERAL DEVIATION OF A CAPSULORHEXIS

If a capsulorhexis begins to deviate peripheral to its intended path, extreme attentiveness is the first appropriate tactic. Any forces on the capsule should be ceased, and stabilize the anterior segment by adequately deepening and pressurizing the anterior chamber. If the origin of the peripheral movement can be identified, it should clearly be reversed. For example, if the anterior chamber is too shallow, it should be deepened; if the view of the capsule was inadequate, then capsular dyes should be applied. Ideally, the tear should be redirected by folding over the leading edge of the capsule to better control the tear. Although some surgeons have reported pulling the capsule in the opposite direction of the tear, which presumably should bring the tear centrally, I have not tried this maneuver.

If the tear has already extended to the zonules, surgeons should avoid further manipulations in that area. It is probably wiser to start the tear in the opposite direction and complete from the opposite rotation. Some surgeons advocate one or more additional radial breaks in the CCC in such cases to reduce the direct forces on the one break point. Surgeons should perform hydrodissection with extreme caution, and, if attempted, remove some of the OVD moved to shallow the anterior chamber before the hydrodissection wave so that if the pressure within the bag increases, the lens will be more likely to come forward, rather than the posterior capsule splitting posteriorly.

WHEN THE CAPSULORHEXIS IS TOO SMALL

If the CCC is too small, the surgeon can carefully enlarge it by making a small tangential incision in the CCC and peeling an additional small amount off the margin in a spiral. Surgeons can repeat this maneuver as needed, remembering that although it is a bit challenging to enlarge the opening, reducing its aperture is impossible. I typically prefer to wait until after posterior chamber IOL placement to enlarge a CCC.

SUMMARY

The capsulorhexis remains among the most crucial step in the complex cataract case, both for safe removal of the lens material and for ultimate fixation of the implanted lens. The components of a complex capsulorhexis can be highly variable, yet, with meticulous attention to technique, most of these problems can be overcome, even in the most difficult cases. The surgeon should always keep in mind the balance of all hydrostatic and mechanical forces on the capsular bag, how these forces are unique to a given case. and how they can be manipulated either by altering the hydrostatic pressures or the mechanical stresses applied to the capsule to achieve an intact capsulorhexis with the greatest degree of safety. Prudent use of an appropriately chosen OVD and/or capsule-expanding or fixating device can aid the surgeon in this endeavor. ■

This article originally appeared in the October 2007 issue of CRSToday.

CHAPTER 15

How to Avoid an Errant Tear

ROSA BRAGA-MELE MEd, MD, FRCSC

Continuous curvilinear capsulorhexis (CCC) is one of the most important steps for successful phacoemulsification and IOL implantation.[1] The main cause of an errant capsular tear is a shallowing of the anterior chamber, with a subsequent excursion of the rhexis' peripherally along the path of least resistance. Thus, the surgeon should ensure that the anterior capsule is flat during the entire CCC procedure. This article describes measures to follow to complete a successful surgery.

SURGICAL STEPS

Incisions

First, the surgeon needs to ensure that the speculum or drape is not causing any unnecessary pressure on the orbit and thereby shallowing the chamber. Next, he should make sure a proper main incision is constructed so that the chamber does not inadvertently shallow when the wound is decompressed. A surgeon needs to make a good shelved, self-sealing wound that is constructed appropriately for the type of eye that he is treating. If the surgeon is operating on an eye that is very myopic or long, he should make the main incision slightly shorter than average (about 2 mm) to prevent putting undue pressure on the wound with the Utrata forceps. This step is important, because the chamber tends to be deep and one needs to angle down to reach the capsule. Alternatively, a longer-than-average incision will help stabilize the chamber in a more hyperopic or shorter eye.

Injecting Viscoelastic

It is necessary to be certain that the anterior chamber is completely filled with viscoelastic, either dispersive or cohesive, before performing the rhexis. Refill the anterior chamber with viscoelastic as necessary. If the chamber is particularly shallow, the surgeon may opt for a visco-adaptive viscoelastic such as Healon5 (Advanced Medical Optics, Inc., Santa Ana, CA) to aid in the deepening and stabilizing of the chamber. Of note, when performing a CCC with Healon5, the rhexis tends to want to turn inward, and thus an errant tear is less likely to occur. The surgeon should account for this and lead the rhexis in the direction needed more frequently or use a small amount of balanced salt solution directly on top of the rhexis as described by Steve A. Arshinoff, MD, FRSCS, of Toronto (ultimate soft-shell technique).[2]

Managing the Rhexis

It is imperative to regrasp the rhexis frequently with any procedure, at least every 90° or less, and the surgeon must ensure that he is holding it close to the edge of the flap on the free edge. Viscoelastic can also be used to direct the leading capsular flap into an optimal direction and position.

If the pupil is small or the iris is floppy and the surgeon decides that iris hooks or pupil rings need to be used, it is easier to insert these devices before commencing the rhexis.

Capsular Staining

If the lens is hypermature or white, a surgeon may want to use a capsular staining dye to guarantee visibility of the anterior capsule during the procedure. Out of the many staining techniques described,[3] I prefer to use trypan blue in a small aliquot painted directly onto the anterior capsule underneath some viscoelastic. Also, if there appears to be any positive pressure produced by the contents of a hypermature lens, it is beneficial to decompress the lens with a 25-gauge needle inserted into the anterior capsule prior to beginning a CCC in order to avoid the Argentinean flag sign (ie, capsule tearing centrally end to end).[4] In this case, surgeons can also tamponade the capsule with Healon5.

CONCLUSION

The key to avoiding a rhexis tear is to recognize and avoid running into problems and to use an armamentarium of techniques and technologies available to make performing a capsulorhexis a success. If one follows the steps reviewed previously, you should be able to avoid or effectively deal with any potential problems during CCC. ■

This article originally appeared in the October 2007 issue of CRSToday.

1. Gimbel HV, Neuhann T. Development, advantages, and methods of the continuous circular capsulorhexis technique. *J Cataract Refract Surg.* 1990;16:31-37.
2. Arshinoff SA. Capsular dyes and the USST. *J Cataract Refract Surg.* 2005;31:259-260.
3. Dada V, Sharma N, Sudan R, et al. Anterior capsule staining for capsulorhexis in cases of white cataract: comparative clinical study. *J Cataract Refract Surg.* 2004;30:326-333.
4. Chan DD, Ng AC, Leung CK, Tse RK. Continuous curvilinear capsulorhexis in intumescent or hypermature cataract with liquefied cortex. *J Cataract Refract Surg.* 2003;29:431-434.

CHAPTER 16

The Errant Capsulorhexis Tear

CHRISTOPHER S. CONNOR, MD

An anterior capsulotomy is the capsular incision necessary to permit removal of the nucleus and cortex. It should be capable of preserving the integrity of the capsular bag against the asymmetric forces that occur during phacoemulsification and IOL implantation. By maintaining symmetry of the capsular bag after IOL implantation, the anterior capsulotomy should confine the haptics and prevent IOL subluxation due to delayed contractile forces. The continuous curvilinear capsulorhexis, developed concurrently by Drs. Gimbel and Neuhann in 1986,[1] was a landmark advance because it achieved both of these goals. It has led to safer phacoemulsification and to improved postoperative IOL centration.

The anterior capsule is a homogeneous basement membrane that is made up of collagen-like protein. It has elastic properties without being composed of elastic fibers. The underlying epithelial cells are loosely adherent. Finally, the anterior capsule has a smooth surface contour except at the equator, where the zonules attach. These properties of the anterior capsule allow a multidirectional continuous curvilinear capsulorhexis to occur. However, these same characteristics can lead to misdirected and errant tears.

THE TEAR DILEMMA

A smaller diameter capsulorhexis is easier to control than a larger one. For most patients, a capsulorhexis diameter measuring 0.5 mm to 1 mm smaller than the IOL optic diameter is preferred. The IOL generally remains well centered postoperatively in this situation. However, in eyes that have weakened zonules or an excessively hardened nucleus, it is preferable to have a capsulorhexis diameter that is 0.5 mm to 1 mm larger than the optic. This will allow for cataract removal techniques that minimize stress to the already weakened zonules. As the capsule contracts postoperatively, the IOL will remain centered. Avoid making a capsulorhexis that matches the optic diameter because the IOL can "pea pod" off-center as the capsulorhexis and capsular bag contract postoperatively.

ASSESS ZONULE STRENGTH

How does the surgeon know if the zonules are weak at the onset of the capsulorhexis? It is necessary to execute a "zonular strength assessment" every time a capsulorhexis is performed. The surgeon, with whatever instrument is used to initiate the capsular puncture, should "jiggle" the lens diaphragm slightly to determine zonular strength. If the zonules appear strong, then the capsulorhexis can be the standard size of 0.5 mm to 1 mm smaller than the optic diameter. If the assessment shows a generally loose lens diaphragm, then the capsulorhexis should be 0.5 mm to 1 mm larger than the optic. Finally, if the zonular strength assessment shows an asymmetric weakness, the rhexis should still be 0.5 mm to 1 mm larger than the optic, but placed off-center and away from the possible dehiscence. The IOL optic will better align and center up with the capsulorhexis when the haptic is oriented toward the quadrant of zonular weakness.

Why is a larger diameter capsulorhexis more difficult to control? The primary reason is that the anterior capsular contour slopes away more dramatically from the surgeon's instrument as one moves toward the periphery. As it spirals peripherally, the capsulorhexis tear can suddenly encounter a zonular attachment that can act as a straight edge, sending the tear out to the capsular fornix and possibly around and through the posterior capsule.

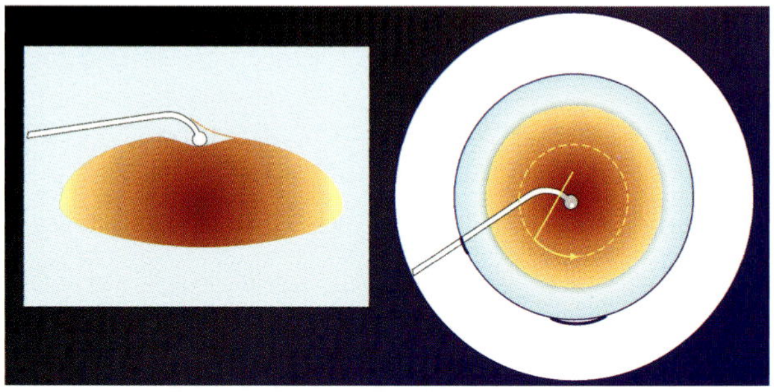

Figure 1. The ball-tip of a wand manipulator flattens the anterior lens dome during a touchdown maneuver.

Once an errant tear starts to extend radially, the surgeon should appreciate that it becomes much harder to control as the tear approaches the periphery. This is because the anterior capsular dome, and thus the base of the tear, drops away from the tip of the tool (forceps) that is controlling it. This is much like giving a dog too much lead on its leash. One cannot control the errant dog or the errant tear when there is too much "leash" ahead of one's grip. Understanding this principle that errant tears run "downhill" and away from the forceps tips dictates the following preventive measures:

1. Avoid lifting the capsular flap during the capsulorhexis.
2. Keep the capsule forceps low to the anterior lens surface and forward to the base of the tear.
3. Lead the tear much like one pulls a wagon in a circle by its handle. Think of the tearing motion as being more of a "peeling" action.
4. Utilize capsulorhexis forceps, such as the Connor Peeler (Rhein Medical, Tampa, FL), that have forward facing tips. Tips with this orientation facilitate a peeling action, rather than the lifting motion that downward facing forceps tips promote.
5. Regrasp frequently—at least at every quarter hour of circumference—to optimize control of the base of the flap.

THE DOWNHILL CHALLENGE

A lifting movement can cause the base of the tear to advance downhill and out toward the periphery. Certain patients present with what I would call a "downhill challenge." These eyes have an unusually steep anterior capsular dome that predisposes them to having an errant capsulorhexis tear occur. Children, young adults, and hyperopes fall into this category. A swollen, intumescent lens, or eyes with posterior pressure will be a challenge for the same reason, namely, the presence of a steep anterior capsular dome.

A steeper anterior lens curvature produces an unwanted effect similar to that of lifting the flap upward. The base of the tear runs downhill and away from the point of control. By anticipating this

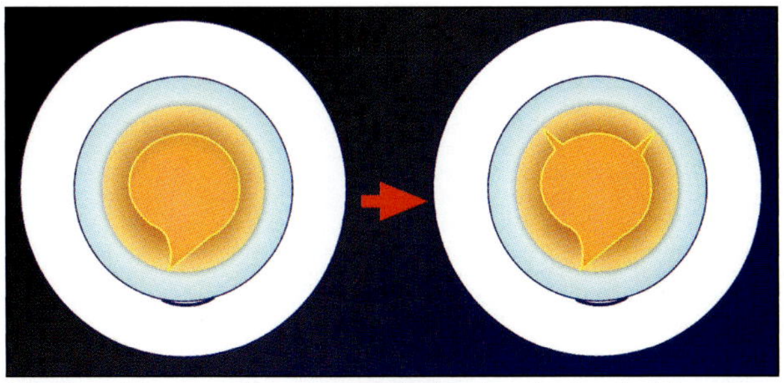

Figure 2. The equidistant capsulorhexis-relaxing incisions are 120° apart from the initial rim split.

lens configuration, one can negate the downhill slope of the dome. I call this a "touchdown" maneuver. The surgeon employs the fellow hand to flatten the steep anterior lens dome as the capsulorhexis is being performed. A blunt-tipped instrument, such as a Connor Wand manipulator (Rhein Medical), is used to depress the central lens surface just under the initiated capsulorhexis flap. This reverses the chamber shallowing caused by posterior pressure and helps flatten the anterior lens dome. The capsulorhexis is then completed around this centrally placed tool (Figure 1).

THE MIGRATING CAPSULORHEXIS TEAR

Suppose the surgeon has followed the previously mentioned precautions, and the capsulorhexis tear still wants to migrate peripherally? First, he or she should deepen the anterior chamber with a cohesive viscoelastic. Next, I suggest maneuvering the errant flap into a peeling orientation. Tilt the eye to grasp the flap at its base and from a forward position. If the misdirected tear does not turn around, employ a touchdown maneuver with the fellow hand. This technique of depressing the central lens surface with a wand manipulator to counter posterior pressure and flatten the anterior capsule contour will often allow the recovery of an errant capsulorhexis.

Tilting the eye enables the surgeon to better control the base of the flap by utilizing a forward peeling position. If an errant tear cannot be "rescued," do not try to reinitiate the capsulorhexis with a new tear proceeding in the opposite direction. This will produce a teardrop-shaped capsulotomy, in which the iris conceals the full extent of the radial tear. During phacoemulsification, this capsulorhexis "split" could very well extend around the capsular fornix and through the posterior capsule, which could possibly result in a dropped nucleus. Instead, use a cystotome to offset the forces transmitted to this weakened area by making numerous relaxing incisions in the capsule for 90°. These multiple puncture incisions should begin adjacent to the radial tear and as far out as one can visualize. After one quarter hour, or 90°, regrasp the capsule and finish the rhexis. The capsular bag will be able to sustain the forces necessary to remove the cataract and still allow the surgeon to knowingly insert the IOL within the bag.

If the surgeon inadvertently cuts the intact capsulorhexis rim during phacoemulsification, he or she should immediately stop and refill the anterior chamber with a thick, cohesive viscoelastic. I recommend using fine-tipped scissors to make two additional relaxing incisions in the capsulorhexis approximately 120° away from the accidental tear. Elevate the nucleus out of the capsular bag by injecting either fluid or viscoelastic. Finally, sandwich the nucleus with viscoelastic and complete the emulsification at the iris plane. The surgeon can still place the IOL within the salvaged capsular bag (Figure 2).

ADDITIONAL STRATEGIES

The intumescent lens presents even greater challenges with capsulorhexis because of the intralenticular opening pressure. With the first break into the anterior lens capsule, whether by needle or forceps, a rapid lateral extension can occur. A two-staged decompression technique has been suggested in the past using a small bore needle to reduce the lens pressure. A more controlled and reproducible method involves using the phaco tip to make the initial punch entry into the anterior capsule. The vacuum of the tip decompresses the intumescent lens. A cystotome or scissors reinitiates the rhexis at the punch entry with the curvilinear capsulorhexis easily being performed in a now flattened anterior capsular dome. The punch entry is incorporated within the completed capsulorhexis.

Finally, if a posterior capsular rent occurs during phacoemulsification, whether centrally or as a result of a radiating anterior capsular cut, employ the same principles as mentioned previously. Remember that because tears always run downhill, make the posterior capsule concave with a thick, cohesive viscoelastic before attempting a posterior capsulorhexis with long-tipped forceps. Perform this step as soon as the posterior capsule defect is recognized and before continuing with phacoemulsification, cortex removal, or lens implantation. Completing a posterior capsulorhexis salvages the integrity and strength of the capsular bag, permitting in-the-bag implantation of an IOL. ■

This article originally appeared in the March 2002 issue of CRSToday.

1. Gimbel HV, Neuhann T: Development, advantages, and methods of the continuous circular capsulorhexis technique. *J Cataract Refract Surg.* 1990;16:31-37.

CHAPTER 17

Retrieval Maneuver for CCC Tear-Out

BRIAN LITTLE, MD

One of the most disheartening ways to start any phaco operation is with a tear-out of the capsulorhexis. It happens to every surgeon at some point, and retrieving a tear-out is always a technical challenge that, unfortunately, is all too often unsuccessful. This article describes a simple yet highly effective technique for salvaging this situation. It works reliably even when the tear has gone out into the zonules, and it can retrieve tears that appear impossible to recover by any other

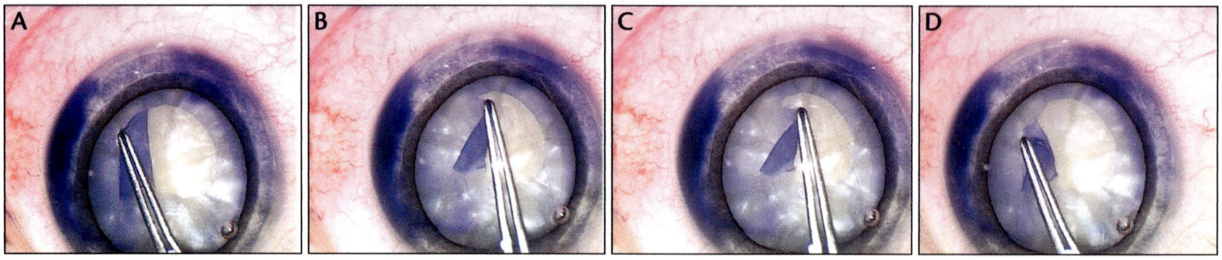

Figure 1. The use of trypan blue stain highlights the basic steps of the technique. The flap is folded forward as the capsulorhexis is constructed (A). The flap is unfolded and grasped (B). The flap is pulled backward to redirect the tear centrally (C). The flap is refolded forward, and the tear is continued (D).

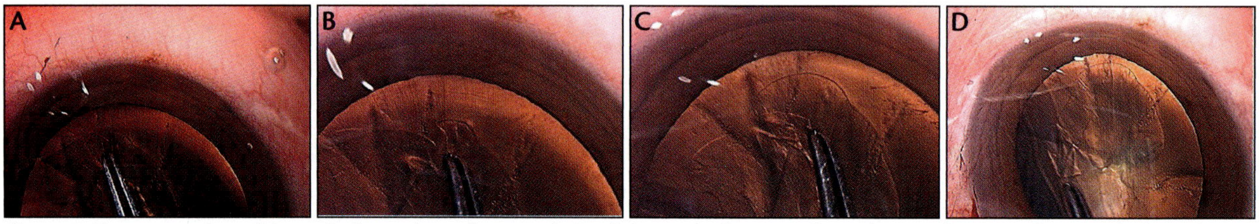

Figure 2. Demonstration of the technique where the capsulorhexis is torn in the area of zonular attachments. The capsulorhexis has inadvertently torn into the zonules (A). The flap is unfolded, grasped, and pulled backward (B). Backward traction on the flap has redirected the tear (C). The capsulorhexis is continued in the standard fashion (D). (Reprinted with permission from Little BC, Smith JH, Packer M. "Little" capsulorhexis tear-out rescue. *J Cataract Refract Surg.* 2006;32:1420-1422.)

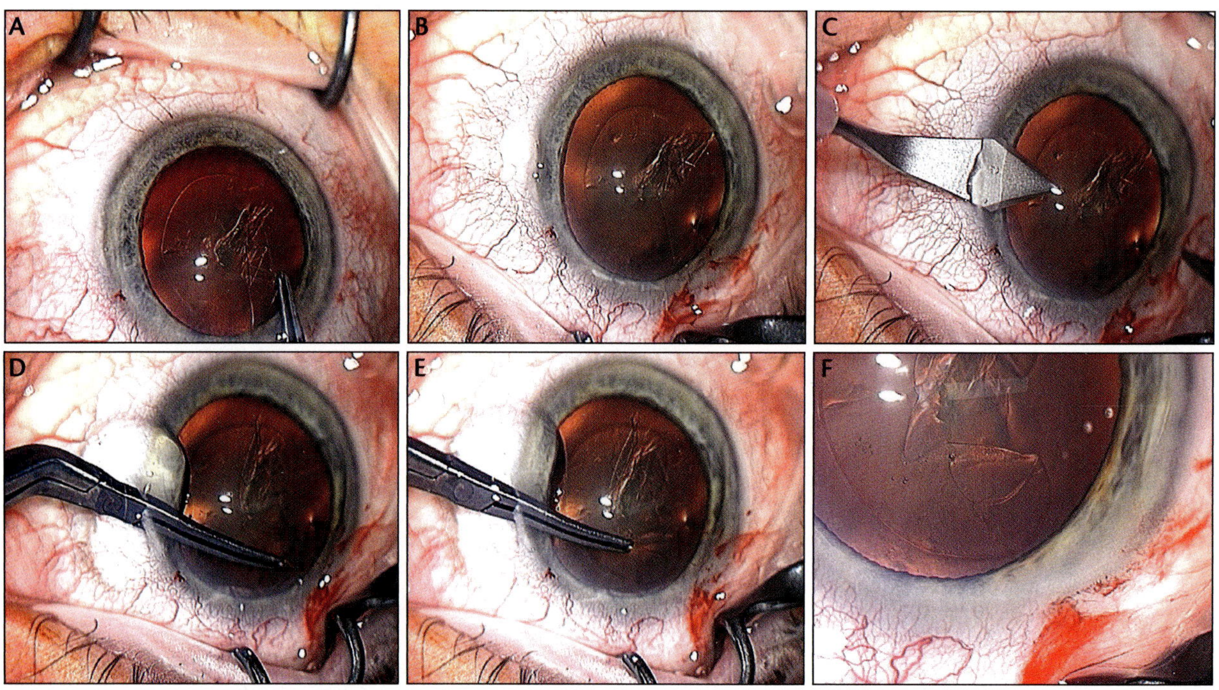

Figure 3. The surgeon demonstrates the use of a new paracentesis to obtain optimal positioning for redirecting the tear. The capsulorhexis is tearing out (A). The forceps are removed from the eye, and the tear-out is examined (B). A new incision is made across from the position of the tear-out (C). The apex of the flap edge is grasped and pulled backward from the direction of the tear (D). The tear is redirected centrally (E). The surgeon demonstrates the capsulorhexis U-turn (F). (Reprinted with permission from Little BC, Smith JH, Packer M. "Little" capsulorhexis tear-out rescue. *J Cataract Refract Surg.* 2006;32:1420-1422.)

means. This procedure will hopefully prove to be a useful addition to your personal library of surgical rescue maneuvers.

PREVENTION

As with all surgical complications, the concept that prevention is better than cure applies here without exception. Surgeons can avoid a tear-out of the rhexis in nearly all cases just by using an adequate amount of appropriate ophthalmic viscosurgical device (OVD) to keep the chamber deep throughout creation of the rhexis.

In the case of significant positive vitreous pressure with a tendency for aggressive chamber collapse, there are a few helpful strategies that surgeons can employ. You can use one of the higher-molecular-weight

KEY POINTS OF THE RHEXIS RESCUE TECHNIQUE

- Fill the chamber completely with viscoelastic before any attempt at retrieval.
- If necessary, make a second stab incision at the position that allows the optimal angle of approach for applying traction on the flap.
- Unfold the flap of the anterior capsule and flatten it against the lens (instrumental or viscomanipulation).
- If visibility of the capsule edge is compromised, use trypan blue to visualize the edges of the tear.
- Refill the chamber immediately before attempting retrieval.
- Use only rhexis forceps; do not attempt this technique with a needle cystotome because the directional control is inadequate, and the needle tip is likely to tear the flap.
- Grasp the flap as near to the root of the tear as possible.
- Apply traction in the horizontal plane of the capsule and do not lift it forward.
- The initial pull should be circumferentially backward, and while holding the flap in tension, pull more centrally to initiate the tear, which will then propagate toward the center.
- The big mystery is how much force can be safely applied—the answer is as much as you feel safe using, and you will better understand this concept as you become more experienced. If in doubt, abandon the technique and use an alternative recovery method.

cohesive OVDs such as Healon5 (Advanced Medical Optics, Inc., Santa Ana, CA) to perform the rhexis through a sideport using a needle cystotome or microcoaxial forceps, or use an infusion of OVD through a syringe that is held in the nondominant hand through the sideport.

The other principle for prevention is early recognition of a threatening situation while it is still retrievable, before it develops into a full-blown complication. As soon as there is even the slightest hint of the rhexis migrating out peripherally, surgeons should immediately stop and then refill the chamber to flatten the anterior lens surface. This rapid response is usually sufficient to maintain control of the tear.

SURGICAL TECHNIQUE

Once a surgeon feels he has lost control, he should stop all activity in order to calmly assess the situation and decide on a surgical strategy. With a rhexis tear-out, the primary aim is to prevent its posterior propagation around the equator and through the posterior capsule. In my practice, this happens surprisingly infrequently, possibly due to the criss-crossed insertions of the zonules offering an interwoven web of resistance and blocking extension of the tear. Having acknowledged that it has happened, the next step is for the surgeon to completely fill the chamber with an OVD before making any attempt to rescue the rhexis.

The surgeon needs to redirect the tear centrally back to its original path. The most efficient way of doing this is to unfold the anterior capsule flap and lay it flat against the lens cortex. Using forceps, the trick is then to hold the flap near the root of the tear and pull it back circumferentially in the direction from where it came, applying the force in the plane of the capsule, to put it under tension. While holding the flattened flap under tension, the surgeon should then direct traction more centrally to initiate the retrieval of the tear. Resolution of the tangential and central vector forces redirects the tear predictably toward the center of the pupil. The flap can now be refolded and the rhexis safely continued in the usual manner.

Three contrasting cases are illustrated (Figures 1 through 3). In the rare event that the capsule refuses to tear easily and the entire lens is pulled centrally, surgeons should abandon the rescue maneuver to avoid a wraparound tear of the capsule. Alternative recovery techniques such as completing the capsulotomy from the opposite direction, making a relieving cut in the flap edge and continuing in the same direction, or resorting to a can-opener technique are all appropriate options. ■

The article was adapted with permission from Little BC, Smith JH, Packer M. "Little" capsulorhexis tear-out rescue. J Cataract Refract Surg. *2006;32:1420-1422; and Little BC. Rescuing Capsulorhexis Tear-Out.* Cataract & Refractive Surgery Today. *2007;2:2:30-31.*

This article originally appeared in the October 2007 issue of CRSToday.

CHAPTER 18

Single Radial Tear in the Rhexis

LISA BROTHERS ARBISSER, MD; DAVID F. CHANG, MD; UDAY DEVGAN, MD; AND BONNIE AN HENDERSON, MD

LISA BROTHERS ARBISSER, MD

Controlling the capsular dome and properly directing the shear vector by regrasping the edge noting any errant direction within 1 or 2 mm can prevent tears in almost every case. Rescuing an errant tear with centripetal force applied to the crux of the tear or completing a continuous curvilinear capsulorhexis (CCC) from the opposite direction almost always results in success. In the following paragraphs, I explain how I proceed in the rare case of an unavoidable radial tear.

The key in managing the tear is to "cement" the edges of the tear in close approximation to each other and avoid anterior-posterior displacement or rotational forces throughout the case.

After covering the tear with a dispersive ophthalmic viscosurgical device (OVD), causing the two edges of the tear to approximate into a semblance of the intact position, I pack the dispersive in place with cohesive OVD stabilizing the chamber and inspect it by retracting the iris to see the extent of the tear. Tears naturally stop at the zonular attachments just anterior to the equator where the interdigitating fibrillar elements fortify the delicate capsule. If the tear extends beyond the equator, I consider converting to an extracapsular technique without external pressure.

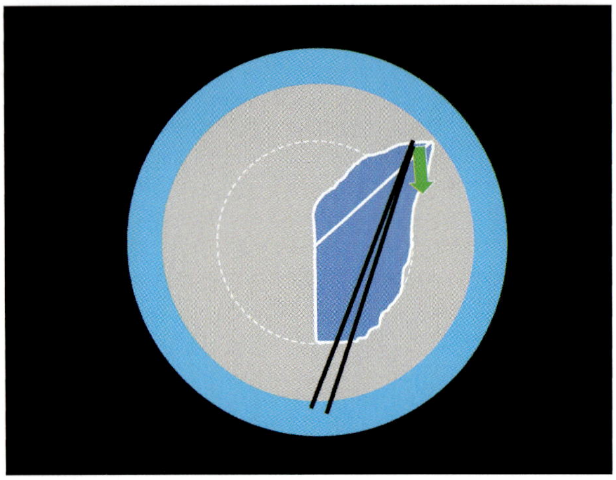

Figure 1. In step one of Dr. Little's method, the surgeon unfolds the capsule back and lays it down flat. The dashed line is the intended capsulorhexis.

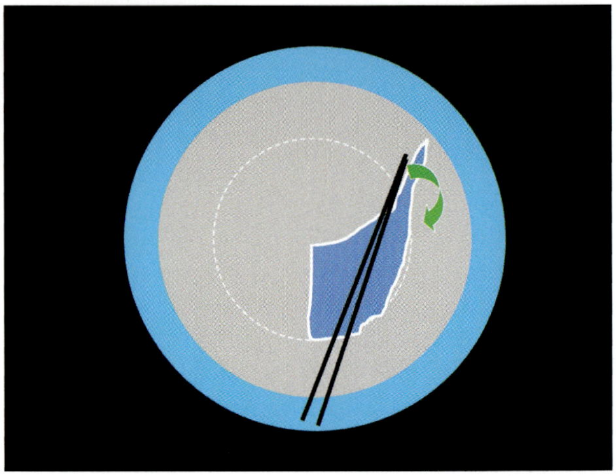

Figure 2. In step two, the surgeon pulls backward and curves in to retrieve the capsulorhexis.

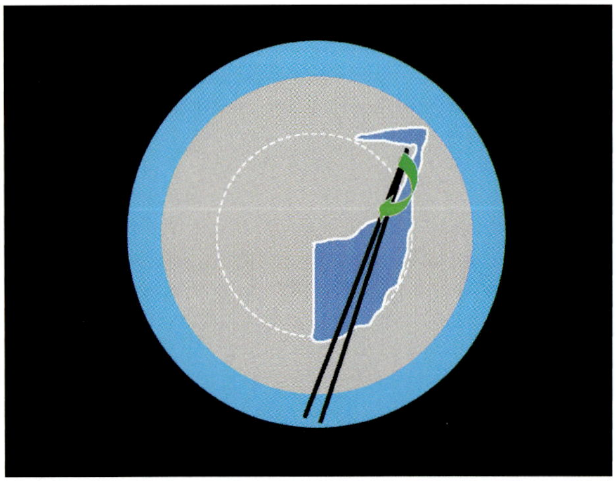

Figure 3. In step three, the surgeon pulls centrally to bring the edge of the capsulorhexis back to the desired size.

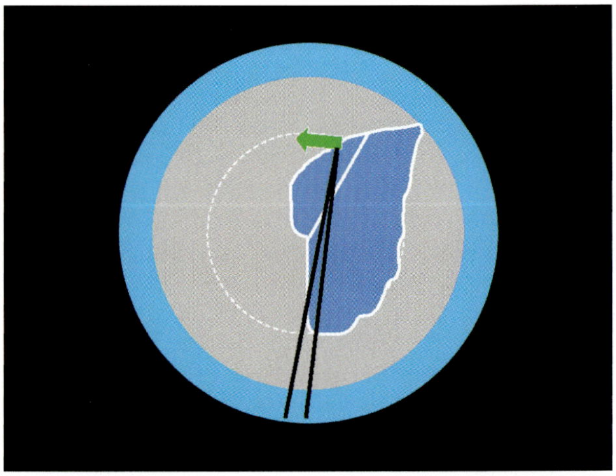

Figure 4. In step four, the surgeon resumes the usual method of creating a capsulorhexis.

As long as the tear stops at the zonules, I will proceed with hydrodelineation without cortical cleaving hydrodissection. This process frees the nucleus from adhering to the bag, allowing nucleus rotation while maintaining an intact rim of epinucleus to hold the edges of the capsular tear in place, which discourages extension.

Next, I introduce the phaco tip with the bottle at a very low level to avoid the distension of the anterior chamber. In a myopic or vitrectomized eye, I place my chopper under the edge of the pupil and lift the iris off the anterior capsule before I step on the pedal, all of which prevents retropulsion of the iris. I slowly raise the bottle to the usual height while in foot position one; flow is established in foot position two to prevent wound burn before I initiate ultrasound. I then perform my usual vertical chop technique. Dispersive OVD must be kept over the tear, however, and I replace it through the sideport if necessary. I advise surgeons to avoid capsule torque by using a slow and gentle, two-handed technique to turn the nucleus as required to access and remove it. Once I extract the endonucleus, I remove the epinucleus if it is free or left in place via I/A. I avoid chamber shallowing by replacing the chopper with a cannula filled with balanced salt solution and irrigating through the sideport while exchanging the phaco tip for the I/A tip.

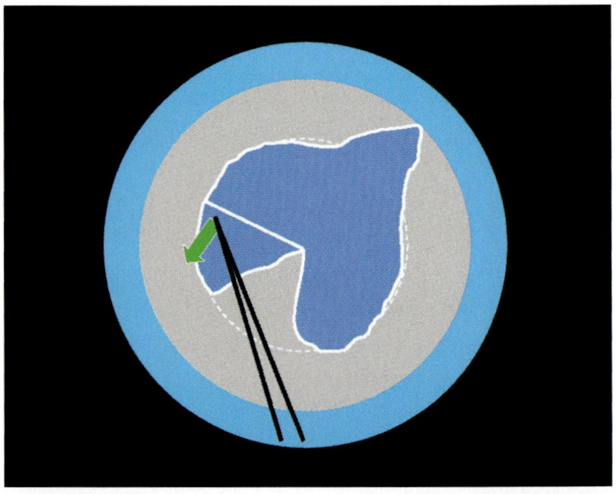

Figure 5. In step five, the surgeon finishes the capsulorhexis.

I leave the cortex adjacent to the tear last. If it is recalcitrant, the surgeon can remove it manually with a dry technique under cohesive OVD. Once the bag is empty, tissue relationships are maintained with cohesive OVD. A one-piece acrylic IOL is most valuable in my opinion because it can be placed as a very compact package with haptics folded on the optic, it opens without pent-up energy, and its forces are evenly distributed when the haptics unfurl. I orient the haptics to avoid their escaping through the tear. The tackiness of the lens ensures that it will stay put, and the material is least likely to induce fibrosis with time. If I thought it were necessary to place a three-piece lens, I would use bimanual insertion without dialing the IOL into place, and I would consider a cut on the opposite side of the capsule if the forces of the haptics distorted the capsule tear. These steps are not necessary with a one-piece acrylic IOL. I irrigate the incision prior to OVD removal so there will be no shallowing of the chamber when I take out the I/A tip.

I would not attempt to clean the posterior chamber of the OVD. Carbonic anhydrase inhibitors immediately postoperatively prevent IOP spikes.

In my experience, these eyes generally benefit from the same rapid and uneventful recovery as a routine case.

DAVID F. CHANG, MD

If a peripheral capsulorhexis tear that cannot be rescued occurs, one must consider any other surgical comorbidities in deciding upon a surgical strategy. If there is a brunescent nucleus with weak zonules and a small pupil, converting to a manual extracapsular cataract procedure may be prudent. With a brunescent nucleus and normal zonules, making two additional anterior capsule relaxing incisions 120° away from each other may reduce the chance for a wraparound posterior capsular tear. If the nucleus is reasonably soft, I usually opt to complete the rest of the capsulorhexis from the opposite direction, prior to performing phaco in the presence of the single anterior capsular tear.

The maneuver most likely to extend a radial anterior capsular tear into the posterior capsule is the rotation of either the nucleus or IOL. When rotating either structure with a single instrument, we must first push it against the equator of the capsular bag to establish countertraction before applying torque. In my opinion and experience, this is the moment at which a wraparound tear occurs. Therefore, emulsifying the nucleus without rotating it is the key objective when proceeding with phacoemulsification in this situation. Gentle hydrodissection and hydrodelineation will not extend the anterior capsule tear, and in fact, these steps are critically important if one is to remove both the endonucleus and the epinucleus without rotation. The advantage of horizontal phaco chop is that one can initiate the first two chops/fractures without rotating the nucleus. The first fragment that is created is lifted out of the capsular bag. Especially if the endonucleus is small enough, the remaining hemi-sections can be elevated out of the bag with the phaco tip or the horizontal chopper.

Following cortical cleanup, the bag should be filled with an OVD. The capsulorhexis will take on a teardrop appearance because of the radial tear. One can easily inject a single-piece hydrophobic acrylic lens without applying any haptic force against the capsular equator. If this IOL design is not available, however, one could safely place a three-piece IOL inside the capsular bag. The key is to avoid forcefully decentering the optic and haptic toward the quadrant where the capsulorhexis is torn. One can accomplish this step by first directing the lead haptic into the anterior chamber rather than into the capsular bag. This technique allows me to rotate the trailing haptic into the bag while all decentering forces are applied to the anterior chamber angle. The second haptic is rotated into the bag by decentering the optic away from the capsulorhexis tear. The haptics are oriented 90° away from the location of the radial capsulorhexis tear. The advantage of completing phacoemulsification in the presence of a single capsulorhexis tear is that the intended IOL can still be placed inside the capsular bag with a low risk of decentration. IOL placement into the ciliary sulcus is still an option, but it carries a higher risk of a refractive surprise or of postoperative decentration due to insufficient overall length.

UDAY DEVGAN, MD

When the capsulorhexis radializes, it can turn a routine case into a challenging situation with a higher risk of intraocular complications. If the capsulorhexis can be retrieved and completed in a continuous manner, surgeons can avoid these problems to successfully finish the case.

The main culprit in a radialized capsulorhexis is a flat anterior chamber and loss of viscoelastic. When there is posterior pressure, or if I distort the incision and allow egress of the viscoelastic, then the anterior lens capsule becomes more curved, and the rhexis tends to roll downhill toward the zonules. By reinflating the anterior chamber with viscoelastic, I can redeepen it and flatten the anterior lens capsule, thus facilitating capsulorhexis retrieval.

Although traditional force vectors can be used to lead the capsulorhexis back toward the center of the lens capsule, this maneuver is often difficult to perform through my sub–3-mm incisions. Use of paracentesis incisions, along with 23- or 25-gauge capsule forceps, can allow better instrument positioning to redirect the capsulorhexis centrally.

I owe a debt of gratitude to Brian Little, FCRS, FRCOphth, of London, for his technique of capsulorhexis retrieval, which is simple and yet very effective. It involves unfolding the capsule back and placing it flat. The next step is to pull backward and then curve in to redirect the tear centrally. Continue pulling centrally to bring the capsulorhexis edge back to the desired size. Now, a normal method of capsulorhexis creation can occur, and the procedure is finished (Figures 1 through 5).

I consider Dr. Little's method for capsulorhexis retrieval invaluable in many difficult situations. My recommendation to surgeons is that the next time they encounter a single radial tear, they should reinflate the anterior chamber with a cohesive viscoelastic and use Dr. Little's method.

BONNIE HENDERSON, MD

If the surgeon manages a small radial tear properly, creating a complete continuous capsule opening is still possible. The first important step is to determine why the radial tear occurred. Is the patient uncomfortable and squeezing the lid speculum? Is there posterior pressure?

After investigating and correcting any of the possible causes, as the next step, I inflate the anterior chamber with the proper amount and type of viscoelastic solution. The anterior chamber should be inflated enough to flatten the lens diaphragm without over inflating. I choose a type of viscoelastic based on my goal for the surgery. A dispersive, highly retentive form, such as chondroitin sulfate, will maintain the chamber better, whereas the cohesive form, such as sodium hyaluronate, allows for easier handling of the capsular flap.

Once the anterior chamber is deepened with viscoelastic solution, I grasp the middle of the inverted capsular flap rather than at the peripheral base of the tear. Grasping the flap at the peripheral base can cause the radial tear to extend further out to the periphery. Once I grasp the flap, I attempt to change the direction of the tear by gently pulling tangentially at first, then turning centrally toward the center of the pupil. It is important to keep the forceps in the same area slightly anterior to the plane of the anterior capsule and to not lift toward the cornea.

If the radial tear cannot be easily redirected, I do not continue. Instead, I leave the tear alone and use a cystatome to restart a capsulorhexis at the same beginning position and tear in the opposite direction to meet at the radial tear. I tear a larger capsule opening to incorporate the radial tear into the new capsule opening. When restarting the capsulorhexis, I ensure that the configuration of the new opening is heart-shaped. This arrangement allows me to craft a new flap without creating a fresh extension and, consequently, a point of weakness.

If I cannot incorporate the radial tear into the new capsulorhexis, and if the radial tear is still present, I carefully hydrodissect and hydrolineate the lens without prolapsing it out of the capsular bag. I remove the center nucleus using a chopping technique with minimal rotation of the lens. Once the center nucleus is removed, I carefully extract the outer epinuclear layer without causing undue stress on the capsule. In the presence of a radial tear, it is best to avoid over rotating the lens, which increases the chance of extending the small tear. When removing the epinucleus and cortex, I leave the area closest to the radial tear until last. Remember to strip the cortex toward the radial tear rather than away from the tear. ■

This article originally appeared in the October 2007 issue of CRSToday.

CHAPTER 19

Torn Anterior Capsule

RICHARD TIPPERMAN, MD; WILLIAM J. FISHKIND, MD; LISA BROTHERS ARBISSER, MD; AND MARC MICHELSON, MD

CASE PRESENTATION

Early in the phacoemulsification of a nucleus, a tear in the anterior capsule becomes identifiable 180° away from the incision site. Please comment on your strategy for completing the remaining steps of the procedure, including your IOL preference and insertion technique.

RICHARD TIPPERMAN, MD

Of primary concern is the potential posterior extension of the anterior radial tear, a problem that could lead to dislocation of the nucleus into the vitreous cavity. Three main factors will influence the management of this situation: (1) the density of the lens; (2) the size of the capsulorhexis; and (3) the experience of the surgeon.

Obviously, increasing the lens' density or decreasing the capsulorhexis' size will both make managing the subsequent surgery more difficult. If an inexperienced surgeon is not comfortable with completing phacoemulsification, one option is simply to convert to a "beer can" type of capsulorhexis and then to perform a manual nuclear-expression extracapsular procedure.

Several approaches may be used to complete phacoemulsification. If the lens is not too dense, then the surgeon can sculpt a large central bowl and use the phaco needle to engage and pull the rim of the nucleus into the pupillary space. The nucleus can then be rotated, and the surgeon may repeat this maneuver at multiple locations. As high vacuum brings the individual nuclear quadrants into the center of the work space, it will be possible to fracture the material from the remaining nucleus without putting undue stress on the anterior radial tear.

In denser lenses, one can employ either a divide and conquer or a chopping technique, as long as these maneuvers are performed away from the region of the capsular tear. During the sculpting of a groove, the phaco tip should be directed away from the region of the tear. Once the groove is sufficiently deep, the surgeon should rotate the lens 90° away from the tear in order to complete cracking without adding stress to the region of the tear. A similar approach may be used with a chopping technique.

A single-piece Acrysof lens (Alcon Laboratories, Inc., Fort Worth, TX) is ideal in these situations. The lens can be inserted directly into the capsular bag while its haptics are still folded. The surgeon then orients the lens such that its haptics will expand 90° away from the anterior radial tear. This step will allow completely atraumatic implantation. The capsular bag will seal down and essentially shrinkwrap the IOL, thus providing excellent long-term centration of the lens.

It may also be helpful for less experienced phaco surgeons to realize that large numbers of phaco cases were completed in the 1980s and early 1990s in the presence of multiple radial tears/can-opener capsulotomies.

WILLIAM J. FISHKIND, MD

Radial tears of the anterior capsule commonly occur. In my surgeries, they happen at a rate of approximately 1%. They are most common when the nucleus is hard and the capsulorhexis is relatively small, but the tears may also extend from a notch in the capsulorhexis.

After the identification of a radial tear, it is imperative to prevent it from extending through the equator of the capsular bag and into the posterior capsule. The tear could then become large and be associated with vitreous loss. Thereafter, the anterior capsule might become too unstable to allow the fixation of an IOL in the ciliary sulcus.

For these reasons, I would stop phacoemulsification immediately

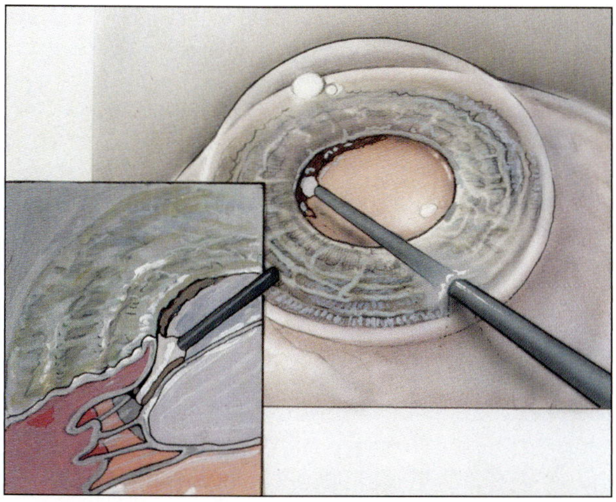

Figure 1. A dispersive OVD is placed within and above the capsular bag to isolate the tear. (Reprinted with permission from Fishkind WJ, ed. *Complications in Phacoemulsification: Avoidance, Recognition, and Management*. 1st ed. New York, NY: Thieme Medical Publishers; 2002.)

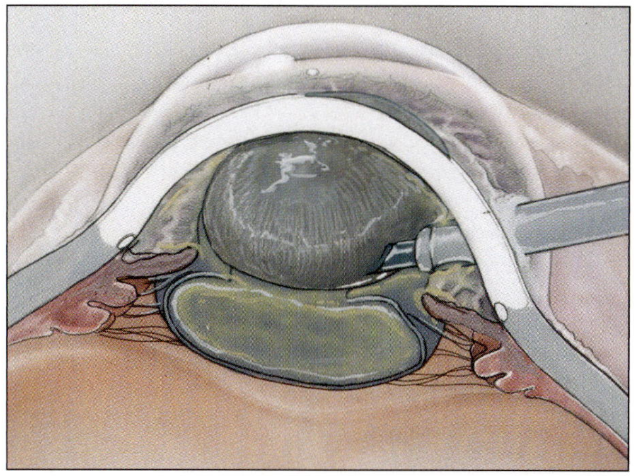

Figure 2. The nucleus is elevated to the plane of the iris and emulsified with a dispersive OVD above and below it. (Reprinted with permission from Fishkind WJ, ed. *Complications in Phacoemulsification: Avoidance, Recognition, and Management*. 1st ed. New York, NY: Thieme Medical Publishers; 2002.)

upon recognizing the radial tear. Before removing the phaco tip, I would fill the anterior chamber with a dispersive ophthalmic viscosurgical device (OVD) in order to prevent the vitreous from moving anteriorly upon the removal of the phaco tip and thus enlarging the tear. Next, I would inject a dispersive viscoelastic above and within the capsular bag, between the nucleus and the bag's equator, in the region of the tear (Figure 1). Because the anterior capsule is not intact, there will be little resistance to the nuclear material moving forward into the anterior chamber.

I would perform phacoemulsification in the anterior chamber and either use a chopping technique or carousel the nucleus without placing pressure on the capsular bag (Figure 2). I would replace the dispersive OVD within the capsular bag as necessary during phacoemulsification to keep the bag full and stable and thus prevent an extension of the tear.

After emulsifying the nucleus, I would perform I/A starting with the subincisional cortex and working toward the area of the anterior capsular tear. I would remove the cortex tangentially but, when approaching the tear, pull toward the tear so as not to extend it. Prior to removing the phaco and I/A tips, I would fill the anterior chamber with an OVD in order to prevent anterior movement of the vitreous.

If the capsule tore posteriorly but no vitreous presented, I would implant the IOL in the sulcus. If the tear extended and vitreous loss occurred, a pars plana, bimanual vitrectomy would be necessary.

Next, I would inject the IOL into the anterior chamber, anterior to the iris. If the posterior capsule is intact, the lens should be placed gently into the OVD-filled bag, perpendicular to the tear in the anterior chamber. If the posterior capsule were torn, the IOL (with a suitably adjusted power) should be placed into the ciliary sulcus, perpendicular to the rent.

The early recognition of tears in the anterior capsule and an attention to detail will allow the successful management of the complication and excellent surgical outcomes.

LISA BROTHERS ARBISSER, MD

Upon identifying a tear in the anterior capsule, I would fill the chamber with a dispersive OVD through the sideport incision, withdraw my phaco tip, and inspect the extent of the tear by retracting the iris if necessary. Assuming that the tear does not extend beyond the zonules, I would change my phaco parameters to low flow settings, lower the bottle of BSS, and continue with my usual vertical chop technique but with cautious and minimal rotational force. All the while, I would monitor the tear and keep it in place by maintaining compartmentalization with the OVD over this area. If the tear has extended beyond the zonular insertion, I would use a supracapsular technique.

Great care would be necessary to avoid engaging the edges of the tear during the aspiration of the cortex. If there were any resistance due to poor hydrodissection around the area of the tear, I would use a dry manual technique under a cohesive viscoelastic without irrigation to aspirate the cortex in this area. This approach should provide the most control and prevent forces that might extend the tear.

I would choose a single-piece acrylic IOL, my usual lens, and place it in the bag. Because there is no pent-up energy in this lens as it unfolds, the IOL can be safely implanted in cases such as this one and maneuvered without difficulty before it has unfolded completely so that its haptics are not located in the area of the tear. This lens will stay put and will not cause asymmetric forces in the postoperative period. If only a three-piece lens were available, I would use a bimanual insertion technique and avoid dialing the lens into the bag. I would also make a small radial cut in the anterior capsule, 180° away from the tear, to balance forces and lessen the chance of asymmetric capsular fibrosis, which could lead to decentration of the IOL. Plate haptic lenses would never be appropriate under these circumstances.

I would not remove viscoelastic from the posterior chamber under the IOL in my usual way. Instead, I would constrict the pupil with Miochol-E (Novartis Ophthalmics, Inc., Duluth, GA) after smoothing out the edge of the tear, which the overlying iris would support during aspiration of the OVD from the anterior chamber. Due to the likelihood of residual OVD, I would use an antihypertensive medication to prevent a spike in IOP during the immediate postoperative period. I would expect an uncomplicated postoperative course with an excellent result in this case.

MARC MICHELSON, MD

Upon recognizing the tear, my first thought would be, "no big deal." Not long ago, all phacoemulsification was performed with a can-opener capsulotomy and approximately 15 to 20 radial tears in the anterior capsule. Most of those cases were completed without any tears extending into the posterior capsule.

The advent of the continuous curvilinear capsulorhexis applied a higher technical standard to the cataract operation; in fact, some IOLs require an intact anterior capsulorhexis for insertion. In addition, phaco techniques using high flow and vacuum may place additional stress on an already weakened capsulorhexis, thereby precipitating a potential posterior capsular tear.

In this case, I would attempt to redirect any procedural stressors away from the tear. I routinely use Healon5 (Advanced Medical Optics, Inc., Santa Ana, CA) during phacoemulsification. I would ensure that there was an adequate amount of the OVD in the anterior chamber and add more if necessary in order to apply some increased pressure from the anterior chamber posteriorly against the anterior capsule. This pressure would help stabilize the anterior capsule by prohibiting the development of posterior pressure that could force an extension of the tear. Attempts to hydrodissect with BSS should be abandoned. I would modify fluidics by lowering the aspiration rate to the low 20s, decreasing vacuum to 150 mmHg, and proceeding with phacoemulsification at a slower rate. I would also attempt to perform the phacoemulsification at least 1 to 2 clock hours away from the tear and avoid placing the phaco tip near the tear.

If the nucleus does not rotate well within the bag, I would lower the phaco energy and perform an in situ emulsification until the nucleus breaks away freely from the capsular bag. I would not hesitate to remove nucleus from beneath the tear but would do so slowly and cautiously. After nuclear removal, the challenge would be to aspirate the remaining cortex. I usually do not modify my I/A settings, but I would strive to avoid aspirating the torn flap.

If cataract removal could be completed successfully with an intact posterior capsule, I would implant a three-piece silicone or acrylic IOL. I would avoid a single-piece or plate-style lens. My lens of choice is the Alcon Acrysof SN60WF (Alcon Laboratories, Inc.), owing to how little stress it places on the capsule as it gently unfolds. If I were to use a three-piece IOL, I would allow the implant's leading haptic to unfold in the anterior chamber in order to reduce the hazard of a haptic's sweeping across the inside of the bag as the IOL unfolded and expanding the tear. The unfolded lens could then be guided into the bag with little stress to the anterior capsule. ■

This article originally appeared in the March 2005 issue of CRSToday.

CHAPTER 20

Pearls for Sizing the Capsulorhexis

DAVID F. CHANG, MD; STEVEN DEWEY, MD; RICHARD TIPPERMAN, MD; AND R. BRUCE WALLACE III, MD

DAVID F. CHANG, MD

The capsulorhexis is generally considered the most important step in cataract surgery. A continuous curvilinear capsulorhexis (CCC) provides numerous surgical advantages,[1] and a continuous curvilinear capsular edge reduces the chance of a capsular tear occurring during surgery. Like an elastic waistband, the capsulorhexis will stretch—rather than tear—in response to surgical forces. A continuous edge is necessary to perform cortical cleaving hydrodissection, and it facilitates cortical cleanup as well as the placement of both haptics into the capsular bag. It also converts the anterior capsule into a contingency platform for IOL support should the posterior capsular tear.

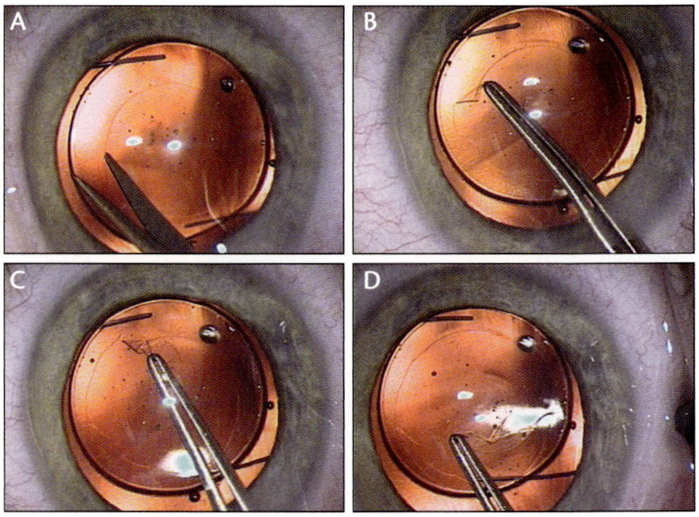

Figure 1. A small-diameter capsulorhexis is enlarged with forceps after creating a new flap with an oblique microscissors cut (A–D).

The postoperative advantages of a properly sized capsulorhexis are equally important. As the capsular bag contracts, it prevents pea-podding (ie, the escape of either haptic).[2,3] Asymmetric capsular forces resulting from an eccentric CCC can cause delayed optic decentration. Continuous circumferential overlap of the IOL's optic edge will produce a capsular shrink-wrap effect, whereby the posterior capsule is kinked by the optic edge—a major factor in the prevention of posterior capsular opacification (PCO).[4,5] This overlap will also lessen any edge dysphotopsias as it opacifies over time. Finally, such continuous overlap of the optic's edge is the only way to attain consistency in the axial IOL position from case to case. Being able to accurately predict this effective lens position is a critical factor in calculating the proper IOL power for emmetropia.

It follows that a capsulorhexis with a diameter extending beyond the optic edge in some or all areas loses these advantages. Posterior lens epithelial cell migration will occur in any region

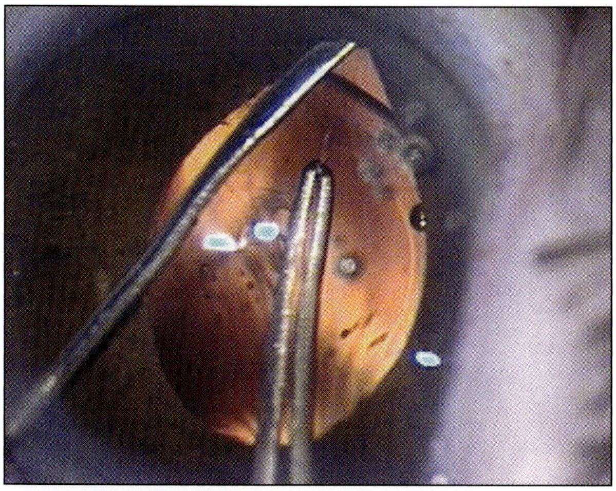

Figure 2. A Lester hook is used to retract the iris to better view the IOL's optic edge.

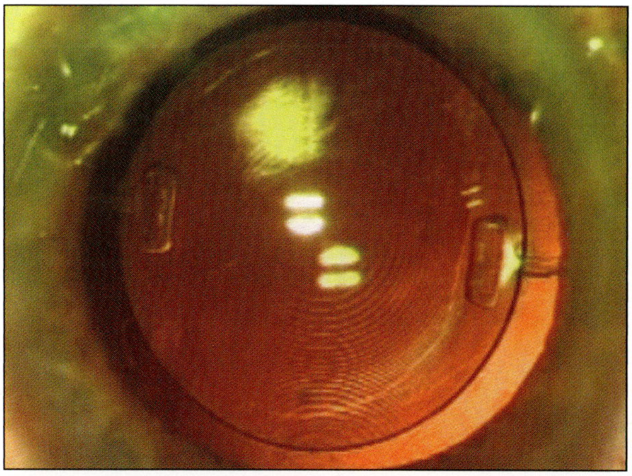

Figure 3. With a 6-mm-optic IOL, making a central 5.0- to 5.5-mm anterior capsulotomy results in a 360° capsular overlap.

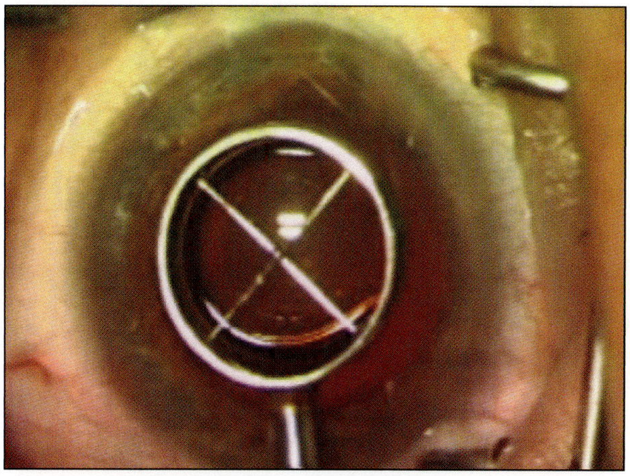

Figure 4. A capsulotomy diameter mark is placed on the central cornea with a 6-mm optic zone marker.

where the posterior capsule is not kinked by the optic's edge.[5] Over time, slight optic decentration may result from asymmetric capsular contractile forces. Finally, as the posterior capsule tenses postoperatively, the optic may be slightly more anteriorly displaced wherever it is not restrained by a taut capsulorhexis edge, resulting in a myopic shift.

What are the disadvantages of a capsulorhexis with a diameter that is too small? In addition to impeding surgical steps such as the removal of subincisional cortex, a small-diameter CCC may also create postoperative problems. The increased load of lens epithelial cells on the back of the anterior capsule can increase inflammation, cause anterior capsular fibrosis and opacification, and result in excessive contraction of the capsulorhexis and capsular bag,[6-8] leading to zonular damage or dehiscence and optic decentration.[9,10] With sufficiently weakened zonules, visually significant capsulophimosis or subluxation of the bag-IOL complex can occur.[7,11] Finally, excessive anterior capsular opacification can impair visualization of the peripheral retina.

Given the importance of obtaining a proper capsulorhexis diameter, it is ironic that this is one of the only cataract surgical steps that technology has not yet improved. We continue to use a low-tech, manual method to perform the tear with a needle and/or forceps. The intended diameter is estimated visually. Individual variability in anterior segment and pupil diameter and corneal magnification make it difficult to precisely size the capsulorhexis. Parallax occurring with movement of the globe makes it difficult to judge the symmetry and centration of the evolving capsulotomy.

My personal solution for sizing the capsulorhexis is to plan on performing it in two stages when necessary (Figure 1). As I make the primary capsulorhexis, I try to err on the small side, because the diameter can always be enlarged, but not reduced. I take a moment to assess the appropriateness of the CCC diameter after IOL implantation. Frequently, the size and centration are fine, but it is surprising how often the CCC is slightly eccentric to the center of the optic. Sometimes, a perfectly round CCC becomes ovoid following implantation due to the directional stretch of the stiff three-piece haptics. This is a sign of zonular laxity and insufficient centrifugal tension in the areas perpendicular to the haptic axis.

In either situation, or if the overall diameter is too small, I enlarge the capsulorhexis by making an oblique cut with a pair of scissors and grasping the resulting flap with capsular forceps (Figure 1A and B). The cut should be oblique, rather than radial, so that the resulting flap is more inclined to tear in a circumferential direction. The flap is then maneuvered with capsular forceps under a generous amount of ophthalmic viscosurgical device. Curved Uthoff-Gills capsulotomy scissors with blunt tips (Katena K4-5126; Katena Products, Inc., Denville, NJ) have the perfect shape for creating an initial curved cut to either side of the phaco incision. If the pupil is small enough to conceal the optic's edge, it can be locally retracted with a Lester hook (Figure 2). In some cases, I only trim a part of the remaining anterior capsular rim where it is excessively wide. Other times, I re-tear the entire 360° circumference of the opening (Figure 1).

Executing the second-stage enlargement may be easier than the primary capsulotomy for several reasons. Following removal of the cataract, the red reflex is improved, and there is no convexity to the anterior capsule to promote radial extension of the tear. The optic provides a perfect visual template for resizing the CCC's diameter. Finally, in cases of weak zonules, the presence of the three-piece haptics or a capsular tension ring increases outward tension on the capsular bag, improving control over the direction

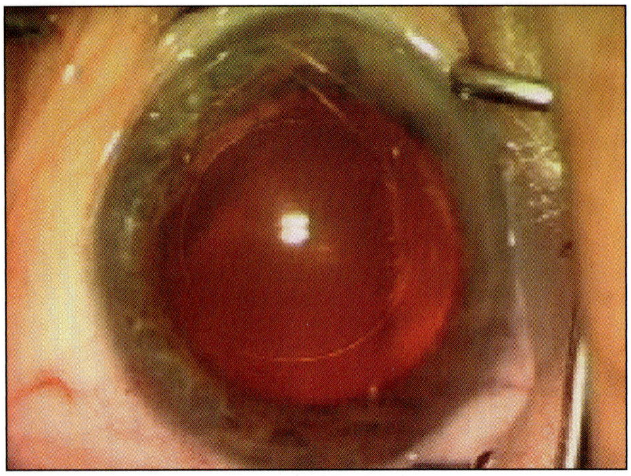

Figure 5. The resulting capsulotomy diameter mark on the cornea serves as a guide for creating the capsulorhexis.

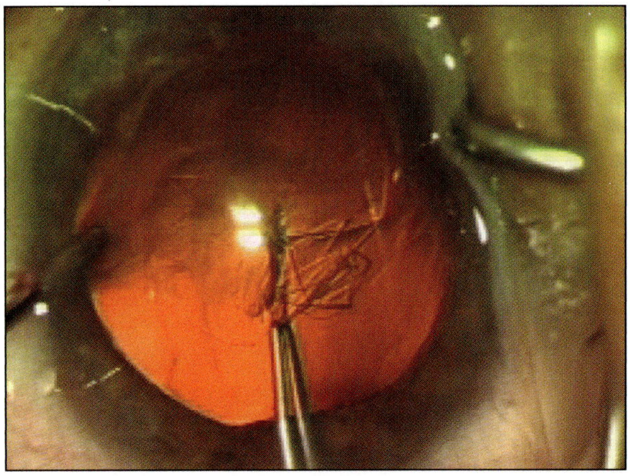

Figure 6. The tear is made just inside the capsular diameter mark with modified Utrata forceps.

of the tear. Should the tear escape peripherally, it is reassuring that no subsequent surgical steps would extend the tear posteriorly. The IOL should not be rotated in this situation, however, for this reason.

Although in most cases, enlargement of a smallish capsulorhexis is not absolutely necessary, I encourage the mastery of this technique. With multifocal IOLs, achieving a symmetric capsulorhexis that completely overlaps the optic's edge is particularly important. There is even less margin for CCC diameter error with accommodating IOLs such as the Crystalens (Eyeonics, Inc., Aliso Viejo, CA). With dynamic accommodating designs such as the Visiogen Synchrony ICL (Visiogen, Inc., Irvine, CA), if the CCC's diameter is too large, it may allow the anterior optic to partially protrude through the capsulotomy. Too small of an opening, however, may cause capsulophimosis or excessive capsular fibrosis that may strain the zonules, stiffen the bag, and incapacitate the accommodative mechanism. Initially erring on the small side, with the option to enlarge it when and where necessary, is the only 100% reliable way I have to attain a perfectly sized capsulorhexis diameter.

Finally, comfort with this maneuver is important if there is difficulty steering the flap during the primary capsulorhexis. Whether the cause is poor visibility, patient movement, a shallow chamber, or weak zonules, the surgeon can make a smaller diameter opening to increase control and to better avoid a peripheral extension. The diameter can be secondarily enlarged after the IOL has been implanted.

STEVEN DEWEY, MD

A properly sized capsulorhexis is an absolute must for standardizing the results of cataract surgery. In routine cases, overlapping the edge of the optic by 0.5 to 1 mm will result in a consistent lens position from case to case. It also has the benefit of driving the sharp posterior edge of an IOL into the posterior capsule and reducing the potential for PCO. In less routine cases, an intact capsulorhexis allows for optic capture to secure the IOL, even if the posterior capsule is completely absent.

Sizing the capsulorhexis can be challenging. The variability of pupil dilation and corneal diameter may make it difficult to consistently create the proper opening, and therefore, the easiest method is the most direct. Prior to loading the IOL into the insertion device, simply hold the lens over the surgical field and mentally establish the relative size of the optic to the size of the eye.

Several techniques have been developed to gauge the proper capsulorhexis size. R. Bruce Wallace III, MD, of Louisiana, advocates the use of an optical zone marker to effectively provide a size guide *(see Dr. Wallace's description on the following page)*. Barry S. Seibel, MD, of Los Angeles, created capsulorhexis forceps with a millimeter marker on the shaft as an intraocular gauge. This product is manufactured by Microsurgical Technology (Redmond, WA) and easily works with either a standard or bimanual incision.

Instrumentation inherently creates different-sized openings, and this appears to be related to the tangential forces applied as the capsule is torn. A bent needle, which holds the flap closer to the tear, creates a smaller capsular opening. Forceps, which grasp the capsule farther from the tear, will generally create a larger opening.

Although I prefer a 0.5- to 1.0-mm overlap of the anterior capsule on the optic, more overlap is also acceptable, as long as the surgical technique can accommodate removing the nucleus and cortex through a smaller opening. To keep my capsulorhexis size smaller, I generally prefer a dispersive ophthalmic viscosurgical device to flatten the capsule, and I use a bent needle. In cases of poor visualization or loose zonules, the forceps provide extra control. Of course, a larger capsulorhexis is appropriate when the situation warrants, such as when dealing with a very dense cataract or in cases of zonular laxity where an endocapsular approach should be abandoned.

RICHARD TIPPERMAN, MD

Creating an appropriately sized capsulorhexis is critical for achieving excellent clinical results with presbyopia-correcting IOLs. Regardless of the IOL, a consistent capsulorhexis size will improve predictability of the IOL power calculation.

A specific capsulorhexis size is ideal for maximizing an optic's exposure, centration, and movement with an accommodating IOL. If the capsulorhexis is too small with a true multifocal IOL (ie, simultaneous vision), the amount of light able to travel through the peripheral portion of the IOL is restricted, thereby limiting the light energy transmitted from this portion of the lens. A variety of techniques that aim to create a specific-sized capsulorhexis have been described. The following is an approach that has worked well in my clinical practice.

At the start of surgery, I ask the patient to fixate on the microscope light, and I try to center a 6-mm radial keratotomy optical zone marker on the reflection from the microscope light. Placing the optical zone in this fashion creates a 6-mm circular indentation on the patient's cornea that is roughly centered on his visual axis. I then begin the tear of my capsulorhexis and bring it out until it is in line with the inner edge of the mark from the optical zone marker.

At this point, if the pupil is round and symmetric, I no longer need to shift my focus between the anterior capsule and the corneal dome where the optical zone marker is visible. I simply mentally note the distance between the capsulorhexis' edge and the iris sphincter and then complete the tear for the full 360°. I try to maintain this constant distance for the entire capsulotomy.

This is a simple technique using readily available instrumentation that provides for a consistent capsulorhexis size. Surgeons often find that shifting their fixation from the corneal dome to the anterior capsule while trying to bring the tear around can be cumbersome at best. At worst, this maneuver will lead to unpredictable sizing or difficulty with completing the capsulorhexis. Using the corneal marker to create a landmark for the peripheral border of the tear and then completing the capsulorhexis with a different constant landmark in the anterior capsular plane (ie, pupillary margin) makes consistent sizing of the capsulorhexis much simpler.

R. BRUCE WALLACE III, MD

A well-centered and properly sized anterior capsulotomy plays an important role in achieving successful visual outcomes after cataract or lens-based refractive surgery. Many studies have credited the reduced rate of PCO to an anterior capsular overlap of the periphery of the IOL's optic.[12-14] Sequestering the optic also improves implant power prediction with more reliable lens constants for IOL calculation formulas, and creating an anterior capsular shelf allows for easier insertion of an IOL in the ciliary sulcus, if indicated.[12]

In 2003, I described a method to consistently create a well-centered and properly sized capsulorhexis.[12] After placing the capsulotomy diameter mark, the surgeon has a visual template to guide the location and proper diameter of the capsulotomy (Warren E. Hill, MD, oral communication).[15] For instance, if a 6-mm optic IOL is to be implanted, making a central 5.0- to 5.5-mm anterior capsulotomy will result in a 360° capsular overlap of the peripheral IOL (Figure 3).

At the beginning of the procedure, the surgeon places a 6-mm optical zone mark on the central cornea (Figures 4 and 5). I have learned that parallax from the surgical microscope can cause minor decentration of the capsulotomy. A rule of thumb is to shift the mark slightly to the left for a right-eye-dominant surgeon and to the right for left-eye dominance. During the capsulotomy, bring the initiated flap to just inside the cornea mark, and slowly complete the capsulotomy. Always stay just inside the circular mark on the cornea. Due to corneal magnification, the resulting capsulotomy should measure 5.0 to 5.5 mm. An easy way to gauge the IOL's centration and size is to evaluate the capsular coverage of the 6-mm IOL optic after implantation.

Because I routinely utilize topical anesthesia for lens surgery, I like to stabilize the globe when performing these measures. I place a blunt-tip cyclodialysis in the sideport incision before making a tear in the central capsule with a bent 25-gauge needle. I guide the tear temporally to the edge of the capsulotomy diameter mark and complete the circular capsulotomy with modified Utrata forceps (Figure 6). Sharp-tipped capsular forceps may be used for the entire procedure; however, they need to be replaced when the tips become dull. Replacing the autoclavable stainless steel 25-gauge bent needle is less costly.

Refractive cataract surgery and lens-based refractive surgery have moved to center stage. These procedures will continue to grow in popularity with aging baby boomers. Any step we can take to improve IOL power accuracy and reduce complications such as PCO will help us become more successful in achieving the desired results for our patients. ■

This article originally appeared in the October 2007 issue of CRSToday.

1. Gimbel HV, Neuhann T. Development, advantages, and methods of the continuous circular capsulorhexis technique. *J Cataract Refract Surg.* 1990;16:31-37.
2. Assia EI, Legler UF, Merrill C, et al. Clinicopathologic study of the effect of radial tears and loop fixation on intraocular lens decentration. *Ophthalmology.* 1993;100:153-158.
3. Ram J, Apple DJ, Peng Q, et al. Update on fixation of rigid and foldable posterior chamber intraocular lenses. Part I: Elimination of fixation-induced decentration to achieve precise optical correction and visual rehabilitation. *Ophthalmology.* 1999;106:883-890.
4. Ram J, Pandey SK, Apple DJ, et al. Effect of in-the-bag intraocular lens fixation on the prevention of posterior capsule opacification. *J Cataract Refract Surg.* 2001;27:367-370.
5. Nishi O, Nishi K, Wickstrom K. Preventing lens epithelial cell migration using intraocular lenses with sharp rectangular edges. *J Cataract Refract Surg.* 2000;26:1543-1549.
6. Hansen SO, Crandall AS, Olson RJ. Progressive constriction of the anterior capsular opening following intact capsulorhexis. *J Cataract Refract Surg.* 1993;19:77-82.
7. Davison JA. Capsule contraction syndrome. *J Cataract Refract Surg.* 1993;19:582-589.
8. Joo CK, Shin JA, Kim JH. Capsular opening contraction after continuous curvilinear capsulorhexis and intraocular lens implantation. *J Cataract Refract Surg.* 1996;22:585-590.
9. Hayashi K, Hayashi H, Nakao F, Hayashi F. Anterior capsule contraction and intraocular lens decentration and tilt after hydrogel lens implantation. *Br J Ophthalmol.* 2001;85:1294-1297.
10. Hayashi H, Hayashi K, Nakao F, Hayashi F. Anterior capsule contraction and intraocular lens dislocation in eyes with pseudoexfoliation syndrome. *Br J Ophthalmol.* 1998;82:1429-1432.
11. Jahan FS, Mamalis N, Crandall AS. Spontaneous late dislocation of intraocular lens within the capsular bag in psuedoexfoliation patients. *Ophthalmology.* 2001;108:1727-1731.
12. Ravalico G, Tognetto D, Palomba MA, et al. Capsulorhexis size and posterior capsule opacification. *J Cataract Refract Surg.* 1996;22:98-103.
13. Hollick EJ, Spalton DJ, Meacock WR. The effect of capsulorhexis size on posterior capsular opacification: one-year results of a randomized prospective trial. *Am J Ophthalmol.* 1999;128:271-279.
14. Apple DJ, Peng Q, Visessook N, et al. Eradication of posterior capsule opacification: documentation of a marked decrease in Nd:YAG laser posterior capsulotomy rates noted in an analysis of 5416 pseudophakic human eyes obtained postmortem. *Ophthalmology.* 2001;108:505-518.
15. Wallace RB. Capsulotomy diameter mark. *J Cataract Refract Surg.* 2003;29:1866-1868.

CHAPTER 21

New Technology for Sizing the Continuous Curvilinear Capsulorhexis

H. BURKHARD DICK, MD, AND ADOLFO PENA, MD

The success of the continuous curvilinear capsulorhexis at reducing complications and providing satisfactory refractive outcomes depends on its centration, location, and size. Studies have demonstrated that the capsulorhexis' diameter should be small enough to overlap 360° of the IOL optic's periphery to reduce the risk of posterior capsular opacification (PCO)[1-3] and that the overlapping configuration may prevent PCO more effectively than the design of the IOL's edge.[4]

A prototypic system could help surgeons create optimally sized capsulorhexes and thus reduce the risk of postoperative PCO.

THE CAPSULORHEXIS' EFFECT ON PCO

Large capsulorhexes (6 to 7 mm in diameter) have been associated with greater rates of PCO and less acute visual outcomes than those with smaller diameters (4.5 to 5.0 mm).[2] Conversely, too small a capsulorhexis could cause phimosis of the anterior capsule,[5,6] decrease vision, block the surgeon's view of the peripheral fundus, or neutralize the benefits of aspheric IOLs. At this time, the functional success and diameter of a continuous curvilinear capsulorhexis depends entirely on the surgeon's ability and experience. The risk of intraoperative complications arising from unsuccessful capsulorhexes increases for complicated cases (eg, intumescent cataracts, small or large eyes, intraoperative floppy iris syndrome, or weak zonules) performed by inexperienced surgeons.[7]

IMPROVING THE CAPSULORHEXIS' FORMATION

To assist inexperienced surgeons and promote the consistent formation of the continuous curvilinear capsulorhexis, Michel Perez, MD, of Dijon, France, and Dr. Dick have developed in conjunction with Carl Zeiss Meditec AG (Jena, Germany) an interface-module (data-injection) system (DIS) that projects a reference ring through the operating microscope's light source onto the anterior capsule.[8,9] Surgeons can use the projected image to guide their placement and execution of the capsulorhexis (Figure 1).

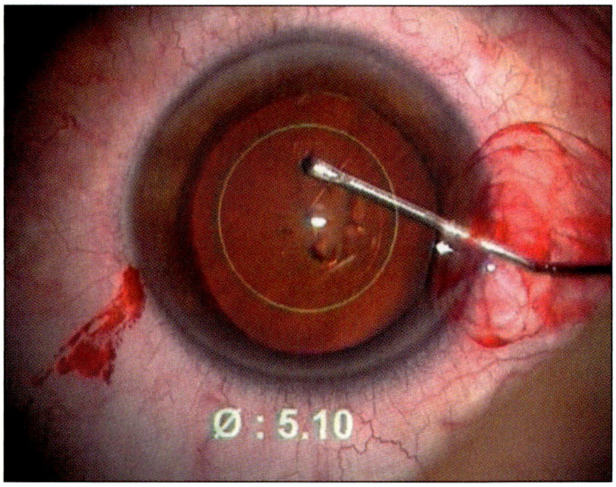

Figure 1. This intraoperative view shows a 5.1-mm–diameter green ring projected onto the anterior capsule by the DIS. An active eye tracker follows ocular movements and maintains the ring's proper position on the capsule.

The DIS consists of an OPMI VISU 140 surgical microscope (Carl Zeiss Meditec AG), the DIS module that projects the ring onto the capsule through the microscope, and a video camera mounted between the microscope's tube and the DIS module. The patient's preoperative biometric data (ie, axial length and anterior chamber depth) are stored on a personal computer, and a display control unit forwards the data to the DIS module. From the display control unit, surgeons can modify the operative parameters, including the planned diameter of the capsulorhexis, the corneal radius, and the anterior chamber depth. Other options allow users to change the size and color of the projected ring as well as the focal length of the main objective in order to increase depth of focus.

If the surgeon decides to magnify the microscope's image intraoperatively, the DIS' program automatically maintains the projected ring's correct size (Figure 2). The DIS also employs an active eye tracker that captures 12 to 25 images per second. These images are sent to the module to keep the projected ring in the correct position on the anterior capsule. After the capsulorhexis' creation, pushing a button on the display screen discontinues the projected ring.

THE DIS IN ACTION

To evaluate the effectiveness of the DIS, investigators at the University Eye Clinic of the Knappschafts-Krankenhaus in Bochum-Langendreer, Germany, randomized 96 eyes of 96 patients to undergo unilateral clear corneal cataract surgery with and without the device (data on file at the Study Coordination Center, Ruhr University Eye Hospital, Bochum, Germany). The capsulorhexis' targeted size in both groups was 5.1 mm.[10]

In addition to using an Engel spatula (Geuder AG, Heidelberg, Germany) to measure the capsulorhexes' horizontal and vertical diameters intra- and postoperatively, the investigators evaluated the size of the openings with the computer-assisted Evaluation of Posterior Capsule Opacification 2000 system (available from Manfred Tetz, MD, in Berlin). They also measured subjects' UCVA, BSCVA, manifest refraction, keratometry, axial length, and anterior chamber depth pre- and postoperatively. The investigators analyzed these data to determine if the difference in the capsulorhexes' diameter or scatter around the target diameter was statistically significant.

The eyes in both groups had similar baseline and postoperative UCVAs, keratometric readings, spheres, astigmatism, refractions, and axial lengths, and they received comparably powered IOLs.

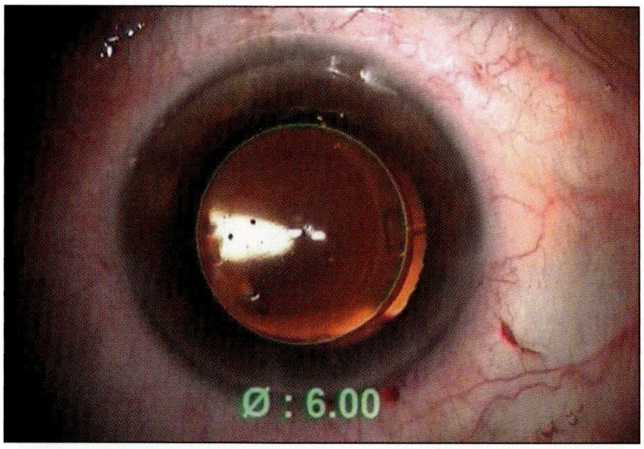

Figure 2. As the surgeon uses the foot pedal of the OPMI VISU 140 surgical microscope to zoom in on the eye, the DIS automatically verifies the projected ring's position and size. Here, a 6-mm ring is positioned exactly on the outer rim of a Tecnis silicone IOL's optic (Advanced Medical Optics, Inc., Santa Ana, CA).

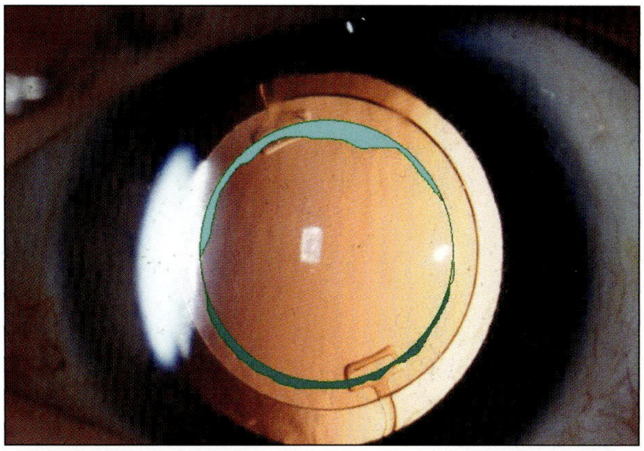

Figure 3. The bright blue area in this analysis of a pseudophakic eye with the Evaluation of Posterior Capsule Opacification 2000 system indicates that the capsulorhexis is smaller than its targeted diameter. The dark green area indicates that the capsulorhexis is larger than the targeted diameter.

The mean depth of the anterior chamber was 3.15 and 3.38 mm in the DIS and control groups, respectively (Wilcoxon rank-sum test [P=.079]). The investigators did not find statistically significant differences in the capsulorhexes' mean diameters or in the deviation from the targeted size (5.1 mm) between the groups.

The scatter around the diameter of the capsulorhexes differed between the groups. Intraoperatively, more capsulorhexes in the DIS group (92%) had horizontal diameters within the reference zone's normal range (4.9 to 5.3 mm, P<.001 [Fisher's exact test]) than in the control group (27%). Postoperatively, 83% of the capsulorhexes in the DIS group were within the reference zone's normal range (4.9 to 5.3 mm) versus 21% in the control group.

Although the capsulorhexes' diameters changed postoperatively, mostly due to smaller values, the differences in scatter between the treatment groups were smaller. The same tendency, however, persisted (P=.002 for horizontal and P≤.001 for vertical diameter [Fisher's exact test]). Furthermore, after dividing the groups according to whether the anterior chamber depth was less than or greater than 3 mm, the same tendency in scatter persisted between both groups intra- and postoperatively for the capsulorhexes' horizontal and vertical diameters (Mantel/Haenszel method [P≤.002]). The Evaluation of Posterior Capsule Opacification 2000 system showed no difference between the treatment groups in terms of the capsulorhexes' area (Wilcoxon rank-sum test [P=.344]) (Figure 3).

CONCLUSION

The diameters of the capsulorhexes created by experienced surgeons using the DIS were more accurate in relation to the scatter around the reference zone than those created without the DIS. We believe that the DIS, which is scheduled to be incorporated into the next generation of OPMI Lumera Surgical Microscopes (will be available in Europe and the US; Carl Zeiss Surgical, Oberkochen, Germany), could be useful for training residents and fellows, and it could be a helpful tool for optimizing postoperative outcomes after phacoemulsification. The DIS will enlarge the surgical portfolio of every cataract surgeon. ■

This article originally appeared in the January 2008 issue of CRSToday.

1. Ravalico G, Tognetto D, Palomba M, et al. Capsulorhexis size and posterior capsule opacification. *J Cataract Refract Surg.* 1996;22:98-103.
2. Hollick EJ, Spalton DJ, Meacock WR. The effect of capsulorhexis size on posterior capsular opacification: one-year results of a randomized prospective trial. *Am J Ophthalmol.* 1999;128:271-279.
3. Apple DJ, Peng Q, Visessook N, et al. Eradication of posterior capsule opacification: documentation of a marked decrease in Nd:YAG laser posterior capsulotomy rates noted in an analysis of 5,416 pseudophakic human eyes obtained postmortem. *Ophthalmology.* 2001;108:505-518.
4. Smith SR, Daynes T, Hinckley M, et al. The effect of lens edge design versus anterior capsule overlap on posterior capsule opacification. *Am J Ophthalmol.* 2004;138:521-526.
5. Davison JA. Capsule contraction syndrome. *J Cataract Refract Surg.* 1993;19:582-589.
6. Joo CK, Shin JA, Kim JH. Capsular opening contraction after continuous curvilinear capsulorhexis and intraocular lens implantation. *J Cataract Refract Surg.* 1996;22:585-590.
7. Martin KR, Burton RL. The phacoemulsification learning curve: per-operative complications in the first 3000 cases of an experienced surgeon. *Eye.* 2000;14 (pt 2):190-195.
8. Dick HB. The 4th C: customized CCC. Film presented at: The ASCRS Symposium on Cataract, IOL and Refractive Surgery; April 16, 2005; Washington, DC.
9. Dick HB. Perfecting the capsulorhexis using data injection: prospective trial. Paper presented at: The ASCRS Symposium on Cataract, IOL, and Refractive Surgery; March 20, 2006; San Francisco, CA.
10. Tetz MR, Auffarth GU, Sperker M, et al. Photographic image analysis system of posterior capsule opacification. *J. Cataract Refract Surg.* 1997;23:1515-1520.

CHAPTER 22

Anterior Capsular Contraction Syndrome

PRISCILLA PERRY ARNOLD, MD

The specific description of anterior capsular contraction syndrome was published in 1993, following the widespread adoption of the continuous curvilinear capsulorhexis (CCC).[1-4] Unfortunately, this acceptance proves that every medical advance—which the CCC certainly represents—has potentially negative, unanticipated results. Anterior capsular contraction syndrome is a peculiarly frustrating circumstance because the progressive constriction of the capsule that thwarts a "perfect" surgical procedure is seemingly out of the surgeon's control. Extreme phimosis of the anterior capsule's opening can obscure vision (Figure 1), the distortion of the capsule can affect the IOL's position and function, and the progressive contraction can directly result in zonular dehiscence, thus leading to capsular/IOL complex dislocation. Concern about capsular contraction and opacification is of even more importance now in the setting of presbyopia-correcting IOLs. Achieving perfect lens centration, preventing any later tilt or distortion, and maintaining pristine optical quality are all paramount in meeting the heightened expectations of both surgeons and patients in this setting.

PATHOLOGY

It is important to understand the pathology of capsular contraction syndrome. Its etiology—as opposed to that of posterior capsular epithelial cell migration—involves anterior, cuboidal lens epithelial cell metaplasia with myofibroblastic transformation. The altered cells contain smooth muscle actin, and contraction occurs in the resultant fibrous membrane. Anterior capsular opacity and shrinkage usually occur much earlier than posterior capsular opacification (PCO) (eg, within the first 3 to 6 months postoperatively). Studies have shown that some opacity and shrinkage probably occur after every case of cataract extraction.[5-7]

RELATED MEDICAL CONDITIONS

Several medical conditions can predispose patients to the development of significant anterior capsular contraction syndrome. The best known and probably most commonly encountered of these conditions is pseudoexfoliation. Other pathologies include a history of uveitis, retinitis pigmentosa, high myopia, myotonic dystrophy, advanced age, and trauma (including ocular surgery). Subtle zonular damage, which most likely occurs from previous surgery such as trabeculectomy or vitrectomy, allows for progressive changes after cataract extraction in some cases. Diabetes mellitus is sometimes implicated in this condition as well, although this relationship appears to be less direct. It is certain, however, that zonular disease or trauma is closely associated with the problem of pathologic capsular contraction. Also, instability of the blood aqueous barrier appears to be an inciting factor in pathologic capsular contraction. A history of any of these situations should alert the surgeon to approach the procedure with caution and consider surgical techniques.[8-11]

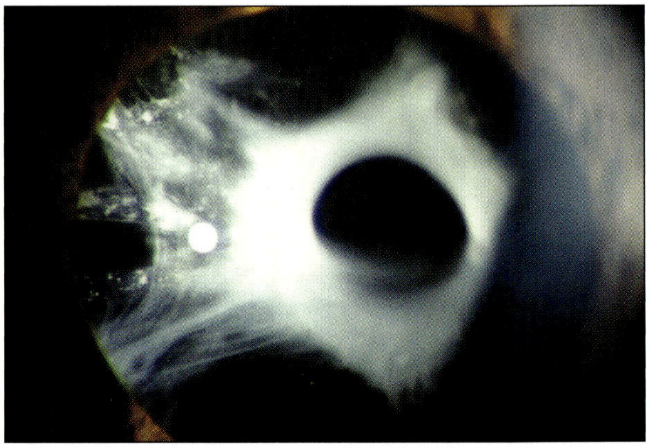

(Courtesy of Garry Condon, MD.)

Figure 1. Extreme anterior capsule phimosis.

CREATING A LARGE CCC

Surgically, it would be logical that creating a larger CCC opening would address the concern of progressive contraction. Although a larger opening does not eliminate the contraction effect, a wider visual aperture adds a margin for retaining good unobstructed vision, even with some degree of capsular phimosis. I advise that surgeons pay particular attention to making the CCC as large as possible (within limits of the IOL's optic margin) in situations of known increased risk.

REMOVING ANTERIOR LENS EPITHELIAL CELLS

Investigators have shown conclusively that careful removal of the anterior lens epithelial cells reduces anterior capsular opacity and constriction. Although there may be a trade-off due to a reported increased tendency toward PCO with the removal of the anterior lens epithelial cell removal, this exchange would seem worth the extra effort in conditions such as pseudoexfoliation. Such maneuvers at times are difficult in the setting of obvious zonular weakness, but surgeons should attempt them.[12,13] Care must be taken not to create stress on the zonules, especially in areas of dehiscence, and curettes or diamond-finished tips, which polish the anterior capsule, are probably preferable in this setting, rather than using an I/A handpiece, which may place tension on the capsule and zonule.

IOL DESIGN AND MATERIALS

Many researchers have analyzed the influence of the IOL's design and material on capsular behavior. Anterior capsular contraction occurs most frequently and is most pronounced in patients with silicone-plate IOLs. In consideration of lens optic material alone, silicone has higher anterior chamber contraction rates than acrylic.[14-17] Investigators have also studied haptic material and found that prolene haptics are more often associated with the syndrome than PMMA haptics. Studies' results vary in terms of whether three-piece or single-piece acrylic IOLs have the lowest overall rate of contraction. Furthermore, having a square-edged optic design is more important for preventing PCO than for influencing the anterior capsule's behavior. Surgeons should carefully consider those patients at risk for the syndrome of capsular contraction before selecting a presbyopia-correcting IOL.[14-17]

CAPSULAR TENSION RINGS

With the introduction of capsular tension rings (CTR), surgeons expected these devices to prevent contraction of the capsular bag. There is evidence that a CTR centers the capsular bag despite weak zonules, stabilizes the IOL's position in the bag, and is effective in controlling severe capsular contraction.[18-23] Experience has shown, however, that a nonsutured CTR does not guarantee protection against progressive zonular dehiscence occuring, especially in cases of pseudoexfoliation (Figure 2). Surgeons are now reporting complications of subluxation or dislocation of the IOL/bag complex years after what appeared to be stable surgery using CTRs.[18-23] Currently, there is reason to consider utilizing only sutured CTRs or capsular tension segments for high-risk patients, with the caveat that the device's insertion itself is traumatic to the zonular support.

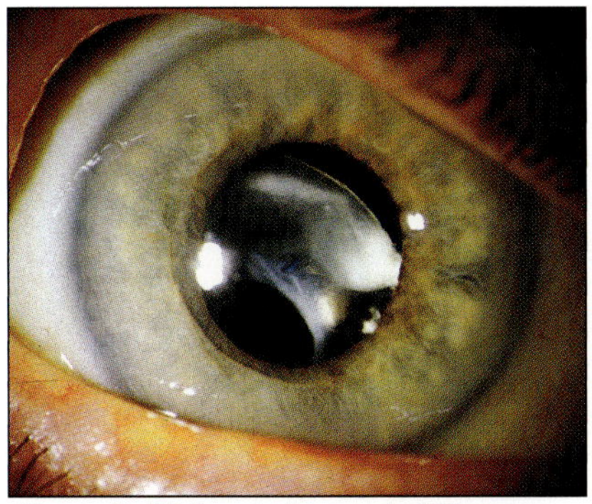

(Courtesy of Garry Condon, MD.)

Figure 2. Dislocated capsule/IOL complex in an eye with pseudoexfoliation.

CLINICAL FOLLOW-UP

One of the best forms of prevention against capsular contraction syndrome after the appropriate surgical precautions have been observed is the clinical follow-up of patients who are at an increased risk for the condition. As mentioned previously, the risk of the most aggressive form of this syndrome is highest in the first 3 to 6 months after cataract surgery. The first evidence of this problem is seen either by direct visualization of the capsule at the slit lamp or by changes in the IOL's position and resultant shifts in refraction. If surgeons note apparent contraction of the anterior capsular opening, they should perform relaxing radial incisions around the margin of the capsulorhexis with an Nd:YAG laser. If done early enough, this treatment will usually alleviate the capsular force on the lens implant and zonules.[24]

In some cases of capsular contraction syndrome, the thickened fibrotic tissue may become so dense that radial incisions are impossible. In this instance, surgeons can use an Nd:YAG laser to release the ring of capsular tissue from around the phimotic opening. Uncommonly, the contraction creates such severe deformity that surgeons should remove and replace the IOL. In addition, there is high risk of capsular dislocation and vitreous loss, and surgeons will likely place the replacement IOL in the sulcus, rather than in the badly distorted, fibrotic bag. Preparation for this worst-case scenario is prudent in surgical planning when faced with the aforementioned challenges.[25-29]

The problem of progressive zonular dehiscence despite all preventative efforts is the most serious complication of capsular contraction syndrome, although investigators have reported that dehiscence can occur without evidence of pathologic contraction. In either case, this complication demands surgical intervention. If evidence of capsular/IOL instability is identified, the surgeon should consider placing scleral sutures. This process is complicated and not without risks, but it is less hazardous than "rescuing" the entire bag/lens complex from the vitreous. The procedure is beyond the scope of this article, but it is elegantly described by Ahmed et al.[27] For these cases, surgeons should prepare to enlist the participation of a posterior segment specialist if necessary.

CONCLUSION

The preparations and actions that will best help surgeons avoid capsular contraction syndrome include knowledge of the syndrome, awareness of high-risk conditions, selection of the appropriate IOL, consideration of CTRs, segments, and suture placement, meticulous surgery including capsular lens epithelial cell cleanup, and vigilant observation of the patient for early detection and intervention. These strategies will help avoid the most serious complications of anterior capsular contraction syndrome, which can confound the surgical outcome, leaving both the physician and patient disappointed. ■

This article originally appeared in the October 2007 issue of CRSToday.

1. Gimbel HV, Neuhann T. Continuous curvilinear capsulorhexis (letter). *J Cataract Refract Surg.* 1991;17:110-111.
2. Hanson S, Crandall A, Olson R. Progressive constriction of the anterior capsular opening following intact capsulorhexis. *J Cataract Refract Surg.* 1993;19:77-82.
3. Davison JA. Capsule contraction syndrome. *J Cataract Refract Surg.* 1993;19:582-589.
4. Masket S. Postoperative complications of capsulorhexis. *J Cataract Refract Surg.* 1993;19:721-724.
5. Caporossi A, Casprini G, Toss GM, et al. Histology of anterior capsule fibrosis following phacoemulsification. *J Cataract Refract Surg.* 1998;24:1343-1346.
6. Kurosaka E, Ando I, Kato K, et al. Fibrous membrane formation at the capsule margin in capsule contraction syndrome. *J Cataract Refract Surg.* 1999;25:930-935.
7. Werner L, Pandey S, Escobar-Gomez M, et al. Anterior capsule opacification: a histopathological study comparing different IOL styles. *Ophthalmology.* 2000;107:463-471.
8. Gallagher SP, Pavilack MA. Risk factors for anterior capsule contraction syndrome. *J Cataract Refract Surg.* 1999;25:1356-1361.
9. Werner L, Pandey S, Apple DJ, et al. Anterior capsule opacification: correlation of pathologic findings with clinical sequelae. *Ophthalmology.* 2001;108:1675-1681.
10. Abela-Formanek C, Amon M. Uveal and capsular biocompatibility of hydrophilic acrylic, hydrophobic acrylic, and silicone intraocular lenses. *J Cataract Refract Surg.* 2002;28:50-61.
11. Kato S, Suzuki T, Hayashi Y, et al. Risk factors for contraction of the anterior capsule opening. *J Cataract Refract Surg.* 2002;28:109-112.
12. Sacu S, Menapace R, Wirtitsch M, et al. Effect of anterior capsule polishing on fibrotic capsule opacification: three-year results. *J Cataract Refract Surg.* 2004;30:2322-2327.
13. Hanson R, Rubinstein A, Sarangapani S, et al. Effect of lens epithelial cell aspiration on postoperative capsulorhexis contraction with the use of the Acrysof intraocular lens. *J Cataract Refract Surg.* 2006;32:1621-1626.
14. Hayashi K, Hayashi H, Nakao F, Hayashi F. Reduction in the area of the anterior capsule opening after polymethylmethacrylate, silicone, and soft acrylic intraocular lens implantation. *Am J Ophthalmol.* 1997;123:441-447.
15. Nishi O, Nishi K, Akura J. Speed of capsular bend formation at the optic edge of acrylic, silicone, and poly(methyl methacrylate) lenses. *J Cataract Refract Surg.* 2002;28:431-440.
16. Wallin T, Hinckley M, Nilson C, Olson RJ. Single- vs three-piece truncated hydrophobic acrylic intraocular lenses. *Am J Ophthalmol.* 2003;136:614-619.
17. Hayashi K, Hyashi H. Intraocular lens factors that may affect anterior capsule contraction. *Ophthalmology.* 2005;112:286-292.
18. Cionni R, Osher R. Management of profound zonular dialysis or weakness with a new endocapsular ring designed for scleral fixation. *J Cataract Refract Surg.* 1998;24:1299-1306.
19. Jehan F, Mamalis N, Crandall A. Spontaneous late dislocation of intraocular lens within the capsular bag in pseudoexfoliation patients. *Ophthalmology.* 2001;108:1727-1731.
20. Waheed I, Eleftheriadis H, Liu C. Anterior capsular phimosis in eyes with a capsular tension ring. *J Cataract Refract Surg.* 2001;27:1688-1690.
21. Moreno-Montanes J, et al. Complete anterior capsule contraction after phacoemulsification with acrylic intraocular lens and endocapsular ring implantation. *J Cataract Refract Surg.* 2002;28:717-719.
22. Masket S, Osher R. Late complications with intraocular lens dislocation after capsulorhexis in pseudoexfoliation syndrome. *J Cataract Refract Surg.* 2002;28:1482-1484.
23. Scherer M, Bertelmann E, Rieck P. Late spontaneous in-the-bag intraocular lens and capsular tension ring dislocation in pseudoexfoliation syndrome. *J Cataract Refract Surg.* 2006;32:672-675.
24. Jardim D, Soloway B, Starr C. Asymmetric vault of an accommodating intraocular lens. *J Cataract Refractive Surg.* 2006;347-350.
25. Battacharjee H, Bhattacharjee K, Das D. Management of a posteriorly dislocated endocapsular tension ring and a foldable acrylic intraocular lens. *J Cataract Refract Surg.*

2004;30:243-246.
26. Moreno-Montanes J, Heras H, Fernandez-Hortelano A. Surgical treatment of a dislocated intraocular lens-capsular bag-capsular tension ring complex. *J Cataract Refract Surg.* 2005;31:270-273.
27. Ahmed I, Chen, S, Kranemann C, Wong DT. Surgical repositioning of dislocated capsular tension rings. *Ophthalmology.* 2005;112:1725-1733.
28. Lim M, Jap A, Wong E. Surgical management of late dislocated lens capsular bag with intraocular lens and endocapsular tension ring. *J Cataract Refract Surg.* 2006;32:533-536.
29. Deka S, Deka A, Bhattacharjee H. Management of posteriorly dislocated endocapsular tension ring and intraocular lens complex. *J Cataract Refract Surg.* 2006;32:887-889.

CHAPTER 23

Does the Capsulorhexis Affect Refractive Outcomes?

WARREN E. HILL, MD

Consider the following scenario. You have a demanding, high-profile patient who expects a perfect refractive outcome. Everyone in your office is anxious to meet his expectations, so you and your staff double-check his preoperative K-readings, scrutinize the measurement of his axial length, and carefully calculate the power for your favorite IOL. All of the parameters line up and seem to make sense. To your delight, the surgery goes well, and the patient's UCVA is 20/20 at his first postoperative visit. You and your staff indulge in a well-deserved round of self-congratulations.

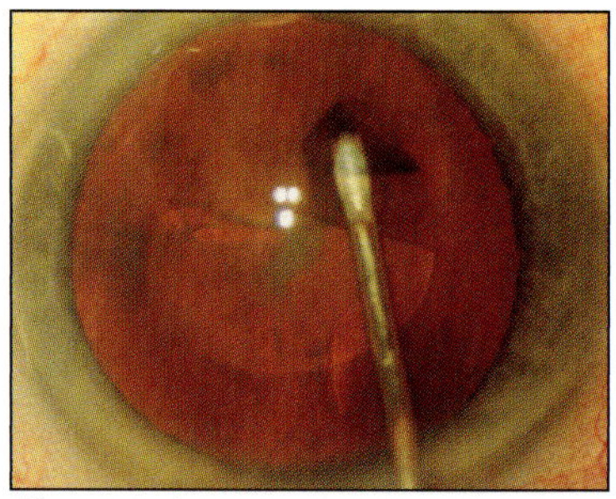

Figure 1. A surgeon uses a 25-gauge cytotome to create a continuous curvilinear capsulorhexis. To ensure the symmetric shrinkage of the capsule around the IOL's optic and to prevent tilt and decentration, the surgeon should create a round and centered capsulorhexis that is slightly smaller than the optic of the IOL.

Several months after surgery, however, the same patient returns stating he is unhappy with his vision. His UCVA measures 20/60, and a manifest refraction shows a -1.25 D myopic shift in his refractive error.

You and your staff are now scrambling for answers. A double-check of the patient's axial length and K-readings shows that all of your measurements were correct. A recalculation of the IOL's power with multiple formulas also confirms your original results. What is going on with this patient?

REMEMBER RELATIVE POWER

In the case described above, the most likely cause of the decline in the patient's uncorrected postoperative vision is an excessively large capsulorhexis. If the capsulorhexis is larger than the implanted IOL's optic, the forces exerted on the lens by the contraction of the capsular bag may shift the IOL anteriorly and increase its effective power.

We should always remember that in a two-lens system consisting of the cornea and an IOL, the IOL's effective power inside the pseudophakic eye is not absolute, but relative. For example, a +21.00 D lens (the power listed on the lens' box) will add that exact amount of power to the eye only if it remains in the position assumed by the formula used to calculate its strength (ie, at the plane of the zonules and completely confined within the capsular bag.) If a formula miscalculates the IOL's position by 0.50 mm and the optic ends up 0.50 mm more posterior to the cornea's principal plane, a +21.00 D IOL would produce only +20.00 D of correction.

Conversely, if a formula miscalculates the position of a +21.00 D IOL by 0.50 mm and the optic ends up 0.50 mm more anterior to the cornea's principal plane, then the lens would act as if it were a +22.00 D IOL. I always account for this effect by decreasing an IOL's power when it is implanted in the ciliary sulcus versus the capsular bag.[1]

ACCOUNT FOR CAPSULAR CHANGES

To ensure that an IOL's position in the capsular bag matches that anticipated by the formula used to calculate its power, the capsulorhexis should be round, centered, and smaller than the IOL's optic (Figure 1).

At the conclusion of the case, the optic should be centered directly beneath the capsulorhexis. Careful placement of the IOL allows the capsular bag to uniformly "shrink-wrap" around the lens' optic and maintain its proper centration.

The creation of centered, round capsulorhexes also encourages consistent refractive outcomes. Irregularly shaped and decentered capsulorhexes can contract asymmetrically, thereby exerting uneven forces on the IOL's optic and leading to decentration and tilt. Because the performance of new aspheric and pseudoaccommodative IOLs is particularly sensitive to their position in relation to the center of the pupil, decentration and tilt of these lenses can decrease their visual performance.

CONCLUSION

With any form of lens exchange, patients are increasingly demanding refractive perfection, and correctly configuring the capsulorhexis is no longer optional. Achieving good refractive outcomes with cataract surgery not only requires the correct calculation of the IOL's power but also the proper formation of the capsulorhexis.[2] Therefore, every part of cataract surgery, excluding the placement of limbal relaxing incisions, should be directed toward preparing the capsular bag for the IOL's implantation. ■

This article originally appeared in the October 2007 issue of CRSToday.

1. Fang JP, Hill WE, Wang L, Chang V, Koch DD. Advanced intraocular lens power calculations. In: Kohnen T, Koch DD, eds. *Essentials in Ophthalmology: Cataract and Refractive Surgery.* 2nd ed. Berlin, Germany: Springer-Verlag; 2006:31-46.
2. Hill WE. Highly accurate IOL calculations. *Cataract & Refractive Surgery Today.* 2006;6:3:82-86.

CHAPTER 24

Six Tips on Hydrodissection Technique

DAVID F. CHANG, MD

Because the topic of hydrodissection receives relatively little attention compared to phacoemulsification and IOL insertion techniques, I believe it is the most underrated step of cataract surgery. A properly developed hydrodissection fluid wave must travel behind the nucleus along the internal posterior capsular surface. In addition to permitting endonuclear rotation, such a wave also facilitates epinuclear and cortical cleanup by loosening their adhesion to the capsule. There are several tips that will help surgeons attain these three important goals.

TIP NO. 1

One of the most common mistakes cataract surgeons make is to initiate hydrodissection while the anterior chamber is overinflated with viscoelastic. Hydrodissection is easier if the eye is somewhat soft and if the anterior chamber has been partially emptied. Of course, this condition is at odds with the preceding capsulorhexis step in which a generous amount of viscoelastic is desirable.

Using viscoelastic to deepen the chamber and flatten the anterior capsular convexity makes controlling the developing capsulorhexis tear much easier. However, by exerting downward pressure against the nucleus, overfilling the AC with viscoelastic increases the resistance that the posteriorly directed hydrodissection wave must overcome. By limiting the escape of injected fluid through the incision, it can also lead to excessive deepening of the AC during the hydrodissection maneuver. It is therefore advisable to burp out some viscoelastic immediately prior to initiating hydrodissection. This can be accomplished by pressing the shaft of the hydrodissection cannula against the incision floor just prior to the injection. Partially emptying the AC will permit the nucleus to rise anteriorly away from the posterior capsule upon separation.

TIP NO. 2

Fear of "blowing out" the capsule causes many residents to be overly timid with the injection pressure. Because the volume of fluid that can be injected into the anterior chamber is limited, it must be injected rather quickly and decisively in order to generate sufficient hydrostatic force. The force is proportional to the rate of flow and the cannula resistance. Either a 30- or 27-gauge cannula (Figure 1A through C) provides sufficient resistance to generate the necessary force. A 3-mL syringe is small enough to provide good tactile feedback regarding the rate of flow. Increasingly larger syringes provide less and less tactile feedback.

TIP NO. 3

Although it is possible to rupture the posterior capsule with hydrodissection, nuclear/capsular block is a prerequisite. As a dense nucleus elevates, it may totally seal off the capsulorhexis from below. This prevents any fluid from escaping the capsular bag, and continued infusion can inflate the bag enough to cause posterior capsule rupture.[1] The surgeon may not be aware of this complication until he inserts the phaco tip. At this point, the high infusion pressure will expand the rent, and the nucleus will drop before or during the initial sculpting stroke. To avoid this complication, terminate the injection once the nucleus "pops up." Resist the temptation to continue injecting until the hydrodissection wave has completely crossed behind the nucleus. Instead, stop and reposit the nucleus posteriorly—thus breaking the nuclear/capsular block—before continuing with a second injection wave.

TIP NO. 4

I. Howard Fine, MD, of Eugene, Oregon, has taught us to orient the fluid stream along the inner capsular surface by tenting the anterior capsule slightly upward with the cannula tip.[1] A wave that hugs the inner capsular surface will produce a slower advancing fluid front with scalloped edges (Figure 1B and C). These characteristics indicate the resistance that is encountered as the wave shears through the cortical capsular adhesions. If the wave moves so quickly that the surgeon cannot track the advancing edge, this may indicate that he achieved hydrodelineation instead of hydrodissection (Figure 2A). Hydrodelineation will permit endonuclear rotation, but the epinucleus and cortex will remain adherent to the capsular bag. Some surgeons have advised leaving your thumb off the plunger until the cannula tip is positioned properly. Otherwise, if even a tiny amount of fluid is trickling out, it may prevent the tip from actually tenting up the capsule just prior to the definitive injection.

Because both hydrodissection and hydrodelineation will permit

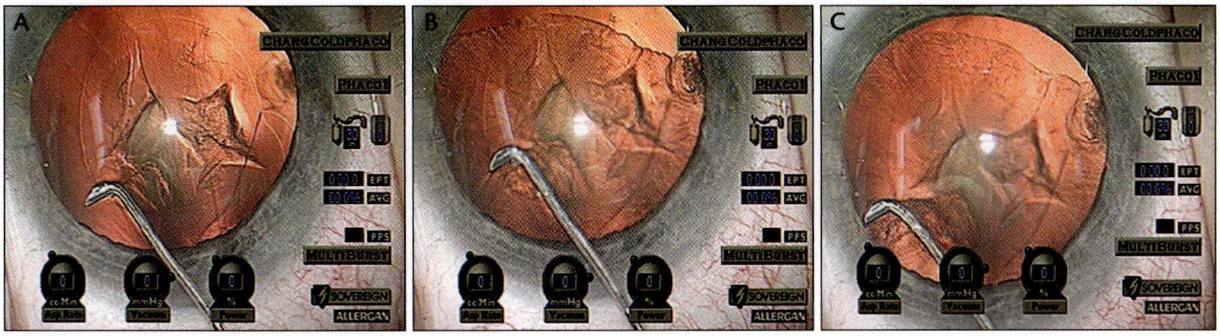

Figure 1. The Chang right-angled cannula tip is placed under the proximal CCC edge (A). The propagating hydrodissection wave has a scalloped, advancing edge (B and C).

the surgeon to rotate a moderately dense endonucleus, he can confirm proper hydrodissection only once the epinucleus and cortex are removed. A loosened epinucleus will flip when aspirated. If the anterior shelf continues to break off, the surgeon can rotate the epinucleus to bring a fresh anterior shelf to the contraincisional quadrant. In contrast, an adherent epinucleus does not rotate or flip, and the distally aspirated sections eventually break off. This leaves a proximal adherent remnant with nothing to grab onto, and increases the risk of aspirating/tearing the posterior capsule with the phaco tip.

Dr. Fine describes the principle of cortical cleaving hydrodissection whereby the loosened cortex can be entirely aspirated with the phaco tip.[1] However, even if the surgeon chooses not to attempt this maneuver, the degree to which the cortex has been loosened is evident during conventional automated I/A. For example, a mailing label easily separates in one piece from its waxed paper backing. However, once applied to a cardboard box, it becomes difficult to remove as a single piece. After one strip prematurely shreds and breaks off, we must again struggle to regrasp a new area. The difference is in the strength of the adhesion. The tendency of loosened cortex to come out easily in sheets, as opposed to small adherent strips, is particularly advantageous in the subincisional area. Again, the risk of aspirating or rupturing the posterior capsule is greater if the cortex remains strongly adherent.

TIP NO. 5

A hydrodissection wave frequently fails to travel completely across the posterior capsule. Given the importance of preferentially loosening the subincisional cortex, it is therefore logical to initiate the hydrodissection wave from the subincisional anterior capsular rim. A partially incomplete wave that started from the contraincisional fornix will leave the subincisional cortex maximally adherent.

I advocate a right-angle hydrodissection cannula tip, because, like a right-angle I/A tip, this configuration can access the proximal 180° of capsular rim (Figure 1A). A straight cannula can access the distal 135° of capsular rim, and a J-shaped cannula is limited to the subincisional 90° of capsular rim.

TIP NO. 6

I prefer to sever the last remaining capsular attachments by using the cannula tip to rotate the nucleus within the bag prior to phaco. The previously mentioned short, right-angle tip works well at engaging the peripheral anterior nuclear surface and rotating it with circular raking motions (Figure 2B, C, and D). The surgeon can readily perform additional hydrodissection if necessary. The Chang hydrodissection cannula (Katena Products, Inc., Denville, NJ, and Mastel Precision, Rapid City, SD) has a dull point at the tip to further facilitate this maneuver. This reusable, 27-gauge cannula has a short, right-angled tip that is flattened to create a slightly fan-shaped fluid stream, and to more snugly nestle beneath the proximal anterior capsular rim (Figure 1A). A disposable version is available through Oasis Medical, Inc. (Glendora, CA).

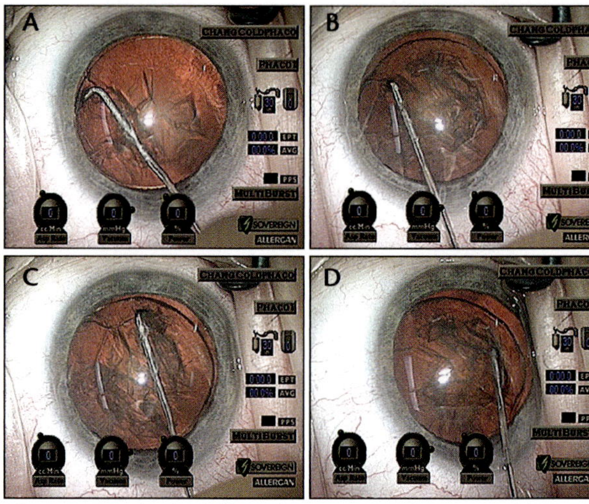

Figure 2. The hydrodelineation wave produces a "golden ring" sign (A). Use a circular raking motion with the pointed tip to spin the nucleus counterclockwise (B-D).

FINAL THOUGHTS

Because we are limited to a single incision in phacoemulsification, cortical cleaving hydrodissection greatly facilitates removing the nucleus, epinucleus, and cortex. Without rotation, we cannot otherwise safely access subincisional nucleus and epinucleus. Overly adherent subincisional cortex carries increased risk. Therefore, successful hydrodissection improves our efficiency, reduces the risk of posterior capsular rupture, and by cleaving the cortical attachments, reduces the rate of posterior capsule opacification.[2,3] By optimizing our technique and instrumentation, we can reliably achieve these benefits on a consistent basis. ■

This article originally appeared in the September 2002 issue of CRSToday.

1. Miyake K et al. New classification of capsular block syndrome. *J Cataract Refract Surg.* 1998;24(9):1230-1234.
2. Fine IH. Cortical cleaving hydrodissection. *J Cataract Refract Surg.* 1992;18:508-512.
3. Peng Q, Apple DJ, Visessook N, Werner L, et al. Surgical prevention of posterior capsule opacification. Part II. Enhancement of cortical clean up by focusing on hydrodissection. *J Cataract Refract Surg.* 2000;26:188-197.
4. Vasavada AR, Singh R, Apple DJ, et al. Efficacy of hydrodissection step in the phacoemulsification for age related senile cataract. *J Cataract Refract Surg.* 2002;28(9):1623-1628

CHAPTER 25

Avoiding and Managing Complications From Hydrodissection

WILLIAM J. FISHKIND, MD

The hydrosteps are a significant but often overlooked portion of the phacosurgical procedure. Although hydrodelineation is straightforward, hydrodissection is associated with complications that can compromise the patient's zonular structure and capsular bag.

CAUSATIVE FACTORS OF COMPLICATIONS

Conventional Hydrodissection

If the surgeon fails to place the irrigating cannula far enough peripherally, hydrodissection will occur between the layers of cortex, and a dense layer of cortex will remain adherent to the posterior capsule. This situation places unnecessary stress on the zonules and possibly the ciliary body during I/A, and it will extend the time required for I/A. In the presence of a torn posterior capsule, traction on the capsular bag can enlarge the rent and/or rupture the vitreous face. The technique described here is termed *conventional hydrodissection.*

Errant Placement of the Cannula

Although unusual, it is possible inadvertently to place the irrigating cannula beneath the iris, but on top of the anterior capsule. As a result, fluid is injected within the zonules, over the vitreous face, and into the posterior capsule. The fluid will cause the anterior chamber to become shallow, as occurs with a fluid misdirection syndrome. This situation most often occurs in the presence of small pupils.

INCOMPLETE HYDRODISSECTION

If the irrigating fluid does not pass completely around the epinucleus and cortex, some of this material will remain attached to the capsular bag (Figure 1). The lens will therefore not rotate freely, and attempting rotation may (1) stretch or tear the zonules or (2) create a rent in the capsular bag. In cases of pre-existent zonular weakness, the problem is magnified.

Additionally, without adequate cortical cleavage, epinuclear and cortical remnants usually adhere to the capsular bag at the equator. When the surgeon performs phacoemulsification and pursues the equatorial material, he may accidentally aspirate the equatorial bag while in the process of aspirating epinucleus and cortex adhering to the capsular bag. That action can disrupt the zonules, may lead the surgeon to phaco through the equatorial bag, and may tear the posterior capsule.

A Small Capsulorhexis and a Large Nucleus

In patients with large nuclei, creating a small capsulorhexis can result in capsular block (Figure 2). When the surgeon injects fluid beneath the anterior capsule and behind the nucleus, the vector forces created by the large nucleus and small capsulorhexis cause the nucleus to float forward and block the egress of fluid around or underneath the anterior capsule. The fluid builds up quickly

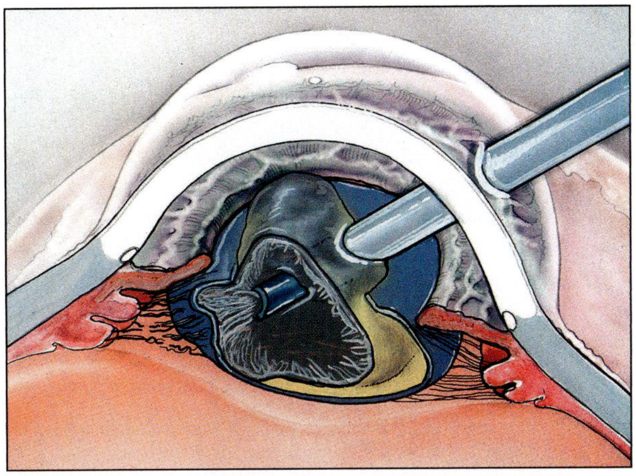

Figure 1. When hydrodissection is incomplete, the cortex remains attached to the capsular bag. Phacoemulsification can aspirate cortex and the attached capsular bag, either tearing the zonules or creating a rent in the capsule. (Reprinted with permission from Fishkind WJ, ed. *Complications in Phacoemulsification: Avoidance, Recognition, and Management*. 1st ed. New York, NY: Thieme Medical Publishers; 2002.)

within the capsular bag and causes it to blow out either anteriorly or posteriorly, depending on where the weakest point of the capsule is located.

Similarly, rapidly injecting a large amount of hydrodissecting fluid, even in the presence of a smaller, softer nucleus, can cause fluid to accumulate so quickly that a relative pupillary block occurs and, again, tears the capsule.

AVOIDANCE PEARLS

Cortical Cleaving Hydrodissection

There are several reasons to switch from conventional hydrodissection to cortical cleaving hydrodissection (Figure 3). The latter technique is performed peripherally in order to cleave cortex from the capsular bag, a situation that allows the entire endonucleus, epinucleus, and cortical complex to rotate freely within the bag. The surgeon then separates the endonucleus from the epinucleus and cortex via hydrodelineation. This step permits a two-procedure phacoemulsification. First, the surgeon emulsifies the endonucleus. If performed with a protective shell of epinucleus, this process will prevent sharp fragments (particularly an issue with hard nuclei) from tearing the posterior capsule during potential surge. Next, the surgeon removes the epinucleus and cortex using lower settings to minimize surge, to remove the material more completely, and to minimize the need for I/A.

In the presence of a torn posterior capsule, cortical cleaving hydrodissection facilitates the removal of cortex without enlarging

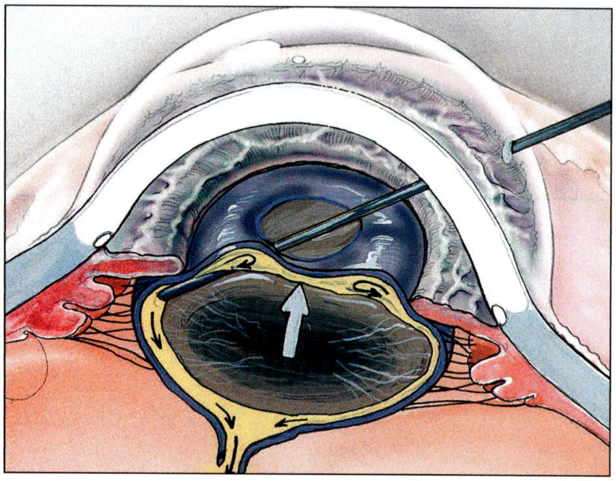

Figure 2. A large dense nucleus and small capsulorhexis cause fluid to fill the space behind the nucleus. As the nucleus floats anteriorly, it may seal the anterior capsule. The resultant vector forces prevent fluid egress, and the increase in fluid pressure then blows out the posterior capsule. (Reprinted with permission from Fishkind WJ, ed. *Complications in Phacoemulsification: Avoidance, Recognition, and Management*. 1st ed. New York, NY: Thieme Medical Publishers; 2002.)

the tear because the cortex adheres less to the capsular bag. If the patient's zonules are weak, cortical cleaving hydrodissection eases the removal of the epinucleus and cortex and avoids both tearing more zonules and disrupting the capsular bag. The complications of both forms of hydrodissection are similar.

Additional Tips

To avoid accidentally placing the irrigating cannula on top of the anterior capsule, the surgeon should carefully watch the instrument's progression to ensure that it passes below the capsule, particularly in the presence of small pupils.

If the nucleus is large and hard, it is sensible to create a larger capsulorhexis (eg, 5.50 to 5.75 mm) and use a 6.00-mm lens implant, rather than make a 4.00-mm capsulorhexis. If the capsulorhexis created is too small, enlarging it prior to performing hydrodissection can avert the potential problem of capsular block. The surgeon may need to use a vital stain of the anterior capsule to extend the capsulorhexis. Additionally, he should judiciously perform hydrodissection behind the nucleus. It is important to watch the fluid wave to ensure that excessive amounts of fluid do not build behind the nucleus, a situation that can cause capsular block.

MANAGEMENT ADVICE

Errant Fluid Injection

When a misplaced cannula injects fluid over the anterior capsule so that it fills the space between the vitreous face and lens nucleus, the surgeon will notice the problem as the anterior chamber suddenly becomes shallow and the lens, capsule, and iris move anteriorly. At this point, he must determine whether a suprachoroidal effusion/hemorrhage or a variant of a fluid misdirection syndrome has occurred. First, he should halt the procedure and feel the globe in order to ascertain its firmness. Generally, the globe will be firm due to the presence of excess fluid in the vitreous. The next step is to decompress the anterior chamber slightly and wait 5 to 10 minutes. If the globe remains firm, then it probably has suffered a choroidal effusion or hemorrhage. With a variant of a fluid misdirection syndrome, the fluid will regain equilibrium within the eye during the waiting period. Once the eye has stabilized, the surgeon again performs careful hydrodissection while the cannula is properly positioned.

A vitreous tap is an alternative to the waiting period and may also be appropriate for a case in which the eye has not softened adequately but the surgeon strongly suspects fluid misdirection. To perform the tap, the surgeon uses an MVR blade to make a small stab incision through the pars plana 3.0 to 3.5 mm posterior to the limbus. Next, he uses a 27-gauge cannula to gently withdraw between 0.1 and 0.3 cc of liquid vitreous. If the eye becomes firm again after the tap, there is probably a suprachoroidal hemorrhage.

Obviously, the surgeon is free at any point to use an indirect ophthalmoscope to examine the retina for a choroidal effusion or hemorrhage. An alternative is to use the handheld lens created by Robert Osher, MD, of Cincinnati (Osher 78 D Maxfield; Ocular Instruments, Bellevue, WA).

Adherent Epinucleus and Cortex

The endpoint of cortical cleaving hydrodissection is that the surgeon sees the fluid wave pass behind the entire nucleus to the opposite side. When the nucleus rises within the capsular bag, it indicates that fluid is collecting behind the lens. The surgeon then presses down on the nucleus to force the fluid trapped behind it to travel around the equator, thereby lysing all peripheral cortical-nuclear connections. He applies this pressure first on one side of the nucleus and then again in a location 180° opposite. These steps should ensure a freely rotating nucleus. If the nucleus does not turn freely, then the hydrodissection was incomplete, and the surgeon should repeat the procedure.

If repeated or full hydrodissection is impossible, the surgeon must exercise greater care during phacoemulsification so as not to stress the zonules or approach the equatorial cortical material too closely. A nick in the anterior capsule or a discontinuous capsulorhexis (eg, one that extended toward the equator and had to be finished from the other side) are good reasons not to complete hydrodissection. The addition of too much fluid will cause a capsular tear that extends to the equator or, worse, into the posterior capsule. Another reason surgeons might hesitate to complete hydrodissection is poor visualization due to a small pupil. Additionally, some might forego complete dissection in cases of preexisting weak zonules caused by earlier zonular trauma, zonular tears, or pseudoexfoliation. Although it is difficult to hydrodissect and fully rotate the nucleus in these cases, I believe they actually require extra hydrodissection. If the surgeon can continue to work carefully until the nucleus is completely free within the capsular bag, then emulsifying the endonucleus, epinucleus, and cortex will be easier and less likely to further damage the zonules.

A Torn Capsule

Whether caused by incomplete hydrodissection leading to a torn equatorial bag, a discontinuous capsulorhexis, or a capsular block, the end result may be a torn capsule. The surgeon must then choose whether to convert to extracapsular surgery or to complete the case with phacoemulsification. The decision depends on his level of comfort when performing phacoemulsification in the presence of a torn capsule.

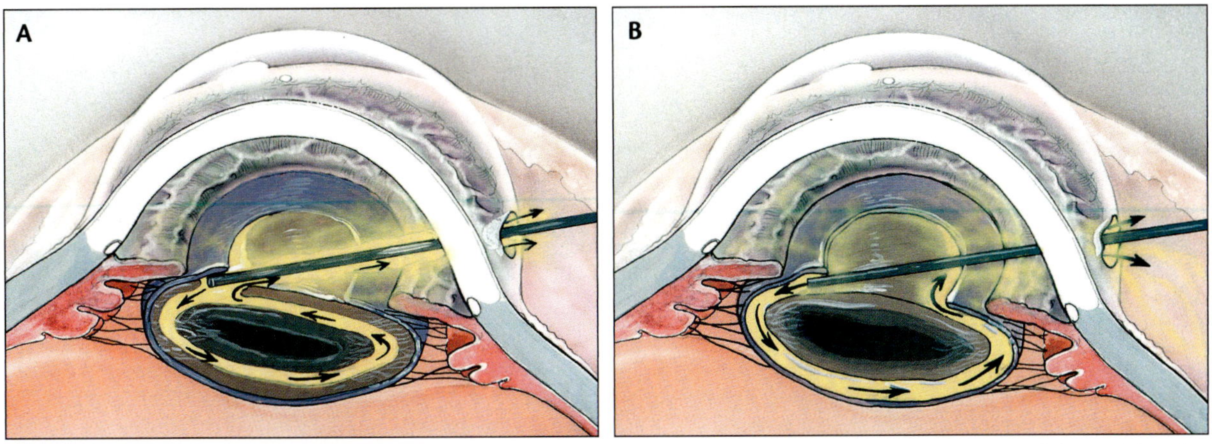

Figure 3. During conventional hydrodissection, the surgeon places the cannula within the layers of cortex, and the peripheral cortex therefore remains attached to the capsular bag (A). By contrast, in cortical cleaving hydrodissection, the surgeon places the cannula immediately under the anterior capsule and advances it halfway between the edge of the capsulorhexis and the equator. Next, the surgeon gently and steadily injects BSS (Alcon Laboratories, Inc., Fort Worth, TX) toward the equator until the fluid wave passes to the opposite equator (B). (Reprinted with permission from Fishkind WJ, ed. *Complications in Phacoemulsification: Avoidance, Recognition, and Management*. 1st ed. New York, NY: Thieme Medical Publishers; 2002.)

In this situation, many surgeons use a dispersive viscoelastic (Viscoat; Alcon Laboratories, Inc.) to elevate the nucleus to the level of the iris, close the phaco wound, and open an extracapsular wound through which to deliver the nucleus. I prefer to continue with phacoemulsification. First, I inject a dispersive viscoelastic behind the nucleus in order to secure it and over the nucleus to protect the endothelium. I call this maneuver a Viscoat sandwich. If I believe that the posterior capsule has blown out due to a posterior capsular block, I often enlarge the anterior capsulotomy so that I may float the nucleus up to the level of the iris. I emulsify the nucleus over a Sheets Glide. I try to keep the nucleus in one piece and emulsify it with a carousel technique.

CONCLUSION

Often overlooked as an important prerequisite to successful phacoemulsification, the hydrosteps are vitally important. When performed well, good cortical cleavage will make the entire phacoemulsification procedure safer and more efficient. It will also shorten the time needed for I/A and increase its safety. Finally, in the presence of a torn posterior capsule, thorough cortical cleavage will facilitate the removal of residual cortex without placing additional stress on the damaged capsule.

An awareness of the fundamentals of hydrodissection and the gentle, cautious performance of the procedure can avert complications. It is well worth the time and effort to master this technique. ■

This article originally appeared in the March 2003 issue of CRSToday.

CHAPTER 26

Review of Top Phaco Innovations

ROBERT H. OSHER, MD

Every year, Dr. Osher chairs the "What's New" symposium in New York City and the "Cutting Edge" symposium at the AAO Annual Meeting. This article presents Dr. Osher's evaluation of innovations from 2007.

CATEGORY 1: MICROSCOPES

The OPMI Lumera microscope from Carl Zeiss Meditec AG (Jena, Germany) is extraordinary. The resolution is unprecedented, and the depth of field is dramatic. The stereo coaxial illumination provides a brilliant homogeneous red reflex during the capsulorhexis, I/A, the lens' implantation, and the ophthalmic viscosurgical device's (OVD) removal. I would award the Lumera the title of top innovation of the year.

CATEGORY 2: PHACO MACHINES

Both Advanced Medical Optics, Inc. (Santa Ana, CA), and Bausch & Lomb (Rochester, NY) introduced new machines in 2007. The Whitestar Signature System (Advanced Medical Optics, Inc.) features elliptical transverse emulsification, which is in response to the success that Alcon Laboratories, Inc. (Fort Worth, TX), has had with torsional ultrasound. The Stellaris Vision Enhancement System (Bausch & Lomb) has been designed for the transition to sub-2-mm surgery and is compatible with the Akreos lenses (not available in the US; Bausch & Lomb). The wireless foot switch and the option to select either a peristaltic or Venturi pump on the fly are significant innovations.

CATEGORY 3: PHACO TIPS

Two new phaco tips gained attention this past year. The Dewey Radius tip from MicroSurgical Technology (Redmond, WA) has a blunt edge and reportedly offers additional capsular protection. The Osher tip from Alcon Laboratories, Inc., is designed for the surgeon who wants to perform torsional ultrasound but is uncomfortable with the more extreme curve of the Kelman tip. My tip (no financial interest) has a gentle curve, with the bevel opening on the same side as the curve. Takayuki Akahoshi, MD, of Tokyo also independently developed a similar tip. Since 70% of phaco surgeons worldwide prefer a straight tip, this tip should facilitate the transition to torsional ultrasound. The award-winning film from Teruyuki Miyoshi, MD, of Fukuyama, Japan, clearly demonstrates the enhanced efficiency of torsional ultrasound.

CATEGORY 4: IOL INJECTORS

The winner in this category was the Isert Injector from Hoya (not available in the US; Frankfurt, Germany). The lens, preloaded on the reusable injector, never comes into contact with handling instruments or the environment outside the eye. The award-winning film from Hiroko Bissen-Miyajima, MD, of Tokyo emphasizes that the ocular surface is often contaminated during cataract surgery.

CATEGORY 5: IOLs

In the US, Alcon Laboratories, Inc., has swept this category with its introduction of the aspheric AcrySof Restor and the AcrySof Toric lenses. The improved resolution and reduction of the glare circle are impressive on the optical bench. Because the lens can be injected through a 2.2-mm incision, the surgeon does not induce undesirable astigmatism, according to the work of Samuel Masket, MD, of Los Angeles. However, it fails to correct preexisting cylinder, and my European colleagues are fortunate to have the multifocal toric IOLs from Carl Zeiss Meditec AG (which purchased Acri.Tec GmbH) and Rayner Intraocular Lenses, Ltd. (East Sussex, United Kingdom) (both IOLs not available in the US). Refractive cataract surgeons have enthusiastically embraced the introduction of the toric lens, even though the method of identifying the steepest axis leaves room for improvement. Eyeonics, Inc. (Aliso Viejo, CA), with its new Crystalens 5-O, and Visiogen, Inc. (Irvine, CA), with its dual-optic Synchrony (not available in the US), continue to attract an enthusiastic following.

CATEGORY 6: DEVICES

The modification of the Morcher capsular tension ring (CTR; Morcher GmbH, Stuttgart, Germany) by Bonnie Henderson, MD, of Boston to have eight indentations to facilitate cortical removal demonstrates continued innovation in CTR technology. The Capsular Anchor (Hanita Lenses, Kibbutz Hanita, Israel), designed by Ehud I. Assia, MD, of Kfar Saba, Israel, is also exciting. Unfortunately, it may take years for the FDA to approve these products. In 1993, my younger associate, Robert J. Cionni, MD, of Cincinnati and I implanted the first CTRs in the US; it required 11 years before the standard CTR was approved. The other device that created excitement at the 2007 AAO Annual Meeting in New Orleans was the Malyugin ring and inserter (MicroSurgical Technology) for the management of small pupils.

CATEGORY 7: OVDs

As part of the settlement in the lawsuit with Alcon Laboratories, Inc., Advanced Medical Optics, Inc., gained the right to package and market a combination of OVDs. Years prior to the introduction of DuoVisc (Alcon Laboratories, Inc.), I had suggested this idea to Hakan Edstrom, President of the US division of Kabi Pharmacia (Upsala, Sweden). The concept was vetoed in Sweden, and the rest of the story is history. Advanced Medical Optics, Inc., plans to add Healon D, a new dispersive agent, to its existing family of Healon, Healon GV, and Healon5. It is anticipated that the surgeon will be able to select two OVDs in separate carpules for any given case.

CATEGORY 8: SURGICAL KNIVES

Becton, Dickinson and Company (Franklin Lakes, NJ) has set the new standard in blade safety. With increasing concerns about spreading HIV, hepatitis, prion disease, etc., surgeons and OR personnel have rapidly accepted the protective safety shield placed on an assortment of ophthalmic surgical knives.

CATEGORY 9: INSTRUMENTS

Every surgeon has encountered a case in which intraocular scissors or forceps function poorly, because the angle of the blades seems to be in the wrong plane or meridian. For this reason, I designed a unique set of intraocular scissors and forceps with interchangeable tips (no financial interest in the products) with Geuder AG (Heidelberg, Germany) and with Duckworth & Kent, Ltd. (Hertfordshire, United Kingdom) and Bausch & Lomb (Rochester, NY). Compatible with microincisional surgery, the blades have been angled to cut either a vertical or a horizontal plane along different meridia.

Two additional instruments have created much interest. Bong-Hyun Kim, MD, of South Korea has developed an intraocular mirror that allows the surgeon to visualize structures in the angle and in the posterior chamber. Manfred R. Tetz, MD, of Berlin has developed a new device for measuring the anterior chamber diameter and another device for separating the arms of the Artisan and Artiflex (Ophtec, Groningen, the Netherlands; marketed as the Verisyse and Veriflex [Advanced Medical Optics, Inc.] in the US) haptic for easier implantation.

CATEGORY 10: BUGS AND DRUGS

Advanced Vision Care (Woburn, MA) has introduced SteriLid, an antiseptic foam that kills 99% of all bacteria within 1 minute of contact. Two antibiotics drew a great deal of attention at the recent AAO Annual Meeting: AzaSite from Inspire Pharmaceuticals, Inc. (Durham, NC), and Iquix from Vistakon Pharmaceuticals, LLC (Jacksonville, FL). AzaSite is 1% azithromycin, a broad-spectrum topical agent with a dosing regimen of twice a day for the first 2 days and once daily thereafter. Iquix is unpreserved 1.5% levofloxacin, the highest available concentration for a topical fluoroquinolone.

Xibrom, produced by Ista Pharmaceuticals (Irvine, CA), completed its phase 3 FDA clinical trials for a higher-concentration, once-daily formulation of this potent anti-inflammatory agent. As interest in intracameral antibiotics continues to grow, the strong safety performance of moxifloxacin created excitement at the AAO Annual Meeting.[1]

To conclude, 2007 has been a banner year for new products in cataract surgery. Our specialty is predicting continued innovations in 2008. ■

This article originally appeared in the February 2008 issue of CRSToday.

1. Lane SS, Osher RH, Masket S, Belani SL. Evaluation of the safety of prophylactic intracameral mixofloxacin in cataract surgery patients. Poster presented at: The 2007 AAO Annual Meeting; November 10-13, 2007; New Orleans, LA.

CHAPTER 27

Improving Surgical Safety With Modern Phaco Technology

Strategies With the Whitestar Signature System

DAVID F. CHANG, MD

We cataract surgeons and our patients continue to benefit from ongoing improvements in phaco technology. Because cataract surgery is already such a fast and efficient operation, we are primarily interested in new technologies that can expand our margin of safety—particularly in eyes with dense nuclei and weak zonules. Historically, our three main safety-related concerns with phacoemulsification have been (1) thermal damage to the incision, (2) endothelial trauma associated with prolonged ultrasound time, and (3) capsular rupture due to postocclusion surge.

Incision burns are most likely to occur with the higher power levels and prolonged ultrasound times needed for brunescent lenses. Increasing the stroke length of the vibrating phaco tip generates more frictional heat as well as more phaco power. The thicker nuclear emulsate can admix with a highly retentive ophthalmic viscosurgical device (OVD) to form a viscous plug that clogs the phaco tip or aspiration line. If fluid outflow is blocked, then the gravity-fed inflow of irrigation also ceases. With neither the inflow nor the outflow of fluid to cool it, a phaco tip in continuous mode will instantaneously burn the cataract incision.

The loss of endothelial cells is also much greater with brunescent nuclei, the size and density of which require increased phaco time and energy for emulsification compared with standard cataracts. In my opinion, it is the increased particulate turbulence occurring with brunescent nuclear fragments that causes the most damage to endothelial cells. Rigid nuclear pieces drawn by aspiration to the phaco tip do not mold and conform as well to its opening. This and the added stroke length of higher ultrasound power settings increase the chatter and turbulence of nuclear particles within the anterior chamber.

Finally, there are several reasons why posterior capsular rupture is more common with rock-hard nuclei. The added rigidity and girth of the nucleus more directly transfers instrument-related forces to the capsule and zonules, and there is far less of an epinuclear shell to cushion the movements of the endonucleus. We typically maximize vacuum levels to improve holding power in these cases, but this increases the risk of postocclusion surge. A lax posterior capsule due to weak or deficient zonules will trampoline more easily toward the phaco tip, making even a minor or momentary degree of surge precarious.

Fortunately, all three major manufacturers provide us with bona fide advances in their latest machine platforms that address the

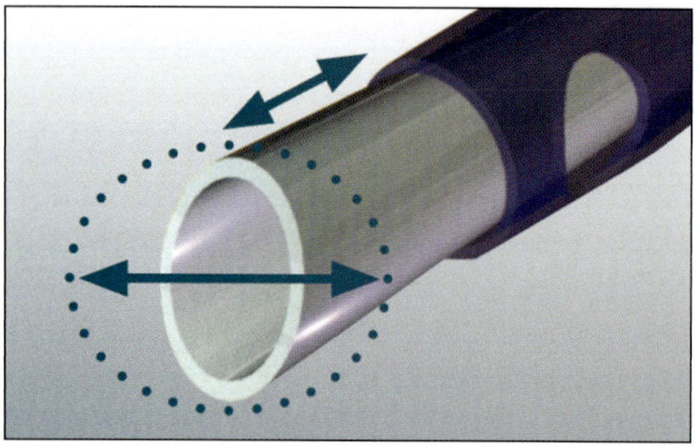

Figure 1. Illustration of the phaco tip's transverse elliptical path combined with some longitudinal axial motion.

three problems I have outlined. This article highlights specific safety features that users of the Whitestar Signature System (Advanced Medical Optics, Inc., Santa Ana, CA) should understand and deploy.

POWER MODULATIONS: WHITESTAR AND ELLIPS

This decade has brought two major advances in ultrasound technology, starting with the launch of Whitestar hyperpulse power modulation with the Sovereign system (Advanced Medical Optics, Inc.) in 2001. Shortening the pulse's duration allows us to significantly increase the frequency of ultrasound pulses. In addition, the ability to decrease the duty cycle produces a major reduction in cumulative ultrasound time. These changes significantly reduce the production of heat and the total ultrasound energy delivered by the phaco tip, and they practically eliminate the risk of wound burn. As well illustrated by the ASCRS award-winning videos of Teruyuki Miyoshi, MD, that used ultra-high-speed digital photography, alternating each ultrasonic pulse with rest periods of "off" time diminishes the repelling force of the vibrating phaco tip. This in turn reduces the chatter and turbulence of small lenticular particles at the phaco tip that would otherwise bombard the corneal endothelium.

The second major advance was the OZil Torsional handpiece (Alcon Laboratories, Inc., Fort Worth, TX), which replaces the axial movement of a traditional phaco needle with the sideways oscillation of a bent Kelman tip. Dr. Miyoshi's videos also showed that eliminating longitudinal repelling forces at the phaco tip dramatically improved followability and reduced the chatter of fragments. Advanced Medical Optics, Inc., has built on this concept by blending some longitudinal movement with a transverse elliptical path of the phaco tip (Figure 1). Ellips Transversal Ultrasound retains some longitudinal motion in order to improve the tip's ability to cut dense nuclear material. Although I have only limited personal experience with torsional phacoemulsification, Ellips seems to provide comparable benefits with a straight phaco tip, which is my strong preference for phaco chop (Figure 2). This is the single most exciting feature of the Whitestar Signature System.

I now routinely combine Ellips with variable Whitestar ICE Technology (Advanced Medical Optics, Inc.), but I use a higher, foot-pedal–controlled duty cycle that I can vary from 60% to 90%. The higher duty cycle compensates for the overall reduction in the tip's axial motion. The enhanced followability that characterizes Ellips Transversal Ultrasound is the most dramatic and obvious when used on dense nuclei. The reduced endothelial trauma in eyes with brunescent lenses is apparent in the form of clearer corneas on postoperative day 1, a well-acknowledged hallmark of phacoemulsification using nonlongitudinal ultrasound.

MICROPHACO TIP

Moving from a 19-gauge to a 20-gauge phaco tip is one strategy that all of us can use to enhance safety regardless of the brand of phaco machine. This single modification reduces the size of the incision, decreases surge, lessens the chance of accidental aspiration of the iris or capsule, and makes it easier to pluck thin or crumbling nuclear fragments from the capsular fornices. The last advantage stems from the fact that the smaller tip becomes occluded without having to penetrate too deeply into the nucleus. The narrower lumen restricts flow, reduces surge, and prevents material from rushing in as fast as through a needle with a shaft of standard diameter. Like an I/A tip with a smaller opening, a microphaco tip provides us with greater control over which tissue is or is not aspirated. Slowing things down in this way helps when we want to guard against snagging the capsule, such as when aspirating epinucleus or thin nuclear pieces abutting the peripheral capsular bag.

Counterbalancing these advantages are several tradeoffs. A microphaco tip increases nuclear chatter because of its smaller "mouth," and its restricted flow lengthens the time needed to remove a bulky nucleus. The smaller surface area of the tip's opening also reduces the effective holding power for any given vacuum level. Fortunately, we can solve the followability problem by chopping the nucleus into smaller pieces and combining Ellips and variable Whitestar power modulations to virtually eliminate chatter. Improved pump technology enables us to safely use higher aspiration flow and vacuum to compensate for the other factors. It is therefore possible to reap the benefits of a smaller phaco tip regardless of whether we perform coaxial or biaxial phacoemulsification, and yet using a microphaco tip is the most overlooked safety modification that we surgeons can make.

ENHANCED FLUIDICS

The Whitestar Signature System's pump is a measurable improvement over that of the Sovereign. Experiments in cadaveric eyes by Randall Olson, MD, were able to measure surge associated with a variety of vacuum levels using different machines with the same experimental eye. These studies have provided quantitative confirmation of the improved chamber stability that we perceive clinically. I also strongly advocate using two optional but important safety features of the Signature's Fusion Fluidics pump: passive automatic reflux and the antisurge algorithm (discussed later).

We are much more likely to aspirate a lax posterior capsule during cortical cleanup in eyes with weak zonules. All phaco machines provide active auto reflux, whereby pressing a foot switch reverses flow in the aspiration line. Doing so expels ensnared material, such as the posterior capsule, from the aspirating port. Passive auto reflux is a safety option of both the Signature and the Sovereign that automatically refluxes the port at every transition from foot position 2 to 1. We surgeons instinctively make this change as soon as the capsule is aspirated, and this wonderful safety feature immediately expels the capsule for us. I select this indispensable option for all cases.

ANTISURGE ALGORITHM

I believe that postocclusion surge is still the most common cause of posterior capsular rupture occurring during nuclear

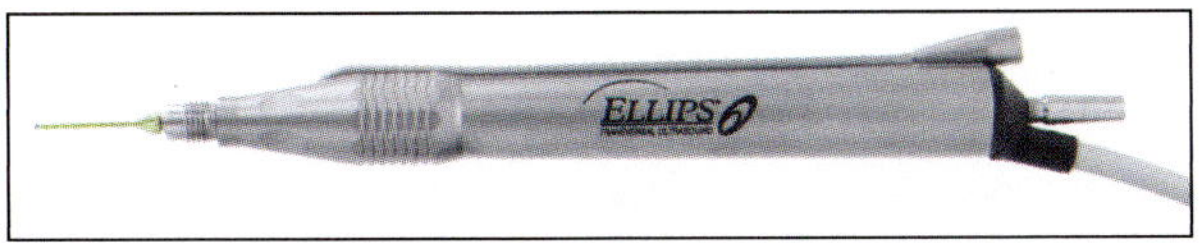

Figure 2. The Ellips Transversal Ultrasound handpiece with a straight 20-gauge phaco tip (infusion sleeve removed).

emulsification. The Diplomax machine (Advanced Medical Optics, Inc.) was the first to offer the occlusion mode feature, which we could program to automatically change ultrasound and fluidic parameters once the phaco tip became occluded or unoccluded. I always thought, however, that it would be much safer if we could drop the vacuum immediately before a break in occlusion. When using higher vacuum levels, this decrease would significantly reduce surge and improve chamber stability.

In response to this suggestion, the Fusion Fluidics pump technology has an antisurge algorithm to accomplish just this result. The pump's onboard computer recognizes occlusion and proactively reverses the pump to actively step down the vacuum before the break in occlusion occurs. I use the antisurge algorithm during emulsification of chopped fragments, when breaks in occlusion are happening repeatedly. Like a car's antilock braking system, the antisurge algorithm automatically reduces the vacuum level after a predetermined interval to prevent surge as the fragments are evacuated. The algorithm tries to automate and duplicate what an experienced surgeon could do with a dual linear foot pedal once the tip became occluded. High vacuum is first used to maximize holding power, but we would then lower the vacuum with the dual linear foot pedal before delivering phaco power to clear the phaco tip.

CONCLUSION

Advances in phaco technology continue to improve our ability to manage the most challenging cataracts. Although such sophistication comes at the expense of simplicity, understanding and properly configuring our phaco technology deliver better performance while improving safety. ■

Strategies With the Stellaris Vision Enhancement System

ELIZABETH A. DAVIS, MD

Enhancing safety in phacoemulsification requires optimizing fluidics and reducing the amount of ultrasound energy delivered. Several new phaco systems represent improvements in these areas over previous platforms. This article focuses on the Stellaris Vision Enhancement System (Bausch & Lomb, Rochester, NY).

TRANSITION TO MICROINCISIONAL CATARACT SURGERY

I have been performing cataract surgery with the Stellaris Vision Enhancement System for approximately 2 years. I had been a longtime user of Bausch & Lomb's Millennium microsurgical system, with which I performed coaxial surgery through an incision of 2.8 to 3.0 mm. One of the factors motivating my switch to the Stellaris was that it has several new features that enhance surgical safety and efficiency. Additionally, the system is capable of microincisional cataract surgery, which I was anxious to incorporate into my practice. The significance of the benefits of smaller incisions (reduced astigmatism, enhanced chamber stability, and a lower risk of leaking wounds and infection) was clear to me. Based upon many of my colleagues' experience, however, I was not enthusiastic about bimanual microincisional surgery for numerous reasons. The procedure seemed fraught with challenges in fluidics, chamber stability, and prolonged surgical time. It also demanded a significant change in technique. Although the Stellaris Vision Enhancement System may be used for biaxial surgery, the opportunity to perform microincisional surgery in a coaxial fashion was what I found particularly attractive.

I started with a standard 3.0-mm coaxial procedure but then was pleasantly surprised to experience a seamless transition to 1.8-mm coaxial surgery. I did not have to make any substantial changes to my surgical technique aside from adjusting to the use of a microincisional capsulorhexis forceps instead of a Utrata model.

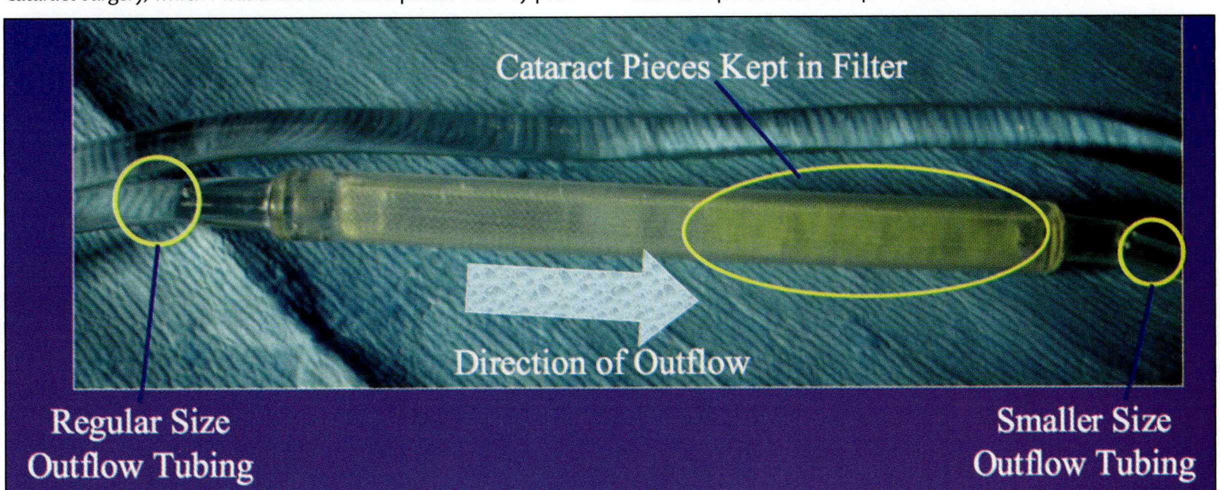

(Courtesy of Uday Devgan, MD.)

Figure 1. The Stellaris Vision Enhancement System's restrictive outflow tubing.

HIGH VACUUM AND TUBING

In terms of enhancing my technique, I have found the Stellaris' high vacuum settings (up to 600 mm Hg) beneficial. I usually employ very high vacuum for supracapsular surgery, and, even at 600 mm Hg, the chamber remains extremely stable. This technology can be combined with flow-restrictive tubing that prevents postocclusion surge at high vacuum levels (Figure 1). A mesh filter located in the tubing traps particles and prevents clogging.

A simple but ingenious new feature of the Stellaris Vision Enhancement System is the connection of the infusion tubing to the handpiece via a luer lock. This setup prevents the dangerous loss of inflow and chamber collapse that can occur if the tubing disengages from the handpiece during surgery.

FLOW MODULE

Although I prefer the vacuum module, the Stellaris Vision Enhancement System has a flow module available that can function in either a flow or vacuum mode. This feature not only allows multiple surgeons with different pumping preferences to use the same machine, but it also permits a single surgeon to toggle between flow and vacuum mode during a single case to enhance efficiency at various stages of nuclear removal. The flow module also uses an electrical pump, which eliminates the need for external compressed gases and the associated tanks.

POWER MODULATION

The Stellaris' power modulation represents another improvement on the Millennium. Because the former delivers up to 250 pulses per second with adjustable duty cycles, the surgeon may use waveform modulations in pulse or burst modes. The ultrasound power can also be turned on for as little as 2 milliseconds at a time. I like the Stellaris' power modulation, because it can adapt to the type of cataract or the stage of the phaco procedure.

PHACO HANDPIECE AND FOOT PEDAL

The new titanium handpiece features six crystals versus four in most other systems. As a result, the Stellaris' handpiece is more ergonomic and comfortable, and it has spared me a fatigued wrist at the end of a long surgical day.

As with the Millenium cataract extraction system, the Stellaris' foot pedal is dual linear, which gives me on-the-fly control of power and either vacuum or flow. I have particularly enjoyed this feature, which allows me to alter surgical parameters instantaneously as events occur intraoperatively. Additionally, the foot pedal is now wireless, which eliminates one of the cords across the OR floor.

CONCLUSION

The Stellaris Vision Enhancement System's enhanced fluidics, chamber stability, and power modulation improve efficiency and reduce the use of phaco energy. I encourage other surgeons to try microincisional cataract procedures on this system. They can perform bimanual or coaxial surgery and use either the vacuum or flow module. I am convinced they will not face a difficult transition but will, like me, find their surgical performance and efficiency enhanced. ■

Strategies With the Intrepid Micro-Coaxial System

TERRY KIM, MD

The goals of microincisional cataract surgery are to minimize surgically induced astigmatism, hasten wound healing, and reduce the risk of a leaking wound and infection. The Intrepid Micro-Coaxial System, using both the Infiniti Vision System and the OZil Torsional handpiece (all from Alcon Laboratories, Inc., Fort Worth, TX), represents a fully integrated line of equipment and instruments specifically designed to maximize the safety and efficiency of microincisional coaxial phacoemulsification through a 2.2- or 2.4-mm incision.

OZIL TORSIONAL TECHNOLOGY

Systems that use conventional longitudinal ultrasound incorporate the forward and backward motion of the phaco tip, analogous to the movement of a jackhammer, to emulsify the lens. OZil Torsional ultrasound represents a breakthrough. The side-to-side oscillatory motion of the phaco tip is amplified to shear lenticular material, which results in more efficient emulsification by almost eliminating the repulsion caused by the cutting of nuclear tissue. As a result, the surgeon will notice less repulsion and increased followability of lenticular material, which mean a lesser dependence on the high vacuum levels needed with longitudinal ultrasound to overcome repulsion. Surgical efficiency also increases. Moreover, whereas 50% of the stroke (ie, the backward stroke) is wasted energy with longitudinal ultrasound, torsional ultrasound uses 100% of the stroke to shear nuclear material while also reducing frictional movement within the incision. As a result, torsional ultrasound achieves higher thermal safety than modulated longitudinal ultrasound.

For microincisional coaxial phacoemulsification, the Intrepid's MicroSmooth Ultra irrigation sleeve (Alcon Laboratories, Inc.) protects the wound against thermal/mechanical stress and provides sufficient flow that the bottle need not be excessively high, as with some other phaco systems.

THE INTREPID FLUID MANAGEMENT SYSTEM

The Intrepid Fluid Management System (Alcon Laboratories, Inc.) uses very low-compliance aspiration tubing to minimize the risk of postocclusion surge and to increase the stability of the anterior chamber without requiring additional irrigating flow. Stable fluidics is essential during both routine and complex cataract surgery through a small incision, because surge and increased turbulence in the anterior chamber can heighten the risk of intraoperative complications. The Intrepid Fluid Management System allows the surgeon a sufficient range of vacuum levels during microincisional coaxial phacoemulsification with incisions as small as 2.2 mm and a bottle less than 110 cm high. The bottom line is a safer cataract procedure.

MONARCH III IOL DELIVERY SYSTEM

The Monarch III IOL delivery system with the D Cartridge (Alcon Laboratories, Inc.) completes the microincisional system by permitting the IOL's safe, controlled implantation through an unenlarged 2.2-mm incision. Compared with the C cartridge, the D cartridge has a nozzle with a 33% smaller tip and a 0.5-mm larger

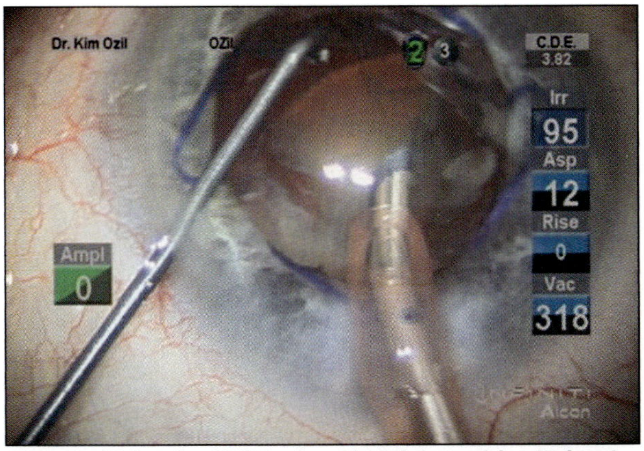

Figure 1. Using the OZil Torsional handpiece with a Malyugin ring (MicroSurgical Technology, Redmond, WA), Dr. Kim performs phaco chop on a dense nucleus.

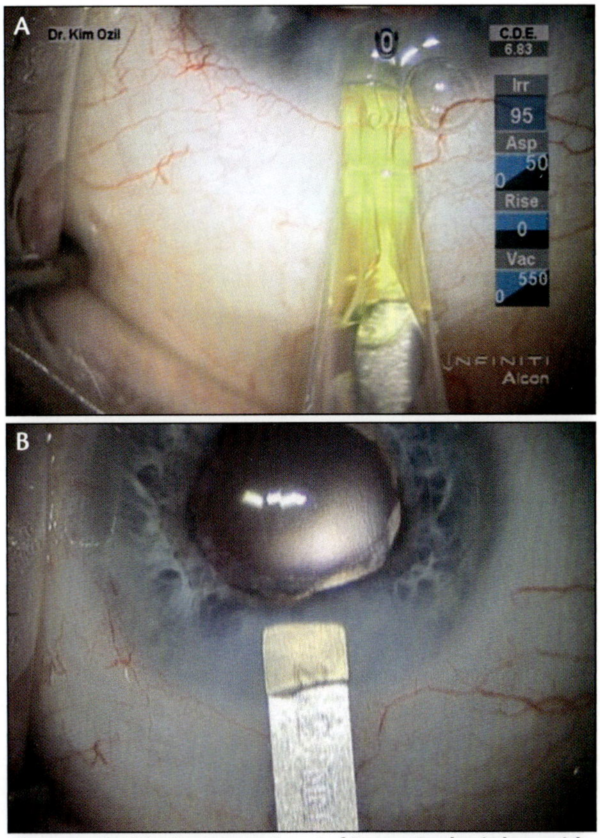

Figure 2. Dr. Kim inserts an AcrySof Restor Aspheric lens with the Monarch III IOL delivery system with a D cartridge (A). He confirms a 2.2-mm incision size with an incision gauge at the conclusion of the case (B).

opening. The aspheric design and material properties of the AcrySof IOLs (Alcon Laboratories, Inc.) complement this injector; their thin optics are made of high-quality hydrophobic acrylic material, and their single-piece design facilitates in-the-bag implantation. Easier, more consistent delivery of the IOL decreases stress on the corneal incision.

PERSONAL EXPERIENCE

I have been using the Alcon Intrepid Micro-Coaxial System routinely for all of my phaco procedures for more than 2 years. The incision's proper construction and architecture are increasingly important as they grow smaller. Shorter tunnels and shallow wounds (resulting in tears at their edges) leave the incision more vulnerable to mechanical stress during phacoemulsification and I/A, and they increase the likelihood of a leaking wound that will require suturing.[1]

One of the steeper learning curves in transitioning to a 2.2-mm incision occurs during the capsulorhexis. The smaller incision limits the movement of a standard capsulorhexis forceps. As a result, the surgeon must grasp the capsulorhexis' edge more frequently and torque/angulate the forceps more often to complete the tear. After a few cases, I became accustomed to these maneuvers and found the need to switch to a microcapsulorhexis forceps unnecessary.

With the 0.9-mm Mini-Flared Kelman tip with a 45° bevel (Alcon Laboratories, Inc.), I routinely use 100% torsional ultrasound with a vacuum setting of 350 mm Hg, an aspiration flow rate of 35 mL per minute, and a bottle height of 100 cm. I particularly notice the benefits of torsional ultrasound with denser lenses: the enhanced followability and decreased anterior chamber turbulence have been impressive (Figure 1).

I have used the Monarch III IOL delivery system with the D cartridge to implant the full line of single-piece AcrySof IOLs, including the AcrySof IQ, the AcrySof Toric, and the AcrySof Restor Aspheric as well as high-powered spherical IOLs such as a 34.00 D monofocal AcrySof IOL. Regardless of the lens used, its delivery through a 2.2-mm incision has been consistently easy with a wound-assisted technique, which is my preference (Figure 2). I have found that these incisions seal completely after stromal hydration without the need for a suture, even in atypical cases such as after trabeculectomy or pars plana vitrectomy, and they are astigmatically neutral.[2]

LABORATORY AND CLINICAL STUDIES

A number of studies have confirmed the safety and efficiency of the Intrepid Micro-Coaxial System using the Infiniti Vision System, OZil Torsional technology, and the Intrepid Fluid Management System.[3-6] My colleagues and I conducted a series of laboratory and clinical studies examining the wound's architecture and integrity after phaco procedures performed using the Intrepid system. The results of these investigations have consistently supported the positive safety profile of phacoemulsification with a 2.2-mm microincision and torsional ultrasound.[7,8]

In an ex vivo study using human eye-banked eyes, my colleagues and I analyzed the effects of different OZil settings (ie, 100% torsional ultrasound or 70% torsional/30% longitudinal ultrasound) through a 2.8- or 2.2-mm incision. Surgical parameters—including vacuum, aspiration, and bottle-height settings—were constant for all procedures. Gross and histopathologic examination as well as findings on optical coherence tomography and scanning electron microscopy revealed no differences in the corneal wound's architecture or integrity among all groups. Compared with longitudinal ultrasound, torsional and mixed torsional/longitudinal ultrasound did not adversely affect these incisions.[7]

We recently performed a contralateral eye study in 30 human patients with bilaterally similar cataracts in order to compare the differences in various intraoperative and clinical parameters after phacoemulsification using 100% torsional ultrasound.[8] The procedure was performed through a 2.8-mm incision in subjects' right eye (with a 0.9-mm tapered Kelman tip with a 30° bevel and the standard Infiniti Fluid Management System) and a 2.2-mm incision in their left eye (with a 0.9-mm Mini-Flared Kelman tip with a 45° bevel and the Intrepid Fluid Management System). We chose these tips to maximize the fluidic performance for the corresponding size of incision. The surgical techniques (ie, prechop, horizontal chop, etc.) and settings (ie, vacuum, aspiration, and bottle height) were similar for each patient. The parameters we studied included the accumulated usage of ultrasound energy, the usage of balanced salt solution, the change in central corneal thickness (on postoperative day 1), and the change in endothelial cell count (at postoperative month 6). Of these, the only two that showed a statistically significant difference in favor of the 2.2-mm incision were the amount of ultrasound energy used (cumulative dissipated energy) and the change in the endothelial cell count. Based on these results, we concluded that microincisional phacoemulsification with a 2.2-mm incision, the 45° beveled Mini-Flared Kelman tip, 100% torsional ultrasound, and the Intrepid Fluid Management System is a safe and effective procedure that may offer favorable clinical and intraoperative benefits to our patients.

CONCLUSION

The Intrepid Micro-Coaxial System includes the 2.2-mm ClearCut metal keratome blades, OZil Torsional ultrasound, the Intrepid Fluid Management System, the Monarch III IOL delivery system with the D cartridge, and the line of AcrySof Aspheric IOLs. This platform offers the latest integrated technology specifically designed to enhance the safety and efficacy of modern cataract surgery. ■

This article originally appeared in the November 2008 issue of CRSToday.

1. Ernest PH, Fenzl R, Lavery KT, Sensoli A. Relative stability of clear corneal incisions in a cadaver eye model. *J Cataract Refract Surg.* 1995;21:39-42.
2. Masket S. Surgically induced astigmatism with 2.2 mm clear corneal incisions. Paper presented at: The ASCRS Symposium & Congress on Cataract, IOL, and Refractive Surgery; March 18, 2006; San Francisco, CA.
3. Vasavada AR, Raj SM, Patel LM, et al. Evaluating intra-operative performance and post-operative outcome of torsional versus longitudinal phacoemulsification: a prospective, randomized, masked clinical trial. Paper presented at: The XXV Congress of the ESCRS; September 8-12, 2007; Stockholm, Sweden.
4. MacDonald SM. Comparison of traditional phacoemulsification and torsional phacoemulsification. Paper presented at: The ASCRS Symposium & Congress on Cataract, IOL, and Refractive Surgery; May 1, 2007; San Diego, CA.
5. Aguilera-Zarate F, Garcia-Quinones D. Comparing outcomes of microcoaxial torsional vs standard torsional and traditional phaco in the emulsification of cataracts. Paper presented at: The ASCRS Symposium & Congress on Cataract, IOL, and Refractive Surgery; April 28, 2007; San Diego, CA.
6. Ahmed IK, Teichman JC, Tam DY. Clear corneal incisional morphology with torsional versus longitudinal phacoemulsification: prospective randomized controlled clinical and imaging study. Paper presented at: The ASCRS Symposium & Congress on Cataract, IOL, and Refractive Surgery; April 8, 2008; Chicago, IL.
7. Jun B, Berdahl JP, Kuo A, Kim T. Corneal wound architecture and integrity after OZil and mixed phacoemulsification: evaluation of standard and microincisional coaxial techniques. Poster presented at: The XXV Congress of the ESCRS; September 8-12, 2007; Stockholm, Sweden.
8. Berdahl JP, Jun BK, DeStafeno JJ, Kim T. Comparison of the OZil Torsional handpiece through microincisional and standard clear corneal cataract wounds. *J Cataract Refract Surg.* In press.

CHAPTER 28

The Influence of New Technology

WILLIAM J. FISHKIND, MD; STEVEN DEWEY, MD; ROBERT J. CIONNI, MD; ALAN S. CRANDALL, MD; AND UDAY DEVGAN, MD

WILLIAM J. FISHKIND, MD

The past few years have brought the introduction of noteworthy new phaco technologies that have altered the way we surgeons analyze and execute the procedure. To better understand these advances, we must partition phacoemulsification into its components of power and fluid. The former is characterized as the combined effect of cavitational and jackhammer energy (the debate over the role of cavitational energy is beyond the scope of this discussion).

The fluidic element of the procedure includes the management of vacuum and flow. When the fragment is adjacent to the phaco tip during emulsification, it obstructs the inflow of fluid and allows vacuum to increase to the preset maximum (defined as occlusion). The instant of occlusion is a critical dividing point in the procedure. The act of removing the fragment can therefore be divided into preocclusion phacoemulsification, occlusion, and postocclusion phacoemulsification (Figure 1A).

In the past, we performed the majority of the procedure with occlusion inevitably followed by postocclusion phacoemulsification. Every occlusion resulted in a surge, which we came to accept, albeit unhappily.

Micropulse phacoemulsification is a revolutionary power modification composed of extremely short bursts of phaco power, for use even with hard nuclei. This technology and torsional phacoemulsification have shown us that we can emulsify the fragment near the tip without total occlusion. As a result, there is rarely an occlusion or surge. If we perform phaco chop, we create multiple fragments early in the procedure. We remove these fragments with low amounts of power in stable anterior chambers (Figure 1B).

If we take an expansive look at the new phaco technologies, their major effects are to permit the phacoemulsification of fragments in the preocclusion phase and therefore avert postocclusion surge.

STEVEN DEWEY, MD

Six years ago, the introduction of the original Whitestar micropulse technology (Advanced Medical Optics, Inc., Santa Ana, CA) ushered out the remnants of traditional longitudinal phacoemulsification by significantly reducing chatter, turbulence, and instability of the chamber seen with older phaco systems. With the latest Whitestar ICE technology (Advanced Medical Optics, Inc.) upgrade, three features now transform the micropulse power delivery: micropulse shaping; variable duty cycle power delivery; and chamber automated stabilization environment (CASE; Advanced Medical Optics, Inc.).

The benefits of the original Whitestar Technology in reducing effective phaco time are well known.[1] My own measurements

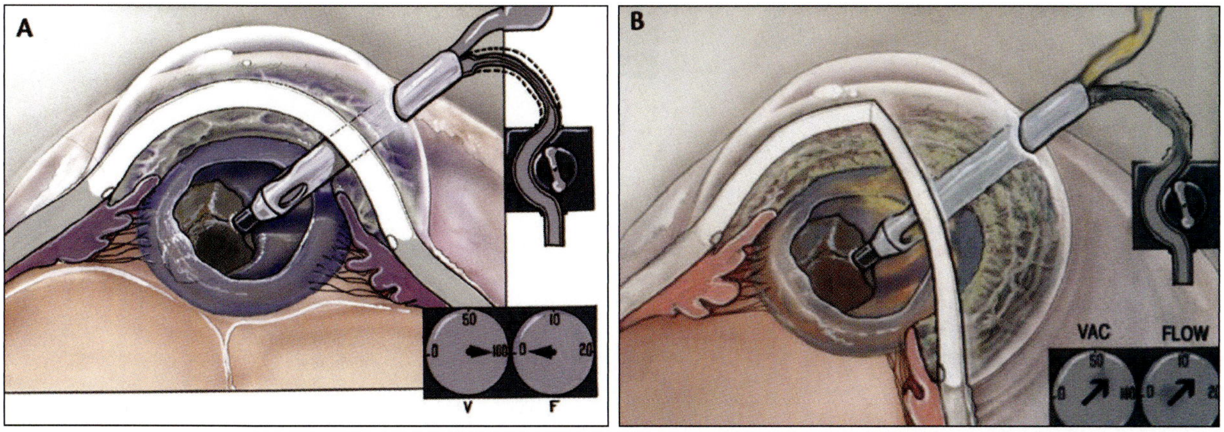

Figure 1. The fragment occludes the phaco tip.There is full vacuum and no flow.When phaco power is energized, the fragment is emulsified, resulting in greater outflow through the phaco tip than inflow, a situation that inevitably leads to surge (A).The fragment is near the phaco tip but does not occlude it.There is always partial vacuum and flow.Without occlusion, there is no surge, and the anterior chamber remains deep (B). (Reprinted with permission from Fishkind WJ, ed.Complications in *Phacoemulsification: Avoidance,Recognition,and Management.*1st ed. New York,NY:Thieme Medical Publishers; 2002.)

comparing Whitestar generations show further gains with the ICE technology. Using a nonstop horizontal chop, my effective phaco time has decreased by 40% for a 2+ nuclear sclerotic cataract and by 20% for a 3+ cataract. By reviewing digital video, I can measure the time from the phaco needle's insertion to its removal. I find my phaco needle is a few seconds more efficient with the Whitestar ICE technology than the original technology.

To understand how my surgical efficiency improved, I wanted to evaluate how the equipment interacted with my technique. While reviewing hundreds of surgical videos using the Whitestar ICE technology, I observed virtually no surge, turbulence, or chatter; far less bouncing of the chamber; and impressive followability of particles.

I believe the Whitestar ICE technology allows me to attack the point of occlusion instead of hesitantly engaging the material. I use vacuum much more effectively to shear the nucleus apart and achieve occlusion prior to applying power. As occlusion breaks, I no longer depend on my response with the foot pedal to release vacuum and prevent surge or on my placement of a second instrument against the capsule to prevent its engagement with the tip. Instead, I work as comfortably with the last quadrant as I did the first. This technology allows me to remove the nucleus efficiently without having to anticipate the limitations of the equipment.

ROBERT J. CIONNI, MD

Just when I think that cataract removal technology cannot improve further, something revolutionary knocks my socks off. The introduction of Ozil torsional phacoemulsification (Alcon Laboratories, Inc., Fort Worth, TX) is one of the most impressive advances that I have witnessed during the last decade.

Traditional phacoemulsification is characterized by a longitudinal motion of the phaco tip along its long axis. The forward striking movement of the sharp metal tip emulsifies the nucleus of the cataract. This force, however, also encourages the movement of nuclear material away from the tip, thereby requiring higher vacuum levels and aspiration rates as well as power modulations to keep nuclear material from chattering away. Additionally, because the tip only cuts with a forward movement, the 50% of the time that it is moving backward is wasted energy that generates potentially harmful heat.[2]

Torsional phacoemulsification is characterized by an oscillatory motion around the long axis of the phaco tip. This motion generates sufficient energy to emulsify the nucleus but has several advantages over traditional longitudinal ultrasound. First, the oscillatory motion does not encourage the chattering of lenticular material.3 Followability is therefore markedly improved. Second, torsional phacoemulsification emulsifies in both the to and fro directions and thereby does not waste energy. The rotational movement induces less frictional heat at the incision as well. The net result is lower energy delivered and less risk of thermal damage to the incision (data on file with Alcon Laboratories, Inc.).

I have found that the best-performing tip for Ozil torsional ultrasound is the tapered Kelman tip (Alcon Laboratories, Inc.) through a 2.7- to 3.0-mm incision. With traditional longitudinal ultrasound, a strong holding force is needed to prevent lens chatter, and a high aspiration rate is needed to improve followability. With Ozil torsional phacoemulsification, I decrease the vacuum from 500 to 350 mm Hg and the aspiration rate from 40 to 25 mL/min. Because the vacuum level and aspiration rates are lower, I can also decrease the bottle's height to 90 cm without inducing volatility in the chamber. Finally, I no longer need to rely on power modulations and simply set the torsional amplitude on linear continuous control. These settings work well with chopping or dividing techniques.

Torsional ultrasound has increased my safety profile for cataract removal while simplifying my technique so much that it feels like cheating.

ALAN S. CRANDALL, MD

Phacoemulsification has progressed since its introduction more than 40 years ago by Charles Kelman, MD. Technical advances such as the continuous curvilinear capsulorhexis have improved outcomes. Understanding the lens' anatomy led to different techniques of disassembly (including divide and conquer and various forms of chopping) that have improved the safety of the procedure and reduced the risk of capsular rupture.

New phaco software to increase surgical safety has included measures to reduce surge and pulse and burst modes to decrease the energy delivered. A better understanding of the combination of aspiration flow, vacuum, and ultrasound power with all the available phaco units has increased procedural safety and improved outcomes. Research into alternate methods for removing the lens (eg, lasers and water jets) has yet to replace traditional phacoemulsification, however.

Traditional phacoemulsification uses longitudinal motion of the phaco tip to emulsify the lenticular material. The frequency of the tip varies with different units from the middle 20,000s to 46,000 cycles per second. Heat is produced with this motion, and fluid is used to lower the risk of burns to the cornea and iris. With the longitudinal motion of the tip, there is a repulsive force that can decrease the efficiency of the procedure. Part of the art as well as the science of the phaco procedure is using various modes, flows, and phaco powers to effectively remove cataracts of different hardness safely and with the least amount of energy and fluid. Alterations to phaco tips have allowed further variations in technique.

In the 1990s, the Neosonix tip (Alcon Laboratories, Inc.) had a 2° oscillation along with longitudinal phacoemulsification, but the oscillation was very slow at a few oscillations per second. The theory was that the movement would help prevent occlusion, so it was helpful in divide and conquer techniques or anytime that nuclear material was being removed due to improved flow.

Torsional phacoemulsification involves an ultrasonic torsional motion (33,000 cycles/sec) that significantly improves the followability of nuclear material. The technology can use variations such as pulse and burst modes to further reduce potential heat-related complications and surge. The Ozil handpiece permits surgeons to use longitudinal (traditional) phacoemulsification for hard nuclei or for their comfort during the transition to full-time torsional phacoemulsification.

The torsional motion reduces friction at the incision,4 which should lower the risk of wound burn. The small phaco tip (0.9 mm) and the torsional motion work well for 2.2-mm microincisional phacoemulsification.

I currently use Ozil torsional phacoemulsification almost exclusively. The followability of nuclear fragments allows me to reduce vacuum to 300 mm Hg and aspiration flow to 38 mL/min. I am still learning about the intricacies of the new technology and how to use the system most efficiently.

UDAY DEVGAN, MD

The current phaco platforms have successfully made the use of phaco power modulations the standard of care. This decrease in phaco energy has resulted in less endothelial cell damage, a near-zero rate of phaco wound burns, and patients happy with their clear corneas and minimal inflammation immediately after surgery. The new machines have not significantly decreased the rate of posterior capsular complications, however, because the inadvertent rupturing of the capsule is most often due to issues of fluidics and not ultrasonic power.

The next frontier for safety and efficiency in cataract and IOL surgery is the delicate balance of fluidics within the confines of the anterior segment. As surgeons transition to refractive cataract surgery, they require an increased level of stability, followability, efficiency, and, most importantly, safety to deliver the expected outcomes for patients. Fluidic balance is the key.

The Stellaris Vision Enhancement System (FDA approved; Bausch & Lomb) delivers a superb balance of fluidics. The system includes new-generation fluid pumps, customized control software, options for advanced surgical control, and high-vacuum restrictive phaco tubing. The results are rock-solid stability of the anterior chamber during surgery, an efficient phaco procedure with magnetic followability, and a large margin of safety. I have found that the fluidic control and balance are outstanding and fully integrated into a true next-generation system. Whether the surgeon favors a bimanual or coaxial approach, flow-based or vacuum-based surgery, a divide-and-conquer or phaco chop technique, the Stellaris Vision Enhancement System delivers the performance and fluidic control that empowers ophthalmologists and benefits the patient. ■

This article originally appeared in the March 2007 issue of CRSToday.

1. Fishkind W, Bakewell B, Donnenfeld ED, et al. Comparative clinical trial of ultrasound phacoemulsification with and without the WhiteStar system. *J Cataract Refract Surg.* 2006;32:45-49.
2. Zacharias J. Jackhammer or cavitation: the final answer. Film presented at: The ASCRS/ASOA 2006 Symposium & Congress; March 17-22, 2006; San Francisco, CA.
3. Solomon K. Creating a fluidics model: a new paradigm. Paper presented at: The ASCRS/ASOA 2006 Symposium & Congress; March 2006; San Francisco, CA.
4. Mackool RJ, Mackool RJ Jr. Lens removal/torsional phacoemulsification: advantages of nonlinear ultrasound. Paper presented at: The ASCRS/ASOA 2006 Symposium & Congress; March 18, 2006; San Francisco, CA.

CHAPTER 29

Phaco Machine Settings

WILLIAM J. FISHKIND, MD; R. BRUCE WALLACE III, MD; BONNIE AN HENDERSON, MD; D. MICHAEL COLVARD, MD; UDAY DEVGAN, MD; DONALD N. SERAFANO, MD; Y. RALPH CHU, MD; ELIZABETH A. DAVIS, MD; AND JAMES P. GILLS, MD

WILLIAM J. FISHKIND, MD

During the last few years, manufacturers have introduced phaco machines that are strikingly superior to and more refined than previous units. Even those that have been in service for a number of years are eligible for several upgrades. I asked several surgeons which machine and phaco settings they use and what their phaco settings are.

I myself presently use the Sovereign cataract extraction system (Advanced Medical Optics, Inc., Santa Ana, CA) and a 19-gauge 0° phaco tip. My preferred technique is quick chop. I have four settings programmed into the machine (Table 1). I use "phaco 1" solely for the hardest cataracts and only to embed the tip and chop. Once I have completed numerous chops, I switch to "phaco 2" to mobilize and remove the fragments. I generally rely on "phaco 3" to remove softer nuclear/cortical material and epinucleus. Rarely, I employ "phaco 4" for a soft nucleus. All of the settings are designed to enhance partial occlusion phacoemulsification and to minimize surge.

TABLE 1. Dr. FISHKIND'S SETTINGS				
	Aspiration Rate, mL/min	Vacuum, mm Hg	Power	Whitestar Pulse Setting
Phaco 1 hard chop				
Unoccluded	26 linear	350 panel	40%	F/b
Occluded	26 linear	220 threshold	40%	D/I 31%, CD 43%, CB 60%, DB 67%
Phaco 2 soft chop				
Unoccluded	24 panel	275 linear	25%	CL 20%, CF 33%, CD 43%, DB 67%
Occluded	26	220	25%	CL 20%, CF 33%, CD 43%, DB 67%
Phaco 3 epinuclear				
Unoccluded	26 panel	280 linear	15%	CL 20%, CF 33%, CD 43%, DB 67%
Occluded	26 panel	200	15%	CF 4 long pulses per second
Phaco 4 slow				
Unoccluded	24 panel	315 linear	10%	C/N
Occluded	24	215	10%	C/N
Note: with the Sovereign cataract extraction system.				

TABLE 2. Dr. WALLACE'S SETTINGS						
Phase	Submode	Power	Pulses per Second	Duty Cycle	Bottle Height, cm	Vacuum, mm Hg
Sculpting	1	0 to 45%	250	50%	85	0 to 50
	2	0 to 60%	250	50%	85	0 to 60
	3	0 to 60% continuous			85	0 to 50
Segment removal	1	10% to 28% dual linear	50	40%	108	0 to 390
	2	10% to 40% dual linear	50	40%	108	0 to 390
	3	0 to 12% dual linear	50	40%	108	0 to 390
Epinuclear	1	0 to15% continuous			100	0 to 325
Note: with the Stellaris Vision Enhancement System. Submode 1 for standard nuclei, 2 for dense nuclei, and 3 for soft nuclei.						

TABLE 3. Dr. COLVARD'S SETTINGS			
Setting	Aspiration Rate (mL/min)	Vacuum Limit (mm Hg)	Power
Phaco 1 (sculpting)	22	60	60%
Phaco 2 (segment removal)	35	350	60%
Phaco 3 (epinucleus)	35	180	20%
Note: with the Sovereign Compact.			

R. BRUCE WALLACE III, MD

I favor the new Stellaris Vision Enhancement System (Bausch & Lomb, Rochester, NY). Its enhanced fluidics have improved surgical safety. Although the flow-based option performs well, I prefer to use the vacuum system. I have found it to be amazingly responsive, which gives me greater confidence in cases of small pupils, shallow anterior chambers, and dense nuclei. Because the Stellaris anticipates changes in pressure in the anterior chamber, I am able to use higher vacuum levels than on earlier phaco machines. My program includes three settings (Table 2). The dual linear foot pedal allows me to use mostly phacoaspiration on the downstroke of the pedal and more phaco power, when needed, through my foot's movement outward. Using this phaco system, I am able to perform coaxial phacoemulsification through a microincision of 1.8 mm.

BONNIE AN HENDERSON, MD

I primarily use the Infiniti Vision System with the Ozil

Dr. Henderson's Settings

Dr. Henderson favors the Infiniti Vision System with the Ozil Torsional handpiece (Alcon Laboratories, Inc., Fort Worth, TX).

Soft lenses
Sculpting
- Ozil amplitude—85% (all torsional, no longitudinal), linear pedal control
- Vacuum—90 mm Hg, linear pedal control
- Aspiration—24 mL/min, fixed pedal control
- Bottle height—95 cm

Chop/quadrant removal
- Ozil amplitude—80% (all torsional), linear pedal control
- Vacuum—400 mm Hg, fixed pedal control
- Aspiration—35 mL/min, fixed pedal control
- Bottle height—105 cm

Medium lenses
Sculpting
- Ozil amplitude—85% (all torsional), linear pedal control
- Vacuum—100 mm Hg, linear pedal control
- Aspiration—24 mL/min, fixed pedal control
- Bottle height—95 cm

Chop/quadrant removal
- Ozil amplitude—80% (all torsional), linear pedal control
- Vacuum—400 mm Hg, fixed pedal control
- Aspiration—35 mL/min, fixed pedal control
- Bottle height—105 cm

Dense lenses
Sculpting
- Ultrasound longitudinal power, 35% linear, 10% on time, 22 pulses per second, combined with Ozil amplitude, linear 100%, 90% Ozil on time
- Vacuum—90 mm Hg, linear pedal control
- Aspiration—24 mL/min, fixed pedal control
- Bottle height—95 cm

Chop/quadrant removal
- Ultrasound longitudinal power, 40% linear, 5% on time, 10 pulses per second, combined with Ozil amplitude, linear 100%, 95% Ozil on time
- Vacuum—400 mm Hg, fixed pedal control
- Aspiration—35 mL/min, fixed pedal control
- Bottle height—105 cm

Torsional handpiece (Alcon Laboratories, Inc., Fort Worth, TX). I prefer the 0.9-mm 45° miniflare ABS tip when I employ a microcoaxial approach, because I feel it delivers the best irrigation flow and provides increased protection against surge. I find that this combination allows me to perform safe, effective phacoemulsification for all types of lenses. It is possible to remove cataracts of all densities with a single phaco setting due to technological improvements in the forms of (1) aspiration bypass systems that prevent the buildup of heat, (2) stiffer tubing that maintains the chamber's stability, and (3) linear and fixed pedal settings that enhance surgeon control. Nevertheless, I vary the parameters for lenses of different grades (see *Dr. Henderson's Settings*). I mainly use the stop-and-chop technique.

D. MICHAEL COLVARD, MD

Over the years, I think I have tried virtually every phaco technique I have ever seen or read about, and I have taught myself the same lesson over and over again. The best way to ensure that the cornea will be crystal clear on the day after surgery is to stay away from it. Techniques that tend to bring the nucleus into the anterior chamber are faster but not as gentle to the cornea as those that encourage the surgeon to stay below the iris plane.

Except for very soft lenses, which I can subluxate above the iris by means of hydrodissection and then simply aspirate, I perform a central groove and then a series of vertical and/or horizontal chops, as described originally by Paul Koch, MD.[1] The groove, which is cracked before chopping, allows me to chop at lower vacuum levels. Much more importantly, the groove provides an empty space below the iris plane where I can safely perform phacoemulsification. Denser nuclei need to be chopped into smaller segments, but the basic phaco parameters I use are the same for all cases. My surgery center has several Sovereign Compact units (Advanced Medical Optics, Inc.), and I am extremely happy with this system. I use Whitestar pulse settings (Advanced Medical Optics, Inc.), and, regardless of the density of the nucleus, I never seem to need more than 60% of the machine's phaco power. Table 3 shares my parameters.

UDAY DEVGAN MD

I use several different phaco machines at a private surgical center as well as at the Olive View UCLA Medical Center to teach ophthalmology residents. The newer phaco platforms are far better than their predecessors. If you are using a machine that is a few years old, you owe it to yourself to test drive the newer models.

I prefer large-bore phaco needles for dense cataracts, because they allow for more efficient phaco aspiration of the nuclear material. On the new Stellaris Vision Enhancement System, I prefer the MicroFlow Plus needle in combination with the high-vacuum tubing, and I like using a phaco pulse mode. The concept of increasing the phaco power level for dense cataracts is well known. In addition, I increase the duty cycle of the pulse mode as the nuclear density increases, with as low as 20% for a soft lens and as high as 80% for a brunescent one. I keep the pulse rate high (between 80 and 120 pulses per second), which I feel provides better followability and less risk of built-up heat at the phaco tip (Table 4).

For dense cataracts, my main advice is carefully to modulate the phaco power, to recoat the corneal endothelium periodically with viscoelastic, and to take your time. If you are using a phaco machine from the previous generation such as the Millennium microsurgical system (Bausch & Lomb), you can still implement some of these techniques to improve surgery on dense cataracts. With the Millennium, you can program a variable duty cycle and a wide range of power modulation parameters, although not quite up to the range available on the Stellaris. Older phaco machines may have a tendency for more fluidic imbalance and surge, so it is advisable to use more conservative settings, including lower flow and vacuum and perhaps a higher bottle.

DONALD N. SERAFANO, MD

I use the Infiniti Vision System with the Ozil Torsional handpiece for cataracts of all grades. Ozil with a 45° mini-flared Kelman tip can emulsify a cataract of any grade with only a setting of basic continuous torsional ultrasound and moderate fluidic settings. Because torsional ultrasound almost eliminates repulsion and increases thermal safety, I do not change my phaco parameters

TABLE 4. Dr. DEVGAN'S SETTINGS

	Phaco Parameters			Fluidic Parameters		
Nucleus' Grade	Power Level	Pulse Rate (pulses per second)	Duty Cycle	Bottle Height, cm	Vacuum, mm Hg	Aspiration, mL/min
I	5% to 10%	80 to 120	20%	100	300 to 500	35 to 50
II	10% to 20%	80 to 120	40%	100	300 to 500	35 to 50
III	20% to 40%	80 to 120	60%	100	300 to 500	35 to 50
IV	40% to 60%	80 to 120	80%	100	300 to 500	35 to 50
Note: with the Stellaris Vision Enhancement System using a MicroFlow Plus Needle, peristaltic pump, and high-vacuum tubing.						

TABLE 5. Dr. SERAFANO'S SETTINGS

Phase	Amplitude	Vacuum	Aspiration Flow Rate
Prephacoemulsification	20% linear	180 mm Hg fixed	30 mL/min linear
Sculpting	100% linear	90 mm Hg linear	22 mL/min fixed
Quadrant	100% linear	400 mm Hg fixed	38 mL/min fixed
Epinuclear	20% linear	320 mm Hg linear	32 mL/min linear
Note: for a 2.75-mm incision with Ozil continuous torsional ultrasound on the Infiniti Vision System.			
Phase	**Amplitude**	**Vacuum**	**Aspiration Flow Rate**
Prephacoemulsification	20% linear	180 mm Hg fixed	30 mL/min fixed
Sculpting	100% linear	90 mm Hg linear	22 mL/min fixed
Quadrant	100% linear	350 mm Hg fixed	38 mL/min fixed
Epinuclear	20% linear	320 mm Hg linear	28 mL/min linear
Note: for an incision smaller than 2.40 mm with the Infiniti Vision System.			

based on the density of the nucleus.

Instead, I base my phaco parameters on the steps of the procedure (Table 5). For instance, just before phacoemulsification, I establish flow by using moderate fluidic settings with a very low torsional amplitude. The sculpting phase is nonocclusive with continuous linear torsional ultrasound and moderate fluidics. In the quadrant phase, I only adjust to a higher vacuum setting with a slight modification in minimum ultrasound. During this phase, I use continuous Ozil torsional ultrasound but adjust the linear amplitude to start at 20%.

I do, however, slightly change my parameters based on the size of the incision. For instance, I have certain settings for my standard 2.75-mm phaco incision. I reduce vacuum somewhat for microcoaxial phacoemulsification, in which the incisions are 2.40 mm or smaller, to compensate for the decreased flow. I use the Intrepid Fluid Management System (Alcon Laboratories, Inc.), which reduces my need to adjust my settings or the bottle's height when adopting microcoaxial phacoemulsification.

Y. RALPH CHU, MD

I currently prefer the Whitestar Signature System with Fusion Fluidics (Advanced Medical Optics, Inc.). I use the phaco flip setting for the majority of cataracts. I generally use a 19-gauge phaco tip, but I employ a Dewey Radius phaco tip (MicroSurgical Technology, Redmond, WA) for soft nuclei. For dense nuclei, I prefer a phaco tip with a chiseled edge such as the Chu Chisel (Mastel Precision, Inc., Sioux City, SD). Table 6 shows my settings, including those for when a grooving method is necessary. For extremely hard nuclei, I sometimes incorporate a second mode of phaco flip, which includes Advanced Chamber Stabilization Environment technology (Advanced Medical Optics, Inc.). This feature is particularly helpful in situations requiring high vacuum. My fourth phaco setting is low flow, which I find extremely useful in patients who are taking tamsulosin or in those with small pupils. This setting effectively maintains the chamber's stability and thus minimizes the turbulence in the eye that could disrupt the iris.

ELIZABETH A. DAVIS, MD

Phaco energy—although useful for emulsifying nuclear material—can create inflammation, cause corneal edema and the loss of endothelial cells, and damage other intraocular structures. Minimizing phaco energy is therefore important in cataract surgery. In

TABLE 6. DR. CHU'S SETTINGS

Setting	Aspiration Rate, mL/min	Vacuum	Power, %	Whitestar Pulse Setting	Pump Ramp, %	Bottle Height, cm
Phaco 1 Phaco Flip	36	250 L	50	16/24, 14/16,12/11 10/8 Variable Whitestar 1	70, 70	85
Unoccluded						
Pulse Shaping	1% to 12%	0 to 70%				
CASE Vacuum	N/A					
Phaco 2 Grooving	20	40 L	65	7/3, 70% duty	70, 70	55
Pulse Shaping	1 to 12%	0 to 70%				
CASE Vacuum	N/A					
Phaco 3 Phaco Flip With CASE	36	325 L	50	16/24, 14/16,12/11 10/8 Variable Whitestar 1	70, 70	85
Unoccluded						
Pulse Shaping	1% to 12%	0 to 70%				
CASE Vacuum (used)		250 CASE vacuum	290 mm up	75 mm down	time 500 milliseconds	
Phaco 4 Tamsulosin Low Flow	24	200 L	50	16/24, 14/16,12/11 10/8 Variable Whitestar 1	70, 70	60
Unoccluded						
Occluded						
CASE Vacuum	N/A					

Note: with the Whitestar Signature System with Fusion Fluidics. CASE = Advanced Chamber Stabilization Environment (CASE) technology.

addition to the use of power modulations to reduce total energy, one can also employ high vacuum so that aspiration, rather than ultrasound, evacuates lenticular particles. High vacuum levels can only be achieved safely when fluidics are optimized and postocclusion surge is avoided.

I prefer a high-vacuum supracapsular approach. Working in the iris plane minimizes capsular complications and, in eyes with small pupils or floppy irides, enhances visualization. By combining the Stellaris Vision Enhancement System with high-resistance outflow tubing such as Bausch & Lomb's Stable Chamber tubing or Cruise Control from STAAR Surgical Company (Monrovia, CA), I am able to use aspiration alone, without phaco energy, in at least 80% of my patients (see *Dr. Davis' Settings*). I also enjoy performing sub-2-mm coaxial surgery on this phaco system and have used both the flow module (which allows me to switch between flow and vacuum control even within a single case) and the vacuum module with success.

TABLE 7. DR. GILLS' SETTINGS

Phase	Pulses per Second	Torsional Amplitude	Percentage or Burst on Time	Aspiration Flow Rate	Vacuum Limit
Sculpting	0	35% linear	0	23 mL/min fixed	350 mm Hg linear
Quadrant	0	85% linear	0	20 to 40 mL/min linear	370 mm Hg fixed
Epinuclear	10	75% linear	75% on time	30 mL/min linear	300 mm Hg linear

Note: with the Infiniti Vision System, Ozil Torsional handpiece, and a bottle height of 105 cm.

DR. DAVIS' SETTINGS

Dr. Davis favors the Stellaris Vision Enhancement System from Bausch & Lomb (Rochester, NY).

Vacuum Mode Using the Advanced Flow System
- 300 to 400 mm Hg dual linear vacuum
- 1% to 30% ultrasound power, 50 pulses per second, 60% duty cycle
- Bottle height of 125 cm
- I/A
- 0 to 550 mm Hg
- Bottle height of 125 cm

Flow Mode Using the Advanced Flow System
- 40 mL/min flow
- 350 to 450 mm Hg vacuum
- 1% to 30% ultrasound power, 50 pulses per second, 60% duty cycle
- Bottle height of 125 cm
- I/A (vacuum mode)
- 0 to 550 mm Hg
- Bottle height of 125 cm

Above setting combined with Stabile Chamber tubing (Bausch & Lomb) or Cruise Control tubing (STAAR Surgical Company, Monrovia, CA).

JAMES P. GILLS, MD

I use the Infiniti Vision System with the Ozil Torsional handpiece, a 45° Kelman mini-flare tip, and a phaco chop/divide-and-conquer surgical technique.

For soft lenses, I use the lowest settings (Table 7). I typically start with a horizontal chop and will frequently cut off or use modulated torsional power, because so much of the soft material is vacuumed with moderate or little use of ultrasound.

To address lenses of medium density, I switch to a divide-and-conquer approach and, providing the visualization is good, use a combination of vertical and horizontal chop. In the event of poor visualization, I attempt a quick chop, sculpt out the central part of the nucleus, divide it, and fragment the lens into six or eight pieces prior to its removal. I frequently use this approach in the eyes of patients taking tamsulosin.

For hard lenses, I employ slightly higher flow and vacuum settings; I sometimes use 100% continuous torsional ultrasound to perform a vertical chop with a sharply pointed manipulator. When creating these pie-shaped divisions, I take extra care not to chop the anterior capsule during phacoemulsification. I divide the lens into eight, 12, or 16 pieces using a combination of vertical and horizontal chop. ■

This article originally appeared in the September 2008 issue of CRSToday.

1. Koch PS, Katzen LE. Stop and chop phacoemulsification. *J Cataract Refract Surg.* 1994;20:566-570.

CHAPTER 30

Phaco Myths and Reality

RANDALL J. OLSON, MD

Because phaco machines play an important role in refractive cataract surgery, it is incumbent upon us to understand the differences as well as the full spectrum of parameters between the available platforms. My group and I have published seven studies on phaco systems, and following is a review of the primary lessons I have learned from studying these machines.

Myth No. 1: Percent power is an appropriate way to compare different platforms.

Percent power is not equivalent across the phaco platforms, nor are one machine's parameters comparable to another's. A study that my colleagues and I published in the *Journal of Cataract & Refractive Surgery*[1] compared the percent power of four phaco machines: the Millennium Microsurgical System (Bausch & Lomb, Rochester, NY), the Infiniti Vision System (Alcon Laboratories, Inc., Fort Worth, TX), the Series 20000 Legacy Cataract System (Alcon Laboratories, Inc.), and the Sovereign System with WhiteStar technology (Advanced Medical Optics, Inc., Santa Ana, CA). We determined each system's percent power when working with its phaco tip in water alone versus with their tips working in water with a 200-gram weight placed on the end (to simulate a dense nuclear fragment). The purpose of the study was to see how the machines adjusted their power outputs in different environments.

We tested each phaco system at 20% to 100% linear power in 20% increments, but each one used more power when its tip was working with the load versus unweighted (Table 1). The

Millennium has the lowest kilohertz but ran the hottest, which means it has the longest stroke length. Its percent power did not change much with the load, nor did the Sovereign's.

The Legacy had the most change in percent power, and the Infiniti's change was moderate. The Legacy's power system works like a car's cruise control, adjusting the amount of power to maintain its stroke length in different environments. So, if the phaco tip suddenly encounters a hard nuclear fragment, the Legacy will surge the power without the surgeon's increasing pressure on the foot pedal. Indeed, we found a statistically significant difference in wound burn between the machines in another study.[2]

The Millennium had the least amount of wound burn, followed by the Sovereign (the two were statistically similar), and the Legacy had statistically significantly more than the other two. We did not have enough data on the Infiniti to include that system in this comparison.

Myth No. 2: Peristaltic systems create vacuum only after occlusion and vacuum are allowed to build.

I think this myth is the most pervasive and troublesome for surgeons. It is true that Venturi systems have active vacuum to produce flow, but we wanted to examine the belief that peristaltic systems have no vacuum in the unoccluded state. This is an important argument to understand, because many surgeons have concerns about active vacuum's not releasing an unintended object. Also, many physicians wonder whether active vacuum causes damage if it is set too high. Peristaltic systems offer a chance to pull the phaco tip free if necessary.

To determine each system's true flow rates, we compared the mL/min that the machines indicated versus what they really produced. We found errors in flow rates of up to 17% in general, and some of more than 20% when STAAR Cruise Control (STAAR Surgical Company, Monrovia, CA) was used. For example, the Sovereign machine set to 40 mL/min with Cruise Control produced a flow of only 32 mL/min. In fact, we found it difficult to achieve more than 35 mL/min in any phaco system we tested with Cruise Control.

When we tested the machines' actual vacuum power, we found errors of up to 23%. For instance, ABS, the bypass port at the phaco tip's end, decreased the actual vacuum by an average of 12.1%. Thus, on top of what error may be in the system, ABS produces an additional error of 50 to 60 mm Hg at high vacuum levels.

Our findings on flow and vacuum rates were critical to determining each phaco system's true, unoccluded vacuum. At 32 mL/min actual flow, the Sovereign's unoccluded vacuum was 57.7 ±5.3 mm Hg, and 140 mm Hg with Cruise Control, which is more vacuum at this flow than the Millennium system using Venturi vacuum (Table 2)! Therefore, it is a myth that a peristaltic pump system provides no vacuum without occlusion, at least at most of the parameters we use today. In fact, a peristaltic device may have more active unoccluded vacuum than a Venturi device with a flow restrictor like Cruise Control. This is worth remembering when approaching the capsule and iris, because that amount of unoccluded vacuum can produce enough energy to damage the capsule or iris. The way each phaco system responds to different situations factors into how to control surge with each one.

Myth No. 3: Postocclusion surge is largely tame and nearly equivalent for all current phaco machines. Postocclusion surge is one of ophthalmologists' biggest enemies to avoiding complications. A machine builds kinetic energy when its tip is occluded. Breaking occlusion creates a relatively rapid evacuation of fluid inside the eye, and that trampolining or loss of depth in the anterior chamber can cause an instantaneous break in the capsule. Therefore, controlling surge is a critical safety issue.

Having determined each system's true vacuum power, we could adjust them to equalize their power output. We also had to know each one's actual flow, because flow is related to surge. The higher the flow, the greater the surge.

These data appear in an article that is to be published in the *American Journal of Ophthalmology*. We used a bottle height of 75 cm, 20-gauge phaco tips, and a flow rate of 24 mL/min. We used 430 mm Hg/min vacuum power (the highest vacuum we could guarantee for all the machines in this testing). The Millennium peristaltic system surged the least, at approximately 50 µm. The Sovereign was second, with 110 µm of surge, the Infiniti had 153 µm of surge, and the Legacy had 317 µm. These were highly statistically significant with tight standard deviations. The Millennium Venturi, however, almost completely collapsed the anterior chamber at that power. At over 2 mm, we could not quantitate its surge, because the chamber collapsed so much that it pulled away from our measuring device.

Our next test produced results that I did not expect. Using the same parameters, we switched to using 19-gauge phaco tips. The Sovereign's surge increased by 140%, and the Infiniti's by 200%. In particular with the Millennium Venturi, Cruise Control was extremely powerful in decreasing the overall surge. The Millennium peristaltic system did not show a statistically or clinically significant change in surge: it went from 47 to 42 µm. The Sovereign went from 110 to 147 µm. The Millennium Venturi (tested at 400 mm Hg and 125 cm bottle height, because the higher parameter was still not safe), however, went from more than 2 mm to 210 µm. Its surge went from a dangerous to a safe parameter. Also, at 400 mm Hg, the Millennium Venturi had a flow of approximately 90 mL/min. Remember that flow and vacuum are inseparable in a Venturi system, and the Cruise Control dropped the flow down to 60 mL/min—a great combination that makes this Venturi system much safer.

A FEW OTHER FINDINGS ABOUT SURGE

Adjusting ABS had no impact on the Infiniti system but improved the Legacy by 66%. Thus, it seems that ABS is not important if internal surge protecting systems are present. Increasing the bottle height to 125 cm improved surge on the Infiniti by only 37% and on the Legacy by 70%. Obviously, the machines use different tactics to control surge. Using 40 mL/min of flow increased surge

TABLE 1. COMPARISON OF PERCENT POWER

Machine	Water Load	Water plus 200 gm	Ratio of the two
Millennium	5.67+/-0.51	6.80+/-0.80	1.20
Sovereign	4.59+/-0.70	5.65+/-0.72	1.23
Infiniti	2.79+/-0.62	3.96+/-0.31	1.42
Legacy	1.99+/-0.49	4.27+/-0.76	2.15

TABLE 2. COMPARISON OF UNOCCLUDED VACUUM AT 32 ML/MIN

Machine	Vacuum (unoccluded)o
Sovereign	57.7+/-5.3 mm Hg
Sovereign - CC	140.4+/-0.6 mm Hg
Infiniti	66.4+/-0.5 mm Hg
Legacy	70.1+/-1.5 mm Hg
Mill - P	88.9+/-2.6 mm Hg
Mill - V	104.7+/-0.0 mm Hg

in the Legacy by 60% but in the Infiniti by only 20%. These findings show that the Infiniti phaco system is much more forgiving in regard to surge than the Legacy, and that the other machines are as good or better than the Infiniti. Surge is the real barrier to better outcomes, particularly for refractive cataract patients. ■

This article originally appeared in CRSToday's *February 2007 Best of Source supplement.*

1. Payne M, Georgescu D, Waite AN, Olson RJ. Phacoemulsification tip vacuum pressure: comparison of 4 devices. *J Cataract Refract Surg.*2006;32:8:1374-1377.
2. Bradley MJ, Olson RJ. A survey about phacoemulsification incision thermal contraction incidence and causal relationships. *Am J Ophthalmol.*2006;141:1:222-224.
3. Floyd MS, Valentine JR, Olson RJ. Abstract fluidics and heat generation of Alcon Infiniti and Legacy, Bausch & Lomb Millennium, and Advanced Medical Optics Sovereign phacoemulsification systems. *Am J Ophthalmol.*2006;142:3:387-392.

CHAPTER 31

Comparing Phaco Technologies in a Teaching Hospital

TAL RAVIV, MD

My affiliation with the New York Eye and Ear Infirmary in Manhattan, where I perform cataract surgery on my private practice patients and teach ophthalmology residents, has given me a unique opportunity to compare a wide range of phaco platforms. The Infirmary's ASC-like OR houses most of the current phaco machines, including the WhiteStar Signature Phacoemulsification System (Advanced Medical Optics, Inc., Santa Ana, CA), the Stellaris Vision Enhancement System, the Millennium Microsurgical System (both by Bausch & Lomb, Rochester, NY), and the INFINITI with OZil Torsional ultrasound (Alcon Laboratories, Inc., Fort Worth, TX). During the past 12 months, I have used and compared different machines almost weekly as I move between the facility's ORs. I do not find this burdensome; rather, I truly enjoy testing and optimizing the newest phaco technologies to benefit my patients. Furthermore, I am better able to demonstrate the latest technologies to the Infirmary's residents.

In general, new-generation machines continue to evolve the science of phacoemulsification. In the past 3 years, all of the platforms have benefited from improved fluidics that feature greater programmable settings, advanced sensors, low-compliance tubing, and overall improved efficiency. On the phaco energy side, power modulations such as hyperpulse with variable duty cycles have become standard, offering better followability, a safer thermal profile, and the ability for micro-incisional phacoemulsification. With traditional longitudinal ultrasound, these power modulations decrease chatter and improve surgical cutting efficiency.

TORSIONAL PHACO

Paradigm Shift

I believe that the most exciting advance in phaco energy delivery since manufacturers introduced modulated power is Alcon's INFINITI with OZil Torsional ultrasound. When the INFINITI was first introduced, I was also using the Millennium Microsurgical system and the Sovereign WhiteStar with ICE (Advanced Medical Optics, Inc.), and I thought all three systems were very good. I liked the speed, agility, and dual-linear control of the Millennium; its Venturi fluidics allowed for safe and efficient segment removal. The Sovereign's power modulations and occlusion mode did a lot of work behind the scenes to optimize phaco energy output. Admittedly, I was not initially enamored of this machine's nonlongitudinal technology. I thought the INFINITI with Torsional ultrasound was an excellent platform that worked well and had very good followability, but it did not particularly stand out to me.

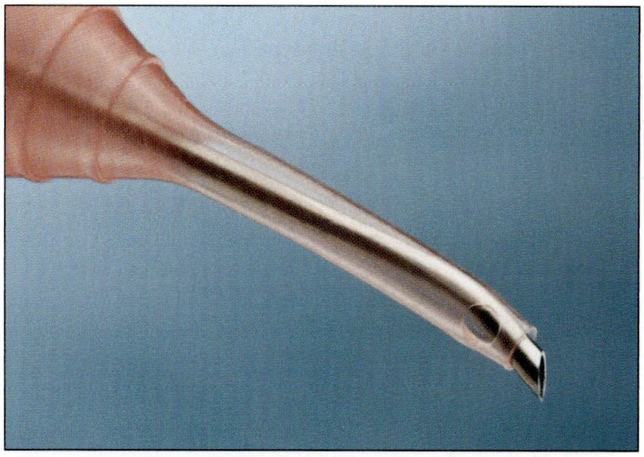

Figure 1. The Kelman 45° mini-flared tip enhances torsional cutting efficacy and puts torsional phaco "on steroids."

My opinion changed dramatically when I recently switched phaco tips from the standard 30° tapered to the newer 45° mini-flared tip (Alcon Laboratories, Inc.) (Figure 1). It is hard to believe what difference a tip can make, but the results were very positive.

"Extreme Nuclear Breakdown Efficiency"

Instead of pounding or hammering the nucleus head-on, the INFINITI's OZil tip oscillates side to side, creating a much more powerful shearing force. The wider angle of the 45° mini-flared tip

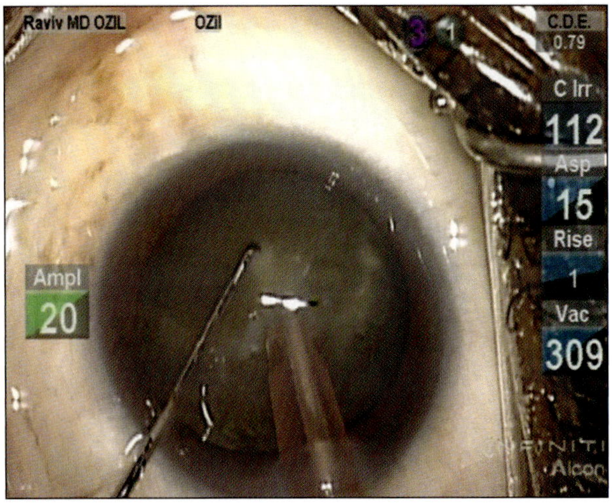

Figure 2. The author demonstrates a 2.2-mm quick-chop maneuver using OZil Torsional to impale the nucleus.

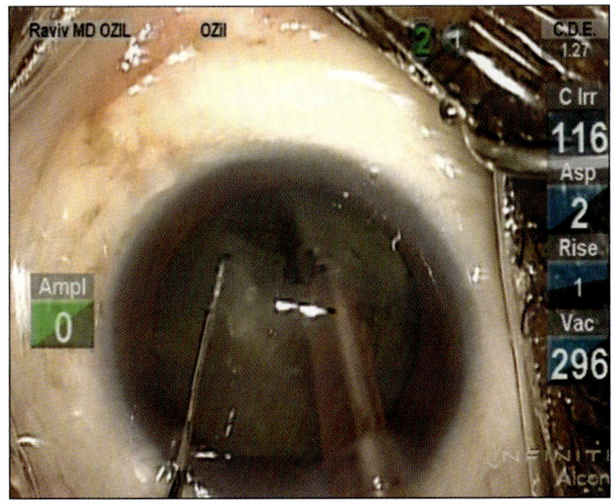

Figure 3. After occlusion with maximum vacuum, the author returns the torsional power to zero and chops the nucleus into two halves.

provides greater surface area contact for this shearing action, which creates extreme nuclear breakdown efficiency—even more than with the compressional force of longitudinal ultrasound.

The difference between the two forces can be illustrated by an unrelated example—a block of ice. In one scenario, a dense block of ice is easily broken down to ice crystals by an ice shaver. The alternative would be to break it into chunks with a hammer or ice pick. With the hand ice shaver, the block stays still as it is gently grated down. Conversely, with a hammer, the energy is distributed throughout the entire ice block, which shakes with each strike. Similarly, in the eye, torsional ultrasound minimizes chatter/repulsion, and the perfectly constructed and angled tip can actually cut more effectively than with longitudinal energy.

Clinically, without any meaningful repulsion, once a nuclear fragment nears the 45° Kelman tip, it just folds itself into the handpiece and disappears. Furthermore, whereas I experienced some clogging with the 30° tip, the 45° OZil tip does not become clogged; the surgeon simply moves it close to any nuclear piece, and it will attract, shear, and crumble material effortlessly. With such efficient nuclear breakdown, I find that I actually need less manipulation with my second instrument, which I normally utilize to reposition nuclear pieces at the tip. Torsional ultrasound actually requires less skill on the surgeon's part, because he or she does not have to emulsify around the edges of nuclear segments to avoid stagnation and clogging, the way we have learned to do with traditional longitudinal ultrasound.

Power Modulations Unnecessary

The efficiency of the INFINITI Torsional platform negates the need for power modulations, in my opinion. I love the power modulations such as hyperpulse, variable duty cycle, etc., that make longitudinal phacoemulsification more efficient. I expected the INFINITI console's power modulations to similarly enhance the torsional technology, but it actually slowed down phacoemulsification. The pulse action introduces a pause to the shearing process that is unnecessary and counterproductive to OZil's efficiency. The OZil Torsional technology is almost a new paradigm for phacoemulsification.

The 45° mini-flared tip not only provides increased surface area for torsional phacoemulsification to work, but also a larger amplitude of movement per oscillation. I consider the jump in performance from the OZil 30° tapered tip to the 45° mini-flared angled tip to be equal to the difference between traditional longitudinal and torsional phaco technology. It is just that dramatic.

Decreased Fluidic and Power Settings

I noticed that besides not needing hyperpulse, the OZil Torsional handpiece does not need high flow and vacuum rates. I was able to decrease these settings to approximately two thirds of what I had been using with longitudinal ultrasound without losing efficiency. This option is a tremendous benefit for surgeons, as it reduces total fluid usage in the eye and further lessens the chance of postocclusion surge, thus making the procedure safer and more efficient overall.

Since switching to the new tip, I have not had to mix in more than 5% longitudinal ultrasound to the torsional ultrasound. In fact, I have typically been using a maximum of 80% torsional power to emulsify 1 to 4+ nuclei. When I first used the system with the 30° tip, I programmed combination settings for nuclear densities of 1, 2 and 3, 4, but I have since found that I needed fewer settings. Now, my settings are for grades 1 and 4, and the latter mixes in about 5° longitudinal ultrasound. I recently scheduled a 5+NS black cataract that ordinarily I would not have dreamt of attempting with a pure torsional setting. The 45° mini-flared tip handled this cataract with aplomb, even without longitudinal ultrasound. Although it did take some patience, the tip did not get clogged, and the lens was safely emulsified—chatter free.

TECHNIQUE

Having always used a straight phaco tip with other platforms, switching to the angled Kelman 45° tip was my only minor learning curve with the INFINITI system. I now utilize it the same way as a straight tip. On occasion, if the eye's chamber is very shallow, I may turn the OZil handpiece on its side. I use one of two techniques, either a supracapsular or a quick-chop technique. Like divide-and-conquer, quick chop produces four nuclear quadrants, an approach in which torsional ultrasound excels in efficiency (Figures 2 and 3). In the supracapsular technique, which I use for soft and intermediate lenses, I skip the initial grooving and go right into emulsification (Figure 4). I have found that the OZil handpiece is very efficient in that technique as well.

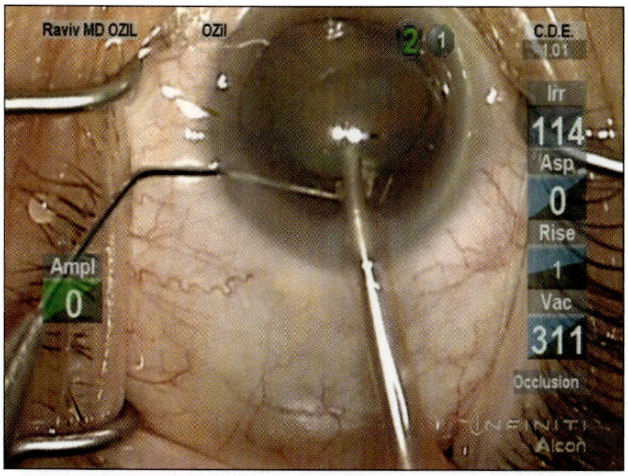

Figure 4. The author uses the Kelman 45° tip sideways in this shallow chamber at the start of a supracapsular technique.

Micro-Incisional Phaco

One other very important benefit to the 45° mini-flared tip is its ready adaptability to coaxial micro-incisional cataract surgery (C-MICS). By simply switching the traditional Micro sleeve to the Ultra sleeve (both from Alcon Laboratories, Inc.), surgeons can maintain all of the power and safety benefits of OZil through a 2.2-mm incision. The flared tip shaft design is constructed to allow maximum irrigation flow with the Ultra sleeve. I have used OZil with C-MICS with excellent results, without needing to change my vacuum or flow settings. I simply increase my bottle height for the 2.2-mm incision to maximize irrigation flow. Practically speaking, there is minimal-to-no learning curve when switching from 2.75-mm phacoemulsification.

Certainly, aside from the benefits of OZil, micro-incisional cataract surgery is the clear future direction of phacoemulsification. With 2.2-mm surgery, we can achieve a more minimally invasive procedure with less astigmatism, less iris prolapse, and maybe even a slightly lower risk of endophthalmitis. The ability to match a full spectrum of IOLs through the micro-incision, including aspheric, toric, and presbyopic lenses, makes the Alcon platform currently a leader in C-MICS in the US.

CONCLUSION

Torsional phacoemulsification, especially with the 45° mini-flared tip, represents a significant advancement in phaco energy delivery. Although I continue to use the Stellaris and the Signature and enjoy the unique attributes of the differing technologies, OZil changes the paradigm. Simply said, it makes phaco surgery easier, and by allowing lower fluidic and power settings, it also increases surgical safety. ■

This article originally appeared in CRSToday's *April 2008 supplement.*

CHAPTER 32

The Stellaris Vision Enhancement System

TERENCE M. DEVINE, MD

With its new Stellaris Vision Enhancement System (FDA approved, commercial launch in United States planned for April 2007) (Figure 1), Bausch & Lomb (Rochester, NY) has designed an integrated phaco platform with advanced technology and precise instrumentation that will facilitate surgeons' transition to the newer microincisional phaco techniques. The system's unique fluidics, power modulation, and precise controls are optimized for any of three phaco approaches: standard coaxial; bimanual sleeveless microincisional; and microcoaxial (through a 1.8-mm incision).

ABOUT THE SYSTEM

When I joined the Stellaris development team 3 years ago, our goal was to imagine and build the phaco machine of the future. To that end, we solicited input from 200 ophthalmic surgeons and 40 nurses worldwide. The resultant phaco platform has an array of high-tech capabilities and a modular design that will allow easy upgrading in the future.

The Stellaris also addresses some practical issues that the survey respondents said impeded surgical efficiency with earlier phaco machines. For instance, the system's wireless foot control reduces clutter in the OR and is responsive and precise. A six-crystal titanium handpiece is small, light, and shaped to avoid fatiguing the surgeon's hand. A locking infusion line connector means no surprise disconnection during surgery and thus prevents a loss of infusion and the chamber's collapse.

Surgeons may choose either vacuum- or flow-based fluidics. The totally electric system for vacuum-based fluidics exceeds the performance of Bausch & Lomb's Venturi system and no longer requires external compressed gases. In addition, the Stellaris features improved fluidics sensing and control, which permit the use of vacuum as high as 600 mm Hg. Optional high-vacuum, flow-resistant tubing incorporates a mesh filter to capture lenticular particles larger than 0.3 mm before they can reach the lumen of the evacuation line. The tubing thus maintains the chamber's stability.

The Stellaris features advanced power modulations with hyper-pulse settings of up to 250 pulses per second and duty cycles with on times as low as 2 milliseconds. Square-wave and waveform modulation may be used with the pulse or burst mode.

The system's 18-inch, high-resolution screen with advanced graphic and animated displays is intuitive to use and designed to enhance operational efficiency. An optional window on the screen shows real-time video of the surgery and thus eliminates the need for a second monitor for the surgeon's assistant. The Stellaris' internal modularity facilitates upgrades and speeds technical service, and the system has an online capability for diagnostics or preventative maintenance.

THE NEEDLE AND SLEEVE

One year after joining the Stellaris design team, I began a parallel project working on the new needle and sleeve combination that would be optimal for microcoaxial phacoemulsification. My initial experiences with the Stellaris and a prototypic sub–2-mm needle/sleeve combination suggested that the microcoaxial approach might be a simple, easily learned way for surgeons to transition to using smaller incisions. Unlike with bimanual sleeveless microincisional surgery, I could not discern any difference from my standard coaxial cases.

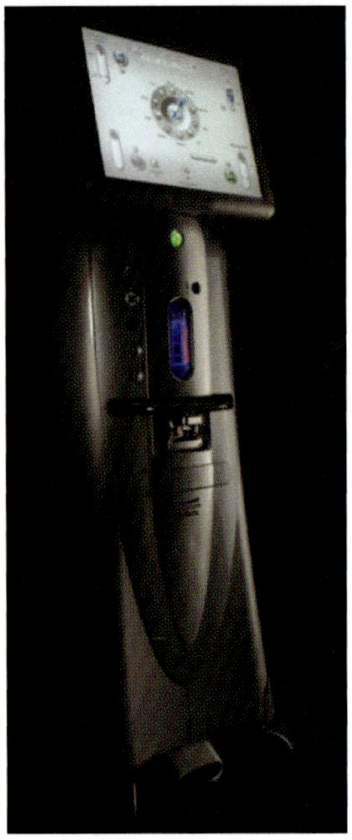

Figure 1. The Stellaris Vision Enhancement System.

Our aims were as follows. We wanted to eliminate the learning curve for surgeons transitioning to microincisional phacoemulsification. We also wanted to make the microcoaxial method compatible with any surgical technique (eg, chopping, divide and conquer, phaco flip, supracapsular phacoemulsification). In addition, we wanted to make microcoaxial surgery compatible with either high or low flow and high or low vacuum, according to the surgeon's preference. Finally, we sought to eliminate the need for excessively high or pressurized infusion bottles.

Using computer-modeling software, we determined the minimum needle lumen that could maintain excellent followability, vacuum holding force, and aspiration. Then, we reduced the thickness of the needle's wall while preserving the instrument's structural integrity. Next, we modeled the minimum clearance needed between the needle and sleeve to deliver a safe volume of infusion in high-vacuum cases. The sleeve's wall was thinned, and its ports were redesigned to deliver more infusion laterally for improved followability at the needle's tip.

On October 30, 2006, I performed the first eight human phaco procedures with the Stellaris. Half were microcoaxial cases using a needle/sleeve of the computer-optimized design (Figure 2). I performed two of the microcoaxial cases with flow-restrictive tubing and vacuum of 600 mm Hg. I performed the other six cases (four coaxial, two microcoaxial) at 300 mm Hg vacuum. The bottle's height was 125 cm for all eight cases. I performed cortical cleanup through the 1.8-mm incision with a standard 0.3-mm I/A handpiece fit with a microcoaxial sleeve. There was excellent chamber stability using linear vacuum of up to 600 mm Hg. Measurements of all the incisions after I/A revealed no stretching. The new machine and needle performed flawlessly. There were no complications, and all surgical parameters were evaluated as excellent.

CONCLUSION

With the Stellaris, surgeons have the option of choosing microcoaxial phacoemulsification as a simple alternative to bimanual sleeveless surgery. I myself favor the microcoaxial approach to

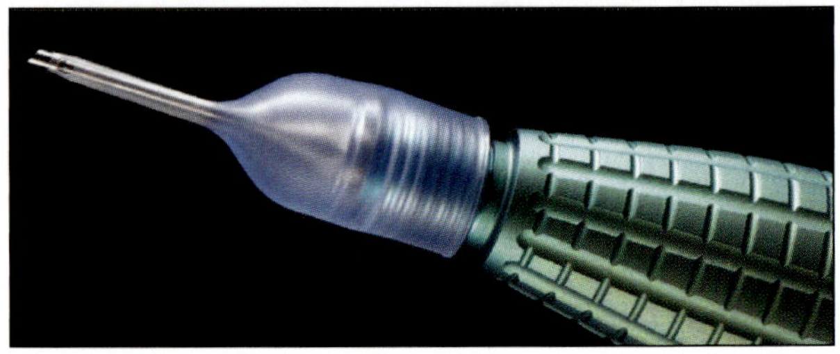

Figure 2. The Stellaris' needle and sleeve were optimized for microcoaxial phacoemulsification.

sub–2-mm surgery, because it offers the advantages of a smaller sideport incision (0.5 mm or less), a sleeve-protected needle, and less incisional stress and distortion than bimanual sleeveless surgery.[1] These factors are all important to improving the seal of the incision and potentially reducing the risk of postoperative leakage and endophthalmitis.

It is noteworthy that the ASCRS white paper in September 2006 discussed the association between clear corneal incisions and postoperative endophthalmitis. The paper's authors concluded that wound architecture is the most significant potential risk factor.[2] Paul Ernest, MD, had earlier demonstrated that square tunnel incisions are more resistant to deformation and leakage than rectangular tunnels.[3] Stress placed on the incision during surgery might prevent the tight closure of a clear corneal wound, which could allow contaminants and bacteria to enter the eye. One study by Mikhail Boukhny, MD, showed that a sleeveless phaco needle produces five-and-a-half times more stress on the incision than one with a sleeve.[1] In addition, the ASCRS white paper noted that the sideport incision must also be recognized as a possible source of contamination.[2] With bimanual sleeveless phacoemulsification, this wound is usually approximately 1.5 mm long and is subject to stress from the infusion chopper.

Microcoaxial phacoemulsification eliminates many of the aforementioned concerns. A 1.8-mm clear corneal incision results in a square tunnel through which it is easy to work. In addition, the infusion sleeve minimizes stress on the incision, thereby improving its seal and eliminating the need for a separate incision for the IOL. Finally, the surgeon may construct the sideport incision as a 0.5-mm square, and it will not be subjected to stress, because choppers or nucleus rotators may be made smaller if they do not need to deliver infusion. Compared with bimanual sleeveless phacoemulsification, I also find that the microcoaxial instruments are easier to maneuver in the eye, and I have greater flexibility in my choice of technique and fluidics.

As more surgeons have an opportunity to evaluate the Stellaris microcoaxial platform, the development of many alternative fluidics settings and power modulations is likely, and they should further improve patients' safety and surgical outcomes. ■

This article originally appeared in the March 2007 issue of CRSToday.

1. Boukhny M. Incision stress comparison in conventional microincision cataract surgery and coaxial phacoemulsification. Paper presented: The ASCRS/ASOA 2005 Symposium & Congress; April 19, 2005; Washington, DC.
2. Nichamin LD, Chang DF, Johnson SH, et al; American Society of Cataract and Refractive Surgery Cataract Clinical Committee. ASCRS White Paper: what is the association between clear corneal cataract incisions and postoperative endophthalmitis? *J Cataract Refract Surg.* 2006;32:1556-1559.
3. ErnestÊP, KiesslingÊLA, LaveryÊKT. Relative strength of cataract incisions in cadaver eyes. *J Cataract Refract Surg.* 1991;17:668–671.

CHAPTER 33

Whitestar Signature With Fusion Fluidics

WILLIAM J. FISHKIND, MD

I strive to preserve the safest and most stable surgical environment for my patients. For that reason, I am always eager to test new phaco technologies. In general, the trends in this area are focused on using less energy with more power modulations. Lowering the amount of energy entering the anterior chamber during surgery decreases the chances of damaging the blood/aqueous barrier and reduces postoperative inflammation. Upgrades to the Infiniti Vision System (Alcon Laboratories, Inc., Fort Worth, TX), the Millennium microsurgical system (Bausch & Lomb, Rochester, NY), and the Sovereign with Whitestar technology (Advanced Medical Optics, Inc., Santa Ana, CA) push toward preocclusion phacoemulsification, the ability to emulsify the nucleus without occlusion.

Recently, I have had the opportunity to work with the Whitestar Signature System with Fusion Fluidics (Advanced Medical Optics, Inc.) (Figure 1). I have found it easy to use and customize, and the unit optimizes intraoperative safety to help maximize surgical outcomes. The system features a number of significant improvements on the original unit. A notable example is the Fusion Dual Pump Fluidic system, which provides improved irrigation and higher flow and vacuum capabilities under the control of the company's proprietary Occlusion Mode and Advanced Chamber Stabilization Environment (CASE) technology. These functions work together to better stabilize the anterior chamber. Details on the Whitestar Signature System with Fusion Fluidics follow.

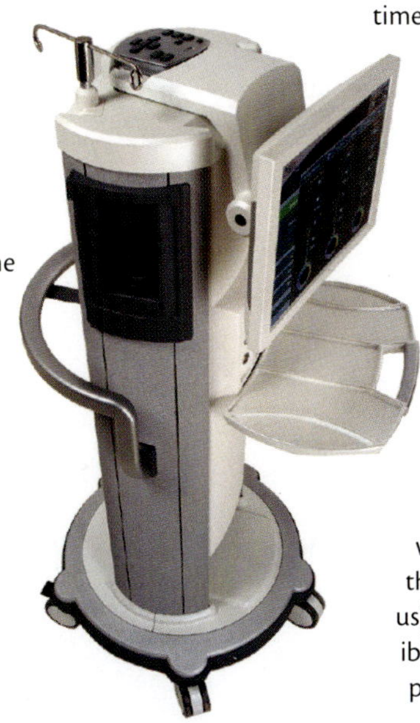

Figure 1. The Whitestar Signature System with Fusion Fluidics.

FUSION FLUIDICS AND ADVANCED CASE TECHNOLOGY

Micropulsed phaco technology can be programmed to halt occlusion surge, which causes a sudden shallowing of the anterior chamber that may lead to tears in the capsule and vitreous face. I consistently perform phaco procedures that use preocculusion phacoemulsification, because it increases safety. The upgrades of the Whitestar Signature System are of significant help in this area. The machine sets limits over parameters the surgeon could not control previously. For example, by eliminating inadvertent occlusion, the Advanced CASE technology protects the anterior chamber. Designed for enhanced chamber stability, this automatic control monitors vacuum during phacoemulsification and gives surgeons the ability to choose their occlusion threshold and adjust it as needed. I can vary my rise times individually and change the timing on the pump to speed up or slow down to suit the surgery. During phacoemulsification, the Advanced CASE function actually reduces vacuum when occlusion occurs, maintains particle-holding power, and resets the maximum vacuum when occlusion ceases.

What I find particularly beneficial about the Advanced CASE technology is that it is easy to use during surgery. I can select the threshold where it begins to function and the duration of time for occlusion to occur as well as when the vacuum will drop and for how long. Using the four variable settings, I can set the technology for the parameters that work best for me and customize the surgery to the circumstances (eg, dense cataract, dark nucleus). Advanced CASE technology offers me the flexibility necessary to accommodate the cataract, the patient, and my own surgical technique.

NEWLY DESIGNED PUMPS

New pumps on phaco systems are what I call *hybrids.* The Whitestar Signature System is the only phaco platform that allows the surgeon to use a peristaltic or a Venturi pump, a choice that provides flexibility during surgery. The phaco machine's aspiration capabilities include a peristaltic flow of up to 60 mL/min, a peristaltic maximum vacuum of 650 mm Hg, and a Venturi vacuum of up to 600 mm Hg. In addition, the Whitestar Signature System features

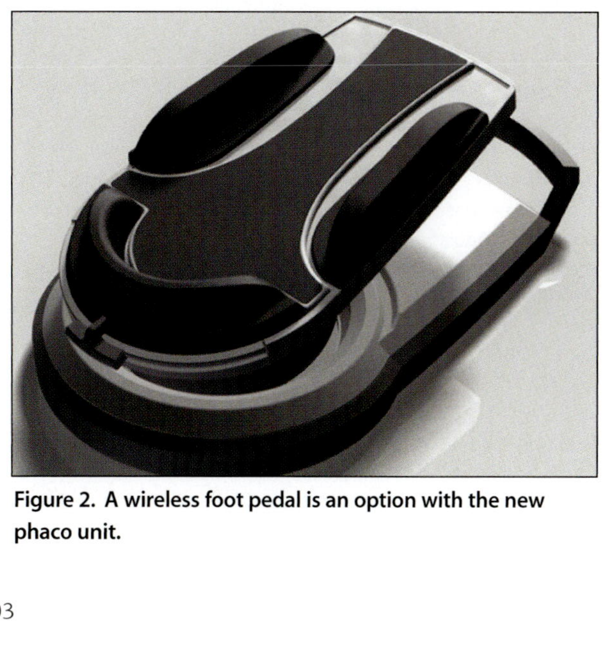

Figure 2. A wireless foot pedal is an option with the new phaco unit.

improved irrigation with a bottle height of up to 106 cm without extension.

Thus far, I have found the unit's Fusion Fluidics pumps to be quite responsive. They demonstrate strong tuning and more recognition of internal fluctuations in pressure compared with the Sovereign cataract extraction system (Advanced Medical Optics, Inc.). The processing unit of the machine provides a virtual representation of the internal chamber, recognizes changes in vacuum and flow, and makes continuous adjustments accordingly.

ADDITIONAL FEATURES

I have found moving between menus on the Whitestar Signature System's touch screen to be user friendly and simple, and the wireless foot pedal (Figure 2) reduces the number of cords below the operating table. In addition, the system primes quickly, which saves a significant amount of time in surgery. Overall, I find the system to be much easier to use than many other phaco machines because of its intuitive operation and extensive number of individualized options.

CONCLUSION

Modifications to the original Whitestar platform have improved procedural efficiency and lessened the amount of power delivered to the anterior segment. The benefits of the Whitestar Signature System include enhanced stability of the anterior chamber, a lower incidence of torn posterior capsules and other complications, and improved outcomes. ■

This article originally appeared in the March 2007 issue of CRSToday.

CHAPTER 34

Power Modulations Come of Age

TAL RAVIV, MD

After a decade of fluidic advancements such as enhanced pump function, anterior chamber pressure sensing, less compliant tubing, and microprocessor controls, new digitally driven, rapidly cycling, and programmable microbursts of phacoemulsification have heralded the age of the power modulations. First introduced by Advanced Medical Optics, Inc. (Santa Ana, CA), on its Sovereign cataract extraction system with Whitestar Technology in 2001, advanced power modulations such as hyperpulse technology have recently been adapted by both Alcon Laboratories, Inc. (Fort Worth, TX), in its new Infiniti system and by Bausch & Lomb (Rochester, NY) for the Millennium microsurgical system's Custom Control Software (CCS) upgrade.

By rapidly cycling micropulses of phaco energy with variable duty cycles, the surgeon gains three key advantages: (1) better phaco efficiency, the ability to achieve the same cutting power with less total phaco energy; (2) a decreased heat buildup and risk of thermal injury; and (3) enhanced followability with less chatter due to the better balance between phaco repelling forces and the flow/vacuum attractive forces. These three factors allow for a better, safer cataract surgery, and they are responsible for surgeons' recent movement toward bimanual microincisional phacoemulsification.

A byproduct of the novel power modes is new, sometimes confusing nomenclature. This article attempts to clarify what the newest power modulations mean, what they actually do, and how those of different systems compare.

THE BASICS

Continuous phacoemulsification preceded traditional pulse, which was followed by burst mode and then hyperpulse with a variable duty cycle. The way to understand these modes is to break each one down to its basics. Aside from continuous phacoemulsification, all of the power modes are essentially combinations of phaco-on periods followed by phaco-off periods. The percentage of phaco-on time to total time is called the *duty cycle.*

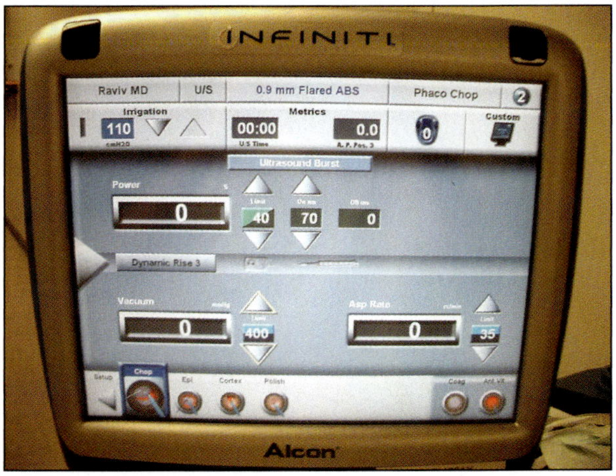

Figure 1. The Infiniti's phaco chop memory setting is programmed to linear power burst mode.

PULSE

With traditional pulse (which in the original software of all three platforms was limited to a maximum of 10 to 20 pulses per second), the duty cycle was fixed at 50%. A setting of four pulses per second therefore meant that each pulse interval was 250 milliseconds long, comprising a 125-millisecond phaco-on and 125-millisecond phaco-off period. Increasing the pulse rate to 10 would decrease the pulse interval to 100 milliseconds (50 milliseconds phaco-on and 50 milliseconds phaco-off). No matter the pulse setting (from two to the previous limit of 20), the phaco power was always on 50% of the time (a 50% duty cycle). With pulse mode chosen, foot position three on the footswitch controlled linear power with a fixed phaco-on and phaco-off interval.

BURST MODE

Burst mode was the first power modulation to indirectly allow variation of the duty cycle. In traditional burst mode, the phaco-

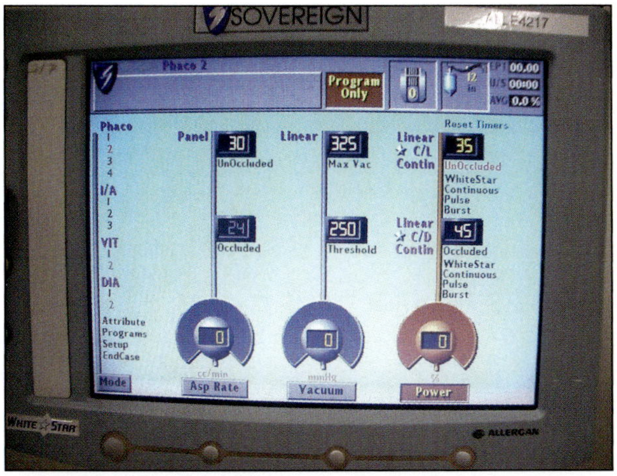

Figure 2. Occlusion mode on the Sovereign allows for automatic shifting to a second group of settings once a preset threshold vacuum is reached.

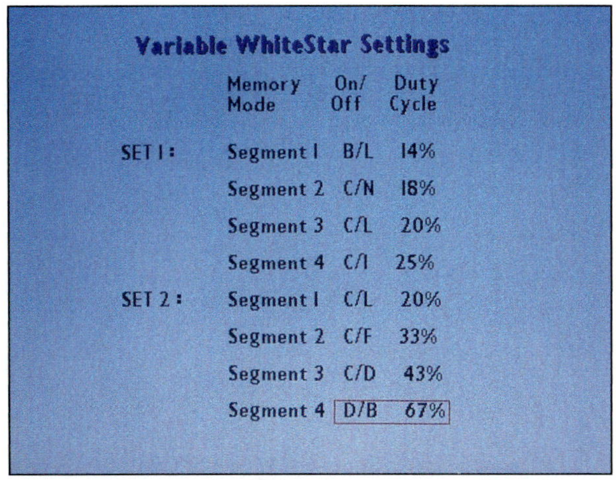

Figure 3. The Sovereign Whitestar 6.0 software allows the surgeon to cycle through preset duty cycles by depressing the foot pedal.

on time is preset, and the phaco-off time was linearly controlled or decreased with foot position three. Phaco power remained constant in all positions of foot position three. For example, the Millennium's CCS software allows the surgeon to set a phaco-on period of between 4 and 600 milliseconds. The phaco-off time is variably controlled with foot position three. Starting at the beginning of foot position three, the cycle interval becomes progressively shorter than 1,200 milliseconds as the pedal is depressed. At full pedal excursion, the phaco-off period goes to zero, and the equivalent of continuous phacoemulsification is achieved. Burst mode fixes the phaco power and phaco-on time but effectively allows the surgeon to vary the duty cycle. If, for example, the burst-mode phaco-on time is preset to 300 milliseconds, then the duty cycle goes from 25% (300 milliseconds phaco-on with 900 milliseconds phaco-off) at the top of foot position three all the way to 100% at full foot pedal depression.

PREPROGRAMMED POWER MODES

On all three companies' systems, the newest hyperpulse power modulations allow surgeons to choose variable duty cycles as well as newer pulse settings of 100 pulses per second and beyond. By preprogramming different combinations of settings, ophthalmologists can employ unique power modulations for different lens densities or disassembly techniques. For example, one may approach soft nuclei with lower overall phaco energy settings such as a power of 30%, a frequency of 60 pulses per second, and a low duty cycle of 10% to 40%. Hard nuclei can be approached with 40% power, 30 pulses per second, and a duty cycle of 40% to 50%.

Similarly, different power modulations are advantageous for different stages of the procedure. Continuous mode works best for sculpting, in which low vacuum settings and a stationary, in-the-bag lens are present. By contrast, short, higher-powered microbursts of energy coupled with longer phaco-off periods avoid repulsion and achieve good impaling ability during quick chopping, which employs high vacuum and requires rapid, strong occlusion (Figure 1). For quadrant removal or other supracapsular techniques, followability is critical and can be enhanced by using a hyperpulse setting in the 50- to 100-pulses-per-second range, with a 25% to 40% duty cycle. Minimizing the percentage of ultrasound and allowing more rapid cycling between the phaco-on and phaco-off periods decreases the repulsive forces and allows the forces of fluidic attraction to predominate. This type of setting creates so-called *magnetic followability*, which minimizes chatter and wasted phaco energy. Many surgeons feel that hyperpulse mode enhances the efficiency of cavitation by preventing the wasteful buildup of cavitation bubbles on top of each other as occurs in continuous mode.

OCCLUSION MODE

Another power modulation, again first introduced by Advanced Medical Optics, Inc., is occlusion mode, which is now also available on the Infiniti (although Advanced Medical Optics, Inc., is seeking an injunction against the phaco power occlusion mode offered by Alcon Laboratories, Inc.). This technology, currently available only with the peristaltic pump (not the Millennium's venturi pump), allows the application of different phaco settings before and after tip occlusion.

On the Sovereign, an occlusion threshold vacuum setting can be programmed that will automatically switch phaco parameters. For example, if the vacuum level is 325 mm Hg, the surgeon can set a threshold vacuum level of 250 mm Hg, which when reached would automatically change to new settings. Typically, postocclusion settings should have a higher Whitestar duty cycle, a higher maximum power, and a lower aspiration flow rate. In Figure 2, power increases from 35% to 45%, the Whitestar duty cycle increases from CL (20%) to CD (43%) (the two-letter nomenclature is explained later), and aspiration flow is decreased from 30 to 24 mL/min. Once a nuclear fragment occludes the port, thus causing the vacuum to rise and exceed the predetermined threshold, the machine switches to more phaco power for greater cutting efficacy and decreases the flow rate to avoid a postocclusion surge. After the occlusion is cleared, the vacuum level drops, and the settings return to their original lower level.

Care must be taken not to increase the power and duty cycle too high in postocclusion mode. Because the tip is occluded and flow is minimal or zero, the tip can heat up very rapidly, potentially causing tissue damage.

The Infiniti system's occlusion mode differs somewhat. Instead

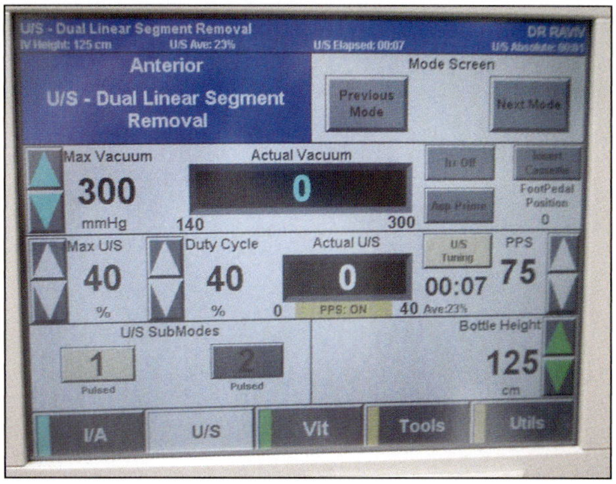

Figure 4. The Millennium's CCS software allows for an adjustable duty cycle, hyperpulse settings of up to 120 pulses per second, and the use of submodes.

of just relying on a threshold vacuum level, it uses a sophisticated algorithm based on irrigation pressure and aspiration vacuum to determine occlusion onset and full occlusion. The Infiniti's postocclusion settings, however, are limited—only allowing for a reduction of power, not the more logical increase in power or duty cycle.

COMPARING THE THREE SYSTEMS

Infiniti

Alcon Laboratories, Inc., increased the maximum pulse rate from 15 pulses per second on its Legacy machine to 100 pulses per second on the Infiniti (a software upgrade to the Legacy called *Everest* allows similar settings). Furthermore, the surgeon can now set the pulse duty cycle (formerly fixed at 50%) from 5% to 95%. This change gives the surgeon predictable and complete control over all phaco-on and phaco-off parameters.

The company also enhanced traditional burst mode (named *fixed burst* on the Infiniti) with linear burst. In this mode, the phaco-on interval is fixed (from 5 to 500 milliseconds), and the phaco-off time—as well as the phaco power—is linearly controlled with the foot pedal (Figure 1). This change allows a dual step-up of duty cycle and phaco power as the surgeon depresses foot position three.

Moreover, the Infiniti system offers the company's proprietary Neosonix technology, which allows for additional sonic oscillatory energy to be added to the ultrasound. Neosonix can now be applied in hyperpulse or any of the burst modes.

Sovereign With Whitestar

Unlike the Infiniti, which allows for numerous combinations of pulse frequency and duty cycle, Whitestar Technology has 10 preset hyperpulse/duty cycle settings from which to choose. The different settings are defined by the fixed period of phaco-on and phaco-off intervals. Advanced Medical Optics, Inc., has clinically validated and chosen the 10 settings to represent a manageable range of options.

Trying to compare the Whitestar settings with the hyperpulse settings of the Infiniti or Millennium can be confusing, due to the different nomenclature used by Advanced Medical Optics, Inc. For example, the lowest duty cycle setting on Whitestar alternates 4 milliseconds of phaco-on followed by 24 milliseconds of phaco-off. The highest duty cycle phaco setting has 8 milliseconds of phaco-on with 4 milliseconds of phaco off. The company uses a two-letter nomenclature for each setting; the letter's order in the alphabet represents a 2-millisecond multiple in time. The first letter represents the phaco-on period, and the second letter the phaco-off. In the first example just given, the setting is dubbed *BL*. *B* is the second letter of the alphabet, and multiplying two by 2 milliseconds yields 4 milliseconds of on time. *L* is the 12th letter, and multiplying 12 by 2 milliseconds represents the 24 milliseconds of off time. The second example is named *DB* (*D* as 4th letter times 2 milliseconds equals 8 milliseconds of on time, and *B* signifies 4 milliseconds of off time).

Some simple calculations are necessary to express the Whitestar BL mode in terms of pulses per second and duty cycle—the adjustable variables on the Infiniti and the Millennium's CCS. With 4 milliseconds on and 24 milliseconds off, the duty cycle is 14% (four divided by 28 equals 0.142), and the pulse frequency is 36 pulses per second (1,000 milliseconds divided by an interval length of 28 milliseconds). Likewise, the DB setting can be mimicked on the other machines with settings of 83 pulses per second and a 67% duty cycle.

The Sovereign allows surgeons to layer one of the 10 preset Whitestar hyperpulse modes on top of a traditional pulse mode called *long pulse*. In other words, a slow, fixed, 75% duty cycle long pulse of five pulses per second (with 150 milliseconds phaco-on and 50 milliseconds phaco-off) is further modulated by having the phaco-on portion comprise hyperpulses instead of continuous phacoemulsification. Combining a Whitestar setting with a long-pulse setting effectively reduces the Whitestar duty cycle by 25%, thus further decreasing the buildup of heat.

The recent 6.0 software upgrade includes the latest power modulation, called *variable Whitestar*. In this mode, the surgeon can customize a set of four different Whitestar settings to be cycled through with depression of the foot pedal in position three (Figure 3). For example, the beginning of foot position three can be set with a low duty cycle mode such as CL (20% duty cycle), and progressive depression can shift to modes CF (33%), CD (43%), and DB (67%). This setup allows the surgeon a bimodal linear increase in phaco power and duty cycle with foot pedal depression so that he may enhance cutting efficiency and total phaco energy when needed. During microincisional phacoemulsification, a set of lower duty cycle settings may be chosen, as seen in set 1 of Figure 3. Keeping the duty cycle below 33% greatly limits the buildup of heat.

Millennium With CCS

The CCS upgrade allows the surgeon to preprogram hyperpulse settings in three modes: hyperpulse; fixed burst; and multiple burst. Multiple burst mode is similar to traditional burst mode (described earlier); the phaco-on time and phaco power are fixed, and the phaco-off time is controlled with the foot pedal. One little modification is the ability to set the maximum (full foot pedal depression) duty cycle at between 50% and 100%, as opposed to traditional burst mode, which is fixed at 100% continuous phacoemulsification at maximal excursion. This capability is useful during bimanual phacoemulsification, where the duty cycle is best kept below 50% to lessen heat.

The new hyperpulse mode is set similarly to the Infiniti's, with a pulse rate of up to 120 pulses per second and an adjustable duty cycle of between 10% and 90% (Figure 4). What is termed *fixed burst mode* on the Millennium's CCS is analogous to the Whitestar method of describing the hyperpulse setting. In this mode, the surgeon sets fixed phaco-on and phaco-off intervals (each is independently set at between 4 and 600 milliseconds). The pulse intervals stay fixed, with linear power control in foot position three. Unlike the 10 preprogrammed combination settings of Whitestar, the Millennium's CCS offers thousands of potential combinations. Again, it is important to realize that, on the Millennium, hyperpulse mode and fixed burst mode can achieve identical phaco-on/off settings—just expressed in different terms.

The Millennium's CCS has personalized "submodes" that allow surgeons to toggle between different preset duty cycle and hyperpulse settings. While in foot position two, the surgeon can kick left to change to a higher duty cycle and pulse rate for a particularly dense piece of nucleus. Up to three different submodes can be programmed per memory setting. The system's proprietary dual-linear foot pedal already allows the surgeon separate linear control of both phaco energy and vacuum. The new submodes are another means of adjusting the duty cycle with the foot pedal.

CONCLUSION

Overall, the newest power modulations add more complexity and sophistication to current phaco systems. Understanding the terminology and properly setting up the new modes are critical to maximizing phaco success. With more efficient energy use, enhanced followability, and better thermal safety, power modulations enhance the surgical experience and outcomes for physicians and patients alike. ■

This article originally appeared in the January 2005 issue of CRSToday.

CHAPTER 35

The Advantages of a Rounded Tip

STEVEN H. DEWEY, MD

For about 1 year, I have had a secret weapon to assist me in refractive lens exchange. I have specifically rounded both the inner and outer edges of the distal tip of a standard, 30° Kelman 19-gauge phaco tip for use in coaxial phacoemulsification. No changes have been made in either my technique or the phaco machine's parameters. For refractive lens exchange, the advantages of a tip without sharp edges are tremendous. Perhaps surprising is how effective the rounded phaco tip (Microsurgical Technology, Redmond, WA) is at removing even dense cataracts.

TESTING A THEORY

My first success in improving capsular safety came in 1993. I began using a J-cannula to flush cortex from regions of poor visualization, especially the subincisional space. This technique avoids the notorious "vacuum break" when I/A occludes the aspirating tip. In April 2001, I tested the efficiency of a J-cannula for irrigating cortex from the subincisional space with the expert assistance of David Apple, MD; Liliana Werner, MD, PhD; Suresh Pandey, MD; and several others at the Storm Eye Institute in Charleston, South Carolina. In three of the Miyake-Apple specimen eyes, I purposefully latched onto the capsule with the J-cannula while aspirating as firmly as I could with a 5-mL syringe. I simply occluded the tip with the capsule while applying aggressive aspiration to the plunger and then dragged the fully occluded tip across the capsule. Despite this aggressive force, the cannula did not break the capsule, and manipulating the cannula did not visibly disrupt the zonules. I reasoned that capsular damage in similar situations requires a cutting feature or effect such as a sharp edge, a simple burr, or cavitation.

POWER MODULATIONS

Micropulses and Cavitation

Approximately 3 years ago, micropulsed phaco technology became available. It is effective at removing a nucleus with less power than previous technologies for many reasons. First, within each duty cycle, the millisecond off periods or rests allow heat to dissipate. Second, these off periods improve the anterior chamber's stability by decreasing the chatter occurring with a nuclear fragment against a phaco tip that is always on. Third, the microbursts of ultrasound create transient cavitation, an effect described by Mark Schafer, PhD,[1] and found to deliver more energy than the stable cavitation created by continuous power.

Despite continuing controversy, I feel the evidence[2] supports cavitation as a major factor in dismantling the nucleus into fragments small enough for efficient aspiration. Although many would dismiss cavitation as secondary to the physical effects of the titanium needle itself, cavitation is a mechanism that erodes ships' propellers and destroys the inner workings of pumps. The multifactorial effects of ultrasound at the end of the phaco needle will make the isolation of a single component a challenge. These microscopic explosions undoubtedly play a significant role in nuclear removal, especially at higher phaco powers for dense nuclei.

I had the idea of rounding the edges of the phaco needle to improve procedural safety with an expected cost of decreased cutting efficiency.

Phaco Technique and Outcomes

I conducted a study in 2002 that compared a form of chopping to a divide-and-conquer approach for nuclear removal.[3] Whether it was a 2+ or 3+ nucleus (on a scale of 1+ to 4+), the chopping technique used only one-third the power of the divide-and-conquer approach. The former reduced my case time by 1 full minute. I was surprised at how many lenses of 2+ nuclear sclerosis vacuum alone could remove and by how many lenses that I had graded clear or 1+ required power for removal, despite their clinical appearance at the slit lamp.

One day postoperatively, patients in the phaco-chop group had clearer corneas, and I felt the micropulsed technology had contributed significantly to these results. After 1 week, however, the two groups of patients were indistinguishable.

As other clinicians and researchers had noted, power usage in phacoemulsification was safe within a rather large range, and less-

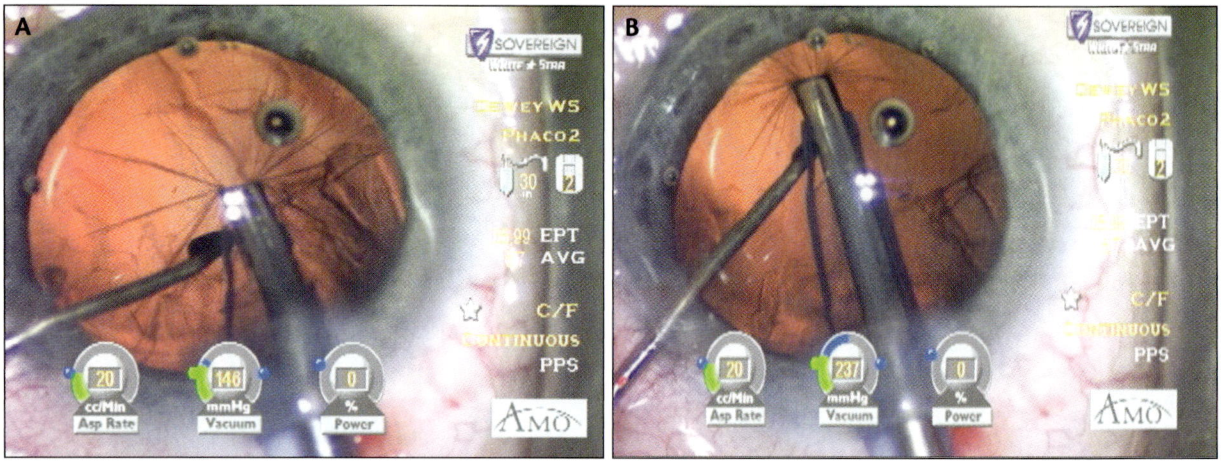

Figure 1. Earlier in the case, Dr. Dewey accidentally aspirated the capsule into the lumen of the rounded needle without incident. Here, he deliberately aspirates the capsule into the lumen of the needle at 146 mm Hg without damage (A). Later in the case, the rounded tip aspirates the posterior capsule and capsulorhexis' edge at 237 mm Hg without damage (B).

ening power simply for the purpose of reducing it did not necessarily improve surgical outcomes, except in the short term. It was then that I had the idea of rounding the edges of the needle to improve procedural safety at a modest cost to efficiency due to decreased phaco power. These results confirmed for me that a modest increase in power (eg, from decreasing cutting efficiency by rounding the phaco needle) was unlikely to lessen the safety of phacoemulsification for the patient.

RESULTS TO DATE

Since July 2004, I have performed well over 500 cases with the rounded tip, and the difference in power usage compared with a sharp tip has been virtually unnoticeable. As I had observed before, several lenses that I had considered to be clear at the slit lamp required phaco power for their removal. Other patients' cataracts required less power than I had expected.

Moving from refractive lens exchange into the true cataract category, I found no difference in power usage for 2+ nuclear sclerosis whether I used a rounded or a sharp tip. For 3+ cataracts, the differences in power are a bit more apparent, with the sharp tip being 20% to 30% more efficient.

BENEFITS OF A ROUNDED TIP

The advantages of a phaco needle with a rounded tip are more than theoretical. With passive contact, this tip has no sharp edge that can damage the ocular structures it touches—whether the iris, the capsule, or the incision. Occasionally during insertion, a sharply edged needle may catch on the internal structure of the incision. This problem is less frequent with a rounded needle. Of greater significance, incidental contacts of the rounded tip with the anterior capsule or capsulotomy's edge have not yet resulted in a radial tear of the anterior capsule.

During surgery, the rounded tip has grabbed both the iris and capsule during aspiration and left no signs of damage to either. At first, I incidentally aspirated the capsule while going after residual cortex without damaging the capsule. Since then, I have purposefully aspirated the capsule into the needle during a handful of cases without resulting damage (Figures 1 and 2). I thus confirmed my earlier work on cadaveric eyes and dispelled (for me, at least) the myth of the vacuum break due to a fundamental weakness in the average capsule. Of course, capsules do not all have the same

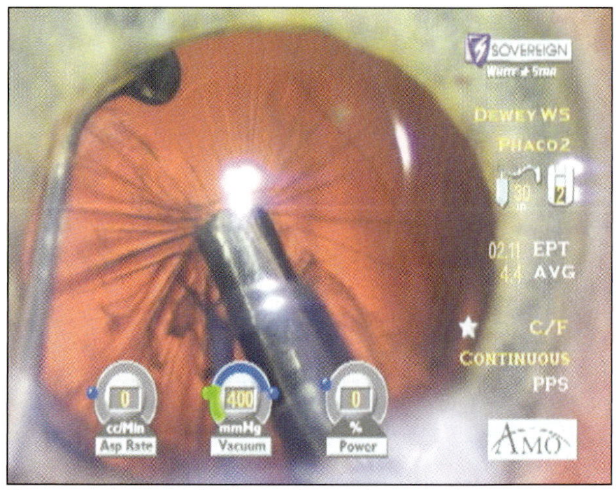

Figure 2. A 0° rounded tip aspirates the capsule to a maximum of 400 mm Hg without damage.

intrinsic strength, and zonules are not all equally resilient. Based on my experience, however, I think of the rounded edge as I think of my bicycle helmet. The margin of safety either one provides me with amply merits its use. I certainly do not test the safety of the rounded tip on every capsule, just as I do not test my helmet's ability to resist impact on every ride I take.

Even without a sharp tip, the phaco needle can damage tissue, or it would not be useful for removing the nucleus. On occasion, the iris may enter the lumen of the needle, usually when it has cored through a piece of nucleus before the surgeon eases off the foot pedal. A pleasant and unexpected benefit of the rounded tip is that it does not damage the iris during a brief grab, even with ultrasound applied (Figure 3). Previously, I would observe a characteristic notching created in the sphincter of the iris by a sharp-edged tip. Although the rounded tip can disrupt a bit of pigment during an incidental grab with ultrasound applied, the pupil remains nicely round (pathological irides, such as floppy irides, undoubtedly will remain a challenge).

CAUTIONS

Three times in my experience, the capsule has touched the rounded tip and occluded it while I was in foot position 3. Twice,

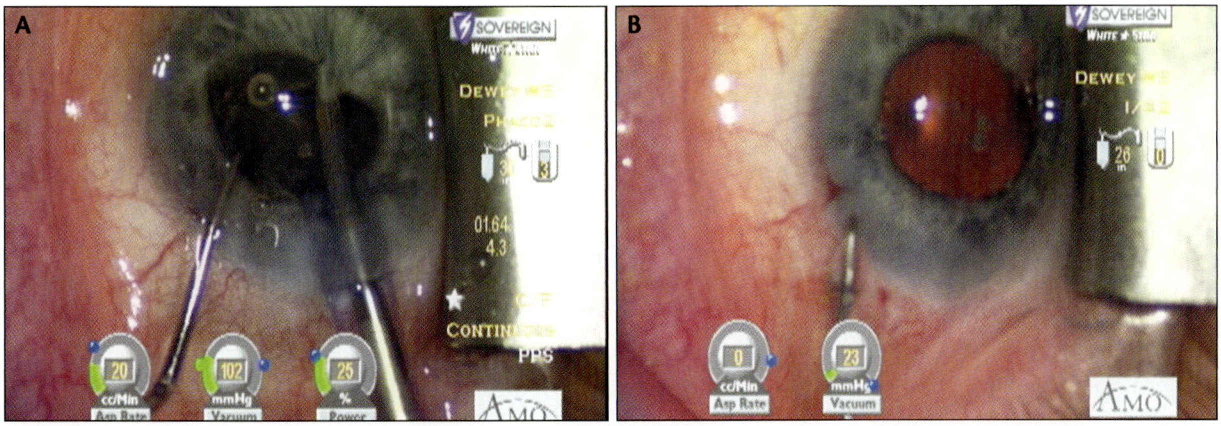

Figure 3. The iris is accidentally grabbed during phacoemulsification with 25% power and 102-mm Hg aspiration (A). The iris sphincter appears to be undamaged, but a mild loss of stroma is visible in the region of the aspirated iris. Unlike the characteristic notching seen with a sharp-edged needle, this patient's pupil remains functionally and cosmetically intact (B).

the capsule was released without injury. Unfortunately, the overlay for the Sovereign cataract extraction system (Advanced Medical Optics, Inc., Santa Ana, CA) was not properly set up to record the power used at that time, although I expect it was fairly low because I was easing off the foot pedal. In one case, the capsule bounced into the tip of the needle with the phaco power at 14%, according to the overlay, and ruptured. The case involved a dense posterior subcapsular cataract in a patient with significant pseudoexfoliation and 20/200 vision. Intriguingly, the capsulotomy that the tip created was round.

It is important to note that the rounded needles change shape over time. In the case of the ruptured capsule, a restriction in the availability of rounded phaco tips had me using needles I no longer considered safe due to burrs. Titanium flows with the tip's movement and leads to the formation of burrs. I have been told anecdotally that the linear marks appearing on a phaco needle after several uses are due to contact with other metal items during surgery. Although I am certain that metal-to-metal contact will worsen the process, these marks appear on the tips and sides of the rounded needles after a dozen or so uses without any observable instrument in the cases I reviewed. At what point these burrs are large enough to break the capsule by mere contact needs research.

CONCLUSION

As far as I can tell, a sharp-edged phaco tip is of no benefit in eyes with soft nuclei. Rather, it can cause significant damage to the capsule, the iris, and even the incision. Rounding the tip's edge improves procedural safety without sacrificing the efficiency of nuclear removal or requiring a change in surgical equipment or technique. For firm lenses, the difference in power usage becomes evident, but whether it will result in a significant clinical difference remains to be seen. Were it not to provide the basis for a comparative study, I would have given up a sharp tip for any case of less than 4+ nuclear sclerosis in favor of the safety that the rounded edge provides. ■

This article originally appeared in the October 2005 issue of CRSToday.

1. Schafer ME. Cavitation generation and cavitational effects in phacoemulsification. Paper presented at: The ASCRS/ASOA Symposium on Cataract, IOL and Refractive Surgery; April 13, 2003; San Francisco, CA.
2. Packer M, Fishkind WJ, Fine IH, et al. The physics of phaco: a review. *J Cataract Refract Surg.* 2005;31:424-431.
3. Dewey SH. Transitioning to chop: nonimpaling technique. Paper presented at: The ASCRS/ASOA Symposium on Cataract, IOL and Refractive Surgery; April 15, 2003; San Francisco, CA.

CHAPTER 36

Phaco Chop Techniques: Horizontal Versus Vertical Chop

DAVID F. CHANG, MD

Several different variations of the chopping technique have evolved since Kunihiro Nagahara, MD, gave his original presentation at the 1993 ASCRS meeting. Conceptually, these can be divided into two main categories.[1] I call the classic Nagahara technique *horizontal chopping,* because the instrument tips move toward each other in the horizontal plane during the chop. In vertical chopping, the two instrument tips move toward each other in the vertical plane in order to create the fracture. Although David Dillman, MD, later popularized the name "phaco quick chop," the "phaco snap and split" technique, developed by Hideharu Fukasaku, MD, was the first incarnation of this concept.

All chopping techniques utilize manual instrument forces to segment the nucleus, thereby replacing the ultrasound power otherwise needed to sculpt grooves. Such energy efficiency is possible

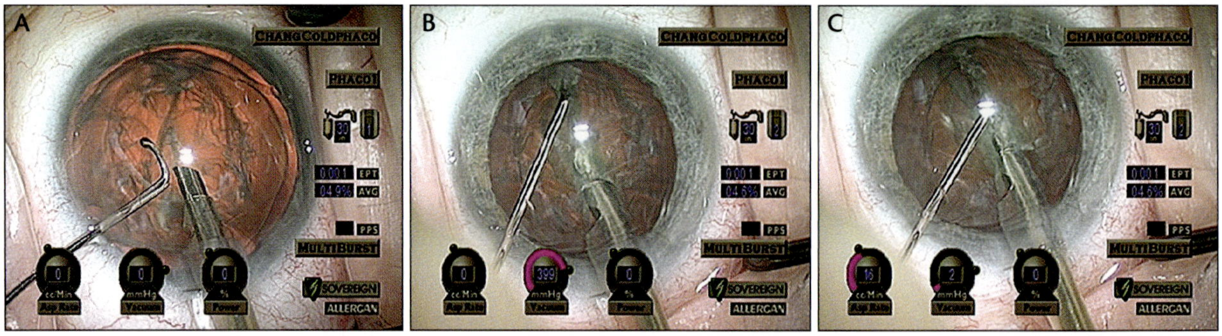

Figure 1. The modified microfinger horizontal chopper (Katena-Chang combination chopper) (A). The chopper hooks the equator beneath the anterior capsule (B). Initiating a horizontal chop as the nucleus is fixated with 400 mm Hg of high vacuum (C).

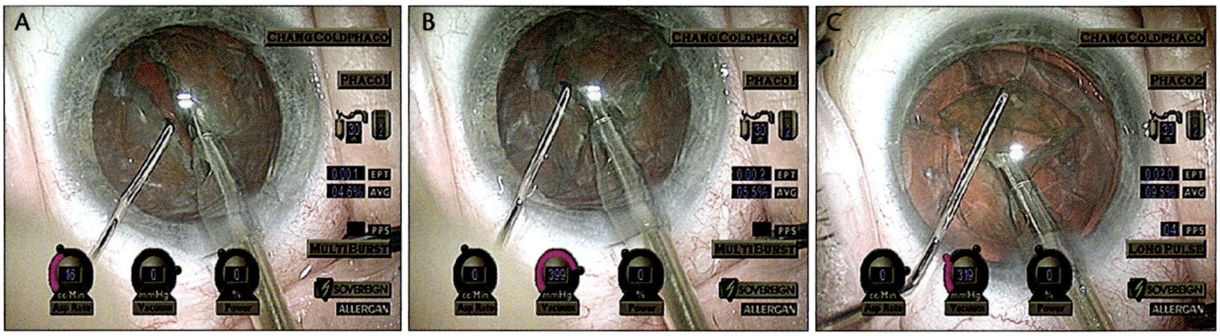

Figure 2. Sideways separating the instrument tips to bisect the nucleus (A). After the second chop, the pie-shaped piece is elevated with high vacuum (B). The elevated fragment is subchopped with the horizontal technique (vacuum at 320 mm Hg) (C).

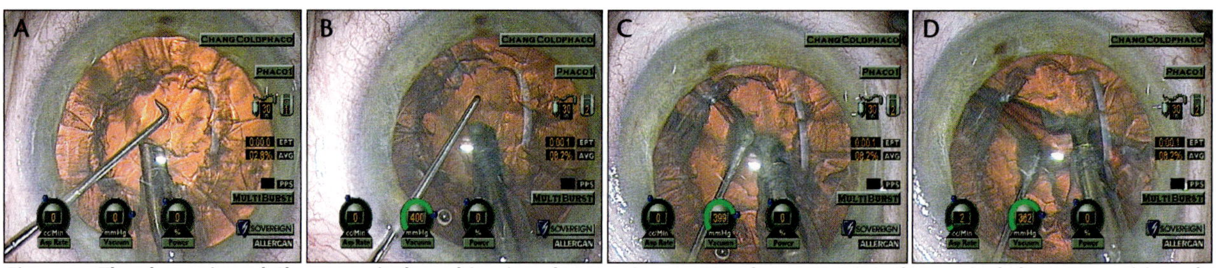

Figure 3. The sharp-tipped Chang vertical combination chopper (Katena Products, Inc.) (A). The vertical chopper positioned after the phaco tip has impaled the nucleus with 400 mm Hg vacuum (B). The vertical chopper penetrates into the nucleus, generating the fracture (C). The sideways separation of the instrument's tips bisects the nucleus (D).

because the lamellar orientation of the lens fibers creates natural fracture planes within the hardened nucleus that are exploited by the chopping maneuver.

The surgeon eventually elevates these smaller nuclear segments into the supracapsular space for phaco-assisted aspiration at a safe distance from the posterior capsule. I believe that phaco chop provides the same advantages as supracapsular phaco flip—efficiency, safety, and reduced stress on the capsular bag—without the difficulty of prolapsing the entire nucleus out of the bag in one piece.

ADVANTAGES FOR CHALLENGING CASES

During sculpting, the capsular bag fixates the nucleus. In comparison, chopping applies much less force against the zonules because the phaco tip secures the nucleus, and the manual instrument forces are directed centripetally against each other. This difference in zonular stress is particularly evident when comparing chopping and sculpting from the Miyake-Apple viewpoint in cadaver eye surgery.

During chopping, the critical instrument maneuvers are primarily kinesthetic, and are performed with the chopper tip. The surgeon does not need the red reflex to visually gauge the depth of the instrument tips, which is advantageous when dealing with mature cataracts. Because the phaco tip is relatively stationary and always remains in the central 2- to 3-mm pupillary zone, phaco chop is an excellent technique for small pupil cases.

In addition to improved efficiency, the features of reduced phaco power, reduced zonular stress, decreased reliance on the red reflex, and the supracapsular location of emulsification all serve to enhance safety. These universal benefits of both horizontal and vertical phaco chop are particularly important for complicated cases such as brunescent nuclei, white cataracts, loose zonules, capsulorhexis tears, and small pupils.

HORIZONTAL PHACO CHOP

Following the capsulorhexis and hydrodissection, hydrodelineation is performed in order to define and separate the epinuclear shell. After the surgeon fragments and removes the endonucleus, he aspirates and flips the remaining epinuclear shell as the final step. In horizontal chop, the chopper tip must hook the equator of the endonucleus peripherally beneath the anterior capsule. Several steps and principles that help the surgeon to properly place the chopper tip are discussed in the following paragraphs.

There are numerous horizontal chopper designs, but all feature an elongated tip, which is blunt to avoid capsule perforation. A relatively long tip is necessary in order to transect thicker, brunescent nuclei, and the inner cutting surface of the tip may be sharpened for this purpose. I prefer a modified Lieberman Microfinger (the Chang Combination Chopper; Katena Products, Inc., Denville, NJ) for horizontal chopping because its slender, curved tip is ideally shaped for hooking and cupping the lens equator (Figure 1A). Typical right-angled chopper tips do not conform as well to the natural contour of the equator and can result in more distention of the peripheral capsular bag.

The surgeon first aspirates the central anterior epinucleus with the phaco tip in order to better estimate the size of the endonucleus and the amount of separation between the endonucleus and the capsular bag. The chopper tip touches the central endonucleus, and maintains contact as the surgeon passes it peripherally beneath the capsulorhexis edge. This ensures that the tip stays inside the bag as it descends and hooks the endonucleus peripherally (Figure 1B). Because the chopper tip drops into and occupies the epinuclear space, it does not overly distend or stretch the capsular bag fornix. Although not approved for use in the US, capsular dye improves visualization of the capsulorhexis for this step and is a useful teaching adjunct.[2,3]

Once it has hooked the nuclear equator, the surgeon may use gentle palpating motions with the chopper to confirm that the tip is internal and not external to the capsular bag. Next, the surgeon deeply impales the nucleus with the phaco tip. The phaco tip should be directed downward and positioned as proximally as possible in order to maximize the nuclear mass encompassed between the two instrument tips. The surgeon pulls the chopper tip directly toward the phaco tip, and upon contact, moves the two tips slightly apart (Figure 1C and 2A). This separating motion propagates the fracture across the entire nuclear diameter.

If the surgeon has not positioned the phaco and chopper tips deep enough, the chop will not succeed. The thicker and denser the endonucleus, the deeper the chopper tip must pass. The tendency to elevate the chopper tip during the chop arises from a fear of perforating the posterior capsule. Instead of dividing the nucleus, this may merely score the superficial nuclear surface.

The surgeon rotates the nucleus in a clockwise direction and repeats the maneuver in order to create a pie-shaped fragment. He then elevates this fragment out of the bag using high vacuum (Figure 2B). Once he chops and evacuates the first heminucleus, there is enough room to pull the second heminucleus to the center of the bag. The surgeon can then perform subsequent chops without having to place the chopper beneath the anterior capsule.

VERTICAL PHACO CHOP

In the case of denser nuclei, a horizontal chopper must exert a greater compressive force in order to fracture the nucleus along its natural lamellar cleavage plane. In contrast, vertical chopping utilizes a shearing force to split the nucleus into pieces. The vertically chopped edges appear sharp, like pieces of broken glass, because there is no crushing force involved.

Whereas a horizontal chopper moves centripetally inward from the periphery, the surgeon uses the vertical chopper like a spike to impale downward into the nucleus just anterior to the centrally buried phaco tip. This action creates the fracture line that is propagated farther posteriorly when he separates the embedded instrument tips (Figure 3B, C, and D). All vertical chopper designs have a short, sharpened tip that is able to penetrate the nucleus (Figure 3A). If the chopper tip is too dull, it will displace the fragment from the phaco tip instead of incising into it.

The key to a successful vertical chop is to impale the phaco tip as deeply into the central nucleus as possible (Figure 3B). Like spearing a potato, the tip must gain enough purchase to be able to lift the entire nucleus upward. By immobilizing the nucleus against the incoming sharp chopper tip, the surgeon generates enough shearing force to fracture the material. High vacuum is invaluable for vertical chop, which requires a maximally strong purchase. With brunescent lenses, burst mode helps to maintain a tight seal around the phaco tip, which is a prerequisite for accessing high vacuum.

COMPARING CHOPPING TECHNIQUES

In horizontal chop, sequentially removing each newly created fragment provides the chopper with increased working space within the capsular bag. Because there is no need to hook the equator with vertical chopping, I prefer to fragment the entire nucleus in situ before removing any pieces when employing this method. Like interlocking puzzle pieces, the adjacent segments add stability to the portion being chopped.

Vertical chopping requires a nucleus that is brittle enough to be snapped in half. Therefore, horizontal chopping is better suited for the softer nucleus. I prefer vertical chopping for brunescent nuclei because it is more consistently able to fracture through the leathery posterior plate. However, if mobile brunescent pieces must be subdivided, horizontal chopping is more effective as this maneuver traps and compresses the fragment between the two instrument tips (Figure 2C).

Horizontal and vertical chopping are complementary variations offering different advantages but common benefits. I utilize both chopping techniques routinely depending on the nuclear density. With dense lenses, I may employ both strategies during the same case, and I designed the Chang double-ended combination chopper (Katena Products, Inc.) to provide both tips on a single instrument. ■

This article originally appeared in the September 2002 issue of CRSToday.

1. Chang DF: Converting to Phaco Chop: Why? Which technique? How? *Ophthalmic Practice.* 1999; 17(4):202-210.
2. Horiguchi M, Miyake K, Ohta I, Ito Y: Staining of the lens capsule for circular continuous capsulorhexis in eyes with white cataract. *Arch Ophthalmol.* 1998;116:535-537.
3. Melles G, de Waard P, Pameyer J, Beekhuis W: Trypan blue capsule staining to visualize the capsulorhexis in cataract surgery. *J Cataract Refract Surg.* 1999;25:7-9.

CHAPTER 37

Why We Prefer Bimanual Microincisional Phacoemulsification

I. HOWARD FINE, MD; RICHARD S. HOFFMAN, MD; AND MARK PACKER, MD

With bimanual microincisional phacoemulsification, we are able to achieve nearly watertight conditions and an almost completely closed system. We are using smaller incisions, which are inherently safer, and we have improved followability because the fluid enters the eye from one side and leaves through the other. This flow avoids creating competing currents around the phaco tip, such as in coaxial phacoemulsification. In addition, the incoming irrigation flow can be used as a tissue manipulator, which aids in directing tissue to the phaco tip. We use the incoming fluid stream to facilitate flipping the epinucleus after purchasing its rim and roof in the distal quadrant with the phaco tip and achieving vacuum on the roof and rim.

We believe that the anterior chamber is much more stable with bimanual microincisional phacoemulsification than with coaxial phacoemulsification. In fact, in a couple of instances when we tore the posterior capsule, the constancy of the irrigation high up in the anterior chamber allowed us to reach down into the bag of the posterior capsule and remove material with the phaco tip. With coaxial phacoemulsification, the incoming fluid would have gone down into the capsular bag along with the phaco tip, almost certainly extending the tear. Also, subincisional cortex has long been recognized as more accessible with bimanual microincisional instruments.

ANCILLARY TECHNIQUES

Bimanual microincisional phaco instrumentation and technology have led to innovative spin-offs, of which we have been able to take advantage. The capsulorhexis forceps enables us to be safe and precise in difficult and challenging cases, especially in the presence of compromised zonules or subluxated cataracts, because there is no loss of viscoelastic or shallowing of the chamber during creation of the capsulorhexis. With a large incision and standard forceps, the chamber is quite unstable. In addition, we have been able to utilize bimanual microinstruments for intraocular cautery (Figure 1), with an irrigating handpiece coming in through one side of the eye and a microincisional cautery entering through the other sideport incision. We are able to identify bleeding points by pinching the irrigation tubing, thus allowing the bleeding to commence, and then to perform cautery under direct visualization.

ZONULAR DIALYSIS OR SUBLUXATED CATARACTS

Bimanual microincisional phacoemulsification is invaluable in the presence of zonular dialysis or subluxated cataracts because we are able to switch hands. If the zonular dialysis is toward the left side, we can use the phaco tip in our left hand and the irrigating chopper in our right hand (Figure 2). With vacuum and flow activated, movement of the lenticular material is toward the area of dialysis or weakened zonules rather than away from it (with the possibility of extending the dialysis). Posteriorly subluxated cataracts can be more easily brought up into the anterior chamber and phacoemulsified bimanually rather than coaxially. Bimanual microincisional refractive lens exchange allows us to hydroexpress the lens out of the capsular bag and carousel it in the plane of the capsulorhexis, where we remove the lens with vacuum and no phaco energy (Figure 3). This is a minimally invasive, very safe procedure that is mandatory in a refractive practice.

INCISIONS

We use incisions that are approximately 1.0 mm internally and 1.2 mm externally, and, with our new irrigating choppers, we are

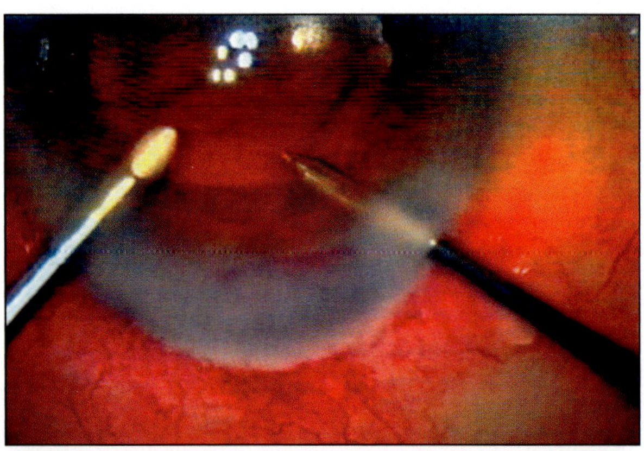

Figure 1. The authors use bimanual microinstrumentation to facilitate intraocular cautery. An irrigating handpiece is inserted into one side of the eye (left) while a microincisional cautery is placed through the sideport incision on the other side of the eye (right).

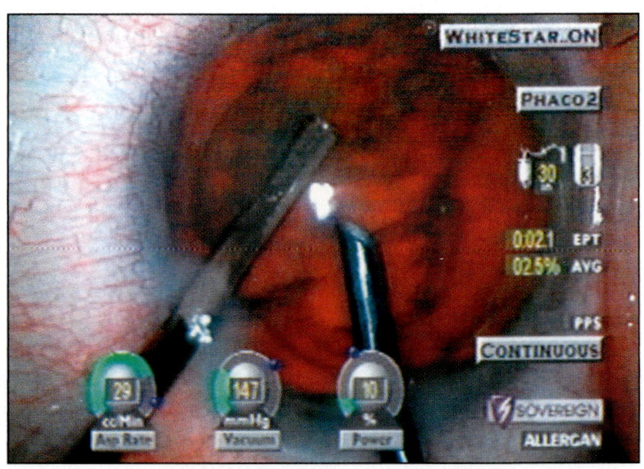

Figure 2. When faced with a patient with zonular dialysis in the left side of his eye, bimanual microincisional phacoemulsification enables the surgeon to switch phacoemulsification to his left hand and irrigation to his right hand.

TABLE 1. PERCENTAGE OF EYES WITH CLEAR CORNEAS 2 TO 24 HOURS POSTOPERATIVELY*

Machine	Coaxial Results	Bimanual Results
Series 20000 Legacy with Neosonix (Alcon Laboratories, Inc., Fort Worth, TX)	98%	100%
Millennium with Phaco Burst (Bausch & Lomb, Rochester, NY)	100%	100%
Staar Sonic Wave (Staar Surgical Company, Monrovia, CA)	95%	100%
Sovereign phaco system with Whitestar Technology (Advanced Medical Optics, Inc., Santa Ana, CA)	100%	97%

*P>.05 *for all comparisons*

TABLE 2. PERCENTAGE OF EYES WITH A UCVA OF 20/40 OR BETTER 2 TO 24 HOURS POSTOPERATIVELY

Machine	Coaxial Results	Bimanual Results
Series 20000 Legacy with Neosonix	96%	93%
Millennium with Phaco Burst	100%	95%
Staar Sonic Wave*	74%	100%
Sovereign phaco system with Whitestar Technology	94%	95%

*P<.01

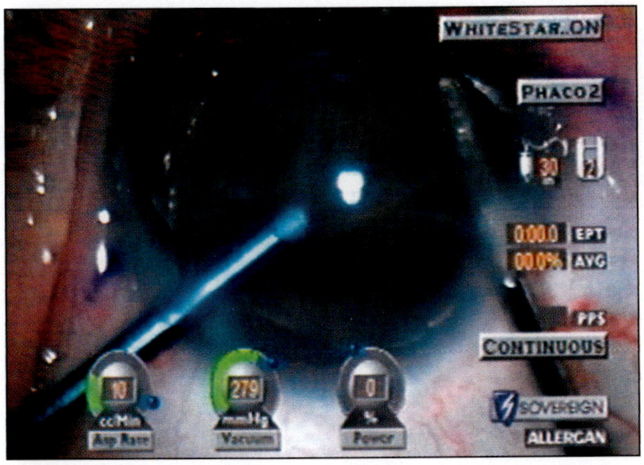

Figure 3. The authors feel that bimanual refractive lens exchange is a safe procedure. Vacuum, rather than phaco energy, is used to remove the lens.

able to insert our instruments comfortably into the eye and to maintain stable chambers. Power modulations allow us to optimize the parameters of all phaco machines available in the United States and to perform bimanual microincisional phacoemulsification with each of them.

We recently compared our bimanual microincisional outcomes to our coaxial phaco outcomes using chi-square analysis and found that our results are as good or better with the former procedure in patients with clear corneas (Tables 1 and 2).

The incision for implanting the IOL is placed between the two sideport incisions, because the manipulation of these microincisions stretches them a little and they will seal much better than if they are not enlarged for IOL implantation. We are commencing trials of the Thinoptx IOL (Thinoptx, Abingdon, VA) and injectable IOLs, such as the SmartIOL (Medennium Inc., Irvine, CA), both of which are inserted through microincisions. We will continue to use an incision between the two sideports, however, until we have a lens that will pass through the unenlarged sideport microincision.

CONCLUSION

Many surgeons say that they will wait to perform bimanual microincisional phacoemulsification until they have a lens that can pass through a microincision. This decision reminds us of the early 1980s when we were trying to convert people to phacoemulsification and their response was, "What is the point? You have to enlarge the incision anyway to put in an IOL." The point is that phacoemulsification is a better procedure than extracapsular extraction, and bimanual microincisional phacoemulsification is superior to coaxial phacoemulsification. ■

This article originally appeared in the September 2004 issue of CRSToday.

CHAPTER 38

Pearls for Cortical Cleanup

GERALD J. ROPER, MD

The informed cataract surgeon approaches the removal of lens cortex with the familiar adage in mind, *last but not least.* Successfully removing the lens requires meticulous surgical handling of even the last cortical fiber. Complications during this portion of the cataract procedure result in significant associated comorbidities. Most excellent surgeons constantly remind themselves of the basic elements of their refined procedure, which are outlined in this article.

SOMETIMES OVERLOOKED

The complexity of the human eye commands the utmost respect, especially when it is being surgically altered. During the cortical-removal phase of lens extraction, this level of respect must be maintained. For example, your initial attention is always directed toward an analysis of the characteristics of the eye tissues you are manipulating that identify potential complications, as well as human factors that may affect your choices and behavior.

Despite the imminent danger in the sharp tip of the phaco needle, remind yourself not to let your guard down the moment you remove the instrument from the eye. The work is certainly not yet finished. Even at the outset, prudent surgeons constantly work to focus their attention on the issues at hand. Cortical removal is greatly enhanced by the perfection of the preceding steps. An intact capsulorhexis and protection of the entire zonulocapsular support apparatus are perhaps the most important issues in long-term success for the patient.

During each step, remain focused on factors that could make or break a successful procedure. Give immediate consideration to the quality of visualization, which is profoundly important in removing lens cortex. When visualization is poor, the implications for the entire procedure are grave. Cortical whitening may be associated with weak zonules, fragile capsules, an expanded capsular bag, and poor visibility, which can negatively affect all phases of surgery (so be ready to use a capsular dye). Polar subcapsular cataracts are a harbinger of a weak or open posterior capsule. Small pupils equal restricted visualization and, likely, weak zonulocapsular support, with all of its attendant challenges.

Several factors during nuclear extraction affect the cortical-removal phase. Mature, dense nuclei—especially in the presence of a thin, fragile anterior capsule—have implications for zonulocapsular stability, visualization, and, ultimately, the behavior of the lens cortex during its attempted removal. One useful technique for cortical removal is to use the phaco handpiece to carve the anterior cortex and epicortex into a circular opening, just inside the edge of the capsulorhexis. This maneuver enhances the visibility of the capsulorhexis' edge when the phaco needle is in the eye and thus prevents the inadvertent disruption of the anterior capsule. The technique also clears cortex from the central path so that the phaco tip is less likely to pull cortex (and capsule) during nuclear and epinuclear removal. As always, the early recognition of and response to a damaged capsulorhexis or posterior capsule are key.

EARLY CORTICAL MANAGEMENT

You are managing cortex even before the I/A instrument enters the eye. This phase of the procedure depends on hydrodissection and hydration. Hydrate the cortex as completely as possible. Avoid high fluid volumes and velocities but persist with smaller volumes at a controlled, constant rate or in pulsations. Laminar and intralaminar cleavage facilitate nuclear mobility, improve visualization, loosen cortex for clean stripping, and spare the lens capsule and zonules. When in doubt, repeat these steps.

During nuclear removal, reassess the condition of the cortex and epicortex. If thorough hydrodissection and cleavage techniques have failed to prepare the cortex appropriately for safe removal, do not despair! While the final heminuclear fragment remains in the eye during phacoemulsification, you can use it as a third instrument to separate epinucleus. Rotating a heminuclear fragment around the bag's equator can free unwanted epinucleus and friable, pasty, adherent cortex, thereby promoting cleaner, safer, and less stressful cortical stripping. The nucleus also supports the bag and facilitates the distribution of BSS during hydrodissection. Proceed with care and use slow hydrodissection. Your aim is to hydrate cortex and lift epinuclear and epicortical planes, without fragmenting the cortex into fine shards. Do not attempt to power-spray large cortical segments out of the bag with BSS, or you may fragment the cortex into strings that are difficult to remove.

MANAGE THE I/A INSTRUMENT CAREFULLY

Reinflate the anterior chamber and capsular bag with BSS through the sideport incision before initially inserting the I/A instrument. The IOP and anatomic configuration of the anterior segment will return to a more physiologic state. The capsule will remain back, away from the I/A tip during its insertion, and visualization will be enhanced for better safety. If the epicortex needs to be lifted or hydrated further, the BSS cannula can help, as mentioned earlier.

Inspect the I/A tip immediately after its insertion, before beginning cortical cleanup. The 0.3-mm aspiration aperture should be smooth and free of burrs or other threats to the capsule. A silicone-tipped I/A cannula may be even more gentle than other designs and spare an incarcerated posterior capsule. The equipment's function is the surgeon's responsibility, so do not forget to check it!

Focus your microscope just posterior to the capsulorhexis for maximum visualization of the capsule anteriorly and posteriorly. The better the depth of field of the microscope, the better your visualization. A spray of faint radial lines interrupting the red reflex may be the earliest indication of an inadvertently grasped posterior capsule. In such a case, immediately release aspiration and vacuum and kick the reflux button on the foot pedal.

CORTICAL I/A SPECIFICS

Gently strip cortex in an anterior-to-posterior direction while avoiding aspiration until after the segment is clear. Large numbers of persistent, fine cortical fibers often remain when cortex is not properly stripped. Purchase and hold a generous amount of the anterior cortical leaflet near the capsulorhexis by means of carefully controlled aspiration and vacuum, then strip the largest possible sheet of cortex to reduce fragmentation. A straight I/A tip may offer the greatest freedom of rotation for grasping cortex.

Whenever possible, remove subincisional cortex early. The remaining cortex will provide some support for the capsular bag while you enlarge the incision and reach downward into the subincisional zone.

A compromised capsule or zonules require a different cortical cleanup strategy. Avoid traction near the area of compromise. Never strip cortex radially from weak zonules or a capsular rent. Instead, start away from and move toward the defect. If you note that the zonules are compromised, move the i/A instrument toward and tangential to the area of zonular weakness. Support the inside of the equatorial bag with a curved instrument in your opposite hand or consider using capsular/iris hooks, a capsular tension ring, or the lens implant's haptics for additional support. When required, manual I/A with a 27-gauge cannula (on a 3-mL syringe with no filter) under viscoelastic may be safest.

Consider polishing the capsule directly. Sweep the 0.3-mm aspiration port across the posterior capsule, face down, on low aspiration and vacuum to thoroughly clean residual lens material and free cortical wisps. Fine cortical threads will release the posterior capsule and extend from the equatorial bag, where you may grasp them against the anterior capsule's lip for removal.

Occasionally, you may wish to place the IOL in the capsular bag despite the presence of residual cortical fragments. The IOL's optic serves as a barrier between the I/A tip and a dangerously undulating posterior capsule. Also, the lens' haptics can provide some zonular support, but you can rotate them away from the cortex being removed so as not to bind it. The presence of the IOL and the viscoelastic used to support the bag during the lens' implantation will aid in the manual aspiration of tenacious subincisional cortex with a J-shaped, 27-gauge cannula.

Brief, pulsating jets of BSS through a 30-gauge cannula identify and free lingering, wispy cortical fibers. A jet directed behind the IOL's optic and into the bag's fornix will displace viscoelastic, hydropolish remaining lens cortical cells, and free wispy cortical segments from the fornix for removal. The small aperture of the 30-gauge cannula may enable you to grasp the smallest remaining cortical threads more effectively.

CONCLUSION

The long-term health of the eye depends on the complete, careful extraction of lens cortex. Mind the hints that the eye gives to you during all phases of the cataract procedure. The surgeon who maintains a back-to-the-basics approach will likely go home happy. ■

This article originally appeared in the September 2005 issue of CRSToday.

CHAPTER 39

Removing Subincisional Cortex

STEVEN H. DEWEY, MD

The removal of subincisional cortex remains a challenge in cataract surgery that, ironically, seems to increase in magnitude as refinements in technique improve the outcome of the procedure. Obviously, the greatest impediment is the natural configuration of our instruments for working directly in front of the incision, with that section of cortex tucked neatly beneath it. Longer tunnel incisions seal well, which decreases the likelihood of endophthalmitis and improves astigmatic stability, but they sequester the subincisional space to an even greater extent than shorter incisions. Smaller capsulotomies that overlap the optic's edge decrease posterior capsular opacification, improve refractive stability, and probably decrease dysphotopsia. They also provide another barrier to accessing cortex in the subincisional space, however. The question, then, is how can one best attack subincisional cortex?

HYDRODISSECTION

I. Howard Fine, MD, of Eugene, Oregon, deserves credit for advancing the concept of hydrodissection as a means of improving both nuclear and cortical removal during phacoemulsification. Although I have had great success using this technique to remove the cortex opposite the incision after phacoemulsification, I still find that a considerable amount of subincisional cortical material remains. The problem is that the wave of fluid must pass along a very precise plane between the cortex and capsule, and the cortex frequently adheres more to the capsule than to itself. As a result, the wave permeates deep into the lens while the subincisional cortex remains intact and adherent.

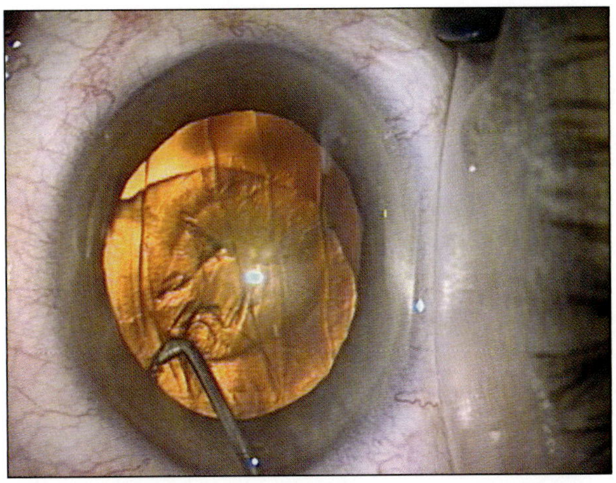

Figure 1. Hydrodissection effectively separates the subincisional cortex from the capsule prior to standard phacoemulsification. The fluid wave is clearly visible as the crescent arcing from the 9:30- to the 3:30-o'clock positions. One may use the angled tip of the cannula designed by Dr. Chang to grip and rotate the nucleus with great efficiency.

If one wishes consistently to ease the removal of the subincisional cortex, then performing hydrodissection in the subincisional space first makes sense. Using a simple J-cannula in this manner can free the subincisional cortex and leave the stubborn cortex opposite the incision to be removed by standard, automated I/A. Unfortunately, this technique is not always as successful as one would like. A more useful instrument than the J-cannula in this region is the hydrodissection cannula angled at 90° that David Chang, MD, of Los Altos, California, designed (Chang right-angled cannula; available from Katena Products, Inc., Denville, NJ, and Mastel Precision, Inc., Rapid City, SD) (Figure 1). This instrument has the advantage of hydrodissecting in the subincisional space and then rotating the nucleus without additional manipulations.

BIMANUAL I/A

Once the nucleus has been extracted, probably the best way to remove cortex using simple I/A devices is with a bimanual technique. Angled I/A cannulas have been in use for quite some time, but they require the placement of an aspirating tip into a region of poor visibility. "Steerable" I/A enjoyed a brief stint as the new technology. Although instruments of this type have largely been relegated to back-room storage, they did demonstrate that the surgeon can successfully use a soft, silicone I/A tip to remove cortex in a poorly visualized area. Compared with reusable instruments, this choice is the most expensive on a per-case basis of those discussed in this article, because the tip can only be safely used for relatively few surgeries. Video demonstrations of this soft tip incidentally grabbing the capsule without damage are certainly compelling, however.

Bimanual techniques allow the alternation of I/A handpieces between the two incisions. For visualization, this technique has significant benefits, because one may use the irrigating handpiece to retract the iris and capsule as needed to perform aspiration in the subincisional space (this technique cheats a bit, because the true subincisional space changes as the instruments alter positions). I frequently have problems with "oar-locking" when attempting this maneuver. Kenneth Rosenthal, MD, of Great Neck, New York, developed a Vespa incision, which is essentially shaped like a wasp or an hourglass. His innovation was to make the external and internal ostia of the microincision for bimanual phacoemulsification larger with a narrower intervening waist. This construction has dramatically reduced the incidence of oar-locking during manipulation of the instruments for removing subincisional material.

MY TECHNIQUE

As an alternative or supplement to aspiration techniques, my approach to subincisional cortex has been relatively different. Instead of aspirating, I knock loose the subincisional cortex with irrigation. This approach has the distinct advantage of being able to free up smaller strands of cortex that are too small to be aspirated by a standard handpiece. At first, I found my technique to be a matter of improved convenience. I was inspired, however, by the work of David Apple, MD, of Salt Lake City early in this decade regarding the correlation between retained cortex after cataract surgery and increased rates of posterior capsular opacification. Using Miyake-Apple specimens, we found my technique to be consistently successful at thoroughly removing cortex to the equator.[1]

In essence, I use a J-cannula to irrigate the cortex, not just out of the subincisional space, but even opposite the incision. With vigorous hydrodissection, I find that little cortex remains after cataract surgery. It is typically a thin layer that is relatively easily stripped away with irrigation, but it is perhaps too thin to aspirate successfully. I use a 26-gauge McIntyre-Binkhorst J-cannula on a 5-mL syringe loaded with BSS. This cannula has a specific flaring of the J-tip that is not parallel to the cannula's shaft. After placing the tip of the cannula against the capsule, I flush the cortex out of the capsule and, in most cases, out of the eye in one simultaneous motion.

For me, this technique has been irreplaceable, and I use the J-cannula in at least 80% of my cases on any given day. Usually, this approach allows complete cortical removal, especially of the subincisional material, within 25 seconds from the removal of the phaco handpiece.

CORTEX AND LENS IMPLANTATION

Whether to remove the cortex before or after implanting the IOL remains controversial. Implanting the IOL first protects the posterior capsule, especially if one is using a standard, angled I/A cannula. The disadvantage is that the IOL and its haptics can be a physical barrier to removing cortex. An older technique from Harry Grabow, MD, of Tampa, Florida, involved placing the viscoelastic cannula under the layer of cortex that remained after nuclear removal. By inflating this space with viscoelastic, he could separate the cortex from the capsule and then place the IOL in this space prior to cortical removal. Of course, one can rotate the IOL to dislodge the cortex at the equator as needed. The older, rigid, single-piece IOLs with PMMA haptics were particularly well suited to this task. The advances in foldable lens technology (eg, three-piece designs and flexible, single-piece designs) make this technique a bit less successful.

CONCLUSION

Subincisional cortex presents several challenges, many of which are of the surgeon's own creation. Consistency is the goal, and the best strategy in removing this material is an individual approach based on one's own talents and preferences. Much like other problems in medicine, the diversity of available solutions points to the absence of consensus on a single solution. ■

This article originally appeared in the September 2005 issue of CRSToday.

1. Dewey SH, Apple DJ, Werner L. Cortical removal by J-cannula irrigation to reduce posterior capsule opacification. Video presented at: The AAO Annual Meeting; November 11-14, 2001; New Orleans, LA.

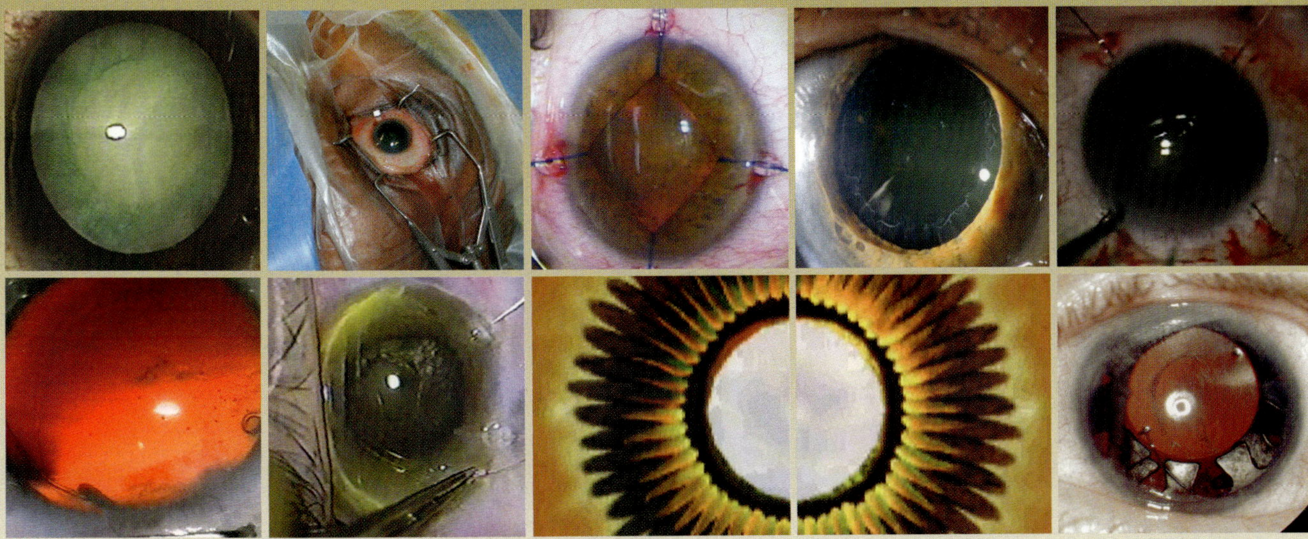

STRATEGIES FOR COMPLICATED CASES

MATURE CATARACTS

IFIS AND SMALL PUPILS

TRAUMA AND WEAK ZONULES

COMPLICATED CATARACTS AND COMORBIDITIES

CHAPTER 40

Confronting the White Cataract

ROBERT H. OSHER, MD, AND JAMES M. OSHER, MS

Like the great white shark, the white cataract can cause catastrophe in the deep. Clinically, the generic white cataract may be divided into four types, which may be differentiated by careful biomicroscopy. The longstanding, mature white lens often has a golden nuclear hue and hard consistency. White cortical cataracts are characterized either by spoking, clefting, corticocapsular adhesions or by diffuse anterior and/or posterior cortical opacification. The swollen intumescent cataract, usually observed in younger patients, shows abundant vacuoles often associated with a white posterior subcapsular opacity. Finally, the liquefied, milky cortex of the Morgagnian cataract may actually permit the nucleus to sink within the capsular bag.

Managing elevated endocapsular pressure and improving intraoperative visualization can turn the surgical course for a white cataract into smooth sailing.

ELEVATED ENDOCAPSULAR PRESSURE

Historically, two difficulties that have plagued surgeons when removing white cataracts are unanticipated elevations of the endocapsular pressure that can cause the tear to run peripherally and compromised visualization of the capsulorhexis. Increased endolenticular pressure is most problematic in younger patients with a swollen cortex or in cases of liquefied Morgagnian cataracts. Perhaps the most graphic example of capsular extension secondary to the endolenticular pressure appeared in the video, *The Argentinean Flag Sign*,[1] which depicted a visible white cortex beneath a torn capsule bordered by the blue color of an intact, dye-stained anterior capsule (Figure 1).

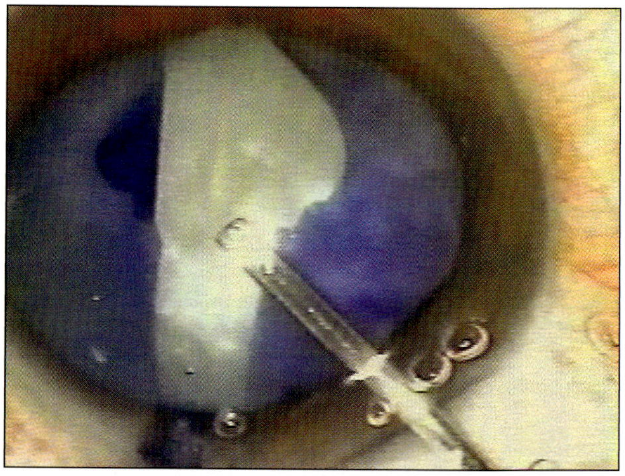

Figure 1. The Argentinean flag sign shows white cortex through the tear, bordered by the blue-stained anterior capsule. (Reprinted with permission from Perrone D, Albertazzi R. The Argentinean flag sign. *Video Journal of Cataract and Refractive Surgery*. 2001;Vol 17:Issue 1.)

Several researchers investigating the issue of increased endocapsular pressure have attempted to puncture the central anterior capsule with a 27-gauge needle in order to aspirate some lens material.[2-4] Although this maneuver seemed to lower the endocapsular pressure, the investigators abandoned it, because it could interfere with the capsulorhexis. The technique was more helpful with the Morgagnian cataract, because the surgeon could almost completely aspirate the liquefied cortex and replace it with a more stable viscoelastic agent. A more predictable method for neutralizing endocapsular pressure was using a viscoelastic agent to flatten the lens dome and retard the capsule's tendency to run downhill. Ophthalmologists who had preferred to create the capsulorhexis with a needle often found it easier to control the edge more precisely with a forceps in any of these white cataracts. Still, the successful completion of the capsulorhexis has remained technically difficult for many surgeons.

VISUALIZATION

Capsular Dyes

Compromised visualization is the other challenge surgeons face with all white cataracts. Methods for dealing with this problem include the use of air,[5] diathermy,[6] high magnification, and oblique illumination.[7] The first strategy to work well involves staining the capsule. Reports detail the use of fluorescein,[8] autologous blood,[9] and indocyanine green (ICG),[10] but a real breakthrough occurred when Gerrit Melles, MD, PhD, of Rotterdam, the Netherlands, and his colleagues described the use of trypan blue.[11] This dye possesses superior staining characteristics (Figure 2), although several physicians have claimed that it increases capsular fragility, as did Ehud Assia, MD, of Kfar Saba, Israel, in a personal conversation (2001).

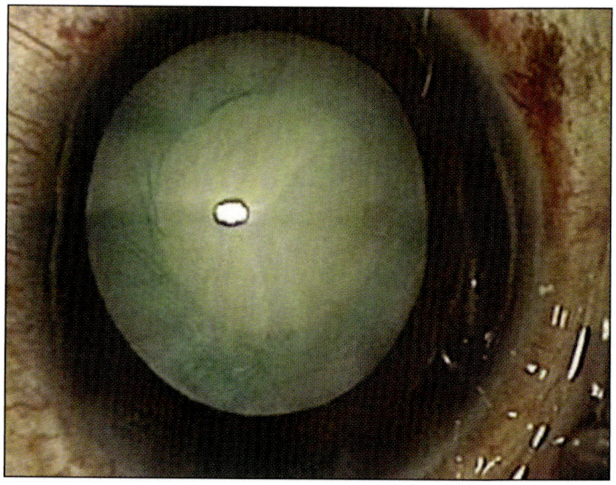

Figure 2. Trypan blue greatly improved the visibility of the capsulorhexis.

US surgeons face a regulatory hurdle with trypan blue. Because the FDA classified the dye as a drug, many US companies consider the cost of bringing it to market to be prohibitive. Whereas ICG may be used off label for an approximate price of $70, trypan blue costs the equivalent of a mere $10 in Europe and less than $5 in

South America. Trypan blue would improve surgeons' outcomes in cases of white cataracts,[12] and some US surgeons value the dye enough to purchase it internationally.[13]

Three-Step Surgical Technique

A three-step technique facilitates capsular staining with either ICG or trypan blue while avoiding misdirection of the dye and its accumulation in dense pockets within the viscoelastic material.[14] First, the anterior chamber is filled with Healon 5 (Pfizer Inc., New York, NY). Gently placing a small amount of BSS (Alcon Laboratories, Inc., Fort Worth, TX) onto the surface of the lens creates a fluid monolayer by elevating the Healon 5 into the dome of the chamber. After introducing the capsular dye into the BSS monolayer, we use a specially designed cannula with a posteriorly placed hole (Duckworth and Kent Ltd., Hertfordshire, England) to paint dye onto the anterior capsule. Thus far, in approximately 100 cases, this technique has resulted in consistent, safe, uniform staining of the capsule.

CONCLUSION

We liken the capsulorhexis to the first letter of the alphabet; if A goes awry, then B is bad, C is catastrophic, and D is disastrous. In cases of white cataracts, if the capsulorhexis is unsuccessful, significant complications may follow. The surgeon who neutralizes elevations in endocapsular pressure and who possesses a good technique for staining the capsule can avert a disaster in the deep and instead enjoy a good day of fishing. At the 2008 annual meeting of the American Academy of Ophthalmology, I was invited to review the Argentinean Flag Sign described by Perrone and Albertazzi for the Spotlight Session. In researching the literature, I was fortunate to review a video entitled, "The Getting Rid of the Argentine Flag," by Carlos Figueiredo. Dr. Figueiredo beautifully illustrated the increased endolenticular pressure secondary to cortical liquefaction not only in the anterior but also in the posterior cortical compartment. Because of a nuclear block between the two compartments, simply decompressing the anterior cortical compartment does not equalize the pressure gradient that causes the nucleus to be projected forward which leads to peripheral extension of the capsulorhexis tear. The posterior compartment must be decompressed by simply retro placing or rotating the nucleus which Dr. Figueiredo refers to as "posterior voiding."

It is worth remembering that this risk does not exist in the hard white cataract or in the Morgagnian cataract. The crucial five steps in preventing this complication in the patient with an intumescent white cataract are as follows: (1) Use a highly retentive OVD like Healon 5 to create a higher pressure in the anterior chamber; (2) Stain the anterior capsule with a dye to optimize visualization; (3) Perform a small capsulorhexis; (4) Decompress the posterior cortical space by either retro placing or rotating the nucleus; (5) Enlarge the capsulorhexis as needed with a microscissors and microforceps. By adhering to these principles, Argentina can shed its association with a dreaded complication and can resume its admired reputation for the world's best beef and tango! (Addendum from December 2008) ■

This article originally appeared in the November 2003 issue of CRSToday.

1. Perrone D, Albertazzi R. The Argentinean flag sign. *Video Journal of Cataract and Refractive Surgery.* 2001;Vol. 17:Issue 1.
2. Osher RH. The anterior capsulotomy techniques and complications. *Video Journal of Cataract and Refractive Surgery.* 1985;Vol. 1:Issue 1.
3. Cionni RJ, Buratto L, Osher RH. The White Cataract. *Video Journal of Cataract and Refractive Surgery.*1992;Vol. 7:Issue 2.
4. Metz G. Lens-induced glaucoma. *Video Journal of Cataract and Refractive Surgery.* 1986;Vol. 2:Issue 3.
5. John M. The anterior capsulotomy. *Video Journal of Cataract and Refractive Surgery.* 1996;Vol. 12:Issue 1.
6. Krag S, Thim K. The anterior capsulotomy. *Video Journal of Cataract and Refractive Surgery.* 1996;Vol. 12:Issue 1.
7. Basti S, Guallapalli R. The anterior capsulotomy. *Video Journal of Cataract and Refractive Surgery.* 1996;Vol. 12:Issue 1.
8. Hoffer KJ, McFarland JE. Intracameral subcapsular fluorescein staining for improved visualization during capsulorhexis in mature cataracts. *J Cataract Refract Surgery.* 1993;19:566.
9. Cimetta DJ, Gatti M, Lobianco G. Haemocoloration of the anterior capsule in white cataract CCC. *Eur J Implant Refract Surg.* 1995;7:184-185.
10. Horiguchi M, Miyake K, Ohta I, Ito Y. Staining of the lens capsule for circular continuous capsulorhexis in eyes with white cataract. *Arch Ophthalmol.* 1998;116:535-537.
11. Melles GR, de Waard PW, Pameyer JH, Hoadijn Beekhuis W. Trypan blue capsule staining to visualize the capsulorhexis in cataract surgery. *J Cataract Refract Surg.* 1999;25:7-9.
12. Dada T, Ray M, Bhartiya P, Vajpayee RB. Trypan-blue-assisted capsulorhexis for trainee phacoemulsification surgeons. *J Cataract Refract Surg.* 2002;28:575-576.
13. Osher RH. FDA or DWR? *Video Journal of Cataract and Refractive Surgery.* 2001;Vol. 17:Issue 4.
14. Osher RH, Marques D, Marques F. A 3-step technique for staining the anterior lens capsule with indocyanine green or trypan blue. *J Cataract Refract Surg.* 2004;30(1):13-16.

CHAPTER 41

Trypan Blue Versus Indocyanine Green

DAVID F. CHANG, MD

Staining the anterior capsule with dye is by far one of the most important advances in the management of complicated cataracts. With the FDA's recent approval of trypan blue, US surgeons are finally able to capitalize fully on this strategy (Figure 1). More than 5 years of worldwide experience has demonstrated that capsular staining is safe and effective for cataract surgery. Safety, however, depends on the specific dye used and its formulation. Uttley et al[1] reported on four eyes in which intraocular methylene blue, used for capsular staining, resulted in corneal decompensation that eventually required penetrating keratoplasty.

A HISTORY OF CAPSULAR STAINING

In 1998, Fritz[2] published a report on the use of sodium fluorescein dye to stain the anterior capsule for cases of mature cataract. Unfortunately, because of its small molecular size, fluorescein did not remain confined to the anterior chamber but diffused into both the lens and the vitreous.

Horiguchi et al[3] first published a report on the use of 0.5% indocyanine green (ICG) to stain the anterior capsule in 1998. They reported on a randomized, prospective study of 20 consecutive, mature, white cataracts in which one-half of the eyes received ICG dye and the other half did not. There were no statistically significant differences in laser flare-cell photometry, endothelial cell loss, or postoperative IOP spikes. Since it is only approved for choroidal angiography, lyophilized ICG (Akorn, Inc., Buffalo Grove, IL) is sold and packaged with a solvent that, because it is intended for IV injection, is of an inappropriate pH and osmolality for the anterior chamber. For this reason, Horiguchi et al mixed the dye using BSS Plus (Alcon Laboratories, Inc., Fort Worth, TX) and the supplied solvent in a 9:1 ratio. The OR personnel must be careful either to warm or vigorously shake the mixture in order to fully dissolve the ICG powder. Otherwise, large, undissolved particles will remain suspended in the solution.

In 1999, Melles et al[4] published their use of 0.1% trypan blue dye to stain the anterior capsule in a series of 30 patients with mature cataracts. As with the aforementioned study by Horiguchi et al, there was no clinical evidence of increased inflammation, corneal endothelial impairment, or elevated IOP, but there was no control group. After receiving CE Marking that year, trypan blue 0.06% has been distributed internationally by DORC International BV (Zuidland, the Netherlands) as Vision Blue. Because it is specifically intended for capsular staining, Vision Blue is packaged in an appropriately small vial of solution that is formulated for intraocular use and requires no mixing.

LABORATORY AND CLINICAL STUDIES

Laboratory and animal studies have supported the safety of both ICG and trypan blue. ICG was shown to be nontoxic in rabbits and was safely used to count cells on human donor keratoplasty buttons.[5] Investigators reported similar findings with trypan blue, which was used to examine the endothelium in more than 32,000 donor corneas by the Dutch National Eye Bank.[4] To gain CE Marking in Europe, Gerritt Melles, MD, employed a standard cytotoxicity study with cultured fibroblasts to evaluate four different dyes: trypan blue; ICG; methylene blue; and gentian violet. Trypan blue had the best score with the lowest toxicity (data on file with DORC International BV).

Since these initial reports, ophthalmic surgeons have adopted both of these dyes worldwide for capsular staining. For example, Vision Blue has been available in 60 countries, with approximately 700,000 units sold by DORC International BV prior to the dye's US release. There are no published reports of anterior segment complications directly attributable to either dye. One prospective, randomized, controlled study found no difference in endothelial cell loss when trypan blue was used.[6] Even so, there has been concern that ICG, when used for peeling the internal limiting membrane, may be toxic to the retinal photoreceptors and may cause new visual field defects.[7] A recent study in vitrectomized rabbits found no retinal toxicity from the commercially available 0.06% concentration of trypan blue.[8] Trypan-blue staining of an expandable hydrophilic acrylic IOL has been reported, however.[9,10] This particular lens model has the highest water content of the hydrogel class.

With respect to efficacy, the benefit of improved visualization of the capsule is clinically obvious, but one randomized study demonstrated that better visualization improves a surgeon's ability to complete the capsulorhexis in mature cataracts. Dada et al[11,12] randomized 50 eyes to capsular staining with five different agents (10 eyes each): 0.1% trypan blue; 0.001% gentian violet; 0.5% ICG; 2% fluorescein; and autologous hemocoloration. The first three dyes provided superior visualization of the capsule and higher success rates in completing a capsulorhexis with no cases of extended capsular tears. The last two groups both had poorer visualization of the capsulorhexis and an extension rate of 20%.

In 2000, I reported on one of the first clinical comparisons of ICG and trypan blue for capsular staining.[13] Trypan blue provided a significantly darker and more intense staining of the capsule (Figure 1), particularly helpful qualities when other complicating factors such as corneal edema are present. In addition, trypan blue provided more persistent, longer-lasting staining of the anterior capsule (Figure 2). This attribute greatly facilitates nuclear emulsification in mature white and brown lenses, where poor visualization makes the disruption of the capsulorhexis with the phaco tip or chopper more likely. As reported from a retrospective study,[14] I performed ICG staining in 18 consecutive mature white cataracts between June 1998 and October 1999, and, in the US and abroad, I used trypan blue in 16 cases of consecutive mature lenses between November 1999 and November 2000. I performed a planned, can-opener capsulotomy for extracapsular cataract extraction for one eye in each group. I successfully completed a capsulorhexis in 15 of 17 eyes and 15 of 15 eyes stained with ICG and trypan blue dye, respectively, that subsequently underwent phacoemulsification. Both dyes provided excellent visualization of the capsule and were not associated with complications. Staining with trypan blue was definitely more intense and persistent.

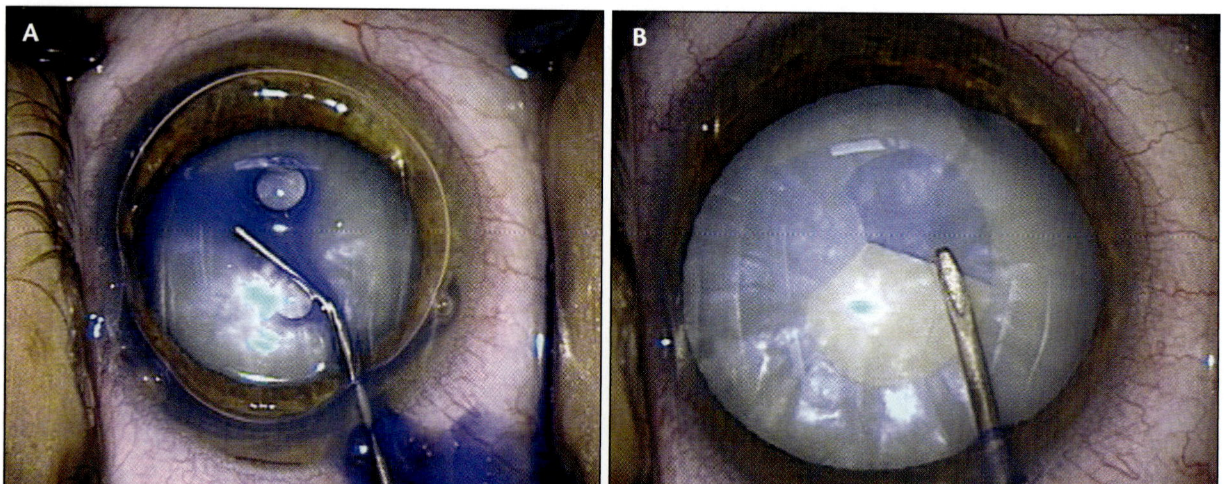

Figure 1. The surgeon injects trypan blue by means of a No. 30 cannula on a tuberculin syringe beneath an air bubble (A). The blue stain contrasts with the white cortex during the capsulorhexis step (B).

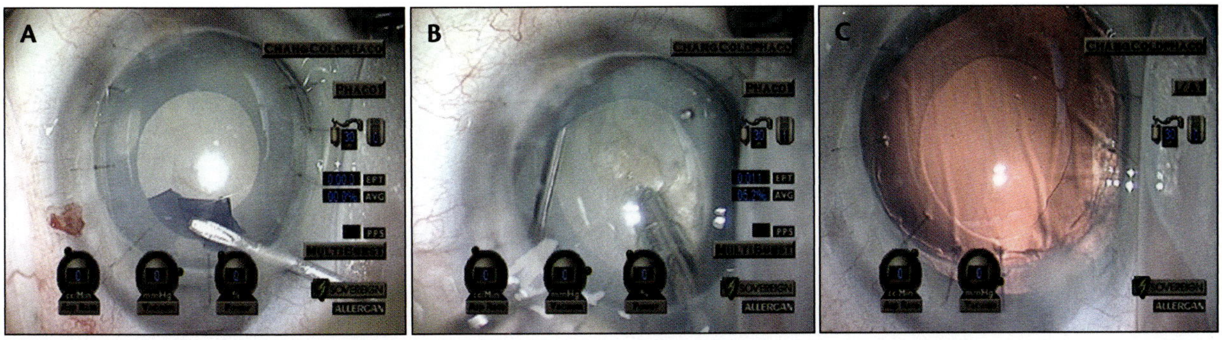

Figure 2. This eye has a mature, white cataract. The intense staining with trypan blue is advantageous when corneal clarity is suboptimal, such as after a penetrating keratoplasty (A). Persistent staining helps the surgeon to judge the placement of a horizontal chopper (B). Visible staining of the capsule with trypan blue persists even after the completion of phacoemulsification (C).

CLINICAL INDICATIONS

In addition to the white cataract, capsular dye should be considered whenever the red reflex is compromised.[15] Examples include corneal scars or edema, dense anterior cortical spokes, a mature brown nucleus, vitreous hemorrhage, and asteroid hyalosis. Trypan blue is superior for the brunescent lens in particular (Figure 3), because ICG does not provide adequate color contrast with this hue of nucleus. The enhanced visibility of a capsulorhexis' edge stained with trypan blue is also very helpful when removing traumatic cataracts, for which the surgeon must place capsule retractors or capsular tension rings. Others have reported on dye-aided anterior and posterior capsulorhexes in pediatric cataracts.[16-18]

Another underused application of capsular dye is for teaching phaco techniques.[19,20] Not only can staining help beginning residents find and grasp the anterior capsular flap, but it is particularly valuable for any surgeon learning new phaco techniques such as phaco flip or phaco chop. With the latter method, a stained capsulorhexis' edge helps the transitioning surgeon to avoid overly distending it with the chopper's shaft or misplacing the horizontal chopper's tip peripherally, outside the capsular bag (Figure 2B).

Finally, surgeons sometimes find the capsular flap unexpectedly difficult to visualize when performing the capsulorhexis. It is important to recognize that one can stop and perform capsular staining even after the capsulorhexis has been initiated,[21] because the dye preferentially stains the capsule and not the cortex.[22] When irrigating out the dye in this situation, it is important not to allow the chamber to become shallow, or the tear may extend peripherally.

STAINING TECHNIQUES

Many surgeons continue to inject capsular dye beneath an air bubble, as originally described by Horiguchi et al[3] and Melles et al[4] (Figure 1A). The ophthalmologist fills the anterior chamber with air using a 30-gauge cannula inserted through a tiny paracentesis. He then draws several drops of dye into a tuberculin syringe and places them on the anterior capsular surface by means of the same cannula. Although the dye is not toxic to the endothelium, the bubble prevents excessive dilution and helps to confine the dye to the capsular surface. After waiting at least 10 to 15 seconds, the surgeon can easily irrigate out the dye with BSS before injecting viscoelastic.

Laureano and Coroneo[23] suggested simply omitting the air bubble. Takayuki Akahoshi, MD, has described an alternate technique

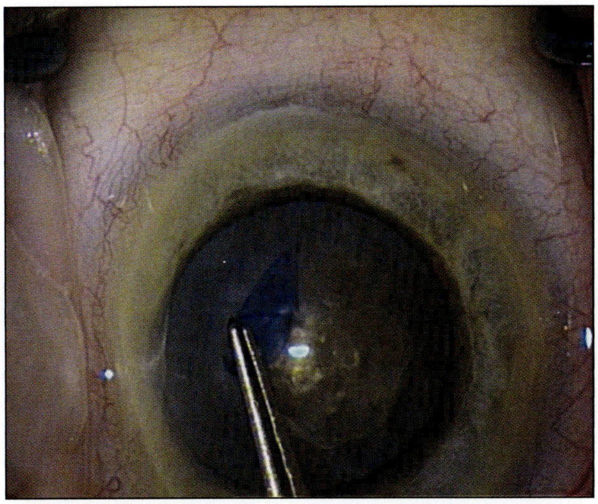

Figure 3. Brunescent nuclei require dark staining for adequate contrast.

of mixing ICG with viscoelastic (see Dr. Akahoshi's article in this issue), and Kayikicioglu et al[24] have used a similar viscoelastic-mixing technique with 0.4% trypan blue. Finally, Robert Osher, MD, has popularized the technique of isolating a puddle of dye on the anterior capsule beneath a partition of cohesive or viscoadaptive viscoelastic (eg, Healon 5 [Advanced Medical Optics, Inc., Santa Ana, CA]).[25] This method intensifies the staining compared with the bubble technique in which the bubble's meniscus and surface tension displace the dye from the central anterior capsular surface.

CONCLUSION

Both ICG and trypan blue have been safely and successfully used to enhance visualization of the anterior capsule. Unlike ICG, trypan blue does not require mixing, and it provides superior, more prolonged capsular visualization. Now that trypan blue is the first and only product to receive FDA approval for capsular staining, it is clearly the dye of choice. ■

This article originally appeared in the March 2005 issue of CRSToday.

1. Uttley SA, Lawrence MG, Hardten DR, et al. Methylene blue-associated corneal decompensation. Poster presented at: The AAO Annual Meeting; November 11, 2001; New Orleans, LA.
2. Fritz W. Fluorescein blue light-assisted capsulorhexis for mature or hypermature cataract. *J Cataract Refract Surg.* 1998;24:19-20.
3. Horiguchi M, Miyake K, Ohta I, Ito Y. Staining of the lens capsule for circular continuous

capsulorhexis in eyes with white cataract. *Arch Ophthalmol.* 1998;116:535-537.
4. Melles G, de Waard P, Pameyer J, Beekhuis W. Trypan blue capsule staining to visualize the capsulorhexis in cataract surgery. *J Cataract Refract Surg.* 1999;25:7-9.
5. McEnerney JK, Peyman GA. Indocyanine green: a new vital stain for use before penetrating keratoplasty. *Arch Ophthalmol.* 1978;96:1445-1447.
6. Van Dooren BT, de Waard PW, Poort-van Nouhuys H, et al. Corneal endothelial cell density after trypan blue capsule staining in cataract surgery. *J Cataract Refract Surg.* 2002;28:574-575.
7. Kanda S, Uemura A, Yamashita T, et al. Visual field defects after intravitreous administration of indocyanine green in macular hole surgery. *Arch Ophthalmol.* 2004;122:1447-1451.
8. Veckeneer M, van Overdam K, Monzer J, et. al. Ocular toxicity study of trypan blue injected into the vitreous cavity of rabbit eyes. *Graefes Arch Clin Exp Ophthalmol.* 2001;239:698-704.
9. Werner L, Apple DJ, Crema AS, et al. Permanent blue discoloration of a hydrogel intraocular lens by intraoperative trypan blue. *J Cataract Refract Surg.* 2002;28:1279-1286.
10. Bisol T, Rezende RA, Guedes J, Dantas AM. Effect of blue staining of expandable hydrophilic intraocular lenses on contrast sensitivity and glare vision. *J Cataract Refract Surg.* 2004;30:1732-1735.
11. Dada VK, Sharma N, Pangtey MS, et al. Comparison of various anterior capsular staining methods for capsulorhexis in white cataracts. Paper presented at: The AAO Annual Meeting; November 12, 2001; New Orleans, LA.
12. Dada VK, Sharma N, Sudan R, et al. Anterior capsule staining for capsulorhexis in cases of white cataract: comparative clinical study. *J Cataract Refract Surg.* 2004;30:326-333.
13. Chang DF. Capsule staining and mature cataracts: a comparison of indocyanine green and trypan blue dyes. *Br J Ophthalmol* [serial online]. 2000 June. Available at http://bjo.bmjjournals.com/cgi/content/full/84/8/DC1. Accessed January 31, 2005.
14. Chang DF. Clinical comparison of ICG and trypan blue dye for mature cataract. Paper presented at: The ASCRS/ASOA Symposium on Cataract, IOL and Refractive Surgery; April 30, 2001; San Diego, CA.
15. Pandey SK, Werner L, Vroman DT, Apple DJ. Dye-enhanced anterior capsulorhexis: surgical techniques, guidelines, and recommendations for surgeons. *Comp Ophthalmol Update.* 2003;4:179-185.
16. Wakabayashi T, Yamamoto N. Posterior capsule staining and posterior continuous curvilinear capsulorhexis in congenital cataract. *J Cataract Refract Surg.* 2002;28:2042-2044.
17. Guo S, Caputo A, Wagner R, DeRespinis P. Enhanced visualization of capsulorhexis with indocyanine green staining in pediatric white cataracts. *J Pediatr Ophthalmol Strabismus.* 2003;40:268-271.
18. Saini JS, Jain AK, Sukhija J, et al. Anterior and posterior capsulorhexis in pediatric cataract surgery with or without trypan blue dye: randomized prospective clinical study. *J Cataract Refract Surg.* 2003;29:1733-1737.
19. Werner L, Pandey SK, Escobar-Gomez M, et al. Dye-enhanced cataract surgery. Part 2: learning critical steps of phacoemulsification. *J Cataract Refract Surg.* 2000;26:1060-1065.
20. Dada T, Ray M, Bhartiya P, Vajpayee RB. Trypan-blue-assisted capsulorhexis for trainee phacoemulsification surgeons. *J Cataract Refract Surg.* 2002;28:575-576.
21. De Waard PW, Budo CJ, Melles GR. Trypan blue capsular staining to "find" the leading edge of a "lost" capsulorhexis. *Am J Ophthalmol.* 2002;134:271-272.
22. Singh AJ, Sarodia UA, Brown L, et al. A histological analysis of lens capsules stained with trypan blue for capsulorrhexis in phacoemulsification cataract surgery. *Eye.* 2003;17:567-570.
23. Laureano JS, Coroneo MT. Crystalline lens capsule staining with trypan blue. *J Cataract Refract Surg.* 2004;30:2046-2049.
24. Kayikicioglu O, Erakgun T, Guler C. Trypan blue mixed with sodium hyaluronate for capsulorhexis. *J Cataract Refract Surg.* 2003;27:970.
25. Marques DM, Marques FF, Osher RH. Three-step technique for staining the anterior lens capsule with indocyanine green or trypan blue. *J Cataract Refract Surg.* 2004;30:13-16.

CHAPTER 42

Trypan Blue and Healon 5

ROBERT H. OSHER, MD

Since the independent reports of Horiguchi et al[1] and Melles et al,[2] who introduced indocyanine green and trypan blue, respectively, for staining the anterior capsule, I have been a vocal advocate of capsular dyes. There is no question that capsular dyes increase the safety of performing the capsulorhexis in cases of white cataract. A patient with a dark brunescent cataract or an anterior cortical cataract may also benefit when the visibility of the capsule is enhanced. Although the original reports favored the use of trypan blue beneath an air bubble, I never enjoyed as much control as when performing the capsulorhexis beneath Healon 5 (Advanced Medical Optics, Inc., Santa Ana, CA). Unfortunately, injecting a dye when an ophthalmic viscosurgical device (OVD) is present in the anterior chamber can result in an "inkblot," which will interfere with visualization. Moreover, the additional resistance of the OVD may force the dye back through the zonules and cause a loss of the red reflex.

This article describes my three-step technique for capsular staining.

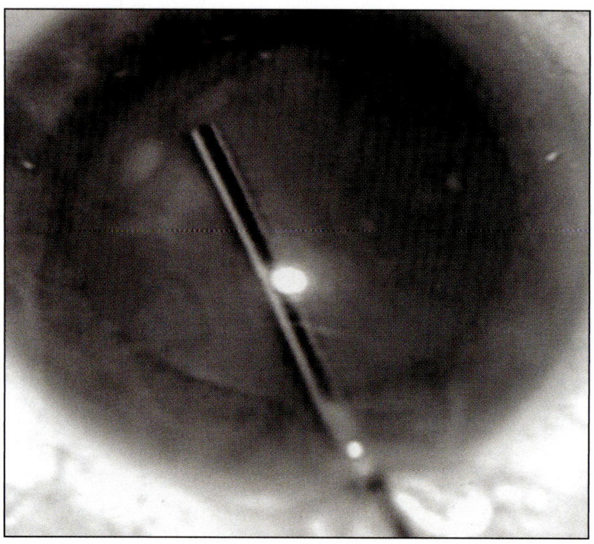

Figure 1. The author fills the anterior chamber with Healon5.

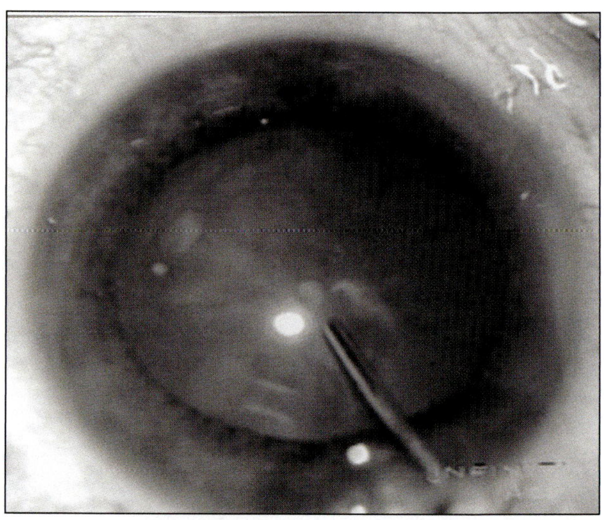

Figure 2. The author injects BSS through a 27-gauge cannula onto the anterior capsule.

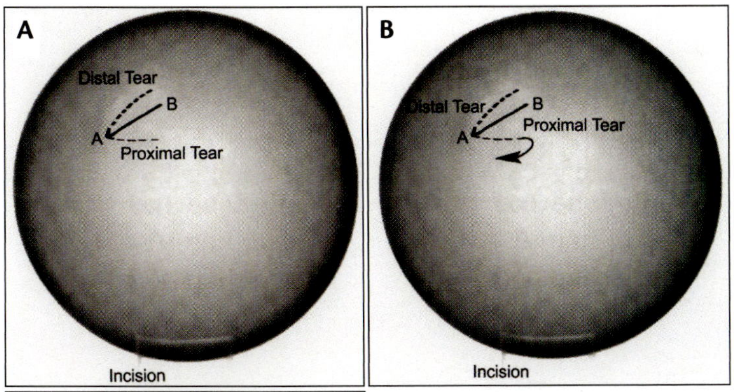

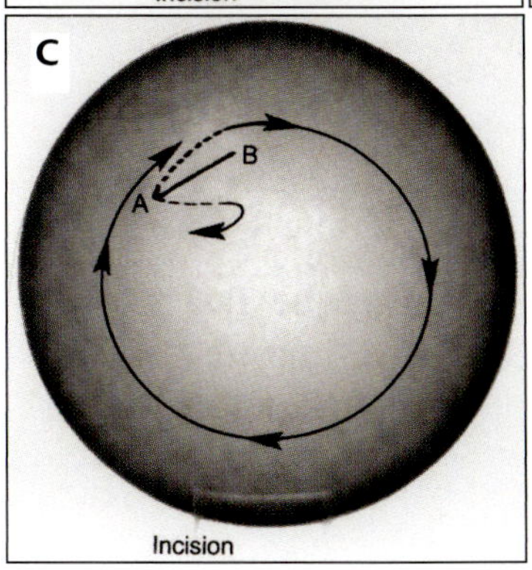

Figure 5. The surgeon makes a slash from A to B with a needle to create a <-shaped aperture (A). While redirecting the proximal tear to create the safety edge, the surgeon uses the distal tear for the leading edge of the capsulorhexis (B). The surgeon completes the capsulorhexis in a clockwise fashion (C).

HOW IT WORKS

The three-step technique allows the surgeon to create the capsulorhexis beneath the OVD with the clearest possible view. First, I fill the anterior chamber with Healon 5 (Figure 1). Next, I gently inject balanced salt solution through a 27-gauge cannula directly onto the anterior capsule (Figure 2). This monolayer of fluid lifts the Healon 5 into the chamber's dome while creating a wafer-thin fluid medium into which the trypan blue can easily be distributed onto the surface of the lens. A special cannula with a hole on its posterior surface (MMP203; Duckworth & Kent Ltd., Hertfordshire, England) facilitates the precise placement of the capsular dye onto the anterior capsule (Figure 3). If some extra dye accumulates within the anterior chamber and compromises visualization, I can easily irrigate it away and replace the volume with a bit more OVD. In the vast majority of cases, the three-step technique alone will offer a surgeon clear visualization (Figure 4) and enable one to complete the capsulorhexis with excellent control by means of either a bent needle or a forceps in combination with a variety of capsulorhexis techniques.

I prefer the same bent 22-gauge needle that I have used since 1986, unless the zonules are loose, in which case I will use a forceps. I call my favorite capsulorhexis technique the *safety capsulorhexis*, because it offers me a second edge to use if I encounter a problem with the initial one. I start the capsulorhexis approximately 160° opposite to the incision by creating a midperipheral, left-to-right slash with the bent tip of the 22-gauge needle, which raises a <-shaped flap (Figure 5A). Turning around the proximal edge with the needle (essentially a U-turn) makes the edge point to my left (Figure 5B). I then direct the distal edge clockwise 360° and complete the capsulorhexis outside of the proximal safety edge (Figure 5C).

CONCLUSION

Regardless of the technique or the choice of instrument, performing the capsulorhexis safely has never been easier than with the three-step method for capsular staining. Capsular dyes give surgeons an advantage when critical visualization is compromised. ■

This article originally appeared in the March 2005 issue of CRSToday.

1. Horiguchi M, Miyake K, Ohta I, Ito Y. Staining of the lens capsule for circular continuous capsulorhexis in eyes with white cataract. *Arch Ophthalmol.* 1998;116:535-537.
2. Melles GR, de Waard PW, Pameijer JH, Beekhuis WH. Trypan blue capsule staining to visualize the capsulorhexis in cataract surgery. *J Cataract Refract Surg.* 1999;25:7-9.

CHAPTER 43

Tips for Capsular Staining

MINAS CORONEO, MD, MS, MSc, FRACS, FRANZCO

The development of VisionBlue capsular dye (Dutch Ophthalmic Research Corporation International BV, Zuidland, the Netherlands) represents a significant advance in capsular staining, and, as a consequence, the safety of cataract surgery. As a result, usage has gained in popularity with sales of approximately 2 million units to date in mid-2007. The superior capsular visualization achieved with this dye was noted in its development and was later confirmed by other investigators.[1,2] Several techniques for the application of VisionBlue have been described;[3-5] however, my minimalist technique[6,7] is effective and adds little time to the procedure.

STAINING TECHNIQUE

I drain a small amount of aqueous from the eye via the paracentesis port before injecting the dye. This action induces a relative pupillary block that confines the dye to the pupillary area, minimizing the risk of dye passing into the posterior segment.[8-10] Thirty seconds after I inject the dye, I introduce an ophthalmic viscosurgical device (OVD) into the anterior chamber via a cannula while placing pressure on the posterior lip of the paracentesis port. Dyed aqueous humor exits the anterior chamber through the port. To minimize the risk of the cannula's tip damaging the anterior capsule, I initially inject a small amount of OVD just inside the paracentesis. This method obviates the need to take an additional step to remove dye and/or OVD from the anterior chamber. Because I avoid using air in the anterior chamber, I reduce the risk of potential toxicity to the endothelium and infection that can occur with

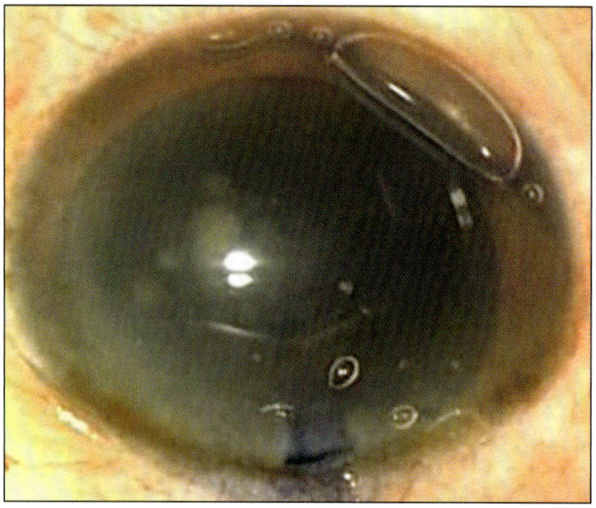

Figure 1. When displaced with an OVD, air bubbles serendipitously placed in the anterior chamber for 30 seconds during surgery leave areas of the anterior capsule unstained in the sections covered by the bubbles on instillation, demonstrating that air retards capsular staining by trypan blue.

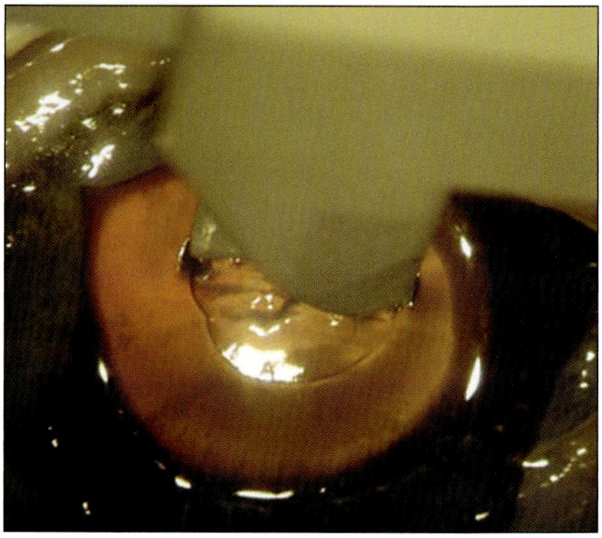

Figure 2. The capsulorhexis is being stretched with a vernier caliper in a cadaveric eye. The capsulorhexis can be stretched from approximately 4 to 10 mm before it ruptures. VisionBlue has no effect on the capsulorhexis' ability to be stretched.

unfiltered air. I have observed that air actually retards capsular staining (unpublished data, 2007; Figure 1). Additional instrumentation, such as a specific cannula designed for "painting" dye onto the capsule is not required.[11]

PRINCIPAL OPHTHALMIC USES

VisionBlue's ability to stain connective tissue and basement membranes is expanding[12-14] its ophthalmic uses and indications (See *Indications for Capsular Staining*). During cataract surgery, it (1) enhances capsular visualization for the safe completion of the capsulorhexis (the critical step in cataract surgery); (2) stains the anterior capsule, highlights the capsulorhexis, and provides a landmark during the remainder of the procedure; and (3) helps surgeons achieve a perfectly centered capsulorhexis that overlaps the IOL's optic by 0.5 to 1 mm[15] or to create a "re-rhexis"[16] in cases of severe capsular phimosis.

Apart from issues relating to decentration, a perfect capsulorhexis may be a critical determinant of final IOL power,[17] because the IOL's final position in the capsular bag is determined in part by the size of the capsulorhexis.[18] These days, in part due to technological advances, patients do not just desire highly accurate refractive outcomes, but they also expect them. The simple "low-tech" method of achieving a perfectly sized capsulorhexis with the aid of VisionBlue is a very effective strategy for meeting patients' expectations.

In my opinion, it is possible to create a properly sized and centered capsulorhexis by using the position of the IOL's edge in the capsular bag to execute a "re-rhexis" after the IOL's placement. This step is greatly facilitated by staining the capsule with trypan blue, because the stain increases the contrast between the IOL's and the capsulorhexis' edges.

As we begin to perform refractive lensectomies on younger patients and implant more multifocal and accommodating IOLs, we need to be aware that long-term capsular contraction can affect the results of these procedures. Creating optimally sized capsulorhexes during the initial surgery can reduce the risk of poor outcomes.

I believe that VisionBlue can be used in every surgery and have made this approach my standard practice. Cataract surgery is a critical lifetime event for patients that can be compared with flying. A take-off into a clear sky does not necessarily mean the continuation of good weather. Similarly, corneal haze or other complications can make an apparently routine surgery technically demanding. Although skill and experience usually result in a safe outcome, staining the capsule blue makes the procedure safer. Introducing VisionBlue during cataract surgery takes little time and adds relatively minimal cost to the procedure.

SAFETY ISSUES

In the initial search for a safe dye for intraocular use, investigators quickly determined that anionic (acidic) dyes such as trypan blue are less injurious to ocular tissue than cationic (basic) dyes.[19] This inherent safety factor should be remembered in a commercial climate in which claims of toxicity are sometimes poorly documented.

The safety of trypan blue has been demonstrated by long-term studies[20] as well as by its use in eye bank corneas to determine endothelial cell viability prior to transplantation. For more than 30 years, the exclusion of trypan blue has remained a standard test of cellular viability and is used extensively in ophthalmic research.[21]

Although some investigators have suggested that trypan blue decreases the tear strength of the capsulorhexis,[22] no data exist to support this claim. The stiffness of porcine capsules may increase after photosensitization in the presence of trypan blue;[23] however, this effect is unlikely to be clinically significant. My colleagues and I recently demonstrated[24] that VisionBlue does not decrease the tear strength of the capsulorhexis' margin in an in vitro human eye model (Figure 2). There was no significant difference in the "stretchability" of the capsulorhexis' opening with or without VisionBlue.

Of interest was a 4-mm capsulorhexis that could be stretched to approximately 10 mm before it ruptured.[24] One report suggests the dye had in vitro toxicity to porcine endothelial cells,[25] but controls for the solution's toxicity were inadequate, and the postmortem time for eyes used was not reported. Endothelial safety is consistent with clinical experience and earlier clinical studies.[26] Keep in mind that there is also a report of permanent staining of a hydrogel IOL.[27]

Recent outbreaks of toxic anterior segment syndrome remind us that we need to be vigilant about the potential toxicity of the agents we introduce into the eye.[28] VisionBlue, however, appears to have an excellent track record. Some patients developed marked intraocular inflammation after they were exposed to trypan blue,[29] but in these cases, the surgeons used generic preparations of the dye. According to Dutch Ophthalmic Research Corporation International BV, VisionBlue is currently the only ophthalmic dye produced following the FDA's good manufacturing practices and is the only one that contains a highly purified form of trypan blue. The literature reports contamination in dyes prepared in eye banks[30] and compounding pharmacies, which suggests that surgeons should avoid using trypan blue from these sources. For additional safety, surgeons should know that VisionBlue has a shelf life of 2 years.

CONCLUSION

Using VisionBlue to stain the capsule during cataract surgery improves the procedure's safety. The technique described herein is safe, easy, effective, does not require extra instrumentation, and adds minimal time to the procedure. VisionBlue also helps surgeons create "perfect" capsulorhexes, conferring short- and long-term benefits on the outcome of cataract surgery. ■

This article originally appeared in the October 2007 issue of CRSToday.

INDICATIONS FOR CAPSULAR STAINING

Although the initial ophthalmic application for VisionBlue was to improve the visualization of mature cataracts during phacoemulsification, its indications have expanded to include any eyes with compromised red reflex and less obvious conditions such as:

- White/brown cataract or cortical cataract with a predilection for the nasal quadrant;
- Corneal opacity[1-3] or ocular surface disease;[3,4]
- Vitreous opacity;[5]
- Pigmented fundus; and
- Traumatic cataract.[6]

VisonBlue is also useful for:

- Creating anterior and posterior capsulorhexes in pediatric cases;[7-9]
- Training residents[10-12] and assisting surgeons as they transition to advanced procedures such as phaco chop (the identification of the capsulorhexis' edge is important during these procedures);
- High-risk cases including pseudoexfoliation and true exfoliation;[13]
- Cases in which the zonules are compromised or when a surgeon is operating on a patient's second eye after his first eye developed an intraoperative complication (VisionBlue can assist in identifying anteriorly inserted zonules);[14]
- Open-sky techniques;[15]
- The removal of capsular plaque;[16]
- Resolving complications such as "lost" or errant capsulorhexes;[17] and
- Managing miscellaneous difficult cases.[18]

1. Bhartiya P, Sharma N, Ray M, et al. Trypan blue assisted phacoemulsification in corneal opacities. *Br J Ophthalmol.* 2002;86:857-859.
2. Titiyal JS, Sinha R, Sharma N, Vajpayee RB. Dye-assisted small incision cataract surgery in eyes with cataract and coexisting corneal opacity. *Eye.* 2006;20:386-388.
3. Gregory ME, Bibby K. Dye-assisted small incision cataract surgery in an eye with cataract and coexisting corneal scarring and epithelial disease. *Eye.* 2007;21:299-300.
4. Kuchenbecker J, Vorwerk C, Mawrin C, Behrens-Baumann W. Trypan-blue-assisted anterior continuous curvilinear capsulorhexis in a case of ocular pemphigoid. *Ocul Immunol Inflamm.* 2006;14:313-315.
5. Yamamoto N, Ozaki N, Murakami K. Trypan blue- and endoillumination-assisted phacoemulsification in eyes with vitreous hemorrhage during combined cataract and vitreous surgery. *Ophthalmologica.* 2005;219:338-344.
6. Kazem MA, Behbehani JH, Uboweja AK, Paramasivam RB. Traumatic cataract surgery assisted by trypan blue. *Ophthalmic Surg Lasers Imaging.* 2007;38:160-163.
7. Brown SM, Graham WA, McCartney DL. Trypan blue in pediatric cataract surgery. *J Cataract Refract Surg.* 2004;30:2033.
8. Saini JS, Jain AK, Sukhija J, et al. Anterior and posterior capsulorhexis in pediatric cataract surgery with or without trypan blue dye: randomized prospective clinical study. *J Cataract Refract Surg.* 2003;29:1733-1737.
9. Sharma N, Balasubramanya R, Dada VK, Vajpayee RB. Efficacy of trypan blue in posterior capsulorhexis with optic capture in pediatric cataracts. *BMC Ophthalmol.* 2006;6:12.
10. Sharma N, Bhartiya P, Sinha R, Vajpayee RB. Trypan blue assisted phacoemulsification by residents in training. *Clin Experiment Ophthalmol.* 2002;30:386-387.
11. Akman A, Akova YA. Trypan-blue-assisted capsulorhexis for trainee phacoemulsification surgeons. *J Cataract Refract Surg.* 2003;29:861-862.
12. Dada T, Ray M, Bhartiya P, Vajpayee RB. Trypan-blue-assisted capsulorhexis for trainee phacoemulsification surgeons. *J Cataract Refract Surg.* 2002;28:575-576.
13. Rossiter J, Morris A. Trypan blue vital staining of the anterior lens capsule in the management of cataract in true exfoliation of the lens capsule. *Eye.* 2005;19:809-810.
14. Chen SD, Glover N, Patel CK. Trypan blue staining of anteriorly placed zonules in patients with pigment dispersion. *J Cataract Refract Surg.* 2004;30:2462-2463 (author reply, 2463).
15. Ozkiris A, Arslan O, Cicik E, et al. Open-sky capsulorrhexis in triple procedure: with or without trypan blue? *Eur J Ophthalmol.* 2003;13:764-769.
16. Sharma N, Gupta V, Vajpayee RB. Trypan-blue-assisted posterior capsule plaque removal. *J Cataract Refract Surg.* 2002;28:916-917.
17. de Waard PW, Budo CJ, Melles GR. Trypan blue capsular staining to "find" the leading edge of a "lost" capsulorhexis. *Am J Ophthalmol.* 2002;134:271-272.
18. Lee GA, Hann JV, Braga-Mele R. Phacoemulsification in anterior megalophthalmos. *J Cataract Refract Surg.* 2006;32:1081-1084.

1. Chang DF. Capsule staining and mature cataracts: a comparison of indocyanine green and trypan blue dyes. *Br J Ophthalmol.* 2000;84:809-936.
2. Sturmer J. Cataract surgery and the "Blue Miracle". *Klin Monatsbl Augenheilkd.* 2002;219:191-195.
3. Ozturk F, Osher RH. Capsular staining: recent developments. *Curr Opin Ophthalmol.* 2006;17:42-44.
4. Jacobs DS, Cox TA, Wagoner MD, et al. Capsule staining as an adjunct to cataract surgery: a report from the American Academy of Ophthalmology. *Ophthalmology.* 2006;113:707-713.
5. Goldman JM, Karp CL. Adjunct devices for managing challenging cases in cataract surgery: capsular staining and ophthalmic viscosurgical devices. *Curr Opin Ophthalmol.* 2007;18:52-57.
6. San Laureano J, Coroneo MT. Crystalline lens capsule staining with trypan blue. *J Cataract Refract Surg.* 2004;30:2046-2049.
7. Coroneo M. Retrospective on staining with trypan blue. *Cataract & Refractive Surgery Today.* 2005;5:3:49-51.
8. Birchall W, Raynor MK, Turner GS. Inadvertent staining of the posterior lens capsule with trypan blue dye during phacoemulsification. *Arch Ophthalmol.* 2001;119:1082-1083.
9. Gaur A, Kayarkar VV. Inadvertent vitreous staining. *J Cataract Refract Surg.* 2005;31:649.
10. Chowdhury PK, Raj SM, Vasavada AR. Inadvertent staining of the vitreous with trypan blue. *J Cataract Refract Surg.* 2004;30:274-276.
11. Marques DM, Marques FF, Osher RH. Three-step technique for staining the anterior lens capsule with indocyanine green or trypan blue. *J Cataract Refract Surg.* 2004;30:13-16.

12. Cheung LM, Wilcsek GA, Francis IC, Coroneo MT. Staining of the tenon capsule with trypan blue during enucleation surgery. *Arch Ophthalmol.* 2005;123:1125-1126.
13. Balestrazzi E, Balestrazzi A, Mosca L, Balestrazzi A. Deep lamellar keratoplasty with trypan blue intrastromal staining. *J Cataract Refract Surg.* 2002;28:929-931.
14. Jackson TL, Kwan AS, Laidlaw AH, Aylward W. Identification of retinal breaks using subretinal trypan blue injection. *Ophthalmology.* 2007;114:587-590.
15. Pandey SK, Apple DJ, Werner L, et al. Posterior capsule opacification: a review of the aetiopathogenesis, experimental and clinical studies and factors for prevention. *Indian J Ophthalmol.* 2004;52:99-112.
16. Arora R, Shroff D, Chauhan D, Narula R. Trypan-blue-assisted "re-rhexis" for smooth in-the-bag exchange of a calcified intraocular lens. *J Cataract Refract Surg.* 2006;32:215.
17. Hill WE. Highly accurate IOL calculations. Pearls for achieving consistent outcomes. *Cataract & Refractive Surgery Today.* 2006;6:3:82-86.
18. Cekic O, Batman C. The relationship between capsulorhexis size and anterior chamber depth relation. *Ophthalmic Surg Lasers.* 1999;30:185-190. [Erratum in: *Ophthalmic Surg Lasers.* 1999;30:714.]
19. Grant WM, Schuman JS. *Toxicology of the Eye.* 4th ed. Springfield, IL: Charles C. Thomas; 1993.
20. Norn MS. Per operative trypan blue vital staining of corneal endothelium. Eight years' follow up. *Acta Ophthalmol (Copenh).* 1980;58:550-555.
21. Werner L, Yeh O, Haymore J, et al. Corneal endothelial safety with the irradiation system for light-adjustable intraocular lenses. *J Cataract Refract Surg.* 2007;33:873-878.
22. Olson RJ. Strategies for complicated lens surgery, Part 1: advanced cataract and pseudoexfoliation syndrome. *American Academy of Ophthalmology Focal Points.* 2005;23:1-10.
23. Wollensak G, Sporl E, Pham DT. Biomechanical changes in the anterior lens capsule after trypan blue staining. *J Cataract Refract Surg.* 2004 ;30:1526-1530.
24. Coroneo MT, Pandey SK. Capsulorhexis integrity is unaffected by trypan blue: an in vitro study in human eyebank eyes. Poster presented at: The ARVO Annual Meeting. April 30, 2007; Fort Lauderdale, FL.
25. Hisatomi T, Enaida H, Matsumoto H, et al. Staining ability and biocompatibility of brilliant blue G: preclinical study of brilliant blue G as an adjunct for capsular staining. *Arch Ophthalmol.* 2006;124:514-519.
26. van Dooren BT, de Waard PW, Poort-van Nouhuys H, et al. Corneal endothelial cell density after trypan blue capsule staining in cataract surgery. *J Cataract Refract Surg.* 2002;28:574-675.
27. Werner L, Apple DJ, Crema AS, et al. Permanent blue discoloration of a hydrogel intraocular lens by intraoperative trypan blue. *J Cataract Refract Surg.* 2002;28:1279-1286.
28. Mamalis N, Edelhauser HF, Dawson DG, et al. Toxic anterior segment syndrome. *J Cataract Refract Surg.* 2006;32:324-333.
29. Wu L, Velasquez R, Montoya O. Non-infectious endophthalmitis associated with trypan blue use in cataract surgery. *Int Ophthalmol.* 2007;Jul 19 [E-pub ahead of print].
30. Morel PC, Roubi N, Talon DR, Bertrand X. Contamination of trypan blue with *Burkholderia cepacia* in a cornea bank. *Infect Control Hosp Epidemiol.* 2003;24:198-201.

CHAPTER 44

Phacoemulsification of the High-Risk Lens

TAL RAVIV, MD

Long-standing, mature cataracts frequently present many challenges simultaneously. One or two complicating factors are sufficient to increase the difficulty of cataract surgery, and four or more risk factors may be present in cases of advanced cataract. The overripe lens is commonly associated with a small pupil, a super-dense nucleus, a shallow anterior chamber, and shaky zonules.

Surgeons need to plan ahead for the difficulties they are likely to encounter in high-risk cases. A small mistake or unplanned move early in the case can snowball into a serious, multifaceted complication. This article elucidates the techniques and technology available to confront the probable challenges of mature cataracts and to prevent escalating complications. I find that the three keys for success in hypermature lenses are (1) constructing a capsulorhexis that is as large as possible, (2) deepening the chamber by means of a 25-gauge vitrectomy, when indicated, and (3) using a vertical chopping technique (also known as *quick chop*) for nuclear disassembly.

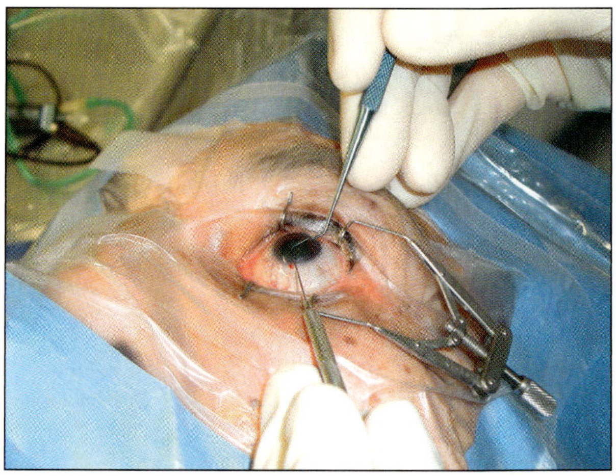

Figure 1. An angled Kuglen hook provides access below a prominent brow during bimanual pupillary stretching.

LARGE CAPSULORHEXIS

Although the sizing of the capsulorhexis varies from surgeon to surgeon (and in many instances from case to case), bigger is definitely better with a hypermature lens. A large (greater than 6mm), continuous, central capsulorhexis has a number of advantages. First, locating the capsulorhexis' edge toward the periphery greatly reduces the likelihood of inadvertent capsular damage by the phaco tip due to poor visibility. Second, a large capsulorhexis allows quadrant or segment removal to proceed without capsular trapping or increased zonular stretching. Finally, and most importantly, in case of trouble, a large capsulorhexis will allow the dense nucleus to prolapse out of the capsular bag for capsule-free phacoemulsification.

In order to construct a large capsulorhexis, one must overcome difficulties such as a small pupil, a shallow chamber, iris prolapse, and poor capsular visibility. Unless one plans to perform a blind capsulorhexis under the iris, prudent pupillary expansion is necessary. Enlarging the pupil can be done in a number of ways: with an all-in-one pupil dilator such as the Beehler (Moria, Antony, France); a pupil-expansion ring; manual pupillary stretching; or iris hooks (older techniques such as multiple macrosphincterotomies or sector iridectomies are less practical, because they result in the permanent loss of pupillary anatomy and function). A shallow chamber and close endothelial proximity to the iris make the insertion of the relatively large Beehler or the placement of a pupil expansion ring risky. Manual pupillary stretching is therefore the procedure of choice. Iris hooks can also work well and may be relied upon as a backup at any point in the case.

Another trick for creating a large capsulorhexis is to start with a

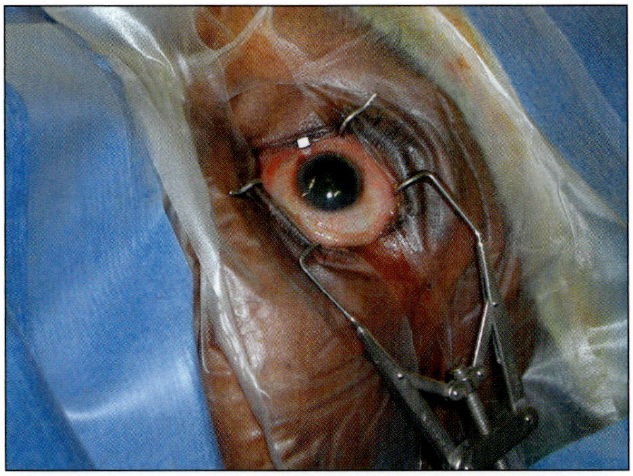

Figure 2. The entry-site alignment cannula lines up the openings in the conjunctiva, Tenon's capsule, and sclera. It thereby facilitates the 25-gauge instrument's access to the posterior segment.

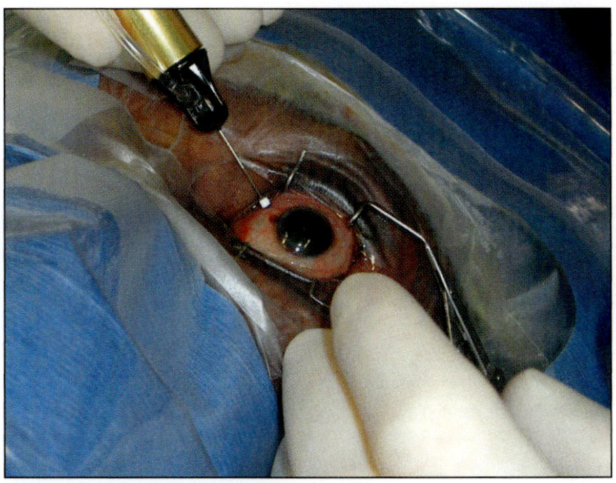

Figure 3. The high-speed vitrectomy cutter is easily inserted through the cannula for the 25-gauge PPV.

smaller, more controllable capsulorhexis. When coming around to finish the capsulorhexis, overlap the starting point and continue the tear around again at a wider diameter. With intralenticular pressure resolved, removing the circumferential ribbon of capsule on the second pass will be much easier and allow the creation of a large capsulorhexis, even in a challenging case.

PUPILLARY STRETCHING

The location and construction of the incision should facilitate pupillary management. For a temporal clear corneal approach, the two paracenteses should be placed 45° to either side of the main incision in order to allow the instruments plenty of leverage to stretch in all meridians. This placement also enables the surgeon to easily switch to iris hooks later in the case, if necessary, by creating two more paracenteses 90° apart.

Stretching is best accomplished with two smooth Kuglen hooks. At least one of the hooks, if not both, should have an angled handle to allow easy access beneath the brow (Figure 1). Stretching works by breaking the fibrotic pupillary margin/sphincter complex—in essence, a microsphincterotomy. To achieve the maximal effect, the surgeon should use the Kuglen hooks to stretch two opposite pupillary edges all the way to the angle and hold them there for a few seconds. Typically, stretching in the four cardinal directions is sufficient. Viscoelastic injection can then clear the iris pigment and keep the pupil enlarged. Healon 5 (Advanced Medical Optics, Inc., Santa Ana, CA) or Viscoat (Alcon Laboratories, Inc., Fort Worth, TX) are quite retentive and tend to be efficacious for this step. Using too much viscoelastic can lead to iris prolapse, however.

IRIS PROLAPSE

Iris prolapse from the incision is not uncommon in complex cases. The complication results from a number of anatomic variables, including a shallow chamber, a floppy iris, a posteriorly placed entry incision, and diverse pressure dynamics. Prolapse can cause pain (in topical anesthesia cases), lead to iris depigmentation and atrophy, complicate instrument entry through the wound, and alter the pupil's size and shape, thereby affecting visibility. If the iris prolapses early in the case, it is likely to have "memory" and prolapse repeatedly throughout the surgery. Preventing and managing iris prolapse is critical to good visibility and a complication-free procedure.

The iris will prolapse initially either during the capsulorhexis or, more commonly, during hydrodissection. Prolapse occurs when the closed system of the anterior chamber is disrupted, such as during instrument insertion. Similarly, once the surgeon has passed the phaco sleeve through the incision, thus re-establishing the closed system, the iris will remain controlled.

Preventing iris prolapse depends on careful wound construction and management of the IOP dynamics. The paracentesis should be narrow and parallel to the iris surface. The clear corneal wound should begin as temporally as possible, with an intrastromal tunnel that is approximately 2 mm in length. A shorter tunnel will predispose the eye to iris prolapse, whereas a longer tunnel will cause the oar-locking of instruments and visually significant corneal striae.

Understanding the pressure dynamics of iris prolapse is critical to managing the complication without frustration. In conjunction with the aforementioned anatomic variables, prolapse can only occur when the pressure inside the anterior chamber is greater than the atmospheric pressure outside. In such an instance, when an instrument breaches the self-sealing wound, fluid (aqueous or viscoelastic) exits the eye and sweeps out the iris in a susceptible case. The surgeon must maintain the equilibrium in pressure between the anterior chamber and outside. One suggestion is to avoid overfilling the anterior chamber with viscoelastic initially. Also, during hydrodissection, the surgeon should angle the cannula diagonally across the wound (and above the subincisional iris) while simultaneously pressing down on the posterior lip. When fluid is injected, displaced viscoelastic and fluid exit the eye instantaneously, before pressure has built up.

Once prolapse has occurred, it is tempting to place more viscoelastic in the chamber and push the iris back inside. Paradoxically, doing so actually increases the anterior chamber pressure and can lead to aggravated prolapse. Depressurizing the anterior chamber by depressing the paracentesis can equalize the pressure and cause the iris to pull itself into the eye. Although this technique works for most cases of iris prolapse due to increased anterior chamber pressure, it will not work in the rare instance of increased posterior pressure. The vitrectomy technique outlined later in this article can help in such a case.

If persistent iris prolapse hinders capsulorhexis creation despite the techniques just described, it may be necessary to close the incision and perform the capsulorhexis via the paracentesis. Once the closed system is re-established, viscoelastic may be used to deepen and dilate the already stretched pupil. The surgeon may create the capsulorhexis in a controlled fashion with either a cystotome or, preferably, a microcapsulorhexis forceps.

CAPSULAR VISIBILITY

Visualization is critical to achieving a large capsulorhexis. Even if the cataract is not white, dense lenses typically obscure the red reflex. Capsular staining with either indocyanine green or trypan blue (where available and approved) should be used. The dye should be injected after pupillary enlargement (under air, viscoelastic, or both), although the dye may be placed at any time, even in the middle of the capsulorhexis procedure, if necessary. If visualization remains poor due to coexisting corneal clouding or opacity, a coaxial vitrectomy light pipe can be helpful. The surgeon should turn off the microscope light and place the light pipe perpendicular or oblique to the limbus.

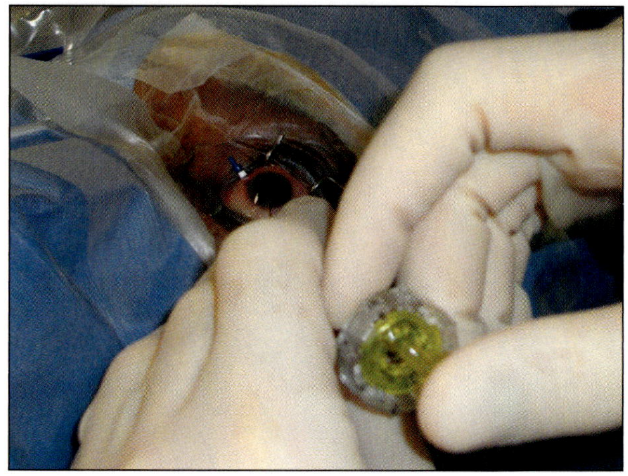

Figure 4. After vitrectomy and chamber deepening, the blue plug seals the cannula as the phaco procedure commences.

SHALLOW-CHAMBER MANAGEMENT

In most cases, placing viscoelastic in the eye provides adequate chamber depth, but this step may not be sufficient in eyes with extremely thick lenses. In the presence of severe anterior chamber shallowing (my threshold is less than two corneal thicknesses centrally), one should resort to a limited pars plana vitrectomy (PPV). This step can dramatically improve the chamber depth and IOP dynamics. For the anterior segment surgeon, the most effective manner in which to perform the PPV is with the 25-gauge, sutureless, transconjunctival vitrectomy system (TSV25) on the Millennium microsurgical system (Bausch & Lomb, Rochester, NY). The TSV25 system allows for safe and efficient vitrectomy, especially for the purpose of chamber deepening. No conjunctival dissection, cautery, or scleral suturing is necessary. That only one port is required further simplifies the process.

The location of the sclerotomy depends on exposure. For a temporal approach, a supra- or infranasal spot allows the easiest access. The TSV25 system uses an entry-site alignment cannula over a 25-gauge trocar. The surgeon inserts the trocar/cannula unit transconjunctivally, 4 mm from the limbus, at the beginning of the case, when the eye is firmest. The trocar is then removed, but the cannula is left in place for easy instrument insertion and removal (Figure 2). After placing a 25-gauge, high-speed vitrectomy cutter through the cannula into the vitreous cavity, the surgeon performs a minimal core vitrectomy with settings of 1,500 cuts/min and vacuum of 500 mm Hg (Figure 3). After chamber deepening, the vitrector may be removed and the cannula sealed with the plug provided. Phacoemulsification may then proceed (Figure 4). Further vitrectomy may be performed at any time, if necessary. After completing phacoemulsification and IOL insertion, the surgeon employs a forceps to remove the cannula and the plug as a unit and uses a Weck cell sponge to slide conjunctiva over the sclerotomy site. The 25-gauge sclerotomy is self-sealing and requires no sutures.

The TSV25 system is efficient, elegant, and also highly efficacious. With this technology, performing a limited PPV is simple, takes only a few additional minutes, and can transform a difficult case into a manageable one.

EFFICIENT NUCLEAR DISASSEMBLY

Preferred Technique

Of all the elements addressed so far, a large capsulorhexis is the most important by far when preparing to disassemble a superdense nucleus on loose zonules. Even with suboptimal pupillary dilation, vertical chopping or quick chop is the procedure of choice for nuclear disassembly.

Quick chopping has numerous advantages over disassembly techniques such as divide and conquer. In vertical chopping, the phaco tip and chopper remain within the central 2 to 3 mm of the eye during the entire case, a positioning that allows safe phacoemulsification even if pupillary constriction occurs. The phaco tip stays at a safe depth throughout quick chop (unlike the grooving technique) and never approaches the posterior capsule. Chopping is also friendlier to the zonules. Because the forces used in chopping are equal and opposite, they balance each other out and minimize zonular stress.

Vertical chopping of a hypermature nucleus differs slightly from chopping a cataract of regular density. Hydrodelineation is not possible in most cases. Because the multiple layers of a dense nucleus typically become one, the usual epinuclear cushion is lacking. Also, the density of the nucleus may require numerous chops instead of the typical three. Chopping the nucleus into smaller pieces will facilitate its removal.

A leathery posterior plate is present in certain dense red or brown cataracts that prevents the complete separation of the chopped segments. In such cases, it is best to phacoemulsify and debulk the anterior aspect of the segments and to leave the tenuous posterior plate intact. A viscoelastic cannula may then be placed behind the plate to elevate it from the posterior capsule for final emulsification.

Sources of Trouble

During phacoemulsification, further problems such as zonular dehiscence or capsular compromise may occur. After identifying such a complication, one should cease phacoemulsification and reform the chamber with Viscoat via the sideport incision before removing the phaco tip in order to prevent chamber fluctuation. At this point, it is important to tamponade any prolapsing vitreous with Healon 5 or Viscoat. Further intracapsular manipulation of the nucleus is very risky, and the case must be converted to a supracapsular or capsule-free procedure. A large capsulorhexis is of real benefit in these instances, because it permits the use of this escape maneuver.

One method for elevating the lens out of the bag through the capsulorhexis opening is to inject viscoelastic behind the lens to prolapse the nucleus completely above the anterior capsule. If a large portion of the lens remains, the surgeon may need to elevate it with a spatulated nucleus manipulator by sweeping under the anterior capsular rim and behind the lens. Once the lens is free from the confines of the capsule, placing Viscoat in front of and behind it will provide capsular and endothelial protection. The surgeon should emulsify the lens in one piece in a carousel fashion while supporting it underneath with the second instrument.

Intentionally prolapsing the nucleus out of the compromised capsular bag resembles the conversion to an extracapsular, large-incision procedure, except that the latter involves a large, uncontrollable incision. Although converting to an extracapsular procedure can be safely accomplished, I believe maintaining a closed system is critical in complicated situations with capsular compromise and vitreous prolapse. Using the aforementioned technique can help re-establish control of an errant case and achieve excellent results.

CONCLUSION

Phacoemulsification has become the procedure of choice for even the most hypermature cataracts. With a meticulous, stepwise approach that combines advanced technical skills and the newest technologies, surgeons can transform a feared, complex cataract surgery with multiple risk factors into an anticipated challenge. ■

This article originally appeared in the October 2004 issue of CRSToday.

CHAPTER 45

Phacoemulsification of the Mature Nucleus

PRISCILLA PERRY ARNOLD, MD; LISA BROTHERS ARBISSER, MD; JOHN D. HUNKELER, MD; AND D. MICHAEL COLVARD, MD

INTRODUCTION

Whether brown or black, the nuclear mature lens often presents a challenge to the cataract surgeon. In this article, experts share their pearls for managing these difficult cases.

THE BROWN CATARACT

Priscilla Perry Arnold, MD

One of the most important aspects of any successful cataract surgery, including dealing with a hard (dense) nucleus, is surgical planning. At the time of the preoperative examination, your attention to detail sets the stage for the ultimate outcome.

In addition to the dense nuclear sclerosis, note other complicating factors, including endothelial dystrophy, a shallow anterior chamber, a pre-existing bleb, the presence of exfoliation, or evidence of previous trauma or inflammation. Any of these conditions, especially in combination with a hard nucleus, may necessitate an alteration of your routine procedure.

Consider whether circumstances indicate that peribulbar anesthesia would be a more appropriate choice than topical anesthesia. Achieve maximal pupillary dilation for surgery by whatever technique is necessary. Ordinarily, pharmacologic, viscoelastic, or stretching maneuvers are adequate. In rare circumstances, hooks or expander rings may be required. Be prepared for this instance.

Select the viscoelastic with properties best suited to the case and any special challenges—whether for protecting the cornea, maintaining space, or tamponading the vitreous. Tailor your choice to the challenge.

Plan to use the phaco technique most effective for the circumstances and your own experience (whether a dividing or chopping process). Modulate the machine's parameters to minimize intraocular energy. Also, select the IOL material and design based on the situation anticipated but predetermine a back-up lens.

At the time of surgery, proceed deliberately and methodically. Speed is the enemy in any difficult situation. Adequate visualization coupled with safe and effective surgical manipulation will result in the best outcome for the patient.

Lisa Brothers Arbisser, MD

When operating on an eye with a hard nucleus, retract the sleeve of the phaco tip as far as possible without allowing irrigation into the incision's tunnel in order to avoid collapsing the chamber. The retracted sleeve will expose approximately 2 mm of the phaco needle to permit its adequate entry into the nucleus. This technique allows a vertical chop without sculpting and creates a fault line in the nucleus that results in two hemispheres. The exposed phaco needle functions as a "dipstick," which measures how deeply it penetrates the lenticular material. Knowing that the average lens is 4.6 mm thick for a 60-year-old gives assurance of the needle's safe depth when plunged to the level of the sleeve.

THE BLACK CATARACT

John D. Hunkeler, MD

When faced with a dense nucleus, I use the stop-and-chop nucleofractis technique combined with a technique pioneered by Howard Gimbel, MD, of Loma Linda, California, called *posterior pole exploration*. The term describes a very short ultrasound phacoemulsification with a compact linear groove aiming toward the posterior pole of the lens. The narrow groove allows efficient emulsification to set the stage for a cleavage plane that will extend through all the layers of the nucleus.

I use the following steps with a dense nucleus. After hydrodissection (without hydrodelineation), I loosen the nucleus and compact cortex from the capsular bag, as apparent by rotation of the material within the capsular bag. With ultrasound, I complete a short, central but deep groove. The ultrasound and dissection point toward the posterior pole of the lens through the deeper nuclear layers and compact cortex. I pay less attention to the lateral, peripheral nuclear layers and epinucleus at this time. My arrival at the posterior pole of the nucleus is indicated by a dramatic improvement in the red reflex, in addition to my judgment that the clarity is adequate to achieve nuclear fracture through the posterior plate of the nucleus and the lateral peripheral layers in that meridian.

Using the nucleus rotator and the exposed tip of the phaco needle, I create two new heminuclear fragments. The remaining heminuclear fragment can be dealt with using the same instrument for horizontal chopping or a more conventional chopping instrument for vertical chopping. Regardless, four to six fragments are created for emulsification in the safe zone in the center of the pupil. As a result, the hybrid procedure of divide and conquer and phaco chop can effectively remove the dense nucleus prior to cortical cleanup.

Occasionally, the leather-like posterior aspect of the peripheral nuclear fibers is not cleaved. In this situation, further ultrasound dissection to enhance the red reflex and thin the posterior plate will allow nuclear cracking through this posterior plate. With a dense nucleus, there is often a need to grasp and regrasp nuclear fragments. In an additional maneuver, the bevel of the phaco tip can be pointed either laterally or posteriorly to minimize cavitational energy directed toward the endothelium. I will add an ophthalmic viscosurgical device (OVD) as needed to protect the endothelium and enhance safety.

To optimize the surgical outcome, microburst phacoemulsification and a focus on grasping and chopping to create smaller fragments will further reduce the total amount of energy, thus promoting the safe and effective removal of dense nuclear material.

The technique described requires a precise, intact capsulorhexis. With dense nuclei, a larger capsulorhexis is preferred. Improved visualization of the capsule is key and may be achieved through staining with either trypan blue or indocyanine green dye. The need for capsular staining is obvious when the red reflex is absent.

D. Michael Colvard, MD

My approach is informed by two observations. The first is that the truly rock-hard nucleus is almost invariably associated with a tissue-thin capsule and very fragile zonules. The second is that, unlike most contemporary cases, for which the refractive outcome defines success, the elderly patient with a ruby red cataract is invariably happy just to see again. This patient is unlikely to be upset by 0.50 to 1.00 D of postoperative cylinder.

Occasionally, I am pleasantly surprised that the nucleus is not as dense as it appeared upon slit-lamp examination and the phaco procedure can be completed safely. I use trypan blue to stain the capsule and a dispersive OVD to protect the endothelium. I divide the nucleus into quadrants with deep grooves and then chop the quadrants. If the first four or five passes with the phaco device do not seem to make a dent in the nucleus, however, I do not hesitate to convert to a standard extracapsular procedure.

The one pearl I have for surgeons who do not perform extracapsular cataract extractions very often is to use the OVD to lift the huge nucleus out of the fragile capsule without placing stress on the zonular system. I make several radial cuts in the capsulorhexis' margin and enlarge the incision. If I have made any kind of notch in the anterior surface of the nucleus, I place my chopper through the sideport, direct it nose down in the notch, and slide the nucleus inferiorly toward the patient's feet. Simultaneously, I use the OVD cannula to press gently on the posterior lip of the primary incision. The chamber partially shallows, and the proximal edge of the nucleus rises above the iris margin.

I then engage the nucleus just under its equator with the OVD cannula and inject viscoelastic beneath the lens. As I gently fill the capsular bag, I lift and rotate the large nucleus into the anterior chamber. The nucleus can then be spun out of the eye with a Sinskey hook without placing any stress on the capsule or the zonules whatsoever. ■

This article originally appeared in the June 2005 issue of CRSToday.

CHAPTER 46

Techniques for IFIS

BY DAVID F. CHANG, MD

Benign prostate hyperplasia (BPH) causes poor urinary outflow due to an enlarged prostate. Flomax (Boehringer-Ingelheim Pharmaceuticals, Inc., Ridgefield, CT) is an alpha-blocker that improves urinary outflow by relaxing the smooth muscle in the prostate and the bladder's neck. There are three alpha-1-blocker receptor subtypes, alpha-1 A, B, and D. Flomax is specific to the alpha-blocker 1A, which is the predominant subtype in the prostate and the iris dilator muscle. The nonspecific blockers such as Hytrin (Abbott Laboratories Inc., North Chicago, IL), Cardura (Pfizer Inc., New York, NY), and Uroxatral (Sanofi-Aventis, Bridgewater, NJ) can also cause Intraoperative Floppy Iris Syndrome (IFIS), although much less severely. Because Flomax is more urospecific and causes less postural hypotension than most nonspecific agents, it is the most commonly prescribed drug for treating BPH symptoms. Unfortunately, cessation of this and other alpha-blocking drugs does not prevent IFIS.[1]

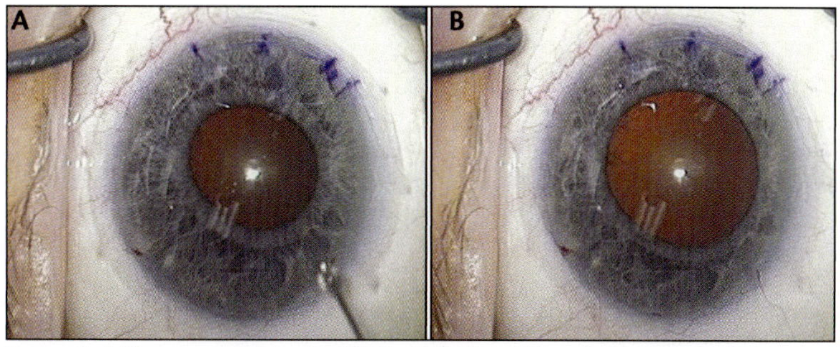

Figure 1. A Flomax patient with IFIS both before (A) and after (B) the intracameral injection of epinephrine (1:1,000 bisulfite-free,mixed 1:3 with balanced salt solution).

MANAGING IFIS

Severity Scale

In order to manage IFIS, you must understand and recognize that there is a continuum of severity that varies between different patients and even between the two eyes of the same patient.[2] Mild IFIS is characterized by good pupillary dilation, slight billowing of the iris, and no significant miosis or prolapse. If there is also intraoperative miosis (eg, > 2 mm decrease in pupil diameter), I characterize this as moderate IFIS. Severe IFIS has billowing, miosis, and a strong tendency for iris prolapse (Figure 1). Because pupillary stretching is ineffective, there are three primary types of management strategies that can be used alone or in combination: pharmacologic; viscoadaptive; or mechanical restraining devices. For me, the choice of what techniques to use depends on the severity of the IFIS, and familiarity with all three methodologies is therefore beneficial.

Viscoadaptive Stretching

Popularized by Robert Osher, MD, and Douglas Koch, MD, the viscoadaptive ophthalmic viscosurgical device (OVD) Healon5 (Advanced Medical Optics, Inc., Santa Ana, CA) is very effective for IFIS, because it can mechanically dilate the pupil and also forms an impenetrable barrier to iris prolapse. The caveat is that you must use low aspiration flow and vacuum settings so that the Healon5 is not immediately withdrawn from the eye. I first try to chop the nucleus into multiple fragments within in the capsular bag. This allows me to delay the phaco-assisted aspiration of the mobilized pieces in the supracapsular plane, at which point the Healon5 will also start to be aspirated. If the pupil begins to constrict during this step, you simply add more Healon5. If the nucleus is soft, high vacuum is generally not needed. During cortical I/A, the principle is to keep the phaco tip in the peripheral fornices of the bag, where you can constantly reocclude it with more cortex to avoid removing the OVD. If you have limited experience with Healon5, do not try it in IFIS eyes until you have mastered the nuances of its use in routine cases. For example, Healon5 changes the mechanical dynamics of flap manipulation during the capsulorhexis. It must also be aspirated from behind the IOL's optic to avoid a postoperative pressure spike.

Pharmacologic Strategies

Administering atropine preoperatively, as advocated by Samuel Masket, MD, may help hold a mild-to-moderate IFIS pupil open if it is well dilated to begin with. However, my preferred pharmacologic approach is to inject 1:1,000 bisulfite-free epinephrine diluted 1:3 with plain balanced salt solution (BSS Plus [Alcon Laboratories, Inc., Fort Worth, TX] works fine, also), as suggested by Joel Shugar, MD.[3] Richard Packard, BSc, FRCOphth, and David Allen, BSc, FRCOphth, of the UK, have also published on the efficacy of using intracameral phenylephrine, which is not available in the US.[4] These alpha agonists will further dilate the pupil in a mild-to-moderate IFIS case. More importantly, they increase the dilator's smooth muscle tone, which reduces or even eliminates the iris' floppiness and tendency to prolapse. Injecting epinephrine is a great rescue technique when IFIS is not recognized until after completion of the capsulorhexis and hydrodissection. Placing iris retractors is more difficult and risky at this point because of poor visibility of the capsulorhexis' edge, and I would therefore try intracameral epinephrine as a first step in this situation. I now use intracameral epinephrine with every potential IFIS case, unless I know that I will be using iris hooks.

The combination of Healon5 and epinephrine works well if the pupil does not dilate enough after the intracameral injection of epinephrine. The epinephrine will increase the iris' rigidity, while Healon5 viscomydriasis can facilitate the capsulorhexis.

Pupillary Expansion Devices

If the pupil hardly dilates in a Flomax patient, you should antici-

TABLE 1. IFIS SEVERITY (FLOMAX)	
Chang Multicenter Study (N=167)	
Severity	Percentage of cases
No IFIS	10%
Mild	17%
Moderate	30%
Severe	43%

Chang DF, Osher RH, Wang L, Koch DD. A prospective multicenter evaluation of cataract surgery in patients taking tamsulosin (Flomax). Ophthalmology. 2007 (In press).

pate severe IFIS, because the dilator muscle is not responding at all. Another clue of greater IFIS severity is noticeable billowing of the iris as you first inject intracameral lidocaine. In these cases, you should consider using iris retractors.

I place the iris retractors in the diamond configuration.[5] Through a separate paracentesis that I make immediately behind the clear corneal incision, I place a subincisional retractor that pulls the iris down and beneath the phaco tip. In contrast, the traditional square configuration of the hooks' placement tents the iris up in front of the incision. The nasal retractor also gives great exposure for placing the chopper. Fortunately, the IFIS pupil is usually very elastic and can be maximally stretched without damaging the iris sphincter. In contrast to eyes with pseudoexfoliation or on miotics, the IFIS pupil is not fibrotic, which is why it does not respond well to stretching.

Some surgeons prefer to use a pupil expansion ring as an alternative to iris hooks, although some experience is needed because they are difficult to position if the pupil is very small or if the anterior chamber is shallow. I prefer reusable retractors that are made from 4–0 Prolene (Katena Products, Inc., Denville, NJ, and FCI Ophthalmics, Inc., Marshfield Hills, MA) instead of 6–0 nylon, because the former are easier to manipulate and also sturdy enough to be autoclaved and reused, which makes them very cost effective.

Because they guarantee a large pupil that will not constrict, I use iris retractors in IFIS eyes whenever I am concerned about visibility or other concomitant risk factors, such as a dense nucleus or pseudoexfoliation. If you are dealing with a one-eyed patient or plan to implant a presbyopia-correcting IOL, the security of a widely expanded pupil may well be worth the extra time needed to place retractors. With practice, using iris retractors will add a negligible amount of time to your procedure's overall duration.

STUDY

Because patient history obviously forewarns about IFIS, complication rates should be based on whether the syndrome was anticipated or unanticipated. Retrospective studies in which eye surgeons could not anticipate IFIS have reported higher rates of surgical complications in Flomax patients.[1] A prospective, multicenter study I conducted with nine colleagues evaluated the complication rate in 167 consecutive eyes in Flomax patients when the medication history was known in advance of the procedure.[2] Table 1 shows the severity of the IFIS. The surgeons used one of the three previously discussed categories of strategies, either alone or in combination, and the rate of vitreous loss and posterior capsular rupture was 0.6%. In short, the study showed that experienced surgeons who knew about their patients' history with Flomax preoperatively and were able to use these IFIS management strategies had very low complication rates. This was the basis for the joint AAO/ASCRS/AUA (American Urological Association) public press release in August 2006 that reported that these drugs were still safe to prescribe and take, as long as the ophthalmologist was informed. ■

This article originally appeared in CRSToday's *February 2007* Best of Source *supplement.*

1. Chang DF, Campbell JR. Intraoperative floppy iris syndrome associated with tamsulosin (Flomax). *J Cataract Refract Surg.* 2005;31:664-673.
2. Chang DF, Osher RH, Wang L, Koch DD. A prospective multicenter evaluation of cataract surgery in patients taking tamsulosin (Flomax). *Ophthalmology.* 2007 (In press).
3. Shugar, JK. Intracameral epinephrine for prophylaxis of IFIS [letter]. *J Cataract Refract Surg.* 2006;32:1074-1075.
4. Manvikar S, Allen D. Cataract surgery management in patients taking tamsulosin. *J Cataract Refract Surg.* 2006;32:1611-1614.
5. Oetting TA, Omphroy LC. Modified technique using flexible iris retractors in clear corneal surgery. *J Cataract Refract Surg.* 2002;28:596-598.

CHAPTER 47

Intracameral Epinephrine for IFIS Prophylaxis

BY JOEL K. SHUGAR, MD, MSEE

Chang and Campbell's report of intraoperative floppy iris syndrome (IFIS) associated with the use of tamsulosin[1] is one of the landmark discoveries of this decade in the field of cataract surgery. The syndrome is characterized by a floppy, billowing iris that exhibits progressive miosis during cataract surgery, has a propensity to prolapse through all surgical incisions and into the phaco port, and is unresponsive to pupillary stretching.

Tamsulosin is a systemic alpha-1 adrenergic antagonist that has gained widespread popularity among urologists for treating the symptoms of benign prostatic hypertrophy. A significant proportion of men presenting for cataract surgery, therefore, are taking or have taken the drug. Tamsulosin's effect upon the iris is likely due to a blockade of the iris dilator muscle's alpha-1 adrenergic receptors. This effect often appears to be irreversible and of rapid onset. I have observed severe IFIS in patients with only a short history of using the drug who had discontinued it more than 1 year prior to surgery.

The initial suggestions for managing IFIS were to use Healon5 (Advanced Medical Optics, Inc., Santa Ana, CA) and/or iris hooks or pupillary rings. Although effective, these modalities involve

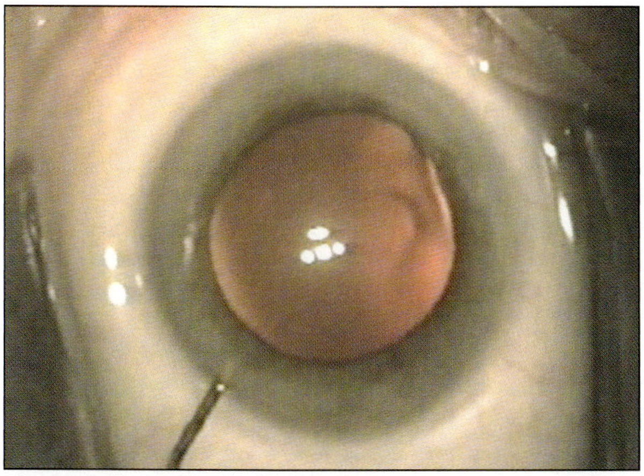

Figure 1. The author instills epi-Shugarcaine in the eye of a patient taking tamsulosin. A previously placed arcuate keratotomy is co-linear with the pupillary margin.

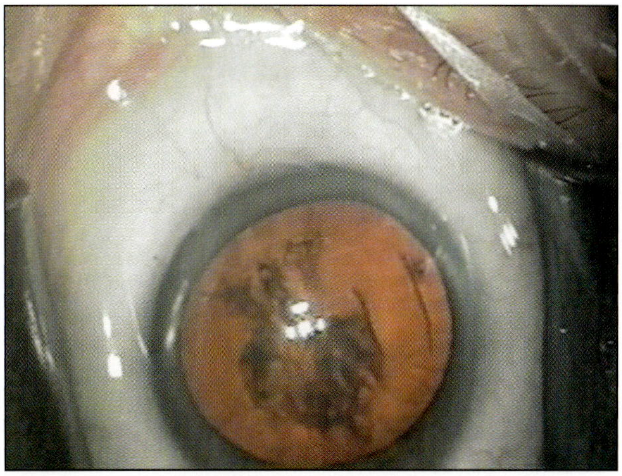

Figure 2. In the same eye, the author has completed the capsulorhexis and hydrodissection. The pupil has dilated an additional 2 mm, and the arcuate keratotomy is now well within the pupillary margin.

altering one's surgical technique. They also typically add time and expense to the case, and they raise the possibility of complications. For example, residual Healon5 has been associated with severe postoperative pressure spikes, especially likely in the hands of surgeons who use it infrequently. The use of iris devices can lead to iatrogenic capsular tears, sometimes progressing to nuclear loss into the vitreous cavity (S. Rooney, MD, written communication, January 2006).

An optimal solution for managing IFIS would neither involve a change in surgical technique nor pose additional risk to the patient. Ideally, it would also use materials that are already readily available in most ophthalmic ORs. I searched for a pharmacologic agent to fulfill these criteria. Because tamsulosin blocks the alpha-1 adrenergic receptors of the iris dilator muscle, it seemed plausible that this blockade could be overcome by flooding the receptors with an intracameral administration of their natural agonist, epinephrine.

THE MIXTURE

The endothelial toxicity of epinephrine has decreased in recent years thanks to the introduction of a sulfite-free, preservative-free 1:1,000 solution (American Reagent Laboratories, Inc., Shirley, NY). It has been shown to cause much less corneal edema than earlier sulfite-containing solutions.[2] I measured the pH of this medication, however, and found it to be 3.13. In order to raise the pH enough for safe intracameral injection, I diluted one part of the stock solution with three parts Shugarcaine. The pH of the resultant mixture measured 6.90, well above the minimum safe threshold of 6.50.[3]

Shugarcaine is 4% unpreserved lidocaine (Abbott Laboratories, Inc., North Chicago, IL) diluted 1:3 with BSS Plus (Alcon Laboratories, Inc., Fort Worth, TX), which produces a 1% lidocaine solution with a pH of 6.97. I developed this mixture when my use of stock 1% lidocaine—the pH of which measures from 6.10 to 6.33—caused corneal edema in my cataract patients. Since I published this formulation,[4] many ophthalmologists have adopted it. There has not been a single report of an adverse effect in the many thousands of cases in which Shugarcaine has been employed.

In the spring of 2005, I began using the mixture of epinephrine and Shugarcaine (which was dubbed *epi-Shugarcaine*) in patients with a history of taking tamsulosin. Because the solution also contains the intracameral anesthetic I routinely use, there was no need for me to change my surgical technique. I administer an initial injection of approximately 1 mL prior to instilling a viscoelastic (Figure 1). In my experience, the iris' flaccidity typically resolves within a few seconds, and 1 to 2 mm of additional mydriasis occurs during the next several minutes (Figure 2). It is my usual practice to repeat the intracameral injection of an anesthetic after completing phacoemulsification. If the patient used or is using tamsulosin, I instill the epinephrine-containing mixture.

In whole milliliter quantities, the formulation for epi-Shugarcaine is to mix 9 mL of BSS Plus with 3 mL of 4% preservative-free lidocaine and 4 mL of 1:1,000 bisulfite-free epinephrine.

RESULTS

My experience with epi-Shugarcaine has been uniformly positive.[5] To date, I have used it in more than 30 patients with a history of taking tamsulosin, and each case has been routine with no IFIS encountered. I did not administer the epinephrine-containing solution during surgery on the first eyes of two patients, and severe IFIS ensued, although I noted no IFIS on the second eyes in which epi-Shugarcaine was used. Per the suggestion of Samuel Masket, MD, of Los Angeles, I premedicated the first few eyes in which I used epi-Shugarcaine with atropine. For the past year, I have omitted the atropine and have not encountered any IFIS.

In June 2005, I suggested using the formulation in a posting on the ASCRS Eye Mail Cataract Group. Since then, about 10 ophthalmologists have reported their experiences with this mixture on the Eye Mail list, and all have been positive. Several surgeons have described patients who exhibited severe IFIS in their first eye (operated on without epinephrine) and required the use of iris hooks and/or Healon5. In contrast, those patients' second eyes, in which the epinephrine mixture was used, did not pose unusual surgical difficulty. Additionally, several surgeons employed epinephrine in the middle of a case that had already progressed to severe IFIS. They reported that the medication aborted the IFIS and made the remainder of the case routine.

The interviews I have given in other publications have raised awareness of epi-Shugarcaine.[6,7] Since then, I have received feedback from a multitude of other ophthalmologists regarding the use of this mixture. All have found it to be efficacious, and no adverse effects have been reported. Only one surgeon who did not use atropine with epi-Shugarcaine has encountered IFIS (S. Masket, MD, written communication, June 2006). A small subset of patients, therefore, might benefit from preoperative atropine and/or might subsequently require additional adjunctive techniques such as iris hooks or Healon5.

Epi-Shugarcaine is my preferred form of prophylaxis against IFIS, because I do not use epinephrine without mixing it with the Shugarcaine formulation. In routine cases, surgeons may use lidocaine to dilate the pupil without the need for adjunctive agents,[8] so lidocaine may add to the efficacy of the epinephrine mixture.

I often receive inquiries about substituting plain balanced salt solution for BSS Plus. Although some surgeons have reported success with this variation (R. Schultz, MD, written communication, June 2006), I prefer BSS Plus because I initially inject the mixture prior to instilling a viscoelastic. I have measured the pH of epi-Shugarcaine formulated with plain balanced salt solution and found it to be 6.67, and I found the pH of bisulfite-free epinephrine diluted 3:1 with balanced salt solution to be 6.75. Plain balanced salt solution therefore may safely be used as a dilutant if BSS Plus is unavailable.

Other surgeons have recommended the use of intracameral phenylephrine. A review of the literature suggests that epinephrine has more potency at the alpha-1 adrenergic receptor,[9,10] and phenylephrine's longer duration of action gives rise to concerns about potential anterior segment ischemia.

CONCLUSION

Epi-Shugarcaine has thus far proven to be safe and effective in IFIS prophylaxis. The combined experience of many surgeons suggests that this formulation will obviate the need for other techniques to expand a small pupil in the vast majority of cases. For eyes in which measures such as iris hooks are necessary, administering epi-Shugarcaine may decrease the severity of IFIS and will not interfere with the adjunctive techniques. I therefore advocate epi-Shugarcaine as the preferred agent for IFIS prophylaxis in all patients with a history of using tamsulosin. ■

This article originally appeared in the September 2006 issue of CRSToday.

1. Chang DF, Campbell JR. Intraoperative floppy iris syndrome associated with tamsulosin. *J Cataract Refract Surg.* 2005;30:664-673.
2. Slack JW, Edelhauser HF, Helenek MJ. A bisulfite-free intraocular epinephrine solution. *Am J Ophthalmol.* 1990;110:77-82.
3. Gonnering R, Edelhauser HF, Van Horn DL, Durant W. The pH tolerance of rabbit and human corneal endothelium. *Invest Ophthalmol Vis Sci.* 1979;18:373-390.
4. Shugar JK. "Shugarcaine" lessens burning sensation. *Ocular Surgery News.* January 1, 1998;16:1:1,13.
5. Shugar JK. Intracameral epinephrine for prophylaxis of IFIS [letter]. *J Cataract Refract Surg.* In press.
6. Kent C. Stopping the flopping: managing IFIS. *Review of Ophthalmology.* March 2006;13:3:13.
7. McDonald JE. Eye Mail insights: IFIS, epinephrine, and pH measurements. *EyeWorld Magazine.* February 2006;11:2:2-3.
8. Cionni RJ, Barros MG, Kaufman AH, Osher RH. Cataract Surgery without preoperative eyedrops. *J Cataract Refract Surg.* 2003;29:2281-2283.
9. Ohkobu K, Chiba S. Responses of isolated canine ophthalmic and ciliary arteries to vasoactive substances. *Jpn J Ophthalmol.* 1988;31:627-634.
10. Green K, Lollis G. Response of the isolated rabbit ciliary epithelium to adrenergic drugs following superior cervical ganglionectomy. *Curr Eye Res.* 1982;1:217-222.

CHAPTER 48

Atropine and Epinphrine for IFIS

BY SAMUEL MASKET, MD

Generally associated with the systemic use of alpha-1A blockers for improved urinary bladder function, intraoperative floppy iris syndrome (IFIS) was well defined by Chang and Campbell,[1] and it can represent an increased risk of cataract surgical complications. A subsequent, multicenter investigation, however, demonstrated that a number of strategies can reduce the likelihood of complications to normal or nearly normal levels. These methods include the use of iris hooks or pupillary ring devices and/or the alteration of fluidic inflow in combination with the use of highly retentive viscoagents. Additionally, I have advocated administering atropine sulfate 1% eye drops for 2 or 3 days prior to surgery. Recently, I have combined the use of this topical drug with intracameral epinephrine for more effective prophylaxis.

ATROPINE: WHY AND HOW?

Given that the manifestations of IFIS may include a poorly dilating pupil and progressive intraoperative miosis in the presence of a weakened iris dilator muscle, it is logical to employ the strongest iridoplegic agent available. This reasoning is particularly strong, because cyclopentolate and tropicamide have failed to obtain and maintain pupillary dilation in cases of IFIS.

I instruct patients with IFIS to administer atropine 1% t.i.d. for 2 days prior to surgery and again on the day of surgery. I emphasize the need to continue the systemic alpha-1A blocker, most often tamsulosin, because the use of atropine may increase patients' risk for acute urinary retention should the alpha blocker be discontinued. The chief effect of atropine is its prevention of intraoperative, progressive miosis—particularly because pupillary stretching methods are of no help or are contraindicated. Should the combined effects of atropine and other routine mydriatic agents provide an amply sized pupil for surgery, it is generally unnecessary to employ other strategies. In those rare instances that pupillary dilation is not sufficient for surgery, I employ disposable iris hooks in a diamond or pentagonal configuration.

ADDING INTRACAMERAL EPINEPHRINE

Recently, I began combining the aforementioned regimen with intracameral, unpreserved epinephrine in a 1:2500 dilution, in keeping with the method of Joel Shugar, MD.[2] In my view, the synergy of atropine and epinephrine is more effective than either agent alone, and the relatively strong concentration of epinephrine seems capable of stimulating the weakened dilator muscle. I have had limited experience (two cases), however, with the use of epinephrine alone. The patients did not report their use of tamsulosin until during their procedures, and I needed additional strategies for managing IFIS.

In all but one of the approximately 20 cases in which I had combined atropine and epinephrine, surgery was routine. The exception involved an 88-year-old, blue-eyed male whose pupillary diameter was less than 2 mm after the administration of atropine and epinephrine as well as the routine application of additional mydriatics. In this case, my use of iris hooks made the surgery otherwise routine.

CONCLUSION

Several strategies have evolved for managing IFIS, and they are complimentary rather than competitive. I employ a pharmacologic approach preoperatively and at the outset of surgery. If those agents prove inadequate, I may then apply other methods of my choosing, because the use of dilating agents does not preclude the application of other strategies. For that reason, I strongly advocate a pharmacologic approach as the initial strategy for managing IFIS. I reserve the use of iris hooks and other methods for the rare cases in which the medications are insufficient. ■

This article originally appeared in the September 2006 issue of CRSToday.

1. Chang DF, Campbell JR. Intraoperative floppy iris syndrome associated with tamsulosin (Flomax). *J Cataract Refract Surg*. 2005;31:664-673.
2. Shugar, JK. Intracameral epinephrine for prophylaxis of IFIS [letter]. *J Cataract Refract Surg*. 2006;32(7):1074-1075.

CHAPTER 49

Phenylephrine for IFIS

BY RICHARD B. PACKARD, MD, FRCS, FRCOPHTH

In 2004, Chang and Campbell[1] first described a new cause of small pupils and erratic intraoperative behavior of the iris. They called it the *intraoperative floppy iris syndrome* (IFIS) and attributed its cause to the use of tamsulosin, a drug indicated for the treatment of benign prostatic hypertrophy (BPH). Since their original description, there have been a number of letters in response[2-13] describing IFIS in patients with a history of taking a variety of other drugs, including less receptor-specific treatments for BPH and other therapies that block alpha adrenergic receptors. In addition, it has been found that drugs that block alpha adrenergic receptors, even if taken for a short length of time, can induce IFIS in some patients.[14] Although IFIS is not a universal result in all who have taken the aforementioned drugs, there may be a rapid and permanent effect on the iris muscle. What causes the floppy iris is unknown because there is no histology available on the syndrome.

Since the original article about IFIS was published, several surgical maneuvers have been described to minimize the effects of the syndrome.[15,16] The idea behind these procedures is to stabilize the iris and prevent its egress from the eye or into the phaco tip. Iris hooks, various combinations of viscoelastics, pupillary rings, and bimanual microincisional cataract surgery have all been suggested. I have pursued a different method when treating IFIS, however, based on a pharmacological approach using a diluted solution of preservative-free phenylephrine. The use of this drug can improve pupillary size when injected intracamerally in cataract patients.[17]

THE PROSTATE AND THE IRIS

The main cause of IFIS is tamsulosin.[1] By specifically blocking the alpha-1a adrenergic receptors that are found in the prostate, this drug minimizes the contraction of the enlarged muscle fibers in the gland. The action of tamsulosin enables BPH sufferers to delay prostate surgery for a long period. Unfortunately, the iris contains similar receptors, which are also targeted by this drug. As stated earlier, some but not all patients taking tamsulosin experience an abnormally functioning iris—particularly regarding the dilator pupillae—that leads to the lack of tone and poor dilation.

PHARMACOLOGICAL APPROACH

For some years, I have used a diluted solution of preservative-free phenylephrine (Minims phenylephrine 2.5%; Chauvin Pharmaceuticals Ltd., Surrey, UK) in eyes with an unsatisfactorily dilated pupil. In the majority of my small-pupil patients, unless they had synechiae that required breaking, I would enhance the pupil's dilation to a useful size. After becoming aware of IFIS, it seemed logical for me to try phenylephrine. In my first case, the patient was taking tamsulosin and had a poorly dilated pupil. Intracameral phenylephrine not only enlarged the pupil but, more importantly, increased the iris' tone sufficiently to minimize its billowing and lower the risk of its prolapse through the surgical incisions. Since then, all of my patients with a history of using tamsulosin or similar medication routinely receive intracameral injections of phenylephrine.

Part of a class of chemicals called *sympathomimetics*, phenylephrine is a strong stimulator of alpha adrenergic receptors, which include all the alpha-1 receptors that are blocked by tamsulosin. Thus, it seems that, although all cataract surgery patients on tamsulosin or similar drugs for BPH will receive topical phenylephrine preoperatively, the effect of this ophthalmic drug on the relevant iris receptors is minimal dilation at the most. Intracamerally injected agonists overwhelm these receptors to achieve a response. Other receptors in the iris may react to this injection as well, but I do not know thatfor certain. In some cases, the iris' response only lasts for a few minutes, and then another injection of phenylephrine is required to redilate the pupil. For patients who are currently taking or who have received tamsulosin or similar drugs, I have not had to resort to any other surgical procedure to avoid difficulty with or a complication related to their floppy irides.

HOW TO PREPARE AND USE INTRACAMERAL PHENYLEPHRINE

I add seven drops of 2.5% phenylephrine to 1 mL of balanced salt solution and then draw the mixture up into a syringe. I intracamerally inject the phenylephrine after making the initial stab incision but prior to using any viscoelastic. Mydriasis visibly improves with the intracameral injection, even in eyes that have received numerous topical mydriatic drops. Colleagues have expressed concerns to me about the effect of intracameral phenylephrine on the cardiovascular system. Their concerns are unfounded, however, because the pulse rate and blood pressure are not affected by the direct use of this drug on the iris, according to the observations of my anesthetist. Often, both the pulse rate and blood pressure are reduced intraoperatively as a patient relaxes from his initial anticipation of the procedure.

CONCLUSION

Now that ophthalmologists are aware of IFIS and the number of medications in general use that may cause it, a careful account of each patient's past medical and drug history becomes very important. After establishing that a patient may be at risk for IFIS, it is prudent to anticipate problems and take proper precautions. To me, this means having a couple of single-dose containers of phenylephrine 2.5% for appropriate dilution and intracameral use. ■

This article originally appeared in the September 2006 issue of CRSToday.

1. Chang DF, Campbell JR. Intraoperative floppy iris syndrome associated with tamsulosin. *J Cataract Refract Surg.* 2005;31:664-673.
2. Chang DF, Campbell JR. Reply: Intraoperative floppy iris syndrome associated with tamsulosin. *J Cataract Refract Surg.* 2005;31:2240.
3. Kershner RM. Intraoperative floppy iris syndrome associated with tamsulosin. *J Cataract Refract Surg.* 2005;31:2239; author reply 2239-2240.
4. Nguyen DQ, Sebastian RT, Kyle G. Intraoperative floppy iris syndrome associated with tamsulosin. *J Cataract Refract Surg.* 2005;31:2240; author reply 2240.
5. Lawrentschuk N, Bylsma GW. Intraoperative 'floppy iris' syndrome and its relationship to tamsulosin: a urologist's guide. *BJU Int.* 2006;97:2-4.
6. Nguyen DQ, Sebastian RT, Philip J. Intraoperative floppy iris syndrome associated with tamsulosin. *BJU Int.* 2006;97:197.
7 Kaplan SA. Intraoperative floppy iris syndrome associated with tamsulosin. *J Urol.* 2006;175:2213.
8. Tiwari A. Tamsulosin and floppy iris syndrome in benign prostatic hyperplasia patients. *Expert Opin Investig Drugs.* 2006;15:443-446.
9. Schwinn DA, Afshari NA. Alpha1-adrenergic antagonists and floppy iris syndrome: tip of the iceberg? *Ophthalmology.* 2005;112:2059-2060.
10. Osher RH Association between IFIS and Flomax. J Cataract Refract Surg. 2006;32:547.
11. El-Ghatit AM. Association of IFIS and vasodepressor medication. *J Cataract Refract Surg.* 2006;32:546-547.
12. Parmar B, Qatarneh D, Claoue C. Alpha antagonists in cataract surgery. *J Cataract Refract Surg.* 2005;31:2241; author reply 2241.
13. Pringle E, Packard R. Antipsychotic agent as an etiologic agent of IFIS. *J Cataract Refract Surg.* 2005;31:2240-2241; author reply 2241.
14. Michel M, Okutsu H, Noguchi Y, et al. In vivo studies on the effects of alpha1-adrenoceptor antagonists on pupil diameter and urethral tone in rabbits. Naunyn Schmiedebergs *Arch Pharmacol.* 2006;372:346-353.
15. Modi S. Discovisc versus Healon5: clinical results of cataract surgery in complicated tamsulosin cases. Paper presented at: The ASCRS/ASOA Symposium on Cataract, IOL and Refractive Surgery; March 18, 2006; San Francisco, CA.
16. Chang D, Fine IH, Masket S, et al. Terminating IFIS complications. Paper presented at: The ASCRS/ASOA Symposium on Cataract, IOL and Refractive Surgery; March 21, 2006; San Francisco, CA.
17. Gurbaxani A, Packard R. Intracameral phenylephrine to prevent floppy iris syndrome during cataract surgery in patients on tamsulosin. *Eye.* 2007;21(3):331-332.

CHAPTER 50

Improving the Iris' Behavior

BY ROBERT H. OSHER, MD; FREDERICO F. MARQUES, MD; DANIELA M. MARQUES, MD; AND JAMES M. OSHER, MS

Healon5 (Advanced Medical Optics, Inc., Santa Ana, CA) is a retentive viscoadaptive agent with a high molecular weight that has both dispersive and cohesive properties. Because of this ophthalmic viscosurgical device's (OVD) capability to cause viscomydriasis and add pseudotonia by mechanically displacing and immobilizing the iris, we undertook a study to determine whether Healon5 can widen and maintain pupillary dilatation, improve the iris' behavior, and reduce the complication rate in patients using Flomax (Boehringer-Ingelheim Pharmaceuticals, Inc., Ridgefield, CT).[1]

When Chang and Campbell[2] first reported that intraoperative floppy iris syndrome (IFIS) is associated with Flomax, they encountered a 12.5% incidence of torn posterior capsules. Suboptimal pupillary dilatation, a billowing iris, and a constricting pupil characterized these cases. According to the literature, a suboptimal pupil is conducive to intraoperative complications in patients with pseudoexfoliation syndrome.[3] It is likely that the pupil's behavior contributes to the difficulties encountered by the surgeon performing cataract surgery on an eye with IFIS.

STUDY: CATARACT SURGERY IN FLOMAX PATIENTS

We evaluated 25 eyes of 19 patients with a history of Flomax use who underwent cataract surgery. We used a retrospective video review to evaluate the effect of using Healon5 on viscomydriasis, the suppression of billowing and prolapse of the iris, intraoperative and postoperative complications, and early, uncorrected vision after surgery. Viscomydriasis occurred consistently and ranged from mild to dramatic (1 to 3mm) dilatation. The average diameter of the pupil before the administration of Healon5 was 5.82 mm, which increased to 7.21 mm after the viscoelastic's injection. Injecting additional Healon5 could reverse pupillary constriction. Both billowing and prolapse of the iris were markedly improved by the use of slow-motion phaco parameters.[4] Complications were rare—one torn posterior capsule and one significantly bruised iris. On postoperative day 1, 23 eyes (92%) achieved a UCVA of 20/40 or better.

THE EFFECTS OF HEALON5

Viscomydriasis

We have found that Healon5 produces excellent viscomydriasis by its mechanical dilatation of the pupil while it adds "tone" to the floppy iris in virtually every case.[5] Injecting enough Healon5 to create a concave configuration to the iris widens the pupil and markedly reduces billowing of the iris. As soon as the Healon5 escapes or is removed, however, a marked change in the iris' behavior occurs, including pupillary constriction, dramatic shimmering, and billowing.

Iris Prolapse

The tendency for iris prolapse also diminishes when Healon5 is present in the anterior chamber. Because the atonic iris is sensitive to any pressure gradient, the iris seeks the aspiration port or the incision (or both). Initially, injecting Healon5 directly onto the subincisional iris displaces it away from the incision and prevents the iris from leaping into the incision as the viscoelastic fills the remainder of the anterior chamber. In only three cases (12%), the iris actually prolapsed into the incision at the beginning of the surgery. We managed these cases by aspirating Healon5 to lower the

IOP with a 25-gauge cannula inserted through the stab incision. Then, we could sweep the iris out of the main incision with the same cannula. After repositioning the iris, we re-injected Healon5 onto the subincisional iris until it became concave. We could then introduce a bent, 22-gauge needle for the capsulorhexis.

Capsulorhexis

Healon5 reduces the tendency for the edge of the capsulorhexis to extend toward the periphery, because it flattens the anterior curvature of the lens' dome. By slowing the speed of the capsulorhexis, Healon5 enhanced the surgeon's control of the tear. If the ophthalmologist prefers to perform a quicker capsulorhexis, a forceps is more effective than a bent needle. Regardless of the device selected, the wider pupil and the deeper chamber afforded by the Healon5 are more conducive to a successful capsulorhexis in IFIS. Hydrodissection and hydrodelineation may flush out some of the Healon5. Refilling the chamber is recommended by Dr. Osher, because diluted or fractured Healon5 will not maintain the pupil's size or retard billowing of the iris as well as replacing the OVD. If the fluid wave causes the iris to move visibly toward the incision, it is easier to insert the phaco tip without irrigation. Once the tip is inside the anterior chamber, irrigation can be safely initiated.

Phacoemulsification

Slow-motion phacoemulsification using low parameters and a low bottle height has proven effective in retaining OVDs.[5] The emulsification of the nucleus begins with the embedding of the ultrasound tip bevel down into the anterior cortex. Only lenticular material can be removed when the bevel is down. Raising the vacuum to 250 mm Hg should prevent obstruction of the tip and thus avoid thermal consequences. As soon as a groove or divot appears in the lens, the surgeon may reduce the vacuum to 40 mm Hg and rotate the bevel upward to allow precise sculpting and deepening of the groove in the nucleus while the overlying Healon5 is undisturbed. Next, the surgeon divides the nucleus into hemispheres and chops it into quadrants while raising the vacuum to 180 mm Hg for complete nuclear removal. Healon5 may be re-injected for additional pupillary dilatation or for the posterior displacement of the iris. Certainly, lower levels of vacuum and flow require less infusion pressure, which further reduces billowing and prolapse of the iris.

Cortical Removal and Vacuuming the Posterior Capsule

Although it is possible to retain the OVD during cortical removal, the Healon5 is easily engaged and aspirated when the vacuum is set at 400 mm Hg. Therefore, the surgeon should depress the foot switch only when the port is embedded in the most proximal anterior cortex. During cortical stripping within the bag, the surgeon must release the foot pedal the instant the cortex disappears into the port of the I/A tip. It is less important to keep the OVD in the eye if vacuuming the central posterior capsule, because pupillary dilatation is not critical for this step. Moreover, the low vacuum and bottle height are less conducive to iris prolapse. Re-injecting Healon5 to retroplace the subincisional iris before refilling the capsular bag should precede the injection of the IOL. The viscomydriasis will reveal the edge of the capsulorhexis while confirming that the cortex has been completely removed.

IOLs

Healon5 facilitates the implantation of a single-piece acrylic IOL, because the haptics remain folded, simplifying the lens' placement and maneuverability. Healon5 also absorbs the kinetic energy of an unfolding three-piece silicone or acrylic lens.

Posterior Capsular Rupture and Tear

In contrast to the Chang and Campbell study, which reported a 12.5% incidence of posterior capsular rupture, we encountered this complication in only one eye (4%). In this case, the surgeon neglected to refill the anterior chamber with Healon5 during the phacoemulsification, and the pupil constricted to 3mm. A peripheral tear was identified during the removal of the Healon5 after the IOL had been placed into the bag. Even after reviewing the video, we do not know how and when the tear in the posterior capsule occurred. The surgeon performed a brief anterior vitrectomy "dry" beneath Healon5, and the IOL remained well centered within the capsular bag. This patient attained a UCVA of 20/25 on the first day following the vitrectomy.

POSTOPERATIVE OUTCOMES AND ACTIONS

Complications

Postoperative complications were infrequent. Only one patient had a cosmetic iris bruise measuring 2 mm in diameter as a result of intraoperative iris prolapse. Three (12%) eyes had an IOP of between 30 and 35 mm Hg on the first postoperative day, and they were treated with a topical beta-blocker, a prostaglandin inhibitor, and a carbonic anhydrase inhibitor. All IOPs were normal at the 1-week visit, and no patient experienced any pressure-related consequences. Because the IOP can rise in any eye with residual OVD within the chamber, we attempted to remove the Healon5 completely in every case by means of a two-compartment technique described by Manfred Tetz, MD.[6] When the vacuum is 450 mm Hg, it is possible to aspirate Healon5 rapidly and completely because of its cohesive behavior at high sheering rates.

Administration of Additional Drug Therapies

During the OVD's removal, the dramatic billowing of the iris serves as a reminder that IFIS is present. Intracameral acetylcholine chloride seems to have an exaggerated effect of rapidly constricting the pupil, which further minimizes the risk of iris prolapse. We routinely instill a drop of pilocarpine and brimonidine at the conclusion of surgery as prophylaxis against an increase in IOP. Some patients also receive latanoprost, timolol, or even oral acetazolamide when they have a history of glaucoma, ocular hypertension, pigment dispersion syndrome, pseudoexfoliation, or trauma or if they have a positive family history of glaucoma.

By the 1-week postoperative visit, all eyes had an UCVA of 20/40 or better. Although one patient experienced an intraoperative complication of a torn posterior capsule, no patient in our series developed a significant postoperative complication such as prolonged corneal edema, persistent iritis, infection, cystoid macular edema, glaucoma, or retinal tear/detachment.

CONCLUSION

By mechanically widening the pupil and by reducing the tendency for the iris to prolapse and billow, Healon5 appears to be an ideal OVD for managing IFIS in the patient with a history of using Flomax. Although the added difficulty of operating on patients with IFIS cannot be underestimated, we have achieved excellent surgical outcomes by performing meticulous slow-motion phacoemulsification and using Healon5. ■

This article originally appeared in the September 2006 issue of CRSToday.

CHAPTER 51

Viscoadaptive Devices and Modified Phaco Parameter in IFIS: an Update

BY DOUGLAS D. KOCH, MD

Several excellent concepts and surgical approaches have been devised for managing intraoperative floppy iris syndrome (IFIS) in patients who are taking or have taken tamsulosin (Flomax; Boehringer Ingelheim Pharmaceuticals, Inc., Ridgefield, CT) for benign prostatic hypertrophy. I have operated on approximately 20 eyes with IFIS in the past year and have developed a modified technique that safely supports the iris during phacoemulsification without iris hooks. I combine a "moderate motion" phaco technique with the use of ophthalmic viscosurgical devices (OVDs), such as Healon5 (Advanced Medical Optics, Inc., Santa Ana, CA) and Duovisc (Provisc and Viscoat; Alcon Laboratories, Inc., Fort Worth, TX). My approach is an extension of the wonderful low-flow concept that Robert Osher, MD, of Cincinnati introduced many years ago. I use higher settings than Dr. Osher originally proposed, however, and thus may move through the procedure more efficiently and quickly and use less phaco power than I might need with lower settings.

TECHNIQUE

I begin every case by injecting a topical intracameral anesthetic, making the incision, and then injecting the OVD into the anterior chamber. If the pupil's size is normal, I begin with a soft shell technique using a combination of Viscoat and Provisc (as Duovisc). For small pupils, I inject Healon5. This OVD does an excellent job of dilating pupils affected by IFIS, because the iris tissue has little resistance to the mechanical force that Healon5 exerts. Equally valuable is the way in which it tamponades the iris. The iris acts much more normally during phacoemulsification once this OVD is in place.

When operating on eyes into which I initially injected Duovisc, I first evaluate the iris' behavior during the capsulorhexis and hydrodissection. If I do not see any signs of IFIS, I continue with the soft shell approach.

If I observe signs of IFIS such as a floppy iris or pupillary constriction, however, I inject Healon5 centrally and over the surface of the iris. The OVD dilates the pupil and enables me to proceed with phacoemulsification. At this stage in the procedure, it is essential to use settings that are low enough to retain the Healon5 in the eye. I have found that, if I keep my flow rate at approximately 20 mL/min and my vacuum level below 350 mm Hg, the Healon5 almost always remains in the eye.

Managing IFIS cases with Healon5 requires modifying one's phaco technique. For a surgeon who relies upon vacuum to pull forward and extract nuclear material, the operation can be more tedious. I happen to be comfortable using a modified stop-and-chop technique that relies on mechanical nuclear disassembly. After splitting the nucleus, I mechanically break off pieces using little or no vacuum. I do so by placing the horizontal chopper peripheral to the equator of the lens, positioning the phaco tip deep against the wall of the heminucleus to provide counter pressure, and then simply cleaving off fragments mechanically. I find it useful to leave the chopper in the split to hold adjacent nuclear material away as I use vacuum and phacoemulsification to extract the first nuclear fragment.

In most cases, enough of the OVD remains in the eye to control the iris during emulsification. However, if the pupil starts to constrict, I simply re-inject Healon5 to redilate the pupil.

Because Healon5 is quickly aspirated from the eye by higher flow and vacuum, I sometimes inject the Viscoat component of Duovisc into the angle of the anterior chamber before beginning I/A. This precaution tamponades the peripheral iris and minimizes or eliminates the iris' tendency to prolapse toward the incisions. Viscoat usually does not prevent the pupil from constricting, but that does not present a problem. Because I use a bimanual technique in eyes with IFIS, I can comfortably work through a pupil as small as 3mm to remove the cortical material.

At this point in the procedure, I redilate the pupil and inflate the capsular bag by injecting more Healon5. I then insert the IOL and place the coaxial or bimanual aspirating tip beneath it in order to remove the OVD entirely.

It is during those last moments of I/A and occasionally during the final removal of the Healon5 that the floppy iris may billow. Keeping the bottle's height at a reasonable level and moving expeditiously will avoid problems.

INCORPORATING OVDs INTO CATARACT SURGERY

I recommend that surgeons new to using a viscoadaptive OVD begin by employing it in routine cases in order to become acquainted with its intraoperative characteristics. Some tips for using Healon5 during phacoemulsification follow.

Capsulorhexis

Because of the resistance created by the remarkable viscosity of Healon5, I forego my usual technique of creating the capsulorhexis with a bent needle. Specifically, I find that Healon5 makes it harder to fold the capsule over and control it using a bent needle. For that reason, I typically start the capsulorhexis with a bent needle and then complete it with a forceps.

Hydrodissection

During hydrodissection, one must ensure that there is a path for outflow of the injected fluid from the eye. Healon5 can block fluid egress, theoretically increasing the risk of blowing out the posterior capsule. As I enter the anterior chamber with my cannula, I move it around a bit to create a path for the fluid to escape. I inject the balanced salt solution more slowly and in smaller quantities than normal and ensure that there is not any unusual distension of the anterior chamber itself.

OVD's Removal

I can easily visualize the Healon5 and thus ensure its complete removal. Moreover, the OVD has great followability at high flow and vacuum rates. Occasionally, a fragment of the OVD is chopped off or becomes isolated. More typically, however, one can extract all of the Healon5 at once upon initiating its removal.

The critical point is to remove all the Healon5 from beneath the IOL. Actually, regardless of what OVD I use, I always place my aspiration tip beneath the IOL at the end of the case to ensure that I do not leave any viscoelastic in the capsular bag.

CLOSING THOUGHTS

In complicated cases of IFIS, I have found that the combination of Healon5, Viscoat, modified phaco parameters, and bimanual I/A enables me to remove cataracts safely and comfortably and to prevent injury to the iris. New OVDs, such as Discovisc (Alcon Laboratories, Inc.), may also prove useful in these cases. It is easy to learn these techniques through practice in everyday cases. I routinely teach them to my residents so that they can effectively manage eyes with IFIS. The availability of OVDs with different characteristics greatly enhances our ability to handle these difficult cases. ■

This article originally appeared in the September 2006 issue of CRSToday.

CHAPTER 52

The Modified Use of OVDs for IFIS

BY STEVE A. ARSHINOFF, MD, FRCSC

Ophthalmic viscosurgical devices (OVDs) are unique tools in anterior segment surgery. The ophthalmologist can select OVDs based upon their classification[1] to create a physical environment to facilitate the management of almost any surgical problem.[2] Best known and most frequently used are the soft shell and ultimate soft shell techniques, for which variations to manage specific problems have been described.[3-9]

Chang and Campbell[10] brought to ophthalmic surgeons' attention intraoperative floppy iris syndrome (IFIS), associated with the systemic administration of the alpha-A1 adrenoceptor antogonist tamsulosin (Flomax; Boehringer Ingelheim Pharmaceuticals, Inc., Ridgefield, CT) for benign prostatic hypertrophy. The condition presents a challenging and ever more common surgical problem to cataract surgeons. Chang and Campbell described the clinical, intraoperative, diagnostic triad of (1) fluttering and billowing of the iris stroma caused by ordinary intraocular fluid currents, (2) a propensity for iris prolapse through the phaco and/or sideport incisions, and (3) the progressive constriction of the pupil during surgery. These signs are accompanied by suboptimal pupillary dilation in response to preoperative mydriatic protocols. In addition, pupillary stretching techniques are ineffective due to the floppy, easily stretched nature of the pupillary margin, instead of the fibrosis seen in other cases of pupillary miosis refractory to protocols for dilation.

The degree of IFIS varies considerably among patients taking similar doses of tamsulosin for about the same time. Chang and Campbell recommended the intraoperative use of iris hooks or other mechanical devices for pupillary dilation. They noted, however, that a failure to recognize IFIS before the performance of the capsulorhexis might make the use of these instruments difficult. Although they stated that they found Healon5 (Advanced Medical Optics, Inc., Santa Ana, CA) to be useful in IFIS, Chang and Campbell did not mention the use of more elaborate, multiple-OVD techniques. The approach described herein, which I call *IFIS SST-USST,* follows directly from soft shell and ultimate soft shell methodology.[11]

METHODS AND RESULTS

Illustrated schematically in Figure 1, the IFIS SST-USST consists of sequential steps to prevent expected problems before they occur. First, I make very tight incisions. Incisional leakage encourages the floppy iris to prolapse through the main and sideport incisions. I make a 1-mm sideport incision with the Arshinoff sideport diamond knife (Diamond Surgical Products, Thornville, OH).

I leave 1% nonpreserved Xylocaine (AstraZeneca LP, Wilmington, DE), intracamerally injected through the sideport, in the eye for at least 1 minute before proceeding. Doing so slightly improves pupillary dilation.

When fashioning the primary clear corneal phaco incision, I try to lengthen the tunnel such that the internal corneal entry is slightly central to the pupillary margin, no matter how small the pupil is. The pupils in severe IFIS cases are almost always 5 to 6 mm in diameter, regardless of how many dilating drops they have received. These pupils also tend to constrict as surgery progresses.

I fill the anterior chamber to approximately 75% to 80% with Viscoat (Alcon Laboratories, Inc., Fort Worth, TX) via the phaco incision while making sure the OVD covers the peripheral iris. Next, I inject Healon5 onto the surface of the anterior lens capsule, into the center of the anterior chamber, so that it pushes the Viscoat upward and outward until the pupil stops dilating. It is important that the boundary of the Healon5/Viscoat be at the pupillary margin. It will later serve as a boundary to fracture, and the OVDs will help to keep the iris stable and the pupil dilated throughout surgery. At this point, the anterior chamber should be more than 90% full of OVDs, and the eye should feel slightly firm. This step is a variation of the soft shell technique.

I then slowly inject balanced salt solution or some of the nonpreserved lidocaine (preferable because it will continue to enhance pupillary dilation) under the layer of Healon5, on the surface of the lens capsule. I place the cannula's tip at the very center of the lenticular surface, from which the OVD soft shell becomes elevated. It also creates an aqueous pocket confined to the lenticular surface. This step is a variation of the ultimate soft shell technique, and it reduces the chance of aspirating the Healon5 with the phaco or I/A tip.

Using a bent needle, I perform a routine capsulorhexis that begins at the center of the lens. I keep the diameter of the capsulorhexis smaller than that of the pupil. This sizing will later act to confine fluid flow into an area smaller than the pupil, thus preventing turbulence from impacting the iris and the Viscoat layer, which would permit the pupil to constrict. I perform hydrodissection with very short pulses of balanced salt solution from a 10-mL syringe with a 27-gauge hockey stick cannula.

The careful execution of the aforementioned steps and the placement of the cannula should permit balanced salt solution to circulate around the lens and flow out of the eye, beneath the OVD shell, without disturbing it. If hydrodissection or a later step of the procedure removes part of the shell, the surgeon should reinject Healon5 followed by balanced salt solution to reestablish the shell before proceeding.

The settings for the Infiniti Vision System (Alcon Laboratories, Inc.) or a similar peristaltic machine are adjusted to achieve low turbulence. I use a flow rate of ≤ 20 mL/min, vacuum of ≤ 300 mm Hg, and a bottle height that is 75 to 80 cm above the patient's eye. I employ a linear, continuously variable pulse mode, preferably including Ozil (Alcon Laboratories, Inc.). I use phaco slice and separate, but a similar chopping technique would also work. I make sure that the phaco tip remains beneath the capsulorhexis' edge in order to confine fluid flow to the capsular bag.[12] Aspiration should only be turned on when nuclear material is actively being aspirated in order to minimize disturbance of the shell.

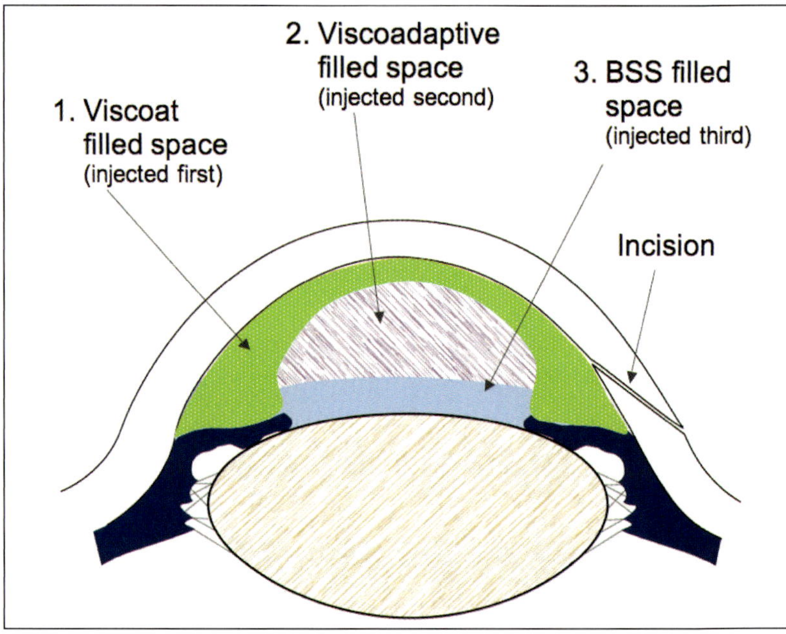

Figure 1. During IFIS SST-USST, the clear corneal incision is as long as reasonably possible so that, when the surgeon imagines depressing the cornea down to the level of the iris, the internal corneal incision is slightly central to the margin of the iris. As a result, iris prolapse is considerably less likely, and balanced salt solution may exit the eye easily without disturbing the OVD shell. After injecting Viscoat followed by Healon5 and then balanced salt solution, the surgeon creates the capsulorhexis with a bent 27-gauge needle and keeps it smaller than the pupil. (Reprinted from Arshinoff SA. Modified SST-USST for tamsulosin-associated intraocular floppy-iris syndrome. *J Cataract Refract Surg*. 2006;32:559-561 with permission from the ASCRS and ESCRS.)

The Healon5 forms the rigid inferior surface of the OVD soft shell, while Viscoat tamponades the iris. As a result, the iris is completely stable throughout the procedure. If the pupil begins to constrict excessively during surgery, it may be necessary to reinject Healon5 followed by balanced salt solution below it. I/A may similarly be accomplished with lower flow and vacuum settings (only occasionally necessary). I implant the IOL using the ultimate soft shell technique.[4]

After the surgeon aspirates the OVD shell at the end of cataract surgery, the characteristic billowing and fluttering of the iris will be observable. Sometimes, it is helpful at the conclusion of the procedure to reinflate the anterior chamber through the primary phaco incision so that no iris tissue becomes trapped in the incision. I then inject 0.1 mL of moxifloxacin 100 µg in 0.1 mL of balanced salt solution into the capsular bag via the sideport incision. Doing so pressurizes the eye and provides antibacterial prophylaxis.

DISCUSSION

Phaco surgery is usually routine, but unusual environmental problems, such as that induced by tamsulosin, do occur. From a structural point of view, the difficulties presented by IFIS are not very different from those associated with absent zonules and prolapsing vitreous, frayed iris strands, or low endothelial cell counts. OVDs allow surgeons to achieve almost any desirable physical environment in the anterior chamber. The IFIS SST-USST is merely one example. A great advantage of this technique is that the surgeon may institute it safely and effectively at any time during the procedure, unlike mechanical pupil dilators.

It is important to understand how and why the IFIS SST-USST works in order to use the technique well. I use Viscoat for the peripheral OVD ring, because I think it is the best low-viscosity, dispersive OVD available. This type of OVD tends to be highly retentive despite the presence of moderate fluid turbulence.[13] The viscoadaptive central layer of Healon5 adds a relatively rigid OVD roof above the surgical space and brings rigidity to the OVD structure that keeps the iris from moving and the Viscoat in place. The layer of balanced salt solution, just over the pupillary space, provides working room for balanced salt solution to circulate during phacoemulsification.

It is important that a viscoadaptive agent be present above the layer of balanced salt solution; excessive mixing would occur if Viscoat were used alone. If the phaco turbulence can be restricted to the capsular bag and this confined area above it, the Healon5 will not be dragged into the phaco tip, and the OVD shell will remain intact throughout the case. The layer of balanced salt solution serves another purpose. When performing hydrodissection, the surgeon depresses the posterior lip of the phaco incision somewhat until the easy egress of aqueous can be obtained from the layer of balanced salt solution, beneath the layer of Healon5 without disturbing it. This technique helps to preserve the OVD shell. The rigid Healon5 bridge is essential to allow IFIS cases to proceed smoothly, and the surgeon may have to reinject Healon5 if the bridge is accidentally disturbed. ■

The use of moxifloxacin described in this article is off label.
This article originally appeared in the September 2006 issue of CRSToday.

1. Arshinoff SA, Jafari M. A new classification of ophthalmic viscosurgical devices (OVDs)–2005. *J Cataract Refract Surg.* 2005;31:2167-2171.
2. Arshinoff SA. Dispersive and cohesive viscoelastic materials in phacoemulsification. *Ophthalmic Pract.* 1995;13:98-104.
3. Arshinoff SA. Dispersive-cohesive viscoelastic soft shell technique. *J Cataract Refract Surg.* 1999;25:167-173.
4. Arshinoff SA. Using BSS with viscoadaptives in the ultimate soft-shell technique. *J Cataract Refract Surg.* 2002;28:1509-1514.
5. Arshinoff S. Using viscoelastics to solve problems in cataract surgery. Video presented at: The ASCRS/ASOA Symposium on Cataract, IOL and Refractive Surgery; April 16-22, 1998; San Diego, CA.
6. Arshinoff SA. Using viscoelastics to manage problems in cataract surgery. In: Fishkind WJ, ed. Complications in Phacoemulsification: Avoidance, Recognition and Management. Thieme: New York; 2002:182-193.
7. Arshinoff SA. The ultimate soft shell technique (USST) and Acrysof Monarch injector cartridges. Letter. *J Cataract Refract Surg.* 2004;30:1809-1810.
8. Arshinoff SA. USST and no cycloplegic drops before cataract surgery. Letter. *J Cataract Refract Surg.* 2004;30:941-942.
9. Arshinoff SA. Capsular dyes and the USST. Letter. *J Cataract Refract Surg.* 2005;31:259-260.
10. Chang DF, Campbell JR. Intraoperative floppy iris syndrome associated with tamsulosin. *J Cataract Refract Surg.* 2005;31:664-673.
11. Arshinoff SA. Modified SST–USST for tamsulosin-associated intraocular floppy-iris syndrome [published correction to title appears in *J Cataract Refract Surg.* 2006;32:1076]. *J Cataract Refract Surg.* 2006;32:559-561.
12. Arshinoff SA. Phaco slice and separate. *J Cataract Refract Surg.* 1999;25:474-478.
13. Arshinoff SA, Wong E. Understanding, retaining, and removing dispersive and pseudo-dispersive OVDs. *J Cataract Refract Surg.* 2003;29:2318-2323.

CHAPTER 53

Discovisc for IFIS

BY SATISH MODI, MD, FRCSC

Like most cataract surgeons, I had occasionally encountered patients with a floppy iris intraoperatively and would note the occurrence in their chart so that I could take precautionary measures with their second eye. The landmark article by Chang and Campbell[1] sensitized me to the interrelation between intraoperative floppy iris syndrome (IFIS) and a patient's use of tamsulosin.

As I sought an effective strategy for managing eyes with IFIS, I found that pupillary dilation with phenylephrine, tropicamide, cyclopentolate, and atropine did not prevent miosis. Nor did pupillary stretching, and I normally shy away from this technique, because it increases my incidence of cystoid macular edema (CME). Other surgeons had advocated viscomydriasis with Healon5 (Advanced Medical Optics, Inc., Santa Ana, CA) and low-flow phaco parameters. Like many cataract surgeons in the US, however, I favor a high-flow phaco technique.

During my training, I was taught to change only one parameter—or as few as possible—when learning a new technique. I therefore set out to determine which ophthalmic viscosurgical device (OVD) was most effective and safe in eyes with IFIS undergoing phaco surgery with high vacuum and aspiration flow parameters. To that end, I compared the supercohesive viscoadaptive Healon5 to the more viscous, dispersive Discovisc (Alcon Laboratories, Inc., Fort Worth, TX). According to my preliminary results, the latter is a better choice.

MATERIALS AND METHODS

My ongoing study prospectively enrolls patients with bilateral cataracts who are using tamsulosin. One eye is randomized to Healon5, and the other receives Discovisc. All eyes undergo pupillary dilation with 2.5% phenylephrine, 1% tropicamide, and 1% cyclopentolate drops, but no mechanical measures are used.

I administer topical anesthesia but will use a block in nervous patients who squeeze their eyelids in order to decrease billowing of the iris during surgery. I create a near-clear biplanar incision. I perform surgery using the Infiniti Vision System (Alcon Laboratories, Inc.) with an aspiration flow rate of 50 mL and vacuum of 500 mm Hg for quadrant removal. During this step, I have found it helpful to put both aspiration and vacuum on linear control. Doing so allows me more control in occluding the phaco tip and moving the nuclear fragment into the pupillary plane for safe emulsification. Finally, using Discovisc to effect a "phacoviscofracture" and elevate an errant nuclear fragment helps tremendously.

For the purposes of the study, I make subjective notes on each pupil's intraoperative behavior and record any complications. Postoperatively, I measure each eye's visual acuity, pachymetry, and endothelial cell count.

RESULTS

To date, I have data on 10 eyes of five patients, with an even distribution to the two OVDs (five eyes with Healon5 and five with Discovisc). The patients ranged in age from 71 to 84 years, and all of them were taking tamsulosin.

Intraoperatively, the iris prolapsed in eight of 10 eyes. Nine eyes exhibited miosis that required viscomydriasis. In those cases, both OVDs performed well. I typically needed two syringes of Healon5, however, because it exited the eye as soon as phacoemulsification began, which led to a recurrence of miosis. Posterior capsular tears occurred in two eyes, both of which were in the Healon5 group. One eye, also in the Healon5 group, experienced iris chafing and burn as well as CME.

Ninety days after surgery, one eye from the Healon5 group had persistent microcystic corneal edema and 20/60- vision. Another eye from the Healon5 group had CME and a visual acuity of 20/40. The remaining eight eyes saw 20/20. One of 10 eyes exhibited a severely chafed iris and persistent CME after phacoemulsification. As mentioned earlier, this eye was in the Healon5 group.

There was no appreciable difference in pachymetry except in the eye with persistent corneal edema. The mean endothelial cell loss was 16.6% in the Healon5 eyes versus 7.5% in the Discovisc eyes.

CONCLUSION

The sample size of my study is small, and further research is necessary. Based on my preliminary results, Discovisc provides longer-lasting viscomydriasis and superior protection for endothelial cells, because it remains in the eye when high-flow phacoemulsification begins. Moreover, when the surgeon uses high aspiration and flow parameters, Discovisc's greater retentiveness means a lower chance of the iris' incarceration in the phaco tip, a decreased incidence of posterior capsular tears, and, hypothetically, less CME. Finally, with my phaco parameters and technique, I usually needed more Healon5 (two syringes) than Discovisc (one syringe).

No single technique is going to work for every eye with IFIS, however, so surgeons must be familiar with multiple strategies for the management of these challenging cases. ■

This article originally appeared in the September 2006 issue of CRSToday.

1. Chang DF, Campbell JR. Intraoperative floppy iris syndrome associated with tamsulosin (Flomax). *J Cataract Refract Surg.* 2005;31:664-673.

CHAPTER 54

Managing IFIS With Iris Retractors

BY DAVID F. CHANG, MD

Intraoperative floppy iris syndrome (IFIS) is most commonly associated with systemic alpha-1 blockers such as tamsulosin (Flomax; Boehringer Ingelheim Pharmaceuticals, Inc., Ridgefield, CT), doxazosin (Cardura; Pfizer Inc., New York, NY), terazosin (Hytrin; Abbott Laboratories Inc., North Chicago, IL), and alfuzosin (Uroxatral; Sanofi-Aventis, Paris, France). A triad of intraoperative signs—iris billowing and floppiness, iris prolapse to the main and side incisions, and progressive miosis—characterizes IFIS and increases the risk of surgical complications when surgeons do not anticipate the condition.[1]

IFIS may be categorized as mild (ample pupillary dilation plus some floppiness of the iris without prolapse or constriction), moderate (some tendency for iris prolapse and some constriction of a moderately dilated pupil), or severe (classic triad and poor preoperative dilation). Of all of the systemic alpha-1 blockers, tamsulosin has the strongest tendency to produce IFIS. The difference may relate to the much higher affinity and specificity of this drug for the alpha-1A receptor subtype present in the iris dilator smooth muscle.[2]

TABLE 1. OVERCOMING HISTORICAL OBJECTIONS TO IRIS RETRACTORS

Objection	Rebuttal
Too costly	Reusable iris hooks are very cost effective.
Time consuming to place	Stiffer 4–0 polypropylene hooks are much easier to handle and manipulate than 6–0 nylon.
Iris sphincter will be torn and damaged	With IFIS, the sphincter is elastic rather than fibrotic. Maximal stretching can therefore occur without excessive trauma to the sphincter muscle.
Iris is tented up in front of the phaco tip	The diamond configuration avoids this problem and the associated iris chafing.
Insufficient surgical exposure	The diamond configuration and the ability to maximally stretch an IFIS pupil provide superb visualization and exposure.

Because the severity of IFIS varies significantly among patients (and even between the eyes of the same patient), it is difficult to conclude whether one surgical technique is superior to another. By gaining experience with several different approaches, surgeons will invariably develop personal preferences. This article focuses on iris retractors.

COMPARING APPROACHES

Stopping tamsulosin preoperatively is of unpredictable and questionable value, as there are many documented cases of IFIS' occurring up to several years following the drug's cessation.[1,2] Preoperatively administered atropine drops (eg, 1% b.i.d. for 3 days before surgery) will maximize cycloplegia. This strategy alone is often insufficient, however, for moderate-to-severe IFIS. Intracameral epinephrine or other alpha agonists can increase the iris' rigidity and prevent the pupil's constriction. Partial-thickness

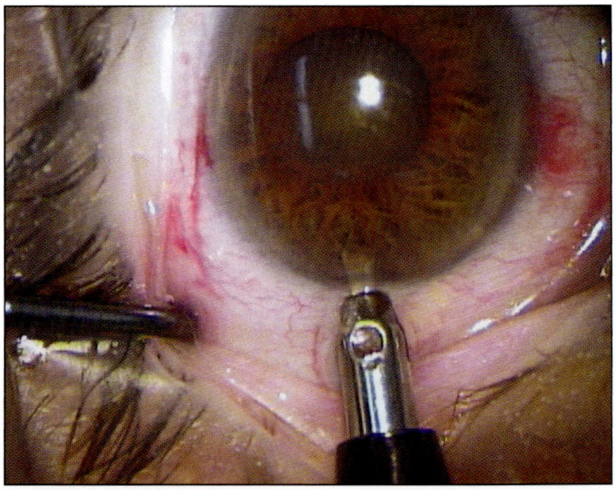

Figure 1. The author makes a separate limbal stab incision just behind the temporal clear corneal incision.

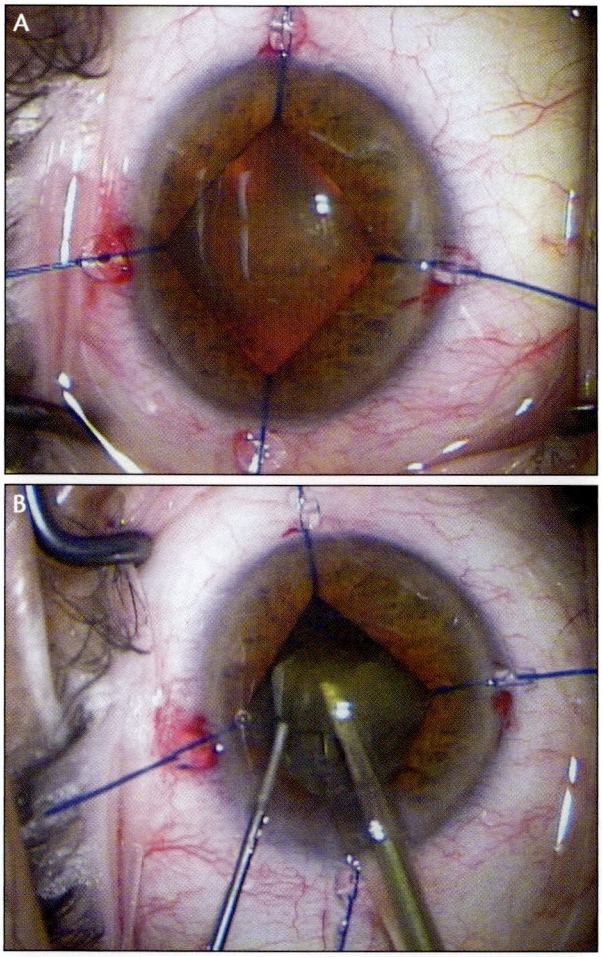

Figure 2. The author places reusable 4–0 polypropylene iris retractors (Katena Products, Inc.) in a diamond configuration, as described by Oetting and Omphroy[4] (A). A subincisional retractor pulls the iris down and away from the phaco tip while maximizing surgical exposure (B).

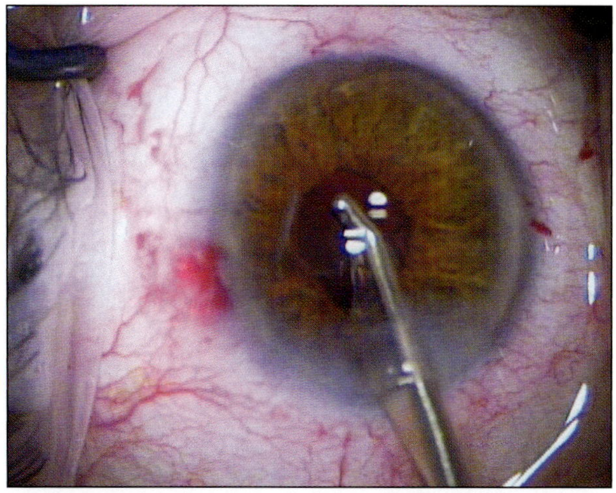

Figure 3. During the removal of viscoelastic and following the withdrawal of the retractors, the iris prolapses, and the pupil immediately constricts.

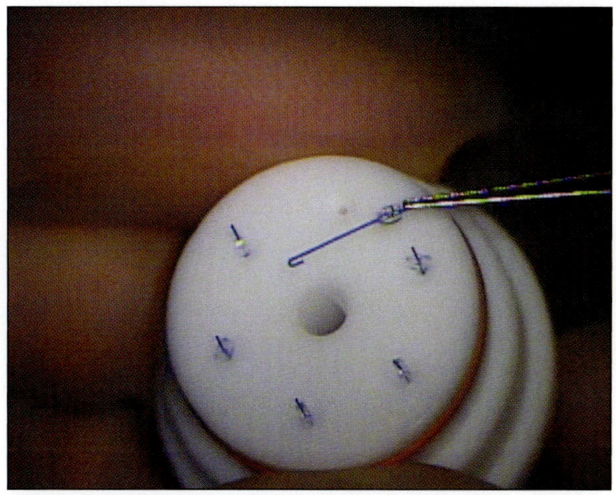

Figure 4. Sterilizing case for reusable iris retractors.

sphincterotomies and mechanical stretching of the pupil are ineffective for IFIS and should be avoided, because they may instead exacerbate the prolapse and miosis.[1]

As general principles, one must be attentive to theincision's proper construction, perform hydrodissection more gently and slowly than usual, and use lower I/A flow parameters if possible. Of all the ophthalmic viscosurgical devices (OVDs), Healon5 (Advanced Medical Optics, Inc., Santa Ana, CA) has particular utility in eyes with IFIS.[2,3] Its maximally cohesive properties are ideal for viscomydriasis and for blocking iris prolapse. To prevent the OVD's premature aspiration, lower flow and vacuum rates (eg, < 26 mL/min and < 175 to 200 mm Hg) are recommended. Even then, supplemental re-injections become necessary as the OVD is eventually aspirated. There is a learning curve for mastering the unique viscoadaptive properties of Healon5, and this IFIS strategy is less suitable if high vacuum settings are needed for a dense nucleus.

Disposable pupil expansion rings are costly but 100% effective. Both the Morcher 5S Pupil Ring (Morcher GmbH, Stuttgart, Germany; distributed by FCI Ophthalmics, Inc., Marshfield Hills, MA) and the Perfect Pupil (Milvella Ltd., Sydney, Australia) are grooved PMMA rings that are threaded alongside the pupillary margin using metal injectors. The surgeon uses a disposable plastic injector to insert the Graether silicone pupil expansion ring (Eagle Vision, Inc., Memphis, TN). All of these rings are more difficult to position if the anterior chamber is shallow or if the pupil is less than 4mm wide. On the other hand, if the pupil is initially too large, the smaller-diameter Morcher and Graether designs will be unable to engage the margin of the iris.

Iris retractors are probably the single most consistent approach that works equally well across the wide range of both IFIS' severity and surgeons' experience (Table 1). They provide another completely reliable strategy for pupillary expansion that can be used regardless of how small or large the starting diameter of the pupil is.

TECHNIQUE

I prefer reusable 4–0 polypropylene retractors (available from Katena Products, Inc., Denville, NJ, and FCI Ophthalmics, Inc.) to disposable 6–0 nylon retractors (available from Alcon Laboratories, Inc., Fort Worth, TX). At 0.15 mm in diameter, the 4–0 retractors are the same size and stiffness as the polypropylene haptic of an IOL. The added stiffness and rigidity, when compared with 6–0 nylon retractors, make 4–0 retractors more durable and easier to manipulate. The 4–0 polypropylene hooks can be autoclaved repeatedly, which makes them more cost effective than their disposable counterparts.

Before initiating the capsulorhexis, I make 1-mm limbal paracenteses in each quadrant, including a separate stab incision just posterior to the temporal clear corneal incision (Figures 1 and 2). In this way, the phaco tip passes through a separate incision directly alongside and above the track for the subincisional retractor. Placing the hooks in this diamond configuration has several advantages.[4] The subincisional hook retracts the iris downward and out of the path of the phaco tip. This configuration also maximizes exposure directly in front of the phaco tip (Figure 2B). The paracentesis incisions may be made with any 1-mm wide diamond or metal blade.

Iris retractors both enlarge and maintain a constant pupillary size throughout the course of surgery. They provide sufficient tension to the iris stroma so that no prolapse can occur. If the pupil is fibrotic, such as with chronic pilocarpine use or longstanding posterior synechiae, overstretching the iris can cause bleeding, tear the sphincter, and result in permanent mydriasis. Fortunately, overextension does not occur with the IFIS pupil, which is so elastic that it readily springs back to physiologic size despite being maximally stretched (Figure 3). Following the IOL's implantation, the iris retractors are removed, rinsed in balanced salt solution, and gently dabbed with an instrument wipe to remove any viscoelastic residue. They are then stored in the autoclavable storage container (Figure 4).

Like pupil expansion rings, iris retractors are much easier to insert prior to the initiation of the capsulorhexis. If the pupil dilates poorly in a patient taking tamsulosin, one should anticipate severe IFIS and consider using these mechanical devices. Often, however, the pupil dilates reasonably well, and it is not until after hydrodissection or during phacoemulsification that the prolapse and miosis occur. Healon5 and intracameral epinephrine are excellent rescue techniques in this situation, where it is difficult to see the edge of the capsulorhexis. If one elects to insert iris retractors at this point, it is useful to lift the pupillary margin with a Lester manipulating hook (Katena Products, Inc.) to avoid engaging the capsulorhexis' margin with the retractors.

CONCLUSION

Eliciting a history of alpha-1 blocker use allows surgeons to anticipate IFIS and to employ a number of varied strategies, either alone or in combination. When I anticipate severe IFIS, such as when the pupil dilates poorly preoperatively, I employ iris retractors because they are 100% reliable in circumventing the problems of IFIS. I also tend to use these devices if there are other concurrent risk factors such as a brunescent lens, pseudoexfoliation, or weak zonules. ■

This article originally appeared in the September 2006 issue of CRSToday.

1. Chang DF, Campbell JR. Intraoperative floppy iris syndrome associated with tamsulosin (Flomax). *J Cataract Refract Surg.* 2005;31:664-673.
2. Chang DF. Intraoperative floppy iris syndrome. In: Agarwal A, ed. *Phaco Nightmares.* Thorofare, NJ: Slack, Inc. In press.
3. Arshinoff SA. Modified SST-USST for tamsulosin-associated intraocular floppy iris syndrome. *J Cataract Refract Surg.* 2006;32:559-561.
4. Oetting TA, Omphroy LC. Modified technique using flexible iris retractors in clear corneal surgery. *J Cataract Refract Surg.* 2002;28:596-598.

CHAPTER 55

Malyugin Ring for Small Pupil Phaco Cases

BY BORIS MALYUGIN, MD, PhD

Patients with small pupils are always challenging for the cataract surgeon. Poor pupil dilation may be observed in cases complicated by pseudoexfoliation (PXF) syndrome, uveitis, posterior synechiae, trauma, or previous intraocular surgery. It may also be associated with local and systemic medications. Inadequate pupil dilation can decrease visualization during all stages of phacoemulsification, compromising surgery and increasing the risk of complications.

Most surgeons decide to mechanically dilate the pupil at the time of surgery if pharmacological agents fail. Unfortunately, there is no general recommendation or universal solution for the problems that small pupils present to cataract surgery; strategies for enlargement greatly depend upon surgical skill, preference, and the individual intraoperative situation.

Several iris retraction devices have been introduced into clinical practice, including the Graether Pupil Expander (Eagle Vision, Memphis, Tennessee), Perfect Pupil Injectable (PPI; Milvella Ltd., Sydney, Australia), and the Morcher Pupil Dilator (Morcher GmbH, Stuttgart, Germany). The main disadvantages of such technologies include their bulkiness and rigidity, making them difficult to insert, remove, and manipulate through a small incision. All of these rings are difficult to position if the anterior chamber is shallow or the pupil is less than 4 mm wide.

Using flexible iris hooks to retract tissue is relatively simple and has therefore been adopted by many surgeons. Multiple incisions for hook insertion are necessary, however, which is the main disadvangate of this technique. If the hooks overstretch the pupil size to more than a 6-mm square, irregular atonic pupils will likely appear postoperatively.

Several years ago, I introduced a new device into clinical practice that facilitates phacoemulsification in eyes with small pupils. This rectangular device, made of 5-0 polypropylene, uses the scroll principle to catch the pupillary margin. It is stretches the pupil to 6 mm wide. The main advantages of this device include gentle and less traumatic fixation of the iris margin and controlled stretching of the pupil. I previously described my surgical technique in the

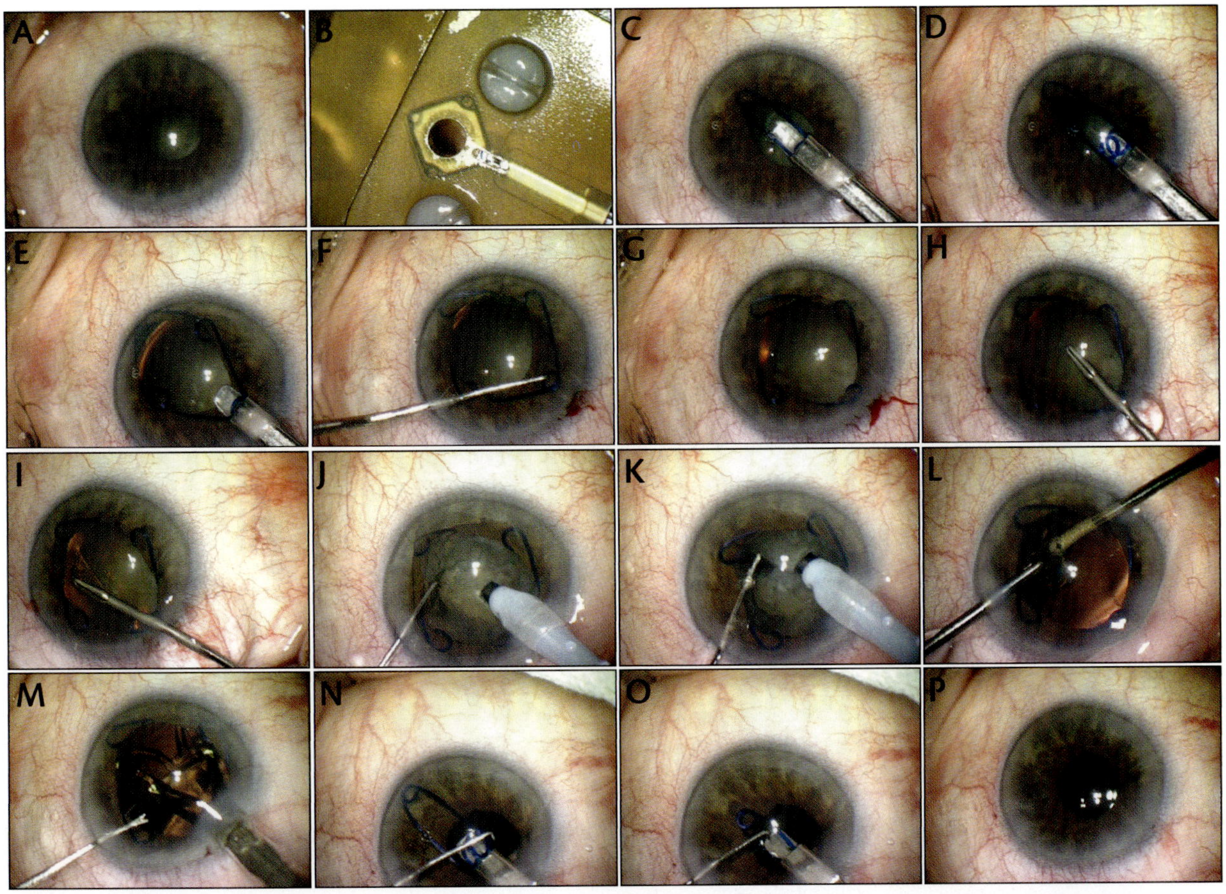

Figure 1. A still-video presentation of one cataract patient complicated by previously operated glaucoma, pseudoexfoliation syndrome, and a small pupil. See text for a detailed description of each step.

April 2007 issue of *CRST Europe* (The IQ-Ring, pages 25-28).

I performed the first implantations of the ring 7 years ago at the S. Fyodorov Eye Microsurgery Complex in Moscow. Since then, the device has undergone several design modifications. Recently, MicroSurgical Technology (Redmond, Washington) has become involved in further developing the device and marketing it in other countries. The current version of this single-use device, the *Malyugin Ring System,* consists of a holder and inserter packaged together with each ring. The inserter is used to withdraw the ring from the holder. It also introduces the ring into the anterior chamber and removes the ring from the eye. I have found that the inserter works very well, and ring implantation and removal is much easier and less traumatic for anterior chamber tissue.

SURGICAL TECHNIQUE

Herein, I present a description and still-video presentation of one cataract patient whose surgery was complicated by a small pupil, previously inoperated glaucoma, and PXF syndrome (Figure 1A).

The ring is loaded into the inserter (Figure 1B). Then, it is inserted through an unenlarged 2.2-mm clear corneal incision at the beginning of phacoemulsification. The tip of the inserter is positioned at the center of the anterior chamber. While pushing on the thumb button, the ring is released from the tip until the distal scroll is engaged with the distal iris (Figures 1C and D). Both lateral scrolls will then start to emerge from the tube of the inserter and simultaneously catch the iris margins (Figure 1E). The proximal scroll is expelled from the cannula/inserter, and the injector is moved proximally until the inserter hook is no longer holding the ring. In this position, the proximal scroll is lying on top of the iris. The inserter is withdrawn from the eye, and an iris hook is used to push the proximal scroll into the pupillary space. The proximal region of the iris margin is engaged (Figures 1F and G).

Once the ring is in position, cataract surgery is performed as usual, including continuous curvilinear capsulorrhexis, hydrodissection, emulsification, cortex removal, and IOL implantation (Figures 1H through M). The Malyugin Ring is then removed from the eye in the reverse order (Figures 1N through P).

I have used the Malyugin Ring System in more than 50 procedures. Clinical trials have shown that it performs as well as if not better than conventional pupil hooks in terms of both safety and efficacy. Additionally, intra- and postoperative complications with the Malyugin Ring were either reduced or comparable to those conventional hooks. Our clinical study demonstrated superior endothelial cell protection and a decrease of hyphemas, fibrinoid reactions, and early postoperative ocular hypertension in the Malyugin Ring group as compared with a group for which iris hooks were used.

CONCLUSION

Adequate transpupillary access to the lens is essential for the success of phaco procedures. We believe that our iris retraction technique with the Malyugin Ring System has many advantages:

- The ring is as effective as conventional iris hooks; however, compared with other commonly used iris retractors, it is friendlier to the eye due to its well-distributed stretching, gentle holding of delicate iris tissue, and the easier and less traumatic implantation. It has no sharp or pointed ends that can damage the eye;

• Equidistant positioning of the loops holds the iris tissue, ensuring correct position of the iris and preventing the effects of an overstretched pupil that are often observed when iris hooks are incorrectly placed;

• The device applies pressure to the iris sphincter over an area, which is wider than iris hooks. It is particularly useful in patients in whom cutting or tearing of the iris tissue should be avoided, especially in the presence of rubeosis, chronic anterior uveitis, or systemic coagulopathy. The iris rim is safely fixed in the ring's loops, and there is no risk of iris aspiration during phacoemulsification;

• Additional incisions are not required. This instrument is inserted through the main incision, thus reducing surgical trauma and minimizing the risk of contamination and postoperative inflammatory reaction. When a square pupil is formed by a conventional iris retractors, the iris can prolapse through the wound. This is particularly true in patients with relatively wide paracenteses or atonic and atrophic irises that seem particularly floppy;

• Sufficient room is available for nucleus fragmentation and removal. The device configuration allows the surgeon to work in the deep lens layers below the iris plane and the square-shaped pupil formed by the ring. This provides enough space for grooving and cutting the nucleus and increases peripheral visualization during the chopping phase; and

• The ring is inserted and removed from the eye with help of an inserter, reducing the risks of contamination and disturbance of the incision architecture and wound integrity.

SUMMARY

Different techniques of nucleus disassembly in small-incision cataract surgery require a wide and unobstructed view of the anterior portion of the lens and the instruments inserted into the anterior chamber. Sufficient manipulability of the instruments is also crucial for the successful completion of surgery. A pupil that fails to dilate makes cataract removal more difficult. The Malyugin Ring System adequately dilates the pupil and prevents iris sphincter damage. The easy-to-insert-and-remove device expands the pupil to 6 mm, protects the iris sphincter during surgery, and allows the pupil to return to its normal shape, size, and function after the operation.

The Malyugin Ring is an important tool in phacoemulsification surgery. Careful intraoperative manipulation and insertion of the ring with liberal use of an ophthalmic viscoelastic device can help prevent complications. After surgery, most of our patients' pupils were almost indistinguishable from their appearance before surgery, and functional activity was preserved.

I consider this new device among the most effective methods to increase the size of even very rigid small pupils during phacoemulsification surgery. The use of this method is highly recommended, as it is likely to reduce postoperative abnormalities in pupil size and function. ■

This article originally appeared in the March 2008 issue of CRSToday Europe.

CHAPTER 56

Weak Zonules

ROBERT H. OSHER, MD

One of the most dramatic triumphs in cataract surgery is surgeons' improved ability to manage a patient with weak zonules. When I was in training at the Bascom Palmer Eye Institute in Miami and at the Wills Eye Hospital in Philadelphia, I learned that a patient with either a congenital or acquired zonular problem was in serious trouble. Yet, removing the entire lens, especially when phacodonesis was absent, and implanting an ACIOL in a young patient seemed like a suboptimal solution. For that reason, I accepted the challenge of tackling the loose lens with phacoemulsification, one of five contraindications to the procedure defined by Charles Kelman, MD, in the mid-1980s. Preserving all, or a portion, of the capsular bag for the fixation of the IOL seemed worth the effort, especially because my phaco equipment was modified to allow the surgeon variable control of the level of ultrasound power, aspiration rate, vacuum level, and bottle height in a technique I named *slow-motion phacoemulsification*.

The method of IOL fixation was often more problematic than removing the loose lens, and I experimented with asymmetric fixation, crimping prolene haptics, and even sewing through the capsular bag. Although the method of IOL fixation was difficult and often frustrating, the surgical results were very favorable when I presented my initial series at the American Intra-Ocular Implant Society in 1986.[1]

EARLY MANAGEMENT OF WEAKENED ZONULES

A trip to Germany in 1992 abruptly changed my thinking. I was awestruck by the presentation by Ulrich Legler, MD, and Bernd Witschel, MD, who were using the capsular tension ring (CTR; Morcher GmbH, Stuttgart, Germany) to re-expand, tauten, and stabilize the compromised capsular bag.[2] One of my previous Fellows, Robert Cionni, MD, and I brought the CTR to the United Sates the following year, and the likelihood of achieving successful endocapsular fixation of the lens markedly improved. In the cases of profound zonular weakness, I developed a method of creating synthetic zonules with prolene sutures around the CTR, an advanced technique that became unnecessary when Dr. Cionni developed his innovative modification of the CTR (not FDA approved).[3] I still cannot believe how great his cases looked!

DIAGNOSTIC METHODS

Identifying Subtle Signs

The outcome of cataract surgery performed in an eye with zonular damage often depends upon the surgeon's preparedness. Minimizing intraoperative complications by modifying the surgical technique and having access to a CTR requires that the surgeon make the initial diagnosis of zonular weakness in the office, rather than in the OR. Phacodonesis, iridodonesis, vitreous prolapse, and an obvious subluxation of the lens make the diagnosis easy. However, the diagnosis of compromised zonules is sometimes only possible if a careful examination reveals any one of a number of more subtle signs that my colleagues and I have identified.[4]

Iridolenticular Gap

The iridolenticular gap sign is based upon the detection of a space between the anterior lens capsule and the border of the iris at the pupil. Usually, these structures appear to be contiguous as the slit lamp's beam passes across the anterior segment. A gap may signify focal zonular loss that has caused a slight posterior tilting of the lens or microsubluxation.

Decentered Nucleus

A decentered nucleus may also signify zonular weakness and can be better detected if the examiner learns to observe the cross-sectional anatomy of the lens with the slit beam. Both the fetal and the adult nucleus appear symmetrically positioned when the patient's gaze is in the primary position. Focal zonular loss may alter the usual symmetry of forces applied to the lens and result in a subtle, but significant, shift of the lens away from the area of zonular compromise.

Focal Iridodonesis

Focal iridodonesis can be observed as a subtle shimmering of the iris that is limited to several clock hours corresponding to adjacent zonular disruption. The loss of the barrier effect of the zonules permits the vitreous gel to move forward and contact the iris. As eye movements cause the gel to quiver, the overlying iris also shimmers.

Vitreous Tension

Lines of vitreous tension may also signify a focal rupture of the zonules. The vitreous probably herniates forward through the zonular opening into the posterior chamber, yet it may not be visible through the pupil. The *anatomy of the invisible,* a phrase coined by Jan Worst, MD, of Haren, the Netherlands, becomes visible as vitreous strands under tension point toward the damaged zonules.

Lens Equator

Another sign of zonular weakness is the visibility of the lens equator when the patient's gaze is eccentric. Indirect ophthalmoscopy may confirm a microluxation of the lens that can be easily overlooked if the examiner only observes the anatomy of the lens in the primary position.

Lens Contour

Changes in the contour of the lens periphery may indicate a loss in zonular tension at the equator. The usual curvilinear shape may appear flat or even seem to be missing a bite if a focal zonular loss allows the elastic forces of the capsule to retract.

CONCLUSION

It is usually true that the examiner will only see what he is seeking! The eye surgeon should always carefully examine the lens with the zonules in mind. Recognizing these subtle signs may provide crucial information about the zonular integrity. ■

This article originally appeared in the April 2005 issue of CRSToday.

1. Osher R. Paper presented at: the American Intra-Ocular Implant Society; Los Angeles, CA; April 7-10, 1986.
2. Witchel B, Legler U. The capsular ring. Video Journal of Cataract and Refractive Surgery [videotape]. 1993;9:4.
3. Cionni RJ, Osher RH, Snyder ME. Modified capsular tension ring use for zonular dialysis. *Ophthalmic Practice.* 1999;17:6:320-322.
4. Marques DMV, Marquess FF, Osher RH. Subtle signs of zonular damage. *J Cataract Refract Surg.* 2004;30:1295-1299.

CHAPTER 57

Preventing Complications in Patients With PXF Syndrome

ALAN S. CRANDALL, MD

Pseudoexfoliation (PXF) syndrome is a systemic and ocular condition in which hyaline material of unknown etiology is deposited onto structures in the eye's anterior segment. The presence of this debris can create problems during phacoemulsification, but surgeons can reduce the risk of complications through a few preventative measures.

WHAT TO LOOK FOR

Telltale signs of PXF syndrome include a classic deposition pattern on the lens (Figure 1) and pigment in the angle on gonioscopy. The most common challenges surgeons face when performing phacoemulsification on affected patients are managing small pupils and maintaining zonular stability.

Patients should undergo a slit-lamp evaluation to rule out zonular instability, phacodonesis, or subtle asymmetry in the depth of their anterior chambers (Figure 2). Any of these abnormalities could portend zonular problems and complicate cataract surgery. Patients with PXF syndrome can experience sudden IOP spikes after pupillary dilation, so surgeons should take steps to avoid this complication.

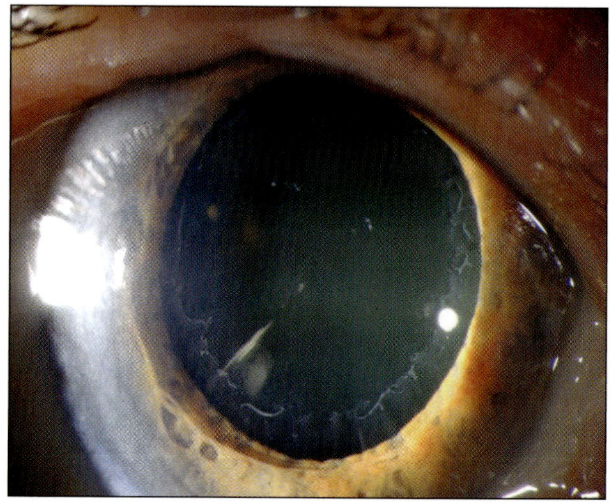

Figure 1. The patient's eye shows a classic deposition of abnormal extracellular tissue. Note the central plaque surrounded by a clear zone and further deposition around the pupillary margin.

DILATING THE PUPIL

Patients' pupils must be large enough to permit the safe creation of the capsulorhexis. Surgeons may use topical mydriatics or mechanical means such as Lester hooks (Katena Products, Inc., Denville, NJ), the Beehler pupil dilator (Moria, Antony, France), the Morcher Pupil Dilator (Morcher GmbH, Stuttgart, Germany; distributed in the United Sates by FCI Ophthalmics, Inc., Marshfield Hills, MA), and the Perfect Pupil Injectable (PPI; Milvella Ltd, Sydney, Australia).

I create my preferred 5.5-mm central capsulorhexis in eyes with PXF through a combination of an adaptive ophthalmic viscosurgical device, such as Healon5 (Advanced Medical Optics, Inc., Santa Ana, CA) or Discovisc (Alcon Laboratories, Inc., Fort Worth, TX), and the Morcher Pupil Dilator. I use the pupil dilator versus a two-handed stretching method, because the device remains in the eye until the end of the procedure and does not tear the iris.

PHACO TECHNIQUES

The phaco techniques I use on patients with PXF syndrome are designed to place minimal stress on weak zonules. I use a Chang Hydrodissection Cannula (Katena Products, Inc.) on a gentle wave setting to dissect the nucleus away from the capsular bag with cortical cleaving hydrodissection. After I rotate the nucleus to ensure it is completely free, I divide it into quadrants with a prechopper. If the nucleus is too hard for prechopping, or if I am working through a particularly small pupil, I use a zonule-friendly vertical chopping technique.

In cases in which debulking or divide-and-conquer is appropriate, I use enough energy to prevent the nucleus from moving during the phaco passes. Choosing the proper duty cycle reduces the amount of energy delivered to the eye and can prevent corneal damage. The surgeon must use enough power to prevent nuclear movement but employ a pulse or burst mode to prevent corneal burns.

The I/A phases of phacoemulsification can be tedious in eyes with PXF and, if not performed carefully, can strip away weak zonules. A bimanual technique may be useful, especially if the patient's pupil is relatively small, because it is easier to get to the subincisional cortex through two sites. Another option is to insert a capsular tension ring (CTR), although there is some debate as to whether the device is necessary in all cases of PXF. CTRs can decrease capsulophimosis and distribute forces to the zonules more equally. Although the devices do not protect against the late dislocation of an IOL, their presence may make it easier to suture the IOL to the sclera if necessary. The placement of these devices can exert stress on the zonules, however, and CTRs can complicate I/A if they are inserted too early. I do not use CTRs in all eyes with PXF syndrome, only in those with clear evidence of zonular weakness. Even then, I only place CTRs as late as safely possible.[1]

POSTOPERATIVE MANAGEMENT

To prevent postoperative IOP spikes, I carefully remove all lenticular fragments and viscoelastic from the eye at the end of surgery. I also start patients on 500 mg of oral acetazolamide for 3 days and, when necessary, release pressure from their eyes through the sideport incision on the day of surgery.

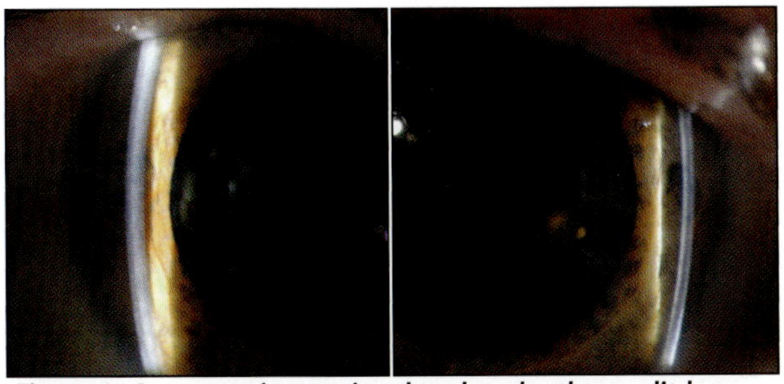

Figure 2. Asymmetric anterior chamber depths on slit-lamp examination suggest zonular weakening in eyes with PXF syndrome.

A long-term complication associated with PXF is the spontaneous subluxation of implanted IOLs.[2] This problem can arise any time between 2 months and 16 years postoperatively, with most cases occurring an average of 8.5 years after the IOL's implantation.

I use several strategies to correct IOL subluxation in patients with PXF. If the patient has plate IOLs, I remove the lenses and replace them with a haptic design. For example, three-piece lenses may be sutured to the sclera or the iris. If the patient does not have glaucoma, and I have to make a large incision to remove his original lens, I may consider implanting ACIOLs, PCIOLs, or foldable IOLs. In general, however, I prefer to use a foldable, iris-fixated, three-piece lens, which I suture to the sclera if the iris is missing or torn. I find that an iris fixation is technically easier, however, and allows me to keep the incision small.

CONCLUSION

When operating on patients with PXF, surgeons should be aware of strategies they can use to prevent IOP spikes after phacoemulsification. Gentle nuclear disassembly, careful cortical cleanup, and the use of devices such as CTRs can reduce the risk of immediate postoperative complications. Fixating nonplate IOLs to the sclera or the iris may help prevent subluxation. ■

This article originally appeared in the July 2008 issue of CRSToday.

1. Ahmed I, Cionni R, Kranemann C, Crandall A. Optimal timing of capsular tension ring implantation: a Miyake-Apple video analysis. *J Cataract Refract Surg.* 2005;31:1809-1813.
2. Jehan F, Mamalis N, Crandall A. Spontaneous late dislocation of intraocular lens within the capsular bag in pseudoexfoliation patients. *Ophthalmology.* 2001;108:1727-1731.

CHAPTER 58

Surgical Management of the Traumatic Cataract

PETER A. ZAKRZEWSKI, MD, AND IKE K. AHMED, MD, FRCSC

A traumatic cataract may develop after various types of ocular insult, including blunt or perforating trauma as well as ionizing, infrared, or ultraviolet radiation.[1] Besides cataract, ocular trauma can also induce lens subluxation and dislocation and cause injuries to the cornea, iris, vitreous, and retina.

In the case of blunt trauma, coup and contrecoup forces on the lens could cause rapid anterior-posterior shortening, leading to abrasion or rupture of the lens capsule with subsequent cataractogenesis. Direct anterior-posterior force also produces equatorial expansion of the lens, which can result in equatorial capsular rupture and zonular dehiscence. Equatorial capsular rupture can further stimulate cataract formation, although zonular dehiscence can lead to lens subluxation or complete dislocation, depending on the extent of zonular incompetence.[2,3] Blunt ocular trauma typically leads to a stellate or rosette-shaped opacification that is axial in location and involves the posterior capsule.[1]

In perforating trauma, direct compromise of the lens capsule by the penetrating object leads to cortical opacification at the site of injury. If the capsular tear is large enough, the entire lens can rapidly opacify, but a cataract caused by a small perforation may become sealed off and remain localized.[4] Contusive forces, as described for blunt trauma, may or may not be present, depending on the agent and mechanism responsible for injury, but they will exacerbate cataract formation if present.

PREOPERATIVE ASSESSMENT

Before performing surgery to manage a traumatic cataract, a detailed preoperative examination is required to identify other pathology that may prevent optimal postoperative visual recovery and to help with the decision of which surgical approach to take. Open-globe injuries and intraocular foreign bodies must be ruled out before surgery.[5,6] Additionally, it is possible that following an episode of intraocular inflammation, a fibrin layer covering the anterior surface of a clear lens may masquerade as cataract. Careful visualization of the exact location of the lens opacification (anterior to or within the lens itself) is important to rule this condition out, thereby preventing unnecessary surgery. This can be difficult,

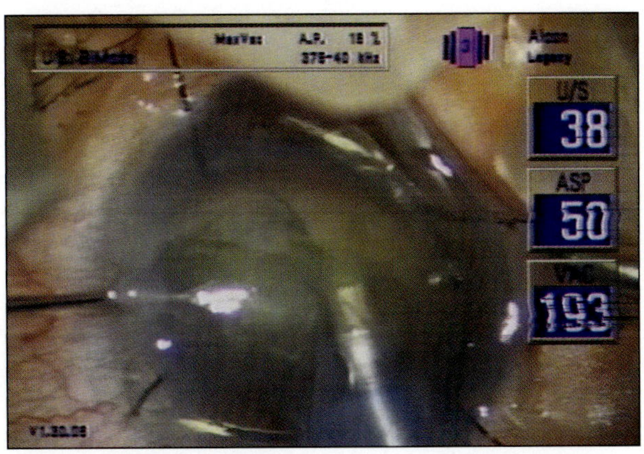

Figure 1. Iris retractors placed at the capsulorhexis' edge can act as artificial zonules during intraoperative maneuvers.

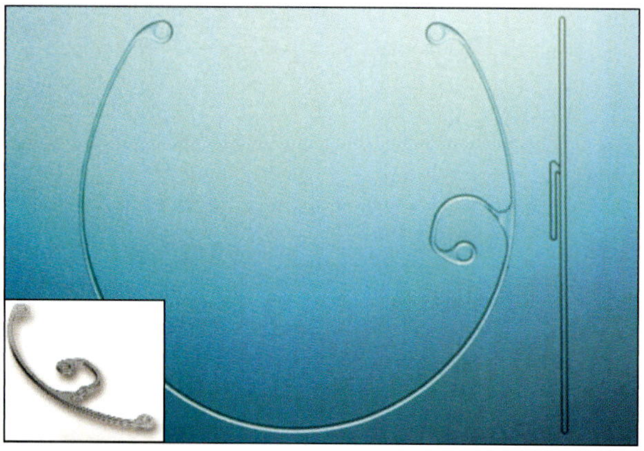

Figure 2. The Cionni-modified CTR can be sutured to the sclera. The CTS, with its 90° arc, can be inserted at a specific site of zonular weakness (inset).

especially with children of whom slit-lamp examination is difficult to perform.[1,7]

Abnormal findings that predict a poor postoperative visual outcome include corneal disease, iridodialysis, a relative afferent pupillary defect, macular scarring, retinal detachment, and optic atrophy.[8] Greven et al[8] found that only 30% of eyes that suffered from contusion injuries had normal preoperative posterior segments; thus, a B-scan is necessary if the posterior pole cannot be visualized. The physician should also examine patients for intraocular inflammation and increased IOP preoperatively and provide appropriate treatment.

In carrying out a thorough lenticular examination, the physician should first determine the type (nuclear, cortical, subcapsular, etc.), location, and degree of lens opacification. Furthermore, a careful assessment for zonular disruption and associated lens subluxation or dislocation is important in deciding which surgical approach to take. Maximal pharmacologic pupillary dilation may be necessary to identify a subtle zonular dialysis. At the slit lamp, the physician should note the degree of zonular dialysis and phacodonesis, as well as the resting position of the lens. Iridodonesis may be the initial clinical sign indicating zonular dehiscence.[1] An anteriorly displaced lens may present with a shallow anterior chamber and requires immediate removal due to the risk of pupillary block.[9] A posteriorly subluxated lens may only be clinically evident during an examination of the patient with a portable slit lamp while he is in a supine position.[7] If available, ultrasound biomicroscopy can be helpful for assessing capsular and zonular integrity.

SURGICAL CONSIDERATIONS

Depending on the clinical situation, the surgical management of a traumatic cataract is performed using either a standard anterior limbal or posterior pars plana approach. An anterior approach is best for a traumatic cataract unless there is complete lens dislocation or capsular rupture with significant lens material incarcerated in the vitreous. The surgeon should perform a standard phacoemulsification cataract extraction using a large capsulorhexis and initiated at the site of greatest zonular stability.[7] Capsular staining with trypan blue in cases of poor visualization (not FDA approved)[10] and generous hydrodissection to avoid stress on the zonules during lens extraction are also important steps.[7] A low-flow, low-vacuum, supracapsular phaco technique is preferred to minimize capsular and zonular stress. If zonular dehiscence and subsequent vitreous prolapse occur intraoperatively, a cutting-aspiration handpiece can be used to remove the vitreous.[7] Subsequent operative steps will depend on the degree of zonular disruption, which will be discussed later.

The posterior approach with vitrectomy and lensectomy is reserved for cases of posterior capsular rupture with vitreous prolapse or a posteriorly dislocated lens.[7]

The degree of zonular dehiscence dictates the management approach for a subluxed or displaced lens. If the dehiscence is small with no vitreous prolapse, extra care should be taken not to stress the zonules; otherwise, routine surgery is appropriate. For a larger zonular disruption, the surgeon should consider the implantation of a capsular tension ring (CTR). For zonular dialysis of up to 150°, the use of a conventional CTR followed by standard phacoemulsification and PCIOL insertion has been highly successful.[11]

The CTR is an open ring made of a single piece of PMMA that is placed inside the capsular bag. The CTR reforms the posterior capsule, and produces a taut capsular equator that protects against aspiration of the capsular fornix, thereby preventing extension of the zonular dialysis during surgical manipulation. It also allows for easier IOL placement, prevents later IOL decentration, and reduces the postoperative incidence of posterior capsular opacification.[11-14]

In the case of surgery to remove a traumatic cataract, the CTR may be implanted before or after phacoemulsification.[11] Although early insertion provides support during phacoemulsification, it may create additional zonular trauma.[15] The use of iris or capsule retractors at the capsulorhexis' edge (Figure 1) or the use of a capsular tension segment (CTS; Morcher GmbH, Stuttgart, Germany [not currently approved by the FDA]) during phacoemulsification are other alternatives that do not induce significant capsular torque during insertion. The CTS (Figure 2) is a partial PMMA ring segment containing an anteriorly offset eyelet through which an iris retractor or suture may be placed.[15]

For more significant or progressive zonular dialysis, the

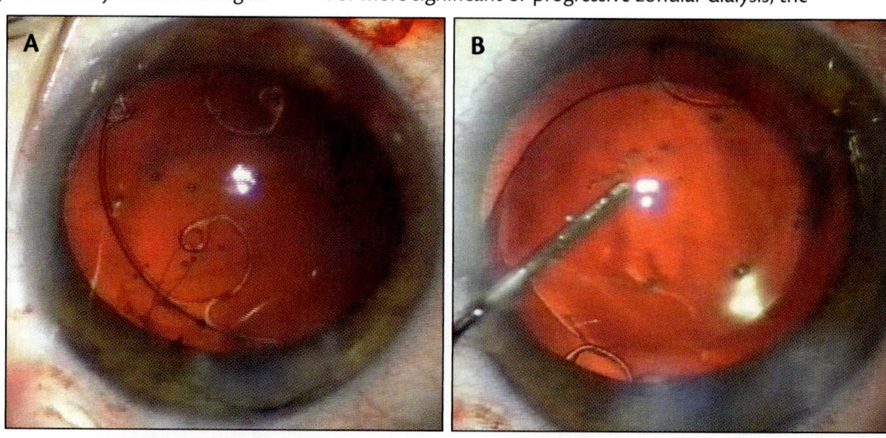

Figure 3. Two CTS devices have been placed in the capsular bag for profound generalized zonular compromise (A). Once sutures have been threaded through the eyelets, a PCIOL can be placed within the capsular bag with optimal centration (B).

Cionni-modified CTR (Morcher GmbH) has been demonstrated to be a useful alternative to the conventional CTR (Figure 2). It can be sutured safely to the sclera without compromising the capsular bag, thus allowing the CTR and capsule to be held in place even in the presence of significant zonular incompetence.[16,17] Alternatively, one or two CTS devices may be used and may also be placed in cases of an anterior capsular tear, incomplete capsulorhexis, or posterior capsular rupture (Figure 3, A and B).

The use of aniridia implant devices such as iris diaphragm rings and iris sector shields is often appropriate in cases of a significant loss of iris tissue. These devices are not FDA approved. Pupilloplasty and/or repair of iridodialysis may also be required.

The choice and positioning of the IOL depends on the degree and location of zonular disruption. In eyes with no zonular disruption and an intact posterior capsule, a standard capsular bag-fixated IOL may be used. With a small area of zonular incompetence, a capsular bag IOL may also be used, but the haptics should be oriented toward the area of incompetence in order to expand and stabilize the capsular bag fully. With more significant zonular disruption, IOL implantation should be combined with CTR or CTS use. In cases of an unsalvageable capsular bag, other IOL options include ciliary sulcus-fixated IOLs, transsclerally sutured PCIOLs, and ACIOLs.[7]

Although the ACIOL has been advocated in special circumstances (elderly patient, good iris support, no evidence of glaucoma, no vitreous in anterior chamber), they should not be used in younger patients because of the increased risk of corneal endothelial injury and glaucoma from further angle injury.[7] Using ciliary sulcus-fixated IOLs in children following traumatic cataract removal resulted in visual outcomes similar to those for capsular bag IOLs but with more complications, in particular uveitis and pupillary capture.[18] Sclerally sutured PCIOLs were not compared directly with capsular bag IOLs but produced good postoperative visual results.[19] The use of multifocal capsular bag IOLs following removal of a traumatic cataract has also been explored. In comparison with standard, monofocal, capsular bag IOLs, the multifocal lenses resulted in improved uncorrected near visual acuity and stereopsis, as well as decreased spectacle dependency.[20]

CONCLUSION

In summary, a traumatic cataract is common after any form of injury to the eye. A thorough preoperative ocular examination is essential to properly assess the eye with a traumatic cataract. The surgical approach, potential use of capsular tension devices, and choice of IOL are all dictated by the inherent integrity of the zonules, lens capsule, and other associated anterior segment structures. Excluding other intrinsic causes of visual dysfunction, an eye with a traumatic cataract is amenable to treatment and has an excellent potential for significant postoperative visual improvement. ■

This article originally appeared in the June 2004 issue of CRSToday.

1. Johns KJ, Feder RS, Bowes Hamill M, et al. *Lens and Cataract. AAO Basic and Clinical Science Course Series.* San Francisco: The Foundation for the American Academy of Ophthalmology, 2001;50-54:213-216.
2. Wolter JR. Coup-contrecoup mechanism of ocular injuries. *Am J Ophthalmol.* 1963;56:785-796.
3. Weidenthal DT, Schepens CL. Peripheral fundus changes associated with ocular contusion. *Am J Ophthalmol.* 1966;62:465-477.
4. Shock JP, Adams D. Long-term visual acuity results after penetrating and perforating ocular injuries. *Am J Ophthalmol.* 1985;100:714-718.
5. Kwitko MR, Kwitko GM. Management of traumatic cataract. *Curr Opin Ophthalmol.* 1990;1:25-27.
6. Irvine JA, Smith RE. Lens Injuries in trauma. In: Shingleton B, Hersh PS, Kenyon KR eds. *Eye Trauma.* St. Louis: CV Mosby; 1991: 126-135.
7. Mian SI, Azar DT, Colby K. Management of traumatic cataracts. *Int Ophthalmol Clin.* 2002;42:23-31.
8. Greven CM, Collins AS, Slusher MM, Grey Weaver R. Visual results, prognostic indicators, and posterior segment findings following surgery for cataract/lens subluxation-dislocation secondary to ocular contusion injuries. *Retina.* 2002;22:575-580.
9. Zaidman GW. The surgical management of dislocated traumatic cataracts. *Am J Ophthalmol.* 1985;22:342-346.
10. Jacob S, Agarwal A, Agarwal A, et al. Trypan blue as an adjunct for safe phacoemulsification in eyes with white cataract. *J Cataract Refract Surg.* 2002;28:1819-1825.
11. Jacob S, Agarwal A, Agarwal A, et al. Efficacy of a capsular tension ring for phacoemulsification in eyes with zonular dialysis. *J Cataract Refract Surg.* 2003;29:315-321.
12. Menapace R, Findl O, Georgopoulos M, et al. The capsular tension ring: designs, applications and techniques. *J Cataract Refract Surg.* 2000;26:898-912.
13. Gimbel HV, Sun R. Clinical applications of capsular tension rings in cataract surgery. *Ophthalmic Surg Lasers.* 2002;33:44-53.
14. D'Eliseo D, Pastena B, Longanesi L, et al. Prevention of posterior capsule opacification using capsular tension ring for zonular defects in cataract surgery. *Eur J Ophthalmol.* 2003;13:151-154.
15. Ahmed, IK, Kranemann CF, Crandall AS. Capsular tension segment: next step in effective management of profound zonular dialysis. Presented at: The ASCRS/ASOA Symposium on Cataract, IOL, and Refractive Surgery Film Festival; April 13, 2003; San Francisco, CA.
16. Ahmed IK, Crandall AS. Ab externo scleral fixation of the Cionni modified capsular tension ring. *J Cataract Refract Surg.* 2001;27:977-981.
17. Moreno-Montanes J, Sainz C, Maldonado MJ. Intraoperative and postoperative complications of Cionni endocapsular ring implantation. *J Cataract Refract Surg.* 2003;29:492-497.
18. Pandey SK, Ram J, Werner L, et al. Visual results and postoperative complications of capsular bag and ciliary sulcus fixation of posterior chamber intraocular lenses in children with traumatic cataracts. *J Cataract Refract Surg.* 1999;25:1576-1584.
19. Chaudry NA, Belfort A, Flynn JW, et al. Combined lensectomy, vitrectomy and scleral fixation of intraocular lens implant after closed-globe injury. *Ophthalmic Surg Lasers.* 1999;20:375-381.
20. Jacobi PC, Dietlein TS, Lueke C, Jacobi FK. Multifocal intraocular lens implantation in patients with traumatic cataract. *Ophthalmology.* 2003;110:531-538.

CHAPTER 59

Conditions and Capsular Tension Rings

DAVID M. DILLMAN, MD

The FDA approved the use of capsular tension rings (CTRs) more than 1 year ago. Surgeons can choose from a variety of these devices, including the Stabileyes CTR (Ophtec BV; Groningen, the Netherlands; distributed in the United Sates by Advanced Medical Optics, Inc., Santa Ana, CA), the CTR (Morcher GmbH, Stuttgart, Germany; distributed by FCI Ophthalmics, Inc.; Marshfield Hills, MA), and the Cionni Morcher CTRs (Morcher GmbH; distributed by FCI Ophthalmics, Inc.). CTRs facilitate cataract surgery performed in the presence of weakened zonules. This article shares what I learned from my first full year of using the Stabileyes CTR.

INDICATIONS FOR USE

It is important to bear in mind that CTRs are appropriate in eyes with a complete anterior capsulorhexis, an otherwise fully intact capsular bag, and weakened zonules. They provide structural support, not surgical miracles. CTRs are actually contraindicated in the presence of an unwanted opening in either the anterior or posterior capsule as well as in the presence of extremely compromised zonules such as those that have lost more than four clock hours of integrity. This article does not discuss devices for cases of extreme zonular deterioration, including the Cionni Morcher CTRs and the Ahmed capsular tension segments (Morcher GmbH; not FDA approved).

SYSTEMIC INDICATIONS FOR CTRs

Compromised zonular strength results from several congenital, endocrinic, and metabolic conditions, including Marfan's syndrome, Marchesani's syndrome, scleroderma, homocystinuria, spherophakia, porphyria, hyperlysinemia, hyperlipoproteinemia, and sulfite oxidase deficiency. I have trouble spelling these, let alone recognizing them. Although I try to be aware of their existence, I do not often see these conditions in Danville, Illinois.

OCULAR CONDITIONS FOR CTRs

Pseudoexfoliation

It is well known that eyes with pseudoexfoliation (PXF) often have weakened zonules and therefore a lax capsular bag. In such eyes, cataract surgery is more challenging, and the risk for intraoperative complications is higher than in healthy eyes. Even if the surgery itself is free of complications, eyes with PXF are at a higher risk for developing postoperative complications such as a decentered IOL and capsular phimosis.

Will every eye with PXF have weakened zonules and a compromised capsular bag? Should every eye with PXF receive a CTR as a matter of routine? I have heard arguments on both sides. At present, I routinely place a CTR in an eye with PXF. If I detect even a hint of weakness in the zonule/bag complex, I place the CTR early, before performing phacoemulsification. Otherwise, I place the device before I insert the IOL.

Previous Ocular Trauma

Surgeons all know to carefully examine preoperatively an eye with a known history of trauma. Even without obvious compromise of the zonule/capsular bag at the time of the slit-lamp evaluation, this complication occurs intraoperatively.

A history of previous ocular surgery is a subset of the category of previous ocular trauma. I am particularly vigilant for eyes that have (1) undergone a vitrectomy (stretched zonules due to a lack of posterior support), (2) had successful filtration surgery for glaucoma (stretched zonules because of a shallow anterior chamber), and (3) undergone "aggressive" RK (ie, with incisions made via the Russian technique that extend all the way to the limbus and/or number more than eight). These eyes may well have endured a micro- or macroperforation with subsequent shallowing of the anterior chamber and stretching of the zonules.

The good news is that CTRs can provide needed support in these cases.

Future Eye Surgery

If it makes good sense to place a CTR in an eye that has undergone a vitrectomy, then perhaps surgeons should consider placing the device in an eye that is going to have a vitrectomy. The most obvious patient group, of course, would be diabetics who are referred for cataract surgery prior to undergoing a vitrectomy as part of the treatment for their diabetic retinopathy. A second group would be patients referred for cataract surgery prior to macular surgery for the treatment of macular holes, epiretinal membranes, etc.

It may be appropriate to consult a retinal surgeon before prophylactically placing a CTR. The retinal specialists with whom I work like having a CTR in place.

Long Axial Length

The amount of a patient's refractive myopia does not always correlate well with his axial length. Steep corneas and nuclear sclerosis can cause myopia in the presence of fairly average axial lengths. I therefore home in on the axial myope. Unusually long eyes have a greater propensity for stretched zonules both intra- and postoperatively. Also, these eyes are perhaps more susceptible to movement of the zonule/capsular bag complex postoperatively and the subsequent influence on the vitreous base. I do not have an absolute number, but I always place a CTR in eyes with an axial length of 26 mm or longer. I individually consider eyes with an axial length of between 25 and 26 mm.

INTRAOPERATIVE FINDINGS

Using CTRs has made me a better observer of intraocular events. Weak zonules can make the capsulorhexis more difficult to start and to complete. They can impede hydrodissection by resisting efforts to spin the lens. They can also hinder the maneuvering of nuclear fragments within the confines of the capsular bag.

In some cases, the zonules are normal at the beginning of the case but weaken as it proceeds. I most expect this problem when I deal with an extremely dense cataract that requires considerable manipulation for its safe removal, and I will often place a CTR into these eyes if I sense that their zonular status has changed.

TIMING THE PLACEMENT OF CTRS

Surgeons new to CTRs often want to know the best time during surgery to place the device. It is easiest to place a CTR into a capsular bag that is nicely distended with a viscoelastic after performing both phacoemulsification and cortical cleanup. The device can only help intraoperatively with these surgical steps, however, when it is located within the capsular bag and not sitting on the stand. I generally place the CTR upon my first inkling that the device may be necessary. ■

This article originally appeared in the November/December 2005 issue of CRSToday.

CHAPTER 60

What Forces Act on the Capsular Bag?

CHRISTOPHER LIU, FRCOPHTH

Recently, my colleagues and I performed a systematic theoretical analysis of the per- and postoperative forces that act on the lens capsular bag. If such forces could be counteracted, we reasoned that the risk of complications could be reduced, especially in high-risk patients. It is important for every surgeon to understand the forces that act on the capsular bag, as well as the devices that will help achieve successful and stable postoperative outcomes. We have found that the use of capsular tension rings (CTRs) is an appropriate option for lowering the amount of force on the capsular bag and managing loose zonules.

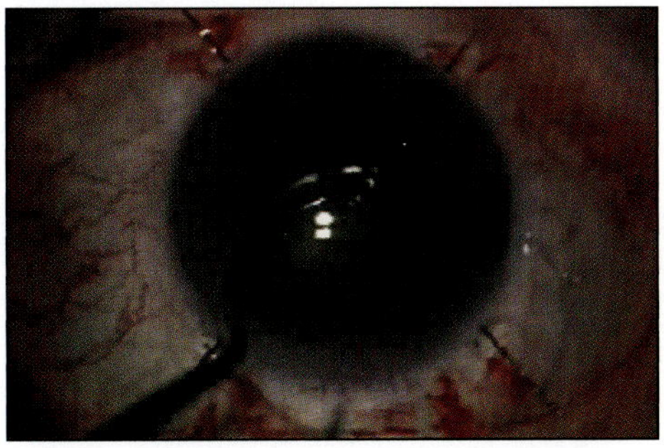

Figure 1. Bimanual insertion of a CTR after hydrodissection.

Our findings indicated that such forces acting on the capsular bag, both perioperatively and postoperatively, include (1) the trampoline effect during collapse and reinflation of the anterior chamber, (2) the capsulorrhexis, which also exerts force on the zonules, (3) phaco probes and second instruments during phacoemulsification, (4) I/A of soft lens matter, (5) insertion of the IOL and dialing it to a position, which may stretch the anterior lens capsule as well as exert forces on the zonules, and (6) long-term contraction of the capsular bag from lens epithelial cell transdifferentiation. This occurs in cases of zonular weakness if the anterior capsulorrhexis is inadequately sized, particularly when silicone IOLs are used.

Several techniques and tricks may counteract the forces exerted onto the capsular bag. First, gentle tissue handling—especially in the case of zonular weakness—is important. Second, try to reduce the long-term bag contraction by only opening the anterior capsular cut to an adequate diameter. Further tricks to reduce the force include supporting the lens capsular bag by using iris retraction hooks and the Mackool Cataract Support System (Duckworth & Kent, Hertfordshire, England); applying the Ahmed Capsular Tension Segment (Morcher, Stuttgard, Germany) to provide pre- and postoperative sectorial capsular support; and using single or multiple CTRs to prevent capsular contraction and capsular bag decentration.

If loose zonules—caused by Marfan's syndrome, pseudoexfoliation, trauma, and iatrogenic causes—are present, then it is more likely that the patient will experience vitreous loss, a dropped nucleus, unopposed capsular bag shrinkage, anterior capsular fibrosis and phimosis, and bag-IOL decentration-subluxation. Surgeons should proceed with caution in these high-risk cases. Their first action must be to ask themselves two questions: (1) In severe cases with few remaining zonules, should the case be referred to a vitreoretinal surgeon? and (2) Should the case be referred to a cataract specialist who is experienced in dealing with complex cases? If you are to proceed with the surgery, aim for long-term centration of the IOL, the absence of anterior capsular phimosis, and no continuing zonular loss, which may lead to subluxation or dislocation of the capsular bag. There are several devices that may help you to reach these goals.

DEVICES

Iris Retraction Hooks

These flexible nylon hooks usually have a colored body so that they may be easily identified. Two popular models are the Grieshaber Iris Retractor (Grieshaber and Co. AG, Kennesaw, Georgia) and the MicroVision Iris Retractor (MicroVision, Inc., Seabrook, New Hampshire). Iris hooks offer many benefits compared with other mechanical methods of pupil dilation, including excellent and stable pupil size. It is also possible to transfer iris hooks to the anterior capsulorrhexis rim. On the other hand, iris hooks require making four extra incisions, and the process is time consuming. Another disadvantage is the expense of the iris hooks.

CTRs

These rings are usually PMMA C-shaped open rings that are designed for in-the-bag implantation. Whether inserted bimanually (Figure 1) or with an injector system, this device maintains the circular shape of the capsular bag. Its function is to help reduce zonular dehiscence and vitreous loss, prevent shrinkage of the capsular bag, and reduce anterior capsular phimosis as well as postoperative IOL decentration and tilt. Several manufacturers offer CTR models. Those that have a square edge also have the added benefit of preventing posterior capsular opacification.

CTRs should be placed as soon as zonular dehiscence or weakness is detected. First, insert iris hooks as necessary onto the intact capsulorrhexis rim. A CTR may be inserted before phacoemulsification of the nucleus or either before or after I/A of soft lens matter. CTRs are especially useful for high-risk cases. Consider using multiple and possibly large-diameter rings for patients with high myopia, pseudoexfoliation, and larger clock hours of zonular dehiscence. If very extensive zonular dehiscence is noted, however, do not insert the CTRs if they do not allow scleral fixation (see the *Variants of the CTR* section in this article for the Cionni Modified CTR). These devices should also be avoided if there is a posterior capsular tear, a subluxated crystalline lens, or if the anterior capsulorrhexis is not intact. If you are planning to use an accommodating IOL, CTRs are contraindicated, because these IOLs require capsular movement.

Several complications may arise with the use of CTRs, including capsular bag decentration or tilt and dislocation of the ring. Furthermore, the capsular tear may be extended if the patient has an imperfect anterior capsulorrhexis, posterior capsular tear, or if the surgeon attempts (1) to enlarge the anterior capsulorrhexis or (2) a primary posterior capsulorrhexis. Use caution when placing the CTR, because inadvertent placement into the sulcus or anterior chamber angle will cause additional complications.

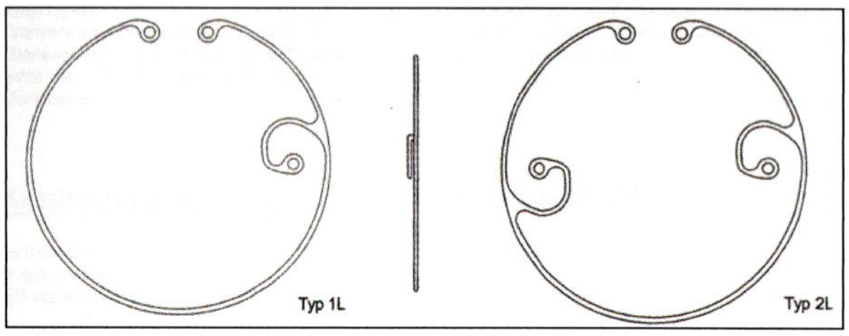

Figure 2. Two of the five available Cionni Modified CTR models.

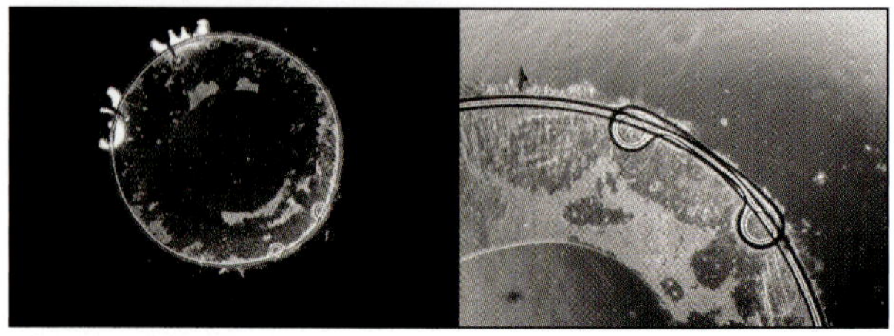

Figure 4. Low-power images of capsular bags following a sham cataract operation and ring insertion.

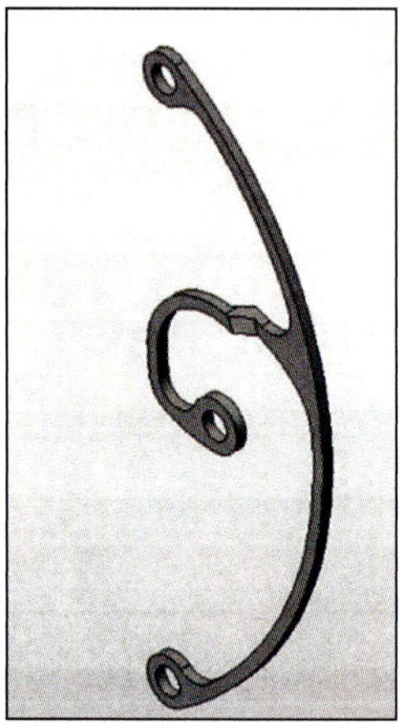

Figure 3. The Ahmed capsular tension segment.

Variants of the CTR

In addition to standard CTRs, there are several variant models on the market, including the Cionni Modified Capsular Tension Ring (Morcher, Stuttgart, Germany) (Figure 2) and the Ahmed capsular tension segment (Figure 3). The last variant has a 5-mm radius of curvature and a third eyelet for an iris hook or suture fixation. It may even be used in the event of a capsulorhexis tear or posterior capsular rent. Some CTRs have a rectangular profile. As previously mentioned, these models prevent posterior capsular opacification. Some models are also foldable and offer a sharp edge and a closed ring.

In conclusion, the importance of counteracting the forces that act on the capsular bag must not be underestimated. Try using a large rhexis. In the presence of zonular weakness, avoid using a silicone IOL. Instead, use one made from materials with low propensity for causing capsular contraction (eg, AcrySof acrylic material [Alcon Laboratories, Inc., Fort Worth, TX]). Additionally, consider employing a device such as iris retraction hooks, capsular tension segment, or CTRs to prevent further complications. CTRs are a wonderful tool to maintain the circular shape of the capsular bag and prevent capsular bag decentration and contraction (Figure 4). ■

This article originally appeared in the November/December 2007 issue of CRSToday.

CHAPTER 61

Implanting the Capsular Tension Ring

HOWARD V. GIMBEL, MD, MPH, FRCSC, AOE, CABES

Surgeons may inject the capsular tension ring (CTR; Morcher GmbH, Stuttgart, Germany) either by inserting it with an injector or by using two forceps to maneuver the device into the eye. Although I like using the injector, forceps are necessary in order to use a modified CTR such as the Cionni Modified Capsular Tension Ring (Morcher GmbH), the colobomas segment ring, and aniridia tension rings, which have appendages. The injector is only useful for the standard CTR.

With the forceps technique, a hook inserted into one of the eyelets of the CTR may help the surgeon to place the final end of the device. A cohesive viscoelastic helps to maintain the chamber and keep the capsular bag open.

INSERTION TECHNIQUE

The insertion technique that I prefer involves placing the first end of the CTR into the capsular bag and moving it out to the equator. I maneuver the device as close to the incision as possible (Figure 1), and then I place a little pressure against the capsular bag to bend the ring before it begins to rotate around the bag. For instance, if the incision is at the 12-o'clock position, rather than engage the capsule with the first end of the ring at the 9-o'clock position, I try to maneuver the end of the ring up toward the

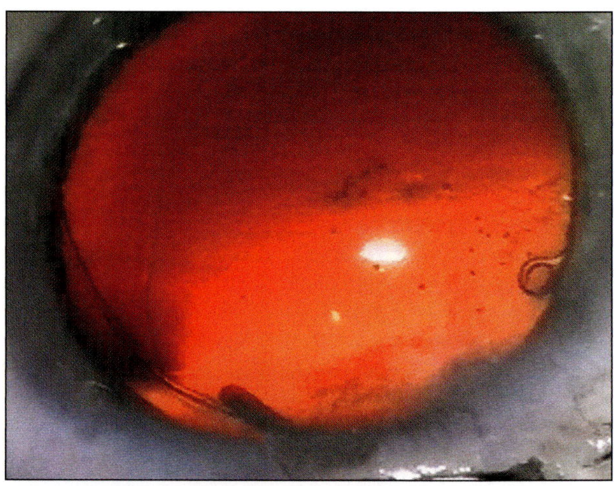

Figure 1. The author maneuvers the CTR into the capsular bag and out to the equator.

11-o'clock position (Figure 2). Before injecting it, I bend the CTR against the capsule to compress the device's curvature so that it will slide around the equatorial area of the capsule. Surgeons may

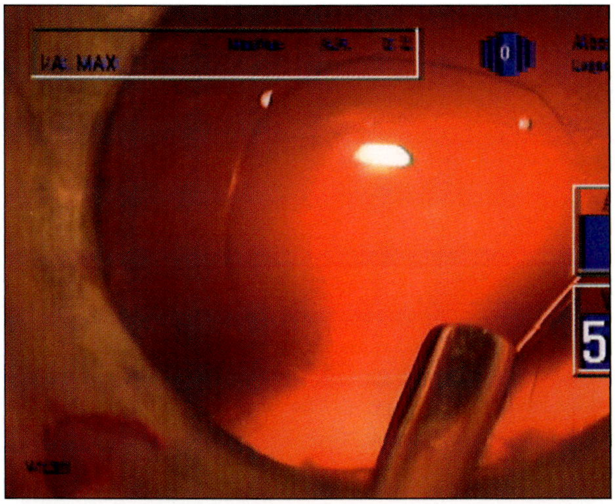

Figure 2. The author pulls the CTR around the capsular bag toward the 11-o'clock position.

also use a Sinskey hook to bend the end of the ring that enters the eye in order to reduce the stress on the equator of the capsular bag.

WEAK ZONULES AND CAPSULAR TEARS

If the zonules are generally weak, then the previously described maneuver may be helpful. In a case of extremely weak zonules, the surgeon may support the capsular bag at the side opposite to where he will place the initial loop against the capsular equator (iris hooks may be used as capsule hooks to support the capsule). If the zonules are weak in only one hemisection because of trauma, then the surgeon should direct the first end of the CTR to the loosest part of the capsular bag in order to exert pressure away from the strongest zonules.

If the capsule tears, I remove the CTR and do not use it (this event is quite unlikely in the presence of an intact CCC). If a capsular tear necessitates explantation of the device, the surgeon may use a Sinskey hook to engage the ring and pull it into the center of the pupil, much like the maneuver of chopping the nucleus in phacoemulsification.

Some cases call for using a CTR although the nucleus and the cortex can be removed safely without it. One such case is that of weak zonules and large striae across the posterior capsule that cause a Maddox rod effect in the vision postoperatively. Eliminating these striae would result in better long-term safety and visual quality.

WHEN TO INSERT THE RING

Some surgeons may wonder whether to implant the CTR before removing the cortex and nucleus as well as before or after placing the IOL. If a patient presents with phacodonesis, which indicates that the zonules are so weak that even removing the nucleus may cause the capsule to collapse, I insert the CTR before I perform phacoemulsification. I also use this approach with traumatic zonulysis, because I find the technique reduces the likelihood of the vitreous' herniating around the area of zonular dehiscence. Inserting the device prior to phacoemulsification, however, does complicate nucleofractis techniques (eg, phaco chop, divide-and-conquer—any technique that splits the nucleus), because the ring does not allow the capsular bag to ovalize (this occurs when the nucleus is split, because the capsular bag has to deform). For that reason, if the zonules seem strong enough to remain intact after the nucleus is removed, then I may extract the nucleus before inserting the CTR.

Cortex removal will also be more difficult if the CTR is already in place, because the ring traps the cortex in the equator. Therefore, if the zonules seem only somewhat loose or are loose in just one quadrant, I may try to strip the cortex, test the capsular support, and proceed as long as there is adequate zonular support. If stripping the cortex places too much stress on the existing weak zonules, however, then I insert the ring and struggle with the cortex removal.

Regarding insertion of the IOL, I have not found advantages with placing the CTR either prior to or after implanting the lens. Generally, I insert the ring before IOL implantation. If striae and ovalization of the capsular bag occur after IOL insertion, however, then the CTR will easily slide by the implant. The order of placement does not seem to matter.

ADDITIONAL CONSIDERATIONS

The FDA recently approved the CTR in three sizes that include pediatric eyes and large eyes that may have a larger lens capsule. Surgeons must select the size of the ring depending on the age of the patient, the size of the eye, and the strength of the capsular support that the patient needs.

In addition to using the CTR to support the capsular bag during cataract surgery, the surgeon may employ a modified tension ring in addition to the first CTR in order to close a coloboma or center the capsular bag. As I mentioned, explanting the first CTR is rather easy and carries little risk if the surgeon prefers that approach. I prefer to leave the CTR in place and add a coloboma or an aniridia ring segment.

A NEW SURGICAL STAPLE?

I believe that the CTR should be used almost routinely in cataract surgery and that someday it will become a component of IOLs, because it eliminates wrinkles on the posterior capsule and the asymmetrical contraction of the capsular bag. Modifications to the CTR that may impede posterior capsule opacification are currently undergoing testing. ■

This article originally appeared in the January 2004 issue of CRSToday.

CHAPTER 62

Capsular Tension Rings Versus Capsule Retractors

DAVID F. CHANG, MD

Loose zonules complicate every step of the cataract procedure.[1-3] Eye conditions associated with weak zonules include pseudoexfoliation, advanced age, trauma, retinopathy of prematurity, and prior intraocular surgery (particularly vitrectomies and trabeculectomies). During nuclear emulsification, poor stability of the capsular bag heightens the risk of capsular rupture. Also, sculpting or rotating the nucleus too forcefully may shear the zonules in the oppositely located quadrants. Fortunately, the intraoperative use of devices such as capsular tension rings (CTRs) and capsule retractors can stabilize the capsular bag during phacoemulsification.

CTRs

Deficient centrifugal zonular tension permits excessive trampolining of the flaccid posterior capsule, either during removal of the last nuclear fragment or during epinuclear and cortical cleanup. The surgeon may accidentally aspirate redundant folds of a lax posterior capsule during I/A or snag them with a capsule polisher. Because the nuclear bulk will mask this situation initially, surgeons must remain vigilant as more nucleus is removed. With the FDA's approval of the Morcher GmbH (Stuttgart, Germany) CTR, United Sates surgeons now have an important new strategy at their disposal for operating in the presence of loose zonules. For preventing capsular rupture during phacoemulsification, the questions now are whether to use the CTR in conjunction with other devices and techniques, and at what point in the procedure to insert it.

PMMA CTRs (Morcher GmbH and OPHTEC BV, Groningen, the Netherlands) partially compensate for a weakened zonular apparatus in several ways.[4-10] Using forceps or a specially designed injector (such as those made by Geuder, AG, Heidelberg, Germany; and OPHTEC BV), a surgeon can insert the ring at any point following completion of the capsulorhexis. In the presence of a focal zonular dehiscence or weakness, the ring redistributes capsular forces to areas of stronger zonular support. However, uniform weakness throughout the entire circumference of the zonular ring will partially negate this advantage.

Another benefit of the CTR is that the centrifugal pressure it applies makes the flaccid capsular bag more taut. This effect reduces redundant capsular folds, forward trampolining of the posterior capsule, and inward collapsing of the capsular fornices toward the aspirating instrument's tip. In the absence of a CTR, the stiff PMMA haptics of a three-piece foldable IOL can provide some of the same benefits during cortical aspiration. In addition, the IOL optic can block a floppy posterior capsule from vaulting toward the I/A tip in the subincisional area.

The final benefit of a CTR becomes evident postoperatively, as the permanently implanted ring counters progressive contractile forces. Centrifugal zonular tension normally resists capsulorhexis shrinkage as the capsular bag contracts. Thus, severe capsulophimosis is always the result of deficient zonular countertraction (although deficient countertraction does not always cause capsulophimosis). Extreme capsular contracture can decenter the IOL and further weaken the remaining zonules.[11] This is likely a factor in pseudoexfoliation cases in which the entire capsular bag dislocates years following the initial surgery.[12,13] There is some evidence that CTRs may also retard posterior capsule opacification by mechanically blocking lens epithelial cell migration.[14]

There are two potential drawbacks to using CTRs. First, if the posterior capsule ruptures, then retrieving the ring may become impossible because it will no longer be safely confined to the bag. Therefore, CTRs should never be inserted if the capsulorhexis or posterior capsule is torn. Second, the CTR traps cortex in the capsular fornix and impedes I/A. For this reason, surgeons should instead consider using capsule retractors to stabilize the bag during phacoemulsification. This approach may allow the surgeon to delay CTR insertion until after cortex removal.

CAPSULE RETRACTORS

In addition to enlarging a small pupil, flexible iris retractors can also be used to support the capsular bag in the presence of extremely loose zonules. John Merriam, MD, of New York first described using these self-retaining retractors through paracentesis openings to hook and fixate the capsulorhexis.[15,16] However, because their hooked ends are short and flexible, iris retractors tend to slip off fairly easily.

Richard Mackool, MD, of Astoria, New York, has designed titanium capsule retractors with hooked ends, which are elongated enough to support the peripheral capsular fornix as well as the capsulorhexis (Figures 1 and 2).[17] In this way, the retractors function like artificial zonules to stabilize the entire bag during phacoemulsification and cortical cleanup. Unlike CTRs, the capsule retractors provide excellent support in the anterior-posterior direction and do not trap the cortex (each retractor applies only point pressure to the capsular fornix without ensnaring the cortex). Called the *capsule support system*, these hooks are available in a reusable (Duckworth and Kent Ltd., Hertfordshire, England) or a single-use design (Impex, Staten Island, NY).

Capsular dye can facilitate proper placement of the retractors. They may be inserted at any surgical stage, including midway through the capsulorhexis step. They stabilize the capsular bag against rotational forces and thereby can aid the completion of the capsulorhexis, hydrodissection, and nuclear rotation. The self-retaining titanium retractors are also strong enough to center and immobilize a capsular bag that is subluxated due to a severe zonular dialysis. As a single strategy for severe zonular deficiency, I believe that capsule retractors are more effective than CTRs at

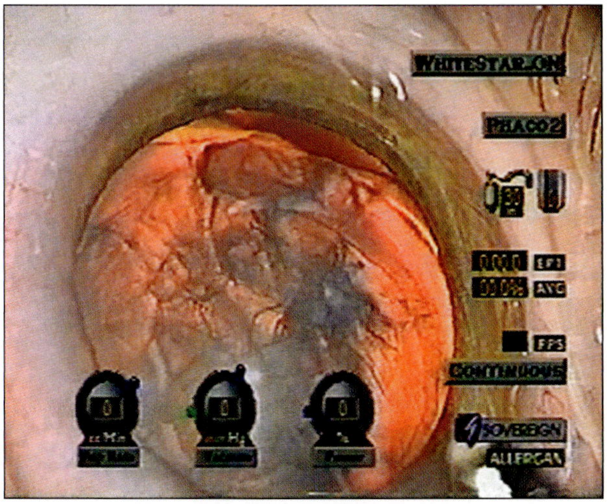

Figure 1. A nasal zonular defect is shown.

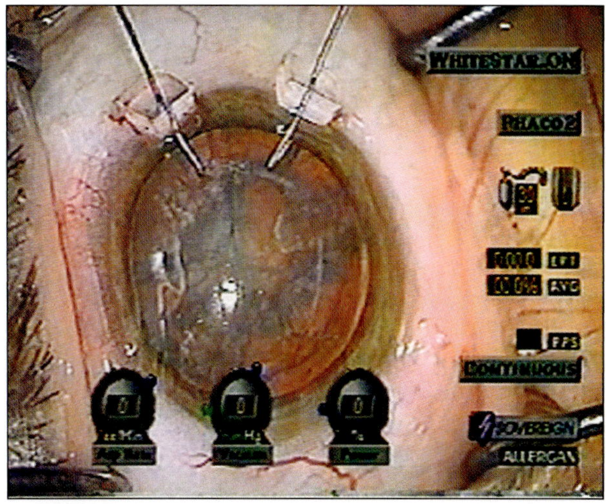

Figure 2. Two Mackool capsule retractors support the nasal quadrant and recenter the bag.

preventing posterior capsular rupture. Because CTRs can only redistribute capsular forces to the remaining intact zonules, the larger the zonular defect is, the less stability CTRs can provide.

Although the tip of the retractor is dull, it is possible for the hooks to tear the capsulorhexis margin during surgery. This is another reason to delay CTR insertion, if possible. Finally, capsule retractors do not solve the problem of permanent capsular bag support for the IOL, and this is when the CTR or the Cionni Modified Tension Ring (Morcher GmbH) is advantageous.[18-20] Ike Ahmed, MD, of Toronto has designed the capsular tension segment (CTS; Morcher GmbH) that merges the concept of a Cionni ring and a capsule retractor. The Ahmed CTS is a partial ring with a hole for temporary or permanent fixation. By hooking this hole, a single iris retractor can support the segment during surgery. Lacking a pointed tip, these broad, segmental retractors will not tear the capsulorhexis during surgery. Postoperatively, the surgeon may either remove them or suture them to the sclera for permanent support.

In conclusion, CTRs provide numerous benefits to surgeons managing challenging cataracts with weakened zonules. However, physicians should consider using capsule retractors to stabilize the capsular bag during surgery in order to delay CTR insertion until after the cortex has been removed. ■

This article originally appeared in the January 2004 issue of CRSToday.

1. Osher RH, Cionni RJ, Gimbel HV, Crandall AS. Cataract surgery in patients with pseudoexfoliation syndrome. *Eur J Implant Ref Surg.* 1993;5:46-50.
2. Fine IH, Hoffman RS. Phacoemulsification in the presence of pseudoexfoliation: challenges and options. *J Cataract Refract Surg.* 1997;23:160-165.
3. Shingleton BJ, Heltzer J, O'Donoghue MW. Outcomes of phacoemulsification in patients with and without pseudoexfoliation syndrome. *J Cataract Refract Surg.* 2003;29:1080-1086.
4. Witschel BM, Legler U. New approaches to zonular cases; the capsular ring. *Audiovisual J Cataract Implant Surg.* 1993;9(4).
5. Nagamato T, Bissen-Miyajima H. A ring to support the capsular bag after continuous curvilinear capsulorhexis. *J Cataract Refract Surg.* 1994;20:417-420.
6. Cionni RJ, Osher RH. Endocapsular ring approach to the subluxed cataractous lens. *J Cataract Refract Surg.* 1995;21:245-249.
7. Gimbel HV, Sun R, Heston JP. Management of zonular dialysis in phacoemulsification and IOL implantation using the capsular tension ring. *Ophthalmic Surg Lasers.* 1997;28:273-281.
8. Masket S, ed. Consultation Section. *J Cataract Refract Surg.* 1998;24:1289-1298.
9. Menapace R, Findl O, Georgopoulos M, et al. The capsular tension ring: designs, applications, and techniques. *J Cataract Refract Surg.* 2000;26:898-912.
10. Gimbel HV, Sun R. Clinical applications of capsular tension rings in cataract surgery. *Ophthalmic Surg Lasers.* 2002;33:44-53.
11. Davison JA. Capsule contraction syndrome. *J Cataract Refract Surg.* 1993;19:582-589.
12. Jahan FS, Mamalis N, Crandall AS. Spontaneous late dislocation of intraocular lens within the capsular bag in pseudoexfoliation patients. *Ophthalmology.* 2001;108:1727-1731.
13. Chang DF. Prevention of bag-fixated IOL dislocation in pseudoexfoliation (letter). *Ophthalmology.* 2002;109:5-6.
14. D'Eliseo D, Pastena B, Longanesi L, et al. Prevention of posterior capsule opacification using capsular tension ring for zonular defects in cataract surgery. *Eur J Ophthalmol.* 2003;13:151-154.
15. Merriam JC, Zheng L. Iris hooks for phacoemulsification of the subluxated lens. *J Cataract Refract Surg.* 1997;23:1295-1297.
16. Lee V, Bloom P. Microhook capsule stabilization for phacoemulsification in eyes with pseudoexfoliation-syndrome-induced lens instability. *J Cataract Refract Surg.* 1999;25:1567-1570.
17. Mackool RJ. Capsule stabilization for phacoemulsification (letter). *J Cataract Refract Surg.* 2000;26:629.
18. Cionni RJ, Osher RH. Management of profound zonular dialysis for weakness with a new endocapsular ring designed for scleral fixation. *J Cataract Refract Surg.*1998;24:1299-1306.
19. Ahmed IK, Crandall AS. Ab externo scleral fixation of Cionni modified capsular tension ring. *J Cataract Refract Surg.* 2001;97:977-981.
20. Cionni RJ, Osher RH, Marques DM, et al. Modified capsular tension ring for patients with congenital loss of zonular support. *J Cataract Refract Surg.* 2003;29:1668-1673.

PREFERRED PHACO TECHNIQUE

Phaco chop significantly reduces the stress that nuclear emulsification places on the zonules and capsule by replacing sculpting and cracking motions with the manual forces of one instrument pushing inward against the other. Because horizontal chopping is particularly effective at avoiding nuclear tilt or displacement, it is my preferred emulsification technique in cases of weak zonules.[1]

1. Chang D. Converting to phaco chop: Why? Which technique? How? *Ophthalmic Practice.* 1999;17:4:202-210.

CHAPTER 63

Does PXF Necessitate a CTR?

ROBERT H. OSHER, MD; I. HOWARD FINE, MD; ROGER F. STEINERT, MD; AND SAMUEL MASKET, MD

There remains a controversy among leading surgeons with respect to the indications for the capsular tension ring (CTR) in the patient with pseudoexfoliation (PXF) undergoing cataract surgery. Although some recommend that every PXF patient have a CTR, others believe that a ring should be inserted only when there is clear evidence of zonular weakness. I am in the latter group for several reasons.

First, the primary defect in PXF is located within the zonules. A ring within the capsular bag just does not seem likely to arrest progressive zonular damage. Advocates of the CTR state that its resistance to contracture of the bag decreases the chance of zonulysis. They add that the device may also make repositioning a dislocated IOL/bag complex easier, which may be true. The facts, however, are that we have operated on many thousands of PXF patients and that IOL/bag dislocation is extremely rare. Is it worth the extra time, effort, and cost to treat all for the sake of a few? While we endorse this prophylactic approach for endophthalmitis, there is an enormous difference in the degree of devastation to the eye when comparing a subluxated IOL to infection.

Moreover, there is a slight downside to implanting the CTR. Brian Little, MD, and colleagues in Sidcup, United Kingdom, have published a case of a CTR inadvertently placed in the anterior chamber.[1] Ricardo Gliken, MD, of Argentina has published on a capsular break during the CTR's insertion.[2] Moreover, Iqbal Ike Ahmed, MD, of Toronto and colleagues have demonstrated the stress on the remaining zonules that can occur during the ring's insertion,[3] which is why the capsular bag must be fully inflated with viscoelastic to facilitate the CTR's safe advancement. A famous European surgeon, who shall remain nameless, told me that he has dehisced the remaining zonules during the CTR's insertion. The complication resulted in the loss of the entire capsular bag. In addition, Lisa Brothers Arbisser, MD, of Davenport, Iowa, has presented a case in which the ring fractured during insertion.[4] Furthermore, the mere presence of a CTR makes cortical removal a bit more difficult.

Certainly, every OR should have a stock of CTRs, because the devices can truly save the day when the surgeon encounters zonular dialysis. The question of implanting a CTR in every PXF eye warrants further discussion, however, and I have invited three of my esteemed colleagues to share their perspectives.

—Robert H. Osher, MD

I. HOWARD FINE, MD

I believe that a CTR should be standard in every patient with PXF. When placed prior to phacoemulsification, but immediately following the capsulorhexis and gentle cortical cleaving hydrodissection, the presence of the ring helps to stabilize the lens during the phaco procedure itself. It also delays capsular phimosis by countering the narrowing forces in the postoperative period.

The biggest advantage of having a CTR in the bag is that it may delay the decentration of the bag/ring/IOL complex as a result of the progressive deterioration of the zonular apparatus. If decentration occurs, one may suture the CTR to the ciliary sulcus to recenter the IOL complex more easily than suturing the haptics to the ciliary sulcus. The technique is noninvasive and atraumatic, and the surgeon may perform the procedure while the IOL is within the capsular bag, whether or not there is a posterior capsulotomy.

ROGER F. STEINERT, MD

Logically, a CTR will reduce the risk of long-term subluxation of the IOL/bag complex in PXF pseudophakia if part of the pathophysiology is progressive contracture of the capsulorhexis. We do indeed see shrinkage of the anterior capsule in cases of late dislocation. We do not know, however, whether this contracture is a cause of progressive zonular loss or only a secondary manifestation of that loss. It is a classic chicken-versus-egg question, and no one knows the answer. Additionally, a CTR is not necessarily benign in asymptomatic, uncomplicated, PXF cataract surgery, because it adds weight to the IOL/bag complex.

The bottom line is that only a long-term, prospective, randomized study can fully elucidate the issue. The other important unknown is natural history. No one knows the rate of late subluxation in uncomplicated surgery. Even if a CTR prevents late subluxation, what rate of this phenomenon justifies the expense and surgical complexity of using the device in every case—1:1,000, 1:100, 1:10?

SAMUEL MASKET, MD

Unfortunately, one cannot rely upon the established literature to help answer whether all cases with PXF syndrome should have a CTR placed at the time of otherwise routine cataract surgery. What is apparent, however, is that a traditional CTR will not reduce the chances for anterior capsular contraction following surgery in most cases of PXF. What, then, would be an advantage? One might speculate that a CTR, if previously placed, would allow the IOL/bag/CTR complex to be easily affixed to the sclera by "lasso" sutures of the ring to the eye wall. Although I have used that technique for a given case, my overall sense is that the number of eyes that would benefit from that maneuver is likely to be low. Moreover, there is no literature available to let us know the rates of complications from inserting CTRs for prophylactic purposes. All in all, I do not consider the costs and risks versus the potential benefits as supporting the routine use of CTRs in all eyes undergoing cataract surgery in the presence of PXF. ■

This article originally appeared in the September 2006 issue of CRSToday.

1. Little BC, Richardson T, Morris S. Removal of a capsular tension ring from the anterior chamber angle. *J Cataract Refract Surg.* 2004;30:1832-1834.
2. Gliken R. *Video Journal of Cataract and Refractive Surgery.* 2001;17(1).
3. Ahmed II, Cionni RJ, Kranemann C, Crandall AS. Optimal timing of capsular tension ring implantation: Miyake-Apple video analysis. *J Cataract Refract Surg.* 2005;31:1809-1813.
4. Arbisser LB. CTR pitfalls. Video presented at: The AAO Annual Meeting; October 17, 2005; Chicago, IL.

CHAPTER 64

The Modified CTR

ROBERT J. CIONNI, MD

The Modified Capsular Tension Ring (CTR; Morcher GmbH, Stuttgart, Germany; distributed in the United Sates by FCI Ophthalmics, Inc., Marshfield Hills, MA) is much like a standard CTR except for the fixation hook attached to the PMMA ring filament. As the device lies inside the capsular bag, this hook rests at a plane anterior to that of the ring so that the hook courses around the capsulorhexis' edge. Passing a suture through an eyelet located at the edge of the fixation hook fixes the ring to the scleral wall.

The Modified CTR is indicated when a standard CTR will not provide sufficient stability to allow phacoemulsification and/or the long-term stability and centration of an IOL implant in the bag. Specifically, the device is appropriate in eyes with more than 180° of zonular dialysis and in cases of marked lens decentration (eg, from trauma or Marfan's syndrome). My advice for success with the Modified CTR follows.

TIMING

The Modified CTR may be placed into the capsular bag at any time after the creation of a continuous, anterior, curvilinear capsulorhexis. As with a standard CTR, the modified device is not appropriate if the capsulorhexis is not intact—for instance, due to a peripheral extension or capsular tear—because the expansile force of the ring can tear the bag further.

Trying to place the Modified CTR before removing the nucleus is challenging, although I have done so many times. The bulk of the nucleus makes it difficult to place the ring without stressing the residual zonules, and the debris in the capsular bag compromises visualization. My advice to surgeons unfamiliar with the device is not to place it until after removing the nucleus.

To stabilize the capsular bag after the capsulorhexis, I recommend grabbing the capsulorhexis' edge with a disposable nylon iris retractor much as one would catch iris tissue to expand a small pupil. This technique will hold the bag still for phacoemulsification.

INSERTING THE RING

After nuclear removal, I like to create a space for the Modified CTR by viscodissecting all of the cortex away from the periphery of the capsular bag. I prefer a dispersive viscoelastic for this maneuver, because some of the agent can ooze from the incision versus the expulsion of a cohesive glob. Before I place the ring in the bag, I preload the fixation hook's eyelet with a suture. I would recommend 9–0 Prolene (Ethicon Inc., Somerville, NJ) or 8–0 Gore-Tex (W.L. Gore & Associates, Inc., Newark, DE).

The Modified CTR is available in three versions. Model 1-L (Figure 1) must be inserted manually, so I use a tying forceps to feed the device into the bag so that the part closest to the fixation hook goes in last. During the insertion of the ring, the fixation hook should catch naturally anterior to the capsulorhexis' edge. If not, the surgeon must manipulate it anteriorly.

The model 2-C is a mirror image of the 1-L, so it may be inserted with an injector (Geuder AG, Heidelberg, Germany; distributed in the United Sates by FCI Ophthalmics, Inc.). I feed the Modified

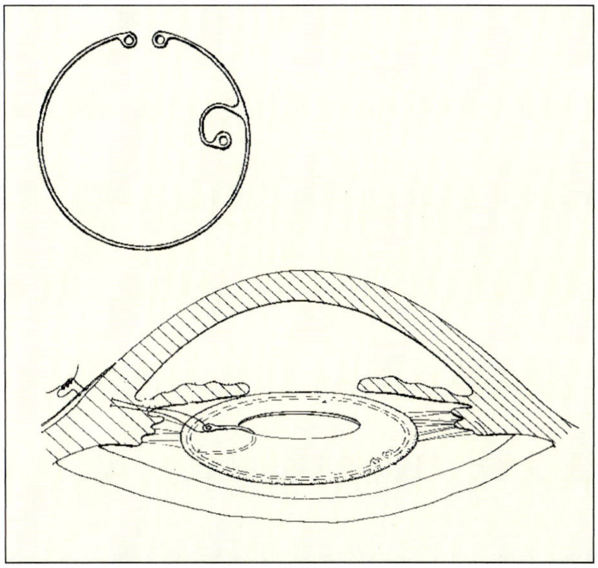

(Courtesy of Morcher GmbH.)

Figure 1. This diagram depicts model 1-L of the Modified CTR and its placement within the capsular bag.

CTR into the injector just up to the point of the fixation hook and then place the shooter through the incision.

The 2-L model has two fixation hooks and is indicated for extremely loose lenses. This is the most difficult version of the Modified CTR to use. I would recommend that surgeons first become familiar with suturing a one-hook model in a few less difficult cases before attempting to use the 2-L.

ORIENTING AND SECURING THE RING

With the Modified CTR in the bag, the next step is to dial the device so that the fixation hook is at the central part of the zonular dialysis. I then use a Sinskey or Y hook to push the device over to the scleral wall in order to determine where the ring should be sutured to center the bag well. I perform a conjunctival peritomy and make a partial-thickness scleral flap at that site.

Next, the needles are passed behind the posterior surface of the iris and in front of the anterior capsule so that they come out through the ciliary body and scleral wall, underneath the scleral flap. I tie them just tightly enough to ensure centration. It is somewhat difficult to bury the knot, which is why I place it under a scleral flap.

Right before placing the IOL, I will inject a cohesive viscoelastic.

CONCLUSION

The availability of the CTR and now the Modified CTR has greatly enhanced cataract surgeons' ability to manage challenging cases. Videos demonstrating the use of the Modified CTR may be found at the AAO's Web site as well as at http://www.fci-ophthalmics.com/videos/cionni_ctr_video.htm. ■

This article originally appeared in the May 2006 issue of CRSToday.

CHAPTER 65

Severe Scleritis, Weak Zonules, and a Rock-Hard Cataract in a One-Eyed Patient

DAVID F. CHANG, MD

I always approach surgery on a complex eye by mentally rehearsing a backup plan in the event of a complication. My most challenging case ever was also my most terrifying, because I could not envision what my backup plan would be.

THE PATIENT'S HISTORY

I first saw this 61-year-old woman in 1997. She had a long history of uveitis and scleritis since the age of 12, which is when she was first diagnosed and managed by Phillips Thygeson, MD. This was complicated by severe secondary uveitic glaucoma. Her left eye underwent cataract surgery in 1984 by one of the leading phaco surgeons in the country. Unfortunately, complications had led to corneal decompensation and severe secondary glaucoma that progressed to optic atrophy and blindness despite all treatment. Her functioning right eye had undergone a successful trabeculectomy in 1977 by H. Dunbar Hoskins, Jr, MD, who, according to the patient, called hers the worst case of scleritis he had ever seen. Her IOP was well controlled in the single digits. As her right cataract became increasingly brunescent and mature, she consulted one of the country's leading phaco surgeons in 1995. His consultation letter described the "formidable anatomic obstacles" and concluded, "There is nothing to be lost by waiting, because the cataract is nearly as hard and fully developed as it will be."

The patient was referred to me by her general ophthalmologist in 1997, because, as a resident of Northern California, she wanted to have her cataract surgery performed close to home. I learned that she was a nationally syndicated writer and an accomplished author of many books who was well known in her field. Although hoping to delay surgery for as long as possible, she was struggling to read and work with 20/400 vision in her only sighted eye.

CLINICAL FINDINGS

Examining this eye with extensive scleromalacia at the slit lamp made my heart stop. The entire superior one-fourth of the cornea had thinned seemingly to the thickness of Descemet's membrane. The corneal and scleral thickness looked to be no more than 100 μm all along the superior 8 clock hours of her limbus. There was a large, thin-walled bleb inferiorly that was rather bullous and encroached onto the peripheral cornea. There was only approximately 3 mm of normal corneal thickness at the inferior-temporal limbus adjacent to the bleb. The pupil did not dilate to more than 3 mm in diameter, and it remained eccentric due to broad inferior posterior synechiae. An ultrabrunescent lens obscured any view of her fundus.

Of the two of us, I am not sure who was more scared, but it might have been me. Because of the limited limbal space, which could barely accommodate a phaco incision, I had no backup plan if there was damaged or inadequate capsular support. Converting to a large incision would be impossible if I encountered complications. The tiny 3-mm wide island of nearly normal peripheral corneal thickness would not allow me to insert an ACIOL. Furthermore, there was insufficient tissue to create a scleral flap anywhere else to suture fixate a PCIOL. Suturing both haptics of a PCIOL to the iris had not yet been described, and it would have been difficult because of her eccentric pupil. Wearing an aphakic contact lens was not an option because of the bullous, thin-walled inferior bleb.

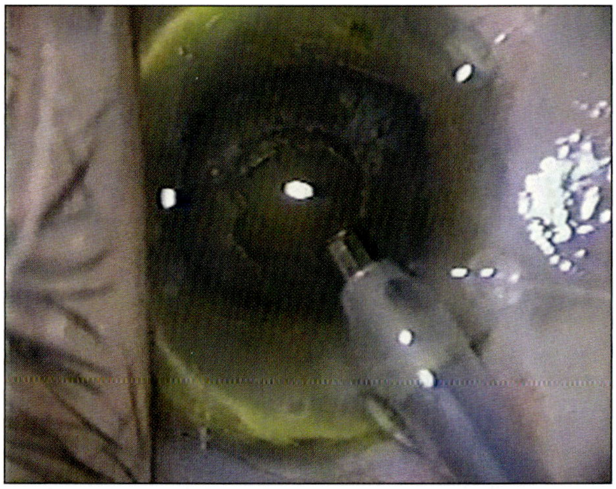

Figure 1. Surgeon's view of the patient's right eye with an inferior bleb, two inferior iris retractors, and the phaco tip placed through an inferotemporal clear corneal incision. There is no red reflex, making visualization of the capslorhexis extremely difficult. Normal corneal thickness disappears at the whitish areas that involve most of the peripheral cornea, beyond which the cornea looks to be no more than 100 μm thick.

There were other potential nightmarish scenarios that I could envision. I knew that a penetrating keratoplasty would be impossible if her corneal endothelium decompensated, and I doubted that a pars plana vitrectomy/lensectomy could be performed in the event that any lens fragments dropped posteriorly. I wondered how I would close the eye if there were any thermal damage to the phaco incision. I was not even sure I could close a sideport incision because of the severe peripheral scleral/corneal thinning.

After we discussed the many risks, I was somewhat relieved when she elected to postpone surgery until she could no longer read with low-vision aids. She returned 12 months later and again 6 months after that before she finally decided to proceed with

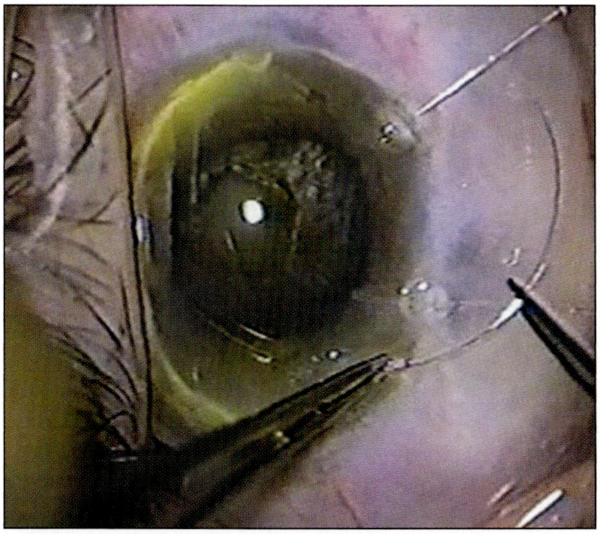

Figure 2. A capsular tension ring (CTR) is manually inserted without an injector. The inability to see the margin of the capsulorhexis makes it difficult to tell whether the CTR is entering the capsular bag. Note the position of the sculpted area showing that the insertion of the CTR is decentering the entire loose lens complex superiorly.

cataract surgery. I had this case on my mind for the ensuing 4 weeks leading up to the date of her surgery in October 1998. Other than a prayer, my only backup plan was to give her aphakic spectacles if the posterior capsule ruptured, and I explained this to her in advance.

SURGERY

Her referring ophthalmologist came to observe her surgery, and she appreciated the moral support. Assuming the posterior sclera to be equally thin as the anterior sclera, I used topical anesthesia to avoid the risks of a retro- or peribulbar injection. I made the 2.6-mm clear corneal incision in the only place possible before encountering the first major problem. Despite lysing the posterior synechiae, inserting two iris retractors inferiorly, and maximizing the microscope's illumination and zoom, I simply could not get enough of a red reflex to see the anterior capsule (Figure 1). Capsular staining with trypan blue dye had not yet been described. The difficulty in puncturing her anterior capsule and the excessive mobility of her lens as I maneuvered the capsular flap indicated that her zonules were extremely loose. I had not expected this. After struggling along at a snail's pace, I thought that I had successfully completed a capsulorhexis, but I could not be absolutely sure.

Following hydrodissection, I was unable to rotate the bulky nucleus within the loose capsular bag. As I began to sculpt a central trough through the brunescent nucleus, I was confronted with a surprising degree of phacodonesis. Despite proceeding very slowly, I got increasingly nervous as the lens jiggled with each phaco stroke. I decided to stop to regroup and ponder my options. After becoming a subinvestigator in Morcher's expanded investigational device exemption study, I had earlier purchased a single CTR (Stuttgart, Germany) from the company to be used in an emergency. Reasoning that desperate times required desperate measures, I decided that now was the time to implant my first CTR. Doing so proved to be extremely difficult, because the pupil was small, I did not have an injector, and I really could not visualize the margins of the capsulorhexis (Figure 2). It was extremely hard to tell if the ring was even entering the bag, and I nervously released the trailing eyelet with mixed feelings of hope and trepidation.

I had heard others speak about how helpful CTRs were for eyes with abnormal zonules. To my dismay, however, there was no reduction in phacodonesis when I resumed sculpting. The idea of using capsule or iris retractors to support the bag had not yet been described, and I did not understand at the time that a CTR can only redistribute instruments' forces to areas of healthy zonules—of which this patient had none. Nevertheless, the naïve notion that the CTR was somehow going to fortify the capsular bag gave me just enough confidence to continue.

After what seemed like an eternity, I eventually succeeded in chopping and removing her nucleus. I accomplished cortical cleanup in the presence of the CTR with great difficulty. I was drenched in perspiration but elated. I filled the loose capsular bag with an ophthalmic viscosurgical device and prepared to inject a foldable IOL. To my dismay, the zonules were so lax that the entire bag bobbed posteriorly away from the approaching IOL. I doubted that I could get the IOL into such a mobile capsular bag and elected to leave it in the ciliary sulcus instead.

OUTCOME

Postoperatively, the eye displayed a large choroidal detachment that persisted for many years, as the IOP remained in single digits. The IOL was slightly decentered within the sulcus but was optically well tolerated thanks to the patient's small pupil. Her BCVA improved to 20/70, and she could happily read J3 with a simple magnifier!

LESSONS LEARNED

No. 1.

As a surgeon, it is much better to be lucky than good. For example, a CTR does not really stabilize the capsular bag intraoperatively if there are 360° of zonular deficiency. Although it probably did nothing to enhance intraoperative safety in this case as I had intended, the CTR fortuitously prevented postoperative capsular contraction with the IOL positioned in the sulcus.

No. 2

We should endeavor to master new technologies. Were I to do this case now (10 years later), I would use VisionBlue dye (DORC International BV, Zuidland, the Netherlands) and a Malyugin pupil expansion ring (MicroSurgical Technologies, Redmond, WA) to avoid the need for multiple paracenteses. Microcoaxial phaco instrumentation would have been ideal for this case, and I would certainly use hyperpulse power modulation with OZil Torsional Ultrasound (Alcon Laboratories, Inc., Fort Worth, TX) or Ellips Transversal Ultrasound (Advanced Medical Optics, Inc., Santa Ana, CA) to minimize heat and endothelial trauma from particulate turbulence.

Finally, I would use polypropylene capsule retractors (eg, Mackool Capsule Support System [FCI Ophthalmics, Inc., Marshfield Hills, MA]) once severe capsulodonesis became apparent. Then, I would implant a CTR (using an injector) in the bag after cortical cleanup to prevent postoperative capsular contraction. I prefer a 13.5-mm long STAAR AQ2010V foldable three-piece IOL (STAAR Surgical Company, Monrovia, CA) for placement in the sulcus. I would consider anchoring one haptic to the iris with a

10–0 Prolene (Ethicon Inc., Somerville, NJ) McCannel suture or suturing both haptics to the iris if the posterior capsule were ruptured. In the event of a dropped nucleus, 25-gauge vitrectomy microinstrumentation would most likely be used.

POSTSCRIPT

I saw this patient several times during her first postoperative year but only twice thereafter. During that second visit in the summer of 2007, we congratulated each other on her 9 years of good visual function and reminisced about how scared we had both been while approaching her cataract operation. Ironically and tragically, she apparently tripped and hit her head on a curb 1 month later, causing a ruptured globe with a spontaneous expulsion of the IOL and much of her iris and vitreous. Her globe was repaired, but she remained limited to counting fingers vision and became very depressed. While preparing this article, I was heartbroken to learn that she had passed away in September 2008 of a possible suicide. Her story is a tragic and sobering reminder of the grave risks we and our patients face whenever we operate on someone's only seeing eye. ■

This article originally appeared in the November 2008 issue of CRSToday.

CHAPTER 66

Combined Cataract and Glaucoma Surgery

RICHARD L. LINDSTROM, MD

A monocular patient with concurrent cataract and glaucoma and a reluctance to undergo ocular surgery not only presented a challenge; her case also led me to significantly change my practice patterns.

THE CASE

Presentation

A 71-year-old white female presented to my office with a complaint of painless, progressive visual loss in her right eye. She was unable to read in bright light with a magnifier and had abandoned driving years ago. She still lived independently, but her family was considering placing her in a nursing home.

The BCVA of her right eye was 20/200 at distance with a refraction of +3.00 +0.75 X 92 and J10 at near with a +3.00 D add. Her pupil and motility and confrontation fields were normal. The IOP in her right eye was 22 mg Hg. A slit-lamp examination revealed dense nuclear and cortical lenticular opacity. She had pseudoexfoliation, and her pupil dilated to only 5 mm. There was no phacodonesis, and gonioscopy exposed an open angle with increased pigmentation. The fundus was normal on direct and indirect ophthalmoscopy except for an enlarged cup. The view on direct ophthalmoscopy was estimated at 20/200.

The patient had a well-fit ocular prosthesis in her left eye socket. The eye had been enucleated some 10 years earlier.

Her laser interferometry visual potential was 20/30 OD. To control her IOP, the patient was taking Travatan Z (Alcon Laboratories, Inc., Fort Worth, TX) at bedtime in addition to Cosopt (Merck & Co., Inc., Whitehouse Station, NJ) and Alphagan P (Allergan, Inc., Irvine, CA) twice daily. Her past medical history was significant for a combined phacoemulsification and trabeculectomy with injections of 5-fluorouracil 10 years earlier. The procedure had been complicated by early hypotony, an inadvertent bleb leak, and, eventually, endophthalmitis that had resulted in the enucleation.

The patient had been followed for years by a skilled comprehensive ophthalmologist. She also saw a glaucoma specialist, who recommended that she undergo phacoemulsification with lens implantation combined with filtering surgery in her left eye. She steadfastly refused additional surgery due to the negative outcome in her right eye.

Surgical Options

The patient and I discussed her options. I advised her that many patients, especially those with pseudoexfoliation and a narrow angle, achieve a significant reduction in IOP simply from the removal of the cataract and placement of a PCIOL. I believed this procedure was an appropriate choice for her. After consulting with her family, she elected to undergo phacoemulsification with lens implantation under topical anesthesia.

The Procedure

After stretching the pupil with Kuglen hooks, I performed phacoemulsification using a tilt-and-tumble subcapsular technique. I injected Viscoat Plus (Alcon Laboratories, Inc.) and Amvisc Plus (Bausch & Lomb, Rochester, NY) twice during the nuclear emulsification. I removed the cortex and placed a capsular tension ring. I then positioned an aspheric lens implant in the capsular bag.

The surgery was uncomplicated, and the patient saw 20/40 1 day postoperatively with mild corneal edema, flare, and cells. Her IOP was 17 mm Hg. The patient eventually achieved 20/30 UCVA and 20/20 BCVA with a manifest refraction of -0.50 +0.25 X 95. Her IOP stabilized at a range of 15 to 18 mm Hg on Travatan Z alone at bedtime, which allowed the patient to discontinue two of her glaucoma medications.

STUDY

This case cemented in my mind that cataract surgery with the implantation of a PCIOL effectively lowers the IOP in many patients. My colleagues and I were motivated by this patient's results and many other similar experiences to study the issue further. Thomas Samuelson, MD; Brooks Poley, MD; Richard Schulze, Sr, MD; and Richard Schulze, Jr, MD; and I decided to look more carefully at the impact of cataract surgery with PCIOL implantation on IOP.

In a retrospective review of 588 patients without glaucomatous damage and another 129 with confirmed glaucoma, we found that patients with preoperative IOP between 23 and 29 mm Hg achieved a 6- to 8-mm Hg reduction in IOP on average after cataract surgery and PCIOL implantation.[1] In addition, cataract surgery with the placement of a PCIOL reduced patients' need for topical glaucoma therapy by 23% among subjects who had been taking antihypertensive medications preoperatively.

Based on the results of our review as well as our clinical experience, we now recommend cataract removal with lens implantation alone to nearly all patients who have cataract and glaucoma. We utilize a clear corneal incision, which spares the conjunctiva for future filtration or tube shunt surgery, if needed.

CONCLUSION

During the past 5 years, my use of combined phacoemulsification and trabeculectomy has fallen to nearly zero from more than 10% a decade ago. The case described herein inspired my more careful evaluation of cataract surgery alone in the glaucoma suspect and glaucoma patient. The result is a significant change in my practice pattern. I now believe that cataract surgery with PCIOL implantation may well be the best glaucoma procedure available today. ■

This article originally appeared in the November 2008 isue of CRSToday.

1. Poley BJ, Lindstrom RL, Samuelson TW. Long-term effects of phacoemulsification with intraocular lens implantation in normotensive and ocular hypertensive eyes. *J Cataract Refract Surg.* 2008;34:735-742.

CHAPTER 67

Combined Glaucoma Procedures

THOMAS W. SAMUELSON, MD

The presentation of coincident cataract and glaucoma is one of the most common clinical challenges facing the anterior segment surgeon. Although the only effective therapeutic intervention for a cataract is surgical, glaucoma may be effectively managed either medically or surgically. When you decide to perform a cataract procedure on patients with glaucoma, therefore, you must also determine whether to continue the medical management of their glaucoma or to perform combined cataract and glaucoma surgery.

Cataract surgery performed alone lowers IOP, at least transiently, in a significant percentage of cases,[1] and the decrease may be more significant than previously appreciated.[2] In addition, recent advances in the medical management of glaucoma have significantly reduced the number of combined glaucoma procedures performed. Despite these considerations, the combined glaucoma procedure remains an extremely important option for some patients, and surgeons must determine the best approach.

WHEN IS A COMBINED PROCEDURE APPROPRIATE?

Although there are exceptions, I prefer coincident cataract and glaucoma surgery in cases of visually significant cataract and

- glaucoma that is poorly controlled despite medical therapy;
- progressive glaucoma in patients who do not comply with prescribed therapy or cannot afford medications;
- progressive glaucoma in patients who are intolerant of medications;
- stable or progressive glaucoma in patients taking three or more glaucoma medications;
- stable, medically controlled glaucoma in patients who choose to reduce or eliminate their need for glaucoma medications;
- far advanced disease with a very aggressive target IOP.

In such cases, the cataract is the primary indication for surgery. That is, an individual with glaucoma has a visually significant cataract requiring surgery. You therefore must decide how to manage the glaucoma. There are also situations in which glaucoma surgery is indicated, and you must decide how to manage the patient's crystalline lens. In many instances, the decision is clear-cut. For example, an obviously cataractous lens in the setting of a planned glaucoma surgery calls for combined surgery. In general, my indications for removing the lens are more liberal in patients scheduled for planned glaucoma surgery. For example, I will remove a marginally significant cataract during a planned trabeculectomy, because I know that the lenticular opacification will likely progress following the glaucoma surgery.

TRABECULECTOMY

After deciding to proceed with combined cataract and glaucoma surgery, you must make several choices regarding management. Although phacoemulsification is clearly the procedure of choice for the lensectomy, there are several options for the surgical management of glaucoma. Each can be combined with cataract surgery.

Coincident phacoemulsification and trabeculectomy remain the gold standard for combined glaucoma procedures. Modern small-incision cataract surgery is an ideal adjunct to trabeculectomy. Debate continues over one-site, single-incision surgery versus separate sites for the trabeculectomy and cataract procedures. Most published studies suggest that one- and two-site surgeries are equally efficacious.[3] I commonly use both strategies, depending on the clinical situation. For example, I consider single-site surgery for eyes with excellent exposure and well-dilated pupils, because this approach is efficient and efficacious and it obviates the need for a corneal suture. I favor two-site surgery, however, for most of my combined procedures. This approach is advisable when exposure is more difficult or if you simply feel less comfortable with cataract surgery from a superior approach.

I also prefer two-site surgery when the pupil fails to dilate well, as with patients taking systemic alpha-1 blockers such as tamsulosin (Flomax; Boehringer Ingelheim Pharmaceuticals, Inc., Ridgefield, CT), those with exfoliation syndrome, or those who have bound-down pupils. In such cases, the clear corneal incision provides a frontal entry into the anterior chamber, and the iris is less likely to prolapse into the wound. When performing clear corneal surgery in the setting of trabeculectomy, I place a suture in the corneal wound, because I cannot be certain that the early postoperative IOP will be sufficient to seal the corneal incision.

Although the early-to-midterm results of trabeculectomy are excellent, the bleb remains vulnerable to the healing whims of the conjunctiva, which often results in late failures. The conjunctiva in its natural state is prone to scarring and contraction, ultimately leading to a failed bleb. Although antimetabolites such as mitomycin C and 5-fluorouracil greatly enhance the success of trabeculectomy, the weakened conjunctiva is more prone to late bleb leaks, hypotony, and, perhaps of greatest concern, late infection of the bleb.

BLEBLESS GLAUCOMA SURGERY

Surgery that lowers IOP independent of a filtration bleb is highly desirable. Such a procedure would eliminate much of the risk and morbidity inherent to traditional bleb-based, transscleral filtration procedures. Viscocanalostomy and nonpenetrating deep sclerectomy are based on this concept. Stegmann inspired a resurgence of interest in viscocanalostomy in the late 1990s.[4] Although his viscocanalostomy is a truly "blebless" procedure, most versions of nonpenetrating deep sclerectomy rely on the presence of a filtering bleb.

Both viscocanalostomy and nonpenetrating deep sclerectomy rely on the flow of aqueous through an exquisitely thin trabeculo-Descemet's membrane. The procedures are technically difficult to perform and, like trabeculectomy, may be prone to late scarring. Accordingly, they have not been widely adopted by surgeons. Nonetheless, nonpenetrating surgery is an acceptable, safe, and effective means of lowering IOP.[5] Procedures of this sort combine well with phacoemulsification.

TRABECULAR BYPASS DEVICES

Renewed interest in procedures involving Schlemm's canal has paved the way for novel, more technologically sophisticated devices that bypass the trabecular meshwork and facilitate the flow of aqueous directly into the canal itself. These stents and shunts are investigational devices that represent the most recent efforts toward blebless glaucoma surgery. Such procedures are based on the premise that the pathology in the physiological outflow system is in the juxtacanalicular portion of the meshwork or within the inner wall itself. By bypassing the proximal trabecular meshwork, these procedures facilitate the flow of aqueous into Schlemm's canal by shunting (Eyepass Glaucoma Implant; GMP Companies, Inc., Fort Lauderdale, FL) or stenting the canal itself (iStent; Glaukos Corp., Laguna Hills, CA).

Another method that is increasingly employed to enhance flow directly into Schlemm's canal is an internal filtration surgery or ab interno trabeculectomy, which uses a device that ablates and aspirates the trabecular meshwork and the inner wall of Schlemm's canal using micro-cautery (Trabectome; NeoMedix Corporation, Tustin, CA). Performed through a clear corneal incision, the procedure combines easily with phacoemulsification.

Other devices such as the Solx Gold Micro-Shunt (not available in the US; Solx, Inc., Waltham, MA) divert aqueous into the suprachoroidal space. During excimer laser trabeculotomy, the excimer laser ablates trabecular tissue to promote the direct communication of aqueous into Schlemm's canal. Although currently investigational, such procedures can be performed at the time of cataract surgery, and they may play an increasingly important role in this setting.

PHYSIOLOGICAL OUTFLOW AND POTENTIAL PITFALLS

The decision to proceed with trabeculectomy or another procedure that completely bypasses the physiological outflow system should not be made lightly. In general, once you choose to bypass the natural outflow system, there is no going back. In all likelihood, such procedures are detrimental to physiological outflow due to underperfusion of the system. For mild or moderate glaucoma, I therefore either perform cataract extraction alone or choose a procedure to enhance conventional outflow. If such a procedure fails, I can then perform a more complete bypass such as trabeculectomy.

Although the concept of bypassing the trabecular meshwork is intriguing and promising, much work remains to be done. Some investigators have expressed concern over the lack of circumferential flow within Schlemm's canal. That is, even if a stent or shunt successfully bypasses the trabecular meshwork, it is generally accepted that the enhanced outflow may be limited to several clock hours surrounding the bypass or perhaps to a single quadrant. As a result, multiple stents or shunts may be needed to lower the IOP adequately. Alternatively, the circumferential flow may be enhanced by microcannulation of the canal with newly developed, investigational techniques such as 360° viscocannulation (iTrack microcatheter; iScience Interventional, Menlo Park, CA). Canaloplasty is gaining acceptance as a viable procedure to lower IOP without the creation of a filtering bleb. Midterm data were recently reported on canaloplasty as a stand-alone procedure and as an adjunct to cataract surgery.[6,7]

ENDOSCOPIC CYCLOPHOTOCOAGULATION

Endoscopic cyclophotocoagulation is another option for the coincident management of cataract and glaucoma. The procedure utilizes a clear corneal incision and is tailor made as an adjunct to cataract surgery, because access to the ciliary processes is greatly enhanced in pseudophakic eyes. Although a prospective randomized trial is not available, the technique has become popular for the management of early, less complex glaucoma as a way of reducing the burden of medical therapy. Although I prefer to lower IOP by enhancing outflow, there may be a role for endoscopic cyclophotocoagulation in the reduction of pressure in select patients.

SUMMARY

The field of glaucoma is in a period of transition, and the surgical options for the simultaneous presentation of cataract and glaucoma continue to evolve and improve. Individualize your decisions on management to the patient and your skill set in order to maximize outcomes and minimize risk. ■

This article originally appeared in the July 2008 issue of CRSToday.

1. Mathalone N, Hyamus M, Neiman S, et al. Long-term intraocular pressure control after clear corneal phacoemulsification in glaucoma patients. *J Cataract Refract Surg.* 2005;31:479-483.
2. Poley BJ, Lindstrom RL, Samuelson TW. Long-term effects of phacoemulsification with intraocular lens implantation in normotensive and ocular hypertensive eyes. *J Cataract Refract Surg.* 2008;34:735-742.
3. Shingleton BJ, Price RS, O'Donoghue MW, Goyal S. Comparison of 1-site versus 2-site phacotrabeculectomy. *J Cataract Refract Surg.* 2006;32:799-802.
4. Stegmann R, Pienaar A, Miller D. Viscocanalostomy for open-angle glaucoma in black African patients. *J Cataract Refract Surg.* 1999;25:316-322.
5. Shaarawy T, Mansouri K, Schnyder C, et al. Long-term results of deep sclerectomy with collagen implant. *J Cataract Refract Surg.* 2004;30:1225-1231.
6. Lewis RA, von Wolff K, Tetz M, et al. Canaloplasty: circumferential viscodilation and tensioning of Schlemm's canal using a flexible microcatheter for the treatment of open-angle glaucoma. Interim clinical study analysis. *J Cataract Refract Surg.* 2007;33:1217-1226.
7. Shingleton B, Tetz M, Korber N. Circumferential viscodilation and tensioning of Schlemm's canal (canaloplasty) with temporal clear corneal phacoemulsification cataract surgery for open-angle glaucoma and visually significant cataract. One year results. *J Cataract Refract Surg.* 2008;34:433-440.

CHAPTER 68

Combined Procedures

BRADFORD J. SHINGLETON, MD

Cataract and glaucoma commonly coexist and present special problems for the ophthalmologist. The risks and rate of complications of cataract surgery are greater in glaucomatous than nonglaucomatous eyes due to miotic pupils, posterior synechiae, peripheral anterior synechiae, the presence of preexisting blebs, and pseudoexfoliation. The lack of consensus as to the best surgical approaches for coexisting cataract and glaucoma is therefore not surprising. Should ophthalmologists perform combined cataract and glaucoma surgery or separate the procedures? If the latter, should phacoemulsification precede glaucoma surgery, or vice versa? If combined surgery is a superior option, is one site or two preferable?

The development of nonfiltering surgeries for IOP control increases the number of glaucoma procedures that can be performed in tandem with cataract surgery. The timing and long-term outcomes of cataract surgery in the setting of glaucoma also remain controversial. This article assesses the benefits and drawbacks of combined cataract and glaucoma surgery, its indications, and its performance.

PROS AND CONS

Among its advantages, combined cataract and glaucoma surgery involves a single trip to the OR and restores patients' vision relatively promptly compared with separate procedures. Compared with cataract surgery alone, patients often require fewer glaucoma medications after combined surgery, and early and long-term postoperative IOP control is often better.[1] In addition, surgeons can administer antimetabolites to enhance the probability of lower IOP postoperatively. Finally, removing the cataract facilitates their assessment of the optic nerve and visual fields.

Unfortunately, combined surgery is associated with more postoperative complications than cataract surgery alone. The problems of a shallow anterior chamber, bleb leak, choroidal effusion and/or hemorrhage, hypotony, infection, dellen, and astigmatism can all be more serious as well. Compared with cataract surgery alone, a combined procedure is more time consuming and is associated with more intense requirements for postoperative care.

INDICATIONS

There are no rigid standards for when combined cataract surgery should be performed, and one cannot be dogmatic about the indications for this approach. Because combined procedures result in better IOP control and reduced requirements for glaucoma medication than phacoemulsification alone, I favor a combined procedure when patients require more than two medicines for satisfactory IOP control. I am similarly inclined if their use of medication is limited by allergy or medical contraindications. I also may choose a combined procedure in young patients and those who have sustained significant glaucomatous visual field loss and cupping. In addition, I tend to prefer this approach in monocular patients or individuals with significant risk factors for glaucoma such as pseudoexfoliation, pigment dispersion, or angle recession. Lastly, combined cataract and glaucoma surgery is indicated in patients unable to tolerate two separate operations due to medical problems limiting the number of trips to the OR.

Cataract surgery alone may be appropriate for an individual whose IOP is adequately controlled and who has sustained no significant glaucomatous visual field loss or cupping. Many patients experience a small but significant reduction in IOP after clear corneal phacoemulsification.[2] A two-staged procedure, with a glaucoma operation preceding the phaco procedure, may be indicated when glaucoma is an immediate threat to vision (eg, markedly increased IOP in patients with active uveitis or neovascularization). Even in the presence of a visually significant cataract, an IOL may not be indicated in patients with high IOPs and active inflammation. The fact that the phacoemulsification performed after glaucoma surgery is often successful makes this approach a reasonable option for certain patients.

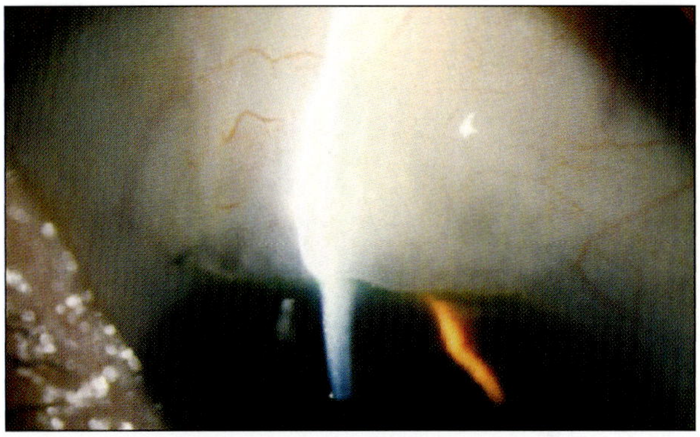

Figure 1. An excellent filtering bleb developed after separate-site combined phacotrabeculectomy.

SEPARATE SITES

Theory

Weitzman and Caprioli have argued that performing phacoemulsification and trabeculectomy at separate sites enhances the development of effective filtration[3] (Figure 1). It also permits cataract surgeons to perform phacoemulsification from a position that most find comfortable—a temporal approach.

Technique

First, the ophthalmologist performs phaco/IOL surgery. A small, clear corneal/limbal incision and foldable IOL are preferable to minimize conjunctival manipulation. I favor a single, buried, 10–0 nylon suture to facilitate early digital pressure and supplemental 5-fluorouracil (5-FU), if needed, during the early postoperative phase.

Next, the surgeon shifts to the superior axis to perform the trabeculectomy. The conjunctival flap is mobilized according to his preference, and intraoperative antimetabolites may be used. The surgeon performs his standard trabeculectomy.

Results

Via an evidence-based review, Friedman et al reported better IOP control with a combined procedure performed at separate sites versus a single one.[1] When comparing single- and two-site combined procedures, my colleagues and I found an equal reduction of IOP, degree of visual improvement, and reduction in medication.[4]

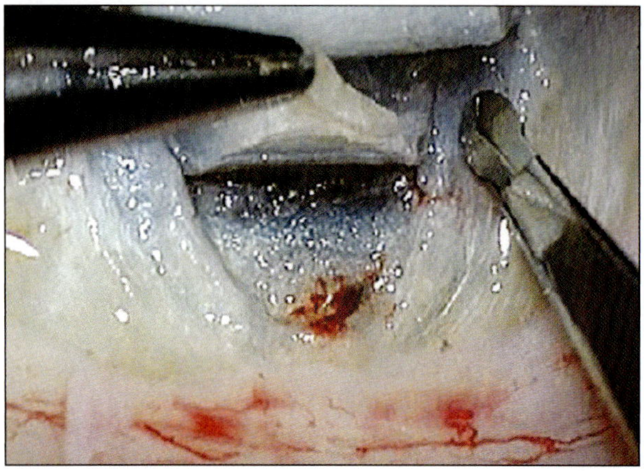

Figure 2. The surgeon mobilized the deep scleral flap to expose Schlemm's canal during combined phacoemulsification and viscocanalostomy surgery.

SINGLE SITE

Theory

A single-incision approach is simple, fast, and effective although potentially less comfortable for the temporally oriented phaco surgeon. An ophthalmologist's choice to perform a single- or separate-site procedure is a matter of preference, but, in all cases, he should make an effort to minimize the manipulation of and trauma to ocular tissue.

Technique

This procedure involves a superior approach, and I favor an inferior, limbal, 6–0 silk positioning suture to facilitate superior exposure of the limbal area. A paracentesis incision permits bimanual phacoemulsification and also enables the testing of filtration outflow at the end of the case. A conjunctival flap is mobilized via a limbus- or fornix-based approach. My colleagues and I found that both limbus- and fornix-based conjunctival flaps are effective for reducing the IOP, developing a bleb, improving vision, and reducing the number of glaucoma medications postoperatively.[5] Most importantly, with a fornix-based flap, one may anticipate more anterior bleb leaks and should closely check for them postoperatively and provide treatment as necessary.

Intraoperative antimetabolites facilitate the reduction of IOP. One may apply topical mitomycin C (0.2 to 0.5 mg/mL) or 5-FU (50 mg/mL) to reduce fibrous proliferation and scarring of the bleb postoperatively.

Scleral flaps can be mobilized in any shape, and the most important factors for IOP control are the thickness of the flap and the tightness of its closure. If I anticipate performing laser suture lysis postoperatively, I favor 10–0 nylon sutures with the knots buried. Releasable sutures are also effective for regulating and modulating aqueous outflow and the development of a bleb.[6-8]

Multiple suture needles and materials can be used for conjunctival closure. For limbus-based flaps, I favor 9–0 Vicryl (Ethicon Inc., Somerville, NJ), 10–0 BioSorb (Alcon Laboratories, Inc., Fort Worth, TX), or 10–0 nylon. Incorporating Tenon's tissue in the closure may enhance its seal. Fornix-based flaps can be closed with wing sutures, horizontal mattress sutures, or running sutures such as those described by Wise.[9] Wing sutures with denudation of the limbal corneal epithelium reduce the number of sutures in the sclerectomy area and may minimize inflammation, but they also may be associated with more leaks and anterior migration of the bleb. Running sutures utilizing a limbal remnant or the Wise closure reduce bleb leaks and the anterior migration of the bleb, but they may be associated with more inflammation because of suture material near the sclerectomy site.

It is important to test filtration and the elevation of the bleb by injecting balanced salt solution via the paracentesis at the conclusion of the procedure. Topical 2% fluorescein strips or a Weck-Cel sponge (Medtronic ENT, Jacksonville, FL) can be used to test for bleb leakage.

Results

In my hands, a single-incision combined procedure without antimetabolites produced a mean IOP reduction of approximately 5 mm Hg at 1 year and decreased the number of glaucoma medications by approximately 75%.[10] The IOP reduction has been sustained for 3 years in these patients, but their need for medication has tended to increase slightly. Intraoperative antimetabolites are associated with lower IOPs postoperatively but also with more postoperative complications. Subconjunctival 5-FU administered postoperatively can also enhance the bleb's development.

OTHER POSSIBLE COMBINATIONS

A host of other glaucoma procedures can be combined with cataract surgery. Surgeons may couple phacoemulsification and the implantation of a tube shunt such as the Ex-Press mini glaucoma shunt (Optonol Ltd., Neve Ilan, Israel), which creates an external filter. Many new shunting devices are currently under development that will permit the surgeon to perform a trabeculectomy with an internal tube shunt, silicone drainage tube, or a gold implant (Solx Gold Micro-Shunt; Solx, Inc., Waltham, MA) in the suprachoroidal space.

Alternatively, one might perform endoscopic cyclophotocoagulation (ECP) along with phacoemulsification. ECP produces modest postoperative reductions in patients' IOPs and needs for glaucoma medication.[11,12] Moreover, ECP does not appear to be associated with the significant inflammation that occasionally occurs after external cycloablative procedures.[11]

Another option is to combine a nonpenetrating deep sclerectomy procedure with cataract surgery (Figure 2). Park et al reported a reduction in IOP of 3.4 mm Hg at 1 year and 3.6 mm Hg at 3 years with viscocanalostomy and cataract surgery.[13] It would be interesting to read an evaluation of the potential combination of phacoemulsification and 360° canaloplasty with the microcannula developed by iScience Interventional (Menlo Park, CA). The device expands the dilation of Schlemm's canal beyond that normally achieved with standard viscocanalostomy and, like the latter procedure, minimizes bleb development. Techniques utilizing collagen (AquaFlow Collagen Glaucoma Drainage Device; STAAR Surgical Company, Monrovia, CA) or hyaluronic acid actually facilitate the egress of aqueous into the subconjunctival space and can be coupled with deep sclerectomy procedures to facilitate bleb development. Surgeons may use antimetabolites intraoperatively with the nonpenetrating deep sclerectomy procedures aimed at creating blebs.

European ophthalmologists have combined cataract surgery with excimer laser trabeculotomy via an *ab interno* approach, although this technology is not approved in the US. Standard trabeculotomy is another option.[14]

It is also worth noting that goniosynechiolysis can be coupled with cataract surgery and chamber-deepening procedures to open preexisting angle closure. My colleagues and I showed this approach to be effective for angle closure of up to 12 months' duration.[15] Finally, Terry described coupling phacoemulsification and holmium laser sclerostomy,[16] and Montgomery and Gills reported combining cyclodialysis with cataract surgery in 1980.[17]

SUMMARY

There have been tremendous advances in combined surgery during the past 4 decades. In the 1970s, intracapsular surgery with a filter was the most common approach, with the filtration procedure typically occurring first. In the 1980s, the trend became extracapsular procedures with simultaneous trabeculectomies. Improvements in viscoelastics and IOLs along with laser suture lysis and releasable sutures enhanced success rates. In the 1990s, phacotrabeculectomy came into its own with the use of small incisions, foldable IOLs, and antimetabolites. In the new millennium, surgeons have become more interested in separating the sites for the combined cataract and glaucoma procedure, and they have a greater appreciation for the effect of phacoemulsification alone on IOP. The use of nonpenetrating deep sclerectomy procedures, some of which avoid a bleb, has also grown extensively.

As cataract incisions shrink further, one may imagine a future in which IOLs enhance the visual field or continuously monitor IOP intracamerally, implants release glaucoma medication, antimetabolites are more effective and safer, photodynamic therapy of the conjunctiva modulates fibroblastic proliferation, and novel nonfiltering surgical procedures reduce bleb-associated problems. ■

This article originally appeared in the July 2008 issue of CRSToday.

1. Friedman DS, Jampel HD, Lubomski LH, et al. Surgical strategies for coexisting glaucoma and cataract. An evidence-based update. *Ophthalmology.* 2002;109:1902-1915.
2. Shingleton BJ, Gamell LS, O'Donoghue MW, et al. Long-term changes in intraocular pressure after clear-corneal phacoemulsification: normal patients vs. glaucoma suspect and glaucoma patients. *J Cataract Refract Surg.* 1999;25:885-890.
3. Weitzman MW, Caprioli J. Temporal corneal phacoemulsification combined with separate-incision superior trabeculectomy. *Ophthalmic Surg.* 1995;26:271-273.
4. Shingleton BJ, Price RS, O'Donoghue MW. Comparison of one-site vs. two-site phacotrabeculectomies. *J Cataract Refract Surg.* 2006;32:799-802.
5. Shingleton BJ, Chaudhry IM, O'Donoghue MW, et al. Phacotrabeculectomy: limbus-based vs. fornix-based conjunctival flaps in fellow eyes. *Ophthalmology.* 1999;106:1152-1155.
6. Johnstone MA, Wellington DP, Zil CJ. Releasable scleral-flap tamponade suture for guarded filtration surgery. *Arch Ophthalmol.* 1993;111:398-403.
7. Cohen JS, Osher RH. Releasable suture in filtering and combined surgery. *Ophthalmol Clin North Am.* 1988;1:187-197.
8. Wilson RP. Technical advances in filtration surgery. In: McAllister JA, Wilson RP, eds. *Glaucoma.* Boston: BU Healthworks; 1986:243-250.
9. Wise JB. Mitomycin-compatible suture technique for fornix-based conjunctival flaps in glaucoma filtration surgery. *Arch Ophthalmol.* 1993;11:992-997.
10. Shingleton BJ, Kalina PH. Combined phacoemulsification, intraocular lens implantation, and trabeculectomy with a modified scleral tunnel and single-stitch closure. *J Cataract Refract Surg.* 1995;21:528-532.
11. Berke SJ, Cohen AJ, Sturm RJ, et al. Endoscopic cyclophotocoagulation (ECP) and phacoemulsification in the treatment of medically-controlled open-angle glaucoma [abstract]. *J Glaucoma.* 2000;9:129.
12. Berke SJ. Phacoemulsification combined with endoscopic cyclophotocoagulation (ECP) in the management of cataract and medically controlled glaucoma: a large, long term study. Paper presented at: The AGS 16th Annual Meeting; March 4, 2006; Charleston, SC.
13. Park M, Tanito M, Mishikawa M, et al. Combined viscocanalostomy and cataract surgery compared with cataract surgery in Japanese patients with glaucoma. *J Glaucoma.* 2004;13:55-61.
14. McPherson SD. Combined trabeculotomy and cataract extraction as a single operation. *Trans Am Ophthalmol Soc.* 1976;74:251-260.
15. Shingleton, BJ, Chang MA, Bellow AR, Thomas JV. Surgical goniosynechiolysis for angle-closure glaucoma. *Ophthalmology.* 1990;97:551-556.
16. Terry S. Combined no-stitch phacoemulsification cataract extraction with foldable silicone intraocular lens implantation and holmium laser sclerostomy followed by 5-FU injections. *Ophthalmic Surg.* 1992;23:218-219.
17. Montgomery D, Gills JP. Extracapsular cataract extraction, lens implantation and cyclodialysis. *Ophthalmic Surg.* 1980;11:343-347.

CHAPTER 69

Combined Phacoemulsification and ECP

STANLEY J. BERKE, MD

Endoscopic cyclophotocoagulation (ECP) safely and effectively lowers IOP.[1-4] This is confirmed by several new, large, long-term studies summarized in this article. Because the surgeon visualizes the ciliary processes directly and can treat them precisely using diode laser energy, the problems of ocular pain, inflammation, hypotony, and visual loss associated with transscleral forms of cycloablation do not occur. The surgeon passes the 18-gauge endolaser probe through the limbus or pars plana to treat virtually any type of glaucoma, regardless of its etiology. I have found that ECP is particularly easy and well suited to lowering IOP and reducing patients' need for glaucoma medications when combined with phacoemulsification in cases of concurrent cataract and medically controlled glaucoma.

HISTORICAL PERSPECTIVE

Using penetrating diathermy, cryotherapy, and, more recently, Nd:YAG and diode lasers, ophthalmologists have been performing transscleral cycloablation for many years. Traditionally, cycloablative procedures have been a last resort for eyes that have undergone multiple failed glaucoma procedures, such as trabeculectomies and the implantation of glaucoma drainage devices, and for eyes that are blind and painful or have very poor visual potential. The downgrade of the procedure was appropriate, because trans-scleral cycloablative procedures are unpredictable. Surgeons cannot visualize the tissue they are ablating, so over- or undertreatments are likely. The procedures are associated with many postoperative complications, including pain, inflammation, visual loss, and phthisis.

ECP is a gentler procedure in comparison to transscleral cycloablation, because surgeons can visualize the tips of the ciliary processes directly and treat them to achieve the desired effect on tissue. ECP does not cause undesirable collateral tissue damage and, therefore, does not cause the complications associated with transscleral cycloablation.[5] Surgeons can perform ECP in eyes with excellent visual potential. Because ophthalmologists can execute ECP with topical/intracameral anesthesia, it is well suited to patients who are monocular or are anticoagulated. In contrast, transscleral diode cyclophotocoagulation requires retrobulbar or peribulbar anesthesia.

PATIENT SELECTION

Surgeons may consider ECP for any patient scheduled for cataract surgery who also requires a glaucoma procedure and is a poor candidate for filtration or drainage device surgery. Two examples are patients who have scarred conjunctivae or those whose

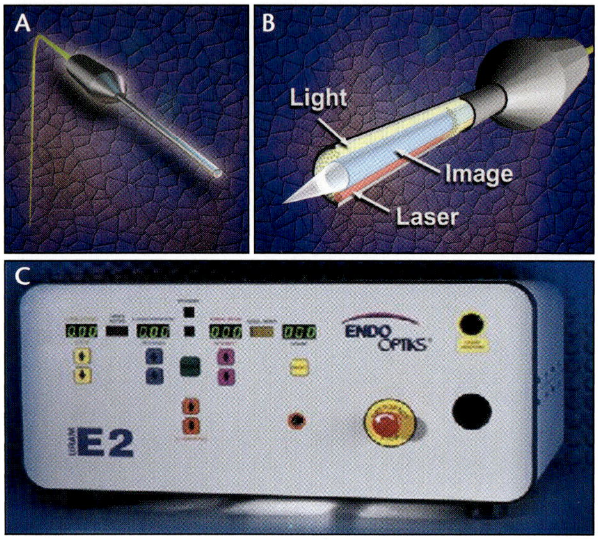

(Courtesy of Endo Optiks.)

Figure 1. Laser endoscope probe (straight) (A, B). E2 Laser and Endoscopy System (C).

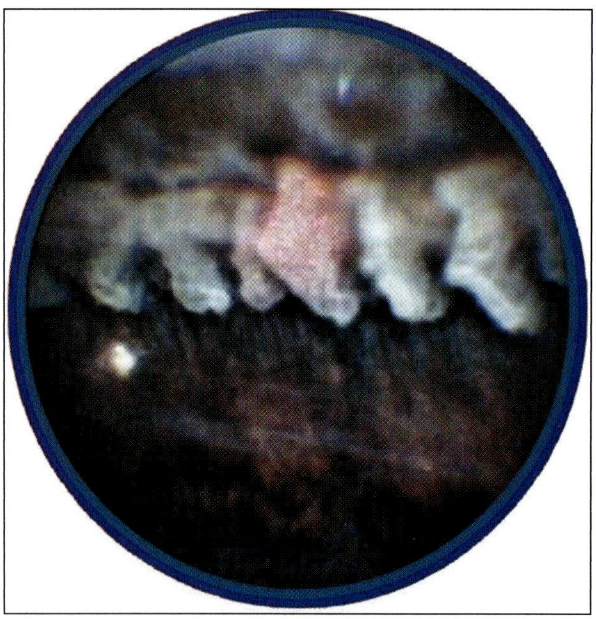

Figure 3. The treated ciliary process is shrunken and white.

contralateral eye has developed complications related to previous trabeculectomy or the bleb.[6]

ECP is preferable to filtration surgery in eyes where an ocular fistula is problematic, such as cases of elevated episcleral venous pressure, intraocular tumor, contact lens wear, or blepharitis.

ECP is much faster and easier than filtering surgery or drainage device surgery, and it involves fewer postoperative visits and additional treatments such as laser suture lysis, bleb needling, 5-fluorouracil injections, etc. ECP may therefore be a good choice for patients who are unable to make frequent postoperative visits or who are unable to cooperate for laser suture lysis, suture removal, or other manipulations of the bleb. Likewise, ECP is an alternative for patients who have had problems with glaucoma drainage devices such as extraocular muscle dysfunction, erosion of the tube or plate, or corneal decompensation.

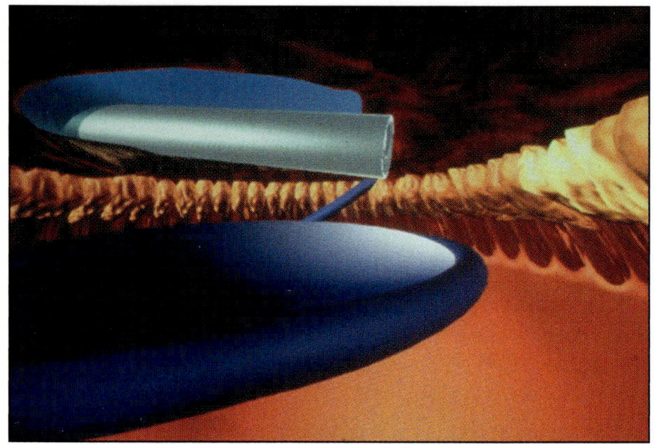

Figure 2. View from behind the iris of endolaser treatment to the ciliary processes with a PCIOL in place.

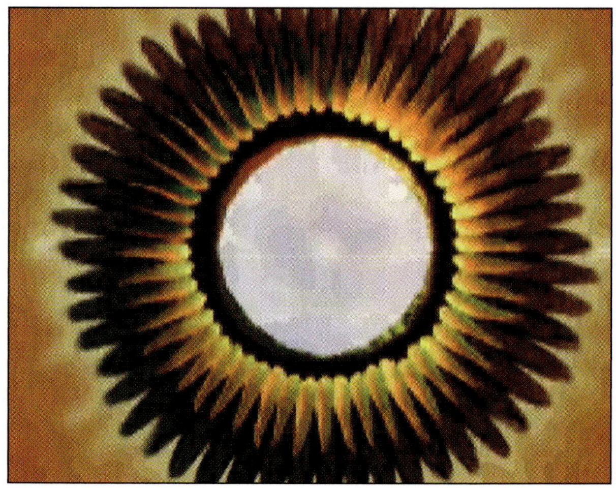

Figure 4. The area of the ECP treatment should be 200° to 360° (a 270° treatment is shown).

TECHNIQUES

The laser endoscope has three fiber groupings: the image; the light; and the laser guide. There is an 18-gauge endoprobe (Figure 1A and B) with a 110° field of view and a depth of focus ranging from 1 to 30 mm. The advantages of the laser endoscope's large diameter are the greater clarity provided by the image bundle and the panoramic field of view that it creates. This feature is especially helpful for the novice endoscopist, because the wide field of view permits simple orientation to the anatomy of the ciliary sulcus and ciliary processes.

The laser endoscope connects to the console (Figure 1C) that contains all of the instruments used for endoscopy—a video camera, monitor, and recorder as well as a light source. Surgeons use a semiconductor diode laser tuned to the 810-nm wavelength. They place the console next to the surgical table and control the progress of the procedure by viewing the video monitor rather than images through the operating microscope.

Surgeons can access the ciliary processes from an incision in the anterior segment in a phakic, pseudophakic, or aphakic eye. They may use a 1.5- to 2.0-mm incision in clear cornea or a scleral tunnel.

Surgeons perform their usual phaco procedure. They may perform ECP before or after inserting the PCIOL. Surgeons should introduce the viscoelastic over the capsular bag, posterior to the iris. This maneuver displaces the capsular bag backward and causes

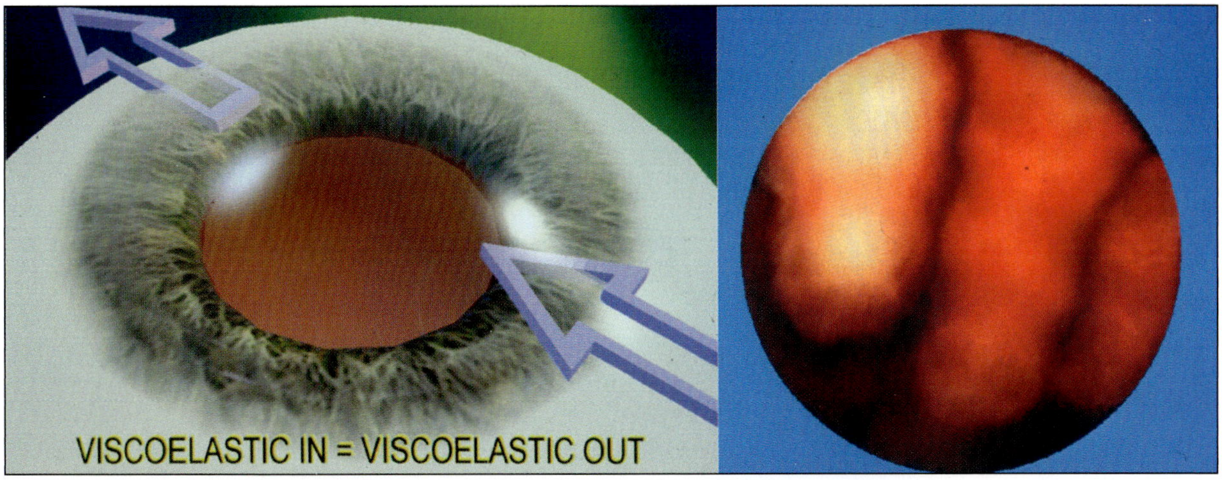

Figure 5. Surgeons should remove all viscoelastic from the eye at the end of the procedure.

the iris to move forward, which provides a clear view of the ciliary processes (Figure 2). A clear corneal incision is preferable for cobined ECP and cataract surgery, because it leaves the superior conjunctiva intact for future filtering surgery.

To me, perhaps the most outstanding quality of ECP is it allows me to deliver laser energy to the ciliary processes on demand in a highly titratable fashion, despite numerous anatomic impediments. The optimal effect on tissue when managing glaucoma is clear. The physical goals of treatment are to whiten the ciliary processes and cause visible shrinkage of the tissue (Figure 3). Surgeons should incorporate the entirety of each process into the treatment zone and, in general, treat 200° to 360° of the ciliary processes (Figure 4). They should avoid the formation of bubbles, pigmentary dispersion, audible popping, photocoagulation of nonciliary processes tissue, and the inclusion of prosthetic material in the treatment zone. At the conclusion of surgery, it is important to remove all of the sodium hyaluronate from the eye to prevent a postoperative increase in IOP (Figure 5).

MY EXPERIENCE

ECP permits visualization and photocoagulation of the ciliary processes in essentially any patient, despite the presence of corneal opacification, a miotic pupil, or previous glaucoma surgery.[1] Laser endoscopy benefits from the advantages of directly viewing the ciliary processes and photocoagulation yet avoids the complications associated with transscleral cyclodestruction.

Since 1998, my partners and I have performed more than 1,000 combined phaco/ECP procedures, primarily in patients with medically controlled glaucoma. We analyzed our first 25 consecutive cases with 1-year follow-up.[2] Treating 180° of the ciliary processes resulted in a mean decrease in IOP of 15% (from 20.2 to 17.2 mm Hg) and a 68% reduction in glaucoma medications (from 1.6 to 0.5). There was no visual loss or significant adverse sequelae postoperatively.

We recently analyzed our long-term phaco/ECP results.[3] We compared 626 consecutive eyes treated with phacoemulsification/ ECP with a similar cohort of 81 eyes that underwent phacoemulsification alone. The follow-up period ranged from 6 months to 5.5 years, with a mean follow-up time of 3.2 years. In the phaco/ ECP group, the mean IOP decreased by 3.4 mm Hg, from 19.1 to 15.7 mm Hg. In the control group, the mean IOP increased 0.7 mm Hg, from 18.2 to 18.9 mm Hg. More significantly, the number of preoperative glaucoma medications decreased from a mean of 1.53 to 0.65 at the end of the follow-up period in the phaco/ECP group but remained unchanged from a mean of 1.20 in the phaco group (Figure 6). There were no serious complications in either cohort, and the rate of cystoid macular edema (CME) was similar in both groups (less than 1%). Another study involving more than 1,000 eyes confirmed our results and showed no difference in angiographic CME between eyes that underwent phacoemulsification/ECP versus phacoemulsification alone (approximately 2% in both groups).[4]

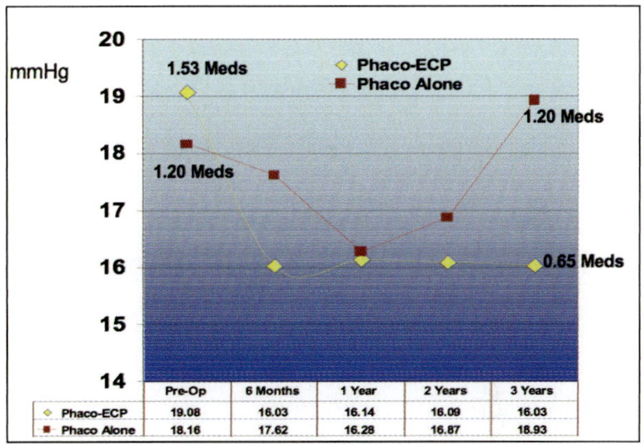

Figure 6. The long-term results of phacoemulsification/ECP.

I still perform phacoemulsification alone and combined phacoemulsification/trabeculectomy on many glaucoma patients undergoing cataract surgery. In an average month, I complete 40 cataract surgeries in which approximately 10 eyes have glaucoma. Of those, I perform phacoemulsification alone on 25%, phacoemulsification/ECP on 50%, and phacoemulsification/trabeculectomy on 25%. Although I evaluate every patient individually, my general rule of thumb is as follows.[7-9]

If a patient with a cataract has mild, well-controlled glaucoma on a single, well-tolerated glaucoma medication, I perform phacoemulsification alone and implant an IOL through a temporal clear corneal incision. This procedure preserves the superior conjunctiva in case trabeculectomy is needed in the future. If the patient has moderate glaucoma and uses two or more glaucoma medications, I perform phacoemulsification/ECP through a clear corneal incision in an effort to lower his IOP and reduce or eliminate his use of glaucoma medications. Last, if a patient has advanced glaucomatous cupping and visual field loss on maximum medical therapy (two or more medications), I perform a phacotrabeculectomy with intraoperative mitomycin C.

CONCLUSION

ECP should not be considered the same as transscleral forms of cycloablation, which are "blind" procedures that can cause a lot of collateral tissue damage and can result in an over- or undertreatment of the tips of the ciliary processes.

ECP may not be indicated for some cataract surgery patients with very mild or very advanced glaucoma. However, it is a safe and effective addition to our armamentarium to treat glaucoma patients with moderate disease on two or more medications. ■

This article originally appeared in the July 2008 issue of CRSToday.

1. Uram M. Ophthalmic laser microendoscope endophotocoagulation. *Ophthalmology.* 1992;99:1829-1832.
2. Berke SJ, Cohen AJ, Sturm RT, et al. Endoscopic cyclophotocoagulation (ECP) and phacoemulsification in the treatment of medically controlled open angle glaucoma. *J Glaucoma.* 2000;9:129.
3. Berke SJ, Sturm RT, Caronia RM, et al. Phacoemulsification combined with endoscopic cyclophotocoagulation (ECP) in the management of cataract and medically controlled glaucoma: a large, long term study. Paper presented at the AGS Annual Meeting; March 6 2006; Charleston, SC, and at the AAO Annual Meeting; November 14, 2006; Las Vegas, NV.
4. The ECP Study Group. Comparison of phaco/ECP to phaco alone in 1,000 glaucoma patients; a randomized, prospective study including fluorescein angiography in all patients in both groups. Paper presented at: The 2002 ASCRS Symposium on Cataract, IOL and Refractive Surgery; June 6, 2002; Philadelphia, PA.
5. Trevisani MG, Allingham RR, Shields MB. Histologic comparison of contact transscleral diode cyclophotocoagulation and endoscopic diode cyclophotocoagulation. *Invest Ophthalmol and Vis Sci.* 1995;36:4.
6. Berke SJ, Bellows AR, Shingleton BJ, et al. Chronic and recurrent choroidal detachment following glaucoma filtering surgery. *Ophthalmology.* 1987;94:154-162.
7. Berke SJ. How ECP compares to other procedures. *Ophthalmology Management.* http://www.ophmanagement.com/article.aspx?article=&loc=archive\2003\march\medtronic\0303medtronic4.htm. Accessed June 23, 2008.
8. Berke SJ. Cyclodestruction as a treatment for glaucoma. *American Academy of Ophthalmology Focal Points.* 2004;22:10:11-14.
9. Berke SJ. Combining ECP and cataract surgery. *Glaucoma Today.* September 2005;3:5:27-28.

CHAPTER 70

Prostaglandin Analogs and Cataract Surgery

ANURAG SHRIVASTAVA, MD, AND KULDEV SINGH, MD, MPH

Given the high prevalence of ocular hypertension and glaucoma in patients undergoing cataract extraction, all cataract surgeons face the question of whether it is safe to use prostaglandin analogs during the perioperative period. The primary concern about this class of drugs in these patients is the possible association between their use and cystoid macular edema (CME). The variability of criteria for defining significant CME[1] along with a lack of understanding as to what causes the condition in some patients but not others makes it difficult to establish a causal association with putative risk factors. This article assesses and summarizes the literature pertaining to such causality and shares our recommendations on how to approach the patient requiring cataract surgery who is receiving prostaglandin therapy.

CASE REPORTS

Several published case reports have demonstrated a temporal association between the use of prostaglandin analogs and CME in pseudophakic patients.[2-7] Some have reported the impressive resolution of CME and prompt visual improvement upon the cessation of prostaglandin therapy in conjunction with the administration of topical steroidal and nonsteroidal anti-inflammatory therapy.[3,4,6-11] Other case reports have been less convincing due to methodological limitations. Case reports and series are clearly not substitutes for well-designed, adequately powered, randomized clinical trials, particularly when the potential impact of study findings on clinical care is significant.

HOW COMMON IS CME FOLLOWING CATARACT SURGERY?

The prevalence of CME after cataract surgery largely depends on how one defines the condition. The term *angiographic CME* refers to the condition as defined and graded by a spectrum of findings on fluorescein angiography.[1] The reported prevalence of CME based upon fluorescein angiography was as high as 30% following extracapsular cataract extraction in one report.[12] The incidence of *clinical CME* (defined ophthalmoscopically by the detection of abnormal cystoid spaces in the macula), however, is much lower. A third criterion for CME relates to the diminution of vision associated with angiographically verified CME. Labeled by some as *clinically significant CME,*[1] its prevalence is reported at between 1% and 5%,[13,14] the variation largely due to preoperative risk factors in the study populations.

The variance in definitions of CME is particularly important when reviewing the literature. The higher rates of angiographic CME relative to clinically significant CME make the former a more attractive endpoint for study design, given that fewer patients are needed to establish causality. Because cataract surgeons hope to satisfy their patients, however, the incidence of clinically significant CME is more relevant to their practice. Strict cause-and-effect relationships are difficult to establish in many areas of medicine, and a rudimentary understanding of a disease process coupled with a less-than-optimal concordance between structural and functional macular changes in CME patients makes this a difficult topic for study.

WHAT CAUSES CME?

Several modulators have been implicated in the causation of CME. These include complement, platelet-activating factor, cytokines, interleukin-6, lysosomal enzymes, vascular endothelial growth factor, and, most notably, products of the arachadonic acid cascade such as prostaglandins (PGE2, etc.).[15] These mediators are thought to cause the breakdown of the blood-aqueous barrier and ultimately the blood-retina barrier, which both contribute to the development of

CME. Pharmacokinetic research has further demonstrated, through the use of radiolabeled prostaglandin esters, that the level of topical medications in the retina and choroid is potentially high enough to affect retinal physiology.[15] A causal relationship between such medications and CME, however, remains difficult to establish.

Hypothetically, the initial insult leading to CME in pseudophakic patients is operative irritation of uveal tissue along with the release of lens epithelial cells.[16] The fact that the prostaglandin analog class of glaucoma medications is thought to work primarily through binding to the prostaglandin F receptor has led many ophthalmologists to postulate that this must be the mechanism of postoperative CME in patients using these medications. Surprisingly, however, one study on the subject revealed that it was not the prostaglandin but rather the drug's preservative that was linked to postoperative CME.[17] The issue of causality with glaucoma medications is clearly more complex than initially theorized.

WHO IS AT HIGH RISK?

Although it is simpler to have a universal preferred practice pattern for patients undergoing cataract surgery, the data indicate that a complex algorithm may be more appropriate for identifying individuals who may develop CME while using glaucoma medications during the period following cataract surgery. Multiple studies have indicated that patients at high risk for CME include those with a history of retinal vein occlusion, diabetes, vitreous loss, uveitis, vitreomacular traction, an epiretinal membrane, aphakia, and an absent posterior capsule (postcapsulotomy or via an intraoperative complication).[14] Given ophthalmologists' knowledge of the pathogenesis of CME and its relationship to increased intraretinal vascular permeability, the list of disease entities linked to this condition is not surprising. Even in such high-risk groups, however, the overall incidence of postoperative clinically significant CME following cataract surgery is generally no more than 5%.[14]

Notwithstanding the lack of proof that the preoperative use of prostaglandins causes CME, it makes sense to consider stopping the agents sometime prior to cataract surgery to minimize the potential risk. How long before the procedure their use should cease and when they should be resumed postoperatively, however, remain widely debated questions. The vast majority of patients undergoing cataract surgery do not have these comorbidities, and the case for preoperatively stopping prostaglandins for a period of time is difficult to justify, particularly because patients are presumably using these agents to lower their IOP to a safe level. The practical question in this debate is not necessarily whether or not prostaglandin analogs and their associated preservatives can lead to CME. Rather, one must ask, does the risk of poorly controlled IOP outweigh the benefits of avoiding a relatively uncommon phenomenon that has not been causally linked to a particular class of drugs?

A survey of the Royal College of Ophthalmologists conducted by Ahad and McKee demonstrated that approximately 60% of the doctors did not stop treatment with prostaglandin analogs for uneventful cataract surgery. Of those who discontinued the drugs, approximately half did so routinely, whereas the other half did so only in high-risk patients. A majority of physicians who stopped prostaglandins did so less than 1 week prior to surgery, and most restarted therapy 30 to 60 days postoperatively, if needed.[18]

THE POSTOPERATIVE USE OF PROSTAGLANDINS

Cataract surgery is arguably the most commonly performed procedure for lowering IOP. Although what happens to the IOP varies widely among patients following phacoemulsification and the implantation of an IOL, a drop in the average IOP has occurred after surgery in almost every examined study population.[19-22] Modern cataract surgery may decrease the need for some or all of the glaucoma medications that a patient has been using. Ophthalmologists therefore may stop prostaglandins at the time of cataract surgery in virtually all patients.

In fact, prostaglandins are actually less than ideal for lowering IOP during the immediate postoperative period. Faster-acting drugs such as alpha adrenergic agonists, beta-blockers, and topical and systemic carbonic anhydrase inhibitors (CAIs)—all of which decrease the production of aqueous humor—are generally preferable. Prostaglandins mediate inflammation, which raises a concern about their use during the postoperative period when ocular inflammation is already present. Although evidence that topical prostaglandins cause or exacerbate inflammation is clearly not overwhelming, most ophthalmologists would agree that using these agents in the early postoperative period is not optimal. A majority of practitioners would also agree that, when necessary during the first few weeks following cataract surgery, patients should use prostaglandins in conjunction with topical nonsteroidal anti-inflammatory agents to minimize the potential risks of both CME and exacerbated postoperative inflammation. The use of topical steroids is, of course, also desirable in such situations.

SUMMARY AND RECOMMENDATIONS

There is no Oxford Level I highest-quality evidence demonstrating harm from the use of prostaglandin analogs prior to or after cataract surgery. The association between these drugs and CME or ocular inflammation remains controversial. Regarding CME, the impact of preservatives also found in other topical glaucoma medications may be more significant than the active components of prostaglandins. Nonetheless, common sense dictates discontinuing prostaglandins perioperatively in patients with preexisting CME or risk factors for developing the condition as well as individuals with other macular diseases for whom the occurrence of CME may have devastating consequences. Similarly, surgeons may wish to avoid prostaglandins in patients undergoing cataract surgery who have a history of ocular inflammatory disease.

We recommend stopping prostaglandins 1 week prior to surgery in high-risk patients when their IOP can be controlled by other agents such as oral CAIs or when their glaucoma is not severe enough to place them at significant risk of ultimate visual deterioration. The 1-week preoperative stopping date is completely arbitrary, as it remains unknown how long the adverse effects (if any) of prostaglandins last following the drugs' discontinuation.

Prostaglandins are our last choice for lowering IOP during the week following cataract surgery for a variety of reasons. Postoperative IOP spikes can generally be controlled by aqueous suppressants such as alpha adrenergic agonists, beta-blockers, or topical and oral CAIs, none of which is a likely mediator of inflammation. If prostaglandins are necessary for controlling IOP in the first 2 to 4 weeks following cataract surgery when ocular inflammation is present, we recommend using adjunctive topical nonsteroidal anti-inflammatory agents, which have not been shown to affect the IOP-lowering response.[21,23,24] Prostaglandins, if needed, are routinely resumed at approximately 1 month following cataract surgery, when they sometimes replace aqueous suppressing therapy.

Cataract surgery provides an opportunity to stop glaucoma medications. In our experience, a substantial proportion of patients who required prostaglandin therapy prior to cataract surgery will not need any glaucoma medications in the long-term postoperative period. When pseudophakic patients require long-term IOP-lowering therapy, however, prostaglandins remain our preferred first-line agents after the first postoperative month. We shorten or extend this timing if patients recover faster or slower than average, respectively, with regard to ocular inflammation after cataract surgery. ■

This article originally appeared in the July 2008 issue of CRSToday.

1. McNamara JA. Macular diseases. In: Ho A, Brown G, McNamara J, et al, eds. *Retina: Color Atlas and Synopsis of Clinical Ophthalmology.* New York: McGraw-Hill; 2003:32-34.
2. Dhingra N, Morgan JE. Pseudophakic cystoid macular edema: 30 months after latanoprost challenge. *Eye.* 2007;21:269-271.
3. Altintas O, Yuksel N, Karabas VL, Demirci G. Cystoid macular edema associated with latanoprost after uncomplicated cataract surgery. *Eur J Ophthalmol.* 2005;15:158-161.
4. Wand M, Gaudio AR. Cystoid macular edema associated with ocular hypotensive lipids. *Am J Ophthalmol.* 2002;133:403-405.
5. Jager M, Jonas JB. Cystoid macular edema associated with latanoprost therapy in a pseudophakic vitrectomized patient after removal of silicone oil endotamponade. *Eur J Ophthalmol.* 2003;13:221-222.
6. Yeh PC, Ramanthan S. Latanoprost and clinically significant cystoid macular edema after uneventful phacoemulsification with intraocular lens implantation. *J Cataract Refract Surg.* 2002;28:1814-1818.
7. Moroi SE, Gottfredsdottir MS, Schteingart MT, et al. Cystoid macular edema associated with latanoprost therapy in a case series of patients with glaucoma and ocular hypertension. *Ophthalmology.* 1999;106:1024-1029.
8. Henderson BA, Kim JY, Ament CS, et al. Clinical pseudophakic cystoid macular edema. *J Cataract Refract Surg.* 2007;33:1550-1558.
9. Arcieri ES, Santana A, Rocha FN, et al. Blood-aqueous barrier changes after the use of prostaglandin analogues in patients with pseudophakia and aphakia: a 6-month randomized trial. *Arch Ophthalmol.* 2005;123:186-192.
10. Miyake K, Masuda K, Shirato S, et al. Comparison of diclofenac and fluorometholone in preventing cystoid macular edema after small incision cataract surgery: a multicentered prospective trial. *Jpn Jl Ophthalmol.* 2000;44:58-67.
11. Asano S, Miyake K, Ota I, et al. Reducing angiographic cystoid macular edema and blood-aqueous barrier disruption after small-incision phacoemulsification and foldable intraocular lens implantation: multicenter prospective randomized comparison of topical diclofenac 01% and betamethasone 0.1%. *J Cataract Refract Surg.* 2008;34:57-63.
12. Gass JD, Norton EW. Follow-up study of cystoid macular edema following cataract extraction. *Trans Am Acad Ophthalmol Otolaryngol.* 1969;73:665-682.
13. Wright PL, Wilkinson CP, Balyeat HD, et al. Angiographic cystoid macular edema after posterior chamber intraocular lens implantation. *Arch Ophthalmol.* 1988;106:740-744.
14. Wand M, Gaudio AR, Shields MB. Latanoprost and cystoid macular edema in high-risk aphakic or pseudophakic eyes. *J Cataract Refract Surg.* 2001;27:1397-1401.
15. Miyake K, Ibaraki N. Prostaglandins and cystoid macular edema. *Surv Ophthalmol.* 2002;47(suppl 1):S203-S218.
16. Nishi O, Nishi K, Imanishi M. Synthesis of interleukin-1 and prostaglandin E2 by lens epithelial cells of human cataracts. *Br J Ophthalmol.* 1992;76:338-341.
17. Miyake K, Ibaraki N, Goto Y, et al. ESCRS Binkhorst lecture 2002: pseudophakic preservative maculopathy. *J Cataract Refract Surg.* 2003;29:1800-1810.
18. Ahad MA, McKee HDR. Stopping prostaglandin analogues in uneventful cataract surgery. *J Cataract Refract Surg.* 2001;30:2644-2645.
19. Kim DD, Doyle JW, Smith MF. Intraocular pressure reduction following phacoemulsification cataract extraction with posterior chamber lens implantation in glaucoma patients. *Ophthalmic Surg Lasers.* 1999;30:37-40.
20. Issa SA, Pacheco J, Majmood U, et al. A novel index for predicting intraocular pressure reduction following cataract surgery. *Br J Ophthalmol.* 2005;89:543-546.
21. Merkur A. Intraocular pressure decrease after phacoemulsification in patients with pseudoexfoliation syndrome. *J Cataract Refract Surg.* 2001;27:528-532.
22. Poley BJ, Lindstrom RL, Samuelson TW. Long-term effects of phacoemulsification with intraocular lens implantation in normotensive and ocular hypertensive eyes. *J Cataract Refract Surg.* 2008;34:735-742.
23. Flach AJ, Jampol LM, Weinberg D. Improvement in visual acuity in chronic aphakic and pseudophakic cystoid macular edema after treatment with topical 0.5% ketorolac tromethamine. *Am J Ophthalmol.* 1991;112:514-519.
24. Rho DS. Treatment of acute pseudophakic cystoid macular edema: diclofenac versus ketorolac. *J Cataract Refract Surg.* 2003;29:2378-2384.

CHAPTER 71

Cataract Surgical Considerations in Diabetics

SAM S. YANG, MD, AND EVERETT AI, MD

The global prevalence of diabetes is estimated to exceed 220 million people by the year 2010[1] and 300 million by the year 2025.[2] Diabetes is the most common risk factor for cataract development in underdeveloped countries.[3] Furthermore, diabetic patients suffer lens opacities at an earlier age than individuals without diabetes. The Framingham Eye Study and the Health and Nutrition Examination Survey showed that the rate of cataract was three- to fourfold higher in diabetic patients who were younger than 65 and up to twofold higher in patients older than 65 compared with patients who were not diabetic.[3] The Wisconsin Epidemiological Study of Diabetic Retinopathy[4] reported that cataract was the principal cause of legal blindness in adult-onset diabetics and the second most common cause of legal blindness after proliferative diabetic retinopathy in those with juvenile-onset diabetes.

Cataract surgery is indicated when a patient's visual function is significantly reduced as a result of lenticular opacity. Surgical intervention may also be indicated if a cataract reduces the ophthalmologist's view of the retina, thus impeding the diagnosis and treatment of diabetic retinopathy.

CONSIDERATIONS IN DIABETIC PATIENTS

Cataract surgery in diabetic patients has been associated with a higher incidence of postoperative complications, including fibrinous uveitis,[5] posterior capsular opacification,[6] neovascularization of the anterior segment,[7] an accelerated progression of retinopathy,[8] and macular edema.[9] Thus, it is important for the surgeon to address the preoperative management of diabetic retinopathy, the impact of surgery on the disease's progression, the appropriate timing of surgery, and the optimal management of postoperative macular edema.

Before initiating surgery, every effort should be made to stabilize diabetic retinopathy with an appropriate laser treatment. The Early Treatment of Diabetic Retinopathy Study (ETDRS) report No. 25,[10] which assessed diabetic patients' visual results after surgical removal of the crystalline lens, found that eyes assigned to early photocoagulation had more favorable outcomes compared with eyes assigned to deferred laser photocoagulation.

Earlier reports have indicated that patients with preexisting diabetic retinopathy who undergo extracapsular cataract extraction have a less favorable visual prognosis due to their developing neovascular glaucoma,[7,11,12] vitreous hemorrhage associated with proliferative diabetic retinopathy,[11] preexisting macular edema,[13] and postoperative macular edema.[8,14,15] Patients with clinically significant macular edema (CSME) or proliferative diabetic retinopathy therefore should receive prompt treatment prior to surgery as recommended by the ETDRS[16] and Diabetic Retinopathy Study.

CATARACT SURGERY'S EFFECT ON DIABETIC RETINOPATHY

The effect of cataract surgery on the progression of diabetic retinopathy is a somewhat controversial topic. The rate of the pathologic condition's postoperative progression may be influenced by a number of variables, including (1) the severity of the preoperative diabetic retinopathy,[5,11,17-20] (2) how long the patient has had diabetes,[17] (3) the adequacy of the patient's glycemic control,[17] and (4) the cataract surgeon's operative techniques.[21]

A review of the literature reveals a wide range in the rate of progression for diabetic retinopathy after cataract surgery, from 15% with experienced surgeons as reported by Mittra et al[19] to more than 70% according to Jaffe et al.[8] In 1992, Jaffe et al[8] conducted a prospective, paired-eye study of 19 diabetic patients that showed a high association between cataract extraction and the asymmetric progression of diabetic retinopathy. The ETDRS report No. 25,[10] which followed 270 eyes, also suggested a trend toward accelerated retinopathy in operated eyes compared with fellow unoperated eyes.

Two small, prospective, paired-eyed studies by Henricsson et al[17] (35 patients) and Squirrell et al[22] (50 patients) showed a similar rate of progression for diabetic retinopathy in both operated and unoperated eyes. In both studies, individuals who experienced postoperative progression of the disease had higher levels of hemoglobin A1C. Based on this information, an effective preoperative glycemic control may be important to preventing the postoperative progression of diabetic retinopathy.

The severity of patients' preoperative diabetic retinopathy also appears to contribute to their risk of postoperative progression. Several studies[19,23,24] have found that diabetic patients without diabetic retinopathy preoperatively showed no increase in the rate of diabetic retinopathy's progression in their operated eye compared with their unoperated one. Clear evidence from prospective and large retrospective studies showed that the preoperative presence of nonproliferative diabetic retinopathy or proliferative diabetic retinopathy is strongly linked with the postoperative progression of diabetic retinopathy.[8,9,15,19,25]

CATARACT SURGERY'S EFFECT ON MACULAR EDEMA

Macular edema is a common cause of poor visual acuity after cataract surgery in diabetics. Because it is difficult to discern between diabetic maculopathy and pseudophakic cystoid macular edema (Irvine-Gass syndrome) in postoperative cataract patients, it is important for ophthalmologists to understand the natural history of macular edema after cataract surgery in order to treat the condition adequately.

In 1992, Pollack et al[9] conducted the first prospective, controlled trial to evaluate the natural history of macular edema in diabetics after cataract surgery. Twenty-two of the 44 eyes developed macular edema. Half of the eyes that developed macular edema improved without laser treatment, and only five eyes required laser treatments. In 1999, Dowler et al[26] reported a 56% incidence of new, clinically detectable macular edema during the first year after surgery, with the peak incidence occurring at week 6. Spontaneous resolution occurred in 50% of the affected eyes within 6 months and in 75% within 1 year after the surgery.

Furthermore, the ETDRS report No. 25 found no long-term increase in macular edema after cataract surgery in diabetics after 4 to 9 years of follow-up.[10] Because these studies suggest that most cases of postoperative macular edema follow a relatively benign course, early laser treatment for all diabetics with postoperative macular edema may not be necessary. Some investigators propose delaying laser treatment for up to 6 months to allow Irvine-Gass syndrome to resolve.[20,26]

The natural history study of macular edema after cataract surgery by Dowler et al[26] showed that eyes with CSME at the time of cataract surgery are more likely to develop persistent CSME throughout the first postoperative year. In these eyes, the angiographic macular fluorescence that developed after the surgery was less likely to resolve spontaneously, and it significantly compromised visual acuity after 1 year.

For eyes with CSME in which lenticular opacity precludes adequate preoperative treatment, the surgeon must examine the retina as soon as he can view it after surgery. Eyes with any CSME present should undergo treatment immediately; conservative management (expecting it to resolve spontaneously) may be inappropriate. Randomized, controlled trials are currently underway to evaluate whether visual acuity may improve from macular laser treatment applied earlier in the postoperative course.

THE TIMING OF CATARACT SURGERY

Studies conducted in the early 1990s recommended a conservative approach to cataract surgery in diabetics due to their limited visual improvement.[8,15,27] In the study by Jaffe et al,[8] only 52% of patients achieved a UCVA of 20/50 or better, and 14% achieved 20/25 or better. Just five of 44 eyes achieved a final UCVA that was more than two lines better than their fellow eye. Pollack et al[15] reported that only 31% of patients achieved a postoperative UCVA of better than 20/40, and the investigators recommended against cataract extraction in patients with diabetic retinopathy until their vision had deteriorated to between 20/100 and 20/200. Schatz et al[27] reported that only 9% of eyes achieved a postoperative UCVA that was better than 20/40. They suggested that patients with diabetes, especially those with any retinopathy present preoperatively, might prefer to defer cataract surgery given these markedly poor postoperative results.

Most recent studies of the postoperative visual outcome of diabetics after cataract surgery report a lower incidence of complications and better visual results compared with the older studies just described.[17,19,21,26,28] Recent evidence that earlier cataract extraction yields fewer complications and better visual outcomes in patients with diabetes may have various explanations, including (1) better preoperative management of retinopathy using the guidelines provided by the ETDRS, (2) improved operative techniques that reduce surgical time and associated complications, and (3) better management of systemic factors such as hyperglycemia and hypertension, as suggested by the Diabetes Control and Complication Study and the UK Prospective Diabetes Study.[28-31]

CONCLUSION

Increasing evidence indicates that the preoperative presence of CSME is the greatest risk factor for poor visual acuity after cataract surgery.[21,26] It therefore may not be appropriate to delay surgery until it is impossible to identify or adequately treat CSME preoperatively. To improve visual outcomes, there is a growing trend among ophthalmologists to intervene with cataract surgery before lenticular opacity prevents their recognition and treatment of retinal thickening. After cataract surgery, many physicians have recommended monitoring diabetics closely for at least 6 months in order to intervene with laser photocoagulation as required to prevent visual loss from diabetic maculopathy and other detrimental sequelae of proliferative diabetic retinopathy.[22,32] ■

This article originally appeared in the August 2005 issue of CRSToday.

1. Amos AF, McCarty DJ, Zimmet P. The rising global burden of diabetes and its complications: estimates and projections to the year 2010. *Diabet Med.* 1997;14(suppl 5):S1-S85.
2. King H, Aubert RE, Herman WH. Global burden of diabetes, 1995-2025: prevalence, numerical estimates, and projections. *Diabetes Care.* 1998;21:1414-1431.
3. Ederer F, Hiller R, Taylor HR. Senile lens changes and diabetes in two population studies. *Am J Ophthalmol.* 1981;91:381-395.
4. Klein BE, Klein R, Wang Q, Moss SE. Older-onset diabetes and lens opacities. The

Beaver Dam Eye Study. *Ophthalmic Epidemiol.* 1995;2:49-55.
5. Hykin PG, Gregson RM, Stevens JD, Hamilton PA. Extracapsular cataract extraction in proliferative diabetic retinopathy. *Ophthalmology.* 1993;100:394-399.
6. Ionides A, Dowler JG, Hykin PG, et al. Posterior capsule opacification following diabetic extracapsular cataract extraction. *Eye.* 1994;8(pt 5):535-537.
7. Ulbig MR, Hykin PG, Foss AJ, et al. Anterior hyaloidal fibrovascular proliferation after extracapsular cataract extraction in diabetic eyes. *Am J Ophthalmol.* 1993;115:321-326.
8. Jaffe GJ, Burton TC, Kuhn E, et al. Progression of nonproliferative diabetic retinopathy and visual outcome after extracapsular cataract extraction and intraocular lens implantation. *Am J Ophthalmol.* 1992;114:448-456.
9. Pollack A, Leiba H, Bukelman A, Oliver M. Cystoid macular oedema following cataract extraction in patients with diabetes. *Br J Ophthalmol.* 1992;76:221-224.
10. Chew EY, Benson WE, Remaley NA, et al. Results after lens extraction in patients with diabetic retinopathy: early treatment diabetic retinopathy study report number 25. *Arch Ophthalmol.* 1999;117:1600-1606.
11. Aiello LM, Wand M, Liang G. Neovascular glaucoma and vitreous hemorrhage following cataract surgery in patients with diabetes mellitus. *Ophthalmology.* 1983;90:814-820.
12. Poliner LS, Christianson DJ, Escoffery RF, et al. Neovascular glaucoma after intracapsular and extracapsular cataract extraction in diabetic patients. *Am J Ophthalmol.* 1985;100:637-643.
13. Straatsma BR, Pettit TH, Wheeler N, Miyamasu W. Diabetes mellitus and intraocular lens implantation. *Ophthalmology.* 1983;904:336-343.
14. Sebestyen JG. Intraocular lenses and diabetes mellitus. *Am J Ophthalmol.* 1986;101:425-428.
15. Pollack A, Dotan S, Oliver M. Course of diabetic retinopathy following cataract surgery. *Br J Ophthalmol.* 1991;75:2-8.
16. Photocoagulation for diabetic macular edema. Early Treatment Diabetic Retinopathy Study report number 1. Early Treatment Diabetic Retinopathy Study research group. *Arch Ophthalmol.* 1985;103:1796-1806.
17. Henricsson M, Heijl A, Janzon L. Diabetic retinopathy before and after cataract surgery. *Br J Ophthalmol.* 1996;80:789-793.
18. Pollack A, Leiba H, Bukelman A, et al. The course of diabetic retinopathy following cataract surgery in eyes previously treated by laser photocoagulation. *Br J Ophthalmol.* 1992;76:228-231.
19. Mittra RA, Borrillo JL, Dev S, et al. Retinopathy progression and visual outcomes after phacoemulsification in patients with diabetes mellitus. *Arch Ophthalmol.* 2000;118:912-917.
20. Benson WE, Brown GC, Tasman W, et al. Extracapsular cataract extraction with placement of a posterior chamber lens in patients with diabetic retinopathy. *Ophthalmology.* 1993;100:730-738.
21. Dowler JG, Hykin PG, Hamilton AM. Phacoemulsification versus extracapsular cataract extraction in patients with diabetes. *Ophthalmology.* 2000;107:457-462.
22. Squirrell D, Bhola R, Bush J, et al. A prospective, case controlled study of the natural history of diabetic retinopathy and maculopathy after uncomplicated phacoemulsification cataract surgery in patients with type 2 diabetes. *Br J Ophthalmol.* 2002;86:565-571.
23. Antcliff RJ, Poulson A, Flanagan DW. Phacoemulsification in diabetics. *Eye* 1996;10(pt 6):737-741.
24. Wagner T, Knaflic D, Rauber M, Mester U. Influence of cataract surgery on the diabetic eye: a prospective study. *Ger J Ophthalmol.* 1996;5:2:79-83.
25. Pollack A, Dotan S, Oliver M. Progression of diabetic retinopathy after cataract extraction. *Br J Ophthalmol.* 1991;75:547-551.
26. Dowler JG, Sehmi KS, Hykin PG, Hamilton AM. The natural history of macular edema after cataract surgery in diabetes. *Ophthalmology.* 1999;106:663-668.
27. Schatz H, Atienza D, McDonald HR, Johnson RN. Severe diabetic retinopathy after cataract surgery. *Am J Ophthalmol.* 1994;117:314-321.
28. Early Treatment Diabetic Retinopathy Study Research Group. Photocoagulation for diabetic macular edema. Early Treatment Diabetic Retinopathy Study report number 1. *Arch Ophthalmol.* 1985;103:1796-1806.
29. Diabetes Control and Complications Trial Research Group. The effect of intensive treatment of diabetes on the development and progression of long-term complications in insulin-dependent diabetes mellitus. *N Engl J Med.* 1993;329:977-986.
30. UK Prospective Diabetes Study Group. Intensive blood-glucose control with sulphonylureas or insulin compared with conventional treatment and risk of complications in patients with type 2 diabetes (UKPDS 33). *Lancet.* 1998;352:837-853.
31. UK Prospective Diabetes Study Group. Tight blood pressure control and risk of macrovascular and microvascular complications in type 2 diabetes: UKPDS 38. *Br Med J.* 1998;317:703-713.
32. Dowler J, Hykin PG. Cataract surgery in diabetes. *Curr Opin Ophthalmol.* 2001;12:3:175-178.

CHAPTER 72

Age-Related Macular Degeneration

RAJA NARAYANAN, MD, AND BARUCH D. KUPPERMANN, MD, PHD

Age-related macular degeneration (AMD) is the leading cause of blindness in individuals over 50 years of age in developed countries.[1-3] The condition was first reported as a clinical entity in 1885 by Otto Haab.[4] Early manifestations of AMD include focal drusen associated with minor visual complaints, but the later stages of the disease result in severe vision loss. The nonexudative or dry form of AMD is approximately 10 times more prevalent than the exudative form, but the latter is the leading cause of blindness from AMD.

PREVALENCE

Various population-based studies have sought to estimate the prevalence of AMD in the general population, including the Framingham Eye Study,[5] the National Health and Nutrition Examination Survey,[6] the Beaver Dam Eye Study,[7] the Rotterdam Study,[8] and the Blue Mountains Eye Study.[9] The prevalence of exudative AMD in the Framingham Eye Study was 1.5%, whereas the dry type of AMD accounted for 90% of all cases. The Beaver Dam Eye Study defined early age-related maculopathy (ARM) as the presence of any drusen (except for hard, distinct drusen) with degeneration of the retinal pigment epithelium (RPE) or increased pigment in the macular area. It defined late ARM or AMD as the presence of geographic atrophy or exudative disease or both. The prevalence of late ARM was 1.6% in this study, and exudative maculopathy in at least one eye was present in 1.2% of the population. The prevalence of late ARM was 7.1% in subjects older than 75 years.

RISK FACTORS

Demographic Factors

All studies indicate that both the prevalence and the incidence of all forms of AMD increase with age. The Framingham Study found a 17-fold increased risk of AMD when comparing the oldest to the youngest age group.[5] Although there was no overall difference in the frequency of AMD between men and women in the Beaver Dam Eye Study, exudative AMD was more common in women 75 years or older compared with men. This subset of women also had approximately twice the incidence of early ARM compared with men in the study.[10] Several studies indicate a genetic factor in the pathogenesis of the disease.[11-14] Those examining the concordance of AMD in monozygotic and dizygotic twins strongly support the role of genetics in the pathogenesis of AMD.[15]

Lifestyle Factors

Most of the epidemiological evidence indicates a strong positive association between dry and wet AMD with smoking.[16-18] Risk grows as pack-years of smoking increase, indicating a dose-dependent relationship. Supplementation with zinc and vitamins A, C, and E helped prevent wet AMD in the Age-Related Eye Diseases Study (AREDS).[19]

Excessive exposure to light can damage the retina. In the Beaver Dam Eye Study, participants exposed to the summer sun for more than 5 hours a day during their teens, in their 30s, and at the baseline examination were at a higher risk of developing increased retinal pigmentation and early ARM by 10 years than those exposed less than 2 hours per day during the same periods.[20] The shorter wavelengths of light pose the greatest hazard to the retinal photoreceptors, because they contain more energy. Exposure to these wavelengths has been called the *blue-light hazard*, because they appear blue to the human eye. It has also been suggested that the removal of the natural lens, as in cataract surgery, should be followed by replacement with a tinted IOL to restore the eye's natural barrier to light radiation.[21]

Cardiovascular Factors

High cholesterol, especially HDL cholesterol[17,22] and oxidized LDL,[23] as well as hypertension[16,18] have been associated with a higher incidence of AMD. In the Macular Photocoagulation Study, there was an increased risk of exudative AMD associated with hypertension in the second eye of individuals with exudative AMD in one eye at baseline.

Ocular Risk Factors

The Macular Photocoagulation Study group described the risk factors for a patient's developing choroidal neovascularization (CNV) in his fellow eye when his opposite eye already has CNV. They include five or more drusen, focal hyperpigmentation, one or more large drusen (>63 µm), and systemic hypertension.[24] Based on the follow-up of patients with juxtafoveal CNV, the 5-year incidence rate for the development of CNV was 87% if all four risk factors were present. Lanchoney et al[25] reported that the 10-year risk of developing CNV in patients with bilateral soft drusen ranged from 8.6% to 15.9%. Hyperopia has a higher association with AMD, whereas darker irides may be protective against AMD.[26,27]

PROTECTIVE MECHANISMS IN THE RETINA AND CRYSTALLINE LENS

Carotenoids, including the xanthophyllic yellow pigments lutein and zeaxanthin, protect the macula from damaging blue light because of their maximum absorption spectrum at the lower wavelengths. By absorbing shorter wavelengths, the xanthophyllic pigments defend the photoreceptors against thermal damage. When molecules within the RPE absorb blue light, however, the formation of free radicals ensues, leading to cellular injury.[28] The crystalline lens is the major protective barrier to near-UV radiation (between 300 and 400 nm). Yellowing of the natural crystalline lens results in a greater absorbance of light of lower wavelengths such as blue light.[29]

Data from the Framingham Eye Study showed that nuclear cataracts were associated with a slightly reduced incidence of mild-to-severe macular changes compared with cortical cataracts.[30] Mild changes were defined as pigmentary changes or fewer than 10 small drusen, whereas moderate-to-severe changes were defined as more than 10 small drusen, large drusen, or hemorrhagic or exudative disease. Cortical cataracts were associated with a slightly increased risk for the development of the macular changes.[31]

Recent analysis of data from the AREDS showed no correlation between cataract surgery and advanced neovascular AMD, although there was a possible risk of advancing geographic atrophy.[31] In a subset analysis of patients in the AREDS who underwent cataract surgery, the risk for developing exudative (neovascular) AMD after cataract surgery was only 1% greater when compared with subjects who did not undergo cataract surgery. Cataract surgery did appear to affect patients' risk for developing geographic atrophy, the form of dry AMD associated with severe vision loss, however. AREDS subjects who underwent cataract surgery had a 47% greater risk of developing poor vision secondary to geographic atrophy compared with those who did not undergo cataract surgery; the *P* value of .05 barely met statistical significance, however, and thus leaves some doubt as to whether the finding was valid.

In a retrospective study of patients with early AMD and extracapsular cataract extraction, progression to wet AMD occurred more often in the pseudophakic than in unoperated eyes.[32] Ophthalmologists' interest in the use of IOLs that have light radiation-blocking mechanisms has increased. Insoluble lens proteins accumulate in the brunescent nuclear cataract, perhaps due to photo-oxidation by UV light. One theory is that this yellow filter protects the retina against blue light in the visible spectrum. If so, replacing this natural filter to high-energy wavelengths with a lens implant could allow damaging near-UV radiation and blue light to reach the retina, depending on the spectral transmittance of the IOL.[33]

Recently, Alcon Laboratories, Inc. (Fort Worth, TX), began marketing the Acrysof Natural lens, an IOL that blocks both UV radiation and blue light.[34] Researchers have demonstrated that yellow-tinted IOLs reduce the death of RPE laden with the lipofuscin fluorophore A2E.[35] Moreover, the incidence of CNV in patients with bilateral drusen and pigmentary changes was much higher in eyes that received untinted IOLs than in phakic fellow eyes.[32]

The use of blue-blocking IOLs has been controversial, however. They may affect color and scotopic vision, especially in the elderly,[36] but no studies to date have been conducted to prove this hypothesis. The decrease in scotopic vision with age has been attributed by some researchers to an age-related reduction in rod phoropter cells[37] and a dysfunction of central visual pathways.[38] Braunstein and Sparrow[39] therefore consider it prudent to use a blue-blocking IOL, because it reduces the transmission of blue light similarly to an adult, cataractous, crystalline lens. Prospective, controlled studies need to be conducted to determine the benefits and effects on color and scotopic vision of these IOLs.

CONCLUSION

Removing the natural crystalline lens after cataract surgery increases the retina's exposure to light of low wavelength and may increase the incidence of macular changes. The relationship between cataract surgery and AMD is not clear, however. A large, multicenter, prospective clinical trial would help to determine the significance. ■

This article originally appeared in the August 2005 issue of CRSToday.

1. Kahn HA, Moorhead HB. Statistics on blindness in the model reporting areas 1969-1970. United States Department of Health, Education and Welfare (NIH). Washington, DC: US Government printing office; 1973:73-427.
2. Wormald R. Assessing the prevalence of eye disease in the community. *Eye.* 1995;9:674-676.
3. Bird AC. Age-related macular disease. *Br J Ophthalmol.* 1996;80:1-2.
4. Haab O. Erkrankungen der macula lutea. *Centralblat Augenheilkd.* 1885;9:384-391. Cited by: Duke-Elder S. *System of Ophthalmology.* Vol 9. London: Kimpton; 1966.
5. Leibowitz HM, Krueger DE, Maunder LR, et al. The Framingham Eye Study monograph: an ophthalmological and epidemiological study of cataract, glaucoma, diabetic retinopathy, macular degeneration, and visual acuity in a general population of 2631 adults, 1973-1975. *Surv Ophthalmol.* 1980;24(suppl):335-610.
6. Klein R, Rowland ML, Harris MI. Racial/ethnic differences in age-related maculopathy. Third National Health and Nutrition Examination Survey. *Ophthalmology.* 1995;102:371-381.
7. Klein R, Klein BE, Linton KL. Prevalence of age-related maculopathy. The Beaver Dam Eye Study. *Ophthalmology.* 1992;99:933-943.
8. Vingerling JR, Dielemans I, Hofman A, et al. The prevalence of age-related maculopathy in the Rotterdam Study. *Ophthalmology.* 1995;102:205-210.
9. Mitchell P, Smith W, Attebo K, Wang JJ. Prevalence of age-related maculopathy in Australia. The Blue Mountains Eye Study. *Ophthalmology.* 1995;102:1450-1460.
10. Klein R, Klein BE, Jensen SC, Meuer SM. The five-year incidence and progression of age-related maculopathy: the Beaver Dam Eye Study. *Ophthalmology.* 1997;104:7-21.
11. Piguet B, Wells JA, Palmvang IB, et al. Age-related Bruch's membrane change: a clinical study of the relative role of heredity and environment. *Br J Ophthalmol.* 1993;77:400-403.
12. Seddon JM, Ajani UA, Mitchell BD. Familial aggregation of age-related maculopathy. *Am J Ophthalmol.* 1997;123:199-206.

13. Hamdi HK, Kenney MC. Age-related macular degeneration: a new viewpoint. *Front Biosci.* 2003;8:305-314.
14. Zareparsi S, Reddick AC, Branham KE, et al. Association of apolipoprotein E alleles with susceptibility to age-related macular degeneration in a large cohort from a single center. *Invest Ophthalmol Vis Sci.* 2004;45:1306-1310.
15. Seddon JM, Cote J, Page WF, et al. The US Twin Study of Age-Related Macular Degeneration: relative roles of genetic and environmental influences. *Arch Ophthalmol.* 2005;123:321-327.
16. Age-Related Eye Disease Study Research Group. Risk factors associated with age-related macular degeneration. A case-control study in the age-related eye disease study: Age-Related Eye Disease Study report number 3. *Ophthalmology.* 2000;107:2224-2232.
17. Tomany SC, Wang JJ, Van Leeuwen R, et al. Risk factors for incident age-related macular degeneration: pooled findings from 3 continents. *Ophthalmology.* 2004;111:1280-1287.
18. Klein R, Peto T, Bird A, Vannewkirk MR. The epidemiology of age-related macular degeneration. *Am J Ophthalmol.* 2004;137:486-495.
19. Age-Related Eye Disease Study Research Group. A randomized, placebo-controlled, clinical trial of high-dose supplementation with vitamins C and E, beta carotene, and zinc for age-related macular degeneration and vision loss: AREDS report no. 8. *Arch Ophthalmol.* 2001;119:1417-1436.
20. Tomany SC, Cruickshanks KJ, Klein R, et al. Sunlight and the 10-year incidence of age-related maculopathy: the Beaver Dam Eye Study. *Arch Ophthalmol.* 2004;122:750-757.
21. Okuno T, Saito H, Ojima J. Evaluation of blue-light hazards from various light sources. *Dev Ophthalmol.* 2002;35:104-112.
22. Van Leeuwen R, Klaver CC, Vingerling JR, et al. Cholesterol and age-related macular degeneration: is there a link? *Am J Ophthalmol.* 2004;137:750-752.
23. Ikeda T, Obayashi H, Hasegawa G, et al. Paraoxonase gene polymorphisms and plasma oxidized low-density lipoprotein level as possible risk factors for exudative age-related macular degeneration. *Am J Ophthalmol.* 2001;132:191-195.
24. Macular photocoagulation study group. Risk factors for choroidal neovascularization in the second eye of patients with juxtafoveal or subfoveal choroidal neovascularization secondary to age-related macular degeneration. *Arch Ophthalmol.* 1997;115:741-747.
25. Lanchoney DM, Maguire MG, Fine SL. A model of the incidence and consequences of choroidal neovascularization secondary to age-related macular degeneration. Comparative effects of current treatment and potential prophylaxis on visual outcomes in high-risk patients. *Arch Ophthalmol.* 1998;116:1045-1052.
26. Age-Related Eye Disease Study research group. Risk factors associated with age-related macular degeneration. A case-control study in the Age-Related Eye Disease Study: Age-Related Eye Disease Study report number 3. *Ophthalmology.* 2000;107:2224-2232.
27. Sandberg MA, Gaudio AR, Miller S, Weiner A. Iris pigmentation and extent of disease in patients with neovascular age-related macular degeneration. *Invest Ophthalmol Vis Sci.* 1994;35:2734-2740.
28. Sparrow JR, Zhou J, Ben Shabat S, et al. Involvement of oxidative mechanisms in blue-light-induced damage to A2E-laden RPE. *Invest Ophthalmol Vis Sci.* 2002;43:1222-1227.
29. Mellerio J. Yellowing of the human lens: nuclear and cortical contributions. *Vision Res.* 1987;27:1581-1587.
30. Sperduto RD, Hiller R, Seigel D. Lens opacities and senile maculopathy. *Arch Ophthalmol.* 1981;99:1004-1008.
31. Guttman C, Ferris FL. No link between cataract surgery, AMD, study shows. *Ophthalmology Times.* 2003 March;28(5). Available: www.ophthalmologytimes.com/ophthalmologytimes/article/articleDetail.jsp?id=47063.
32. Pollack A, Marcovich A, Bukelman A, et al. Age-related macular degeneration after extracapsular cataract extraction with intraocular lens implantation. *Ophthalmology.* 1996;103:1546-1554.
33. Mainster MA. Spectral transmittance of intraocular lenses and retinal damage from intense light sources. *Am J Ophthalmol.* 1978;85:167-170.
34. Niwa K, Yoshino Y, Okuyama F, et al. Effects of tinted intraocular lens on contrast sensitivity. *Ophthalmic Physiol Opt.* 1996;16:297-302.
35. Sparrow JR, Miller AS, Zhou J. Blue light-absorbing intraocular lens and retinal pigment epithelium protection in vitro. *J Cataract Refract Surg.* 2004;30:873-878.
36. Mainster MA. Intraocular lenses should block UV radiation and violet but not blue light. *Arch Ophthalmol.* 2005;123:550-555.
37. Curcio CA, Owsley C, Jackson GR. Spare the rods, save the cones in aging and age-related maculopathy. *Invest Ophthalmol Vis Sci.* 2000;41:2015-2018.
38. Schefrin BE, Tregear SJ, Harvey LO, Werner JS. Senescent changes in scotopic contrast sensitivity. *Vision Res.* 1999;39:3728-3736.
39. Braunstein RE, Sparrow JR. A blue-blocking intraocular lens should be used in cataract surgery. *Arch Ophthalmol.* 2005;123:547-549.

CHAPTER 73

Approaches to a Posterior Polar Cataract

ABHAY R. VASAVADA, MBBS, MS, FRCS, AND SHETAL M. RAJ, MBBS, MS

A posterior polar cataract is a dense white opacity that is situated on the central posterior capsule. It consists of characteristic concentric rings around the central opacity (bull's eye). A posterior polar cataract presents a special challenge to the phaco surgeon because of its predisposition to posterior capsular dehiscence during surgery.[1,2] Osher et al[1] reported a 26% (8/31 eyes) incidence of posterior capsular rupture during surgery in eyes with a posterior polar cataract. We had a rate of 36% (9/25 eyes).[2] Hayashi et al[3] reported 7.1% (2/28 eyes), whereas Lee and Lee[4] reported 11% (4/36 eyes).

To prevent posterior capsular rupture, Osher et al[1] recommended using slow-motion phacoemulsification with a low aspiration flow rate, a low level of vacuum, and infusion pressure. Fine et al[5] avoided overly pressurizing the anterior chamber with viscodissection to mobilize the epinucleus and cortex, Allen and Wood[6] performed viscodissection, and Lee and Lee[4] advocated a lambda technique with dry aspiration. We prefer inside-out delineation.[7] Combined with modern instrumentation, refined surgical strategies, a better understanding of phacodynamics, and cumulative surgical experience, this technique has enabled us to reduce the incidence of posterior capsular rupture to 8% (2/25 eyes).[7]

In our opinion, surgery should be delayed as long as possible and undertaken only if the patient finds it difficult to perform routine activities. We believe that the subsequent paradigm should govern the procedure.

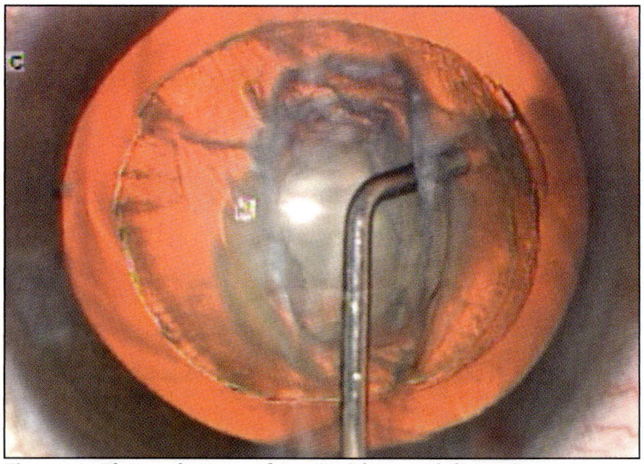

Figure 1. The authors perform inside-out delineation.

COUNSELING

During the preoperative examination, the physician should inform the patient of the possibility of the nucleus' dropping intraoperatively due to a posterior capsular rupture, a relatively long operative time, secondary posterior segment intervention, and a delayed visual recovery. In addition, the surgeon should discuss Nd:YAG capsulotomy for residual plaque[1-3] and emphasize the possibility of preexisting amblyopia, especially in cases of unilateral posterior polar cataract.[3]

ANESTHESIA

Peribulbar anesthesia with oculopressure to soften the globe diminishes intraoperative posterior pressure.[1] With increasing experience, one may use topical anesthesia in a selective manner.

SURGICAL TECHNIQUE

We prefer a closed chamber technique. The contours of the cornea and the globe should be maintained throughout the procedure. Hayashi et al[3] performed phacoemulsification, pars plana lensectomy, or intracapsular cataract extraction, depending on the size of the opacity and the density of the nuclear sclerosis.

THE INCISION

We create a paracentesis with a 15° ophthalmic knife (Alcon Laboratories, Inc., Fort Worth, TX) and inject Provisc (Alcon Laboratories, Inc.). Next, we make a temporal, corneal, single-plane valvular incision of 2.6 mm. A cohesive viscoelastic in the anterior chamber prevents its collapse as well as forward movement of iris-lens diaphragm during surgical entry into the eye. Fine et al[5] cautioned against increasing the pressure in the anterior chamber.

THE CAPSULORHEXIS

Ideally, the capsulorhexis should be no larger than 5 mm. Although a size of 4 mm or less could be detrimental if the surgeon must prolapse the nucleus into the anterior chamber, a larger opening may not leave adequate support for a sulcus-fixated IOL if the posterior capsule is compromised.[2,5]

HYDRO PROCEDURES

Cortical cleaving hydrodissection[8] can lead to hydraulic rupture and should be avoided.[1,2] It is logical instead to perform hydrodelineation to create a mechanical cushion of epinucleus.[2-4,6,9,10] Fine et al[5] performed hydrodissection in multiple quadrants and gently injected tiny amounts of fluid such that the fluid wave could not extend across the posterior capsule.

We employ inside-out delineation to precisely demarcate the central core of nucleus.[7]

INSIDE-OUT DELINEATION

We sculpt a central trench using the slow-motion technique with the Infiniti Vision System (Alcon Laboratories, Inc.). For nuclear sclerosis of grade 3 or less (on a grading system from 1 to 5),[11] our preset parameters are ultrasound energy of 30% to 60% (supraoptimal power), vacuum of 60 mm Hg, an aspiration flow rate of 18 mL/min, and a bottle height of 70 cm. We are careful not to mechanically rock the lens. Injecting a dispersive viscoelastic (Viscoat; Alcon Laboratories, Inc.) through the sideport incision before retracting the probe prevents the forward movement of the iris-lens diaphragm.

We introduce a specially designed, right-angled cannula mounted on a 2-mL syringe filled with fluid through the main incision and place the tip adjacent to the right wall of the trench at an appropriate depth, depending on the density of the cataract. The tip then penetrates the central lenticular substance, and we inject fluid through the right wall of the trench (Figure 1). The fluid traversing inside out produces delineation. A golden ring within the lens indicates successful delineation (Figure 2). If the delineation is incomplete, the surgeon may inject fluid in the left wall of the trench with another right-angled cannula. The trench allows the surgeon to reach the central core of the nucleus. When fluid reaches a desired depth, it will create an epinuclear bowl that will act as a mechanical cushion to protect the posterior capsule during subsequent maneuvers.

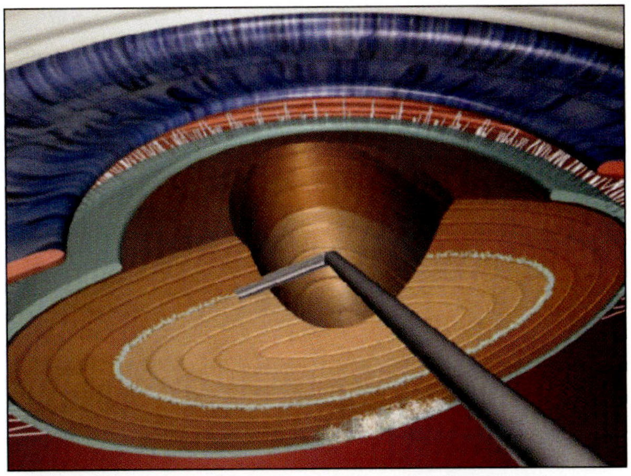

Figure 2. An animated view of inside-out delineation is depicted.

With conventional hydrodelineation, the cannula penetrates the lenticular substance and thus causes the fluid to traverse from the outside inward. It is sometimes difficult to introduce the cannula within a firm nucleus, and the effort can rock and stress the capsular bag and zonules. The surgeon may also inadvertently inject fluid into the subcapsular plane and thereby conduct unwarranted hydrodissection. Inside-out delineation is easy to perform, provides excellent surgical control, reduces stress to the zonules, and precisely demarcates the central core of nucleus.

NUCLEAR REMOVAL

We avoid rotating the nucleus, because this maneuver can rupture the posterior capsule. All of our techniques are geared toward facilitating the removal of the nucleus while it is cushioned by the epinucleus. Bimanual cracking and division of the nucleus involve outward movements and can distort the capsular bag. For nuclear sclerosis greater than +2, we use the technique of step-by-step chop in situ and lateral separation[12] with 40% to 50% ultrasound, vacuum of 150 to 250 mm Hg, an aspiration flow rate of 18 mL/min, and a bottle height of 70 to 90 cm. The resultant fragments are removed with a stop, chop, chop-and-stuff technique.[13]

For less dense nuclei, we aspirate the entire nucleus within the epinuclear shell. We use an aspiration flow rate of 16 mL/min and a vacuum level of 100 to 120 mm Hg. Traction of posterior lenticular fibers and posterior polar opacity during surgery are sufficient to break the weak posterior capsule. Thus, the slow-motion technique reduces turbulence in the anterior chamber.[14] Injecting viscoelastic prior to removing the instrument prevents the anterior chamber from collapsing and the posterior chamber from bulging forward.[2,15]

Lee and Lee[4] described their use of the lambda technique to sculpt the nucleus, after which they cracked along both arms and removed the central piece.

EPINUCLEAR REMOVAL

First, we strip off the peripheral lower half of epinucleus using 30% ultrasound, 80 to 100 mm Hg of vacuum, an aspiration flow rate of 16 mL/min, and a bottle height of 80 to 90 cm. The central area of epinucleus remains attached.[2,5,11] Next, we mobilize the peripheral upper epinucleus (subincisional epinucleus) with gentle,

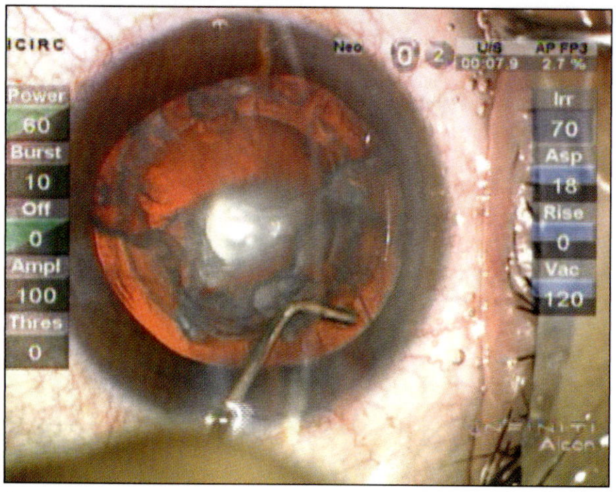

Figure 3. The authors remove the upper half of the epinucleus by means of focal and multiquadrant hydrodissection.

focal, multiquadrant hydrodissection using a right-angled cannula that faces right and left (Figure 3). The fluid wave travels along the cleavage formed between the capsule and lower epinucleus without threatening the integrity of the posterior capsule. Hydrodissection is safe at this stage, because the capsular bag is not fully occupied. In other words, the built-up hydraulic pressure is not sufficient to rupture the posterior capsule. Finally, we aspirate the entire epinucleus, including the central area.

Others have suggested performing viscodissection of the epinucleus by injecting viscoelastic (Healon5 [Pharmacia AB, Stockholm, Sweden][6] or Healon GV [Pharmacia AB] and Viscoat[5]) under the capsular edge to mobilize the rim of epinucleus. The surgeon then removes this rim with a coaxial I/A handpiece. Alternatively, one may perform manual dry aspiration with a Simcoe cannula.[4]

PSEUDOHOLE

At times, the classic appearance suggestive of a defect may be observed in the posterior cortex when the posterior capsule actually remains intact. This phenomenon is known as a *pseudohole*.

CORTICAL REMOVAL

Bimanual, automated I/A using an aspiration flow rate of 20 mL/min and vacuum of 400 mm Hg optimizes surgical control, preserves the anterior chamber, and aids in the complete removal of the cortex. Fine et al[5] reported using coaxial phacoemulsification to protect the posterior capsule with viscoelastic during cortical removal.

POLISHING THE POSTERIOR CAPSULE

We avoid polishing the posterior capsule due to its fragility.[1-3,5,11] The traction produced by polishing an excessively adherent plaque could eventually rupture an otherwise normal posterior capsule. We prefer to perform an Nd:YAG posterior capsulotomy postoperatively when needed.

POSTERIOR CAPSULAR DEHISCENCE

If a defect is present in the posterior capsule, we inject Viscoat over the area before withdrawing the phaco or I/A probe from the eye.[15] Then, we perform a two-port, limbal anterior vitrectomy using a cutting rate of 800 cuts/min, vacuum of 300 mm Hg, and an aspiration flow rate of 25mL/min. Once the anterior chamber is free of vitreous, we aspirate the cortex with bimanual I/A. A posterior capsulorhexis may be performed if the rupture is confined to a small central area.

IOL IMPLANTATION

In eyes with a posterior capsular defect, we implant the IOL in the bag only if we can create a posterior capsulorhexis. If the posterior capsular defect is large, we will place the lens over the anterior capsule in the ciliary sulcus. Although others have suggested capturing the optic through the anterior capsulorhexis,[5,16] we believe optic capture increases inflammation.[17]

After implanting the IOL, we remove viscoelastic by two-port vitrectomy rather than I/A. Vitrectomy aspirates material in a piecemeal and gradual manner, and it reduces the chance of rapidly aspirating vitreous.

We do not suture the main valvular incision but do suture the paracentesis in eyes with a posterior capsular defect. We will periodically evaluate these eyes for retinal break, cystoid macular edema, and raised IOP. ■

This article originally appeared in the April 2005 issue of CRSToday.

1. Osher RH, Yu BC, Koch DD. Posterior polar cataracts: a predisposition to intraoperative posterior capsular rupture. *J Cataract Refract Surg.* 1990;16:157-162.
2. Vasavada AR, Singh R. Phacoemulsification with posterior polar cataract. *J Cataract Refract Surg.* 1999;25:238-245.
3. Hayashi K, Hayashi H, Nakao F, et al. Outcomes of surgery for posterior polar cataract. *J Cataract Refract Surg.* 2003;29:45-49.
4. Lee MW, Lee YC. Phacoemulsification of posterior polar cataracts—a surgical challenge. *Br J Ophthalmol.* 2003,87:1426-1427.
5. Fine IH, Packer M, Hoffman RS. Management of posterior polar cataract. *J Cataract Refract Surg.* 2003;29:16-19.
6. Allen D, Wood C. Minimizing risk to the capsule during surgery for posterior polar cataract. *J Cataract Refract Surg.* 2002;28:742-744.
7. Vasavada AR, Raj SM. Inside-out delineation. *J Cataract Refract Surg.* 2004;30:1167-1169.
8. Fine IH. Cortico-cleaving hydrodissection. *J Cataract Refract Surg.* 1992;18:508-512.
9. Anis AY. Understanding hydrodelineation: the term and the procedure. *Doc Ophthalmol.* 1994;87:123-137.
10. Masket S. Consultation section. *J Cataract Refract Surg.* 1997;23:819-824.
11. Emery JM, Little JH. *Phacoemulsification and Aspiration of Cataracts, Surgical Technique, Complications and Results.* St. Louis, Mo: CV Mosby; 1979: 45-49.
12. Vasavada AR, Singh R. Step-by-step chop in situ and separation of very dense cataracts. *J Cataract Refract Surg.* 1998;24:156-159.
13. Vasavada AR, Desai JP. Stop, chop, chop and stuff. *J Cataract Refract Surg.* 1996;22:526-529.
14. Osher RH. Slow motion phacoemulsification approach. *J Cataract Refract Surg.* 1993;19:667.
15. Osher RH, Cionni R, Burk S. Intraoperative complications of phacoemulsification surgery. In: Steinert RF, ed. *Cataract Surgery: Technique, Complications, and Management.* 2nd ed. Philadelphia, PA: WB Saunders Company; 2004: 469-486.
16. Gimbel HV, DeBroff BM. Posterior capsulorhexis with optic capture: maintaining a clear visual axis after pediatric cataract surgery. *J Cataract Refract Surg.* 1994;20:658-664.
17. Vasavada AR, Trivedi R. Role of optic capture in congenital cataract and IOL surgery in children. *J Cataract Refract Surg.* 2000;26:824-831.

CHAPTER 74

Shallow Anterior Chamber

WILLIAM J. FISHKIND, MD

It is uncommon but disturbing when the anterior chamber becomes shallow during phacoemulsification. Recognizing the complication early helps the surgeon to prevent damage to the endothelium or iris as well as tears in the posterior capsule.

CLASSIFICATION

The anterior chamber may become shallow due to three main causes. First, fluid outflow through the paracentesis or main incision may be excessive, or an overly high flow setting on the phaco machine may pull a large volume of fluid out of the anterior chamber and through the phaco needle. Second, inflow may be insufficient due to either an obstruction in the phaco tip's sleeve or an inadequate bottle height. Third, positive posterior pressure may develop due to (1) mechanical pressure from a tight speculum or drapes or from a retrobulbar hemorrhage; (2) fluid misdirection syndrome; (3) a suprachoroidal effusion; or (4) a suprachoroidal hemorrhage.

If the paracentesis or main incision is leaking excessively (both caused by poor wound construction), the surgeon should tighten either incision with sutures. If the inflow is insufficient, the physician should enlarge the incision to improve flow through the sleeve or raise the infusion bottle.

It is usually easy to correct mechanical causes of a shallow anterior chamber by loosening the speculum or drapes and by watching for a retrobulbar hemorrhage. After eliminating these causes, the surgeon will know that the shallow chamber is due to either fluid misdirection or a suprachoroidal effusion. By placing a finger on the eye, the ophthalmologist will be able to sense if the pressure is elevated and the globe firm, findings that confirm a fluid misdirection syndrome or suprachoroidal effusion/hemorrhage.

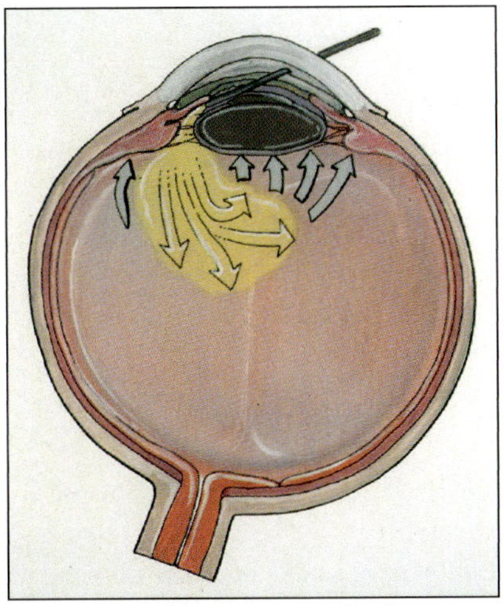

Figure 1 & 2. When irrigation fluid passes through the intact zonules into the vitreous, the result is hydration of the vitreous and a shallowing of the anterior chamber. (Reprinted with permission from Fishkind WJ, ed. *Complications in Phacoemulsification: Avoidance, Recognition, and Management*. 1st ed. New York, NY: Thieme Medical Publishers; 2002.)

FLUID MISDIRECTION SYNDROME

Pathophysiology

Fluid misdirection syndrome occurs when irrigating fluid passes into the vitreous through intact zonules or through a zonular or capsular tear. The zonular/iris diaphragm acts like a one-way valve. Fluid flows into the vitreous and cannot escape, thus causing vitreous hydration, an expanded volume of vitreous, and subsequently elevated pressure in the posterior segment. As this pressure builds, the lens and iris move forward, markedly decreasing the working space in the anterior chamber. If the surgeon proceeds, more fluid will pass into the vitreous, and the problem will worsen (Figure 1).

Risk Factors

Several risk factors are likely to give rise to fluid misdirection syndrome. Anything that disrupts the zonular apparatus may allow fluid to pass into the posterior segment: pseudoexfoliation syndrome, previous ocular trauma, a radial tear in the anterior capsule, zonulysis, and any opening in the posterior capsule. A small pupil and a narrow angle may hide these peripheral capsular defects and thereby delay the surgeon's recognition of fluid misdirection syndrome.

Timing

Fluid deviation can occur during any phase of the operation when the surgeon infuses fluid into the eye. The ophthalmologist must be aware that hydrodissection, phacoemulsification, and I/A can all cause fluid misdirection and positive pressure.

During hydrodissection, the surgeon inadvertently may not place the cannula under the anterior capsule but under it and thus inject fluid directly through the zonules. This error forces injected fluid to pass through the zonules into the vitreous. In another scenario described by Updegraff et al[1] involving small pupils, injected fluid travels under the anterior capsule and elevates the capsule and lens, thereby causing pupillary block. These investigators proposed that the viscoelastic might contribute to an iridocapsular seal by causing the iris to adhere to the capsule and prevent fluid's egress.

Phacoemulsification may force the fluid posteriorly if a dense viscoelastic prevents the adequate anterior circulation of fluid and the bottle is relatively high. This problem occurs when an occult radial capsular tear or small area of zonulysis develops. An intact vitreous face closes the one-way valve that leads to elevated posterior pressure.

During I/A, aggressively attempting to aspirate subincisional cortex can misdirect fluid. A small, iatrogenic, anterior capsular tear can allow the infusion of balanced salt solution into the vitreous, a situation that usually forces the iris up into the incision with positive posterior pressure. Even aspirating the viscoelastic from the eye after placing the lens can lead to balanced salt solution misdirection and a shallow anterior chamber. This phenomenon can occur if the surgeon is intent on removing all traces of viscoelastic behind the IOL and there is a small opening in the zonular-capsular diaphragm.[2]

Diagnostic Tests

An evaluation with an indirect ophthalmoscope or the use of an Osher Emergency Lens to view the posterior segment will reveal a normal periphery that indicates aqueous misdirection, or it may show an elevated choroidal mass, which would indicate suprachoroidal hemorrhage.

Treatment

After verifying that a suprachoroidal effusion/hemorrhage has not occurred, the surgeon can alleviate increased IOP by performing a pars plana vitreous tap. Confirming the diagnosis is imperative; a vitreous tap in the presence of a suprachoroidal effusion/hemorrhage is disastrous, because it dramatically worsens the situation. To perform a tap, one should insert a 23-gauge needle 3 mm posterior to the limbus and direct it toward the central anterior vitreous until one can visualize the needle's tip through the pupil. Slowly withdrawing 0.1 to 0.3 mL of liquid vitreous should deepen the anterior chamber sufficiently to allow the completion of the procedure.

An alternative albeit slower treatment regimen is first to lower rather than raise the bottle to decrease fluid inflow. After intravenously administering Diamox (500 mg in an IV push) (Wyeth Pharmaceuticals, Philadelphia, PA) and/or mannitol (1 to 2 g/kg of a 25% solution), the surgeon should wait approximately 20 minutes for the drug(s) to take effect, the eye to stabilize and soften, and the chamber to deepen. If the globe remains firm and the chamber is still shallow after this treatment, one should suspect a suprachoroidal effusion. In this situation, it is best to interrupt the surgery and complete the procedure a few days to 1 week later.

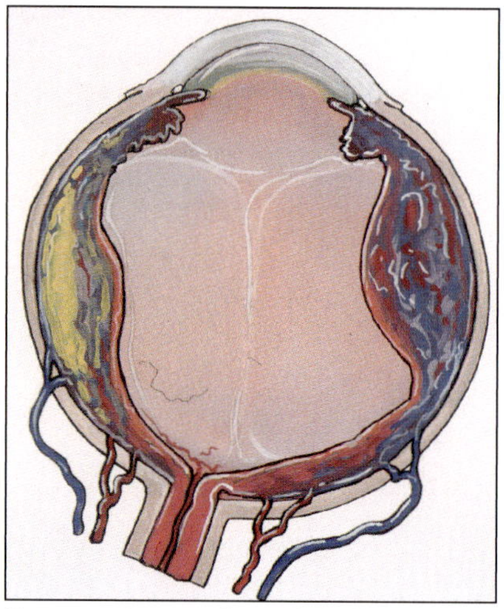

Figure 2. A suprachoroidal effusion appears at left and a suprachoroidal hemorrhage at right. (Reprinted with permission from Fishkind WJ, ed. *Complications in Phacoemulsification: Avoidance, Recognition, and Management.* 1st ed. New York, NY: Thieme Medical Publishers; 2002.)

Suprachoroidal Effusion/Hemorrhage

Suprachoroidal effusion is caused by the rupture of the short posterior ciliary vessels with a subsequent outpouring of plasma and blood into the suprachoroidal space. This complication commonly occurs upon the withdrawal of the phaco or I/A tip. The sudden hypotony thus produced is the driving force for damage to the short, posterior ciliary vessels. Extravasation of plasma into the suprachoroidal space ensues. Subsequently increased IOP limits the total amount of extravasated material, and it effectively tamponades the continued accumulation of fluid and prevents hemorrhage. If the surgeon opens the wound, the resultant hypotony will allow continued effusion and eventually hemorrhage with the resultant extravasation of intraocular contents (Figure 2).

Under no circumstance should the surgeon attempt to convert to an extracapsular cataract extraction, because an enlarged wound will destabilize the eye and allow a suprachoroidal effusion to become hemorrhagic, leading to an expulsive hemorrhage.

Fluid misdirection will generally respond to the treatment previously described. The surgeon can then cautiously proceed with a lower infusion pressure. Because suprachoroidal effusion/hemorrhage will usually not respond to treatment, waiting 24 hours to complete the case is a reasonable and safe compromise.

As with most potential complications, the key to successfully completing cataract surgery in the presence of a shallow anterior chamber is recognizing the problem early, making a sound diagnosis, thoughtfully assessing one's surgical options, and proceeding with a suitable management strategy. ■

This article originally appeared in the April 2005 issue of CRSToday.

1. Updegraff SA, Peyman GA, McDonald MB. Pupillary block during cataract surgery. *Am J Ophthalmol.* 1994;117:328-332.
2. Arnold PN. Positive pressure. In: Fishkind WJ, ed. *Complications in Phacoemulsification: Avoidance, Recognition, and Management.* 1st ed. New York, NY: Thieme Medical Publishers; 2002: 63-74.

CHAPTER 75

Pars Plana Vitrectomy in Nanophthalmos

ROSA BRAGA-MELE, MEd, MD, FRCSC; NASTASIA NIANIARIS; AND EL-KARIM RHEMTULLA, MD, FRCSC

Nanophthalmos is a rare bilateral condition in which the eye is pathologically small but morphologically normal.[1] The combination of a short axial length (15 to 20 mm) and a high ratio of lens-to-eye volume results in severe axial hyperopia, a crowded anterior segment, and angle-closure glaucoma.[2] These eyes are therefore some of the most challenging on which to perform phacoemulsification and IOL implantation.

A crowded anterior chamber coupled with a positive posterior vitreous pressure complicate sequential surgical steps during phacoemulsification. Ophthalmologists may have difficulty constructing the corneal incision due to peripheral iridocorneal proximity and apposition, and they may find the anterior capsulorhexis hard

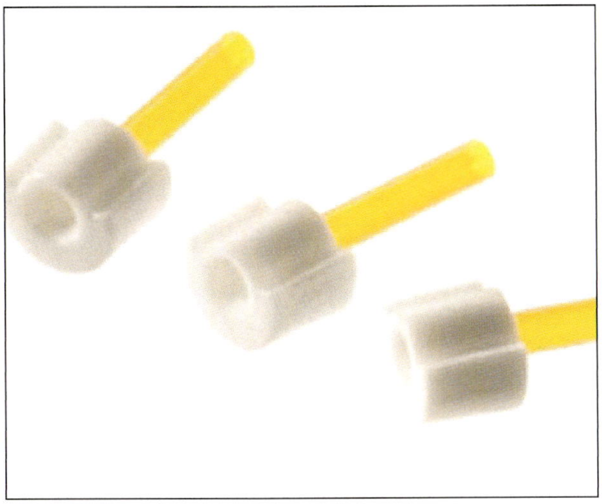

Figure 1. Pictured are the cannulas used during 25-gauge vitrectomy.

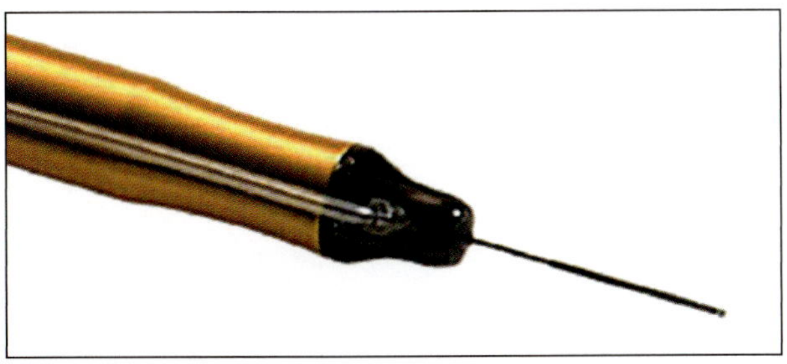

Figure 2. The TSV25 System uses the lightening handpiece with a high-speed electric cutter.

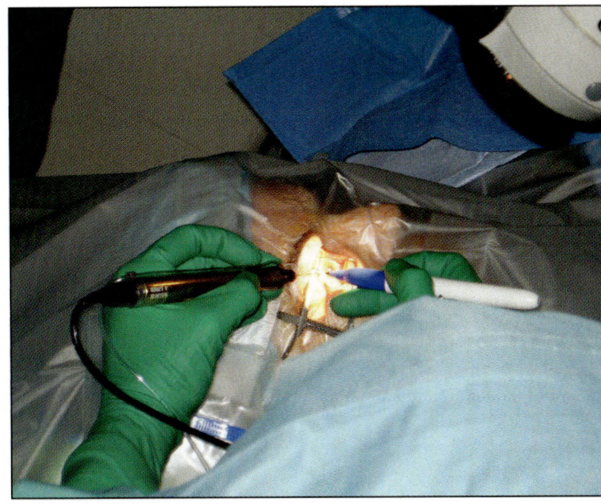

Figure 3. The surgeon marks the cutter with a pen to indicate the length entering the eye.

to control, because the capsule's convexity steers the capsular tears peripherally. Using a forceps in a crowded anterior chamber is tricky. Moreover, the anterior location of the iris leads to its prolapse and contact with instruments, which result in intraoperative pupillary constriction. The close proximity of the phaco tip to the cornea causes endothelial cell loss and corneal edema.[3] In addition, it is challenging to place a piggyback IOL due to the anterior chamber's restricted depth. Intraoperative maneuvers to increase the anterior chamber depth using a viscoelastic substance and elevating the bottle's height can help, but not always.[4,5]

Several strategies have been described for lowering the IOP and shrinking the vitreous prior to cataract surgery in eyes with shallow anterior chambers.[6-9] This article describes a technique for decompressing the vitreous prior to cataract surgery with phacoemulsification by means of a sutureless, 25-gauge, high-speed vitrectomy system (1,500 cuts/min). This approach effectively decompresses the vitreous without conjunctival dissection or scleral suturing. Minimal trauma helps to increase the anterior chamber depth and decrease positive posterior pressure before phacoemulsification.

STEP NO. 1: SMALL-GAUGED PARS PLANA VITRECTOMY

First, we perform a vitreous tap using the Millennium Transconjunctival Standard Vitrectomy 25 (TSV25) System (Bausch & Lomb, Rochester, NY) prior to phacoemulsification. We anesthetize the eye with topical tetracaine 0.5% (Novartis Ophthalmics, Inc., Duluth, GA). After pulling the conjunctiva aside, we introduce a 25-gauge trocar and microcannula transconjunctivally, 3.5 to 4.0 mm posterior to the limbus through the pars plana, as measured with a caliper, and angled down toward the optic nerve. This directionality is important to ensure that the trocar does not contact the posterior capsule.

The trocar forms a continuous bevel with the microcannula to ease the entry of the latter instrument. Referred to as an *entry alignment system*, the 25-gauge cannula (Figure 1) aligns the conjunctival and scleral entry sites, which obviates the need for conjunctival dissection. It is helpful to maneuver the system in a circular motion between one's fingers and to counterbalance the applied pressure by having the patient look toward the entry site.

We remove the trocar and introduce the electric cutter (Figure 2) into the vitreous cavity through the microcannula.[10] It is important to note that, on occasion, one may not be able to visualize the cutter within the eye, either due to a small pupil or dense cataract. In such cases, we recommend using a pen to mark off on the cutter the desired distance at which one wants to enter the eye in order to avoid introducing too much of the instrument into a small eye and perhaps traumatizing the retina (Figure 3).

We aspirate a small amount of vitreous (approximately 0.5 to 1.0 mL) and use no infusion. Throughout the vitrectomy, we monitor the IOP by pressing on the eye with a toothless forceps so as not to remove too much vitreous.[11] After the chamber has deepened, we remove the microcannula from the pars plana and apply pressure to the area. The sclerotomy site need not be sutured, because it is self-sealing.[10,12]

STEP NO. 2: PHACOEMULSIFICATION

We perform phacoemulsification in our usual fashion. If desired, the surgeon may deepen the anterior chamber further with a superviscoelastic agent such as Healon5 (Advanced Medical Optics, Inc., Santa Ana, CA), which has both maximally cohesive and highly retentive properties. We create a continuous curvilinear capsulorhexis and then perform hydrodissection and hydrodelineation. After phacoemulsifying the lens with the quick-chop technique, we piggyback foldable IOL implants with one in the capsular bag and the other in the sulcus.

DISCUSSION

True nanophthalmos is an uncommon condition present in only 20% of cases with short eyes, in which the abnormality is due to short anterior segments.[2] In the remaining 80% of cases, the abnormality is usually a foreshortened axial length due to a shortened posterior segment.[13] Shallow, crowded anterior chambers present one of the most technically challenging situations for cataract surgeons. These severely hyperopic eyes are at high risk of complications,[14] including suprachoroidal hemorrhage.[15] In addition, these eyes commonly develop ocular conditions such as chronic angle closure, pseudoexfoliation with zonular loss, spherophakia, and trauma.[16,17]

As previously described by Chang,[5] combining preoperative mannitol and ocular compression and then administering an intraoperative injection of a viscoelastic agent is often sufficient for deepening the anterior chamber.[5,18] Occasionally, however, the anterior chamber is so shallow that the globe will become excessively firm before the ophthalmologist can inject enough viscoelastic to create sufficient space. In such eyes, an automated pars plana vitreous tap may safely expand the anterior segment to permit routine phacoemulsification and IOL implantation.[5,6,11,19] Another option is a vitreous tap technique that employs a 23- to 26-gauge needle on a 1-mL tuberculin syringe when automated vitrectomy instrumentation is not available.[20]

We have found the small-gauged technique described in this article to be superior to the traditional pars plana vitrectomy (PPV). The 25-gauge system is less traumatic to the eye, and it provides patients with a speedier recovery. Additionally, patients require fewer postoperative drops.[21] Of greater significance, however, are the pre- and intraoperative advantages of the 25-gauge versus the 20-gauge system. Vitreous decompression with the 25-gauge system involves topical anesthesia. In contrast, traditional vitrectomy requires the administration of a retrobulbar local anesthetic.[6] Although effective, retrobulbar anesthesia can cause life-threatening and serious ocular complications such as brainstem anesthesia, retrobulbar hemorrhage, perforation of the globe, injury to the optic nerve, ptosis, and an ocular motility defect.[22,23]

Another disadvantage of the standard 20-gauge system is that the surgeon must perform a conjunctival peritomy. After completing the peritomy, the ophthalmologist must create a 1-mm sclerotomy with a No. 19 microvitreoretinal blade, and the sclerotomy site is closed with sutures at the conclusion of the vitrectomy. Numerous complications are associated with traditional sclerotomy sites, including vitreous incarceration, traction on the retina, entry-site retinal tears, injury to the ciliary body, fibrovascular downgrowth, protruding sutures, wound dehiscence, unstable IOP during closure, and postoperative hypotony.[24]

Because the 25-gauge system reduces the diameter of the incision from approximately 1.0 to 0.5 mm, a conjunctival peritomy is unnecessary. The natural elasticity of the scleral tissues adequately approximates the sclerotomy wound, thus allowing for a completely self-sealing, sutureless procedure. The TSV25 System's microcannula is narrow enough for insertion directly through the conjunctiva and sclera. The small tracts it creates produce self-sealing conjunctival and scleral incisions upon the cannula's removal,[10] thereby avoiding the aforementioned complications associated with traditional sclerotomy sites.[25,26]

The motor-driven TSV25 System uses a vitrector with a high-speed electric cutter, which eliminates the pulsing associated with pneumatic cutters. By creating minimal traction on the vitreous, the system's high cutting rate improves procedural safety and efficacy.[27] The pneumatic cutter causes the duty cycle (ie, the time that the vitrectomy port remains open) to be harder to control as the cutting speed increases. In contrast, the electric cutter allows the ratio to remain 50:50 for successful cutting.[26]

CONCLUSION

We have experienced no complications of vitrectomy, cataract surgery, or corneal decompensation with small-gauged, sutureless PPV in seven eyes of four patients with nanophthalmos. We believe that the TSV25 System represents a simpler, quicker, and less traumatic alternative to the traditional automated approach. By performing a PPV before phacoemulsification, we minimize the risk of intraoperative complications in nanophthalmic eyes while maintaining the safety and advantages of small-incision cataract surgery. ■

This article originally appeared in the February 2008 issue of CRSToday.

1. Brockhurst RJ. Nanophthalmos with uveal effusion. A new clinical entity. *Arch Ophthalmol.* 1975;93:1289-1299; correction 1976;94:583.
2. Singh OS, Simmons RJ, Brockhurst RJ, Trempe CL. Nanophthalmos: a perspective on identification and therapy. *Ophthalmology.* 1982;89:1006-1012.
3. Hayashi K, Hayashi H, Nakao F, Hayashi F. Risk factors for corneal endothelial injury during phacoemulsification. *J Cataract Refract Surg.* 1996;22:1079-1084.
4. Masket S, ed. Consultation section: cataract surgical problem. *J Cataract Refract Surg.* 2000;26:12-20.
5. Chang DF. Pars plana vitreous tap for phacoemulsification in the crowded eye. *J Cataract Refract Surg.* 2001;27:1911-1914.
6. Lu GS. Reduction of intraocular pressure before cataract surgery by ocular compression [in Chinese]. *Zhonghua Yan Ke Za Zhi.* 1988;24:143-145.
7. Honan PR. Preoperative ocular compression. *J Cataract Refract Surg.* 1999;25:607.
8. Masket S, ed. Consultation section: cataract surgical problem. *J Cataract Refract Surg.* 2003;29:12-20.
9. Chan FM, Lee L. Nanophthalmic cataract extraction. *Clin Experiment Ophthalmol.* 2004;32:535-538.
10. Fujii GY, de Juan E Jr, Humayun MS, et al. A new 25-gauge instrument system for transconjunctival sutureless vitrectomy surgery. *Ophthalmology.* 2002;109:1807-1813.
11. Mackool RJ. Pars plana vitreous tap for phacoemulsification in the crowded eye. *J Cataract Refract Surg.* 2002;28:572-573.
12. Chalam KV, Gupta SK, Vinjamaram S, Shah VA. Small-gauge, sutureless pars plana vitrectomy to manage vitreous loss during phacoemulsification. *J Cataract Refract Surg.* 2003;29:1482-1486.
13. Holladay JT, Gills JP, Leidlein J, Cherchio M. Achieving emmetropia in extremely short eyes with two piggyback posterior chamber intraocular lenses. *Ophthalmology.* 1996;103:1118-1123.
14. Masket S, ed. Consultation section: cataract surgical problem. *J Cataract Refract Surg.* 2000;26:1702-1713.
15. Davison JA. Acute intraoperative suprachoroidal hemorrhage in extracapsular cataract surgery. *J Cataract Refract Surg.* 1986;12:606-612.
16. Lowe RF. Causes of shallow anterior chamber in primary angle-closure glaucoma. Ultrasonic biometry of normal and angle-closure glaucoma eyes. *Am J Ophthalmol.* 1969;67:87-93.
17. Ritch R, Schlötzer-Schrehardt U. Exfoliation syndrome. *Surv Ophthalmol.* 2001;45:265-315.
18. Teus MA, Fagúndez-Vargas MA, Calvo MA, Marcos A. Viscoelastic-injecting cystotome. *J Cataract Refract Surg.* 1998;24:1432-1433.
19. Mandic Z, Saric D. Phacoemulsification and pars plana vitreous tap in the crowded eye. Paper presented at: The Deustsche Ophthalmologische Gesellschaft (DOG) meeting; September 2002; Berlin, Germany.
20. Sethi H, Dada T. Pars plana vitreous tap in crowded eyes. *J Cataract Refract Surg.* 2002;28:1897.
21. Puliafito CA, moderator. Evolution of posterior segment micro-incision surgery. *Ocular Surgery News.* August 15, 2003 [monograph, insert].
22. Duker JS, Belmont JB, Benson WE, et al. Inadvertent globe perforation during retrobulbar and peribulbar anesthesia: patient characteristics, surgical management, and visual outcome. *Ophthalmology.* 1991;98:519-526.
23. Hunter DG, Lam GC, Guyton DL. Inferior oblique muscle injury from local anesthesia for cataract surgery. *Ophthalmology.* 1995;102:501-509.
24. Kreiger A. Sclerotomy complications following pars plana vitrectomy. *Br J Ophthalmol.* 2001;85:121-122.
25. Chen JC. Sutureless pars plana vitrectomy through self-sealing sclerotomies. *Arch Ophthalmol.* 1996;114:1273-1275.
26. van Kuijk FJGM, Uwaydat S, Godley BF. Self-sealing sclerotomies in pars plana vitrectomy. *Retina.* 2001;21:547-550.
27. Peyman GA, Livir-Rallatos C, Canakis C, Easley J. A new high-speed pneumatic vitrectomy cutter. *Am J Ophthalmol.* 2002;133:568-569.

CHAPTER 76

Iris Prosthesis/IOL Implantation

KENNETH J. ROSENTHAL, MD

Iris defects occur in a variety of conditions, including congenital aniridia, coloboma, iridocorneal endothelial syndrome, Axenfeld-Rieger syndrome, trauma (surgical and nonsurgical), uveitis, and idiopathic postoperative mydriasis. Many patients have coexisting zonular and capsular abnormalities.[1] Patients with iris and capsular defects present surgical challenges because (1) the anterior segment may destabilize after cataract removal and (2) the implantation of a traditional IOL may cause the patient significant glare, photophobia, and polyopsia. In addition, patients with thin or transparent irides, such as in ocular albinism, chronic inflammation (eg, herpetic uveitis), or trauma may have an exquisite and debilitating sensitivity to light.

The implantation of a masking artificial iris implant can potentially reduce glare and improve patients' visual function. Such devices may also mask the optical aberrations prevalent in the peripheral cornea and eliminate visual competition between focused and unfocused images.

SURGICAL APPROACH

Iris Defect Repair Options

Because every iris defect is unique, the surgical approach must be tailored to the specific situation. Primary repair of an iris defect by means of techniques such as iris sphincterotomy, synechialysis, iris suturing, and cerclage may be adequate in some patients and should be considered before an iris prosthetic implant. However, these other forms of repair may be neither possible nor sufficient in eyes with more extensive iris defects. Overly aggressive iris suturing techniques should be avoided with these cases, because the iris tissue is almost universally abnormal and there is a risk of iatrogenic iridodialysis and hemorrhage, as well as of sequential iris atrophy in areas under tension from suturing. Furthermore, with some iris defects, such as those associated with iridocorneal endothelial syndrome, or in eyes with comorbid conditions, such as retinal abnormalities or glaucoma, the overall success of the procedure may ultimately be compromised by the progression of the disease.

PROSTHETIC IRIS DEVICES

For eyes that have iris defects too extensive for simple repair, a small selection of implantable iris prosthetic devices have been developed that will aid the surgeon in compensating for the deformed or imperfectly functioning iris. Two companies produce these devices on a customized basis. As a participant in the FDA clinical trials for an implant manufactured by Ophtec BV (Groningen, the Netherlands), I have had the opportunity to place a number of these implants.[2] Similar devices are available from Morcher GmbH (Stuttgart, Germany), but they are not FDA-approved and require individual compassionate use exemptions from the FDA. The Morcher implant is available in black only and is made of a rather brittle material. The Ophtec devices are available in multiple colors (Figure 1).

In 1991, Rainer Sundmacher, MD, of Düsseldorf, Germany,[3] developed a PMMA IOL surrounded by an opaque black segment that serves as an artificial iris diaphragm for implantation in patients with iris defects. Peter Choyce, MD, developed and implanted similar designs as early as the 1950s.[4] In patients with absent or inadequate capsular support, this lens is quite useful, although the black optic carrier measures up to 10 mm in diameter (and encompasses varying optic sizes), thus requiring a large incision. Thomas Reinhard, MD, of Düsseldorf, Germany,[3] has shown that these devices provide good visual rehabilitation, although they have been associated with a greater amount of postoperative inflammation and a higher incidence of postoperative pressure elevation when compared to standard extracapsular surgery. This problem

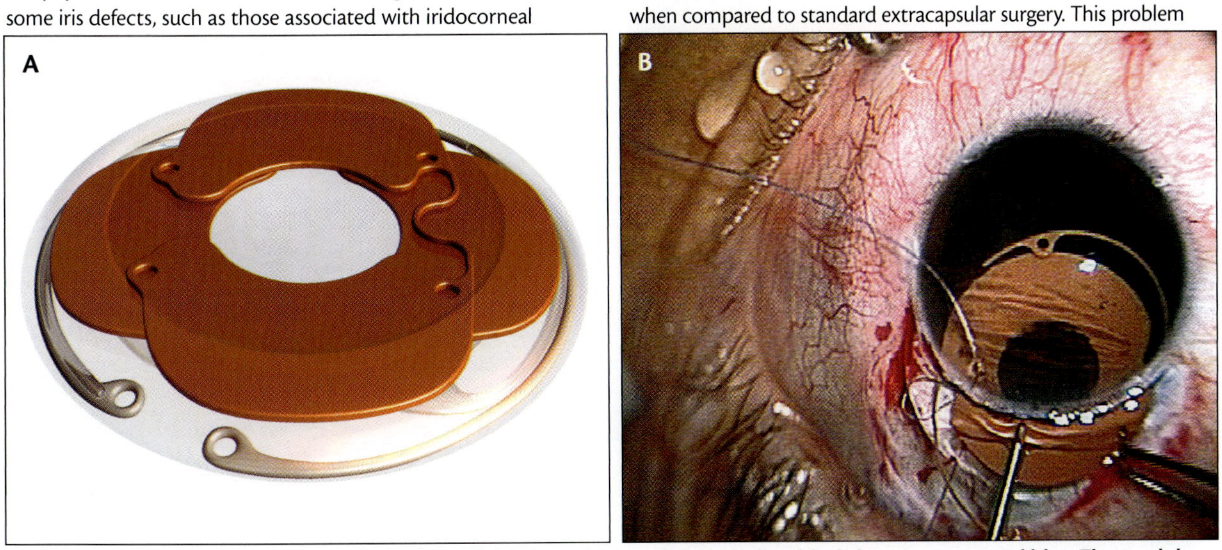

(Courtesy of Ophtec USA.)

Figure 1. The Ophtec Iris prosthetic device is available in multiple colors, including black, brown, green, and blue. The modular Iris Prosthetic System, shown here, is for use in intact capsular bags with or without zonular support (A). The surgical insertion of the Ophtec Model 311 requires a 10- to 11-mm incision (B).

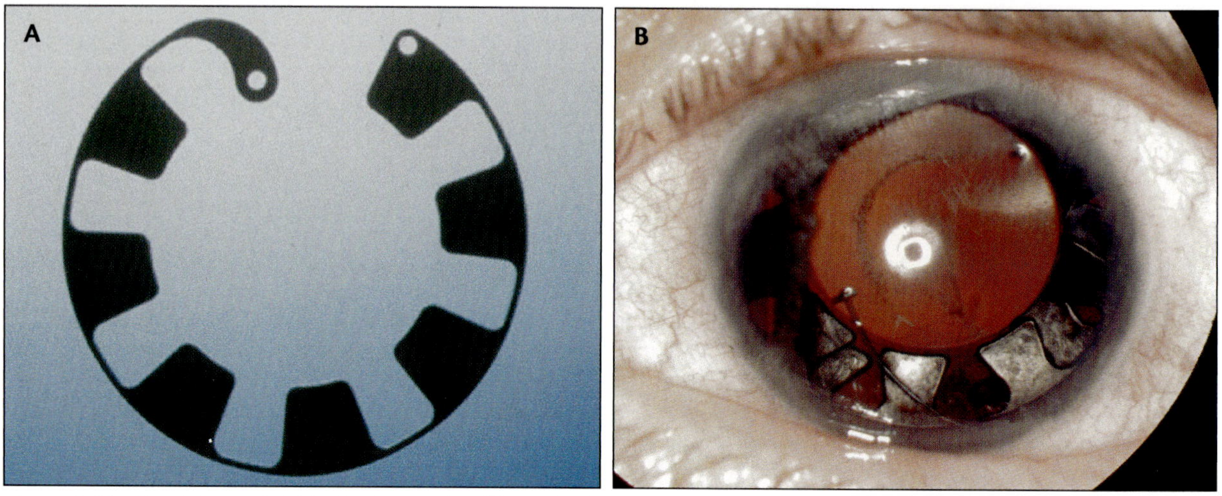

Figure 2. The Rasch Rosenthal Iris Diaphragm ring (A) can be inserted through a 4-mm incision (B).

may relate to the disruption of the blood-aqueous barrier, although it should be pointed out that many of these eyes have other serious defects as well. Robert Osher, MD, and Scott Burke, MD, of Cincinnati have demonstrated similarly favorable results.[5]

STUDY PROGRESSION

Preliminary results of the ongoing Ophtec Iris Prosthetic implant study have been strongly favorable to date.[6] There have been no reported surgical, postoperative or optical complications caused by the device, and there has been no substantial difference in inflammatory response compared with that expected from traditional extracapsular surgery (the device requires an incision larger than 10 mm). All patients reported a subjective improvement in visual quality as well as a reduction in glare and ghosting or other undesired images.

Volker Rasch, MD, of Potsdam, Germany, and I invented a series of aniridia and coloboma aperture rings (Morcher GmbH) designed to be implanted in an intact capsular bag, with or without zonular instability and with a separately implanted IOL (Figure 2).[7] A similar device is available from Ophtec USA (Boca Raton, FL). Because these devices incorporate the properties of a capsular tension ring, they can be used to treat partial capsular instability and iris defects (Figure 3). Michael Snyder, MD, of Cincinnati had suggested that I use a 6.5-mm IOL so that an overlap between the optic and haptic occurs, thereby reducing the potential for optical problems related to the IOL's edge. The devices available from Morcher are black in color, imparted by a proprietary alteration to the PMMA that renders the material very brittle. Therefore, it is necessary to implant the devices gently in order to avoid excessive flexing or torquing, and to have spare devices available in case of breakage. Because a common site of breakage is at the incision, but the ring can be dialed into the anterior chamber and then placed gently into the capsular bag. The Ophtec device is inserted similarly and in conjunction with a capsular tension ring, but it is more flexible and less prone to breakage.

Both companies also produce customized devices that cover only a sector of absent iris. These implants are suitable for the management of coloboma or partial defects such as those seen in iris and ciliary body coloboma or in trauma.

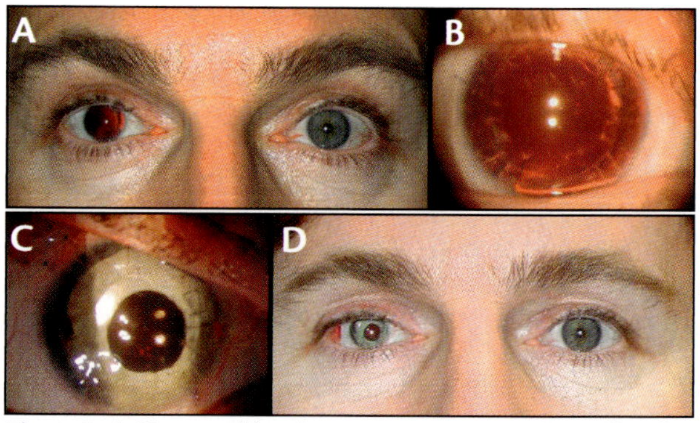

Figure 3. A 49-year-old male, status post–16-cut RK, suffered an expulsive injury to his right eye after being hit with a surfboard. Although the patient underwent corneal transplantation, a vitrectomy to remove retained lens material, and a repair of a retinal detachment, he was left aphakic and aniridic (A). The subsequent implantation of an Ophtec iris prosthesis improved his vision to 20/40 (B). The iris prosthetic implant (C) matched the color of the patient's fellow eye well (D).

CONCLUSION

Capsular instability and iris abnormalities may coexist and remain daunting obstacles to surgical success both during and after cataract surgery. The introduction of capsular fixation devices, which are configured with iris diaphragm attachments, represents a significant step toward improving surgical outcomes. ■

This article originally appeared in the May 2004 issue of CRSToday.

1. Rosenthal KJ. The capsular ring, indications and surgery. Focal Point Module: *American Academy of Ophthalmology*. 2002;20:7.
2. Rosenthal KJ, Osher RH, ed. *Video Journal of Viscosurgery*. Pharmacia. 2002-2003;10.
3. Reinhard T, Engelhardt S, Sundmacher R. Black diaphragm aniridia intraocular lens for congenital aniridia: Long-term follow-up. *J Cataract Refract Surg*. 2000;26:375–381.
4. Choyce P. *Intra-Ocular Lenses and Implants*. London: H.K. Lewis; 1964: 21.
5. Osher RH, Burke SE. Cataract surgery combined with implantation of an artificial Iris. *J Cataract Refract Surg*. 1999;25:1540-1547.
6. Rosenthal KJ. Artificial iris implants: update. Paper presented at: The AAO Annual Meeting; November 17, 2003; Anaheim, CA.
7. Rosenthal KJ. Sutureless phacotrabeculectomy and insertion of an iris diaphragm ring in a patient with the Axenfeld-Rieger Syndrome: first reported case. *Video Journal of Cataract and Refractive Surgery*. 1997;13(2).

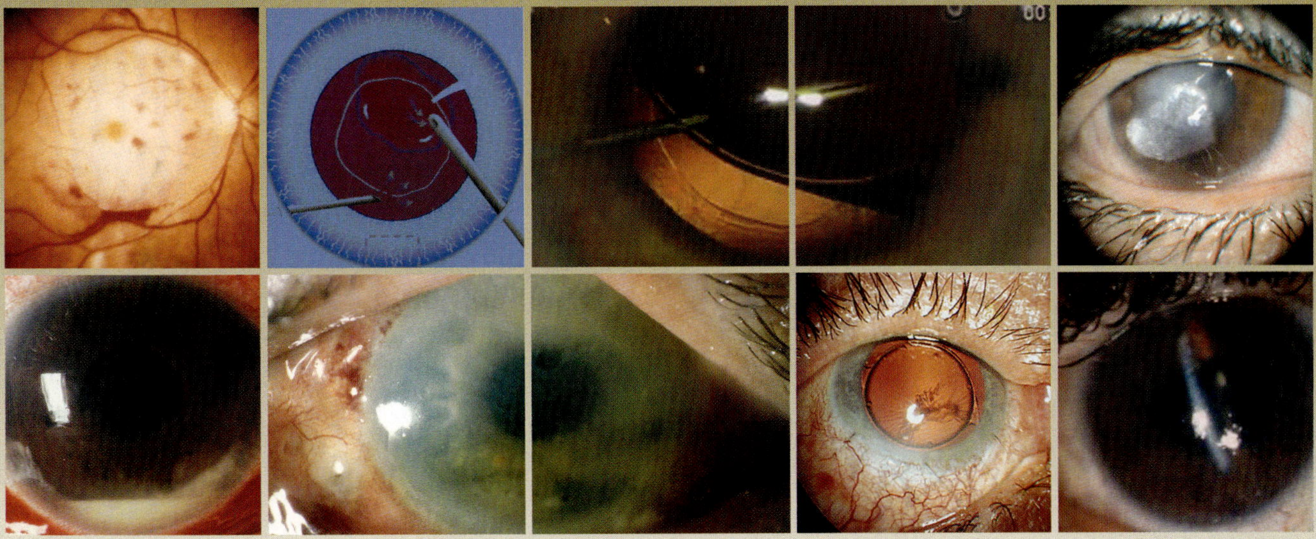

COMPLICATIONS

OPERATIVE COMPLICATIONS

ENDOPHTHALMITIS PROPHYLAXIS

TASS

POSTOPERATIVE COMPLICATIONS

CHAPTER 77

Intraoperative Capsular Block Syndrome

KENSAKU MIYAKE, MD

Capsular block syndrome occurs in eyes with a continuous curvilinear capsulorhexis and is characterized by the accumulation of a liquefied substance within a closed chamber inside the capsule. This pool forms when the lens nucleus, or the PCIOL's optic, occludes the anterior capsular opening created by the continuous curvilinear capsulorhexis. My colleagues and I have proposed a new classification of capsular block syndrome to better understand the etiology of this complication and to provide effective treatment.[1]

Depending on its time of onset, capsular block syndrome can be classified as intraoperative capsular block syndrome (the complication seen at the time of lens luxation following hydrodissection),[2] early postoperative capsular block syndrome (original capsular block syndrome[3,4]), and late postoperative capsular block syndrome (capsular block syndrome with liquefied after-cataract[5,6] or lacteocrumenasia[7]). The etiology of the accumulated substance and method of treatment are different for each type. This article describes the intraoperative capsular block syndrome as a cause of dropped lens nuclei.

CASE REPORTS

No. 1

An 87-year-old female had a nuclear cataract in one eye that had a visual acuity of 20/400 and an axial length of 24.65 mm. My colleagues and I injected 0.1mL of viscoelastic material into the anterior chamber and performed a standard continuous-tear capsulorhexis. Next, we gently injected 0.2mL of BSS between the lens capsule and the lens cortex with a 27-gauge needle, which we placed beneath the anterior lens capsule at the 11-o'clock meridian. After removing the epinucleus, we used the ultrasonic aspiration tip to sculpt the central portion of the nucleus. Immediately after the first sculpting, the entire nucleus dropped into the vitreous cavity.[2]

No. 2

A 75-year-old male presented with a mature nuclear cataract and a visual acuity of hand motion in an eye with an axial length of 27.85 mm. We performed a continuous-tear capsulorhexis and hydrodissection in the same manner as described in the aforementioned case. Immediately after the removal of the epinucleus on the anterior surface, the nucleus slipped down into the vitreous cavity.[2]

No. 3

An 83-year-old female presented with a mature nuclear cataract. She had a visual acuity of hand motion and an axial length of 21.07 mm in this eye. Her contralateral, untreated eye showed evidence of pseudoexfoliation syndrome, including white flakes at the pupillary margin and on the anterior lens capsule. The treated eye, however, disclosed no such findings. We performed a continuous-tear capsulorhexis and hydrodissection. Again, immediately after hydrodissection, the nucleus dropped into the vitreous cavity.

No. 4

An 85-year-old male with a nuclear cataract had a visual acuity of 20/67 in an eye with an axial length of 28.32 mm. Again, we performed a continuous-tear capsulorhexis and hydrodissection. On removal of the epinucleus from the anterior surface, the nucleus descended into the vitreous cavity.

COMMENTS

Intraoperative capsular block syndrome occurs in eyes with a posterior capsular rupture and a luxated nucleus following continuous curvilinear capsulorhexis and hydrodissection. This type of capsular block syndrome is caused by rapid hydrodissection using a large amount of BSS. The eye becomes especially vulnerable when a highly viscous viscoelastic material is injected into the anterior chamber prior to hydrodissection. The phenomenon is common in

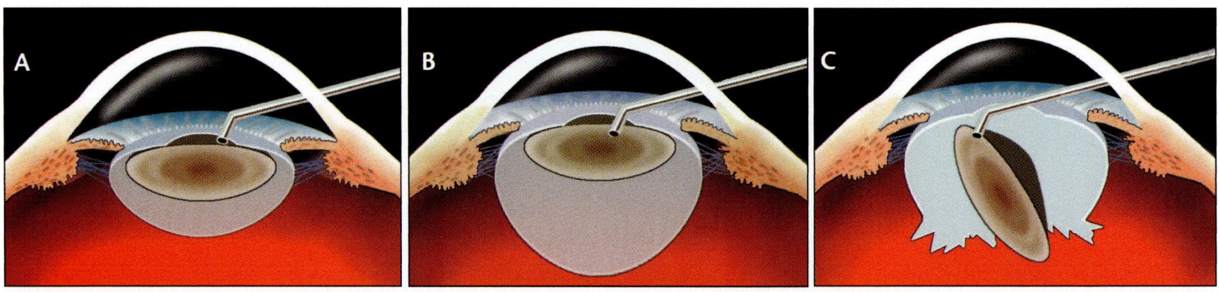

Figure 1. A patient presented with intraoperative capsular block syndrome resulting in posterior capsular rupture and lens nucleus luxation after hydrodissection. The author injected BSS into the lens capsule (A). The lens nucleus occluded the anterior capsular opening created by the continuous curvilinear capsulorhexis. As a result of capsular blockage, the trapped BSS expanded toward the posterior capsule and inflated the entire lens capsule while the anterior chamber became shallow (B). In some cases, the posterior capsule ruptures, and the lens nucleus luxates into the vitreous cavity (C). (Reprinted with permission from Miyake K, Ota I, Ichihashi S, et al. New classification of capsular block syndrome. *J Cataract Refract Surg.* 1998;24:1230-1234.)

eyes with a posterior polar or mature cataract and in those with a long visual axis. The nucleus occludes the anterior capsular opening created by the continuous curvilinear capsulorhexis as a result of capsular blockage, and the trapped BSS expands toward the posterior capsule, which the fluid inflates completely and pushes anteriorly. The anterior chamber becomes shallow, and the IOP rises. In the worst cases, the posterior capsule ruptures, and the nucleus luxates into the vitreous cavity. The BSS that flows into the vitreous cavity through the ruptured posterior capsule may also contribute to an anterior shifting of the capsular bag (Figure 1).

In many eyes with intraoperative capsular block syndrome, the shallow anterior chamber makes it difficult to insert the phaco tip. The nucleus luxates as the epinucleus is removed with an ultrasound tip; in some cases, the luxation of the nucleus occurs during phacoemulsification of the nucleus or during nuclear division. To prevent these complications, hydrodissection should be performed with great caution or avoided in eyes suspected of having a weakened posterior capsule. I also recommend using a large-gauge cannula and depressing the posterior lip of the incision while performing hydrodissection. The latter prevents a high spike in IOP during this phase. ■

This article originally appeared in the April 2005 issue of CRSToday.

1. Miyake K, Ota I, Ichihashi S, et al. New classification of capsular block syndrome. *J Cataract Refract Surg.* 1998;24:1230-1234.
2. Ota I, Miyake S, Miyake K. Dislocation of the lens nucleus into the vitreous cavity after standard hydrodissection. *Am J Ophthalmol.* 1996;121:706-708.
3. Davison JA. Capsular bag distension after endophacoemulsification and posterior chamber intraocular lens implantation. *J Cataract Refract Surg.* 1990;16:99-108.
4. Holtz SJ. Postoperative capsular bag distension. *J Cataract Refract Surg.* 1992;18:310-317.
5. Ota I, Miyake S, Miyake K. Whitish liquefied after cataract: a preliminary report. *Jpn J Ophthalmic Surg.* 1997;10:353-357.
6. Miyake K, Ota I, Miyake S. Liquefied after cataract: a complication of continuous curvilinear capsulorhexis and intraocular lens implantation in the lens capsule. *Am J Ophthalmol.* 1998;125:429-435.
7. Eifrig DE. Capsulorhexis-related lacteocrumenasia. *J Cataract Refract Surg.* 1997;23:450-454.

CHAPTER 78

Lens-Iris Diaphragm Retropulsion Syndrome

ROBERT J. CIONNI, MD

In 1992, Zauberman[1] first described a phenomenon characterized by deepening of the anterior chamber, dilation of the pupil, and bowing of the peripheral iris. In 1994, Wilbrandt and Wilbrandt[2] described this same phenomenon as the *lens-iris diaphragm retropulsion syndrome.* An excessively deep anterior chamber makes cataract surgery more challenging and may cause significant discomfort in patients undergoing phacoemulsification with only topical or intracameral anesthesia. The question, therefore, is how to proceed.

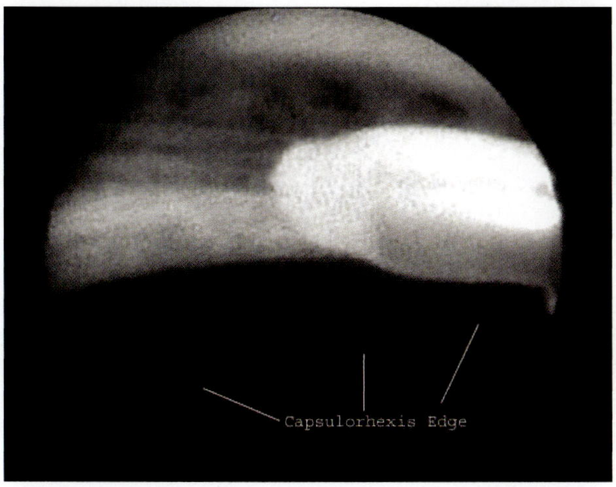

Figure 1. In this endoscopic view of reverse pupillary block, the iris' base is bowed posteriorly.

BACKGROUND

Early management options included (1) lowering the infusion bottle to reduce pressure in the anterior chamber and (2) adding a second infusion line with a chamber maintainer as well as lowering the infusion bottle in order to allow sufficient inflow at a lower pressure. The first option necessitates low flow and vacuum levels to prevent chamber collapse, and it results in a more volatile anterior chamber, which increases the risk of intraoperative miosis, damage to the iris, and posterior capsular rupture. The second option

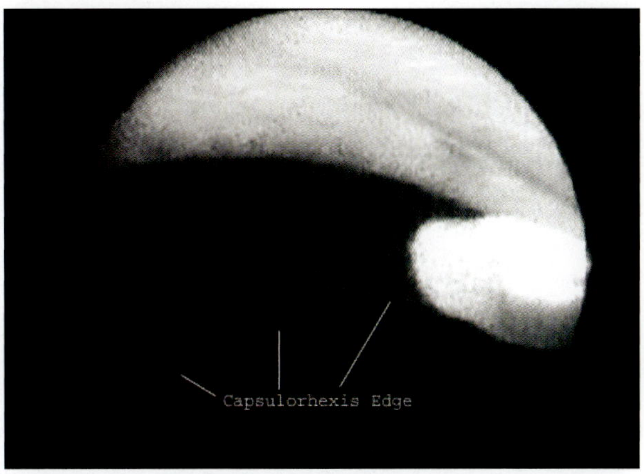

Figure 2. This endoscopic view shows that separating the iris from the anterior capsule with a silicone I/A tip breaks the reverse pupillary block and returns the iris to a more physiologic position and the anterior chamber to a normal depth.

decreases but does not eliminate chamber volatility. It requires a second infusion line, an additional incision, and the extra time involved to set up the chamber maintainer.

Over the last several years, it has become apparent that a reverse pupillary block causes lens-iris diaphragm syndrome, which begins when 360° of iridocapsular contact occurs. As a result of the subsequent pupillary block and infusion into the anterior chamber from an elevated irrigation bottle (high pressure), the iris and lens move posteriorly (Figure 1). In most instances, the zonules and ciliary body are strong enough to resist excessive posterior displacement, but certain conditions allow the iris and ciliary body to move backward, often to dramatic degrees. Some of the conditions that favor marked posterior displacement are youth, myopia, and previous vitrectomy.

MANAGEMENT

After identifying lens-iris diaphragm syndrome due to a reverse pupillary block, the surgeon can manage the complication by separating the iris from the anterior capsule's rim with the I/A tip (Figure 2), the phaco tip, or any available instrument. This step equalizes the pressure between the anterior and posterior chambers. Once this disparity in pressure is eliminated, the iris will immediately return to a more physiologic position, and the chamber will reassume a normal depth. Because the iris root and the zonules both attach to the ciliary body, the lens will also return to a more normal anatomic position.

Any degree of discomfort the patient was experiencing from the syndrome will dissipate when the chamber returns to a normal depth.[3] As this occurs, it is important for the surgeon to realize that the pupil will decrease in size. If the ciliary body has been stretched for a period of time, the pupil may begin to become more miotic, perhaps due to a release of prostaglandins upon stimulation of the ciliary body.

It is also likely that the reverse pupillary block will recur each time the surgeon initiates infusion anteriorly. For this reason, I often place a second instrument between the iris and the anterior capsule before starting infusion to prevent reverse pupillary block in an eye that shows a propensity for lens-iris diaphragm syndrome.

CONCLUSION

I find that certain viscoelastics such as Healon5 (Advanced Medical Optics, Inc., Santa Ana, CA) or generous amounts of Viscoat (Alcon Laboratories, Inc., Fort Worth, TX) make the occurrence of lens-iris diaphragm syndrome more common and more difficult to resolve, because they tend to encourage iridocapsular contact and resist the iris' forward displacement. This syndrome has plagued cataract surgeons for years. Realizing its etiology as a reverse pupillary block allows them to manage the problem easily. ■

This article originally appeared in the April 2005 issue of CRSToday.

1. Zauberman H. Extreme deepening of the anterior chamber during phacoemulsification. *Ophthalmic Surg.* 1992;23:555-556.
2. Wilbrandt HR, Wilbrandt TH. Pathogenesis and management of the lens-iris diaphragm retropulsion syndrome during phacoemulsification. *J Cataract Refract Surg.* 1994;20:48-53.
3. Cionni RJ, Barros MG, Osher RH. Management of lens-iris diaphragm retropulsion syndrome during phacoemulsification. *J Cataract Refract Surg.* 2004;30:953-956.

CHAPTER 79

Vitreous Hydration: Often a Hidden Complication of Cataract Surgery

ROBERTO BELLUCCI, MD

The recent introduction of low-power phacoemulsification surgery opened the way to cold phaco as a safer and gentler way to remove cataracts. In this surgical procedure, the lenticular material is primarily removed by the fluidics, and the phaco power is employed to help the first fragmentation and the removal of harder nucleus fragments. In some instances, as with softer cataracts, the phaco power is not used at all, and only mechanical fragmentation and high vacuum aspiration take place. At the beginning of the phacoemulsification era, fluidics was added to diminish heat and to remove the fragmented material. Now, phacoemulsification is added when the fluidics alone cannot remove hard cataracts (Table 1).

SOLUTIONS, NEW PROBLEMS

This surgical modality offers some solutions, mainly because of the reduced ultrasound use, but also poses new problems of fluidics setting and control. The vacuum level required to remove the lens material with minimal use of ultrasound often exceeds 400 mm Hg,

TABLE 1. PHACO SETTINGS WITH THE MILLENNIUM VENTURI (COMPARED: 2001 VS 2006)

Parameter	2001	2006
Vacuum max (mm Hg)	110	400
Ultrasound power (%)	40 continuous	10 micropulsed
Ultrasound equivalent phaco time (average, sec)	5 to 10	0 to 2
Bottle height (cm)	60	110

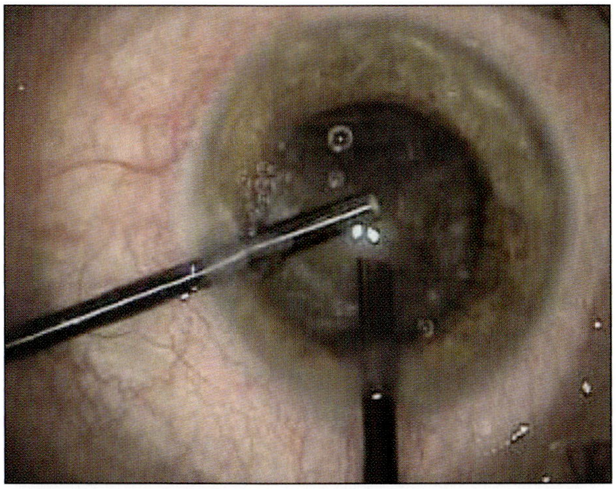

Figure 1. Bimanual phacoemulsification requires tight fluidics control with high pressure in the anterior chamber.

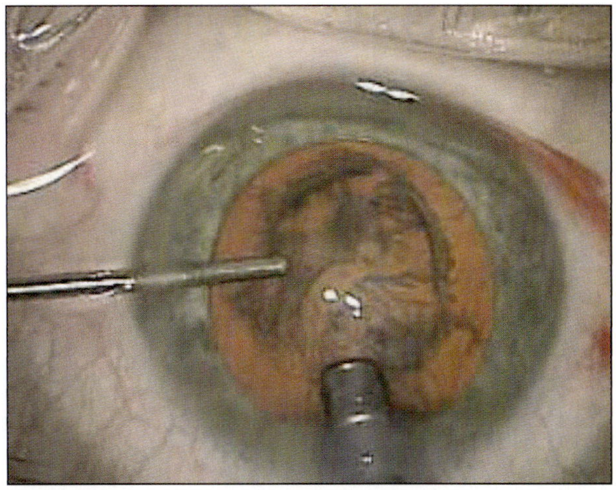

Figure 2. The first-generation Aqualase system involved fast fluid streams within the anterior chamber.

a level compatible with newer phaco machines but one that risks anterior chamber collapse with both pumps operating. With the Venturi pump (Millennium; Bausch & Lomb, Rochester, NY), a large amount of fluid is removed in a short time. With the peristaltic pump, the control of postocclusion surge becomes almost impossible. These difficulties are faced by continuously redesigning the fluidic part of the phaco machines, performing watertight corneal incisions and increasing the irrigation flux.

With some machines, an active air pump pressurizes the irrigation bottle to the desired level to allow the required irrigation in the anterior chamber. Thus, the increased fluid removal due to the high vacuum level (Venturi) or the abrupt postocclusion surge due to the high maximum vacuum selected (peristaltic) is efficaciously counteracted.

Increased bottle height, however, also increases anterior chamber pressure, especially with the watertight incisions that are suggested to avoid fluid leakage. We can easily observe a suddenly deepening anterior chamber occurring during surgery, frequently reduced when aspiration begins. This happens especially with weak zonules, and it is almost always the rule in highly myopic eyes. Increased pressure not only causes visibility loss due to defocusing, but may also promote fluid passing into the vitreous cavity through the zonules. Zonules are permeable to water, especially in older eyes, myopic eyes or in eyes that previously underwent vitreous surgery. The feasibility of pars plana vitrectomy using only anterior chamber irrigation in phakic and pseudophakic eyes has been demonstrated.[1]

DECREASE IN PRESSURE

The sudden decrease of anterior chamber pressure–occurring several times during phacoemulsification with high irrigation–further promotes vitreous hydration. Bimanual phacoemulsification with watertight incisions and lower irrigation ports is at special risk for this complication (Figure 1). This hydration can occur even when the pressure in the anterior chamber is not high but fast fluid streams take place. Large incisions with excessive leakage or the use of the first-generation Aqualase device (Alcon Laboratories, Inc., Fort Worth, Texas) are examples of such risk (Figure 2).

The iris represents a natural barrier against fluid's passage into the vitreous cavity. The iris is apposed to the peripheral lens, especially during earlier phacoemulsification procedures, and the

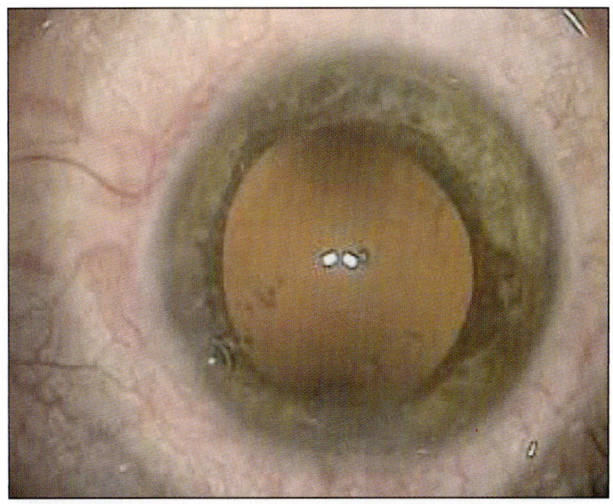

Figure 3. Same case as in Figure 1, showing small cortical fragments within the anterior vitreous, indicating fluid's passage through the zonules.

stimulated dilator muscle keeps the iris adherent. Using epinephrine in the irrigating solution helps dilator muscle contraction, counteracting vitreous hydration. Localized iris lifting with a surgical instrument can help fluid passage through the zonules in selected cases, such as eyes that underwent posterior vitrectomy before cataract surgery.[2] Vitreous hydration could be more evident in the floppy iris syndrome.[3]

THREE CONSEQUENCES

Vitreous hydration has three main consequences. The first is increased difficulty of cataract surgery, especially appearing during the last part of the phaco procedure. Because of posterior pressure due to increased vitreous volume, we find it difficult to enter the anterior chamber with the phaco tip. This problem is often faced by further increasing the bottle height and thus worsening the situation. In addition, small lens fragments pass into the vitreous cavity with irrigation fluid. The fragments can often be seen behind the posterior capsule, floating in the anterior vitreous. Patients frequently complain about increased vitreous floaters following cataract surgery; this may be due to invisible particles of lens material passing into the vitreous (Figure 3). In the worst cases, it can be difficult to implant the IOL, and even heavy viscoelastics may not be adequate to maintain enough space.

To minimize this problem, we should:

- Avoid extreme vacuum levels and–in general–extreme fluidic conditions;
- Avoid local anesthesia, as it can increase posterior vitreous pressure that must be counteracted with a stronger pressure in the anterior chamber;
- Fully dilate the iris with phenylephrine to help pupil block;
- Not pressurize the infusion bottle above the minimum required to maintain a deep enough anterior chamber. I usually start with 80 cm above a patient's head, immediately lowering if possible and especially lowering as phacoemulsification proceeds;
- Avoid watertight incisions to ensure a certain amount of fluid leakage that could reduce pressure spikes and sudden deepening/shallowing of the anterior chamber;
- Employ special care with highly myopic eyes (eyes known to be at risk for zonular distension); and
- Completely avoid high-speed fluid streams in the anterior chamber.

NEW AND EMERGING PROBLEM

Facing the era of refractive lens exchange, we need to recognize and avoid every cataract surgery complication. Vitreous hydration during surgery is a new and emerging problem, and it should be considered a potential complication of all surgeries. Even with a good surgical outcome, the postoperative presence of vitreous floaters is disappointing, both for the patient and for the surgeon. ■

This article originally appeared in the August 2006 issue of CRSToday.

1. One VPPV port for the treatment of epiretinal disorders: slit lamp and new anterior chamber maintainer (ACM). Presented at Vail Vitrectomy 2004. Vail, Colo. March 6-10, 2004.
2. Cheung CMG, Hero M. Stabilization of anterior chamber depth during phacoemulsification cataract surgery in vitrectomized eyes. *J Cataract Refract Surg.* 2005; 31:2055-2057.
3. Chang DF, Campbell JR. Intraoperative floppy iris sindrome associated with tamsulosin. *J Cataract Refract Surg.* 2005;31:664-673.

CHAPTER 80

The Final 2%

J. MICHAEL JUMPER, MD, AND H. RICHARD MCDONALD, MD

Cataract surgeons have many reasons to be proud. With constant refinements in technique and technology, theirs is the most successful of all surgical procedures in medicine. Most studies report an intraoperative complication rate in cataract surgery of less than 2%.[1] The reason to obsess over this final 2% is the same reason that there is a 98% "uncomplicated" rate.

The large volume of cataract surgery worldwide leads to such a rapid pace of innovation that the complications profile reported in the literature often differs from current practice. Regardless, knowing our history helps to avoid those pitfalls and to remind us that each new change or innovation in a surgical procedure may lead to an unforeseen problem. This article provides a brief overview of that final 2% in hopes of reducing that number.

COMPLICATIONS OF ANESTHETIC INJECTION

Anesthesia for cataract extraction has come full circle. Topical cocaine was replaced in the middle 20th century by retrobulbar injection anesthesia. Although the latter provides akinesia and excellent anesthesia, it risks perforation of the globe, injury to the optic nerve, damage to extraocular muscles, brainstem anesthesia, and orbital hemorrhage. Today, with a speedier procedure and greater control of the eye with phaco instruments, the trend of using topical with or without intracameral anesthesia has all but eliminated this risk.

The large-scale transition by cataract surgeons to topical anesthesia means that they now have less experience with the retrobulbar-injection anesthetic technique. We prefer peribulbar injections of anesthetic to retrobulbar injections. Our preferred intraoperative local anesthetic technique for vitreoretinal surgery is an injection into the sub-Tenon's space with a blunt cannula after a small conjunctival/Tenon's cut-down under topical anesthesia.

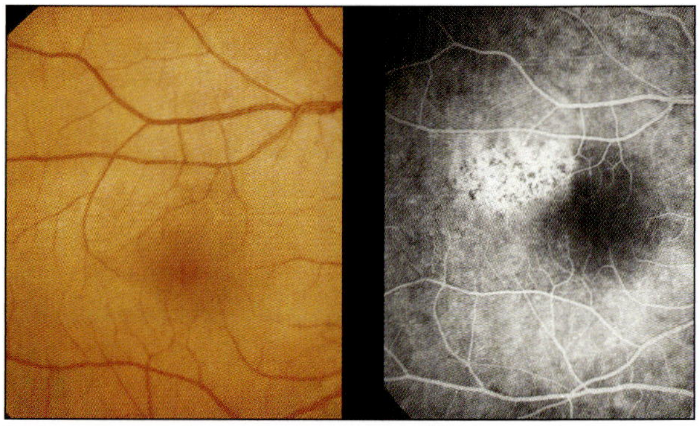

Figure 1. Microscope phototoxicity produces minimal pigmentary stippling, which is only obvious with fluorescein angiography.

MICROSCOPE PHOTOTOXICITY

The first case of retinal phototoxicity undoubtedly occurred shortly after the operating microscope's first use for cataract extraction, although it was nearly 30 more years before this complication was fully recognized.[2] Light toxicity occurs in 3% to 7% of cataract cases. The duration of light exposure correlates with the risk of injury, although phototoxicity has even been reported in cases lasting just 11 minutes.[3] The early finding of deep retinal whitening, with or without serous retinal detachment, resolves during the first 48 hours after surgery, and it is replaced by mottling of the retinal pigment epithelium during the next several weeks. These pigmentary changes may only be visible with fluorescein angiography as a window defect (Figure 1). Patients often complain of a paracentral scotoma but may be asymptomatic. Vision loss can be profound if the injury includes the foveola.

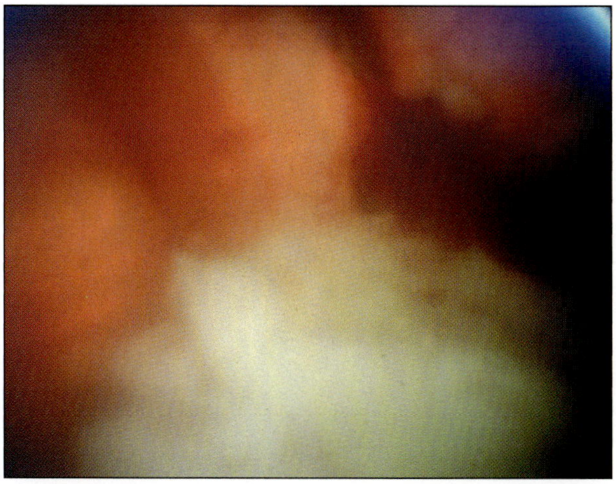

Figure 2. Cataract extraction in a patient with pseudoexfoliation left the lens nucleus and blood in the vitreous cavity.

The most powerful tool in preventing phototoxicity is recognizing that every eye surgeon using any form of illumination may cause this complication. Although no single maneuver has proven 100% effective in avoiding light damage, limiting exposure time and intensity to that which is necessary, using some form of a light shield when possible, and properly filtering the delivered light are simple steps we should all remember.

RETAINED LENS MATERIAL

A primary cause of the final 2% complication rate for cataract surgery is the disruption of the lens capsule or zonules, which can displace lens fragments or the lens implant into the vitreous cavity (Figure 2). This complication occurs more often after phacoemulsification than other forms of cataract extraction. The early recognition of capsular rupture, the use of intracameral viscoelastic, and a careful anterior vitrectomy can prevent excessive traction on the vitreous base and the loss of lenticular fragments into the vitreous cavity. For anterior vitrectomy, we recommend a limbal entry for the vitreous cutter and a separate infusion line, both away from the cataract incision. It is best to avoid heroic maneuvers to rescue a falling lens fragment.

Larger nuclear lens fragments left in the eye are not well tolerated, and surgeons should remove them at a convenient time after the initial cataract surgery.[4] Although even a small amount of lenticular material can cause a severe inflammatory reaction and/or the elevation of IOP, fragments that are less than 20% of the total lens volume may be tolerated in the vitreous cavity and may be carefully observed. Pars plana vitrectomy for retained lens fragments can reduce IOP and improve patients' vision, but the outcome remains guarded because of a higher risk of cystoid macular edema, suprachoroidal hemorrhage, and retinal detachment in these individuals.[5]

Suprachoroidal Hemorrhage

Intraoperative suprachoroidal hemorrhage has become less frequent due to ophthalmologists' transition to small-incision, closed-system cataract surgery.[6] This devastating complication is often preceded by transient hypotony and choroidal effusion. Reported risk factors include advanced age, obesity, glaucoma, high myopia, cardiovascular disease, hypertension, anticoagulation therapy, and intraoperative tachycardia.[7] Surgeons should be aware of the signs of intraoperative suprachoroidal hemorrhage, including a sudden increase in pain, a darkening of the red reflex, a shallowing of the anterior chamber, and a forward prolapse of the posterior ocular structures.

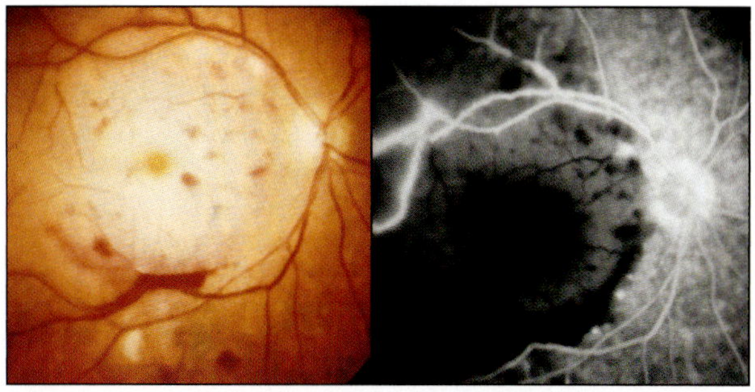

Figure 3. Retinal whitening and a cherry-red spot, which corresponds to a loss of all retinal blood flow, from gentamicin toxicity caused macular infarction.

It is imperative to close the cataract incision rapidly to prevent an expulsive choroidal hemorrhage. Subsequent management strategies are controversial. Some practitioners advocate immediate posterior-drainage sclerotomies in hopes of decreasing IOP and enabling further postoperative drainage. Secondary surgery for further drainage is reserved for those patients with appositional choroidals or macular involvement, and the procedure is timed to coincide with liquefaction of the blood, typically 7 to 14 days postoperatively.

For choroidal drainage, we isolate the rectus muscles with silk ties for better exposure. After placing infusion via the limbus with a self-retaining anterior chamber maintainer, we perform a radial scleral cut-down of 4mm in length, approximately 5mm from the limbus, in the quadrants with hemorrhage. Manipulating the sclerotomy's edges can increase flow and help clear larger clots. We use indirect ophthalmoscopy to verify an adequate removal of blood. The visual prognosis is guarded, especially in those cases requiring reoperation.

Aminoglycoside Retinal Toxicity

Even when properly administered at the intended dose, the intraocular injection of aminoglycoside antibiotics (gentamicin sulfate or amikacin) can lead to macular infarction.[8] Damage is thought to be due to a localized increase in the drug's concentration in the dependent area of the retina, typically the macula (Figure 3). Despite the excellent gram-negative coverage and cost effectiveness of these drugs, we feel that they should never be used in intraocular surgery. Ceftazidime is a safer alternative for endophthalmitis care and infectious prophylaxis.

CONCLUSION

The superior outcomes of modern cataract extraction are the envy of all other ophthalmic surgeons. Constant refinement has, in most cases, made the procedure so painless and rapid that the patient forgets its invasiveness and the potential risks involved. It is our job to gently remind both the patient and ourselves that problems can and do occur. We hope that the final 2% approaches zero with time. ■

This article originally appeared in the August 2005 issue of CRSToday.

1. Masket S, Fine IH, Kidwell TP, et al. Cataract in the adult eye. AAO Preferred Practice Patterns. Washington, DC: American Academy of Ophthalmology; 2001.
2. McDonald HR, Irvine AR. Light-induced maculopathy from the operating microscope in extracapsular cataract extraction and intraocular lens implantation. *Ophthalmology.* 1983;90:945-951.
3. Kleinmann G, Hoffman P, Schechtman E, Pollack A. Microscope-induced retinal phototoxicity in cataract surgery of short duration. *Ophthalmology.* 2002;109:334-338.
4. Kim JE, Flynn HW Jr., Smiddy WE, et al. Retained lens fragments after phacoemulsification. *Ophthalmology.*1994;101:1827-32.
5. Scott IU, Flynn HW Jr, Smiddy WE, et al. Clinical features and outcomes of pars plana vitrectomy in patients with retained lens fragments. *Ophthalmology.* 2003;110:1567-1572.
6. Ling R, Cole M, James C, et al. Suprachoroidal haemorrhage complicating cataract surgery in the UK: epidemiology, clinical features, management, and outcomes. *Br J Ophthalmol.* 2004;88:478-480.
7. Speaker MG, Guerriero PN, Met JA, et al. A case-control study of risk factors for intraoperative suprachoroidal expulsive hemorrhage. *Ophthalmology.* 1991;98:202-209.
8. Campochiaro PA, Lim JI. Aminoglycoside toxicity in the treatment of endophthalmitis. The Aminoglycoside Toxicity Study Group. *Arch Ophthalmol.* 1994;112:48-53.

CHAPTER 81

What Retinal Surgeons Want You to Know

RAHUL PATEL, MD, AND SUBER S. HUANG, MD, MBA

Complications happen to even the most experienced cataract surgeon. Effectively managing intraoperative problems stabilizes the eye, prevents the development of further complications, and prepares the patient for retinal surgery and visual recovery. To this end, you must pay special attention to (1) wound integrity and corneal clarity, (2) the capsulorhexis, (3) the IOL and management of retained intravitreal fragments, (4) postoperative care, and (5) effective communication with patients about complications, management, and expectations.

WOUND INTEGRITY AND CORNEAL CLARITY

In the event of intraoperative complications that may require surgical retinal management, you must seal the wound margin and test its integrity. Using stromal hydration alone may prove inadequate during vitreous surgery. A vertical mattress suture is especially useful in optimizing the wound's integrity in the event of a wound burn.[1] Limbal and sclerocorneal incisions may cause severe chemosis that can interfere with the trocar's placement in 25-gauge pars plana vitrectomy.

Meticulously ensure that no adherent vitreous strands are present at the inner margin of the wound. Gently sweep the wound with a cyclodialysis spatula to check for and relieve vitreous traction. Vitreous incarceration may cause corneal decompensation (reducing clarity for future retinal surgery), and it provides a pathway for exogenous bacteria. Moreover, peripheral retinal traction may lead to retinal breaks, and macular traction from iridovitreal adhesions is a suggested mechanism of cystoid macular edema.[2]

Bullous keratopathy can arise from endothelial dysfunction, elevated IOP, and tears in Descemet's membrane. It requires aggressive treatment. Options for treating tears in Descemet's membrane include observation, the irrigation of the paracentesis wound, the injection of viscoelastic to unroll and reattach Descemet's membrane, the placement of full-thickness sutures, and the use of air or an SF6 gas bubble. Severe corneal opacification may require a delay of retinal surgery or the use of a keratoprosthesis.[1,3]

CAPSULORHEXIS

The ideal size of the continuous curvilinear capsulorhexis has not been established. Zonular integrity, the size of the selected IOL's optic, the cataract's maturity, and the phaco technique are common factors that influence the surgeon's choice on the capsulorhexis' diameter. Nonetheless, a small continuous curvilinear capsulorhexis significantly impairs peripheral retinal visualization.[4] The early detection and accurate localization of all retinal breaks allow their prompt treatment and are critical for successful retinal detachment surgery. Peripheral visualization facilitates laser therapy and the management of retinal vascular disease.

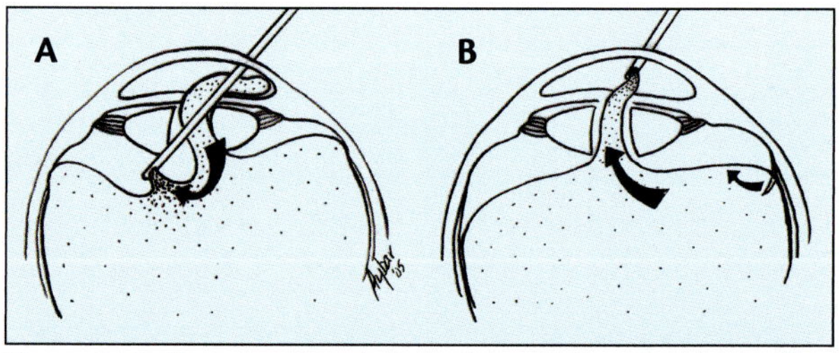

Figure 1. In the correct technique for anterior vitrectomy, the cutter posterior to the iris removes vitreous from the anterior chamber with minimal traction (A). Incorrect technique can produce traction on the vitreous base and a retinal tear (small arrow) (B).

Drawbacks to a large continuous curvilinear capsulorhexis include an increased incidence of posterior capsular opacification and decentered or dislocated IOLs. Moreover, it impedes the surgeon's ability to place a sulcus-fixated IOL in the event of a large posterior capsular tear.[1,4] The benefits of a large (> 6mm), well-centered capsulorhexis in facilitating future retinal examinations and treatment cannot be overstated, however. You must weigh the pros and cons of a larger continuous curvilinear capsulorhexis in patients who may need future retinal care.

SELECTING AN IOL

The ideal lens implant is safe, optimizes the patient's vision, and helps to stabilize the eye. A large continuous curvilinear capsulorhexis allows the placement of an IOL with a large optic, which facilitates visualization of the peripheral retina. Consider larger IOLs in patients with risk factors for retinal detachment, including vitreous loss, high myopia, lattice degeneration, trauma, and a history of retinal detachment/tear.[4] The choice of IOL material also merits careful consideration, especially in diabetic patients or others at risk for future vitrectomy. In 2004, one-third of all IOLs placed during cataract surgery were silicone-based.[5] Silicone IOLs develop fogging from water vapor during air-fluid exchange with intraocular gases such as perfluoropropane and SF6.[6,7] Condensation significantly reduces the ophthalmologist's ability to view the retina during retinal surgery. The use of viscoelastic and manual cleaning of condensation off the IOL are required to improve visualization, but the effect is suboptimal and transient.[6,7]

An acrylic or PMMA lens is recommended for patients who are likely to need vitreoretinal procedures. In cases of retinal surgery requiring silicone oil, droplets may adhere to the posterior surface of a silicone IOL and be difficult to remove, even after removal of the silicone oil. Retained oil may predispose the eye to secondary glaucoma and further diminish visual acuity.[8,9]

MANAGING RETAINED INTRAVITREAL LENS FRAGMENTS

The posterior dislocation of lenticular material into the vitreous is an infrequent but frustrating complication of cataract surgery. Remember that attempts to retrieve dislocated fragments may create retinal traction. During an anterior vitrectomy, the initial cutting and aspiration of vitreous must begin behind the plane of the iris (Figure 1A) to reduce the chance of transpupillary anterior traction on the vitreous base, retinal tear, or retinal detachment (Figure 1B). Refer cases with nuclear fragments that are greater than 25% to 33% of the original lens' size without heroically attempting their retrieval. Observation may be appropriate in cases with smaller fragments (less than 25%). All eyes should undergo aggressive medical therapy.[10,11]

CONTROLLING IOP AND INFLAMMATION

In the event of an intraoperative complication that may require an urgent referral to a retina specialist, immediately work to control the patient's IOP and inflammation. The aggressive use of viscoelastics is common in the setting of a posterior capsular tear with lost nuclear fragments. After inserting the IOL, perform thorough I/A of the eye to ensure the removal of all viscoelastic. The failure to do so will contribute significantly to elevated IOP postoperatively. Uncontrolled IOP worsens corneal clarity and hinders visualization of the posterior segment. Likewise, aggressively treat inflammation to help avoid elevated IOP, prevent cystoid macular edema, reduce pain, and decrease the likelihood of the eye's developing proliferative vitreoretinopathy if a retinal detachment occurs.[12,13]

REFERRAL AND COMMUNICATION

Patients with endophthalmitis or a retained intravitreal lens fragment and coexisting retinal detachment require urgent evaluation and prompt treatment by a posterior segment surgeon. The exact timing of vitrectomy for retained fragments without retinal detachment is less well defined. Margherio et al reported an increased incidence of retinal detachment associated with cases of delayed vitrectomy.[10,14] In another study, 57% of patients who underwent immediate vitrectomy had a final visual acuity of 20/40 or better compared with 78% of those who underwent vitrectomy within 1 week.[10,15] There is no conclusive evidence that vitrectomy performed on the same day of cataract surgery results in a better visual outcome than surgery within 2 weeks.[11,12,15]

Timely and effective communication between you, the patient, and the retinal specialist is vital to ensuring the continuity of care, reassuring the patient, and setting realistic expectations. The discussion and planning of appropriate triage, acute management, and clinical and surgical details, all affect the surgical approach of the retinal specialist. In the setting of a subluxated or dislocated IOL, a knowledge of areas of zonular weakness helps the retinal specialist to place the IOL properly or to avoid dislodging one with tenuous security.[10,12,13] Written documentation of findings and clinical events may be invaluable to the posterior segment surgeon.

Most important is maintaining the patient's trust. The vitreoretinal specialist will be much more able to earn the confidence of one who is well informed. An excellent relationship with the patient will facilitate his visual rehabilitation and minimize medicolegal ramifications that may surface.

SUMMARY

Individualize each patient's surgical plan according to his refractive needs and the ocular findings. Consider techniques that optimize peripheral retinal visualization in patients who are at risk for corneal opacification or peripheral retinal disease or those who may require retinal surgery. If complications occur, recognizing the importance of wound integrity and media clarity and meticulously managing acute events will afford the retinal specialist the best opportunity to provide a rapid and uneventful recovery. Prompt referral and effective communication reassure the patient and enhance the likelihood of a satisfactory outcome. ■

This article originally appeared in the August 2005 issue of CRSToday.

1. Ernest PH, Fine IH, Fishkind WJ. Complications of wound construction and closure. In: Fishkind WJ, ed. *Complications of Phacoemulsification: Avoidance, Recognition, and Management.* New York, NY: Thieme Medical Publishing; 2002:28-35.
2. Harbour JW, Smiddy WE, Rubsamen PE, et al. Pars plana vitrectomy for chronic pseudophakic cystoid macular edema. *Am J Ophthalmol.* 1995;120:302-307.
3. Arbisser LB. Managing intraoperative complications in cataract surgery. *Curr Opin Ophthalmol.* 2004;15:33-39.
4. Tennant MT, Connolly BP. Cataract surgery in patients with retinal disease. *Curr Opin Ophthalmol.* 2002;13:19-23.
5. Health Products Research 2004. PCIOL design in United States: preferred material in U.S. In: Cataract phacoemulsification course materials. Fort Worth, TX: Alcon Laboratories, Inc.; 2004.
6. Eaton AM, Jaffe GJ, McCuen BW II, Mincey GJ. Condensation on the posterior surface of silicone intraocular lenses during fluid-air exchange. *Ophthalmology.* 1995;102:733-736.
7. Carlson AN, Stewart WC, Tso PC. Intraocular lens complications requiring removal or exchange. *Surv Ophthalmol.* 1998;42:417-437.
8. Khawly JA, Lambert RJ, Jaffe GJ. Intraocular lens changes after short- and long-term exposure to intraocular silicone oil. *Ophthalmology.* 1998;105:1227-1233.
9. Kusaka S, Kodama, Ohashi Y. Condensation of silicone oil on the posterior surface of a silicone intraocular lens during vitrectomy. *Am J Ophthalmol.* 1996;121:574-576.
10. Monshizadeh R, Samiy N, Haimovichi R. Management of retained intravitreal lens fragments after cataract surgery. *Surv Ophthalmol.* 1999;43:397-411.
11. Blodi BA, Flynn HW Jr, Blodi CF, et al. Retained nuclei after cataract surgery. *Ophthalmology.* 1992;99:41-44.
12. Fastenburg DM, Schwartz PL, Shakin JL, Golub BM. Management of dislocated nuclear fragments after phacoemulsification. *Am J Ophthalmol.* 1991;112:535-539.
13. Borne MJ, Tasman W, Regillo C, et al. Outcomes of vitrectomy for retained lens fragments. *Ophthalmology.* 1996;103:971-976.
14. Margherio RR, Margherio AR, Pendergast SD, et al. Vitrectomy for retained lens fragments after phacoemulsification. *Ophthalmology.* 1997;104:1426-1432.
15. Tommila P, Immonen I. Dislocated nuclear fragments after cataract surgery. *Eye.* 1995;9:437-441.

CHAPTER 82

Triamcinolone-Assisted Anterior Vitrectomy

SCOTT E. BURK, MD, PhD; ANDREA P. DA MATA, MD; ROBERT H. OSHER, MD; AND ROBERT J. CIONNI, MD

Vitreous gel, transparent by design, is virtually invisible under the operating microscope. Furthermore, it is particularly unwelcome in anterior segment surgery, because it makes surgery more difficult and is associated with a variety of serious intraoperative and postoperative complications such as a dropped lens fragment, corneal edema, cystoid macular edema, retinal detachment, and endophthalmitis.[1-14] Fortunately, meticulous vitreous clean-up can reduce the incidence of many vision-threatening complications associated with vitreous loss.[9] Until recently, however, surgeons had only indirect intraoperative clues to determine if vitreous gel were present in the anterior chamber and, if so, to what extent.

Triamcinolone acetonide (Kenalog; Bristol-Myers Squibb Company, New York, NY) has proven quite useful for visualizing vitreous in the anterior chamber[15] and has become a routine part of our practice for complicated cataracts with large zonular dialyses. To date, we have performed more than 200 cases of triamcinolone-assisted anterior vitrectomy and have not seen a complication attributable to the agent. On the contrary, eyes receiving intracameral triamcinolone have a quieter postoperative course versus those in which the agent is not used.

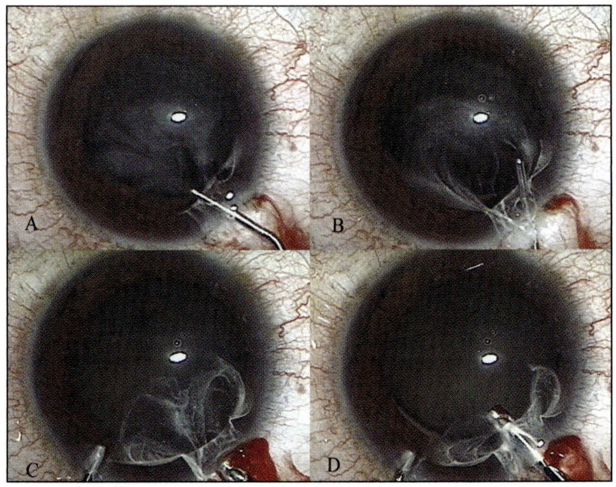

Figure 1. The surgeon injects triamcinolone acetonide into the prolapsed vitreous (A and B) and then performs an anterior vitrectomy (C and D). Note the vitreous present in the wound at the time of injection.

PREPARATION

We continue to prepare triamcinolone as originally described[15] and remove the preservative by a sterile capture-and-wash technique. Our decision is based on a lack of data regarding the intracameral effects of benzyl alcohol, the preservative in Kenalog. Clearly, however, our original washing technique is a bit tedious, particularly when the encounter with vitreous is unexpected or the OR staff is unfamiliar with the technique.

It is therefore not surprising that one of the most common questions regarding intracameral triamcinolone is, "Can the preparation be simplified?" There are actually several options (and wide variation among surgeons) that range from using the agent directly out of the bottle to simple dilution. Others fill a syringe with triamcinolone, stand it inverted until the particles settle, express the vehicle, and resuspend the triamcinolone particles in the desired volume of BSS. In addition, compounding pharmacies sell preservative-free triamcinolone, but it has a limited shelf life.

TECHNIQUE

When asked the best way to use triamcinolone, the answer is not to lose vitreous in the first place. The next best answer is to get lots of practice. Neither reply is practical for most surgeons, who instead must gain insight from the experience of others. Here at the Cincinnati Eye Institute, we typically withdraw 0.2 mL of 40 mg/mL triamcinolone acetonide, then wash and resuspend the agent in 2.0mL of BSS (10X dilution). Much higher concentrations tend to leave too much unbound triamcinolone in the anterior chamber, whereas a larger volume of a lower concentration of triamcinolone tends to distribute the particles more evenly.

Ideally, one injects the agent directly within the substance of the vitreous to obtain maximum visualization. Dusting the surface of the gel works, but only until one has removed the surface, at which point reinjection is necessary. Dr. Burk likes to swirl a little triamcinolone around the anterior chamber to get an overview of the situation. He then buries the cannula's tip within the gel and makes a very controlled injection. It is important to remember that, if the vitreous is near the wound and fluid comes out upon the injection, so will vitreous. Inserting the cannula through the paracentesis often avoids such reflux. Vitrectomy should be performed with a high cutting rate, a low aspiration rate, and separate irrigation. Although not always needed, a pars plana approach can be quite helpful, particularly for vitreous at the site of the corneal incision (Figure 1).

ALTERNATIVES

Realizing that the vitreous gel will capture and hold nearly any particulate matter, some groups are evaluating alternative techniques of vitreous identification. The most notable is 11-deoxycortisol, a steroid precursor without glucocorticoid effects.[16]

Nonetheless, we prefer triamcinolone acetonide because it is readily available, is nontoxic,[17-19] and has a 25-year track record for intraocular use since it was first described in 1980 by Tano et al.[20] In addition, one should not underestimate the role of intracameral triamcinolone in stabilizing the blood-aqueous barrier and minimizing inflammation on postoperative day one in complicated anterior segment cases.

QUESTIONS

To date, two questions about triamcinolone-assisted vitrectomy are unresolved. As mentioned earlier, the first regards the method of preparation and the effects of the benzyl alcohol preservative. The use of preservative-free or washed triamcinolone makes intuitive sense, but we are unaware of any evidence suggesting that the removal of the benzyl alcohol preservative is helpful or necessary.

The second question relates to the probability of steroid-induced glaucoma. It is well known that our vitreoretinal colleagues observe increased IOP after the depot injection of an intraocular steroid. Indeed, the amount of steroid deposited correlates with the percentage of patients experiencing elevated IOPs and with the severity of the rise in pressure.

Although it is certainly possible that an eye will develop glaucoma after undergoing triamcinolone-assisted anterior vitrectomy, we have not observed this complication. Furthermore, the risk of steroid-induced glaucoma seems to be minimal when the surgeon uses a small amount of triamcinolone and then removes most of it along with the vitreous gel that was identified. In summary, we have found triamcinolone acetonide to be safe and quite useful for identifying and removing vitreous. ■

This article originally appeared in the April 2005 issue of CRSToday.

1. Shah DP, Krishnan AA, Albanis CV, et al. Visual acuity outcomes following vitreous loss in glaucoma and diabetic patients. *Eye.* 2002;16:271-274.
2. Tan JH, Karwatowski WS. Phacoemulsification cataract surgery and unplanned anterior vitrectomy—is it bad news? *Eye.* 2002;16:117-120.
3. Ionides A, Minassian D, Tuft S. Visual outcome following posterior capsule rupture during cataract surgery. *Br J Ophthalmol.* 2001;85:222-224.
4. Chitkara DK, Smerdon DL. Risk factors, complications, and results in extracapsular cataract extraction. *J Cataract Refract Surg.* 1997;23:570-574.
5. Berrod JP, Sautiere B, Rozot P, Raspiller A. Retinal detachment after cataract surgery. *Int Ophthalmol.* 1996-1997;20:301-308.
6. Frost NA, Sparrow JM, Strong NP, Rosenthal AR. Vitreous loss in planned extracapsular cataract extraction does lead to a poorer visual outcome. *Eye.* 1995;9(pt 4):446-451.
7. Banker AS, Freeman WR. Retinal detachment. *Ophthalmol Clin North Am.* 2001;14: 695-704.
8. Drolsum L, Haaskjold E. Causes of decreased visual acuity after cataract extraction. *J Cataract Refract Surg.* 1995;21:59-63.
9. Spigelman AV, Lindstrom RL, Nichols BD, Lindquist TD. Visual results following vitreous loss and primary lens implantation. *J Cataract Refract Surg.* 1989;15:201-204.
10. Balent A, Civerchia LL, Mohamadi P. Visual outcome of cataract extraction and lens implantation complicated by vitreous loss. *J Cataract Refract Surg.* 1988;14:158-160.
11. Berger BB, Zweig KO, Peyman GA. Vitreous loss managed by anterior vitrectomy. Long-term follow-up of 59 cases. *Arch Ophthalmol.* 1980;98:1245-1247.
12. Kanski JJ, Ramsay JH. Vitrectomy techniques in the management of complications in cataract surgery. *Trans Ophthalmol Soc UK.* 1980;100(pt 1):216-218.
13. Mamo JG. Late effects of vitreous loss. *Ann Ophthalmol.* 1974;6:935-941.
14. Ruiz RS, Teeters VW. The vitreous wick syndrome. A late complication following cataract extraction. *Am J Ophthalmol.* 1970;70:483-490.
15. Burk SE, Da Mata AP, Snyder ME, et al. Visualizing vitreous using Kenalog suspension. *J Cataract Refract Surg.* 2003;29:645-651.
16. Kaji Y, Hiraoka T, Okamoto F, et al. Visualizing the vitreous body in the anterior chamber using 11-deoxycortisol after posterior capsule rupture in an animal model. *Ophthalmology.* 2004;111:1334-1339.
17. McCuen BW 2nd, Bessler M, Tano Y, et al. The lack of toxicity of intravitreally administered triamcinolone acetonide. *Am J Ophthalmol.* 1981;91:785-788.
18. Hida T, Chandler D, Arena JE, Machemer R. Experimental and clinical observations of the intraocular toxicity of commercial corticosteroid preparations. *Am J Ophthalmol.* 1986;101:190-195.
19. Young S, Larkin G, Branley M, Lightman S. Safety and efficacy of intravitreal triamcinolone for cystoid macular oedema in uveitis. *Clin Experiment Ophthalmol.* 2001; 29:2-6.
20. Tano Y, Chandler D, Machemer R. Treatment of intraocular proliferation with intravitreal injection of triamcinolone acetonide. *Am J Ophthalmol.* 1980;90:810-816.

CHAPTER 83

Early Thoughts on Triesence

ROBERT H. OSHER, MD; LISA BROTHERS ARBISSER, MD; AND TODD GOTHARD, MD

ROBERT H. OSHER, MD

When Triesence (triamcinolone acetonide injectable suspension) 40 mg/mL (Alcon Laboratories, Inc., Fort Worth, TX) was first approved by the FDA, I was fortunate to investigate its capability for visualizing vitreous in a cadaver eye study designed to enhance surgeons' understanding of the dropped nucleus (Figure 1). My colleagues and I deliberately tore the posterior capsule and tested multiple hypotheses by using Triesence in order to determine the role of the vitreous. The results of the study were quite astonishing (RHO, unpublished data, 2008), and the video was awarded prizes at the ASCRS, ESCRS, and AAO 2008 annual meetings. I believe the study would have been much less revealing, however, had we not been so lucky to obtain the Triesence from Alcon Laboratories, Inc.

Vitreous staining in the anterior segment is not new. In fact, Scott Burk, MD, PhD, one of my previous fellows and a current associate, published the concept in 2003.[1] Subsequently, he and his wife, Andrea Da Mata, MD, produced an award-winning video in the ASCRS film competition that also appears in the *Video Journal of Cataract Surgery*.[2] The major advantage of Triesence is that the triamcinolone acetonide is not preserved, which makes it safer in the eye. The suspension can also be prepared quickly should the surgeon encounter an unexpected complication involving vitreous. It is my early opinion that Triesence will become a useful aid to anterior segment surgery.

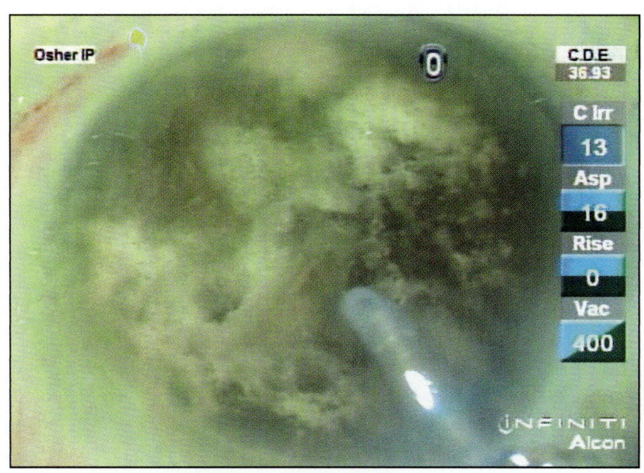

(Courtesy of Robert H. Osher, MD.)

Figure 1. This cadaver eye study shows a nuclear fragment suspended on Triesence-stained vitreous.

LISA BROTHERS ARBISSER, MD

During complicated cataract surgery, or when an anterior vitrectomy is planned in a complex case, vitreous can be a challenge to visualize and therefore to remove properly. Our key goal in these cases is to minimize intraoperative and postoperative traction on the vitreous. Although there is a host of remote signs of vitreous loss such as a peaked pupil and poorly sealing incisions, we now have a valuable tool to assist us in providing the best outcomes for these challenging surgical adventures.

Suggested by Gholam Peyman, MD, for posterior segment surgery and popularized by Dr. Burk for the anterior segment, the particulate identification of prolapsed vitreous with triamcinolone acetate suspension has proven highly effective. The commercially available preparation, Kenalog (Bristol-Myers Squibb Co., Princeton, NJ) is only provided in a preserved vehicle, which works well for the posterior segment. Because the preservatives are not endothelium-friendly, however, Dr. Burk worked out a method to "wash" the Kenalog and resuspend it in balanced salt solution by using filter needles.[1]

Triesence is a time saver and ever at the ready without any preservatives and without the chemical, which may also have toxic potential, that keeps Kenalog dispersed in the suspension. Triesence need not be washed. Like Kenalog, it can be irrigated into the anterior chamber when the surgeon suspects prolapsed vitreous with the effect of throwing a sheet over a ghost; it allows the surgeon to visualize the vitreous. Both products have a beneficial anti-inflammatory therapeutic effect during the postoperative period in addition to their intraoperative diagnostic use. Triesence, which tends to clump more than Kenalog, is best diluted 10 or 15 to one in balanced salt solution. This dilution allows the particles to be individually trapped in the vitreous matrix without a white-out effect, which makes it hard to see the intraocular structures. Like Kenalog, Triesence will rinse out of aqueous and not adhere to viscoelastic but will stick to the vitreous. That allows a critical visual endpoint for anterior vitrectomy and reduces the likelihood that the surgeon will see a strand of vitreous to the incision (an unwanted surprise) at the slit lamp during the postoperative examination.

TODD GOTHARD, MD

I have used Triesence on a number of complex anterior segment cases, and I have found it useful in the determination of both whether vitreous was present in the anterior chamber and when the vitreous was completely cleared during vitrectomy. The suspension can be reinjected several times to help the surgeon ensure vitreal clearance or monitor progress during vitrectomy.

I have found Triesence extremely useful during cases of Descemet's stripping automated endothelial keratoplasty that have positive pressure. I use the solution to determine if vitreous has come forward through a capsulotomy or around the lens.

The cornea is usually edematous in Descemet's stripping automated endothelial keratoplasty cases, and Triesence can facilitate visualization of the vitreous, even with a cloudy cornea.

I use this suspension routinely for all complicated refractive lens exchange procedures that require a vitrectomy. This dye takes the guesswork out of these cases and eliminates the possibility of residual postoperative vitreal strands. Using Triesence is much more convenient than having to filter other commercial preparations and worry about residual preservatives and possible toxic anterior segment syndrome. ■

This article originally appeared in the November 2008 issue of CRSToday.

1. Burk SE, Da Mata AP, Snyder ME, et al. Visualizing vitreous using Kenalog suspension. *J Cataract Refract Surg.* 2003;29(4):645-651.
2. Burk SE, Da Mata AP, Snyder ME, et al. Identifying the vile humor. *Video Journal of Cataract Surgery.* 2002;18(4).

CHAPTER 84

Point/Counterpoint: Should Anterior Segment Surgeons Perform Pars Plana Anterior Vitrectomy?

Yes, this approach may save time and minimize complications.

LOUIS D. "SKIP" NICHAMIN, MD

The single most significant complication today's phaco surgeon faces is a ruptured posterior capsule with vitreous loss. Fortunately, in the setting of small-incision surgery, by adhering to certain fundamental principles and employing proper instrumentation and surgical technique, the ophthalmologist can generally achieve an outcome that differs little from that of an uncomplicated case. I believe that adopting a pars plana approach for the vitrectomy is paramount to achieving such results.

GUIDING PRINCIPLES

The guiding principles for managing a posterior capsular tear with vitreous loss include quickly recognizing the problem, avoiding hypotony, and maintaining a truly closed-chamber environment. Because watertight incisions are therefore essential, the surgeon may employ a much lower flow rate and volume of infusion to reduce intraocular turbulence. To further enhance control of the intraocular environment and reduce vitreoretinal traction, the

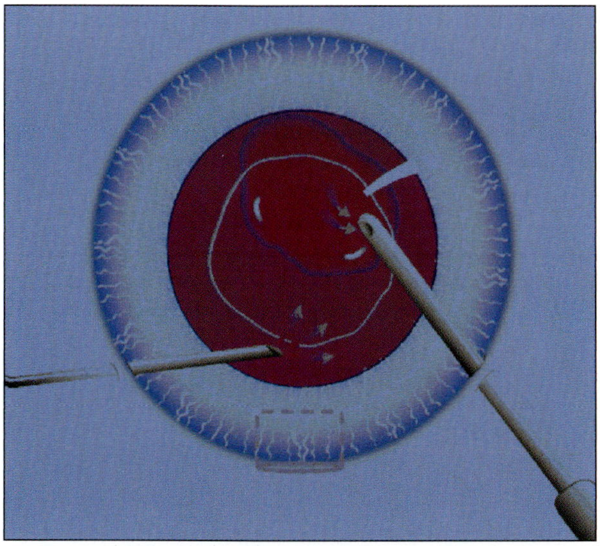

Figure 1. The author performs bimanual vitrectomy through limbal incisions. (Reprinted with permission from Chang DF. *Phaco Chop: Mastering Techniques, Optimizing Technology, and Avoiding Complications*. Thorofare, NJ: Slack Incorporated; 2004.)

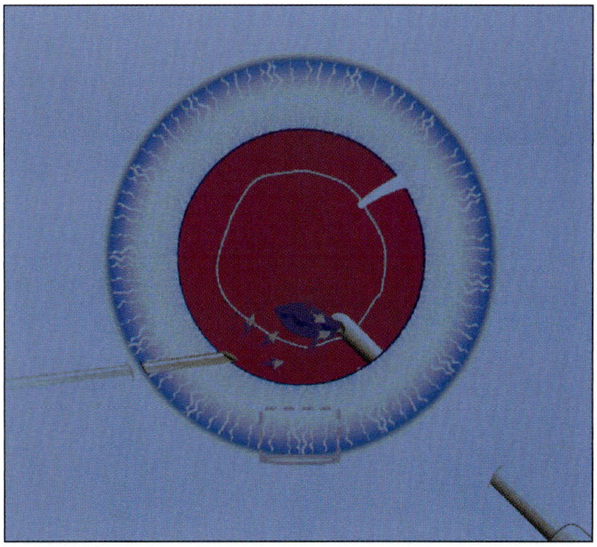

Figure 2. The author performs bimanual vitrectomy with a vitreous cutter placed through the pars plana incision. (Reprinted with permission from Chang DF. *Phaco Chop: Mastering Techniques, Optimizing Technology, and Avoiding Complications*. Thorofare, NJ: Slack Incorporated; 2004.)

surgeon should perform a separated or bimanual vitrectomy. This technique displaces the location and vector force of the infusion from the point where he attempts to delicately remove vitreous. Although a reasonable approach is to place both instruments through limbal incisions (Figure 1), I submit that a much more efficient and potentially safer approach is to perform the vitrectomy through a pars plana incision (Figure 2). This technique allows the surgeon to pull down prolapsed vitreous from the anterior chamber and thereby markedly reduce the amount of vitreous that he removes from the eye. Because working from the limbus to raise vitreous makes finding an endpoint much more difficult, the surgeon often unintentionally removes a considerable portion of the vitreous body and must then deal with a hypotonous eye.

Another significant advantage to working through a pars plana incision is the enhanced access it offers to residual lenticular material. Cortex, epinucleus, and even nuclei of medium density may be removed with the vitrectomy instrument by gradually increasing vacuum and reducing the cutting rate. When addressing vitreous, the surgeon uses the highest cutting rate with the lowest possible vacuum rate that permits tissue removal. This approach achieves more complete cleaning and reduces secondary complications such as increased IOP, inflammation, and cystoid macular edema.

MINIMAL LEARNING CURVE

Obviously, the surgeon must exercise care and effort when learning any new surgical technique, but the pars plana approach is actually quite straightforward. Typically, the surgeon first incises the conjunctiva and applies light cautery at the site of the intended sclerotomy (although some surgeons will incise directly through the conjunctiva). He should avoid the cardinal meridia due to their increased vascularity. Given that the posterior capsule is open, the surgeon may place the infusion through a limbal paracentesis or a second incision in the pars plana. He should select the clock hour of the vitrectomy incision that offers the best access to the remaining lenticular material.

TECHNICAL PARTICULARS

The pars plana is anatomically located 3 to 4 mm posterior to the limbus, so the surgeon usually places the incision 3.5 mm from the limbus, although he may make an adjustment for unusual axial lengths. Depending upon his preference, he creates wounds to accommodate either 19- or 20-gauge instruments. The surgeon should use dedicated, disposable microvitreoretinal blades to create properly sized and therefore watertight incisions for both pars plana and limbal incisions. To create the pars plana incision, the ophthalmologist holds the microvitreoretinal blade perpendicular to the scleral surface and usually orients it in a nonradial fashion. He directs the blade toward the center of the globe with a simple in-and-out motion.

In general, when removing vitreous, the surgeon should use the highest possible cutting rate along with the lowest possible vacuum setting. He may increase vacuum and lower the cutting rate in order to remove remaining lenticular material. The infusion should be minimal, just enough to maintain an adequate volume of the globe.

The surgeon should carefully clean and close the pars plana incision with either 9–0 nylon or 8–0 Vicryl (Ethicon Inc., Somerville, NJ) sutures. Recently, 25-gauge instrumentation has become available that, in some settings, may allow for sutureless surgery. Normal insertion, however, requires a firm globe. Although the surgeon could use these instruments in a complicated setting by creating small incisions with a sharp blade—as opposed to the usual trochar system—they lack tensile rigidity and therefore compromise the ophthalmologist's ability to manipulate the position of the globe.

PRACTICE MAKES PERFECT

Prudence dictates that a surgeon not first perform a pars plana vitrectomy when under duress but rather after carefully studying the technique and practicing it in the laboratory. In this way, he may obtain the most propitious outcome from a daunting complication of cataract surgery. ■

No, they likely lack the necessary training and/or equipment.

J. MICHAEL JUMPER, MD

With the proper training and equipment, anterior segment surgeons are clearly capable of performing pars plana anterior vitrectomy. Why they should not relates to several important aspects of safe vitreous surgery: proper viewing, minimized traction, and a careful inspection of the peripheral retina to identify and treat retinal breaks.

VISUALIZATION

Whereas anterior segment surgery uses coaxial illumination, vitreoretinal surgery mainly employs endoillumination. Intraocular lighting is required because a nonaxial light is often the only way for the surgeon to see the translucent vitreous. Also, coaxial light from the microscope does not penetrate well beyond the iris plane in the best of circumstances, and it is less effective with corneal edema, pupillary miosis, or intraocular hemorrhage—all of which may be encountered in complicated cataract cases. Techniques such as the intracameral injection of triamcinolone acetonide and the use of a fiber-optic light pipe held near the limbus can help the surgeon identify vitreous in the anterior chamber, but these methods are inferior to intraocular illumination.

Also, during pars plana vitrectomy surgery, the surgeon should observe the retina with a contact or noncontact lens system in order to assess and react to the collapse of the eye, a potential problem when aspiration overcomes infusion. Most anterior segment surgeons have little experience with such handheld or microscope-mounted retinal viewing systems.

TRACTION AND INSPECTION

When vitreous is lost during cataract surgery, a retinal tear and detachment may result from increased traction on the retina with the forward movement of the vitreous. This traction can be exacerbated by maneuvers of any kind within the vitreous that are not associated with cutting. Thus, phacoemulsifying lenticular fragments attached to the vitreous and inserting instruments into the vitreous to lift lenticular fragments increase traction as well as the risk of a retinal tear.

The incidence of retinal detachment after vitrectomy (by vitreoretinal surgeons) for retained lenticular fragments is between 6% and 16%.[1] In my experience, large tears can occur with seemingly minimal traction on the vitreous base. Conversely, maneuvers that I would expect to cause a retinal tear often do not. As a result, I routinely inspect the entire retina with indirect ophthalmoscopy and scleral depression in order to identify retinal tears or dialyses. If I identify a retinal break, I treat the surrounding attached retina with a laser or cryotherapy. The early identification of a retinal break is critical to preventing retinal detachment and vision loss. If retinal detachment surrounds the retinal break, further vitrectomy, retinopexy, and fluid-gas exchange with or without scleral buckling are necessary. I feel that anyone who performs a pars plana vitrectomy should at least be able to identify and treat retinal breaks. ORs used by anterior segment surgeons may not have the necessary equipment.

TECHNICAL MODIFICATIONS

Instead of the pars plana approach, I was taught as a resident to perform an anterior vitrectomy by placing the vitreous cutter with its infusing sleeve through the cataract wound and to cut until I no longer saw peaking of the pupil. I now realize that this technique is inefficient and ineffective. First, the infusion sleeve on the cutter makes the instrument's diameter quite large, and the location of the infusion can reduce the cutter's ability to engage vitreous. Second, placing the infusion/cutter through the leaking cataract wound allows more vitreous to flow out of the wound and increases the risk of vitreous incarceration. Third, indirect evidence of vitreous removal (observing the pupil) is no substitute for directly seeing the vitreous.

Separating the infusion from the cutting results in a more effective anterior vitrectomy. One technique is to attach the infusion line to a bent needle, which is inserted into the anterior chamber through the limbus. This approach allows the smaller, sleeveless cutter to enter through a watertight limbal or pars plana incision. The recently developed 25-gauge vitreous cutter has been used for anterior vitrectomy.[2] This potentially important application of the technology may become popular if more phaco machines include 25-gauge vitrectors.

CONCLUSION

Cataract surgery is extremely successful, and the rates of vitreous loss are correspondingly low (1% to 3%).[3] In the 10 to 20 times per year that the busiest anterior segment surgeon would be expected to perform an anterior vitrectomy, he should choose the simplest and safest technique. Although it makes sense to place the vitrectomy cutter through the pars plana, a limbal approach may be equally effective in most cases. The questions, however, that all anterior segment surgeons need to ask themselves are (1) whether they have the training and equipment to do the job safely and effectively and (2) more importantly, do they possess the expertise to identify and treat the retinal breaks that will inevitably occur? ■

This article originally appeared in the April 2005 issue of CRSToday.

1. Scott IU, Flynn HW Jr, Smiddy WE, et al. Clinical features and outcomes of pars plana vitrectomy in patients with retained lens fragments. *Ophthalmology.* 2003;110:1567-1572.
2. Chalam KV, Shah VA. Successful management of cataract surgery associated vitreous loss with sutureless small-gauge pars plana vitrectomy. *Am J Ophthalmol.* 2004;138:79-84.
3. Masket S, Fine IH, Kidwell TP, et al. *Preferred Practice Patterns: Cataract in the Adult Eye.* San Francisco: American Academy of Ophthalmology; 2001.

CHAPTER 85

Is Endophthalmitis on the Rise?

MEHRAN TABAN, MD

Of the numerous advances in the field of cataract surgery during the last half of the 20th century, the introduction of sutureless phacoemulsification using clear corneal incisions has affected the field most significantly. With its efficient technique, minimal rate of surgically induced trauma, shortened operative times, low induction of astigmatism, limited postoperative inflammatory response, and fast postoperative recovery, sutureless, clear corneal cataract extraction has steady gained acceptance among cataract surgeons since its introduction in 1992.[1] In the most recent survey of ASCRS members, Leaming et al[2] reported that the clear corneal incision and the sutureless techniques are preferred by 72% and 92% of US surgeons, respectively.

During the last decade, however, reports have indicated that the incidence of endophthalmitis after cataract surgery may be on the rise, and some have speculated about whether the complication is associated with clear corneal incisions.[3,4] Although the greater rate of infection may primarily be due to increased antibacterial resistance, the absence of a reported increase in endophthalmitis following other intraocular surgeries (penetrating keratoplasty, trabeculectomy, etc.) during this period and the proliferation of aseptic surgical techniques challenge this argument. Other factors therefore must be carefully investigated, and the sutureless clear corneal incision technique remains a possible candidate.

LITERATURE REVIEW AND LABORATORY INVESTIGATION

In 2000, Colleaux and Hamilton[3] reported a two-and-a-half times greater incidence of endophthalmitis following cataract extraction with a sutureless, clear corneal incision relative to a scleral tunnel incision. More recently, Nagaki et al[4] reported an almost sixfold greater risk in endophthalmitis associated with clear corneal incisions compared with sclerocorneal incisions. A recent review of the English-language literature presented at the 2003 AAO annual meeting analyzed more than 200 studies (comprising over 3 million cataract surgeries) that addressed endophthalmitis after cataract extraction between 1963 and 2003.[5] When the study period was split into two sets, prior to and after 1992, a gradual but noticeable increase was apparent after 1992, when the technique of clear corneal incision was introduced. In a comparison of types of incision from 1992 to 2003, a significantly higher risk of endophthalmitis occurred with clear corneal incisions compared to either scleral or limbal incisions (an increase in relative risk of two-and-a-half and three times, respectively).

Two studies conducted in cadaveric rabbit and human eyes may help to explain the etiology of the apparent association between endophthalmitis and clear corneal incisions. One using optical coherence tomography showed the possibility of corneal wound gaping secondary to IOP variations in both human and rabbit eyes.[6] Similarly, investigators using the Miyake viewing technique in cadaveric human eyes showed an ingress of extraocular India ink or fluid following IOP variations.[7] In the latter study, four of seven eyes showed the intraocular presence of ink, after standard external manipulation in three eyes and after IOP variation alone in the fourth. These studies demonstrated a possible mechanism by which microorganisms gain access into the intraocular space during the critical early postoperative period, when the wound has not yet healed.

CONCLUSION

Endophthalmitis remains one of the most feared complications of ocular surgery. Although this review of the literature suggests that the pattern of endophthalmitis after cataract surgery is associated with the introduction and increased use of the clear corneal incision, there is no proof of a causal relationship, and inevitable bias (positive or negative) is evident in the literature. Only a large, multicenter, prospective, randomized study can answer the question of the cause of endophthalmitis after cataract surgery. In the meantime, careful wound construction with a minimal tolerance for wound leakage, the placement of sutures whenever necessary, and continued vigilance in the surveillance of infection are necessary. ■

This article originally appeared in the February 2005 issue of CRSToday.

1. Fine IH. Clear corneal incisions. *Int Ophthalmol Clin.* 1994;34:59-72.
2. Leaming DV. Practice styles and preferences of ASCRS members—2003 survey. *J Cataract Refract Surg.* 2004;30:892-900.
3. Colleaux KM, Hamilton WK. Effect of prophylactic antibiotics and incision type on the incidence of endophthalmitis after cataract surgery. *Can J Ophthalmol.* 2000;35:373-378.
4. Nagaki Y, Hayasaka S, Kadoi C, et al. Bacterial endophthalmitis after small-incision cataract surgery. Effect of incision placement and intraocular lens type. *J Cataract Refract Surg.* 2003;29:20-26.
5. Taban M, Behrens A, Mewcomb RL, et al. Incidence of acute endophthalmitis following cataract surgery or penetrating keratoplasty: a meta-analysis. Paper presented at: The 107th Annual Meeting of the AAO; November 18, 2003; Anaheim, CA.
6. McDonnell PJ, Taban M, Sarayba MA, et al. Dynamic morphology of clear corneal cataract incisions. *Ophthalmology.* 2003;110:2342-2348.
7. Sarayba MA, Taban M, Ignacio TS, et al. Inflow of ocular surface fluid through clear corneal cataract incisions: a laboratory model. *Am J Ophthalmol.* 2004;138:206-210.

CHAPTER 86

Clear Corneal Incisions and Endophthalmitis

I. HOWARD FINE, MD; RICHARD S. HOFFMAN, MD; AND MARK PACKER, MD

There is no doubt that the incidence of infectious endophthalmitis after cataract surgery has increased. Most frequently quoted are the retrospective study by Cooper et al[1] and the prospective study by Nagaki et al.[2] Another certainty is that the use of clear corneal incisions has risen recently. The transition from scleral tunnel to clear corneal incisions involves a learning curve, during which time the surgeon may experience an increased rate of complications. The question to be addressed, therefore, is whether the rising use of clear corneal incisions is causing the increase in cases of endophthalmitis following cataract surgery.

BACTERIAL RESISTANCE

It is important to take into account the change in bacterial resistance to antibiotics (Figure 1). Gram-positive organisms are overwhelmingly responsible for postoperative endophthalmitis: 69% of patients with bacterial endophthalmitis were culture positive, and 94% of the infectious agents were gram-positive organisms.[3] In 1997 and 1998, 100% of the organisms associated with postcataract surgery endophthalmitis were sensitive to the fluoroquinolones then available (Figure 2). By 1999, only 20% remained sensitive, and 100% of those organisms were resistant to the existing fluoroquinolones by 2001.[4] The growing resistance of microorganisms to antibiotics certainly has some bearing on the increased rate of endophthalmitis.

Two Swedish reports[5,6] in 2002 cited the lowest level of endophthalmitis ever despite an increased use of clear corneal incisions. The findings are probably a result of the use of prophylactic intracameral cefuroxime at the close of surgery. These reports provide further evidence of the significant role that antibiotics play in the prevention of bacterial endophthalmitis.

PERSONAL EXPERIENCE

Although we use only clear corneal incisions, we have not encountered a single case of infectious endophthalmitis in more than 9 years and 8,000 cases. Rather than good luck, we believe our experience is due to our attention to detail.

A recent dye study by McDonnell et al[7] in cadaver eyes demonstrated that, in the presence of hypotony, clear corneal incisions tend to draw India ink into the incision. Shingleton et al[8] reported that 20% of the patients examined 2 hours postoperatively had IOPs of less than 10mmHg. Dr. Fine found a 15% similar incidence in his own practice (unpublished data). Of extreme importance is the fact that neither Shingleton et al nor Dr. Fine have experienced an increased incidence of endophthalmitis in spite of immediate postoperative hypotony, which McDonnell et al[7] hypothesized was the cause of an increased incidence of endophthalmitis.

DETAILS THAT MATTER

Preparing the Eye

We apply 5% povidone-iodine (Betadine; Purdue Frederick, Stamford, CT) to the ocular area, and we use Steristrips to evert the eyelashes so that they are flush against the skin and the meibomian gland's orifices are exposed. After draping the eye, we place a wick in the lateral canthus to disallow the pooling of fluid.

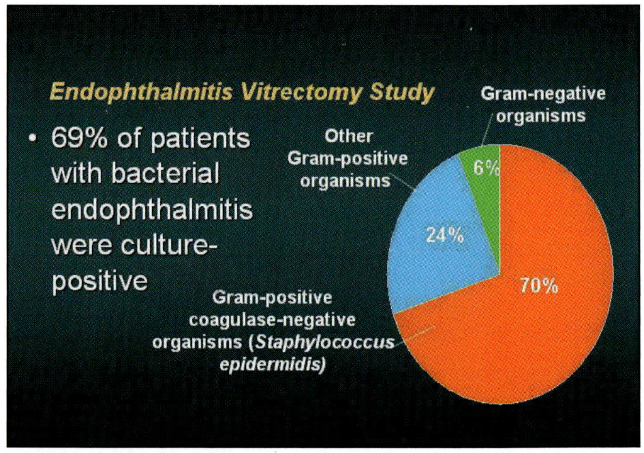

(Courtesy of James McCulley, MD.)

Figure 1. This chart illustrates the types of endophthalmitis encountered after cataract surgery.[3]

Creating the Incision

Rather than incising the steep axis, we create incisions at the temporal corneal periphery in order to address astigmatism and postoperatively neutralize the pressure effects of blinking and gravity. When indicated, limbal relaxing incisions address preoperative astigmatism.

Replacing aqueous with viscoelastic stabilizes the eye and firms the anterior chamber. This technique also permits us to construct incisions reproducibly, because the eye does not become unpredictably distorted due to hypotony.

To create the incision, we applanate the trapezoidal knife against the surface of the globe with the point just anterior to the conjunctival insertion. The knife is advanced in the plane of the cornea for 2 mm and then directed through Descemet's membrane, into the anterior chamber. We then advance the knife until the internal incision's width is the appropriate size, usually indicated by the width of the shoulders of the tip.

We prefer single-plane incisions, which create better architecture for valve structure than do grooved incisions and maximize endothelial pumping, because there is no opening in the corneal-epithelial fluid barrier. We use trapezoidal incisions, which we can enlarge for IOL implantation by advancing the trapezoidal knife farther into the eye without compromising the architecture of the incision. We avoid side-cutting knives, which can alter the incision's architecture and are frequently inaccurate with respect to the final width of the incision. All cataract incisions should be at least 2 mm long and no more than 2.5 to 3.5 mm wide.

Surgical technique is crucial to the incision's integrity. We never

(Courtesy of Francis Mah, MD.)

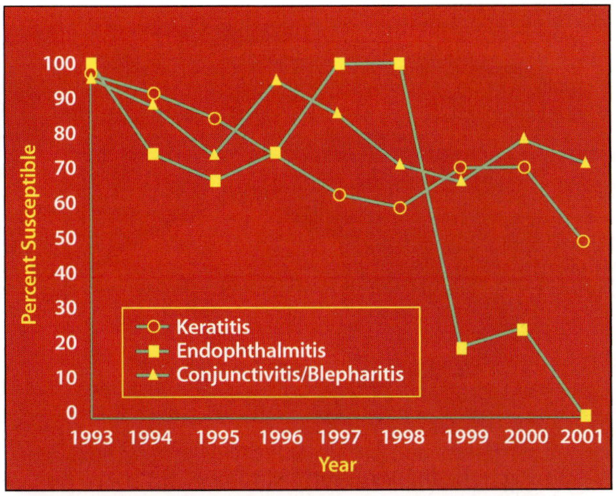

Figure 2. This graph demonstrates the current need for fourth-generation fluoroquinolones and focuses on the in vitro susceptability of *Staphylococcus aureus*.[4]

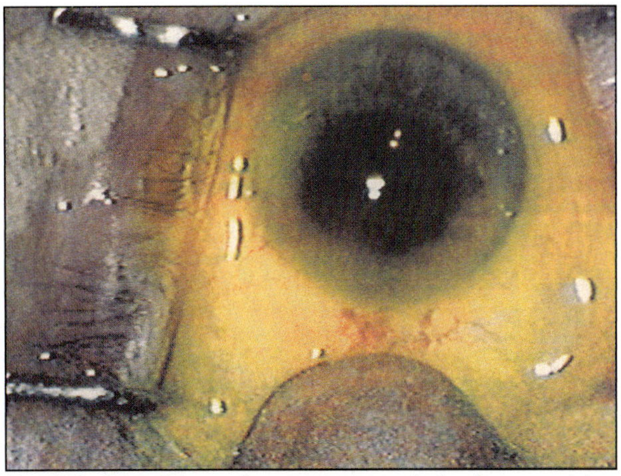

Figure 3. One of the authors tests the seal of a clear corneal incision at the conclusion of surgery.

grasp the superior lip with a forceps, because this instrument can abrade the epithelium and cause a loss of the fluid barrier. Instead, we lift the roof of the incision from its floor with a cannula in order to insert an instrument such as a pupil dilator or an injector for a capsular tension ring. We prefer beveled phaco tips, which we insert bevel down by pushing against the floor of the incision and insinuate into the eye. During phacoemulsification, power modulations protect the eye against thermal injuries, which can compromise the integrity and sealing of the incision.

Implanting the IOL

IOL implantation should occur through adequately and precisely enlarged incisions. Stretching the incision aggressively can negatively affect its ability to seal. When stabilizing the eye with a fixation ring, injection systems are far superior to folding forceps, which require a larger incision and distort the wound further.

Sealing the Incision

We perform stromal hydration of the main and sideport incisions by filling the eye to physiologic pressures or slightly higher without ever overpressurizing the eye. The patient wears a soft contact lens if the epithelium located over the incision is abraded. We suture the incision whenever necessary and always test for leakage. It is important to recognize the importance of endothelial pumping and proper architectural features that allow for mechanical stability. To test for leakage, we place fluorescein stain on the eye and press the posterior lip of the incision with a finger (Figure 3). Many of the studies showing an incision's inability to seal are based on pinpoint pressure.[9,10] This technique is completely nonphysiologic and irrelevant; a patient would have to press on his eye with something the size of a pencil's point. Moreover, pinpoint pressure can cause a paracentesis, although hypersquare, to leak, but no one questions the safety of this type of incision.

Using Antibiotics

Our patients receive a fourth-generation fluoroquinolone q.i.d. for 3 days preoperatively, at least q.i.d. on the surgical day, and q.i.d. for 10 days postoperatively. We believe it would not be unreasonable to administer this antibiotic q2h on the day of surgery and perhaps even on the first postoperative day.

CONCLUSION

Clear corneal incisions offer many benefits, including safety and efficacy, but successful outcomes require a surgeon's attention to detail, as described herein. That stated, ophthalmologists should use the incision that they can perform with the most reproducibly safe results. ■

This article originally appeared in the February 2005 issue of CRSToday.

1. Cooper BA, Holekamp NM, Bohigian G, Thompson PA. Case-control study of endophthalmitis after cataract surgery comparing scleral tunnel and clear corneal wounds. *Am J Ophthalmol.* 2003;136:300-305.
2. Nagaki Y, Hayasaka S, Kadoi C, et al. Bacterial endophthalmitis after small-incision cataract surgery: effect of incision placement and intraocular type. *J Cataract Refract Surg.* 2003;29:20-26.
3. Han DP, Wisniewski SR, Wilson LA, et al. Spectrum and susceptibilities of microbiologic isolates in the Endophthalmitis Vitrectomy Study. *Am J Ophthalmol.* 1996;122:1-17.
4. Kowalski RP, Karenchak LM, Romanowski EG. Infectious disease: changing antibiotic susceptibility. *Ophthalmol Clin North Am.* 2003;16:1-9.
5. Montan PG, Wejde G, Setterquist H, et al. Prophylactic intracameral cefuroxime: evaluation of safety and kinetics in cataract surgery. *J Cataract Refract Surg.* 2002;28:982-987.
6. Montan PG, Wejde G, Koranyi G, Rylander M. Prophylactic intracameral cefuroxime: efficacy in preventing endophthalmitis after cataract surgery. *J Cataract Refract Surg.* 2002;28:977-981.
7. McDonnell PJ, Taban M, Sarayba M, et al. Dynamic morphology of clear corneal incisions. *Ophthalmology.* 2003;110:2342-2348.
8. Shingleton BJ, Wadhwani RA, O'Donoghue MW, et al. Evaluation of intraocular pressure in the immediate period after phacoemulsification. *J Cataract Refract Surg.* 2001;27:524-527.
9. Ernest PH, Lavery KT, Kiessling LA. Relative strength of scleral corneal and clear corneal incisions constructed in cadaver eyes. *J Cataract Refract Surg.* 1994;20:626-629.
10. Ernest PH, Fenzl R, Lavery KT, Sensoli A. Relative stability of clear corneal incisions in a cadaver eye model. *J Cataract Refract Surg.* 1995;21:39-42.

CHAPTER 87

Preventing Endophthalmitis

RANDALL J. OLSON, MD

After a perfectly performed cataract procedure with excellent results on the first postoperative day, it is disheartening when the patient returns with signs of increased inflammation likely to be endophthalmitis (Figure 1). Although cataract surgeons have come a long way in treating endophthalmitis, severe organisms such as *Streptococcus* and *Pseudomonas* species still routinely devastate final visual acuity. Even more benign bacteria will often negatively affect results.

As clear corneal surgery became common practice, the incidence of endophthalmitis increased. Because new approaches or technology are so often greeted by pessimism, it is easy to dismiss critics' complaints as a normal reaction to change. My colleagues and I adopted clear corneal surgery with great enthusiasm, and it became our predominant technique by mid-1996. Clear corneal surgery in combination with topical anesthesia allows for a prompt return of vision without sutures.

Our experience with endophthalmitis is no different than others' in that the complication is rare but often occurs in clusters, making it nearly impossible to gauge the actual incidence. As a result, we began a prospective, quality-control study on endophthalmitis in 1997.

In early 2001, we concluded that our incidence of endophthalmitis was increasing dramatically from a historical rate that we calculated as less than 1 in 1,000 cataract surgeries. We had enough data to know this increase was not simply a cluster of events. Furthermore, we had no cases of endophthalmitis in patients who had corneal-scleral incisions. All of the incidents of endophthalmitis occurred in patients with clear corneal incisions. Nevertheless, we know many ophthalmologists across the country, myself included (I have not had a single case of endophthalmitis after cataract surgery), who state that they have not had a problem with clear corneal surgery during their career. How to make sense of the seeming conflict of data and personal reports was a major and important research step that we decided we must undertake.

CAUSES OF ENDOPHTHALMITIS

Choice of Surgery and Lens

Many studies have suggested an increase in endophthalmitis with clear corneal incisions. Nagaki et al[1] conducted a prospective, randomized, clinical trial comparing the difference between clear corneal and corneal-scleral incisions, the difference between using silicone and acrylic lenses, and the relation of incision and lens type to the incidence of endophthalmitis. This study, which included more than 12,000 surgeries, is definitive in addressing both surgical and lens choices. The results showed a statistically significant increase in the incidence of endophthalmitis in association with clear corneal surgeries (0.29% vs 0.05%; P=.037), but the investigators did not find a difference between silicone and acrylic lenses. It is virtually impossible to refute their study, and the only conclusion that I can make is that clear corneal surgery can dramatically increase the incidence of endophthalmitis. The operative word is *can*, not will.

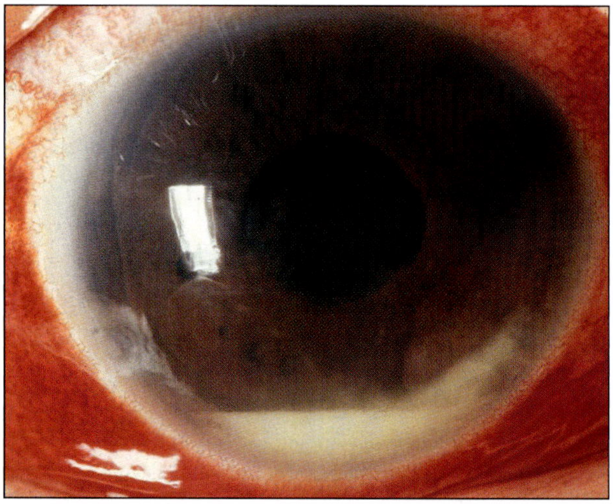

Figure 1. A patient presents with endophthalmitis after cataract surgery.

Cataract Surgery Incisions

In their landmark work, Taban et al[2] studied how wounds behave under pressure using eye-banked eye preparations. They demonstrated that a long incision, which my colleagues and I have always considered the strongest, is very resistant to elevated IOP. However, long incisions can sometimes gape and leak with a low IOP compared with incisions that are more perpendicular to the surface of the eye. The latter type of incision, or short incisions, will leak with an elevated IOP, but they actually seal better with a low IOP. Taban et al[2] studied further and used India ink as a bacterial model because its particle size is similar to that of bacteria. They found that, as the IOP increased, even long incisions resistant to leakage gaped externally and allowed the India ink to enter the wound. Additionally, as the IOP dropped, there was the potential for an internal gape that theoretically could result in bacteria's entering the anterior chamber, although the IOP never dropped to zero and there was never obvious leakage (Table 1). One criticism of this study is that the investigators used dead tissue without living endothelial cells; certainly, if the endothelial pump had been intact, it would have secondarily sealed the wound and possibly avoided some of the leakage associated with their findings.

Clear Corneal Surgery

The study by Taban et al[2] combined with our own results as well as those of Nagaki et al[1] point to the fact that microleaks after cataract surgery are more common in patients who undergo clear corneal surgery, at least some of the time. In addition, the increased risk of leakage with attendant contamination is why some ophthalmologists are seeing more cases of endophthalmitis. A definitive study to prove that thesis would be extremely difficult to create, but the circumstantial evidence seems sufficient.

It is important for ophthalmologists to understand that the risk of endophthalmitis is not guaranteed to be higher with clear

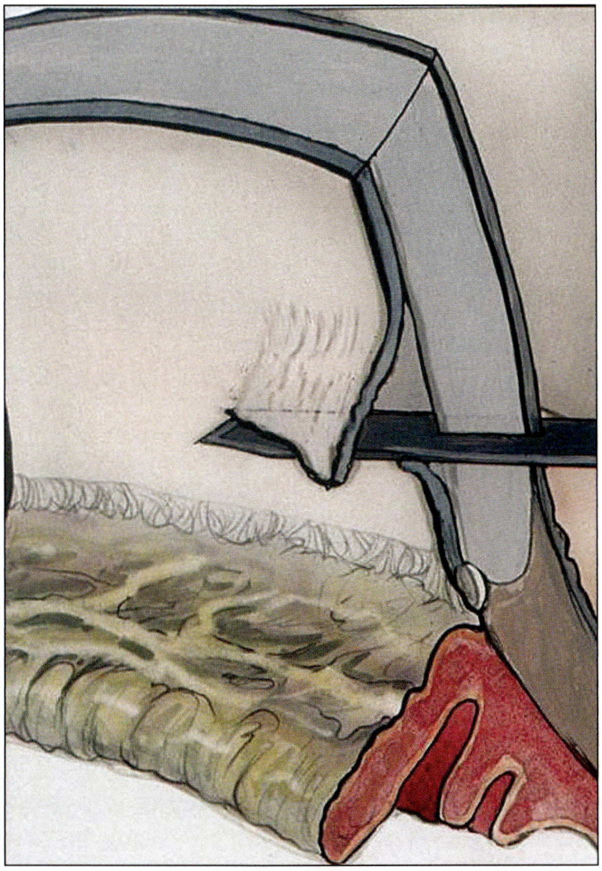

Figure 2. A dull keratome can induce a small, single tear of Descemet's membrane.

corneal surgery but that the incisions themselves are very unforgiving. I believe the reasons why some ophthalmologists have not encountered a rise in their rates of endophthalmitis are their careful attention to detail and their suturing of any marginal wounds, which are more likely to leak than those that are well constructed.

Wounds

Marginal wounds require careful scrutiny. In my experience, they are generally related to a small tear in Descemet's membrane, overstretching and internal tearing, or an external tear, all of which dramatically decrease the IOP/leakage curve.

A small tear in Descemet's membrane can occur at any time during cataract surgery and usually starts at the wound internally and runs back toward the limbus. The tear will leave a portion of Descemet's membrane and endothelium that can flap back and forth during irrigation, but, because it is located under the wound, the tear can often go unnoticed (Figure 2). I always irrigate through the stab incision, because I can often see the torn flap moving as the irrigation passes. Irrigation can frequently bring the torn flap into apposition with the cornea. I believe that all such cases require a suture.

Although some cataract surgeons may consider it overkill, I feel that the closure of the wound requires both a mechanically correct incision and the secondary sealing action of the endothelial pump. As outlined by Taban et al,[2] relying on the mechanical nature of the wound alone is risky. Even though ophthalmologists worry about early elevated postoperative IOP, Shingleton et al[3] clearly showed that significant hypotony (frequently 5 mm Hg) often occurs after surgery. Low pressure is as much a concern as high pressure. A well-constructed wound without an active endothelial pump is a risk I am not willing to take.

Internal tearing or stretching of the wound typically occurs when cataract surgeons force instruments or a lens through a wound that is too small. At the conclusion of surgery, some of the structures may be torn, and the wound may not come together nicely. I do not believe that these indications necessarily require the placement of a suture. If I can easily cause leakage with a little stromal hydration, inflation of the eye, and pressure applied directly behind the wound as well as 180° away, then I will place a suture.

A third problem is an external tear on either side of the incision. This is easily done during the creation of the incision with a diamond blade, either due to torquing or lifting one side of the keratome such that one edge is much shorter than the desired 2.0- to 2.5-mm length. I am convinced that the wound is only as strong as its weakest part. If one side is torn due to surgical maneuvers inside the eye or cut at the beginning of the procedure, then a suture is necessary. As mentioned earlier, if this wound does not automatically and easily seal, I recommend placing a suture.

Stromal hydration can be used to seal the incision. For the wound to seal and the endothelial pump to work, everything must remain in apposition for a period of time. Otherwise, the profound leakage through the wound will overwhelm the endothelial pump, and the wound will continue to leak. Still, surgeons cannot rely too much on stromal hydration, which forces otherwise marginal wounds to close that can leak later. Stromal hydration is a temporary fix.

STUDY

In another study, my colleagues and I randomly analyzed 10% of more than 15,000 consecutive cataract surgeries and compared these with 27 cases of endophthalmitis after cataract surgery during the same timeframe.[4] We found that, if the wound were frankly leaking on the first postoperative day, the risk of endophthalmitis increased more than fortyfold. In fact, with sutureless, clear corneal incisions that leak on the day after surgery (often as a patient blinks), we can see the tears moving in and out of the anterior chamber. I consider such leakage a mandatory reason to put in a suture. These patients need frequent dosing of topical fourth-generation fluoroquinolones and require close observation for the earliest sign of increased inflammation, which should be considered a presumptive diagnosis of endophthalmitis (Table 2).

Eyes with torn capsules or zonules were about 15 times more likely to develop endophthalmitis. This incidence was four times higher than described in the classic study by Javitt et al,[5] who showed that vitreous loss increased endophthalmitis fourfold back when it was standard to suture the incision. Torn capsules and zonules, therefore, warrant a sutured incision and increased surveillance.

The other statistically significant findings of our study relate to the type of antibiotic, when antibiotics were used, and the use of a collagen shield. We switched to fluoroquinolones from aminoglycosides and used only Ciloxan (Alcon Laboratories, Inc., Fort Worth, TX) and Ocuflox (Allergan Inc., Irvine, CA.). We found that the use of Ciloxan increased the risk of endophthalmitis three- to fivefold, which may be related to the inability of ciprofloxacin to penetrate into the anterior chamber. Fortunately, such is not the case for ofloxacin, levofloxacin (Quixin; Santen, Inc., Napa, CA), or

TABLE 1. ATTRIBUTES OF A WOUND LIKELY TO LEAK
Torn and/or detached Descemet's membrane
An unusually stretched wound
A wound difficult to seal
A short distance to the opening at either end of the wound

any of the new fourth-generation fluoroquinolones. This is the first study of which I am aware to give strong, presumptive evidence that antibiotics are important in the prevention of endophthalmitis. It is important to remember that culturing the anterior chamber after cataract surgery will result in a positive endophthalmitis culture 20% to 60% of the time, statistics that have been shown in many studies. Most notable is that the anterior chamber can clear a fairly good sized bacterial inoculum, but the vitreous cannot. Our study results strongly suggest that, if there is enough antibiotic in the eye to eliminate the bacterial inoculum, endophthalmitis can be prevented.

Starting antibiotics on the day of surgery versus waiting until the next day also decreased the risk of endophthalmitis by a factor of three to five. The use of a collagen shield decreased the risk of endophthalmitis three- to fivefold.

All of our findings stood up to the rigor of a multivariate regression analysis and were independently important. In addition to facilitating the delivery of antibiotics to the eye, a collagen shield may provide some support to the wound, much like a bandage contact lens, and may help prevent early leakage. My colleagues and I performed a series of studies, which have been submitted for publication, looking at the use of fourth-generation fluoroquinolones with a collagen shield for the prophylaxis of endophthalmitis. With this approach, gatifloxacin and moxifloxacin demonstrated excellent penetration into the anterior chamber.

TABLE 2. SIGNIFICANT RISK FACTORS ASSOCIATED WITH ENDOPHTHALMITIS IN THE JOHN A. MORAN EYE CENTER ENDOPHTHALMITIS STUDY[4]
Clear corneal incisions
Leaky wound on the first postoperative day
Capsular or zonular trauma
Topical antibiotic that penetrates poorly into the eye
Starting topical antibiotics the day after surgery
Not using a collagen shield

CONCLUSION

Clearly, antibiotic prophylaxis as well as the integrity of the cataract incision are important to the prevention of endophthalmitis. Marshall[6] found that the new Atomic Edge silicon chip blade (BD Ophthalmic Systems, Franklin Lakes, NJ) creates a wound with much greater bursting strength than that created by a diamond. The silicon blade is an example of innovative technology to strengthen sutureless wounds. Other ophthalmologists argue we simply need to go back to using sutures. What is needed are good dialogue and solid studies so we can make progress and minimize this scourge. At the least, we should suture all questionable wounds and frequently use antibiotics that can achieve therapeutic levels in the eye starting right after surgery. ■

This article originally appeared in the February 2005 issue of CRSToday.

1. Nagaki Y, Hayasuku, Kodoi C, et al. Bacterial endophthalmitis after small-incision cataract surgery. Effects of incision placement and intraocular lens types. *J Cataract Refract Surg.* 2003;29;20-26.
2. Taban M, Rao B, Reznik J, et al. Dynamic morphology of sutureless cataract wounds–effect of incision angle and location. *Surv Ophthalmol.* 2004;48:562-572.
3. Shingleton, BJ, Heltzer J, O'Donoghue MW. Outcomes of phacoemulsification in patients with and without pseudoexfoliation syndrome. *J Cataract Refract Surg.* 2003;29:1080-1085.
4. Wallin T, Parker J, Jin Y, et al. A cohort study of 27 cases of endophthalmitis at a single institution. *J Cataract Refract Surg.* In Press.
5. Javitt JC, Vitale S, Canner JK, et al. National outcomes of cataract extraction: endophthalmitis following inpatient surgery. *Arch Ophthal.* 1991;109:1085-1089.
6. Marshall, J. The 2004 Charles D. Kelman innovator's lecture, Developments, Debate and Dilemma: wavefronts and biomechanics. Paper presented at: The ASCRS/ASOA Symposium on Cataract, IOL, and Refractive Surgery; May 3, 2004; San Diego, CA.

CHAPTER 88

Endophthalmitis: Recommendations Based on the ESCRS Study

PETER BARRY, FRCS

The ESCRS endophthalmitis study[1,2] on the prophylaxis of endophthalmitis following cataract surgery with phacoemulsification was designed to answer one fundamental question: do perioperative antibiotics prevent endophthalmitis? If so, investigators also sought to determine how the agents should be administeredÑvia intracameral injection, intensive topical drops, or both?

STUDY DESIGN

The study enrolled 15,971 subjects from 23 clinics in nine European countries. Half of the patients were randomly assigned to receive 1 mg of intracameral cefuroxime in 0.10 mL of normal saline solution at the end of the surgery. Additionally, all patients received, in a randomized, masked fashion, intensive topical levofloxacin or placebo drops commencing 60 minutes before the

TABLE 1. SIGNIFICANT RISK FACTORS FOR PRESUMED ENDOPHTHALMITIS				
Key Risk Factor	*P* Value	Odds Ratio*	95% Confidence Limits for Odds Ratio	
			Lower Limit	Upper Limit
Cefuroxime injection† (present, absent)	.002	4.8	1.8	12.5
IOL optic material (other, silicone)	.002	3.3	1.2	7.1
Site of incision (scleral tunnel, clear corneal)	.021	5.8	1.3	25.4
Levofloxacin perioperative drops† (present, absent)	.462	1.3	0.6	2.8

**Odds ratio after adjustment for age, gender, and other factors within regression model.*
†Study objective factor.

surgery and concluding 30 minutes after its completion. Each patient received a total of five drops.

Because withholding any prophylaxis from the control group was considered unethical, all patients received povidone-iodine preoperatively and topical levofloxacin drops q.i.d. for 6 days beginning on the first postoperative day. The study's objectives were the efficacy of the use of intracameral cefuroxime and intensive perioperative antibiotics versus placebo. The objectives did not include the use of povidone-iodine and routine levofloxacin for 1 week postoperatively. Preoperative antibiotic drops were not used in the conventional sense.

The endpoint was the occurrence of infectious endophthalmitis, either clinically diagnosed or proven. All suspect eyes were subjected to a vitreous/anterior chamber tap for gram stain, culture, and polymerase chain reaction. Investigators considered infection proven if any of these three tests were positive.

INFECTIONS

In the study group that did not receive the perioperative antibiotic, the rate of endophthalmitis was high at 33 per 10,000 patients for presumed cases and 23 per 10,000 patients for proven cases. In the group that received intracameral cefuroxime, the incidence was six presumed cases per 10,000 patients and four proven cases per 10,000 patients. These results represent a fivefold reduction for both presumed and proven cases in patients who received intracameral cefuroxime.

In the group that did not receive intracameral cefuroxime, the investigators found eight staphylococcal and eight streptococcal infections. In the cefuroxime group, there were three staphylococcal and zero streptococcal infections.

VISUAL ACUITY

The final range of visual acuity for the 11 staphylococcal cases ranged from 20/20 to 20/80. No eye incurred legal blindness (ie, 20/200 or less).

For the eyes infected with *Streptococcus*, the final visual acuity range was 20/20 to no light perception. Five eyes in the non-cefuroxime group became legally blind, all due to streptococci.

RISK FACTORS

We analyzed an exhaustive number of potential risk factors. Table 1 shows those factors identified as significant for presumed endophthalmitis. They include a failure to inject cefuroxime (P=.002; odds ratio, 4.8), the use of a silicone as opposed to an acrylic IOL material (P=.002; odds ratio, 3.3), and the utilization of a clear corneal as opposed to a scleral tunnel incision (P=.021; odds ratio, 5.8). Regarding the last factor, only two out of 23 centers in the study routinely used the scleral tunnel incision. Theoretically, therefore, there could be a hospital/center effect, but this is unlikely. A subanalysis of the risk of silicone versus acrylic IOL material is ongoing and will soon be published by the ESCRS Endophthalmitis Study Group.[3] The use of intensive perioperative levofloxacin drops was not shown to be of clinical significance.

THE EFFECT OF INTRACAMERAL CEFUROXIME

The striking outcome of the ESCRS study was the beneficial effect of using 1 mg of intracameral cefuroxime in 0.10 mL of normal saline solution at the end of the surgery. This measure effectively achieved a fivefold reduction in endophthalmitis compared with the group that received no perioperative antibiotics. The 0.3% incidence of endophthalmitis in the latter group was high and surprised us all. We know that retrospective studies showing lower rates of infection are prone to underreporting and that poor results are often unpublished, but this outcome also raises the possibility that preoperative povidone-iodine combined with routine postoperative antibiotic drops q.i.d. for 1 week is not as effective a regimen as originally thought. It certainly appears inadequate compared with the beneficial effects of intracameral cefuroxime.

It is not likely that the ESCRS study will result in a major conversion by ophthalmologists from clear corneal to scleral tunnel incisions, although this has always been my standard practice. Rather, the data will likely result in stricter construction and sealing of the corneal wound for surgeons for whom it is preferred practice.

WHY CEFUROXIME?

My colleagues and I chose cefuroxime for the study, because it is effective against the majority of organisms that cause postoperative endophthalmitis. Importantly, its efficacy and safety have been shown in more than 400,000 Swedish patients.[4,5] The Swedish experience suggested cefuroxime's benefit, and the ESCRS study has proven it.

Although it may always be argued that other intracameral

agents or alternative systems of drug delivery could be superior to cefuroxime, they will require safety studies and clinical trials to prove their superiority. Given the ESCRS study's results, it may well be impossible for any future clinical trial to deny an intracameral antibiotic to participants. A study to evaluate the comparative benefits of the newer fluoroquinolones applied topically versus using cefuroxime intracamerally would require an enormous and expensive trial, and it may be superfluous if intracameral cefuroxime can achieve the endophthalmitis rate of 0.05% that we have shown. Any such planned studies should also consider the ethics of using the newer fluoroquinolones or vancomycin for prophylaxis. Perhaps they should be considered reserve antibiotics for treatment.

SUMMARY

From the results of the ESCRS study, my co-investigators and I believe that intracameral cefuroxime should be adopted worldwide. Its use could save many thousands of eyes from potential blindness due to postoperative bacterial endophthalmitis following cataract surgery with IOL implantation. ■

Cefuroxime is not licensed for intraocular use. An exemption certificate was obtained for the purposes of the ESCRS endophthalmitis study.

This article originally appeared in the April 2007 issue of CRSToday.

1. Seal D, Barry P, Gettinby G, et al. ESCRS study of prophylaxis of post-operative endophthalmitis after cataract surgery: case for a European multicentre study. *J Cataract Refract Surg.* 2006;32:396-406.
2. Barry P, Seal D, Gettinby G, et al. ESCRS study of prophylaxis of post-operative endophthalmitis after cataract surgery: preliminary report of principal results from a European multicentre study. *J Cataract Refract Surg.* 2006;32:407-410.
3. ESCRS Endophthalmitis Study Group. Prophylaxis of post-operative endophthalmitis following cataract surgery: results of the ESCRS multicentre study and identification of risk factors. *J Cataract Refract Surg.* In press.
4. Montan PG, Wejde G, Koranyl G, Rylander M. Prophylactic intracameral cefuroxime: efficacy in preventing endophthalmitis after cataract surgery. *J Cataract Refract Surg.* 2002;28:977-981.
5. Wejde G, Montan PG, Lundstrom M, et al. Endophthalmitis following cataract surgery in Sweden: national prospective survey 1999-2001. *Acta Ophthalmol Scand.* 2005;83:7-10.

CHAPTER 89

Endophthalmitis After Cataract Surgery

RICHARD B. PACKARD, FRCS, FRCOPHTH; RANDALL J. OLSON, MD; ERIC D. DONNENFELD, MD; STEVE ARSHINOFF, MD, FRCSC; FRANCIS S. MAH, MD; TERRENCE P. O'BRIEN, MD; AND SAMUEL MASKET, MD

In a press release on March 13, 2006, the ESCRS announced that the results of its multicenter, prospective, randomized endophthalmitis study showed that intracameral cefuroxime significantly lowered the rate of infectious endophthalmitis. The society deemed the information sufficiently important to alert the global ophthalmic community in advance of the published study. Without details of the study's design and a commercially available intracameral antibiotic, however, ophthalmic surgeons have been left to wonder how to proceed. *Cataract & Refractive Surgery Today* asked several experts for their opinions on the impact and practical implications of this landmark study.

—David F. Chang, MD, Co-Chief Medical Editor

RICHARD B. PACKARD, FRCS, FRCOPHTH

The issue of appropriate prophylaxis to minimize the risk of endophthalmitis after cataract surgery has long vexed ophthalmic surgeons. Most reports on series of patients have either been retrospective or had insufficient numbers to provide genuinely statistically sound data. The ESCRS has just closed its very large prospective study early, because one arm showed a fivefold advantage in terms of the reduced incidence of endophthalmitis. The difference in that arm was the use of intracameral cefuroxime at the end of the operation, a technique that Montan et al[1,2] described in their groundbreaking reports from Sweden. We now have to assess the effect that this information will have on clinical practice for all ophthalmologists who perform cataract surgery.

In King Edward VII Hospital in Windsor, United Kingdom, at the beginning of 2004, my colleagues and I had a cluster of nine cases of endophthalmitis after cataract surgery in 3 months. We reviewed our practices extensively and tried to isolate the cause. Despite looking at the type and site of the incision, the use or not of a topical gel, the subconjunctival injection, etc, we failed to find a single reason for the outbreak. We found no pattern.

Among the changes we instituted was the routine use of intracameral cefuroxime, as prepared by the scrub nurse, for each patient. Since that time, we have performed more than 5,000 cases. Our first incident of endophthalmitis was reported 2 weeks ago. It was culture negative, and the anterior segment cleared in 2 days with some residual vitreous haze, which is dissipating. I would endorse the findings of the ESCRS' study, because, although the rate of endophthalmitis may be higher than previously reported, the difference between the study arms is striking and statistically valid.

RANDALL J. OLSON, MD

Any prospective, randomized clinical trial in association with a treatment for endophthalmitis is a major event. That the ESCRS' trial showed more than a fourfold difference in the rates of endophthalmitis between the use of a topical antibiotic and intraocular cefuroxime is not a result to be taken lightly. I predict

INTRACAMERAL CEFUROXIME

By Richard B. Packard, FRCS, FRCOphth

At the end of surgery, 0.93 mg of cefuroxime in 0.1 mL sterile water for injection is injected into the anterior chamber.

To reconstitute the cefuroxime, my scrub nurse adds 2.5 mL of water for injection to 250 mg of the drug to yield 93 mg/mL or 9.3 mg/0.1mL. She takes 0.1 mL of this solution and adds 0.9 mL of water for injection to get 0.93 mg in 0.1 mL. She then discards 0.9 mL to leave 0.1 mL in a syringe. I inject 0.1mL of the solution into the anterior chamber, preferably the capsular bag, with a 1-mL syringe and a Rycroft cannula. Zinacef is cefuroxime for parenteral use and is manufactured in a sterile crystalline form by Glaxosmithkline (Brentford, United Kingdom).

In a case of suspected allergy to penicillin, the consensus is still to administer cefuroxime intracamerally.

This regimen is based upon the concentration reported by Montan et al.[1]

Editor's note: Although the Prince Charles Eye Unit has been using sterile water to mix cefuroxime without apparent problems, the original methodology published by Montan et al[1] describes the use of 0.9% saline to dissolve and mix cefuroxime.—David F. Chang, MD

1. Montan PG, Wejde G, Koranyi G, Rylander M. Prophylactic intracameral cefuroxime. Efficacy in preventing endophthalmitis after cataract surgery. *J Cataract Refract Surg*. 2002;28:977-981.

that this report will usher in an era when surgeons more frequently use intraocular antibiotics.

Should all ophthalmologists be using cefuroxime intraocularly today, and is not doing so a break from the standard of care, with all of its scary legal ramifications? I do not think so because even the cefuroxime group had an incidence of endophthalmitis of 1:1,370, which is a similar or even higher rate than that of many contemporary surgeons who use topical antibiotics. What is more surprising is the 1:300 incidence of endophthalmitis for the study's control group. Although such a high rate may have been common in the early days of topical antibiotics and an unsutured clear corneal incision, it is unusual for any recent study on the subject of which I am aware.

My colleagues and I examined 27 cases of endophthalmitis in a multivariate analysis[3] and found that starting the antibiotic on the day after surgery increased the incidence of endophthalmitis by a factor of 13.7 (P=.005) compared with antibiosis on the day of surgery. I would therefore expect an investigation like that of the ESCRS to show such a difference if the study group received frequent topical drops right after and on the day of surgery versus on the next day.

Unfortunately, the protocol had the control group start topical antibiotics on the day after surgery. I am not sure that comparing the use of an intraocular antibiotic and a topical drop started on the first postoperative day is the same as comparing the former with antibiotic drops administered on the operative day and the first postoperative day. Furthermore, using an antibiotic that penetrates well into the eye, such as a fourth-generation fluoroquinolone, has kept the incidence of endophthalmitis at the John A. Moran Eye Center in Salt Lake City as low as or better than that of the cefuroxime group in the ESCRS' study.

The future is exciting in that the ESCRS' study definitively shows the importance of antibiotics for preventing endophthalmitis. Due to increasing gram-positive resistance to cephalosporin antibiotics such as cefuroxime, supplementing intracameral fourth-generation fluoroquinolones with frequent topical drops or even an antibiotic-soaked collagen shield is probably the next step for preventing this devastating complication. Regardless, solid studies should demonstrate that surgeons are indeed improving endophthalmitis prophylaxis before they make any changes to the standard of care.

Ophthalmologists who start antibiotics on the day after surgery, however, may find the practice more difficult to defend based on the results of our study[3] and that of the ESCRS. On the other hand, no study to date has proven that intraocular antibiotics are superior to starting appropriate topical antibiotics on the day of surgery.

ERIC D. DONNENFELD, MD

Cataract surgery is one of the most common operations in the US, with approximately 3 million procedures performed annually.[4,5] Modern cataract surgery is a safe and minimally invasive procedure that produces excellent outcomes. Although it is associated with an extremely low incidence of endophthalmitis, the considerable annual surgical volume still produces approximately 4,000 cases of potentially devastating endophthalmitis each year.[6]

The use of intracameral antibiotics at the time of cataract surgery has been a common practice for more than a decade. It makes sense to place the antibiotic into the target tissue of the anterior chamber, a practice that can eradicate or partially treat the potential bacterial inoculum that occurs at the time of surgery and reduce the risk of infection. The first report of successful antibiotic prophylaxis by injection into the anterior chamber was published in the 1970s.[7] Additionally, a number of retrospective studies have suggested that intracameral antibiotics can significantly reduce the risk of infection.[1] Twenty years later, two large series of cataract patients and the usage of infusion fluid containing gentamicin and vancomycin were associated with no cases of endophthalmitis.[8]

The ESCRS' study of intracameral cefuroxime is the latest and by far the most important study to document the significance of intracameral antibiotics in preventing endophthalmitis, because it is the first controlled, double-masked, multicenter study to look at this issue. The next step is a thorough analysis of the data.

An important question that emerges, however, regards exactly what the best antibiotic to use intracamerally is. The appropriate intracameral drug is broad spectrum, bacteriocidal, fast acting, and nontoxic, and it can be supplemented with topical medications. We should all look forward to new research into this important area.

STEVE ARSHINOFF, MD, FRCSC

I have been using prophylactic intracameral antibiotics for every intraocular procedure since 1995. Initially, I used vancomycin 1.0mg/0.1mL balanced salt solution and never had an incident of postoperative endophthalmitis in approximately 5,000 cases. I was concerned about the agent's lack of gram-negative coverage and claims that the intraocular residence time was inadequate for full

INTRACAMERAL GATIFLOXACIN

By Eric D. Donnenfeld, MD

Intracameral gatifloxacin is formulated by diluting intravenous gatifloxacin (Tequin; Bristol-Myers Squibb Company, New York, NY), which is available as 200 mg in 20 mL, with 180 mL of balanced salt solution (9:1 balanced salt solution/gatifloxacin, which results in 200 mg of gatifloxacin in 200 mL or 1 mg/mL). This solution is filtered under sterile conditions using a 0.2-mm filter. A sterile, 26-gauge irrigating cannula is attached to a sterile tuberculin syringe, and the surgeon injects 0.1 mL, which contains 100 µg of gatifloxacin, through the paracentesis incision into the center of the anterior chamber. At my practice, we mix the solution daily and use it for a full day's surgery.

prophylaxis. The risk of inducing resistant bacterial strains through the intracameral or other ophthalmic use of antibiotics is likely insignificant and so did not concern me.[9] The big problem was the introduction in Canada in 2003 of discounted generic vancomycin, which snuck into hospitals and was found to be associated with toxic anterior segment syndrome (TASS). I began to search for a better drug.

Montan et al[1,2] demonstrated, in over 60,000 patients, that intracameral cefuroxime reduced the risk of endophthalmitis by approximately 80%, but it was not level-one evidence. The ESCRS' study is the first level-one evidence conclusively demonstrating that intracameral cefuroxime, used prophylactically, reduces the incidence of endophthalmitis by about 80%, from 1:300 to approximately 1:1,400, when compared with topical levofloxacin alone. My concern with the work by Montan et al[1,2] is that, in the endophthalmitides seen in the patients who received cefuroxime, 90% grew bacteria resistant to cefuroxime. To me, this means that the researchers are proposing the correct route of treatment but the wrong pharmaceutical.

The most broad-spectrum antibiotics currently available are fourth-generation fluoroquinolones, which come as gatifloxacin 0.3% solution preserved with benzalkonium chloride and moxifloxacin 0.5% self-preserved eye drops. My last 1,000 intraocular cases received prophylactic intracameral moxifloxacin 100.0 µg/0.1 mL (1:5 dilution of moxifloxacin with balanced salt solution prepared in a sterile fashion in the OR). I have encountered no infections or untoward side effects. The eyes have been quiet postoperatively, with minimal inflammation. I intend to use this prophylactic regimen for all my intraocular cases. After the ESCRS' report, I believe that using nothing intracamerally may soon leave surgeons open to legal liability if an infection occurs.

At present, further study to determine the optimal drug and dosage for intracameral usage is needed. I would be reluctant to recommend that everyone adopt intracameral prophylaxis in the absence of a detailed analysis of the ESCRS' study and further clarification of the safety of our apparent drugs of choice. At the same time, surgeons must balance the seemingly low risk of intracameral prophylaxis (due to currently unknown potential toxicity, possible diluting errors, and erroneous mixing with sterile water rather than balanced salt solution) with the current alternative of accepting a low but significant rate of continued loss of eyes to endophthalmitis when it appears that we can effectively prevent this complication. Additional study of the issue is urgently needed.

INTRACAMERAL MOXIFLOXACIN

By Steve Arshinoff, MD, FRCSC

I use 0.1 mL of moxifloxacin HCl 0.5% 100 µg/0.1mL at the end of each case. Intracameral moxifloxacin is formulated by diluting the eye drops in a 5:1 ratio with balanced salt solution. Specifically, 2 mL of the drug is drawn into a 10-mL syringe with a sterile needle from a new bottle. Then, 8 mL of balanced salt solution is drawn into the syringe, and the scrub nurse mixes the contents by rotating the syringe in her hands. For each case, she places 0.5 mL into a medicine cup and draws 0.3 mL into a tuberculin syringe. As the final step of surgery, I make the injection through the sideport incision, under the distal edge of the capsulorhexis, and then rapidly exit the eye while ensuring that the globe remains pressurized.

FRANCIS S. MAH, MD

The press release from the ESCRS caused shock waves throughout the ophthalmic community because, on first blush, it seems that the major complication of intraocular surgery could be drastically reduced by completely changing the standard of care to administering intracameral cefuroxime at the end of surgery. Although the results of the study seem dramatic, we should step back and examine whether they make sense in terms of our current knowledge of medications, pharmacokinetics, and pharmacodynamics. In other words, maybe these results are not the end but rather a critical piece of the puzzle that will help lead us to a better way of preventing the devastating complication of postoperative endophthalmitis.

The ESCRS' original prospective protocol called for four groups: (1) intracameral cefuroxime and postoperative levofloxacin; (2) pre- and postoperative levofloxacin only; (3) a combination of intracameral cefuroxime and pre-/postoperative levofloxacin; and (4) neither a preoperative antibiotic nor intracameral cefuroxime, only postoperative levofloxacin. It is important to note that all patients received preoperative povidone-iodine, the only method by consensus to reduce endophthalmitis.

Supposedly, the study was stopped prematurely due to a lack of funding. The organizers combined groups, seemingly arbitrarily, to examine intracameral cefuroxime versus no intracameral cefuroxime. They could just as easily have examined preoperative levofloxacin versus no preoperative levofloxacin, since there were four groups, not two. In other words, the study is not as statistically clean as it looks; there are possible confounders due to the mixing and matching of subsets that were not initially grouped together. The overall rate of endophthalmitis seems high, and it will be interesting to read the peer-reviewed publication to see if we can identify other reasons for the seemingly elevated rate of endophthalmitis.

Regarding the medications used, many ophthalmologists already realize the benefits of the topical fourth-generation fluoroquinolones moxifloxacin and gatifloxacin, including an improved

INTRACAMERAL VANCOMYCIN

By Steve Arshinoff, MD, FRCSC

My technique for formulating intracameral vancomycin (Vancocin; Eli Lilly and Company, Indianapolis, IN) is adapted from one that Howard Gimbel, MD, shared with me in 1995. Ten milliliters of balanced salt solution is added to a 500-mg vial of vancomycin, and the mixture is then warmed in the nurse's hands or on top of a TV monitor to ensure that all of the precipitates dissolve. For two 20-mL syringes, the scrub nurse draws 16 mL of balanced salt solution into the syringe and adds 4 mL of reconstituted vancomycin. For four 10-mL syringes, she draws 8 mL of balanced salt solution and adds 2 mL of reconstituted vancomycin into each syringe. Next, she draws back the plunger and gently tips the needle back and forth to mix the contents and then removes air from the syringe.

The circulator injects the mixture into a 1-mL syringe with a 0.22 µm filter attached. The scrub nurse places a 30-gauge cannula on the end of the 1-mL syringe and pushes the plunger until barely more than 0.1 mL of the mixture remains in the syringe. At the conclusion of surgery, I instill 1mg of vancomycin/0.1mL under the capsulorhexis' edge, into the capsular bag, and around the IOL. I then rapidly withdraw the cannula from the eye.

spectrum of coverage, delayed antibiotic resistance, and better tissue penetration. Would these agents perform better than topical levofloxacin in the prevention of endophthalmitis? Although it seems logically so, we cannot answer that question.

Even though using cefuroxime as the intracameral test drug seems to have been of benefit, it may not have been the best choice, either. Cefuroxime is a second-generation beta-lactam, which provides just average coverage of both gram-positive and gram-negative bacteria. Furthermore, and of more concern, is the fact that the drug has a high rate of resistance; in fact, it would not cover any methicillin-resistant *Staphylococcus aureus*.

Regarding the pharmacokinetics of antibiotics in the anterior chamber, it is generally less than 2 hours. This figure makes sense because the turnover of aqueous humor in the anterior chamber is 1% per minute. Therefore, after 100 minutes, all of the aqueous has been replaced. An elegant study looked at intracameral vancomycin and gentamicin—far superior antibiotics in terms of spectrum of activity.[10] Vancomycin is a time-dependent killer, like cefuroxime, whereas gentamicin has both time- and concentration-dependent killing characteristics. In the study,[10] when *Staphylococcus epidermidis* and *S. aureus* were incubated with both vancomycin and gentamicin for 2 hours, there was no killing of bacteria. Possibly, a better antibiotic to utilize, if a cleaner study of larger magnitude were performed, would be a concentration-dependent killing antibiotic such as a fluoroquinolone. My laboratory and others have been able to show the complete eradication of bacteria within 1 hour of exposure to fluoroquinolones.[11]

Before all 2.5 million cataract patients per year receive intracameral cefuroxime, the potential short- and long-term issues of intracameral antibiotics need to be examined. Who knows if these drugs are associated with diseases such as glaucoma or age-related macular degeneration? Although this scenario may seem far-fetched, who would have thought that systemic, selective NSAIDs would lead to heart disease or that lithotripsy might cause diabetes and hypertension? Then there are the potentially devastating immediate complications of TASS from mislabeling and/or miscalculating the amounts of medications administered intracamerally.

The ESCRS' recent press release regarding the early termination of a bold prospective study on antibiotic prophylaxis for cataract surgery is surprising and warrants closer examination. Before adopting the use of cefuroxime or succumbing to confusion regarding current practices, we should review key aspects of this study and compare them to what we have historically done in the operating suite in order to develop a dynamic scheme for the optimal prevention of postoperative infections.

TERRENCE P. O'BRIEN, MD

Pseudophakic endophthalmitis is a relatively rare but feared and potentially devastating complication of cataract surgery. Hence, ophthalmic surgeons around the world exert considerable effort to prevent its clinical occurrence. The methods aimed at preventing postoperative pseudophakic endophthalmitis are controversial. Moreover, prophylaxis is not treatment, and often the two may be confused in the minds of physicians geared toward the treatment of infection. I commend our colleagues from the ESCRS for undertaking an ambitious, multicenter, multinational study in an attempt to provide evidence-based data comparing topical antibiotics and intracameral cefuroxime in patients undergoing cataract surgery.

The investigators reported postoperative endophthalmitis in the intracameral cefuroxime group (0.07%) and a surprisingly high rate in the control group (0.34%). The findings suggest a highly favorable reduction with intracameral cefuroxime compared with topical antibiotics. The incidence of this complication reported in other European studies varies (0.05% to 0.20%).[12] US cataract surgeons should take note of the ESCRS' study without overly extrapolating the findings to the prevailing situation in this country's ambulatory surgery centers. The ESCRS' study involved levofloxacin in the topical arm rather than the advanced-generation 8-methoxy fluouroquinolone compounds most commonly used in the US that have a greater antibacterial potency and superior aqueous penetration.

Although intracameral injection is indeed a direct delivery route that may be rational for prevention, problems with dilutional errors and toxicity need to be considered, as evidenced by the recent epidemic of TASS. Moreover, the pharmacodynamics of intracameral medications needs careful study, because the turnover rate of the aqueous humor is accelerated after phacoemulsification.

Cases of postoperative endophthalmitis after the use of intracameral cefuroxime is mostly due to a high rate of resistance to this drug among the ocular isolates causing endophthalmitis. Other limitations of cefuroxime include extemporaneous compounding, short-term stability, and hypersensitivity. The ESCRS' study may therefore hint at the right concept (intracameral delivery) without using the most advantageous agent. The study's results suggest that the optimal antibiotic regimen and route of delivery for the prevention of endophthalmitis in cataract surgery require further study.

SAMUEL MASKET, MD

Endophthalmitis remains a serious concern for both patients and physicians. Furthermore, its management represents a significant economic burden in direct and indirect healthcare costs. Given its relative rarity and the many variables in surgical styles, etc, the condition's prophylaxis has been difficult to study.

As one strategy for preventing postsurgical infection, ophthalmic surgeons have often employed intracameral antibiotics, but the evidence that this practice is beneficial has been largely derived from anecdotal case series and/or from survey data.[6] Although recent studies have confirmed a potential anti-infective benefit, the investigations were not controlled.[1,2] The routine use of intracameral antibiotics has therefore been somewhat controversial, because numerous questions about its use remain.

Many surgeons have been concerned that errors in diluting antibiotics for intraocular instillation could harm more eyes than would possibly be saved from infection. Other questions include:

- Which agent(s) is best?
- What is the appropriate dosage?
- What are the potential toxicities?
- Is it best to infuse antibiotic(s) with balanced salt solution, to add a bolus of antibiotic at the close of surgery, or to do both?

Although the answers to some of the questions are a matter of pharmacodynamics, others have not been well studied. Now, with the release of preliminary data from the collaborative, randomized, prospective investigation by the ESCRS, there is seemingly bona fide evidence of the prophylactic benefit of intracameral antibiotics, at least with respect to cefuroxime, a second-generation cephalosporin.

The ESCRS' investigation provided an answer to an important question, but, as to be expected, it generated new queries. Only one topical antibiotic, a third-generation fluoroquinolone (levofloxacin), was investigated, and it was found to offer no statistical benefit against infection when employed in the manner of the ESCRS' study protocol. Would the fourth-generation topical agents (moxifloxacin and gatifloxacin) used more commonly in the US have proven more effective?

The rates of infection in the ESCRS' investigation were alarmingly high; only the group receiving the intracameral cefuroxime displayed a rate of infection that approached those reported in the accepted literature.[6] Greater attention to the incision's construction and closure is clearly warranted.

Is cefuroxime the appropriate agent for intracameral use in the US? Are the offending microbes in this country similar or dissimilar to those in Europe? Would it be more appropriate to consider intraocular doses of fourth-generation fluoroquinolones or other agents?

All in ophthalmology are indebted to the ESCRS for conducting this important investigation. Now, the results must be carefully evaluated, and new investigations, where appropriate, should begin. Heretofore, the FDA has been reluctant to consider new drug applications for prophylactic intraocular antibiotics. We can hope that the evidence from the ESCRS, if accepted as valid, will make the agency more prone to consider such products. Given the chance to produce unit doses of antibiotics, the ophthalmic pharmaceutical industry may be able to provide surgeons with commercially available single doses in order to prevent errors in diluting antibiotics.

At present, surgeons should compare their own rates of infection with those reported by the ESCRS. Should the surgeon's experience be favorable, perhaps no change in prophylaxis is needed. If the surgeon's rates are high, however, then careful attention to all aspects of infection's prevention is warranted, including the use of intracameral antibiotics. ■

All recommendations for antibiotic prophylaxis in cataract surgery are currently off label.

This article originally appeared in the May 2006 issue of CRSToday.

1. Montan PG, Wejde G, Koranyi G, Rylander M. Prophylactic intracameral cefuroxime. Efficacy in preventing endophthalmitis after cataract surgery. *J Cataract Refract Surg.* 2002;28:977-981.
2. Montan PG, Wejde G, Setterquist H, et al. Prophylactic intracameral cefuroxime. Evaluation of safety and kinetics in cataract surgery. *J Cataract Refract Surg.* 2002;28:982-987.
3. Wallin T, Parker J, Jin Y, et al. Cohort study of 27 cases of endophthalmitis at a single institution. *J Cataract Refract Surg.* 2005;31:735-741.
4. Javitt JC, Kendix M, Tielsch JM, et al. Geographical variation in utilization of cataract surgery. *Med Care.* 1995;33:90-105.
5. Solomon R, Donnenfeld ED. Recent advances and future frontiers in treating age-related cataracts. *JAMA.* 2003;290:248-251.
6. Ciulla TA, Starr MB, Masket S. Bacterial endophthalmitis prophylaxis for cataract surgery: an evidence based update. *Ophthalmology.* 2002;109:13-24.
7. Peyman GA, Sathar ML, May DR. Intraocular gentamicin as intraoperative prophylaxis in South India eye camps. *Br J Ophthalmol.* 1977;61:260-262.
8. Gimbel HV, Sun R, DeBroff BM. Prophylactic intracameral antibiotics during cataract surgery: the incidence of endophthalmitis and corneal endothelial loss. *Eur J Implant Refract Surg.* 1994;6:280-285.
9. Ophthalmic moxifloxacin (Vigamox) and gatifloxacin (Zymar). *Med Lett Drugs Ther.* 2004;46:1179:25-27.
10. Gritz DC, Cevallos AV, Smolin G, Whitcher JP Jr. Antibiotic supplementation of intraocular irrigating solutions. An in vitro model of antibacterial action. *Ophthalmology.* 1996;103:1204-1208; discussion: 1208-1209.
11. Kowalski RP, Kowalski BR, Thompson PP, et al. 0.005% benzalkonium chloride (BAK): is it effective in eliminating *Staphylococcus aureus* and *Pseudomonas aeruginosa*? Paper presented at: The OMIG Meeting; October 15, 2005; Chicago, IL.
12. Khan RI, Kennedy S, Barry P. Incidence of presumed endophthalmitis in Dublin for a 5-year period (1997-2001). *J Cataract Refract Surg.* 2005;31:1575-1581.

CHAPTER 90

The Implications of the ESCRS Study

DEEPINDER K. DHALIWAL, MD

The ESCRS study of the prophylaxis of postoperative endophthalmitis after cataract surgery[1] created quite a stir among ophthalmologists. Finally, there was a prospective, randomized, placebo-controlled study demonstrating a benefit of intracameral antibiotics in preventing endophthalmitis. Specifically, the report showed that an intracameral injection of cefuroxime at the end of cataract surgery lowered the risk of endophthalmitis by a factor of five. This landmark study evaluated nearly 14,000 patients from 24 centers in nine European countries. Additional risk factors for endophthalmitis gleaned from the study included clear corneal wounds and silicone IOLs.[2]

Before we surgeons all instruct our surgical nurses to take 750 mg of cefuroxime powder and dilute it to a concentration of 1 mg/0.1 mL of balanced salt solution for our next cataract cases, we need to examine the study closely and understand its implications.

TOPICAL ANTIBIOTICS

Fourth-Generation Fluoroquinolones

The subjects of the ESCRS study were not treated with what we consider the standard of care in the US for surgical prophylaxis, fourth-generation fluoroquinolones, both pre- and postoperatively. Although all patients received preoperative povidone-iodine and postoperative levofloxacin (a third-generation fluoroquinolone), only two of the four groups received preoperative levofloxacin. It has been demonstrated in several studies that the fourth-generation fluoroquinolones, moxifloxacin and gatifloxacin, have an improved spectrum of coverage, higher potency, delayed antibiotic resistance, and better tissue penetration (especially moxifloxacin) when compared with second- and third-generation fluoroquinolones.[3]

An animal study conducted at the University of Pittsburgh[4] showed that topical moxifloxacin could prevent postoperative endophthalmitis in eyes that had been inoculated with *Staphylococcus aureus*. The eyes that did not receive topical moxifloxacin all developed endophthalmitis due to the number of organisms inoculated in the eye. None of the eyes that received topical moxifloxacin before and after inoculation developed endophthalmitis. This striking study illustrated just how powerful topical antibiotics can be in the prevention of endophthalmitis. It showed that a topical agent can penetrate the eye at a high enough concentration to reach therapeutic, bacteriocidal levels. It is unknown what the ESCRS study's results would have been had all patients received pre- and postoperative moxifloxacin or gatifloxacin.

Safety

The greatest advantage of topical antibiotic prophylaxis over intracameral antibiotics is safety. There is no concern of dilutional error, toxic anterior segment syndrome, endothelial toxicity, or the introduction of potentially contaminated substances into the anterior chamber. Antibiotics for intracameral use must be mixed correctly 2,700 times to reduce severe visual loss from endophthalmitis in one patient while avoiding toxic ocular effects in noninfected patients.[5] When mixed in the appropriate concentration, cefuroxime has not demonstrated any toxicity to the corneal endothelium or retina.[6] The pH of the solution is 7.42, and the osmolality is 311 mOsm/kg, well within the suitable range for humans.[5] Also, another study has shown no increased incidence of cystoid macular edema in patients who received intracameral cefuroxime.[7]

An additional issue in regard to an antibiotic's safety is a patient's potential hypersensitivity to the drug. Someone who is allergic to a topical agent will typically have contact dermatitis or conjunctivitis but will not develop an anaphylactic reaction. Patients with hypersensitivity to an intracameral agent, such as cefuroxime, can actually develop systemic anaphylaxis with associated morbidity and possible mortality, as reported by Villada et al.[8] They described a patient with a history of allergy to oral ampicillin who received 1 mg of cefuroxime intracamerally (the same concentration as used in the ESCRS study) at the conclusion of an uncomplicated phaco case. Five minutes later, the patient developed problems breathing and went into hypovolemic shock due to the anaphylactic reaction. Fortunately, the anesthesiologist was present in the recovery room and quickly administered intravenous methylprednisolone, ephedrine, 3 L of Ringer's lactate solution, and antihistamines. The patient recovered from this life-threatening allergic reaction in half an hour but was admitted to the hospital for observation. Referring to this case, Liu et al[9] stated, "conceptually speaking, intracameral antibiotic administration in a patient with a history of antibiotic allergy is highly akin to the direct intravenous route of administration in terms of bioavailability, particularly in the face of a disrupted blood-aqueous barrier during phacoemulsification."

The rate of any hypersensitivity to a cephalosporin such as cefuroxime is reported to be 1% to 3%.[10] The rate of anaphylaxis with cephalosporins is reported to be 0.1% to 0.0001%.[11] With approximately 2.5 million cataract surgeries performed each year in the US, as many as 2,500 patients per year could potentially develop anaphylaxis if every case were performed according to the ESCRS study guidelines and each patient received intracameral cefuroxime. Montan and colleagues[6] continue to use cefuroxime on a wide-scale basis in Sweden by pretreating patients with a history of anaphylaxis to this antibiotic with oral antihistamines. In the ESCRS study, patients were excluded if they were allergic to penicillins and cephalosporins. What if the patient has not been exposed to enough antibiotics, however, to realize a hypersensitivity exists?

Compliance

Topical antibiotic prophylaxis depends on patients' compliance in order to be effective. Intracameral antibiotics have the advantage of being placed into the anterior segment at the conclusion of surgery. Moreover, these agents are effective if they have a sufficiently high concentration for an adequate length of time with a spectrum of activity that encompasses the organisms that enter the anterior chamber during or soon after cataract surgery.

SPECTRUM OF ACTIVITY

The decision to use cefuroxime in the ESCRS study was based on work by Montan et al,[12] who showed a statistically significant reduction in postoperative endophthalmitis in patients who had received intracameral cefuroxime in a prospective, uncontrolled, 3-year survey. Cefuroxime is a second-generation cephalosporin with fair antibiotic coverage against gram-positive organisms and some gram-negative organisms. It has a time-dependent killing action, and its bacteriocidal effect is due to interference with cell wall synthesis. In terms of bacterial susceptibility, cefuroxime has good activity against most *Staphylococcus* and *Streptococcus* species, Escherichia coli, Proteus species, Propionibacterium species, Klebsiella, and Haemophilus influenzae. There are significant gaps in coverage, however. Cefuroxime does not cover methicillin-resistant *S. aureus* (MRSA), some Enterococcus strains, and Pseudomonas. It is important to note that patients from long-term nursing homes were not eligible to participate in the ESCRS study, because this patient population is known to have a greater risk of colonization with resistant strains of bacteria such as MRSA.

A study performed at the University of Pittsburgh showed that moxifloxacin and gatifloxacin provided higher susceptibility to Bacillus, Enterococcus, and gram-negative bacteria than cefuroxime using actual endophthalmitis isolates and equal susceptibility for *Staphylococcus* and *Streptococcus* strains. The researchers concluded that, in regard to the choice of an intracameral agent, fourth-generation fluoroquinolones might provide more broad-spectrum coverage of endophthalmitis-causing bacteria than cefuroxime.[13]

EFFICACY OF CEFUROXIME

Due to the constant turnover of aqueous, the concentration of a drug in the anterior chamber would decrease by one half in 70 minutes, although it might decrease even more rapidly due to quicker aqueous dynamics in the postoperative inflamed eye.[14] A study evaluating the pharmacokinetics of intracameral cefuroxime determined that the concentration declined by a factor of four in 1 hour.[5] Cefuroxime has a slower, time-dependent bacteriocidal action, and, therefore, a certain amount of time must pass before bacteria are killed, even if the concentration of antibiotic is very high. In contrast, agents such as the fluoroquinolones are concentration dependent.

A kinetics of kill study was performed with cefuroxime against staphylococcal ocular isolates.[15] It showed that less than one log kill was achieved in 3 hours. The researchers contrasted this result to the kinetics of kill of moxifloxacin, which showed a greater than three log kill (> 99.9%) after less than 2 hours. This difference may explain the development of endophthalmitis secondary to a cefuroxime-susceptible strain of *S. aureus* in a patient who received intracameral cefuroxime at the end of surgery.[11]

CONCLUSION

The authors of the ESCRS study on the prophylaxis of postoperative endophthalmitis after cataract surgery should be congratulated for undertaking this important task. They designed a partially masked, randomized, placebo-controlled, multinational clinical study to prospectively evaluate the effect of intracameral cefuroxime and/or perioperative topical levofloxacin on postoperative endophthalmitis. Although the total study size goal was 35,000 patients, the study was halted at the end of 2005 after the recruitment of only 13,698 patients, because a clearly beneficial effect from the use of intracameral cefuroxime had been observed.

There are several factors we need to keep in mind before we change our practice patterns in 2007. First, certain groups of patients were ineligible to participate in the ESCRS study, including nursing home patients. In addition, cefuroxime is a slow, time-dependent killer that is ineffective against MRSA, Pseudomonas, and some Enterococcus species. There are several issues of safety with this agent, including reports of severe anaphylaxis. Finally, ESCRS study patients did not receive adjunctive topical fourth-generation fluoroquinolones, which have an improved spectrum of coverage, higher potency, delayed antibiotic resistance, and better tissue penetration compared with the third-generation fluoroquinolone used in the ESCRS study. ■

This article originally appeared in April 2007 issue of CRSToday.

1. Barry P, Seal D, Gettinby G, et al. ESCRS study of prophylaxis of post-operative endophthalmitis after cataract surgery: preliminary report of principal results from a European multicentre study. *J Cataract Refract Surg.* 2006;32:407-410.
2. Barry PJ. ESCRS: study design and results. Paper presented at: The AAO Annual Meeting; November 12, 2007; Las Vegas, NV.
3. Kim DH, Stark WJ, O' Brien TP, et al. Aqueous penetration and activity of moxifloxacin 0.5% ophthalmic solution and gatifloxacin 0.3% ophthalmic solution in cataract surgery patients. *Ophthalmology.* 2005;112:1992-1996.
4. Kowalski R, Romanowski E, Mah F, et al. Topical prophylaxis with moxifloxacin prevents endophthalmitis in a rabbit model. *Am J Ophthalmol.* 2004;138:33-37.
5. Alfonso EC, Flynn HW Jr. Controversies in endophthalmitis prevention. The risk for emerging resistance to vancomycin. *Arch Ophthalmol.* 1995;113:1369-1370.
6. Montan PJ, Wejde G, Setterquist H, et al. Prophylactic intracameral cefuroxime. Evaluation of safety and kinetics in cataract surgery. *J Cataract Refract Surg.* 2002;28:982-987.
7. Gupta MS, McKee HD, Saldana M, Stewart OG. Macular thickness after cataract surgery with intracameral cefuroxime. *J Cataract Refract Surg.* 2005;31:1163-1166.
8. Villada JR, Vicente U, Javaloy J, Alio JL. Severe anaphylactic reaction after intracameral antibiotic administration during cataract surgery. *J Cataract Refract Surg.* 2005;31:620-621.
9. Liu DT, Lee VY, Chan VC, Lam DS. Severe anaphylactic reaction after intracameral antibiotic administration during cataract surgery. *J Cataract Refract Surg.* 2006;32:188.
10≥ Anne S, Reisman RE. Risk of administering cephalosporin antibiotics to patients with histories of penicillin allergy. *Ann Allergy Asthma Immunol.* 1995;74:167-170.
11. Kelkar PS, Li JT-C. Cephalosporin allergy. *N Engl J Med.* 2001;345:804-809.
12. Montan PJ, Wejde G, Koranyi G, Rylander M. Prophylactic intracameral cefuroxime: efficacy in preventing endophthalmitis after cataract surgery. *J Cataract Refract Surg.* 2002;28:977-981.
13. Contreras JE, Kowalski RP, Mah FS, Thompson P. Does cefuroxime provide better in vitro susceptibility that the 4th generation fluoroquinolones and cefazolin? Paper presented at: The OMIG Meeting; November 10, 2006; Las Vegas, NV.
14. Gritz DC, Cevallos AV, Smolin G, Whitcher JP Jr. Antibiotic supplementation of intraocular irrigating solutions. An in vitro model of antibacterial action. *Ophthalmology.* 1996;103:1204-1208.
15. O'Brien TP, Arshinoff SA, Mah FS. Perspective on cefuroxime and the recent ESCRS postoperative endophthalmitis (POE) study. Paper presented at: The OMIG Meeting; November 10, 2006; Las Vegas, NV.

CHAPTER 91

Why I Do Not Use Intracameral Antibiotics

JOHN R. WITTPENN, JR, MD

Some cataract surgeons use intracameral antibiotics as part of their regimen for preventing endophthalmitis, an infrequent but devastating complication of cataract surgery. A recent, population-based review of 477,627 Medicare claims demonstrated that the incidence of endophthalmitis following cataract surgery rose between 1994 and 2001. The study found a rate of endophthalmitis of 1.79 per 1,000 cases in 1994 and a rate of 2.47 cases per 1,000 in 2001, representing a 37% increase in this 8-year period.[1] Ironically, refinements in surgical technique such as clear corneal incisions that allow for sutureless surgery and rapid visual rehabilitation after phacoemulsification may be at least partially responsible for the increased risk of postoperative infection, including endophthalmitis.[2]

Today, surgeons use various strategies to decrease the chances of postoperative infection and the vision-threatening complications of endophthalmitis, but the best regimen or approach remains unproven. Among the several current strategies are (1) the perioperative use of topical antibiotics, usually fourth-generation fluoroquinolones, (2) the intracameral injection of antibiotics at the end of the case, and (3) the use of a combination of intracameral and topical antibiotics. Proponents of the intracameral injection of antibiotics during cataract surgery assert that the practice decreases the rate of endophthalmitis, because it helps to eradicate organisms that enter the eye during or immediately after cataract extraction. Several studies, including a recent report from the ESCRS, appear to support this position.[3]

In my view, however, these recent data do not provide robust support for the superiority of intracameral antibiotics over the perioperative topical antibiotic regimen widely used in the US. First, the ESCRS study did not include in its randomization scheme the use of fourth-generation fluoroquinolones, thus precluding direct comparisons. In addition, the investigators did not address the many risks inherent in the intracameral administration of antibiotics.

TABLE 1. RATES OF ENDOPHTHALMITIS

Study	Treatment Group	Rate
ESCRS (13,698 patients)[3] (Note: all patients had 6 days of levofloxacin q.i.d. beginning 18 to 24 hours after surgery)	No intracameral agent, levofloxacin starting after 18 hours only	0.38%
	Intracameral cefuroxime and levofloxacin starting after 18 hours	0.08%
	Levofloxacin pre- and postoperatively	0.29%
	Intracameral cefuroxime and levofloxacin pre- and postoperatively	0.05%
Moshirfar (20,013 surgeries)[5] (Note: all patients had the study drug 1 hour before and 1 week after surgery/q.i.d.)	Moxifloxacin	0.10%
	Gatifloxacin	0.06%
	Overall rate	0.07%

THE ESCRS STUDY

The ESCRS study evaluated the effects of intracameral cefuroxime on the rate of postoperative endophthalmitis in 13,698 cataract surgery patients.[3,4] This partially masked, randomized, multinational study was conducted at 24 sites throughout Europe, with approximately 72 participating ophthalmologists. Patients were randomized to one of four treatment groups: (1) topical placebo preoperatively and immediately after surgery (no intracameral agent); (2) intracameral cefuroxime 1 mg and topical placebo preoperatively and immediately after surgery; (3) perioperative topical levofloxacin 0.5% (two doses preoperatively and three drops immediately postoperatively); and (4) both intracameral cefuroxime and topical levofloxacin (two doses preoperatively and three drops immediately postoperatively). All patients were treated with povidone-iodine 5% preoperatively and levofloxacin 0.5% q.i.d. postoperatively for 6 days beginning on the morning after surgery.[4]

In the ESCRS study, the lowest rate of endophthalmitis (0.05%) was seen in patients treated with both intracameral and topical perioperative antibiotics immediately pre- and postoperatively. The highest rate (0.38%) occurred in patients who did not receive any perioperative therapeutic. Topical perioperative antibiotics alone had some effect on the rate of endophthalmitis (0.335% vs 0.380%), but they were not statistically significantly better than the no-treatment group. The topical antibiotic used was levofloxacin, a third-generation fluoroquinolone. In the placebo groups, subjects did not receive the drug until at least 18 hours after surgery.

Patients receiving intracameral cefuroxime with or without topical antibiotics had significantly lower rates of endophthalmitis than those not receiving intracameral dosing (P=.002). The rate in both intracameral groups (intracameral only/intracameral with topical pre- and postoperative groups) was 0.073%, whereas the rate in the topical only group was 0.335%. Thus, patients not treated with intracameral cefuroxime had a nearly fivefold greater risk of endophthalmitis than did those who received intracameral dosing.

US STUDY

For comparison, in an evaluation of the two topical fourth-generation fluoroquinolones used in the US to prevent postoperative endophthalmitis, Moshirfar et al[5] found rates similar to the intracameral group rates reported by Barry et al in the ESCRS study.[3] In the retrospective analysis of 20,013 cataract surgeries by Moshirfar,[5] all patients received either gatifloxacin 0.3% with benzalkonium chloride 0.005% (Zymar; Allergan, Inc, Irvine, CA) or moxifloxacin (Vigamox; Alcon Laboratories, Inc., Fort Worth, TX) every 15 minutes, three times, starting 1 hour before surgery; 16,209 patients received prophylaxis with gatifloxacin and 3,804 patients with moxifloxacin. After surgery, patients used the same fluoroquinolone q.i.d. for 1 week beginning on the day of surgery.

A total of 14 individuals developed endophthalmitis, resulting in an overall rate of 0.07%. The rate of endophthalmitis was 0.06% in the gatifloxacin group and 0.1% in the moxifloxacin group. The difference in the rate of endophthalmitis between the two groups was not statistically significant but favored gatifloxacin.[5] Of the 14 patients who developed endophthalmitis, six were diagnosed more than 7 days after surgery. Considering the delayed manifestation of the signs of infection, it is highly unlikely that these infections occurred during the cataract procedure, and intracameral prophylaxis could not have prevented these cases.

Table 1 illustrates the endophthalmitis rates in the studies conducted by the ESCRS[3] and Moshirfar.[5] The incidence of this complication was nearly identical in the gatifloxacin group for Moshirfar and the intracameral cefuroxime/topical levofloxacin perioperative group of the ESCRS study. This similarity suggests that intracameral injection offers little or no benefit over the US regimen of perioperative topical prophylaxis with gatifloxacin. Another interesting comparison may be found in the study by West et al[1] that analyzed records from 1998 to 2001. They showed a rate of endophthalmitis of one in 402 prior to the advent of fourth-generation fluoroquinolones, a lower rate than that seen in the levofloxacin group of the ESCRS study (1:342).

RISK FACTORS FOR ENDOPHTHALMITIS

The Moran Eye Center Endophthalmitis Study was conducted to identify risk factors for the development of bacterial endophthalmitis following cataract surgery.[6] The investigation was based on a retrospective review of 1,525 cataract surgery patients, 27 of whom developed endophthalmitis (approximately 18 of 1,000). The results showed that the timing of the postoperative antibiotic's administration has a dramatic effect on the risk of endophthalmitis (odds ratio: 13.7; P=.005). Waiting to instill topical antibiotics until the day after surgery, as was done in the placebo group of the ESCRS study, increased the risk of endophthalmitis nearly 14-fold compared with starting the antibiotics on the day of surgery, the protocol followed in the study by Moshirfar.

The ESCRS study demonstrated that intracameral dosing has much less impact on the risk of infection than does the timing of antibiotic treatment. This study decreased the risk of endophthalmitis by only fivefold (odds ratio: 4.59; P=.002) compared with the topical antibiotic dosing regimen used in the Moran Eye Center Endophthalmitis Study. Thus, although intracameral antibiotics decrease the risk of endophthalmitis, the actual benefit may be less than the ESCRS study suggests if compared with the optimal perioperative use of topical antibiotics (ie, starting fourth-generation topical drops on the day of surgery).

THE BENEFITS AND RISKS OF INTRACAMERAL ANTIBIOTICS

Surgeons considering the use of intracameral antibiotics need to take into account the many potential risks associated with this approach. Perhaps the greatest risk is administering the wrong concentration. Those antibiotics being considered for intracameral use require correct dilution by an experienced pharmacist to avoid potentially toxic effects, such as toxic anterior segment syndrome (TASS). A recent report by the American Society of Ophthalmic Registered Nurses cited intracameral antibiotics that are "improperly dosed, mixed or injected into the eye" as a possible factor in the recent "outbreak" of TASS.[7]

A further issue is the possibly increased risk of macular thickening and cystoid macular edema following cataract surgery using intracameral antibiotics. Although the ESCRS study failed to find any significant change in final visual acuity in the intracameral groups, it did not look closely at macular thickening. My colleagues and I will report a study at this year's ARVO Annual Meeting in which we found that even small changes (≥ 10 µm) in macular thickening were associated with a statistically significant decrease in contrast sensitivity. The change may not be sufficient to show alterations in mean visual acuity over large populations of patients, but it may have significant effects on certain patients. The potential of increased macular thickening or cystoid macular edema needs careful evaluation before surgeons transition to the routine use of intracameral antibiotics.

FINAL THOUGHTS

The available data do not support the use of intracameral antibiotics over current perioperative prophylaxis with topical fourth-generation fluoroquinolones. The different protocols used in the ESCRS' and US investigations prevent a direct comparison between treatments. At present, the rates of endophthalmitis with perioperatively dosed topical fourth-generation fluoroquinolones are equivalent to intracameral treatments but are without the attendant risks of decreased visual function and increased rates of TASS. Also, the duration of protective effect from intracameral antibiotics is short, probably less than 24 hours. Intracameral antibiotics do not address the significant risk of contamination from the surface of the eye that remains until the surgical wound is healed.

Currently, I prescribe Zymar to my patients undergoing cataract surgery, because laboratory and clinical studies have demonstrated the agent's fast killing properties[8] (also Moss JM, Ta CN, unpublished data to be reported at the ARVO Annual Meeting this year). I instruct patients to begin using the drops 2 days preoperatively and emphasize that they should administer the drug on the day of surgery prior to arriving at the surgery center. They receive Zymar at the conclusion of the cataract procedure and wear a patch and shield for the first 4 postoperative hours.

I recently revised my therapeutic regimen, because six of the 14 cases of endophthalmitis in the study by Moshirfar5 occurred more than 7 days after surgery. Upon removal of their eye patch, patients start administering Zymar q2h until bedtime. They continue using the drug q.i.d. for 1 week if the incision is covered by conjunctiva and for 2 weeks if it is a clear corneal incision. ■

This article originally appeared in the April 2007 issue of CRSToday.

1. West ES, Behrens A, McDonnell PJ, et al. The incidence of endophthalmitis after cataract surgery among the U.S. Medicare population increased between 1994 and 2001. *Ophthalmology.* 2005;12:1388-1394.
2. Cooper BA, Holekamp NM, Bohigian G, Thompson PA. Case-control study of endophthalmitis after cataract surgery comparing scleral tunnel and clear cornea wounds. *Am J Ophthalmol.* 2003;136:300-305.
3. Barry P, Seal DV, Gettinby G, et al; ESCRS Endophthalmitis Study Group. ESCRS study of prophylaxis of postoperative endophthalmitis after cataract surgery: preliminary report of principal results from a European multicenter study. *J Cataract Refract Surg.* 2006;32:407-410.
4. Seal DV, Barry P, Gettinby G, et al. ESCRS study of prophylaxis of postoperative endophthalmitis after cataract surgery. Case for a European multicenter study. *J Cataract Refract Surg.* 2006;32:396-406.
5. Moshirfar M. Endophthalmitis following use of fourth generation fluoroquinolones after uncomplicated cataract surgery: a retrospective, observational case series. *Ophthalmology.* 2007;114(4):686-691.
6. Wallin T, Parker J, Jin Y, et al. Cohort study of 27 cases of endophthalmitis at a single institution. *J Cataract Refract Surg.* 2005;31:735-741.
7. American Society of Ophthalmic Registered Nurses. Interim report identifies several potential sources of recent toxic anterior segment syndrome (TASS) outbreak but no single cause. June 21, 2006. Available at: webeye.ophth.uiowa.edu/ASORN/alerts/tass-6-21-2006.htm. Accessed March 13, 2007.
8. Novosad B, Callegan M. Killing of Streptococcus pneumoniae and Haemophilus influenzae ocular isolates by fourth-generation fluoroquinolones. Poster presented at: The ARVO Annual Meeting; May 1, 2006; Fort Lauderdale, FL

CHAPTER 92

Intracameral Vancomycin: Rationale and Experience

HOWARD V. GIMBEL, MD, MPH, FRCSC

The prevention of endophthalmitis has been the impetus for many innovations in cataract surgery.[1] Although used for more than a decade, intracameral vancomycin for the prophylaxis of postoperative endophthalmitis is challenged by the drug's limited spectrum of activity and pharmacodynamics. Fourth-generation fluoroquinolones may be more effective against both gram-positive and gram-negative bacteria, and their intracameral safety is now being established. This article describes the results my colleagues and I have obtained with the routine, in-the-bag injection of vancomycin for preventing endophthalmitis in 36,047 consecutive eyes over a 16-year period. We previously reported early data and established this strategy's safety regarding corneal toxicity.[2]

PERSONAL EXPERIENCE

James Gills, MD, of Tarpon Springs, Florida, began using vancomycin in irrigating solutions in 1987 (a practice we followed in 1988), and his incidence of endophthalmitis dropped from 0.2% to 0.01%.[3]

In 1990, we started using a therapeutic dose of vancomycin as a concentrated bolus (1 mg of vancomycin in 0.1 mL of balanced salt solution [BSS; Alcon Laboratories, Inc., Fort Worth, TX]) injected under the IOL and into the capsular bag at the end of the case rather than a more dilute solution continuously infused in the irrigating solution. My reasoning was that infection was most likely to start in the aqueous fluid that the IOL sequesters in the bag and that, if the drug were placed in that location, it would not wash out as quickly as it would from the anterior chamber.

I placed incisions on the steep meridian, so there was a mixture of superior scleral tunnel incisions under a limbus-based conjunctival flap and temporal clear corneal incisions. I sutured fewer than 0.5% of the incisions. I started patients on Maxidex or Tobradex (both from Alcon Laboratories, Inc.) drops q.i.d. 1 day preoperatively and had them continue the drops immediately after surgery.

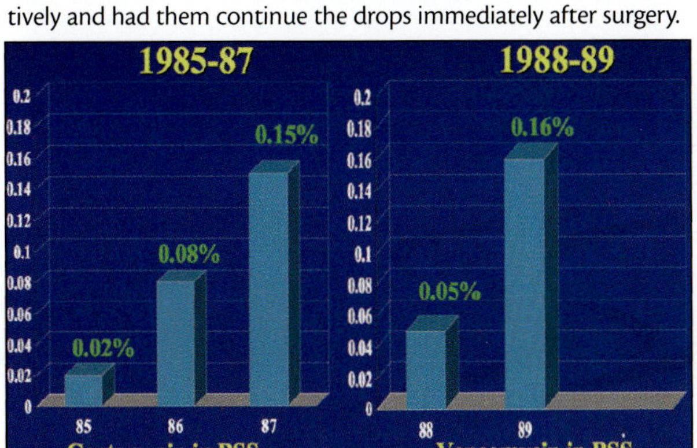

Figure 1. These graphs show the incidence of endophthalmitis at the Gimbel Eye Center prior to the administration of intracameral vancomycin as a bolus under the IOL.

RESULTS

With Garamycin (Schering-Plough Corporation, Kenilworth, NJ) in the irrigating solution (1985 to 1987), the year-to-year incidence of endophthalmitis at the Gimbel Eye Centre in Calgary, Alberta, Canada, ranged from 0.02% to 0.15%. This rate remained relatively unchanged after we replaced vancomycin with Garamycin in the irrigating solution (1988 to 1989) (Figure 1).

In a series of 36,047 consecutive eyes from 1990 through 2006 in which we placed vancomycin as a bolus under the IOL, three eyes developed what was probably toxic endophthalmitis (Figure 2). These patients presented with anterior chamber fibrin but without pain on the first postoperative day. We managed the eyes aggressively with anterior vitrectomy through a posterior capsular capsulorhexis using the original cataract incision and an intravitreal injection of vancomycin 1 mg in 1 mL of BSS. All three eyes were culture negative and regained a BCVA of 20/20.

A fourth eye developed anterior segment inflammation and pain on the second postoperative day, although there was no hypopyon or fibrin. Conservative therapy achieved initial improvement, but then the eye developed a fibrinous veil. It was not managed with the anterior vitrectomy approach like the other three cases. On day 7, the patient was referred to a retinal specialist who, on the eighth day, performed an anterior chamber tap and injected an antibiotic. Visual acuity improved to 20/40, but the recovery was unsatisfactory. Pars plana vitrectomy and antibiotic injection were therefore performed on the 10th postoperative day. The patient's visual acuity 8 weeks later was 20/25. Although cultures were all negative, this case was most likely a low-grade infectious endophthalmitis (Table 1).

Considering all four of these cases, although the first three presented as toxic endophthalmitis, the incidence in this series (at one center) is 4:36,047 or 0.011%.

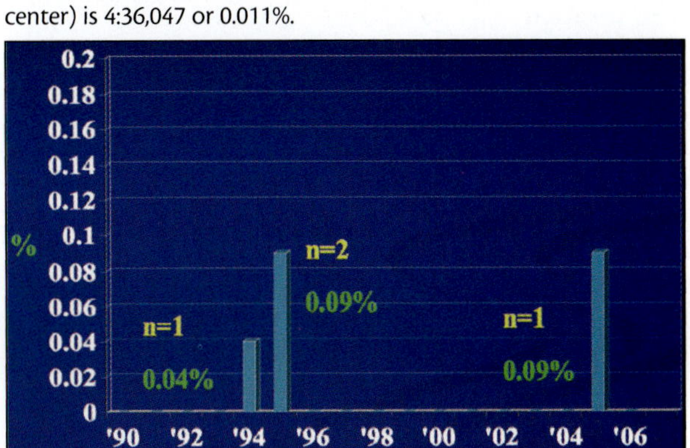

Figure 2. This graph shows the incidence of endophthalmitis (0.01%) in 36,047 consecutive eyes from 1990 to 2006 using intracameral vancomycin as a bolus under the IOL.

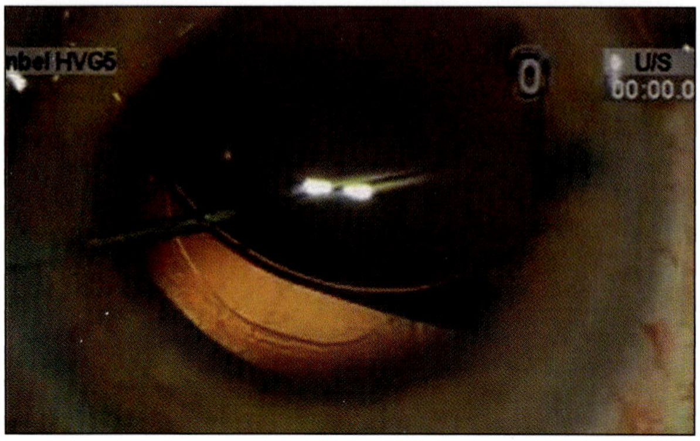

Figure 3. The surgeon injects vancomycin into the bag, under the IOL.

DISCUSSION

Most anterior segment ophthalmologists use broad-spectrum antibiotics either subconjunctivally or intracamerally during surgery. Both in vivo and in vitro studies have shown intracameral vancomycin to be effective for endophthalmitis prophylaxis.[4-8] A number of investigators have suggested that vancomycin used intracamerally can significantly reduce the risk of endophthalmitis.[9-16] A survey conducted by the ASCRS showed that at least 35% of ophthalmic surgeons were using intracameral antibiotics.[17] Of the surgeons surveyed, 80% used vancomycin, and more than 40% used gentamicin.

The AAO-CDC Task Force on Vancomycin Prophylaxis in Ophthalmic Surgery recommends the prudent use of vancomycin in routine cataract surgery because of the potential for resistance to the drug and the lack of evidence for its effectiveness in preventing postoperative endophthalmitis.[18] Recent in vivo and in vitro studies, however, have shown that resistance to vancomycin is unlikely in cataract surgery and that the drug continues to be quite effective in inhibiting bacterial colony-forming units.[9-12]

To determine what constitutes a prudent use of vancomycin, one should consider the pharmacokinetics of the drug. Vancomycin is a time-dependent antibiotic and requires prolonged contact with microbes in the anterior chamber to be effective. When injected at 20 µm per 1 mL of BSS, the antibiotic has a half-life of approximately 2 hours.[14,15] Because aqueous turnover occurs within 1 to 2 hours, vancomycin may be most effective if injected in the bag, under the IOL, with the optic's edge well covered by the anterior capsule (Figure 3). This method of injection should result in a sustained release of vancomycin at therapeutic levels—important because vancomycin is relatively slow at killing organisms and may require 8 to 12 hours to reduce the inocula

The improvement in outcomes in the recent ESCRS study using cefuroxime as a bolus at the end of surgery seems to confirm that a bolus of antibiotic with even a slow kill rate placed in the anterior chamber (where aqueous turnover is shorter than the kill time of the antibiotic) effectively lowers the incidence of endophthalmitis after cataract surgery.[19]

The lower incidence in our series compared with the cefuroxime group in the European series (one per 10,000 compared to six per 10,000) may not be because of the difference in the antibiotic used. Rather, it may be related to a one-center series versus a multicenter study, differences in pre- and postoperative routines, variations in surgical technique (such as the capsulorhexis' diameter compared with the optic of the IOL), whether or not the viscoelastic was removed from under the IOL with the I/A tip placed under the IOL, whether the bolus of the drug was placed under the IOL into the capsular bag or just into the anterior chamber, and the possible additional confounding factor of environmental and host resistance.

Another factor to consider relates to our center's preoperative protocol. Whether diabetic or not, we ask our patients to minimize or eliminate their intake of simple sugars for a few days before and after surgery. The Endophthalmitis Vitrectomy Study found that diabetics tend to have more virulent organisms, to have a higher percentage of gram-negative isolates, and to be culture negative less often.[20]

Although newer broad-spectrum drugs will probably become more commonly used intracamerally than vancomycin, there is little motivation for us to change protocols or drugs when we have not lost an eye or had patients lose vision to less than 20/25 due to infectious or toxic endophthalmitis in 36,047 cataract surgeries. ■

This article originally appeared in the April 2007 issue of CRSToday.

TABLE 1. CASE SUMMARIES OF ENDOPHTHALMITIS

Year	Incision	IOL/OVD	1 Day Postoperatively	Treatment	BCVA	Culture
1994	Scleral 5.5 mm	812A/ Healon GV	4+ cell and flare Hypopyon cell and flare	Posterior continuous curvilinear capsulorhexis Anterior vitrectomy antibiotics	6 days 20/20	Negative
1995	Clear corneal 3.2 mm	SI30NB/ Healon GV	4+ cell and flare Hypopyon 20/70	Posterior continuous curvilinear capsulorhexis Anterior vitrectomy antibiotics	5 weeks 20/20	Negative
1995	Clear corneal 3.2 mm	SI30NB/ Healon GV	4+ cell and flare Hypopyon cell and flare	Posterior continuous curvilinear capsulorhexis Anterior vitrectomy antibiotics	7 weeks 20/20	Negative
2005	Clear corneal 3.2 mm	SA60AT/ Healon5	8 days postoperatively 4+ cell and flare Hypopyon cell and flare	Anterior chamber tap Pars plana vitrectomy antibiotics	8 weeks 20/25	Negative

Note: The 812A lens (Pfizer, Inc., New York, NY); Healon GV, Healon5, and the SI30NB lens (Advanced Medical Optics, Inc., Santa Ana, CA); the SA60AT lens (Alcon Laboratories, Inc., Fort Worth, TX).

1. Gills JP. Filters and antibiotics in irrigating solution for cataract surgery. *J Cataract Refract Surg*. 1991;17:385.
2. Gimbel HV, Sun R, DeBroff BM. Prophylactic intracameral antibiotics during cataract surgery: the incidence of endophthalmitis and corneal endothelial cell loss. *Eur J Implant Refract Surg*. 1994;6:280-285.
3. Gills JP. Pharmacodynamics of cataract surgery. In: Gills JP, ed. Cataract Surgery: The State of the Art. Thorofare, NJ: Slack, Inc.; 1998:19-26.
4. Olson RJ. Reducing the risk of postoperative endophthalmitis. *Surv Ophthalmol*. 2004;49(suppl 2):55-61.
5. Busbee BG. Advances in knowledge and treatment: an update on endophthalmitis. *Curr Opin Ophthalmol*. 2004;15:232-237.
6. Mamalis N, Kearsley L, Brinton E. Postoperative endophthalmitis. *Curr Opin Ophthalmol*. 2002;15:14-16.
7. Benz MS, Scott IU, Flynn HW, et al. Endophthalmitis isolates and antibiotic sensitivities: a 6-year review of culture proven cases. *Am J Ophthalmol*. 2004;137:38-42.
8. Gordon YJ. Vancomycin prophylaxis and emerging resistance: are ophthalmologists the villains? The heroes? *Am J Ophthalmol*. 2001;131:371-376.
9. Seppala H, Al-Juhaish M, Jarvinen H, et al. Effect of prophylactic antibiotics on antimicrobial resistance of viridans streptococci in the normal flora of cataract surgery patients. *J Cataract Refract Surg*. 2004;30:307-315.
10. Ta CN, Chang RT, Singh K, et al. Antibiotic resistance patterns of ocular bacterial flora: a prospective study of patients undergoing anterior segment surgery. *Ophthalmology*. 2003;110:1946-1951.
11. Libre PE, Della-Latta P, Chin NX. Intracameral antibiotic agents for endophthalmitis prophylaxis: a pharmacokinetic model. *J Cataract Refract Surg*. 2003;29:1791-1794.
12. Sobaci G, Tuncer K, Tas A, et al. The effect of intraoperative antibiotics in irrigating solutions on aqueous humor contamination and endophthalmitis after phacoemulsification surgery. *Eur J Ophthalmol*. 2003;13:773-778.
13. Das T, Sharma S, Muralidhar AV; Endophthalmitis Research Group. Effect of vancomycin on Staphylococcus epidermidis adherence to poly(methyl methacrylate) intraocular lenses. *J Cataract Refract Surg*. 2002;28:703-708.
14. Souli M, Kopsinis G, Kavouklis E, et al. Vancomycin levels in human aqueous humour after intravenous and subconjunctival administration. *Int J Antimicrob Agents*. 2001;18:239-243.
15. Mendivil Soto A, Mendivil MP. The effect of topical povidone-iodine, intraocular vancomycin, or both on aqueous humor cultures at the time of cataract surgery. *Am J Ophthalmol*. 2001;131:293-300.
16. Tipperman R. Pharmacologic considerations for cataract surgery. *Curr Opin Ophthalmol*. 2004;15:51-55.
17. Masket S. Preventing, diagnosing and treating endophthalmitis (guest editorial). *J Cataract Refract Surg*. 1998;24:725-726.
18. The American Academy of Ophthalmology information statements page. The prophylactic use of vancomycin for intraocular surgery. A joint statement of the American Academy of Ophthalmology and the Centers for Disease Control and Prevention. Available at: www.aao.org/aao/education/library/information/vancomycin.cfm. Accessed January 14, 2005.
19. Barry P, Seal DV, Gettinby G, et al. ESCRS study of prophylaxis of postoperative endophthalmitis after cataract surgery: preliminary report of principal results from a European multicentre study. *J Cataract Refract Surg*. 2006;32:3:407-410.
20. Results of the Endophthalmitis Vitrectomy Study. A randomized trial of immediate vitrectomy and of intravenous antibiotics for the treatment of postoperative bacterial endophthalmitis. Endophthalmitis Vitrectomy Study Group. *Arch Ophthalmol*. 1995;113:1479-1496.

CHAPTER 93

Prophylaxis With Intracameral Cefuroxime

RICHARD B. PACKARD, MD, FRCS, FRCOphth

Between December 2003 and April 2004, my colleagues and I diagnosed nine cases of infectious endophthalmitis following cataract surgery in our practice. Although we thoroughly investigated all of our procedures and the off-site facility where our instruments are sterilized, we could not determine the cause of this high number of cases in such a short period of time. The surgical cases infected were those of six surgeons of all grades of seniority. They used topical, sub-Tenon's, and peribulbar anesthesia, and they performed both temporal and superior clear corneal incisions.

This article discusses the issues we identified as possible culprits of the outbreak and how we altered our practice to prevent the incidence of infectious endophthalmitis after future cataract surgeries.

INVESTIGATION AND SOLUTIONS

The Sterilization of Instrument Trays

During our investigation, my colleagues and I found that, at the sterilization facility, our instrument trays, due to inadequate vents, would not allow sufficient drying after steam autoclaving by the recently installed, new autoclaving devices. This resulted in some trays' returning to our facility slightly damp. As a solution, we introduced new, custom-designed trays with a much greater area to allow for evaporation at the end of the autoclaving cycle.

Disposable Instruments

We only use our phaco needles once for surgery before discarding them, as recommended by the manufacturers. In order to reduce any further problems with material trapped in lumens, however, we custom-designed disposable bimanual I/A handpieces.

Disinfecting the Wound

Although we had used 5% povidone-iodine preoperatively for each case in question, we now make sure to introduce it before applying any lignocaine gel in patients receiving topical anesthesia. This is done to avoid losing any effectiveness of the antiseptic from its mixing with the anesthetic gel. We also administer a drop of povidone iodine at the conclusion of the case to resterilize the

INTRACAMERAL CEFUROXIME

Use

- Dilute 0.93 mg of cefuroxime in 0.1 mL of water to be injected into the anterior chamber at the end of cataract surgery.

Reconstitution of Cefuroxime

- Add 2.5 mL of water for injection to 250 mg of cefuroxime (results in a mixture of 93.0 mg/mL or 9.3 mg/0.1 mL).
- Take 0.1 mL of this solution and add 0.9 mL of water for injection (results in a mixture of 0.93 mg in 0.1 mL).
- Discard 0.9 mL to leave 0.1 mL in the syringe.
- Inject 0.1 mL of the solution into the anterior chamber with a 1.0-mL syringe and a Rycroft cannula (Ellis Ophthalmic Technologies, Inc., Jamaica, NY).

conjunctival sac and to allow us to ensure that the eye is Seidel negative.

Preoperatively Dosed Ocular Medications

We have switched from the preoperative chloramphenical drops we had previously given immediately before surgery to ofloxacin. This new drug regimen is also followed while the patient is on the operating table, at the end of cataract surgery, prior to the instillation of povidone-iodine. The ofloxacin is continued on the day of surgery four times daily and for 1 week postoperatively. Fourth-generation fluoroquinolones are not yet available in the UK, but, when they do become available, they will probably be incorporated into our regime in place of the ofloxacin.

Intracameral Cefuroxime

Having been aware of the research done in Sweden with intracameral cefuroxime,[1] we decided to add this technique to our regimen at the conclusion of cataract surgery, prior to instilling a drop of ofloxacin and the povidone-iodine wash. The cefuroxime is diluted using the regimen quoted by Montan et al.[1] The nursing staff is responsible for this dilution for each cataract surgery.

CONCLUSION

All surgeons performing cataract surgery at our facility began to use the regimen described herein in May 2004. Since that time, we have had only one case of endophthalmitis after cataract surgery, despite a culture-negative vitreous biopsy. The patient recovered to 20/30 UCVA within 3 weeks of surgery.

Our training unit has five consultants and two associate specialists performing cataract surgery as well as a changing population of five residents in training. Since adopting the new regimen, there have been 15 different operating residents. All surgeons perform clear corneal incisions, albeit with varying skill levels and wound architecture. The incidence of posterior capsular rupture, which is often considered a risk factor for infectious endophthalmitis, has varied between 1% for consultants to 5% for the most junior trainees.

Since May 2004, my colleagues and I have performed more than 7,500 cataract procedures. Our incidence of endophthalmitis is less than 0.013%, much lower than that reported by Montan et al[1] (20 out of 32,180 patients or 0.06%). In the recently published ESCRS endophthalmitis study,[2] the arm using intracameral cefuroxime had an incidence of five out of 6,836 patients (0.073%). In two recent reports of surgery during which intracameral cefuroxime was not utilized, endophthalmitis occurred in 43 out of 8,736 (0.49%) patients and 44 out of 12,362 (0.36%) patients.[3,4] Of course, my colleagues and I cannot say for certain that intracameral cefuroxime has contributed to our low incidence of endophthalmitis after cataract surgery. In light of the Swedish and ESCRS data, however, we believe that surgeons should consider intracameral cefuroxime along with the other measures mentioned herein to minimize postoperative infection. ■

This article originally appeared in the April 2007 issue of CRSToday.

1. Montan PG, Wegde G, Koranyi G, Rylander M. Prophylactic intracameral cefuroxime. Efficacy in preventing endophthalmitis after cataract surgery. *J Cataract Refract Surg.* 2002;28:977-981.
2. Barry P, Seal DV, Gettingby G, et al. ESCRS study of prophylaxis of postoperative endophthalmitis after cataract surgery: preliminary report of principal results from a European multicentre study. *J Cataract Refract Surg.* 2006;32:407-410.
3. Patwardhan A, Rao GP, Saha K, Craig EA. Incidence and outcomes evaluation of endophthalmitis management after phacoemulsification and 3-piece silicone intraocular lens implantation over 6 years in a single eye unit. *J Cataract Refract Surg.* 2006;32:1018-1021.
4. Khan RI, Kennedy S, Barry P. Incidence of presumed postoperative endophthalmitis in Dublin for a 5-year period (1997-2001). *J Cataract Refract Surg.* 2005;31:1575-1581.

CHAPTER 94

Intracameral Moxifloxacin for Antibacterial Prophylaxis in Cataract Surgery

STEVE A. ARSHINOFF, MD

The recent publication of the ESCRS study[1,2] demonstrated the intracameral efficacy of cefuroxime for the prophylaxis of endophthalmitis after cataract surgery. The investigators recommended that surgeons consider intracameral cefuroxime prophylaxis for all cataract procedures.[1,2] The studies validated the intracameral route of antibiotic delivery as effective for antibacterial prophylaxis, but perhaps the investigators involved did not choose the best agent available.[4] The study did have some limitations. Table 1 shows the agents that have been used to date.

I have used intracameral moxifloxacin (Vigamox; Alcon Laboratories, Inc., Fort Worth, TX) for antibacterial prophylaxis in cataract surgery in more than 1,500 cases since October 2004 without any incidence of infection or unwanted side effects. Intracameral Vigamox can be easily prepared from bottles of topical Vigamox by diluting it 5:1 with balanced salt solution (BSS; Alcon Laboratories, Inc.) in the OR. The preparation does not require Millipore filtration, and its yellow color makes confusing it intraoperatively with other coexisting syringes unlikely. The solution's simple use at the end of a case achieves antibacterial prophylaxis and pressurization of the anterior chamber simultaneously. The recent study of Espiritu et al[4] confirms the safety of intracameral Vigamox up to a concentration of 500 µg/0.1 mL (five times the concentration I recommend). This article discusses my prophylactic process with this agent.

MY PREVIOUS EXPERIENCE WITH INTRACAMERAL ANTIBIOTICS

I started using intracameral antibiotics in 1995 with vancomycin 1 mg in 0.1 mL of BSS (recipe received from Howard Gimbel, MD. See Dr. Gimbel's article on page 71) when performing routine, simultaneous, bilateral cataract surgery. I used intracameral vancomycin for about 10 years in every intraocular procedure I performed (approximately 6,000 cases) without any occurrences of postoperative endophthalmitis.

TABLE 1. INTRACAMERAL ANTIBIOTIC PROPHYLAXIS

Class	Drug	Dose (per 0.1 mL)
Complex glycopeptide	Vancomycin	1.0 mg
Cephalosporins	Cefazolin (first-generation) Cefuroxime (second-generation)	1.0 to 2.5 mg 1.0 mg
Fourth-generation fluoroquinolones	Gatifloxacin Moxifloxacin	100 µg 100 µg

Vancomycin does not cover the 5% of reported endophthalmitis cases caused by gram-negative bacteria, and its use requires the relatively complicated dilution of the supplied lyophilized drug and filtering through a Millipore filter. I was afraid that the pharmacy might mix it with sterile water rather than BSS, so I, or the OR's ophthalmic circulating nurse, prepared the solution in the OR. I searched for a better agent, especially after 2002, when Canadian generic preparations of vancomycin began to be substituted in hospitals for the traditional product. Jeff Sher, MD, of Hamilton Health Sciences Centre in Ontario, Canada (verbal communication, summer 2002), discovered that generic vancomycin had been associated with toxic anterior segment syndrome (TASS), and he demonstrated an incompatibility of the drug with BSS. The traditional products were more expensive and therefore avoided by Canadian hospitals.

In January 2004, fourth-generation fluoroquinolones became available, and the self-preserved nature of Vigamox eye drops made the drug an attractive potential intracameral agent. It was also very broad spectrum, could be simply diluted with BSS in the OR, and did not require Millipore filtration. I wanted to know more about the drug's intraocular safety, however, before using it.

Donnenfeld et al performed a study of intracameral prophylaxis for cataract surgery in 40 cases using gatifloxacin 100 µg in 0.1 mL of BSS.5 Frances Mah, MD, from Pittsburgh has reported on intraocular toxicity studies of moxifloxacin that concluded that even full-strength Vigamox (500 µg/mL) was nontoxic to rabbit corneal endothelial cells.6 Moxifloxacin covered all reported endophthalmitis pathogens in both studies.

INTRACAMERAL VIGAMOX

After the 2004 AAO Annual Meeting, I began to use intracameral Vigamox subsequent to receiving appropriate consent from my patients and carefully monitoring each of their eye's postoperative course. Initially, I used 100 µg in 0.2 mL of BSS (50 µg/0.1 mL of BSS; 350 cases), but I changed to 100 µg in 0.1 mL of BSS for the subsequent 1,200+ cases. I have had no incidents of postoperative endophthalmitis or excessive inflammation postoperatively. I continue to routinely use intracameral Vigamox 100 µg in 0.1 mL of BSS for every cataract procedure I perform.

The preparation of Vigamox for intracameral use is simple. A new bottle of Vigamox is opened in the OR. A 10-mL syringe with a 20-gauge needle is used to draw 2 mL of Vigamox into the syringe. The same needle is then inserted into a new 25-mL bottle of BSS, and 8 mL BSS is drawn up into the syringe. This combination yields a 5:1 dilution of the original 500 µg/mL Vigamox to 100µg/mL. Rolling the syringe promotes mixing of the solution, which is already well combined by the turbulence of drawing the BSS up into the syringe after the Vigamox.

A 0.5-mL aliquot of the Vigamox mixture is injected from the same syringe, without changing the needle, into a small medicine

TABLE 2. SCORECARD: BEST DRUG FOR INTRACAMERAL USE

Class of Drug	Glycopeptide	Cephalosporins		Fourth-Generation Fluoroquinolones	
Drug's Name	Vancomycin	Cefazolin	Cefuroxime	Gatifloxacin	Moxifloxacin
Mechanism of action*	(TD) 2	(TD) 2	(TD) 2	(DD) 5	(DD) 5
*Staphylococcus aureus** kill in 3 hours	(< 1 LU) 1	(< 1 LU) 1	(< 1 LU) 1	(> 3 LU) 5	(> 3 LU) 5
Pathogens covered*	3	1	3	5	5
Allergic potential*	5	1	1	5	5
Preparation's complexity*	1	1	1	1	5
Overall score (x/25)	**12**	**6**	**8**	**21**	**25**

**Each attribute scored out of 5.*
TD = time dependent
DD = dose dependent
LU = log unit

cup on each case's scrub table just before it is needed. Next, the scrub nurse draws the solution into a TB syringe. She then attaches a 27-gauge hockey stick cannula to expel any air and all but 0.2 mL of the Vigamox solution. She hands the syringe to me, and I inject 0.1 mL of the Vigamox into the eye through the sideport incision, across the anterior chamber, and under the capsulorhexis' edge. This process bathes the IOL in moxifloxacin, achieving antibacterial prophylaxis and pressurizing the anterior chamber simultaneously, and it is the final step of the procedure. A 0.2-mL Vigamox solution is given to the surgeon, rather than only 0.1 mL, because the extra amount allows the surgeon to expel any air from the cannula before inserting it into the eye.

IN SUMMARY

I currently consider Vigamox to be the most broad-spectrum, simplest, and safest available agent to prepare for intracameral injection (Table 2). Other drugs used intracamerally to date include cefuroxime[1,3,7] and cefazolin,[8,9] for both of which there have reports of anaphylaxis and neither of which is as broad spectrum as Vigamox. As discussed earlier, vancomycin does not cover gram negatives, and gatifloxacin comes preserved with benzalkonium chloride, making it undesirable for intracameral use. If the ESCRS study had used moxifloxacin, I believe the results would have achieved an even more profound reduction of endophthalmitis.

I have used the method described above in over 3,000 surgical cases with no complications and no cases of postoperative endophthalmitis. Others have since proven that full-strength Vigamox straight from the bottle is safe for intracameral use. Thus, the only alteration that I have made to the recipe is that I now have the nurse hand me a TB syringe with 0.5 cc of 100 µg/0.1 ml moxifloxacin. I do not intend to put more than 100 µg (0.1 ml) into the eye, but sometimes extra is useful to hydrate the incisions after the intracameral injection to be sure the wounds seal well and that the moxifloxacin has remained in the eye through the completion of surgery. (Addendum from December 2008) ■

Note: Throughout the article, the author generally used generic names for gatifloxacin and moxifloxacin, except where the drug used and the properties thereby achieved refer to a specific brand of product.

This article originally appeared in the April 2007 issue of CRSToday.

1. Seal DV, Barry P, Gettinby G, et al. ESCRS study of prophylaxis of postoperative endophthalmitis after cataract surgery: case for a European multicenter study. *J Cataract Refract Surg.* 2006;32:396-406.
2. Barry P, Seal DV, Gettinby G. ESCRS study of prophylaxis of postoperative endophthalmitis after cataract surgery: preliminary report of principal results from a European multicenter study. *J Cataract Refract Surg.* 2006;32:407-410.
3. Packard RB, Olson RJ, Donnenfeld ED, et al. Endophthalmitis after cataract surgery. Experts in the field respond to the recent press release from the ESCRS. *Cataract & Refractive Surgery Today.* 2006;6:May:5:28-35.
4. Espiritu CRG, Caparas, VL, Bolinao JG. Safety of prophylactic intracameral moxifloxacin 0.5% ophthalmic solution in cataract surgery patients. *J Cataract Refract Surg.* 2007;33:63-68.
5. Donnenfeld ED, Snyder RW, Kanellopolous AJ, et al. Safety of prophylactic intracameral gatifloxacin in cataract surgery. Paper presented at: The OMIG Meeting; November 15, 2003; Anaheim, CA.
6. Mah Francis S. Which topical fluoroquinolone to use? Paper presented at: The Annual AAO Meeting; October 25, 2004; New Orleans, LA.
7. Montan PG, Wejde G, Koranyi G, Rylander M. Prophylactic intracameral cefuroxime. *J Cataract Refract Surg.* 2002;28:977-987.
8. Garat M, Moser CL, Alonso-Tarres C, et al. Intracameral cefazolin to prevent endophthalmitis in cataract surgery: a 3 year retrospective study. *J Cataract Refract Surg.* 2005;31:2230-2234.
9. Romero P, Mendez I, Salvat M, et al. Intracameral cefazolin as prophylaxis against endophthalmitis in cataract surgery. *J Cataract Refract Surg.* 2006;32:438-441.

CHAPTER 95

The Top Four Errors in Prescribing Antibiotics

DAVID G. HWANG, MD

Much of the impetus for developing the latest group of highly active fluoroquinolones—such as gatifloxacin 0.3% (Zymar; Allergan, Inc., Irvine, CA), moxifloxacin 0.5% (Vigamox; Alcon Laboratories, Inc., Fort Worth, TX), and levofloxacin 1.5% (Iquix; Santen, Inc., Napa, CA)—came from the observation that older ophthalmic fluoroquinolones such as ciprofloxacin (Ciloxan; Alcon Laboratories, Inc.) and ofloxacin (Ocuflox; Allergan, Inc.) had begun to show signs of declining therapeutic efficacy and increasing in vitro resistance.[1] The reasons for this trend include, not just selection pressure caused by human systemic fluoroquinolone use and widespread fluoroquinolone use in US poultry farming, but also selection pressure potentially caused by indiscriminate and incorrect ophthalmic usage.[1]

Ophthalmologists must wisely use the newly available group of fluoroquinolones, which have improved activity relative to the older generations',[2] or these agents will soon meet a fate similar to that of older fluoroquinolones. This article describes the most common errors and misconceptions associated with prescribing antibiotics and highlights new evidence that the proper use of these agents can maximize their efficacy, minimize potential side effects, and limit the development of bacterial resistance.

TABLE 1. GUIDELINES FOR PROPER FLUOROQUINOLONE DOSING
Dose no less frequently than four times daily
Dose only for the required period of time: Bacterial conjunctivitis: 1 week Bacterial keratitis: 2 to 3 weeks Post-LASIK: 3 to 7 days Postcataract surgery: 1 week
Curtail treatment by abrupt discontinuation rather than by tapering

ERROR NO. 1: USING A SLEDGEHAMMER TO SWAT A FLY

Today's powerful, broad-spectrum antibiotics are appropriate for the treatment and prophylaxis of serious infections such as bacterial keratitis, post-LASIK keratitis, and postoperative endophthalmitis. Using these antibiotics as first-line treatment of relatively minor or chronic infections such as blepharitis or uncomplicated conjunctivitis, however, is overkill and can invite the development of resistance.

Not every infectious indication requires the newest antibiotic. Instead, the selection of an antibiotic should be tailored to the type and severity of the infection. In general, older antibiotics with a narrower spectrum can effectively treat less serious ocular infections such as blepharitis and uncomplicated bacterial conjunctivitis. Examples of excellent antimicrobials for these indications include bacitracin for blepharitis and polymyxin B-trimethoprim for uncomplicated bacterial conjunctivitis. Not only are these particular antimicrobials less likely to exert a strong degree of selection pressure that can promote resistance, but they also have the advantage of being considerably less expensive than newer fluoroquinolones.

For most routine, uncomplicated cases of bacterial conjunctivitis, older agents such as polymyxin B-trimethoprim, ciprofloxacin, and ofloxacin have been shown to be generally comparable to the newer fluoroquinolones in effecting a final clinical cure.[3] The more recently introduced fluoroquinolones, however, may be more appropriate when laboratory resistance to first-line agents has been documented or when clinical nonresponsiveness or relapse has been encountered after treatment with a first-line antimicrobial. Furthermore, because fluoroquinolones with better antimicrobial activity may in some cases effect a more rapid microbiological cure than older fluoroquinolones,[4] it may be preferable to use a newer fluoroquinolone as first-line therapy for cases of bacterial conjunctivitis in which rapid bacterial eradication is essential. Examples include patients at risk for secondary infectious complications from bacterial conjunctivitis (eg, those with bullous keratopathy or an avascular filtering bleb) or individuals for whom there is a need to limit horizontal transmission to their contacts at home, school, or workplace.

ERROR NO. 2: IF ONE ANTIBIOTIC IS GOOD, TWO MUST BE BETTER

Another common error is to add unneeded antibiotics to a regimen that already incorporates one of the newer, highly active fluoroquinolones. With few exceptions, as described later, this approach adds no more antibacterial activity or spectrum but instead increases costs and the likelihood of toxicity and noncompliance. Common examples of this prescribing error include using two different fluoroquinolones simultaneously or using a fluoroquinolone in combination with a nonfortified aminoglycoside.

In exceptional cases, the addition of a second agent to a newer fluoroquinolone may be justified for initial treatment or empiric prophylaxis. The prime example is infections for which the suspected pathogens are likely to display fluoroquinolone resistance, such as methicillin-resistant staphylococci or ciprofloxacin-resistant *Pseudomonas*. Although these pathogens can occur in community-acquired infections, they are more common in patients who have been exposed to a hospital environment (eg, healthcare workers[5] or recently hospitalized patients) or who have recently been treated systemically or topically with fluoroquinolones or other broad-spectrum antimicrobials.

Methicillin resistance in staphylococci is frequently associated with the concomitant expression of fluoroquinolone resistance.[6] Although newer fluoroquinolones may show somewhat better activity against methicillin-resistant *Staphylococcus aureus* and *Staphylococcus epidermidis* (MRSA and MRSE, respectively) than the older fluoroquinolones, such activity can be variable. Therefore, infections due to MRSA and MRSE are best treated with vancomycin.

The recommendations for surgical prophylaxis in patients at increased risk for acquiring MRSA and MRSE infections are somewhat different. For intraoperative use in intraocular surgery, vancomycin may be administered via various routes, including intracamerally, subconjunctivally, and in collagen shields. The use of vancomycin delivered intracamerally by injection or via irrigating solutions, however, has been associated with an increased risk of developing clinically significant cystoid macular edema.[7] Using topical vancomycin for perioperative surgical prophylaxis is also problematic because of the lack of a commercially available formulation and the strong association of topical vancomycin use with ocular surface irritation and epithelial toxicity. For these reasons, a reasonable alternative in the subgroup of patients at risk for MRSA and MRSE is to use a topical, commercially available, 8-methoxyfluoroquinolone such as gatifloxacin or moxifloxacin. Although the activity of the 8-methoxyfluoroquinolones against MRSA and MRSE can be variable[2] and is less consistent than that of vancomycin, it is generally superior to the activity of fluoroquinolones such as ciprofloxacin, ofloxacin, and levofloxacin.[8,9]

When treating *Pseudomonas aeruginosa* ocular infections, all of the fluoroquinolones available for ophthalmic use (except for norfloxacin 0.3% [Chibroxin; Merck & Co., Inc., West Point, PA]) provide reasonable coverage for empiric use, but ciprofloxacin may be preferable in more severe, culture-positive cases due to its superior in vitro antipseudomonal activity compared with the other ophthalmic fluoroquinolones. Although data are lacking concerning the potential clinical benefit of combining a fluoroquinolone with a second antipseudomonal drug (such as tobramycin or amikacin), there are some strains for which in vitro testing can show an additional benefit from combination therapy. It therefore may be reasonable to consider adding an aminoglycoside in severe cases of *Pseudomonas* infection. Also, in cases of *P. aeruginosa* infection that occur in the setting of prior topical or systemic treatment with a fluoroquinolone, the possibility of encountering a fluoroquinolone-resistant *P. aeruginosa* strain is greater. For the empiric treatment or prophylaxis of these cases, the inclusion of fortified tobramycin or amikacin in the antibiotic regimen would be prudent.

ERROR NO. 3: IN VITRO = IN VIVO

How would one predict if a particular bacterial pathogen is likely to be resistant or susceptible to a given antibiotic? At first glance, the answer seems simple: one should perform culture and susceptibility testing (eg, Kirby-Bauer disk diffusion assay) and, on that basis, determine whether the pathogen is "susceptible," "intermediate," or "resistant." Yet, relying on such in vitro testing alone in an attempt to predict the clinical response to an antimicrobial is a vast oversimplification and can lead to an erroneous therapeutic strategy.

It is important to remember that the susceptibility breakpoints are based on systemic dosing, not ophthalmic dosing. A pathogen that is deemed resistant to the typical levels of an antibiotic that can be achieved with systemic dosing might be susceptible to the higher levels achievable with topical dosing. Until ocular susceptibility breakpoint criteria are established, clinicians must interpret susceptibility reports with caution. For example, aminoglycoside resistance in *P. aeruginosa* is typically relative and can be overcome by increasing the aminoglycoside concentration. Thus, bacterial keratitis caused by so-called gentamicin-resistant *P. aeruginosa* may in fact respond well to topical gentamicin administration, which can achieve relatively higher concentrations in ocular tissues.[10] Conversely, in vitro susceptibility may not necessarily predict a good clinical response. For example, streptococcal keratitis isolates that are susceptible to ciprofloxacin on in vitro testing frequently respond poorly to ciprofloxacin in vivo.[11]

What can explain the discrepancies between in vitro susceptibility results and clinical response? Certainly, the ocular pharmacokinetic characteristics of the antibiotic in question play an important part. One must take into account a drug's ability to achieve and sustain a desired therapeutic concentration in the tissue or fluid compartment of interest. A drug that is highly active against a particular organism but penetrates poorly into the aqueous might be adequate for treating superficial ocular surface infections, but it would be a poor choice for postoperative endophthalmitis prophylaxis. Nonfortified aminoglycosides, for example, are generally not effective for topical prophylaxis after intraocular surgery, because the anterior-chamber levels of drug achievable after topical dosing are exceedingly low.[12]

Pharmacodynamics is a discipline that attempts to describe how pharmacology, pharmacokinetics, pharmacogenetics, and other factors work together to govern the biological activity of a given drug over time in a living organism. Although the application of pharmacodynamics to ophthalmology (and ocular infectious disease in particular) is still in its infancy, this discipline promises to help clinicians predict whether a treatment regimen is likely to be effective or not and, in the case of antimicrobial therapy, whether such a regimen is likely to promote the development of resistance.

As an example, for fluoroquinolones, there is a dose-response relationship between the tissue concentration of the antibiotic and biological response. In general, the higher the concentration, the better. A higher tissue concentration (relative to the minimum inhibitory concentration [MIC]) translates into better bacterial killing, improved clinical response to infection, and a lower propensity for the development of resistance.[1] In contrast, for cephalosporin antibiotics, bacterial killing is concentration-dependent. Thus, raising the concentration of cephalosporin would have little benefit, but extending the duration of treatment with cephalosporin would be advantageous.

ERROR NO. 4: INCORRECT DOSING

The consequences of inadequate dosing include not only a suboptimal therapeutic effect but also an increased propensity for the development of antibiotic resistance. Examples of dosing regimens that are incorrect include a dosing frequency of less than four times daily, a length of treatment or prophylaxis that extends well beyond the susceptible period for infection, and tapering rather than simply abruptly discontinuing the antibiotic. Table 1 lists some guidelines for proper dosing.

Although researchers have suggested that the ophthalmic use of fluoroquinolones should rarely lead to the development of antibiotic resistance—due to the relatively small amount of fluoroquinolones used as compared with the amounts needed for systemic and veterinary use—there is evidence that incorrect ophthalmic dosing can lead to the rapid development of high-level fluoroquinolone resistance.[1] Insufficiently frequent daily dosing leads to the prolonged exposure of the lid flora to subinhibitory concentrations of fluoroquinolone, a situation that rapidly promotes the development of drug-resistant strains. Indeed, among individuals in whom either ciprofloxacin or ofloxacin was tapered over 4 weeks, the percentage of patients harboring fluoroquinolone-resistant lid flora increased from fewer than 10% before treatment to nearly 40% after 4 weeks of treatment.[1] Furthermore, the majority of these isolates were found to be highly resistant, implying that the bacteria had acquired multiple mutations that were conferring resistance. The fact that the newer fluoroquinolones generally show better activity than their older counterparts does not mean they need not be adequately dosed.

Recent evidence suggests that the optimal target concentration of an antibiotic is not the MIC but a concentration significantly higher than that value. For empiric treatment and prophylaxis, the minimum target value should be the MIC_{90}, not the more commonly reported MIC_{50}. The MIC_{90} designates the concentration of antibiotic at which 90% of tested bacterial strains of a given species are inhibited, and it is generally several times higher than the more commonly reported MIC_{50}, which represents the antibiotic concentration at which 50% of tested bacterial strains of a given species are inhibited. The minimum bacteriocidal concentration is slightly higher yet and designates the antibiotic concentration needed to kill 90% of tested bacterial strains of a given species. Finally, the mutant prevention concentration (MPC) designates the concentration at which the mutational resistance occurs at a frequency of less than 1 in 10^9 or, alternatively, the concentration that is sufficient to prevent the growth of a first-step resistant mutant.[13] According to the MPC hypothesis, keeping the antibiotic concentration at or above the MIC can prevent the development of mutational resistance. The MPC must be determined experimentally for each strain, species, and antibiotic, but, in general for ophthalmic fluoroquinolones, it is three- to fourfold higher than the corresponding MIC. Because a much larger population of bacteria is exposed during treatment than during prophylaxis, the MPC is a more important goal for treatment than for prophylaxis.

Thus, it can be argued that the optimal target concentration for a fluoroquinolone for prophylaxis is the MIC_{90} and the optimal target for treatment is the MPC_{90}. These values may be two- to tenfold higher than the MIC_{50}. Older fluoroquinolones such as ofloxacin and ciprofloxacin typically can maximally achieve only the MIC_{50} in the aqueous humor, even with very frequent dosing (eg, five times in 1 hour). With the newer fluoroquinolones and their enhanced ability to achieve high levels of concentration in target tissues (eg, in the case of levofloxacin 1.5%) and/or significantly lower MICs, reaching the optimal target concentration is easier. Newer fluoroquinolones, if properly dosed, can more readily achieve the tissue concentrations that are necessary to exert the desired antibacterial effect while minimizing the likelihood of the development of resistance.

CONCLUSION

Ophthalmologists are fortunate to have a new group of fluoroquinolones that provide better options for the prophylaxis and treatment of serious ophthalmic infections than older generations.

Incorrectly using these agents, however, could lead to increased risks of suboptimal therapeutic effect, side effects, and antimicrobial resistance. The guidelines presented in this article describe how judicious use, a rational application of susceptibility and pharmacokinetic data, and proper dosing can maximize the therapeutic effect of the newer fluoroquinolones and extend their useful lifetime. ■

This article originally appeared in the February 2005 issue of CRSToday.

1. Hwng DG. Fluoroquinolone resistance in ophthalmology and the potential role for newer ophthalmic fluoroquinolones. *Surv Ophthalmol.* 2004;49(suppl 2):S79-83.
2. Mather R, Karenchak LM, Romanowski EG, Kowalski RP. Fourth generation fluoroquinolones: new weapons in the arsenal of ophthalmic antibiotics. *Am J Ophthalmol.* 2002;133:463-466.
3. Hwang DG. Bacterial conjunctivitis. In: Pepose J, Holland GN, Wilhelmus K, eds. *Infections and Immunity.* St. Louis: CV Mosby; 1996: 799-817.
4. Schwab IR, Friedlaender M, McCulley J, et al, Levofloxacin Bacterial Conjunctivitis Active Control Study Group. A phase III clinical trial of 0.5% levofloxacin ophthalmic solution versus 0.3% ofloxacin ophthalmic solution for the treatment of bacterial conjunctivitis. *Ophthalmology.* 2003;110:457-465.
5. Donnenfeld ED, O'Brien TP, Solomon R, et al. Infectious keratitis after photorefractive keratectomy. *Ophthalmology.* 2003;110:743-747.
6. Venezia RA, Domaracki BE, Evans AM, et al. Selection of high-level oxacillin resistance in heteroresistant *Staphylococcus aureus* by fluoroquinolone exposure. *Antimicrob Chemother.* 2001;48:375-381.
7. Axer-Siegel R, Stiebel-Kalish H, Rosenblatt I, et al. Cystoid macular edema after cataract surgery with intraocular vancomycin. *Ophthalmology.* 1999;106:1660-1664.
8. Marangon FB, Miller D, Muallem MS, et al. Ciprofloxacin and levofloxacin resistance among methicillin-sensitive *Staphylococcus aureus* isolates from keratitis and conjunctivitis. *Am J Ophthalmol.* 2004;137:453-458.
9. Dajcs JJ, Thibodeaux BA, Marquart ME, et al. Effectiveness of ciprofloxacin, levofloxacin, or moxifloxacin for treatment of experimental *Staphylococcus aureus* keratitis. *Antimicrob Agents Chemother.* 2004;48:1948-1952.
10. Ormerod LD, Heseltine PN, Alfonso E, et al. Gentamicin-resistant pseudomonal infection. Rationale for a redefinition of ophthalmic antimicrobial sensitivities. *Cornea.* 1989;8:195-199.
11. Hwang DG, Biswell R, Holsclaw DS, et al. Clinical failures associated with ciprofloxacin monotherapy of streptococcal keratitis. *Ophthalmology.* 1995;102(9A):101.
12. Durmaz B, Marol S, Durmaz R, et al. Aqueous humor penetration of topically applied ciprofloxacin, ofloxacin and tobramycin. *Arzneimittelforschung.* 1997;47:413-415.
13. Blondeau JM, Hansen G, Metzler K, Hedlin P. The role of PK/PD parameters to avoid selection and increase of resistance: mutant prevention concentration. *J Chemother.* 2004;16(suppl 3):1-19.

CHAPTER 96

What are the Best Topical Agents for Prophylaxis?

CHRISTOPHER N. TA, MD

Minimizing the risk of postoperative endophthalmitis requires the elimination of or a significant reduction in the bacterial flora that are found on the ocular surface at the time of surgery and during the immediate postoperative period. The major source of bacteria that cause endophthalmitis is a patient's own eyelids and conjunctiva.[1,2] Applying povidone-iodine at the time of surgery can decrease ocular bacteria.[3-14] Topical antibiotics administered for several days and immediately prior to surgery provide an additional killing of bacteria beyond the effects of povidone-iodine,[7,8,13-16] although a prospective randomized study has yet to prove that the use of topical antibiotics reduces the risk of endophthalmitis. Regardless, almost all ophthalmologists prescribe topical antibiotics for patients undergoing intraocular surgery.

Ophthalmologists also use antibiotics postoperatively to minimize the risk of bacteria's entering the eye via the surgical wound. This is of particular concern with clear corneal incisions, because the wound may not be watertight.17,18 In addition, frequently applying a topical antibiotic may allow the drug to achieve levels in the aqueous that are high enough to kill the bacteria that contaminate the anterior chamber at the time of surgery.[19-29] According to a rabbit study,[30] Vigamox (Alcon Laboratories, Inc., Fort Worth, TX) administered in both the pre- and postoperative period can prevent the development of endophthalmitis following inoculation with *Staphylococcus aureus.*

The ideal topical antibiotics for minimizing the risk of postoperative endophthalmitis must have the following characteristics: broad-spectrum coverage of both gram-positive and gram-negative bacteria; bacteriocidal properties for quick kills of bacteria upon contact; and excellent penetration to achieve intraocular levels that are sufficiently high to kill the offending bacteria.

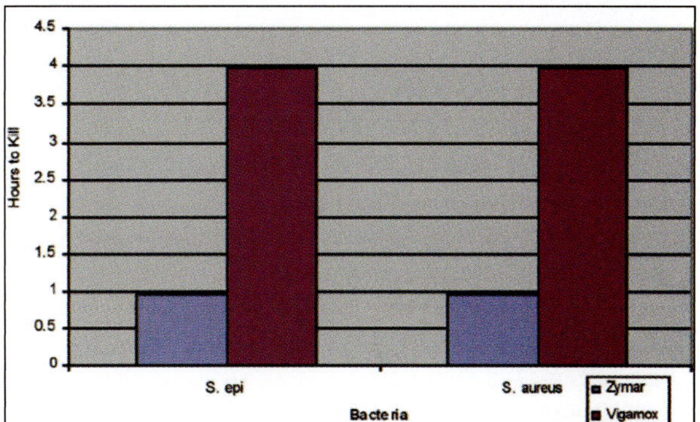

Figure 1. An in vitro laboratory study demonstrating timekill for S. epidermidis and S. aureus. Both bacteria are killed 1 hour following exposure to Zymar, compared to 4 hours for Vigamox.

The agent must also be nontoxic to the ocular surface and cost effective.

Several classes of antibiotics are currently available in the US and include the combination therapy of polymixin B and trimethoprim, the aminoglycosides, and the fluoroquinolones. Many ophthalmic ointments are also available, including erythromycin and the combination therapy of bacitracin and polymyxin B. Of all of these antibiotics, fluoroquinolones, in my opinion, may be the most appropriate antibiotics for endophthalmitis prophylaxis. The greatest advantages of these drugs over other classes of antibiotics are that they provide broad-spectrum coverage, are bacteriocidal and nontoxic, and penetrate the anterior chamber well. In contrast, other antibiotics such as polymixin B and trimethoprim are

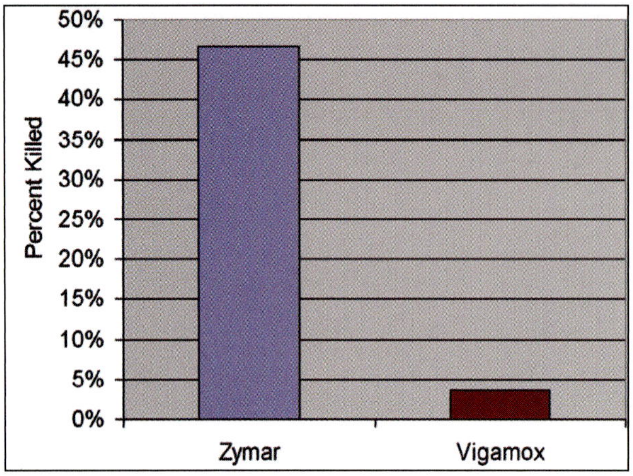

Figure 2. The percentage of bacteria eliminated from the ocular surface following a 1-hour application of antibiotics is shown.

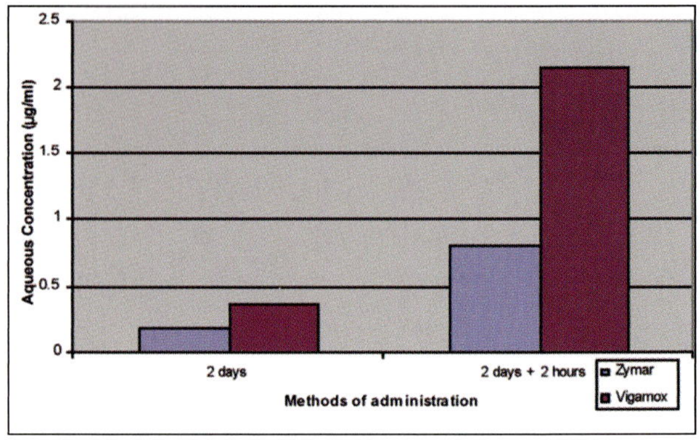

Figure 3. The comparison of the aqueous penetration of Zymar to Vigamox is shown. The study's investigators administered antibiotics q.i.d. for 2 days prior to surgery in one group. In another group, both drugs were given to patients q.i.d. for 2 days, with three additional applications 2 hours immediately before surgery. According to the study, Zymar and Vigamox achieved levels above the minimal inhibitory concentration (MIC) (range, 0.09 to 0.38 μg/mL for most pathogens for the 2-days-plus-2-hours group). (Data adapted from Ong-Tone).[64]

bacteriostatic, and aminoglycosides carry some risk of toxicity.

Among the commercially available topical ophthalmic fluoroquinolones, ciprofloxacin and ofloxacin have limited gram-positive coverage. The newer fluoroquinolonesÑspecifically Quixin (Santen Inc., Napa, CA), Zymar (Allergan, Inc., Irvine, CA), and VigamoxÑhave enhanced activity toward gram-positive pathogens while maintaining broad-spectrum coverage against gram-negative organisms.[31-36] They interfere with both topoisomerase II and IV, and bacterial resistance appears to be lower since mutations of both enzymes are necessary.[32]

After reviewing the published literature for the most desirable properties of commercially available antibiotics, I found some minor differences between them. In general, the three most recently FDA-approved antibiotics (Quixin, Zymar, and Vigamox) are excellent antibiotics. Some of their important characteristics include low resistant rates, high efficacy and kill time, reduced surface toxicity, and effective aqueous penetration. This article discusses the off-label use of the approved products Quixin, Zymar, and Vigamox.

ANTIBIOTIC SUSCEPTIBILITY

Several recently published studies have demonstrated excellent efficacy for Quixin, Zymar, and Vigamox against common ocular pathogens.[33,34,36-42] One potential limitation in susceptibility is that the determination is based on the serum level of the drug and not its tear or aqueous level. For that reason, although an antibiotic may be considered resistant, it may still be effective at killing bacteria given the high level of the medication in the tear film compared with the serum. Another limitation is the variations in resistance pattern based on geographic location. Consequently, a comprehensive study involving multiple sites throughout the US will have much more reliable data than one from a single center. For instance, the Tracking Resistance in the United States Today (TRUST) study[43] is a surveillance report of more than 70,000 isolates that were collected from over 200 institutions since 1999. In this comprehensive study, 99% of Streptococcus pneumoniae remained susceptible to Quixin despite more than 9 years of extensive systemic use. Currently, ocular isolates are collected and analyzed to determine trends in resistance for the commonly prescribed topical antibiotics in the TRUST study.

EFFICACY IN KILLING BACTERIA

Fluoroquinolones as a class effectively kill bacteria, unlike bacteriostatic antibiotics, which inhibit bacterial growth. A fluoroquinolone's efficacy is dependent upon its concentration; the higher the concentration, the greater the kill rate.[44] Frequent dosing of the medication during a short period of time may therefore be more appropriate than infrequent long-term use.

As with any topical antibiotic, the goal is to eradicate the bacteria as quickly as possible. There is some recent evidence suggesting that the preservative benzalkonium chloride (BAK) may have a synergistic effect in improving an agent's kill time.[45-48] A recent in vitro study[45] demonstrated that 0.005% BAK alone or 0.3% gatifloxacin with 0.005% BAK (Zymar) kills Staphylococcus epidermidis and *S. aureus* within 1 hour, compared with 4 hours for 0.5% moxifloxacin alone (Vigamox)45 (Figure 1). Another study demonstrated similar results, with Zymar eliminating all *Staphylococcus* within 60 minutes, whereas 50% of the bacteria treated with Vigamox remained.[46]

Other clinical studies have confirmed the slow kill rate of Vigamox (Figure 2). In a study[47] of 60 patients undergoing intraocular surgery, after a 1-hour application of Vigamox preoperatively, there was no effect on killing bacterial flora on the ocular surface. At baseline, 55% of eyes had positive cultures compared with 53% of the eyes after treatment with Vigamox for 1 hour. In contrast, my colleagues and I will report a study at this year's ARVO Annual Meeting in which a 1-hour preoperative application of Zymar significantly decreased the rate of bacterial contamination of the conjunctiva in patients undergoing intraocular surgery from a baseline of 75% to 40%. These studies suggest that antibiotics preserved with BAK may be much more efficacious in the rapid killing of bacteria compared with antibiotics without BAK. Quixin, which is 0.5% levofloxacin and 0.005% BAK, and Zymar therefore may kill bacteria much quicker than Vigamox.

TOXICITY

In general, fluoroquinolones have an excellent safety profile, which is important given the millions of prescriptions written for this class of drugs every year. A concern with any topical ophthalmic medication is the preservative BAK. A study by Cha et al demonstrated in tissue culture that BAK can cause epithelial cell death that is dependent on concentration and duration of exposure.[47] Although Vigamox does not have BAK, recently published research[49-51] suggests that Vigamox may be toxic to the ocular surface. In a double-masked, prospective study,[48] 28 eyes of 14 patients were randomized to receive either Zymar or Vigamox. The investigators reported that the eyes that received Vigamox had a significantly higher degree of conjunctival injection, discomfort, and corneal epithelial cell loss compared to eyes treated with Zymar. This finding was confirmed by an in vitro study[49] in which the exposure of corneal and conjunctival epithelial cells to different concentrations of Vigamox resulted in poor cellular migration and adhesion. Furthermore, eyes exposed to Vigamox achieved a significant reduction in the production of collagen type IV and fibronectin than eyes exposed to Zymar. Effects on cellular migration, proliferation, and production of collagen and fibronectin are important for wound healing and the health of the ocular surface. These in vitro findings were confirmed by animal studies[50] in which incisions were created in rabbit corneas and exposed to either Zymar or Vigamox. Eyes exposed to Vigamox demonstrated a decrease in collagen IV production, disorganized and slower wound healing, inhibition of cellular proliferation, and a loss of the normal structure of the basal lamina.

In contrast to the aforementioned studies, Burka et al[51] conducted a prospective, masked, randomized study comparing Zymar and Vigamox in patients undergoing PRK. The investigators found that eyes treated with Vigamox healed faster and had smaller epithelial defects compared with those treated with Zymar. Of course, no corneal incision is created during the refractive procedure. In another PRK study,[52] no difference was found with respect to haze, visual acuity, or epithelial healing between eyes treated with Zymar and Vigmox. Finally, Walter and Tyler[53] reported two patients with worsening and persistent corneal ulcers as well as endothelial cell dysfunction while on Vigamox. The patients' conditions resolved after the discontinuation of Vigamox and the initiation of Zymar and corticosteroid treatment.

Adverse side effects are rare with the topical fluoroquinolones. For most patients, Quixin, Zymar, and Vigamox are safe medications. In patients with compromised wound healing abilityÑsuch as those with ocular surface disease, dry eyes, and neurotrophic corneas, among other conditions—the surgeon needs to consider the potentially toxic effects of Vigamox.

AQUEOUS PENETRATION

Occasionally, bacteria can gain access to the anterior chamber during the perioperative period. If this happens, it is important to choose an antibiotic that can penetrate the cornea and achieve levels in the aqueous high enough to eliminate the bacteria. All three of the most recent fluoroquinolones have excellent tissue penetration. Quixin achieves a high drug level in the tear film after a single dose. The peak level was 221.0 µg/mL 15 minutes following the drug's administration, and the level remained above the (MIC) of 2.0 µg/mL for more than 6 hours (6.6 µg/mL).[54] Furthermore, Quixin can achieve levels in the aqueous above the MIC following three to four applications prior to surgery[55-61] Similar studies[62-65] of Zymar and Vigamox demonstrated their excellent penetration into the aqueous humor. In directly comparative studies,[62-65] Vigamox has been shown to have better penetration than Zymar and to achieve higher drug levels in the aqueous humor. Quixin, Zymar, and Vigamox all achieved aqueous levels above the MIC following typical preoperative application.

Figure 3 summarizes the results of a study by Ong-Tone.[64]

IN SUMMARY

Quixin, Zymar, and Vigamox all provide broad-spectrum coverage against both gram-positive and gram-negative bacteria. Thus far, bacterial resistance against these fluoroquinolones is uncommon. As a class, these fluoroquinolones are well tolerated with minimal toxicity, and they penetrate the aqueous humor well.

The choice of antibiotic depends on the clinical situation. To quickly kill bacteria, those drugs preserved with BAK, such as Zymar and Quixin, may be indicated. Vigamox has better penetration into the aqueous humor, however, and may be more appropriate in eyes for which bacterial contamination of the anterior chamber is likely, although some evidence suggests that the drug may impair wound healing.

Based upon the literature mentioned herein, the later generations of topical fluoroquinolones represent the best of the available antibiotics. ■

This article originally appeared in the April 2007 issue of CRSToday.

1. Bannerman TL, Rhoden DL, McAllister SK, et al. The source of coagulase-negative staphylococci in the Endophthalmitis Vitrectomy Study. A comparison of eyelid and intraocular isolates using pulsed-field gel electrophoresis. *Arch Ophthalmol.* 1997;115:357-361.
2. Speaker MG, Milch FA, Shah MK, et al. Role of external bacterial flora in the pathogenesis of acute postoperative endophthalmitis. *Ophthalmology.* 1991;98:639-649; discussion 650.
3. Apt L, Isenberg S, Yoshimori R, Paez J. Chemical preparation of the eye in ophthalmic surgery III: effect of povidone-iodine on the conjunctiva. *Arch Ophthalmol.* 1984;102:728-729.
4. Hale M. Povidone-iodine in ophthalmic surgery. *Ophthalmic Surgery.*1970;1:9-13.
5. Caldwell D, Kastl P, Cook J, Simon J. Povidone-iodine: its efficacy as a preoperative conjunctival and periocular preparation. *Ann Ophthalmol.* 1984;16:577-580.
6. Alp B, Elibol O, Sargon M, et al. The effect of povidone iodine on the corneal endothelium. *Cornea.* 2000;19:546-550.
7. Grimes S, Mein C, Trevino S. Preoperative antibiotic and povidone-iodine preparation of the eye. *Ann Ophthalmol.* 1991;23:263-266.
8. Schmitz S, Dick H, Krummenauer F, Pfeiffer N. Endophthalmitis in cataract surgery: results of a German survey. *Ophthalmology.* 1999;106:1869-1877.
9. Dereklis DL, Bufidis TA, Tsiakiri EP, Palassopoulos SI. Preoperative ocular disinfection by the use of povidone-iodine 5%. *Acta Ophthalmol* (Copenh). 1994;72:627-630.
10. Speaker MG, Menikoff JA. Prophylaxis of endophthalmitis with topical povidone-iodine. *Ophthalmology.* 1991;98:1769-1775.
11. Miño de Kaspar H, Singh G, Egbert PR, et al. Ten-fold reduction of conjunctival bacterial contamination rate using a combined 3-day application of topical ofloxacin and iodine irrigation in patients undergoing anterior segment intraocular surgery. Paper presented at: The ARVO Annual Meeting; May 5, 2003; Fort Lauderdale, FL.
12. Miño de Kaspar H, Chang R, Egbert P, et al. Greater elimination of conjunctival bacteria after preoperative irrigation with 10cc of 5% povidone-iodine. Paper presented at: The AAO Annual Meeting; October 22, 2002; Orlando, FL.
13. Isenberg SJ, Apt L, Yoshimori R, Khwarg S. Chemical preparation of the eye in ophthalmic surgery. IV. Comparison of povidone-iodine on the conjunctiva with a prophylactic antibiotic. *Arch Ophthalmol.* 1985;103:1340-1342. 14. Grimes SR, Mein CE, Trevino S. Preoperative antibiotic and povidone-iodine preparation of the eye. *Ann Ophthalmol.* 1991;23:263-266.
15. De Kaspar HM, Chang RT, Shriver EM, et al. Three-day application of topical ofloxacin reduces the contamination rate of microsurgical knives in cataract surgery: a prospective randomized study. *Ophthalmology.* 2004;111:1352-1355.
16. Ta CN, Egbert PR, Singh K, et al. Prospective randomized comparison of 3-day versus 1-hour preoperative ofloxacin prophylaxis for cataract surgery. *Ophthalmology.* 2002;109:2036-2041.
17. Herretes S, Stark WJ, Pirouzmanesh A, et al. Inflow of ocular surface fluid into the anterior chamber after phacoemulsification through sutureless corneal cataract wounds. *Am J Ophthalmol.* 2005;14:737-740.
18. Taban M, Sarayba MA, Ignacio TS, et al. Ingress of India ink into the anterior chamber through sutureless clear corneal cataract wounds. *Arch Ophthalmol.* 2005;123:643-648.
19. Mistlberger A, Ruckhofer J, Raithel E, et al. Anterior chamber contamination during cataract surgery with intraocular lens implantation. *J Cataract Refract Surg.*1997;23:1064-1069.
20. Dickey J, Thompson K, Jay W. Anterior chamber aspirate cultures after uncomplicated cataract surgery. *Am J Ophthalmol.* 1991;112:278-282.
21. Soto A, Mendivil M. The effect of topical povidone-iodine, intraocular vancomycin, or both on aqueous humor cultures at the time of cataract surgery. *Am J Ophthalmol.* 2001;131:293-300.

22. Samad A, Solomon L, Miller M, Mendelson J. Anterior chamber contamination after uncomplicated phacoemulsification and intraocular lens implantation. *Am J Ophthalmol.*1995;120:143-150.
23. Tervo T, Ljungberg P, Kautiaimen T, et al. Prospective evaluation of external ocular microbioal growth and aqueous humor contamination during cataract surgery. *J Cataract Refract Surg.*1999;25:65-71.
24. Duch-Samper AM, Menezo JL, Hurtado-Sarrio M, et al. Anterior chamber contamination following uncomplicated cataract surgery: comparative results using intravenous imipenem. *Ophthalmic Surg Lasers.* 1996;27:1005-1011.
25. Leong JK, Shah R, McCluskey PJ, et al. Bacterial contamination of the anterior chamber during phacoemulsification cataract surgery. *J Cataract Refract Surg.* 2002;28:826-833.
26. Ariyasu RG, Nakamura T, Trousdale MD, Smith RE. Intraoperative bacterial contamination of the aqueous humor. *Ophthalmic Surg.*1993;24:367-373; discussion: 373-374.
27. Assalian A, Thompson P, St-Antoine P, et al. Anterior chamber fluid contamination after uncomplicated phacoemulsification. *J Cataract Refract Surg.* 1995;21:539-542.
28. Beigi B, Westlake W, Mangelschots E, et al. Perioperative microbial contamination of anterior chamber aspirates during extracapsular cataract extraction and phacoemulsification. *Br J Ophthalmol.* 1997;81:953-955.
29. Ta CN, Egbert PR, Singh K, et al. The challenge of determining aqueous contamination rate in anterior segment intraocular surgery. *Am J Ophthalmol.* 2004;137:662-667.
30. Kowalski RP, Romanowski EG, Mah FS, et al. Topical prophylaxis with moxifloxacin prevents endophthalmitis in a rabbit model. *Am J Ophthalmol.* 2004;138:33-37.
31. Alfonso E, Crider J. Ophthalmic infections and their anti-infective challenges. *Surv Ophthalmol.* 2005;50(suppl 1):S1-S6.
32. Ruiz J. Mechanisms of resistance to quinolones: target alterations, decreased accumulation and DNA gyrase protection. *J Antimicrob Chemother.* 2003;51:1109-1117.
33. Epstein SP, Bottone EJ, Asbell PA. Susceptibility testing of clinical isolates of Pseudomonas aeruginosa to levofloxacin, moxifloxacin, and gatifloxacin as a guide to treating Pseudomonas ocular infections. *Eye Contact Lens.* 2006;32:240-244.
34. Kotlus BS, Wymbs RA, Vellozzi EM, Udell IJ. In vitro activity of fluoroquinolones, vancomycin, and gentamicin against methicillin-resistant Staphylococcus aureusocular isolates. *Am J Ophthalmol.* 2006;142:726-729.
35. Oliveira AD, D'Azevedo PA, Francisco W, Hofling-Lima ALCAHP. In vitro activity of fluoroquinolones against ocular bacterial isolates in Saõ Paulo, Brazil. *Cornea.* 2007;26:194-198.
36. Miño de Kaspar H, Koss MJ, He L, et al. Antibiotic susceptibility of preoperative normal conjunctival bacteria. *Am J Ophthalmol.*2005;139:730-733.
37. Begum NN, Al-Khattaf AS, Al-Mansouri SM, et al. A study of bacterial isolates from corneal specimens and their antibiotic resistance profile. *Saudi Med J.* 2006;27:41-45.
38. Marangon FB, Miller D, Muallem MS, et al. Ciprofloxacin and levofloxacin resistance among methicillin-sensitive Staphylococcus aureusisolates from keratitis and conjunctivitis. *Am J Ophthalmol.* 2004;137:453-458.
39. Miller D, Alfonso EC. Comparative in vitro activity of levofloxacin, ofloxacin, and ciprofloxacin against ocular streptococcal isolates. *Cornea.* 2004;23:289-293.
40. Morrissey I, Burnett R, Viljoen L, Robbins M. Surveillance of the susceptibility of ocular bacterial pathogens to the fluoroquinolone gatifloxacin and other antimicrobials in Europe during 2001/2002. *J Infect.* 2004;49:109-114.
41. Smitha S, Lalitha P, Prajna VN, Srinivasan M. Susceptibility trends of Pseudomonasspecies from corneal ulcers. *Indian J Med Microbiol.*2005;23:168-171.
42. Ta CN, Chang RT, Singh K, et al. Antibiotic resistance patterns of ocular bacterial flora: a prospective study of patients undergoing anterior segment surgery. *Ophthalmology.* 2003;110:1946-1951.
43. Ta CN, Sahm DF, Ingerman A. Levofloxacin susceptibility in multi-drug-resistant S. pneumoniae isolates from the nationwide TRUST surveillance study, 2000-2004. Paper presented at: The ARVO Annual Meeting; May 3, 2006; Fort Lauderdale, FL.
44. Wispelwey B. Clinical implications of pharmacokinetics and pharmacodynamics of fluoroquinolones. *Clin Infect Dis.*2005;41(suppl 2):S127-S135.
45. Kowalski RP, Kowalski BR, Romanowski EG, et al. The in vitro impact of moxifloxacin and gatifloxacin concentration (0.5% vs 0.3%) and the addition of benzalkonium chloride on antibacterial efficacy. *Am J Ophthalmol.* 2006;142:730-735.
46. Eser I, Hyon J, Hose S, O'Brien TP. Comparative antimicrobial efficacy of preserved and preservative-free topical fourth generation fluoroquinolones against various strains o Staphylococcus. Paper presented at: The ARVO Annual Meeting; April 29, 2004; Fort Lauderdale, FL.
47. Cha SH, Lee JS, Oum BS, Kim CD. Corneal epithelial cellular dysfunction from benzalkonium chloride (BAC) in vitro. *Clin Experiment Ophthalmol.* 2004;32:180-184.
48. Kaufman SC, Rusinek C, Salahuddin A, et al. Comparison of the biocompatibility of gatifloxacin 0.3% and moxifloxacin 0.5%. *Cornea.* 2006;25(suppl 2):S31-S44.
49. McDermott M, Wheater M. In vitro comparison of the effects of clinically available ophthalmic solutions of gatifloxacin 0.3% and moxifloxacin 0.5% on human corneal and conjunctival epithelial cell adhesion and migration and on collagen type IV protein expression. *Cornea.* 2006;25(suppl 2):S25-S30.
50. Stern ME, Gao J, Beuerman RW, et al. Effects of fourth-generation fluoroquinolones on the ocular surface, epithelium, and wound healing. *Cornea.* 2006;25(suppl 2):S12-S24.
51. Burka JM, Bower KS, Vanroekel RC, et al. The effect of fourthgeneration fluoroquinolones gatifloxacin and moxifloxacin on epithelial healing following photorefractive keratectomy. *Am J Ophthalmol.* 2005;140:83-87.
52. Yee RW, Setabutr P, Foltermann MO, et al. The effects of topical moxifloxacin 0.5% ophthalmic solution and gatifloxacin 0.3% solution on corneal healing after bilateral photorefractive keratectomy. *Cornea.* 2006;25(9 Suppl 2):S8-S11.
53. Walter K, Tyler ME. Severe corneal toxicity after topical fluoroquinolone therapy: report of two cases. *Cornea.* 2006;25:855-857.
54. Raizman MB, Rubin JM, Graves AL, Rinehart M. Tear concentrations of levofloxacin following topical administration of a single dose of 0.5% levofloxacin ophthalmic solution in healthy volunteers. *Clin Ther.* 2002;24:1439-1450.
55. Healy DP, Holland EJ, Nordlund ML, et al. Concentrations of levofloxacin, ofloxacin, and ciprofloxacin in human corneal stromal tissue and aqueous humor after topical administration. *Cornea.* 2004;23:255-263.
56. Kobayakawa S, Tochikubo T, Tsuji A. Penetration of levofloxacin into human aqueous humor. *Ophthalmic Res.* 2003;35:97-101.
57. Koch HR, Kulus SC, Roessler M, et al. Corneal penetration of fluoroquinolones: aqueous humor concentrations after topical application of levofloxacin 0.5% and ofloxacin 0.3% eyedrops. *J Cataract Refract Surg.*2005;31:1377-1385.
58. Levine JM, Noecker RJ, Lane LC, et al. Aqueous penetration of gatifloxacin and levofloxacin into the rabbit aqueous humor following topical dosing. *J Ocul Pharmacol Ther.* 2004;20:210-216.
59. Mizuki N, Watanabe Y, Miyamoto M, et al. Flomoxef sodium and levofloxacin concentrations in aqueous humor. *Ocul Immunol Inflamm.* 2005;13:229-234.
60. Yamada M, Mochizuki H, Yamada K, et al. Aqueous humor levels of topically applied levofloxacin in human eyes. *Curr Eye Res.* 2002;24:403-406.
61. Yamada M, Mochizuki H, Yamada K, et al. Aqueous humor levels of topically applied levofloxacin, norfloxacin, and lomefloxacin in the same human eyes. *J Cataract Refract Surg.*2003;29:1771-1775.
62. Kim DH, Stark WJ, O'Brien TP. Ocular penetration of moxifloxacin 0.5% and gatifloxacin 0.3% ophthalmic solutions into the aqueous humor following topical administration prior to routine cataract surgery. *Curr Med Res Opin.* 2005;21:93-94.
63. Levine JM, Noecker RJ, Lane LC, et al. Comparative penetration of moxifloxacin and gatifloxacin in rabbit aqueous humor after topical dosing. *J Cataract Refract Surg.*2004;30:2177-2182.
64. Ong-Tone L. Aqueous humor penetration of gatifloxacin and moxifloxacin eyedrops given by different methods before cataract surgery. *J Cataract Refract Surg.*2007;33:59-62.
65. Solomon R, Donnenfeld ED, Perry HD, et al. Penetration of topically applied gatifloxacin 0.3%, moxifloxacin 0.5%, and ciprofloxacin 0.3% into the aqueous humor. *Ophthalmology.* 2005;112:466-469.

CHAPTER 97

Surgical Prophylaxis With Fourth-Generation Fluoroquinolones

PAUL SANGHERA, MD

Many studies have identified that the most common cause of postsurgical endophthalmitis is a result of endogenous ocular surface flora's entering the eye during surgery.[1,2] Thus, even though no randomized clinical trial has been performed to investigate the role of preoperative topical antibiotic prophylaxis, many ophthalmologists still sterilize the ocular surface in order to prevent this devastating intraocular infection.[3]

The theoretical premise behind the use of preoperative topical antibiotics is twofold. The first is to decrease or eradicate the surface organisms, thus preventing intraocular inoculation of these organisms during surgery. The second is to provide a bactericidal level of antibiotic in the anterior chamber before cataract surgery to ensure that any organisms that do enter the eye intraoperatively are killed.

The ideal topical antibiotic should be effective against the many pathogens found on the ocular surface, including the staphylococcal species that are becoming increasingly resistant to commonly used topical medications. The ideal drug should also adequately penetrate the anterior chamber and vitreous to allow for a bactericidal killing level intraoperatively. The levels of this antibiotic should be unaffected by the cataract surgery itself. Finally, it must be capable of preventing endophthalmitis postoperatively should a pathogen enter the eye during surgery. The newest fourth-generation fluoroquinolones, moxifloxacin and gatifloxacin, appear to fulfill the aforementioned criteria and are increasingly becoming the antibacterial drugs of choice in the ophthalmic community. Their wide spectrum of activity, superior ocular penetration with minimal toxicity, and mechanism of action that minimizes the problematic issue of bacterial resistance make them potentially powerful weapons in the battle against endophthalmitis. The following articles were reviewed:

1. *Speaker MG, Milch FA, Shah MK, et al. Role of external bacterial flora in the pathogenesis of acute postoperative endophthalmitis.* Ophthalmology. *1991;98:639-650.*

2. *Han DP, Wisniewski SR, Wilson LA, et al. Spectrum and susceptibilities of microbiologic isolates in the Endophthalmitis Vitrectomy Study.* Am J Ophthalmol. *1996;122:1-17.*

3. *Liesegang TJ. Use of antimicrobials to prevent postoperative infection in patients with cataracts.* Curr Opin Ophthalmol. *2001;12:68-74.*

4. *Van Bambeke F, Michot JM, Van Eldere J, Tulkens PM. Quinolones in 2005: an update.* Clin Microbiol Infect. *2005;11:256-280.*

5. *Mino de Kaspar H, Koss MJ, He L, et al. Antibiotic susceptibility of preoperative normal conjunctival bacteria.* Am J Ophthalmol. *2005;139:730-733.*

6. *Solomon R, Donnenfeld ED, Perry HD, et al. Penetration of topically applied gatifloxacin 0.3%, moxifloxacin 0.5%, and ciprofloxacin 0.3% into the aqueous humor.* Ophthalmology. *2005;112:466-469.*

7. *Hwang DG. Fluoroquinolone resistance in ophthalmology and the potential role for newer ophthalmic fluoroquinolones.* Surv Ophthalmol. *2004;49(suppl 2):79-83.*

8. *Hariprasad SM, Blinder KJ, Shah GK, et al. Penetration pharmacokinetics of topically administered 0.5% moxifloxacin ophthalmic solution in human aqueous and vitreous.* Arch Ophthalmol. *2005;123:39-44.*

9. *Mather R, Stewart JM, Prabriputaloong T, et al. The effect of cataract surgery on ocular levels of topical moxifloxacin.* Am J Ophthalmol. *2004;138:554-559.*

10. *Kowalski RP, Romanowski EG, Mah FS, et al. Topical prophylaxis with moxifloxacin prevents endophthalmitis in a rabbit model.* Am J Ophthalmol. *2004;138:33-37.*

MECHANISM OF ACTION AND SPECTRUM OF ACTIVITY

Quinolones are derived from the parent compound of nalidixic acid, originally designed for antimalarial research.[4] Both moxifloxacin and gatifloxacin are classified as fourth-generation fluoroquinolones due to a fluorine substitution at the C-6 position of their chemical structure, a methoxy group at the C-8 position, as well as larger moieties at the C-1 and C-7 positions. Their activity stems from the formation of complexes with two enzymes crucial in the supercoiling of DNA, DNA gyrase, and topoisomerase IV. The inability of bacteria to supercoil their DNA induces cellular apoptosis. This process results in a surprisingly wide spectrum of activity.

Both moxifloxacin and gatifloxacin have an enhanced spectrum of activity against gram-positives compared to the older fluoroquinolones due to additional chemical alterations to their structures. For example, many isolates of coagulase-negative *Staphylococcus* (which accounts for more than 70% of all cases of endophthalmitis in the Western world) are showing heightened resistance to topical ofloxacin and ciprofloxacin. Many studies have demonstrated that the resistance level of these strains to the newer fluoroquinolones is less than 5%. In addition, this class of medicine also has strong activity against gram-negatives and anaerobes, atypical mycobacteria, and *Chlamydia* species.

ACTIVITY ON OCULAR SURFACE FLORA

Results from in vitro studies have found that the newer fluoroquinolones have excellent activity against ocular flora. De Kaspar et al[5] took baseline conjunctival cultures from 164 eyes of 164 patients prior to anterior segment intraocular surgery and found a total of 124 species of coagulase-negative *Staphylococcus*, 19 cultures of *Staphylococcus aureus*, as well as eight positive cultures for Group D *Streptococcus* species and 11 species of gram-negative rods. Antibiotic susceptibility of the isolates was determined using the Kirby-Bauer disk diffusion technique.

Of the 124 species of coagulase-negative *Staphylococcus*, less than 3% were resistant to either moxifloxacin or gatifloxacin, compared to an ofloxacin resistance rate of 25%. None of the other isolated bacteria was resistant to either of the newer fluoroquinolones, however all eight *Streptococcus* species were resistant to either ofloxacin or ciprofloxacin. There were also 43 isolates of multiresistant bacteria, defined as those organisms resistant to more than five tested antibiotics. Of those organisms, resistance to the two newer fluoroquinolones was less than 10%, whereas for the older ones the resistance rate exceeded 65%.

OCULAR PENETRATION AND INTRAOCULAR CONCENTRATION

Solomon et al[6] instructed 52 patients undergoing cataract surgery to administer one of three different topical fluoroquinolones four times a day for 3 days prior to surgery. A total of 14 patients used moxifloxacin 0.5%, 16 patients received gatifloxacin 0.3%, and 22 patients used ciprofloxacin 0.3% preoperatively. One hour before surgery, patients were asked to use their antibiotic every 15 minutes for a total of three doses. In the OR, before the initiation of surgery, approximately 0.1 mL of aqueous fluid was aspirated using an air cannula needle attached to a tuberculin syringe. The concentration of fluoroquinolone in each sample was determined with reverse-phase, high-pressure, liquid chromatography.

The mean aqueous concentration of moxifloxacin reached 1.31 ±0.46 mcg/mL (range, 0.68 to 2.92 mcg/mL) whereas those of gatifloxacin and ciprofloxacin were 0.63 ±0.30 mcg/mL (range, 0.23 to 1.18 mcg/mL) and 0.15 ±0.11 mcg/mL (range, 0.09 to 0.58 mcg/mL), respectively. The mean aqueous concentrations of both moxifloxacin and gatifloxacin were well above each drug's documented ocular pathogen MIC_{50} of 0.03 to 0.13 mcg/mL and 0.08 to 0.50 mcg/mL, respectively.[7] Only ciprofloxacin's mean concentration fell below its ocular pathogen MIC_{50} of 0.25 to 32 mcg/mL (32 mcg/mL reported for *Streptococcus pneumoniae*).

In a similar study, Hariprasad et al[8] studied the aqueous and vitreous concentrations of moxifloxacin 0.5% in 20 patients undergoing vitrectomy for various reasons, who self-administered topical moxifloxacin either every 2 hours or every 6 hours for 3 days prior to surgery. On the operative day, in addition to maintaining their drop-frequency protocol, a drop of moxifloxacin was administered 15 minutes before the surgery. Aqueous samples were obtained with the collection of 0.1mL via a 30-gauge needle attached to a syringe through a paracentesis. Vitreous samples were collected with the assistance of a vitreous cutter attached to a syringe that obtained 0.2 to 0.3 mL.

Samples were analyzed for moxifloxacin concentration via high-performance liquid chromatography. For both of the dosing regimens of the two previously mentioned studies,[6,8] the aqueous concentration of moxifloxacin exceeded the MIC_{90} for important pathogens causing endophthalmitis. However, only the dosage administered every two hours produced vitreous concentrations that exceeded the MIC_{50} for pathogens such as *Streptococcus epidermidis, S. aureus, S. pneumoniae, Bacillus cereus*, and others.

EFFECT OF SURGERY ON DRUG'S INTRAOCULAR CONCENTRATION

Mather et al[9] investigated the effects of cataract surgery in rabbits on intraocular levels of topical moxifloxacin given for surgical prophylaxis. Thirty-six eyes of 18 rabbits were included in the study whereby both eyes of all rabbits received three drops of moxifloxacin 0.5%, separated by 5 minutes, approximately 1 hour before surgery. Only one eye of each of the rabbits was operated on, with the other eye acting as a nonsurgical control. Surgery consisted of phacoemulsification with a 3-mm clear corneal incision with two nylon sutures to close the surgical wound. At the end of the surgery, both eyes received three drops of moxifloxacin, again, separated by 5 minutes. The rabbits were then split into three groups and euthanized at 30, 60, and 120 minutes postoperatively to compare the levels of moxifloxacin in surgical and nonsurgical eyes. Aqueous and vitreous concentrations were determined by high-pressure liquid chromatography.

Although the aqueous levels of moxifloxacin were higher in the nonsurgical versus the operated eyes, the concentrations in both were at least 200-fold higher than the MIC_{90} for fluoroquinolone susceptible staphylococcal species, and at least fourfold higher than the MIC_{90} for fluoroquinolone-resistant staphylococci. In this study, neither the surgical nor the nonsurgical eyes reached therapeutic vitreous concentrations of moxifloxacin against the most common fluoroquinolone-resistant organisms. However, both were almost equivalent to the MIC_{90} of sensitive staphylococcal species. By inference, these results demonstrate that cataract surgery may not influence the level of intraoperative antibiotic resulting from presurgical prophylaxis.

PROOF OF PRINCIPLE IN THE PREVENTION OF ENDOPHTHALMITIS

Kowalski et al[10] have provided the first proof that newer topical fluoroquinolones may be able to prevent postoperative endophthalmitis in an animal model. Three regimens of topical prophylaxis were used in three groups of 20 rabbits that had anterior chambers challenged with injections of 50,000 colony-forming units of *S. aureus* in 0.025 mL (an amount of pathogen known to reproducibly induce endophthalmitis in the study animals).

In the full-prophylaxis group, 10 rabbits received one drop of moxifloxacin 0.5% every 15 minutes, 1 hour before intraocular injection, for a total of five drops. An additional drop was given immediately after the injection, and four more drops were administered during a 24-hour period.

In the prechallenge-prophylaxis group, 10 rabbits received moxifloxacin every 15 minutes for 1 hour prior to injection, with no additional drug given afterward. In the postchallenge-prophylaxis group, moxifloxacin was only applied immediately after injection in 10 animals and four more times in 24 hours, with no medicine given to any of the rabbits in advance.

In each group, 10 control rabbits (30 in total) endured the same prophylaxis and injection protocol, except saline was substituted for moxifloxacin. All eyes were graded clinically for signs of endophthalmitis at 4, 11, 18, and 22 hours postchallenge. Then, the animals were sacrificed, and samples from their anterior chambers and vitreous were cultured. None of the anterior chamber or vitreous cultures of the 30 rabbits receiving any type of moxifloxacin prophylaxis resulted in bacterial recovery compared with positive cultures from five, three, and six rabbit anterior-chamber cultures in the full-, prechallenge-, and postchallenge-prophylaxis control groups, respectively. Vitreous cultures were positive in three, one, and three of the aforementioned control groups, respectively. Clinical gradings for signs of endophthalmitis showed that rabbits in the full-prophylaxis group had no signs of infection and that postchallenge prophylaxis produced slightly fewer signs than prechallenge prophylaxis.

The investigators concluded that topical prophylaxis with moxifloxacin produces a sufficient bactericidal effect in the eyes of rabbits to prevent endophthalmitis when inoculated with a bacterial load comparable to one that might result if pathogens entered the eye during cataract surgery.

BOTTOM LINE

Fourth-generation fluoroquinolones are readily being accepted in the ophthalmic community as the topical medication of choice in surgical prophylaxis against endophthalmitis. Both moxifloxacin and gatifloxacin are effective in killing ocular surface flora, including gram-positive bacteria resistant to older fluoroquinolones. The newer fluoroquinolones also have excellent intraocular penetration and achieve adequate intraocular bactericidal levels, which were maintained even after cataract surgery in one animal study. Lastly, in vivo, the agents have been proven to eliminate anterior chamber bacterial inoculates similar to those that may occur during cataract surgery, and thus they may combat endophthalmitis postoperatively. ■

This article originally appeared in the August 2005 issue of CRSToday.

CHAPTER 98

Is Resistance to Gatifloxacin and Moxifloxacin Here Already?

DAVID G. HWANG, MD

In the 4 years since their approval by the FDA, gatifloxacin 0.3% (Zymar; Allergan, Inc., Irvine, CA) and moxifloxacin 0.5% (Vigamox; Alcon Laboratories, Inc., Fort Worth, TX) have quickly emerged as the preferred antimicrobials of many ophthalmologists for the prophylaxis and treatment of serious ocular infections.[1] The chief advantages of these agents (sometimes referred to as fourth-generation fluoroquinolones but more precisely and hereinafter termed 8-methoxyfluoroquinolones) compared with older ophthalmic fluoroquinolones such as ciprofloxacin (Ciloxan; Alcon Laboratories, Inc.) and ofloxacin (Ocuflox; Allergan, Inc.) are their enhanced in vitro gram-positive antibacterial activity and favorable pharmacokinetics.[2,3]

Another factor that has encouraged the use of gatifloxacin and moxifloxacin is the well-documented rise in resistance to ciprofloxacin and ofloxacin among ocular isolates.[2,4] Both gatifloxacin and moxifloxacin show better activity against gram-positive isolates compared with ciprofloxacin and ofloxacin.[3] Furthermore, on in vitro testing, the 8-methoxyfluoroquinolones have demonstrated less susceptibility to the development of de novo gram-positive–related resistance in wild-type *Staphylococcus aureus* due to their activity against both bacterial topoisomerase II and IV.[5] On this basis, the first-line use of these agents for prophylaxis and treatment has been suggested as a potential means of forestalling the development of gram-positive resistance.

It thus is perhaps surprising that, in the short time since the introduction of gatifloxacin and moxifloxacin for ophthalmic use, significant rates of in vitro resistance to these fluoroquinolones have already been observed by at least one research group. A recently published study by Miller and colleagues confirmed that resistance to both drugs is prevalent among the ocular isolates responsible for endophthalmitis.[6] These investigators reported that the proportion of coagulase-negative staphylococcal endophthalmitis isolates with in vitro resistance to gatifloxacin and moxifloxacin increased from 3% among historical isolates banked from 1990 to 1994 to 35% among isolates recovered in 2000 to 2004. These data suggest that the rise in resistance to the drugs may have predated their introduction for clinical use. The investigators also reported that the prevalence of cross-resistance to fluoroquinolones was high (ie, isolates that were resistant to ciprofloxacin and ofloxacin were likely to be resistant to gatifloxacin and moxifloxacin).

The findings of the study by Miller and colleagues raise a number of important questions. First, how could resistance have arisen so rapidly, especially given the intrinsic resistance-fighting properties of the 8-methoxyfluoroquinolones? Second, what are the potential clinical implications of this increase in resistance? Finally, what can be done to forestall the further development of resistance to fluoroquinolones?

PRIOR EXPOSURE TO FLUOROQUINOLONES GENERATES LOW-LEVEL RESISTANCE

Resistance to older fluoroquinolones in ocular isolates has been on the rise for some time, dating to before the introduction of gatifloxacin and moxifloxacin.[3] Likely explanations for this trend include not just increasing human systemic use of fluoroquinolones but also the widespread use of these agents in US poultry farming in the recent past. Another potential contributing factor is indiscriminate and incorrect ophthalmic usage of fluoroquinolones.[2]

The increased use of fluoroquinolones generates selection pressure that, over time, enriches an exposed bacterial population for one or more mutations that confer resistance to fluoroquinolones. Depending on the mechanism of such resistance and the bacterial species, these mutations may confer either absolute resistance to gatifloxacin and moxifloxacin or a greatly reduced threshold for the subsequent development of resistance to these agents.

Against gram-negative bacteria, the 8-methoxyfluoroquinolones have no advantage in activity over ciprofloxacin or ofloxacin[3]; accordingly, a Pseudomonas aeruginosa strain that is resistant to ciprofloxacin will be equally resistant to gatifloxacin or moxifloxacin.[7] Clinical and in vitro resistance to gatifloxacin and moxifloxacin has recently been reported in a case of P. aeruginosa keratitis after PRK,[8] and research suggests that the prevalence of gram-negative resistance to fluoroquinolones appears to be rising in systemic isolates.[9]

A SECOND MUTATION CONFERS RESISTANCE TO 8-METHOXYFLUOROQUINOLONES

For gram-positive bacteria, one of the principal (but not exclusive) mechanisms of fluoroquinolone resistance is a mutation to bacterial topoisomerase II (DNA gyrase) and/or topoisomerase IV. Each topoisomerase is made up of separate subunits (A and B), and mutations in either subunit may confer resistance. Whereas

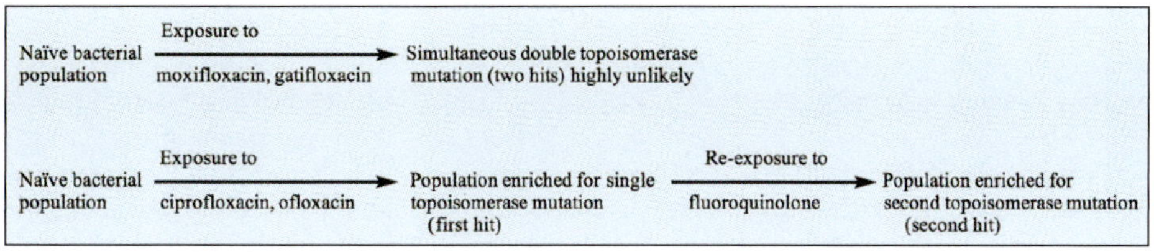

Figure 1. A serial-hit hypothesis may explain resistance to newer fluoroquinolones. Topoisomerase-based resistance in *Staphylococcus* to 8-methoxyfluoroquinolones requires mutations to two different topoisomerase genes.

ciprofloxacin and ofloxacin primarily target topoisomerase IV, the 8-methoxyfluoroquinolones require mutations in both DNA gyrase (encoded by gyrA and gyrB genes) and topoisomerase IV (encoded by grlA and grlB genes) to be rendered inactive. In a na•ve population of wild-type gram-positive bacteria, the likelihood of two such mutations' occurring simultaneously in the same bacterium is extremely low. The situation is quite different, however, in a bacterial population that has had prior exposure to ciprofloxacin and ofloxacin and through such selection pressure has undergone enrichment for mutations conferring fluoroquinolone resistance. In *S. aureus* isolates that have been selected for resistance to older fluoroquinolones, the acquisition of mutations to the topoisomerase IV A subunit gene (grlA) is commonly observed.[10] In this population, resistance to 8-methoxyfluoroquinolones would occur with the acquisition of just one additional mutation in either the gyrA or gyrB gene.

This serial-hit hypothesis to explain the development of 8-methoxyfluoroquinolone resistance is illustrated in Figure 1.

SUCCESSIVE MUTATIONS OCCUR WITH GREATER PROBABILITY

An additional mechanism must be invoked to explain the rapid acquisition of serial mutations in a given bacterial strain, which results in the development of high-level resistance to fluoroquinolones, including 8-methoxyfluoroquinolones. Under optimal conditions, if a given bacterial strain were continuously exposed to a fluoroquinolone concentration in excess of roughly four times the MIC of that strain, the probability of a mutational resistance event would be less than 10-9. At this frequency, the likelihood of even a single mutational resistance event would therefore be expected to be low in the ophthalmic setting, given the relatively low organism burden present in the normal ocular flora and even in active ocular infections.

The threshold antibiotic concentration associated with a spontaneous mutational resistance probability of less than 10-9 is termed the mutant prevention concentration (MPC).[11]

When the tissue concentration of a fluoroquinolone drops to a range below the MPC but above the MIC (this range is termed the mutant selection window), mutations can occur. For fluoroquinolones in particular, the author has demonstrated that the mutational resistance rate increases exponentially, by several orders of magnitude, as the ratio between the antibiotic concentration decreases linearly within the mutant selection window.[2] In the course of normal topical ophthalmic dosing, organisms may be exposed for prolonged durations to concentrations only slightly in excess of the MIC or even to concentrations below the MIC. It is during these intervals that the selection for resistance-conferring mutations can occur with a relatively high probability. Additionally, as each subsequent mutation raises the MIC of the strain further, the ratio between the antibiotic's concentration in tissue and the MIC falls proportionally, and the mutational frequency increases exponentially yet further. Thus, the probability of acquiring each successive mutation increases (Figure 2).

Furthermore, under conditions of antibiotic selection pressure, those isolates with more than one resistance mutation enjoy a strong survival advantage relative to other isolates within a bacterial population. As the number of resistant bacteria rises, so does the likelihood that, within this already resistant subpopulation, there will arise new chance mutations that confer yet greater degrees of resistance to fluoroquinolones.

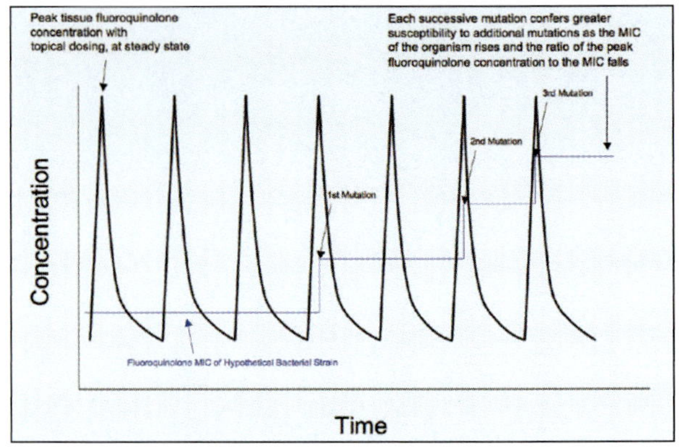

Figure 2. Each subsequent fluoroquinolone mutation is acquired more readily, leading to superresistant bacteria.This theoretical graph shows the development of mutational resistance in a hypothetical bacterial strain exposed to repeated dosing of a topical fluoroquinolone. Each successive mutation confers greater susceptibility to additional mutations as the minimum inhibitory concentration (MIC) of the organism rises and the ratio of the peak fluoroquinolone concentration to the MIC falls.

SUPERBUGS RESULT FROM MULTIPLE MUTATION ACQUISITION

One prediction of the proposed hypothesis is that multidrug resistance may occur as different types of drug-resistant genes are acquired in the process of sequential selection. Because resistance to fluoroquinolones can occur by mechanisms other than an alteration in the topoisomerase target, such as altered permeability or efflux, some of these acquired resistance mechanisms may confer cross-resistance to other antimicrobials. It is therefore interesting to note that exposure to fluoroquinolones has been shown to increase the likelihood of selecting methicillin-resistant strains in a heterogeneous population of *S. aureus*,[12] although a causal mechanistic explanation for this association has yet to be fully elucidated. Conversely, methicillin-resistant staphylococci are also likely to carry multiple fluoroquinolone-resistance genes. A recent study demonstrated that, among methicillin-resistant staphylococcal strains isolated from ocular surface flora, approximately 70% were concomitantly resistant to fluoroquinolones, including the 8-methoxyfluoroquinolones.[13]

A further prediction of the preceding hypothesis is that the acquisition of successive mutations conferring resistance would occur in a runaway fashion, as the probability of acquiring additional mutations rises and the gap in survival advantage between more and less resistant strains within a given bacterial population widens. This process of acquiring further mutations would be expected to stop once the MIC exceeded the peak concentration of antibiotic in tissue, at which point there would be no additional survival advantage to the acquisition of further mutations. This model would therefore predict that (1) resistant isolates obtained after fluoroquinolone selection pressure exerted in vivo would be likely to manifest multiple fluoroquinolone-resistance mutations, rather than just one or two, and that (2) in such strains, high-level resistance to fluoroquinolones would occur, as well as possibly multidrug resistance.

These predictions have been borne out by at least two studies in the ophthalmic literature. I conducted a study of patients given

GUIDELINES FOR THE PROPER DOSING OF FLUOROQUINOLONES

- Dose no less frequently than q.i.d.
- Dose only for the required period of time:
  Bacterial conjunctivitis: 1 week
  Bacterial keratitis: 2 to 3 weeks
  Post-LASIK: 3 to 7 days
  Postcataract surgery: 1 week
- Curtail treatment by abrupt discontinuation rather than by tapering
- Hit hard, get in, and get out

a prolonged postoperative topical dosing regimen of either ofloxacin or ciprofloxacin tapered from q.i.d. to b.i.d. over 4 weeks.[2] At the end of the treatment period, cultures of lid and ocular surface flora were performed. The rates of recovery of fluoroquinolone-resistant ocular flora increased from under 10% prior to exposure to fluoroquinolones to over 30% after exposure. The MIC50 to ciprofloxacin of recovered isolates was in excess of 64 μg/mL, and the MIC50 to ofloxacin was 16 μg/mL, a finding implying that the sequential acquisition of multiple fluoroquinolone-related mutations had occurred. The majority of these resistant isolates also manifested resistance to multiple other antibiotics, including methicillin. In a recently published study by Iihara and colleagues,[14] a high proportion of methicillin-resistant ocular isolates were also found to have high-level resistance to fluoroquinolones, including 8-methoxyfluoroquinolones. Upon genomic analysis of these isolates, more than 60% of the isolates had four or five topoisomerase mutations, 32% had two topoisomerase mutations, and just 5% had only one topoisomerase mutation.

WHAT IS THE CLINICAL SIGNIFICANCE OF IN VITRO RESISTANCE?

In vitro antimicrobial resistance does not always translate into in vivo resistance, particularly if the resistance is low level and the organism burden is modest.[15] In such cases, high tissue levels achieved by adequate ophthalmic dosing may be sufficient to eradicate the relatively modest numbers of low-level resistant organisms. In cases in which high-level resistance is present and/or the organism burden is high, however, the likelihood that the fluoroquinolone will successfully eradicate such resistant organisms in vivo decreases.

Dajcs and colleagues demonstrated in a rabbit model of ofloxacin-resistant staphylococcal keratitis that the initiation of topical moxifloxacin therapy within 9 hours after inoculation successfully treated the infection, but a delay of just 6 hours resulted in reduced efficacy in the treatment of the keratitis.[16] Wilhelmus and colleagues reported that the treatment response to ciprofloxacin experimental keratitis correlated in proportion to the strain's susceptibility to the drug.[17] In another study, Wilhelmus et al described a retrospective analysis of data from clinical trials that found a positive correlation between clinical therapeutic response rates and the quantitative level of ciprofloxacin susceptibility of each of the causative isolates.[18]

Although a confirmation of the finding of rising fluoroquinolone resistance is needed, and further substantiation of the earlier hypothesis will be required, a delay in implementing measures to counter this threat risks disastrous consequences—a rapid rise in fluoroquinolone resistance to the point where the effectiveness of this class of antimicrobials is substantially diminished. Two measures need to be taken by prescribers: (1) limiting their use of fluoroquinolones (perhaps the hardest pill to swallow) and (2) applying optimal strategies for fluoroquinolone dosing and antimicrobial selection, based on pharmacodynamic principles.

THE USE OF AGENTS OTHER THAN FLUOROQUINOLONES

The 8-methoxyfluoroquinolones are considered by many ophthalmologists in the US to be first-line antimicrobials for the treatment and prophylaxis of serious infections such as bacterial keratitis, post-LASIK keratitis, and postoperative endophthalmitis. Nonetheless, there is a surprising lack of clinical data to support the notion that these antimicrobials are clinically superior to older fluoroquinolones or to other antimicrobial agents of a different structural class. In fact, in a recently completed head-to-head comparison of topical levofloxacin and intracameral cefuroxime for surgical prophylaxis in cataract surgery, intracameral cefuroxime proved superior for first-line antimicrobial prophylaxis in intraocular surgery.[19]

Although the merits of topical fluoroquinolones versus intracameral cephalosporins may be the subject of ongoing debate, it is at least clear that not every infectious indication requires the use of fluoroquinolone antibiotics. Particularly for minor, self-limited, or chronic infections such as blepharitis or uncomplicated conjunctivitis, agents other than fluoroquinolones should be considered. Older antibiotics with a narrower spectrum of activity can generally treat less serious ocular infections effectively. Examples of excellent antimicrobials for these indications include bacitracin for staphylococcal blepharitis and polymyxin B-trimethoprim for uncomplicated bacterial conjunctivitis. Not only are these particular antimicrobials less likely to exert a strong degree of selection pressure that can promote resistance, but they also have the advantage of being considerably less expensive than the newer fluoroquinolones.

For most routine, uncomplicated cases of bacterial conjunctivitis, older agents such as polymyxin B-trimethoprim are comparable to the newer fluoroquinolones in effecting a clinical cure. Using one of the newer fluoroquinolones may be appropriate, however, in the exceptional instances in which laboratory resistance to first-line agents has been documented or when clinical unresponsiveness or relapse has been encountered after treatment with a first-line antimicrobial. Furthermore, because fluoroquinolones with better antimicrobial activity may in some cases effect a more rapid microbiological cure than older fluoroquinolones,[20] it may be preferable to use a newer fluoroquinolone as first-line therapy for cases of bacterial conjunctivitis in which rapid bacterial eradication is essential. Examples include patients at risk for secondary infectious complications from bacterial conjunctivitis (eg, those with bullous keratopathy or an avascular filtering bleb) or individuals for whom there is a need to limit horizontal transmission to their contacts at home, school, or workplace.

It is essential to recognize that the hypothesis discussed previously predicts that a strategy of using older fluoroquinolones in preference to the 8-methoxyfluoroquinolones will not result in reduced fluoroquinolone selection pressure but, in fact, may actually increase the likelihood of resistance to 8-methoxyfluoroquinolones. The reason, as previously discussed, is that first-step mutational resistance is much more likely to occur with ciprofloxacin or ofloxacin than with gatifloxacin or moxifloxacin.

Thus, if a fluoroquinolone is needed, an extrapolation from in vitro data would predict that an 8-methoxyfluoroquinolone would have a lower propensity to select for resistant isolates. Further clinical testing, however, is needed to substantiate this prediction.

CORRECT DOSING

Some investigators have suggested that the ophthalmic use of fluoroquinolones should rarely lead to the development of antibiotic resistance, due to the relatively small quantity of ophthalmic fluoroquinolones used compared with the amounts needed for systemic and veterinary use. Incorrect ophthalmic dosing, however, can lead to the rapid development of high-level fluoroquinolone resistance. Insufficiently frequent daily dosing leads to the prolonged exposure of the lid flora to subinhibitory concentrations of a fluoroquinolone, a situation that rapidly promotes the development of drug-resistant strains. The consequences of inadequate dosing include not only a suboptimal therapeutic effect but also an increased propensity for the development of antibiotic resistance.

Examples of regimens that are likely to be less than optimal include a dosing frequency of less than q.i.d., a length of treatment or prophylaxis that extends well beyond the susceptible period for infection, and tapering rather than simply abruptly discontinuing the antibiotic. For example, a 4-week course of topical ofloxacin or ciprofloxacin (q.i.d. for 2 weeks, followed by b.i.d. for 2 weeks) leads to frequent recovery of resistant ocular isolates[2] whereas a 3-day course of ofloxacin given q.i.d. does not result in an increased recovery of resistant isolates.[21]

The fact that the newer fluoroquinolones generally show better activity than their older counterparts does not mean that they need not be adequately dosed. In the absence of available scientific studies needed to create evidence-based guidelines for the proper dosing of ophthalmic fluoroquinolones, the author offers some guidelines for the dosing of these drugs (see Guidelines for the Proper Dosing of Fluoroquinolones). A general principle in the use of ophthalmic fluoroquinolones is to prescribe a sufficiently high dose for the shortest required duration. In other words, hit hard, get in, and get out.

The precise determination of the optimal clinical dosing regimens for 8-methoxyfluoroquinolones will require pharmacodynamic studies relevant to ocular pharmacotherapeutics. Pharmacodynamics is a discipline that attempts to describe how pharmacology, pharmacokinetics, pharmacogenetics, and other factors work together to govern the biological activity of a given drug over time in a living organism. Although the application of pharmacodynamics to ophthalmology (and ocular infectious disease in particular) is still in its infancy, this discipline promises to help clinicians develop antimicrobial dosing guidelines that should improve therapeutic efficacy and even reduce the propensity for the development of resistance.

As an example, for fluoroquinolones, there is a dose-response relationship between the tissue concentration of the antibiotic and biological response. In general, the higher the achieved concentration of fluoroquinolone in the target tissue or fluid, the better. A higher tissue concentration of fluoroquinolone (relative to the MIC) translates into better bacterial killing, an improved clinical response to infection, and a lower propensity for the development of resistance.[2] In contrast, for cephalosporin antibiotics, bacterial killing is dependent on time rather than concentration. Raising the concentration of cephalosporin would therefore have little benefit, but extending the duration of treatment with this agent would be advantageous.

Recent pharmacodynamic evidence from the literature on systemic infectious disease suggests that the optimal target concentration of an antibiotic is not the MIC but a concentration significantly higher than that value. For empiric treatment and prophylaxis, the minimum target value should be the MIC90, not the more commonly reported MIC50. The MIC90 designates the concentration of antibiotic at which 90% of tested bacterial strains of a given species are inhibited, and it is generally several times higher than the more commonly reported MIC50, which represents the antibiotic concentration at which 50% of tested bacterial strains of a given species are inhibited. The minimum bacteriocidal concentration is slightly higher yet and designates the antibiotic concentration needed to kill 90% of tested bacterial strains of a given species. Finally, the MPC designates the concentration at which the mutational resistance occurs at a frequency of less than 10-9 or, alternatively, the concentration that is sufficient to prevent the growth of a first-step resistant mutant.[11]

According to the MPC hypothesis, keeping the antibiotic concentration at or above the MIC can prevent the development of mutational resistance. The MPC must be determined experimentally for each strain, species, and antibiotic. In general, for many fluoroquinolones, it is three- to fourfold higher than the corresponding MIC. Because a much larger population of bacteria is exposed during treatment than during prophylaxis, the MPC may be a more important goal when dosing for treatment than when dosing for prophylaxis.

It can be argued, therefore, that the optimal target concentration for a fluoroquinolone for prophylaxis is the MIC90, whereas for treatment it is the MPC90. These respective values may be two- to 10-fold higher than the MIC50. When using older fluoroquinolones such as ofloxacin and ciprofloxacin, even very frequent dosing (eg, five times in 1 hour) may only produce aqueous humor levels that approximate the MIC50.[22] The MIC90 of the 8-methoxyfluoroquinolones for nonfluoroquinolone-resistant gram-positive species is relatively low, especially in comparison to ciprofloxacin or ofloxacin.[3] This factor, combined with the favorable corneal and aqueous penetration characteristics of gatifloxacin and moxifloxacin, should theoretically result in the ability of the 8-methoxyfluoroquinolones—assuming proper and frequent dosing—to more readily achieve target tissue concentrations that yield the optimally desired antibacterial effect while reducing the propensity for developing resistance.

CONCLUSION

Ophthalmologists have grown increasingly reliant on the newer fluoroquinolones, gatifloxacin and moxifloxacin in particular, as first-line agents in the prophylaxis and treatment of serious ophthalmic infections. The recently reported rise in resistance to these agents, occurring so soon after their introduction, is worrisome. If confirmed, it could require substantial modifications to current antibiotic prescribing patterns. An explanation for these findings may lie in the fact that selection pressure from years of ciprofloxacin and ofloxacin use has resulted in an increasing prevalence of low-level fluoroquinolone resistance. Against this background, the development of multistep mutations that confer 8-methoxyfluoroquinolone resistance is more likely to occur. In the setting of suboptimal dosing of fluoroquinolones, runaway resistance can rapidly develop, leading to high-level fluoroquinolone resistance that is likely to be clinically significant.

Further experimental and clinical work is needed to develop rational strategies for limiting the development of fluoroquinolone resistance. Until such data become available, the recommendations presented in this article may serve as a roadmap for how the judicious, restrained, and reduced use of fluoroquinolones, coupled with appropriate dosing and antimicrobial selection, can maximize the therapeutic effect of the newer-generation fluoroquinolones. Perhaps more importantly, such a disciplined approach may extend the useful lifetime of this important group of ophthalmic antimicrobials. ■

This article originally appeared in the April 2007 issue of CRSToday.

1. Leaming DV. Practice styles and preferences of ASCRS members—2004 survey. Available at: http://www.leamingsurvey.com. Accessed February 3, 2007.
2. Hwang DG. Fluoroquinolone resistance in ophthalmology and the potential role for newer ophthalmic fluoroquinolones. *Surv Ophthalmol.* 2004;49(suppl 2):S79-S83.
3. Alexandrakis G, Alfonso EC, Miller D. Shifting trends in bacterial keratitis in South Florida and emerging resistance to fluoroquinolones. *Ophthalmology.* 2000;107:1497-1502.
4. Mather R, Karenchak LM, Romanowski EG, Kowalski RP. Fourth generation fluoroquinolones: new weapons in the arsenal of ophthalmic antibiotics. *Am J Ophthalmol.* 2002;133:463-466.
5. Ince D, Hooper DC. Mechanisms and frequency of resistance to gatifloxacin in comparison to AM-1121 and ciprofloxacin in Staphylococcus aureus. *Antimicrobial Agents Chemother.* 2001;45:2755-2764.
6. Miller D, Flynn PM, Scott IU, et al. In vitro fluoroquinolone resistance in staphylococcal endophthalmitis isolates. *Arch Ophthalmol.* 2006;124:479-483.
7. Kowalski RP, Dhaliwal DK, Karenchak LM, et al. Gatifloxacin and moxifloxacin: an in vitro susceptibility comparison to levofloxacin, ciprofloxacin, and ofloxacin using bacterial keratitis isolates. *Am J Ophthalmol.* 2003;136:500-505.
8. Moshirfar M, Mirzaian G, Feiz V, Kang PC. Fourth-generation fluoroquinolone-resistant bacterial keratitis after refractive surgery. *J Cataract Refract Surg.* 2006;32:515-518.
9. Gasink LB, Fishman NO, Weiner MG, et al. Fluoroquinolone-resistant Pseudomonas aeruginosa: assessment of risk factors and clinical impact. *Am J Med.* 2006;119:526.e19-526.e25.
10. Kaatz GW, Seo SM. Topoisomerase mutations in fluoroquinolone-resistant and methicillinsusceptible and -resistant clinical isolates of Staphylococcus aureus. *Antimicrob Agents Chemother.* 1998;42:197-198.
11. Blondeau JM, Hansen G, Metzler K, Hedlin P. The role of PK/PD parameters to avoid selection and increase of resistance: mutant prevention concentration. *J Chemother.* 2004;16(suppl 3):1-19.
12. Venezia RA, Domaracki BE, Evans AM, et al. Selection of high-level oxacillin resistance in heteroresistant Staphylococcus aureusby fluoroquinolone exposure. *Antimicrob Chemother.* 2001;48:375-381.
13. Kotlus BS, Wymbs RA, Vellozzi EM, Udell IJ. In vitro activity of fluoroquinolones, vancomycin, and gentamicin against methicillin-resistant Staphylococcus aureusocular isolates. *Am J Ophthalmol.* 2006;142:726-729.
14. Iihara H, Suzuki T, Kawamura Y, et al. Emerging multiple mutations and high-level fluoroquinolone resistance in methicillin-resistant Staphylococcus aureusisolated from ocular infections. *Diagn Microbiol Infect Dis.* 2006;56:297-303 [Epub 2006 June 12].
15. Ormerod LD, Heseltine PN, Alfonso E, et al. Gentamicin-resistant pseudomonal infection. Rationale for a redefinition of ophthalmic antimicrobial sensitivities. *Cornea.* 1989;8:195-199.
16. Dajcs JJ, Thibodeaux BA, Marquart ME, et al. Effectiveness of ciprofloxacin, levofloxacin, or moxifloxacin for treatment of experimental Staphylococcus aureuskeratitis. *Antimicrob Agents Chemother.* 2004;48:1948-1952.
17. Wilhelmus KR. Evaluation and prediction of fluoroquinolone pharmacodynamics in bacterial keratitis. *J Ocul Pharmacol Ther.* 2003;19:493-499.
18. Wilhelmus KR, Abshire RL, Schlech BA. Influence of fluoroquinolone susceptibility on the therapeutic response of fluoroquinolone-treated bacterial keratitis. *Arch Ophthalmol.* 2003;121:1229-1233.
19. Barry P, Seal DV, Gettinby G, et al; ESCRS Endophthalmitis Study Group. ESCRS study of prophylaxis of postoperative endophthalmitis after cataract surgery: preliminary report of principal results from a European multicenter study [Erratum published in *J Cataract Refract Surg.* 2006;32:709]. J Cataract Refract Surg. 2006;32:407-410.
20. Schwab IR, Friedlaender M, McCulley J, et al; Levofloxacin Bacterial Conjunctivitis Active Control Study Group. A phase III clinical trial of 0.5% levofloxacin ophthalmic solution versus 0.3% ofloxacin ophthalmic solution for the treatment of bacterial conjunctivitis. *Ophthalmology.* 2003;110:457-465.
21. Ta CN, He L, Nguyen E, De Kaspar HM. Prospective randomized study determining whether a 3-day application of ofloxacin results in the selection of fluoroquinolone-resistant coagulase-negative Staphylococcus. *Eur J Ophthalmol.* 2006;16:359-364.
22. Durmaz B, Marol S, Durmaz R, et al. Aqueous humor penetration of topically applied ciprofloxacin, ofloxacin and tobramycin. *Arzneimittelforschung.* 1997;47:413-415.

CHAPTER 99

MRSA in Cataract and Refractive Surgery

ERIC D. DONNENFELD, MD

I am passionate about educating ophthalmic providers about the implications of methicillin-resistant *Staphylococcus aureus* (MRSA) and *Staphylococcus epidermidis* (MRSE) for ocular surgery. Here, I share my experience with these organisms to illustrate the consequences of these difficult-to-treat bacterial infections and to highlight their growing threat to public health. Methicillin-resistant staphylococci are currently the most common cause of infection following LASIK, PRK, and cataract surgery.

CASE PRESENTATION

I recently performed PRK to correct moderate myopia on the right eye of a municipal employee who was in his 40s. I decided to treat him with PRK instead of LASIK because corneal topography with the Orbscan (Bausch & Lomb, Rochester, NY) showed an inferiorly decentered apex, inferior steepening, and corneal thinning that could have increased his risk of developing postoperative ectasia.

Immediately after surgery, I instilled prednisolone acetate 1%, gatifloxacin 0.3%, and ketorolac tromethamine 0.4% (all manufactured

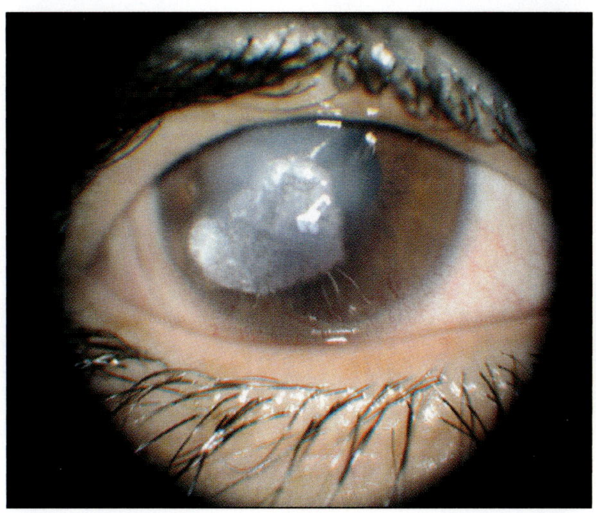

Figure 1. The perforated and MRSA-infected cornea of a PRK patient after he mistakenly discontinued his antibiotic.

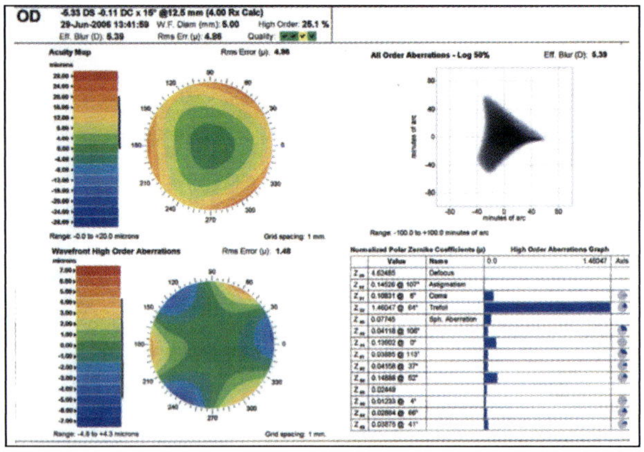

Figure 2. Topography of the patient's eye after undergoing thin-flap LASIK 1 year after a corneal transplant.

by Allergan, Inc., Irvine, CA), into the patient's right eye, and I fitted him with a bandage contact lens. The next day, the patient's endothelium appeared to have healed sufficiently, so I told him to discontinue his NSAID. On day 2, his eye had some pain; by accident, he had stopped using the antibiotic instead of the NSAID. He had a minor corneal infiltrate on his eye, but I saw no evidence of hypopyon or ulceration. I cultured the infiltrate and increased the fluoroquinolone dosing to every 2 hours. We arranged for him to be seen 16 hours later.

On postoperative day 3, I noted that the infiltrate had significantly enlarged, there was iritis, and we were clearly dealing with an infection. I started the patient on vancomycin every half hour and oral doxycycline to prevent collagenase release. I also continued him on gatifloxacin and discontinued the prednisolone acetate. The culture came back 2 days later and revealed MRSA. However, the patient's eye did not improve. He returned on the seventh day with a dense central corneal infiltrate, and I knew he would likely need a corneal transplant. At this point, I thought his condition could not worsen, but I was wrong. When he came back the next day, his cornea had perforated (Figure 1), and I applied cyanoacrylate glue.

A couple months later, I performed a corneal transplant, to which the eye responded very well. One year after the PRK surgery, I removed the transplant sutures, and the eye was -5.00 D with only 0.25 D of cylinder on refraction and 0.10 D of cylinder on aberrometry. The patient's left eye was plano. He was miserable due to the anisometropia and his inability to wear contact lenses.

I chose to perform thin-flap LASIK with a femtosecond laser (Advanced Medical Optics, Inc., Santa Ana, CA) on his right eye to minimize the risk of infection (LASIK's risk of infection is five to eight times less than PRK's[1]). Also, in healthy eyes, the risk of infection is far greater than the risk of ectasia after PRK.[2] The patient's eye did very well after the LASIK surgery; the anisometropia resolved, and his UCVA reached 20/25 (Figure 2).

A PROBLEM GAINING ATTENTION

Unfortunately, the problem posed by MRSA is worse than the public realizes. I maintain that MRSA is the number-one health problem in the US today, and, as a study my colleagues and I published in the *American Journal of Ophthalmology* showed,[3] it may be particularly worrisome for ophthalmology. Of the 14 cases of MRSA we described in our study, 12 occurred in healthcare workers and four in physicians. Physicians and other healthcare workers are colonized by MRSA at an increased rate that puts us at a very high risk of developing infection. More than 50% of all infections in the ICU setting are due to MRSA.[4]

The incidence of MRSA infections is also increasing exponentially in the general population, and this trend is likely to continue, according to the literature.[5] Surgical candidates must understand this risk, as illustrated by a study of endophthalmitis among cataract patients at the University of Pittsburgh. From 1993 to 2004, the university's physicians found that 30% of postoperative infections were caused by MRSA. MRSE accounted for an additional 48% of cases of endophthalmitis. By 2006, MRSA appeared in 60% of their surgical cases, and MRSE—the greatest cause of endophthalmitis—was responsible for three quarters of the endophthalmitis outbreaks.[6] Additionally, the ASCRS Clinical Committee Refractive Surgery Survey[7] cited MRSA as the number-one cause of infection following LASIK and PRK. A study presented at the 2006 ARVO meeting showed that 55% of patients who have endophthalmitis are resistant to generic gatifloxacin and moxifloxacin molecules.[8] Thus, half of the cases of endophthalmitis are not going to respond effectively to the primary antibiotics in use today. With odds like these, our best strategy is to prevent infections before they occur.

CLINICAL IMPLICATIONS

Many clinicians wonder if clinical evidence favors one antibiotic over another for preventing postoperative infections. A study published by Moshirfar et al in *Ophthalmology* in 2007[9] gave the first clinical evidence that cataract patients' incidence of endophthalmitis was approximately 50% lower for those who received gatifloxacin 0.3% compared with moxifloxacin ophthalmic solution 0.5% (Alcon Laboratories, Inc., Fort Worth, TX). This study included 14 cases of endophthalmitis (an overall rate of 0.07%). Importantly, endophthalmitis' average time to presentation is 9.3 days, and the participants in this study were instructed to stop their antibiotics after 7 days. Six cases of endophthalmitis occurred after the drops were stopped and the eyes were left unprotected. When the investigators eliminated these cases, there was a fourfold increase of endophthalmitis with moxifloxacin versus gatifloxacin. Until I see a human endophthalmitis study with different results, I will consider this one the best guide for choosing an antibiotic.

STRATEGIES FOR PREVENTION

Endophthalmitis prevention occurs mainly on the ocular surface. Well-constructed wounds and the use of a suture when necessary are critical for preventing late inoculation of organisms into the eye following surgery, because again, most cases present later than 3 days.

Fortunately, MRSA and MRSE respond brilliantly to the benzalkonium chloride (BAK), a preservative that is added to many ophthalmic medications. A study by Blondeau et al[10] showed that BAK greatly increased an antibiotic's killing effect and reduces the minimal inhibitory concentrations (MICs) to manageable rates versus the generic moxifloxacin and gatifloxacin molecules that lack it. A European study showed a 78% reduction of endophthalmitis with intracameral cefuroxime.[11] Although the study had some flaws, the idea of using antibiotics intracamerally is valid and warrants more research. If you use an antibiotic intracamerally, mix and match: use a broad-spectrum fluoroquinolone on the ocular surface, and use an antibiotic that is specifically effective against MRSA inside the eye.

Also, disinfect the lid well with one of the advanced products available today. The TheraTears SteriLid eyelid cleanser (Advanced Vision Research, Inc., Woburn, MA) is very effective against MRSA. Additionally, the prescription nasal gel mupirocin (Bactroban; GlaxoSmithKline, Research Triangle Park, NC) is a super bacitracin with an FDA-approved indication of effectiveness against MRSA. I apply this to the lid margins of patients known to carry MRSA preoperatively.

CONCLUSION

In summary, we surgeons must do a better job of disinfecting the operative field against infectious organisms. BAK destabilizes cell membranes and enhances the speed of microbial kill. Also, reducing the size of our wounds will greatly minimize the risk of endophthalmitis. Finally, I suggest prescribing antibiotics postoperatively for 10 to 14 days instead of 7, as supported by the Moshirfar study.

MRSA is here to stay as a major health concern. Be aware of it, and remember that prevention is the key. ■

This article originally appeared in CRSToday's *March 2008* Premium Cataract Surgery *supplement.*

1. Donnenfeld ED, Solomon, Holland EJ, et al. Changing trends in infectious keratitis following refractive surgery. Paper presented at: The ASCRS Symposium on Cataract, IOL and Refractive Surgery; April 16, 2005; Washington, DC.
2. Randleman JB, Woodward M, Lynn MJ, Stulting RD. Risk assessment for ectasia after corneal refractive surgery. *Ophthalmology.* 2008;115:1:37-50.
3. Solomon R, Donnenfeld ED, Perry HD, et al. Methicillin-resistant Staphylococcus aureus infectious keratitis following refractive surgery. *Am J Ophthalmol.* 2007;143:4:629-634. Epub 2007 Feb 23.
4. National Nosocomial Infections Surveillance (NNIS) System Report, data summary from January 1992 to June 2002, issued August 2002. *Am J Infect Control.* 2002;30:8:458-475.
5. Kowalski TJ, Berbari EF, Osmon DR. Epidemiology, treatment, and prevention of community-acquired methicillin-resistant Staphylococcus aureus infections. *Mayo Clin Proc.* 2005;80:9:1201-1207.
6. Lab Diagnostic Testing: Bacteria. The Charles T. Campbell Eye Microbiology Lab. Available at: http://eyemicrobiology.upmc.com/Bacteria.htm. Accessed February 1, 2008.
7. Donnenfeld. ED. Cornea clinical committee treatment of infectious keratitis. Paper presented at: The ASCRS Symposium on Cataract, IOL and Refractive Surgery; April 16, 2005; Washington, DC.
8. Major JC, Jr, Flynn Hw, Jr, Miller D, et al. Antibiotic sensitivities and visual acuity outcomes in endophthalmitis caused by methicillin-sensitive (MSSA) versus methicillin-resistant (MRSA) Staphylococcus aureus. Paper presented at: The 2006 ARVO meeting; May 4, 2006; Ft. Lauderdale, FL.
9. Moshirfar M, Feiz V, Vitale AT, et al. Endophthalmitis after uncomplicated cataract surgery with the use of fourth-generation fluoroquinolones: a retrospective observational case series. *Ophthalmology.* 2007;114:4:686-689.
10. Blondeau JM, Borsos S, Hesje CK. Antimicrobial efficacy of gatifloxacin and moxifloxacin with and without benzalkonium chloride compared with ciprofloxacin and levofloxacin against methicillin-resistant *Staphylococcus aureus. J Chemother.* 2007;19:2:146-151.
11. Barry P, Seal DV, Gettinby G, Lees F. ESCRS study of prophylaxis of postoperative endophthalmitis after cataract surgery: preliminary report of principal results from a European multicenter study. *J Cataract Refract Surg.* 2006;32:3:407-410.

CHAPTER 100

Antibiotics in Cataract Surgery

SAMUEL MASKET, MD; ROGER F. STEINERT, MD; AND FRANCIS S. MAH, MD

Endophthalmitis, cystoid macular edema, and corneal decompensation are all serious complications of cataract surgery. Recent innovations in pre-, intra-, and postoperative drug regimens are intended to decrease the incidence of such problems. I asked three respected ophthalmologists to discuss some of these new pharmacologic ideas.

—William J. Fishkind, MD

SAMUEL MASKET, MD

Preventing infection after cataract surgery requires ophthalmologists' attention to four matters. First, they must reduce the number of microbes on the ocular surface and at the lid margins. Doing so may require particular effort when the patient suffers from chronic blepharitis and other conditions. Second, surgeons must avoid intraocular contamination during the cataract procedure by carefully draping the lid margins and eyelashes and by limiting surgical complications, particularly capsular rupture. Third, ophthalmologists must avoid intraocular contamination after surgery through the hermetic sealing and firm stability of the cataract incision. Finally, as a fail-safe, surgeons must destroy any microbes that enter the eye during or after the cataract procedure. It is here that intracameral and topical antibiotics play a significant role.

I employ chemprophylaxis for all four of the aforementioned categories. I instruct patients with blepharitis to cleanse their eyelids and apply bacitracin ointment at bedtime for 1 week, when I recheck their eyelids and lid margins. Assuming this regimen was effective, I then proceed with surgery in my usual fashion.

Very occasionally, I encounter patients who are immunologically incompetent, who have lost an eye to infection after surgery, who have an indwelling Jones lacrimal tube, or who have a prosthetic fellow eye. I would instruct all of these patients to apply bacitracin ointment to their eyelids for 1 week preoperatively and would receive treatment with systemic moxifloxacin 400 mg orally q.d. for 2 days prior to surgery, on the day of surgery, and for an additional 2 days after surgery. Their postoperative course would otherwise be routine.

Because silicone punctal plugs may harbor microbes or allow the formation of a biofilm, I remove them prior to surgery and then treat the patient routinely.

For me, routine preoperative prophylaxis involves topical Vigamox (moxifloxacin hydrochloride 0.5%; Alcon Laboratories, Inc., Fort Worth, TX) q.i.d. 1 day preoperatively and 1 hour prior to surgery in a "cocktail" with an NSAID and viscous anesthetic mixture. I prepare the skin with povidone-iodine 10% and place a 5% concentration on the anesthetized ocular surface.

I add vancomycin 20 mg to the 500-mL BSS (Alcon Laboratories, Inc.) infusate employed during the phacoemulsification. At the close of surgery, after sealing the incision and testing it with fluorescein dye at measured physiologic IOP, I add 50 µL of undiluted Vigamox to the anterior chamber. Using the agent directly from an unopened bottle in this manner is possible, because it has a pH of 6.8 and near isotonicity, and because it is sterile and not preserved. No other currently available product may be used for this purpose. Finally, I instruct patients to apply topical Vigamox q3h on the day of surgery and q.i.d. for an additional 5 days and then to cease its use abruptly so long as there is epithelial sealing of the incisions.

ROGER F. STEINERT, MD

Without firm scientific data, which may never be possible in the arena of endophthalmitis, I use the following regimen for routine cataract surgery based on logic, incomplete science, and my estimation of risks and benefits.

Starting 3 days preoperatively, patients use Zymar (gatifloxacin ophthalmic solution 0.3%; Allergan, Inc., Irvine, CA) and Acular LS (Allergan, Inc.) q.i.d. On the day of surgery, they receive two doses of Zymar approximately 30 minutes preoperatively along with dilating drops. I apply Betadine (The Purdue Frederick Company, Stamford, CT) to the skin around the eye and place 5% Betadine solution on the globe. I do not use an antibiotic in the infusion fluid or intracamerally at the end of surgery. I instill topical Zymar at the end of the procedure.

On the day of surgery, immediately postoperatively, patients receive Pred Forte (Allergan, Inc.), Acular LS, and Zymar q4h. They continue taking these three medications q.i.d. for 1 week. At that point, patients discontinue the Zymar and decrease their dosing of Pred Forte and Acular LS to b.i.d. for the next 2 weeks. They then administer Pred Forte and Acular LS q.d. for 3 more weeks. This therapeutic regimen lasts longer and is more intense than that followed by many cataract surgeons, but it is geared toward the third standard deviation outlier. I almost never have a case of postoperative rebound iritis or cystoid macular edema (CME).

FRANCIS S. MAH, MD

The use of the antiseptic povidone-iodine 5% solution in the conjunctival cul-de-sac prior to surgery is the cornerstone of endophthalmitis prophylaxis.[1]

Although there is no consensus on which antibiotic to use or the method of application in cataract surgery, ophthalmologists generally agree that perioperative antibiotics are the standard of care.[2-6] Outside of ophthalmic surgery, studies have demonstrated the efficacy of antibiotics in the prevention of postoperative infections. In these nonophthalmic surgeries, antibiotics are most efficacious when administered no more than 1 hour before surgery. Moreover, 30 minutes prior to starting the incision is the optimal time to begin intravenous antibiotic prophylaxis.[7] Because there are no clinical trials in ophthalmology helping to guide surgeons as to when to start prophylactic antibiotics, I defer to the general surgical literature and begin topical antibiotics starting 1 to 2 hours prior to surgery.

For ophthalmic procedures, I think it is prudent to use topical antibiotics until the epithelium is intact following cataract surgery. Although tapering steroids and other anti-inflammatory medications is typical, it is important not to taper antibiotics due to the real risk of developing and selecting for bacteria that are resistant.[8] I therefore have patients start using topical antibiotics at least 30 minutes to 1 hour prior to surgery and continue the medication at the full FDA-approved dosage until their epithelium has healed, roughly 3 to 10 days, without tapering the antibiotic.

Factors in the choice of antibiotic include the medications' peak concentrations in the ocular tissues and the minimum inhibitory concentration (MIC) of the key bacteria that cause endophthalmitis.[9] Today's fluoroquinolones generally have the desirable combination of the lowest MICs and the highest concentrations in ocular tissues when used topically.[9] Gatifloxacin and moxifloxacin are the most potent (lowest MICs) and reach the highest concentrations in the cornea and the anterior chamber (highest peak concentrations).[9] It is my opinion that cataract surgeons should use one of these two agents for perioperative cataract surgery prophylaxis.

A study by the ESCRS generated earnest discussion among cataract surgeons regarding the future of prophylaxis.[2] Although the study's results were dramatic, valid criticism of the research includes its use of levofloxacin 0.5% as the topical antibiotic instead of an agent that acquires higher concentrations while providing more potency. Another issue is the study's use of cefuroxime as the intracameral agent instead of a drug that could have better pharmacokinetic and pharmacodynamic characteristics. Further criticism relates to the relatively high rate of endophthalmitis seen in this study (> 1:400 cases) and the potential long- and short-term adverse events, including toxic anterior segment syndrome and anaphylaxis from administering intracameral antibiotics that are not commercially prepared.[2] Although my colleagues and I have conducted some animal studies, I am not currently using intracameral antibiotics of any kind for prophylaxis.

Regarding the prevention of miosis, management of postoperative pain, and control of postoperative inflammation, the peer-reviewed literature demonstrates the superiority of using topical NSAIDs for 3 days prior to surgery compared with 1 day, which in turn is more effective than using the agents only on the day of surgery.[10-12] Considering that CME has a peak incidence of 4 to 6 weeks following routine uncomplicated surgery, it makes sense that an NSAID should be used for at least 6 to 8 weeks to cover the high-risk period. Patients at greater risk (eg, diabetics, uveitics, vasculopaths, and individuals whose surgery was complicated) should probably use prophylactic NSAIDs for at least 8 to 12 weeks. The dosing should never exceed the FDA's recommended frequency, and ophthalmologists should carefully monitor the eyes of all patients who use NSAIDs for more than 4 weeks due to the risk of corneal and scleral melts. These postoperative melts are most likely in patients with neurotrophic keratopathy, severe dry eye disease, and moderate-to-severe ocular surface disease such as blepharitis and meibomitis.[10-12]

Studies have demonstrated the efficacy of diclofenac, ketorolac 0.5%, bromfenac 0.09%, and nepafenac 0.1% in the management of inflammation and pain after cataract surgery.[10-12] In clinical trials, diclofenac and ketorolac were efficacious in the management of CME. The newest NSAIDs, bromfenac and nepafenac, are reportedly more potent and more bioavailable after topical dosing. Nepafenac is the only prodrug.[10-12] Until there are prospective data showing the differences between the available NSAIDs, it makes sense to view the pain management, CME prevention, and anti-inflammatory efficacy as effects of the drug class. Several key differences are the dosing (ranging from b.i.d. to q.i.d.), the formulations (solution vs suspension), and the rate of burning and stinging in the FDA trials (0% to 40%).

Unless they are at high risk of scleral or corneal melts, as mentioned earlier, my patients all begin using a topical NSAID on the day of cataract surgery at the least or, ideally, 3 days preoperatively, and they continue taking the FDA-approved dose for 6 to 8 weeks postoperatively. Those of my patients at high risk of CME after cataract surgery begin using NSAIDs at least 3 days preoperatively and continue them for at least 8 to 12 weeks. ■

This article originally appeared in the March 2008 issue of CRSToday.

1. Speaker MG, Menikoff JA. Prophylaxis of endophthalmitis with topical povidone-iodine. *Ophthalmology.* 1991;98:1769-1775.
2. Barry P, Seal DV, Gettinby G, et al. ESCRS study of prophylaxis of postoperative endophthalmitis

after cataract surgery. *J Cataract Refract Surg.* 2006;32:407-410.
3. Jensen MK, Fiscella RG. Comparison of endophthalmitis rates over four years associated with topical ofloxacin vs ciprofloxacin. Poster presented at: The ARVO Annual Meeting; May 2002; Fort Lauderdale, FL.
4. Masket S. Preventing, diagnosing, and treating endophthalmitis. *J Cataract Refract Surg.* 1998;24:725-726.
5. Fisch A, Salvanet A, Prazuck T; The French Collaborative Study Group on Endophthalmitis. Epidemiology of infective endophthalmitis in France. *Lancet.* 1991;338:1373-1376.
6. Montan PG, Wejde G, Setterquist H, et al. Prophylactic intracameral cefuroxime. Evaluation of safety and kinetics in cataract surgery. *J Cataract Refract Surg.* 2002;28:982-987.
7. Bratzler DW, Houck PM, Surgical Infection Prevention Guidelines Writers Workgroup, et al. Antimicrobial prophylaxis for surgery: an advisory statement from the National Surgical Infection Prevention Project. *Clin Infect Dis.* 2004;38:1706-1715.
8. Mah FS. Fourth-generation fluoroquinolones: new topical agents in the war on ocular bacterial infections. *Curr Opin Ophthalmol.* 2004;15:316-320.
9. Mah FS. New antibiotics for bacterial infections. *Ophthalmol Clin North Am.* 2003;16:11-27.
10. O'Brien TP. Emerging guidelines for use of NSAID therapy to optimized cataract surgery patient care. *Curr Med Res Opin.* 2005;21:1131-1137.
11. Lindstrom R, Kim T. Nepafenac: ocular permeation and inhibition of retinal inflammation: an examination of data and opinion of clinical utility. *Curr Med Res Opin.* 2006;22:397-404.
12. McColgin AZ, Heier JS. Control of intraocular inflammation associated with cataract surgery. *Curr Opin Ophthalmol.* 2000;11:3-6.

CHAPTER 101

What Do I Do?

ELIZABETH A. DAVIS, MD; ROBERT J. CIONNI, MD; ROSA BRAGA-MELE, MEd, MD, FRCSC; ERIK L. MERTENS, MD, FEBO; FRANK A. BUCCI JR, MD; LISA BROTHERS ARBISSER, MD; RANDALL J. OLSON, MD; MARK PACKER, MD; WILLIAM J. FISHKIND, MD; AND JAMES P. GILLS, MD

ELIZABETH A. DAVIS, MD

There are several measures I take to reduce the chance of infection in intraocular surgery. I ask patients to perform lid scrubs, thoroughly remove all eye makeup preoperatively, and refrain from wearing it for 1 week postoperatively. The reuse of mascara and eyeliner makes these products a potential source of bacterial contamination.

Most of my patients receive three topical doses of a fourth-generation fluoroquinolone (Zymar; Allergan, Inc., Irvine, CA) in the 30 minutes preceding their surgery. The minimum inhibitory concentrations of these antibiotics demonstrate broad-spectrum coverage, high penetration, rapid kill rates, and low bacterial resistance. If the patient has a higher-than-average risk of infection, I instruct him to use Zymar q.i.d. for 3 days preoperatively. All patients continue administering this drop q.i.d. for 2 to 3 weeks postoperatively.

Immediately before surgery, I place povidone-iodine 5% in the conjunctival cul-de-sac and carefully prepare and drape the lids. Lashes are taped out of the sterile field with Tegaderm adhesive (3M, St. Paul, MN).

Because I prefer a clear corneal incision, I carefully construct the wound and am extremely meticulous in ensuring a perfect seal at the conclusion of the surgery. If there is any question about the wound's integrity, I place a suture.

I find posterior capsular rupture and vitreous loss to be uncommon with my supracapsular technique. This is important because these two complications significantly increase the risk of endophthalmitis.

At Minnesota Eye Consultants in Bloomington, all five cataract surgeons, including myself, also use 10 mg of vancomycin in a 500-mL bottle of irrigating fluid. We have never had a complication as a result of this intracameral antibiotic and believe it may be partly responsible for the extremely low rate of endophthalmitis at our practice.

ROBERT J. CIONNI, MD

I believe several steps are beneficial in lowering patients' risk for endophthalmitis. First, I strive to decrease the number of bacteria present on the ocular surface, eyelashes, and lid margins by instructing the patient to begin topical antibiotic drops t.i.d. on the day before surgery. I prefer the fourth-generation fluoroquinolone Vigamox (Alcon Laboratories, Inc., Fort Worth, TX), because it is extremely potent and has been shown to reach very high concentrations in the cornea.[1]

I place a drop of 5% povidone-iodine in the conjunctival cul-de-sac approximately 5 minutes before surgery, followed by a standard Betadine preparation (The Purdue Frederick Company, Stamford, CT). Special attention is given to scrubbing the lashes with a Betadine-soaked cotton swab, especially if blepharitis has been noted. The eye is draped (eye drape model 1040; Alcon Laboratories, Inc.), which usually covers the lashes completely. If any lashes remain exposed, they are covered with Steri-Strips (3M).

I place a small amount of Viscoat (Alcon Laboratories, Inc.) on the cornea at the beginning of surgery to keep the tissue moist and clear throughout the procedure. This step obviates the need for repeated drops of balanced salt solution (BSS; Alcon Laboratories, Inc.), which can cause the patient to squeeze his eyes shut and thus allow the lashes to become exposed and release bacteria onto the corneal surface.

At the conclusion of surgery, I hydrate the incision and apply pressure just posterior to the incision to check it for leakage. If any is noted, a 10–0 nylon suture is placed. After removing the drapes, I instill another drop of 5% povidone-iodine in the cul-de-sac in case any bacteria were released by the drapes' removal from the lashes.

After surgery, patients are pulsed with three drops of Vigamox (one drop every 5 minutes) before they are discharged to induce a high concentration of antibiotic in the ocular tissues. They continue using Vigamox t.i.d. for 5 days.

ROSA BRAGA-MELE, MD, MED, FRCSC

It is important to examine all patients prior to surgery for signs of blepharitis or any obstructions of the lacrimal sac. Both of these conditions should be treated preoperatively to decrease the risk of endophthalmitis. For blepharitis, I start patients on lid scrubs and topical antibiotic treatment with a fourth-generation fluoroquinolone 3 days prior to surgery. For an obstruction of the lacrimal sac with reflux, I refer the patient to my oculoplastics colleagues for management prior to cataract surgery.

All other patients receive a topical fourth-generation fluoro-

(Courtesy of Frank A. Bucci, Jr, MD.)

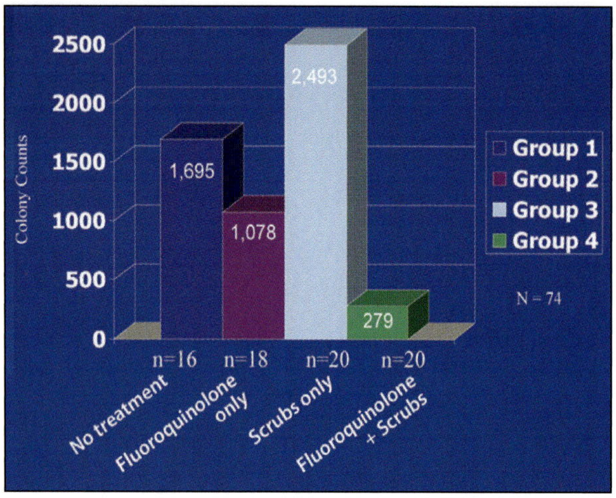

Figure 1. This graph presents the results of preoperative cultures of the ocular surface in a comparative study. (Data adapted from Bucci et al.[2])

quinolone q.i.d. starting 1 day preoperatively and taken every 15 minutes for 1 hour immediately prior to surgery. My antibiotic of choice is Vigamox, because of its broad spectrum of coverage and qualities of penetration.

It is extremely important to perform lid scrubs with 5% Betadine just prior to commencing surgery. I scrub the lids and lashes and insert an aliquot of Betadine into the fornices. I allow the drug to sit for at least 1 to 2 minutes before wiping it off. I then drape the eyelids meticulously with the surgical drape while ensuring the lashes remain pulled back and out of the surgical field.

When starting surgery, I pay particular attention to the wound's construction in order to prevent leakage after surgery and a possible influx of bacteria. I construct a two-stepped, shelved wound in a near clear corneal position, and I make sure that the incision's length is at least two thirds of its width. At the end of the case, I gently hydrate the wounds and ensure their stability with no leakage. If I have any concerns, I will suture the incision. I do not use any intracameral antibiotics, but, at the end of the case, I instill a drop of Vigamox and a mild topical steroid.

Starting immediately after surgery, all patients take Vigamox q.i.d. for a total of 7 days. They also take an NSAID eye drop and a steroid eye drop, both q.i.d. Finally, they receive information on the signs of early endophthalmitis and are instructed either to call the office or to visit the ER if they have any concerns.

ERIK L. MERTENS, MD, FEBO

At their preoperative visit, patients have already commenced treatment for meibomian gland disease in blepharitis. I also instruct them not to wear any cosmetics the day before and the day of surgery.

Patients receive one drop of ocular lomefloxacin 3 mg/mL (Okacin; CIBA Vision, Duluth, GA) 1.5 hours preoperatively, and the dose is repeated every 30 minutes until surgery. While on the operating table, they receive an application of povidone-iodine 10% (Iso-betadine; Viatris, Bad Homburg, Germany) to their eyelids. They are then draped, their eyelids are covered and isolated with Tegaderm, and a lid speculum is inserted. Three minutes before I make the corneal incision, I apply povidone-iodine 5% to the ocular surface.

Meticulous construction of the wound to avoid leakage and to produce self-sealing incisions is also important. When in doubt, I always suture the incision.

At the end of surgery, I instill 5 to 10 mL of vancomycin 6 mg/mL into the anterior chamber. I then administer one drop of lomefloxacin 3mg/mL and a Terracortril suspension (hydrocortisone acetate 17 mg, oxytetracycline 5.7 mg, polymyxine B 11400 IE/g; Pfizer Inc., New York, NY).

The patient's postoperative medications include lomefloxacin 3 mg/mL q.i.d. (starting on the day of surgery) for the first week, a regimen that tapers to one drop per day at 4 weeks postoperatively.

FRANK A. BUCCI, JR MD

My strategy for preventing endophthalmitis can be summarized by my top 10 pearls for preventing intraocular infection.

1. I use a fourth-generation topical fluoroquinolone pre-, intra-, and postoperatively. My choice is Zymar because its penetration levels exceed the minimum inhibitory concentrations for the pathogens that most commonly cause endophthalmitis, just as Vigamox does, but Zymar's speed of kill on the ocular surface is superior to that of Vigamox.
2. I combine a days-prior regimen of topical Zymar with an immediate preoperative pulsing course of therapy.
3. I instruct all patients to perform lid scrubs for at least 2 days prior to their intraocular surgery.
4. I combine the preoperative lid-scrubbing regimen with a days-prior Zymar regimen, which has been shown to be greatly superior to performing lid scrubs alone[2] (Figure 1).
5. Prior to commencing surgery, I apply antiseptics such as povidone-iodine to patients' eyelids, eyelashes, and ocular surface.
6. I use a draping technique that sequesters the lids and lashes from the surgical field intraoperatively.
7. At the conclusion of surgery, I perform stromal hydration of all clear corneal wounds.
8. I administer Zymar immediately postoperatively to replenish corneal and aqueous levels in order to take advantage of the depot effect.
9. I instruct patients to use topical Zymar q.i.d. for at least 1 week postoperatively.
10. I avoid extended low-frequency dosing of topical fluoroquinolones to minimize the development of resistant organisms.

LISA BROTHERS ARBISSER, MD

Surface abnormalities need rehabilitation. I treat lid disease locally and acne rosacea systemically. I will postpone elective surgery if the patient is on systemic steroids that can be tapered in the interest of finding a window for maximum immune competence.

Two days preoperatively, I prescribe a topical fourth-generation fluoroquinolone q.i.d. and have the drug pulsed three times (every 5 minutes) after patients' admission. They are instructed to use a preoperative Eye Scrub (Novartis Ophthalmics, Inc., Duluth, GA) and to wear no makeup.

Before applying lidocaine jelly to the eye, I instill Betadine 5% solution. A Betadine 10% skin preparation is allowed to dry for 3 minutes. I favor double draping by sequestering the lashes and meibomian orifices with a sticky Tegaderm followed by the 10–60 incise drape to minimize touching of the eyelids or the expression of sebum. If any sebum is present after draping, I wash it away with warm BSS, and I coat the cornea with Viscoat for a clear view without repeated corneal irrigation.

At the conclusion of surgery, I confirm watertight clear corneal incisions and verify a dry gutter at normal pressure. I will place a Biosorb 10–0 suture (Alcon Laboratories, Inc.) if the wound architecture is not perfect. I inject 0.2 mL of Vigamox (diluted to 100 µg/mL) into the posterior chamber through the paracentesis and leave a normotensive eye. It is important not to burp the incision during the drape's removal. I instill one drop of Betadine 1.25% into the cul-de-sac. Patients are dosed with a topical fourth-generation fluoroquinolone three times prior to their discharge, and they use the agent every 3 hours while awake until their first postoperative visit. They continue using the drug q.i.d. and an eye shield at bedtime for 1 week.

If the posterior capsule is not intact preoperatively or intraoperatively, I administer a single dose of oral moxifloxacin (Avelox; Bayer Corporation, West Haven, CT) 400 mg preoperatively or immediately postoperatively.

RANDALL J. OLSON, MD

Based upon previous endophthalmitis clinical studies conducted by my colleagues and myself as well as our animal research,3 I have adjusted my profile for cataract prophylaxis according to the following principles. I instruct patients to use a fourth-generation fluoroquinolone q.i.d. for 2 to 3 days prior to surgery. The drug is also administered frequently during the first hour before surgery, and 5% Betadine is applied prior to the placement of any anesthetic gel. I reapply 5% Betadine just prior to starting surgery and carefully use lid drapes to isolate the lid margins.

I am meticulous in the closure of the wound and check its integrity at high and low pressure. When in doubt or for any complicated case, I place a single 10–0 nylon suture. Patients receive three or four drops of a fourth-generation fluoroquinolone immediately after surgery while in the recovery area and then every 1 to 2 hours while awake for the first day. They then use the drug q.i.d. for 2 weeks. Any wound leak on the first postoperative day immediately receives a suture. I will then discuss with the patient the risk of endophthalmitis and instruct him to use the fourth-generation fluoroquinolone q2h for the first week and taper the dosage to q.i.d. for a second week.

My colleagues' and my multivariate analysis3 clearly showed that the greatest risk of endophthalmitis comes from poor antibiosis right after surgery. Also, because any capsular or zonular complication increases the risk for endophthalmitis 17-fold, I suture all such incisions. The highest risk (44-fold) is a leaky wound on the day after surgery, and I feel all such incisions should be sutured and frequent antibiotic drops prescribed.[3]

I have not used intracameral antibiotics, because I do not feel there is evidence showing that they are superior to frequently administered fourth-generation fluoroquinolones right after surgery. The improvement in endophthalmitis shown in the ESCRS study[4] is actually less than the difference in our study comparing the administration of a topical antibiotic on the day after surgery with frequently applied topical fourth-generation antibiotics on the day of surgery.[3]

MARK PACKER, MD

The recent ESCRS study raised questions regarding the use of intracameral antibiotic prophylaxis.[4] It is important, however, to note that procedures were not standardized across all investigators and preoperative topical antibiotics were not generally used. I have instructed patients to use a topical fluoroquinolone q.i.d. for 3 days prior to surgery for 10 years and have never had a case of acute bacterial endophthalmitis (I have had one case of chronic Propionibacterium acnes that was treated successfully with vitrectomy).[5] Povidone-iodine preparation, correct draping, and wound construction have been specifically mentioned as other critical factors in the prevention of infection. Some of the questions about the best practices in this regard may be answered in the final report of the ESCRS study.

A recent ASCRS White Paper specifically considered the role of the clear corneal incision's construction in the prevention of endophthalmitis, and the paper's authors determined that the incision's appropriate design provides adequate prophylaxis.[6] The recent publication by my colleagues and me demonstrating the architecture of clear corneal incisions with optical coherence tomography further supports that an incision in the plane of the cornea with a chord length of at least 2 mm appears to provide advantageous architecture for adequate self-sealing[7] (Figure 2).

Measuring one's own outcomes is crucial to correctly implementing any study's results. At Drs. Fine, Hoffman & Packer in Eugene, Oregon, we have had no cases of bacterial endophthalmitis in approximately 9,000 consecutive operations.

WILLIAM J. FISHKIND, MD

My patients begin taking a fourth-generation fluoroquinolone 3 days before surgery and continue using the drug for 1 week postoperatively to maintain an adequate level to kill organisms. Povidone-iodine 5% is instilled in the operative eye in the preoperative holding area to allow sufficient contact time with the lid margin and conjunctiva. The agent is reapplied during the preparation for surgery, and the lash margin is carefully cleaned and prepared. A barrier drape isolates the lash margin from the operative site.

During surgery, I am careful to avoid the pooling of fluid, which is a potential source of intraoperative contamination. If the eye is deep set, I turn the patient's head to prevent pooling of the BSS. If there is conjunctival chemosis due to a posterior corneal incision, I incise the conjunctiva adjacent to the wound to prevent further chemosis and turn the patient's head to drain fluid.

I create the incision with a diamond blade that is 100 µm thick and 2.75 mm wide (Diamond Stealth Blade; Mastel Precision, Inc., Rapid City, SD). I target a tunnel length of at least 1.75 mm in an effort to produce adequate surface area for secure wound closure. I can then use an appropriate tip/sleeve match for a 19-gauge sleeved phaco tip. The result is a stable anterior chamber during phacoemulsification and the insertion of the IOL without stretching the wound, which facilitates a watertight closure.[7]

JAMES P. GILLS, MD

Throughout my career, I have focused my attention on improving the safety and accuracy of cataract surgery. As a result, I have achieved an infection rate of 1:20,000. I do not attribute it to a single technique or pearl. Instead, it is the cumulative result of several practices that add up to safer surgery.

Using intraocular antibiotics along with cataract surgery is one of the single most important things that can improve safety.[4] At the end of each case, I inject a solution containing vancomycin and ceftazidime into the anterior chamber. I inject the medication rather than place it in the irrigating solution so the patient receives a controlled dosage. This practice has always been somewhat controversial due to a concern over bacterial resistance. The issue is more academic than practical, however, because the antibiotics are

(Courtesy of Mark Packer, MD.)

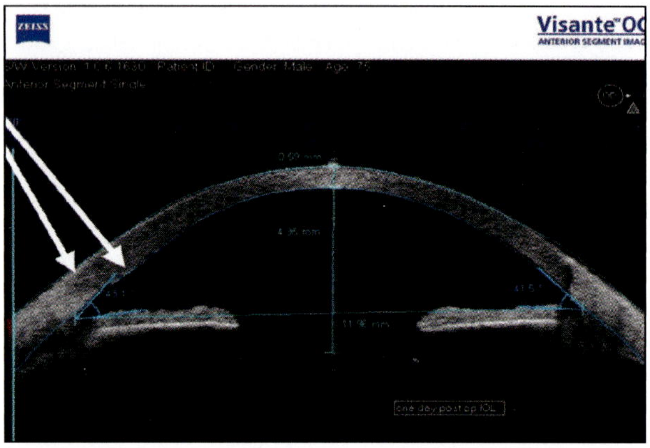

Figure 2. This clear corneal incision is actually curvilinear, not a straight line. It is considerably longer than the chord length originally estimated for the length of the incision. The architecture of the wound allows for a fit not unlike tongue-and-groove paneling, thereby adding a measure of stability to the incision and making it considerably less likely that one surface will slide over the other.

placed inside a closed, sterile container. Although it is difficult to quantify the benefit of intraocular antibiotics, I believe reducing the risk of endophthalmitis justifies their use.

More than 30 years ago, I instituted the use of a 0.2-µm filter for the irrigating solutions.[8] Several years later, there was a series of devastating Paecilomyces lilacinus infections that were caused by contaminated IOLs and solutions.[9-11] Although I was using the same lot of solutions, I did not have a single infection, which I attribute to the use of the filter.

In 1992, I conducted a study in which IOPs were measured at half-hour intervals in the early postoperative period and then at 24 hours.[12] I discovered that, although the patients had firm eyes at the end surgery, some experienced hypotony during the first postoperative half-hour that resolved at 24 hours. Since then, it is part of my standard protocol to measure IOP in the early postoperative period. Any patient with hypotony is patched until the pressure has reached a safe level.

Betadine has always been a critical part of my regimen for controlling infection. The drug works quickly and lasts longer than broad-spectrum antibiotics.[13] Betadine, however, can cause irritation and exacerbate dry eye syndrome following cataract surgery. My colleagues and I measured the pH of our Humco 0.5 Betadine solution (Humco, Texarkana, TX) and discovered that it was approximately 3.5, which is too acidic and likely caused a mildly toxic effect in the cornea. We now balance the pH of the Betadine as follows: 40 mL BSS; 2 mL Betadine; and 1.4 mL sodium bicarbonate 8.4%. This combination yields a solution with a pH of 7.7. Since we began balancing the pH of Betadine, the incidence of dry eye syndrome has been markedly reduced in our patients. ■

This article originally appeared in the April 2007 issue of CRSToday.

1. Robertson SM, Curtis MA, Schlech BA, et al. Ocular pharmacokinetics of moxifloxacin after topical treatment of animals and humans. *Surv Ophthalmol.* 2005;50(suppl 1):S32-S45.
2. Bucci Jr FA, Amico LM, Guerino A, Evans R. The effect of preop lid scrubs and levofloxacin on eyelid and conjunctival cultures prior to cataract surgery. *Invest Ophthalmol Vis Sci.* 2003;44:eabstract 1446.
3. Wallin T, Parker J, Jin Y, et al. Cohort study of 27 cases of endophthalmitis at a single institution. *J Cataract Refract Surg.* 2005;31:735-741.
4. Barry P, Seal D, Gettinby G, et al. ESCRS study of prophylaxis of post-operative endophthalmitis after cataract surgery: preliminary report of principal results from a European multicenter study. *J Cataract Refract Surg.* 2006;32:407-410.
5. Ong-Tone L. Aqueous humor penetration of gatifloxacin and moxifloxacin eyedrops given by different methods before cataract surgery. *J Cataract Refract Surg.* 2007;33:59-62.
6. Nichamin LD, Chang DF, Johnson SH, et al; American Society of Cataract and Refractive Surgery Cataract Clinical Committee. ASCRS White Paper: what is the association between clear corneal cataract incisions and postoperative endophthalmitis? *J Cataract Refract Surg.* 2006;32:1556-1559.
7. Fine IH, Hoffman RS, Packer M. Profile of clear corneal cataract incisions demonstrated by ocular coherence tomography. *J Cataract Refract Surg.* 2007;33:94-97.
8. Gills JP. Prevention of endophthalmitis by intraocular solution filtration and antibiotics. *J Am Intraocul Implant Soc.* 1985;11:185-186.
9. Pettit TH, Olson RJ, Foos RY, Martin WJ. Fungal endophthalmitis following intraocular lens implantation: a surgical epidemic. *Arch Ophthalmol.* 1980;98:1025-1039.
10. Miller GR, Rebell G, Magoon RC, et al. Intravitreal antimycotic therapy and the cure of mycotic endophthalmitis caused by a Paecilomyces lilacinuscontaminated pseudophakos. *Ophthalmic Surg.* 1978;9;54-63.
11. Mosier MA, Lusk B, Pettit TH, et al. Fungal endophthalmitis following intraocular lens implantation. *Am J Ophthalmol.* 1977;83:1-8.
12. Gills JP. Evaluation of early postoperative intraocular pressure in IOL patients with corneal and scleral tunnel incisions. Paper presented at: The ASCRS/ASOA Symposium & Congress; April 12, 1994; Boston, MA.
13. Apt L, Isenberg SJ, Yoshimori R, et al. The effect of povidone-iodine solution applied at the conclusion of ophthalmic surgery. *Am J Ophthalmol.* 1995;119:701-705.

CHAPTER 102

Propionibacterium Acnes Endophthalmitis

RICHARD E. BRAUNSTEIN, MD; NICK MAMALIS, MD; ROBERT KAUFER, MD; AND DANIEL M. MILLER, MD, PHD

CASE PRESENTATION

A healthy 80-year-old female underwent what appeared to be uneventful cataract surgery in her left eye approximately 2 months ago. The surgeon placed a three-piece silicone IOL in the capsular bag. According to the patient, her visual acuity was fine for the first month, but it began to fluctuate and become hazy thereafter. She reported slight pain and redness in her eye as well as photophobia. Treatment with prednisolone q.i.d. reduced her pain but did not enhance her vision. After weeks of no improvement, the patient was referred to you for a consultation.

On examination, the patient's visual acuity measured 20/80 with refraction. Her eye was quiet with minor Descemet's folds, and a capsular plaque located peripherally in the bag (360°) was more intense at the 3- and 9-o'clock positions (Figure 1). No vitreous inflammation or flare and only mild cell were evident. Macular edema was present on the retinal angiogram. An extraction of aqueous from the anterior chamber tested positive for *Propionibacterium acnes*. During that week, her visual acuity decreased to 20/100.

How would you manage this patient?

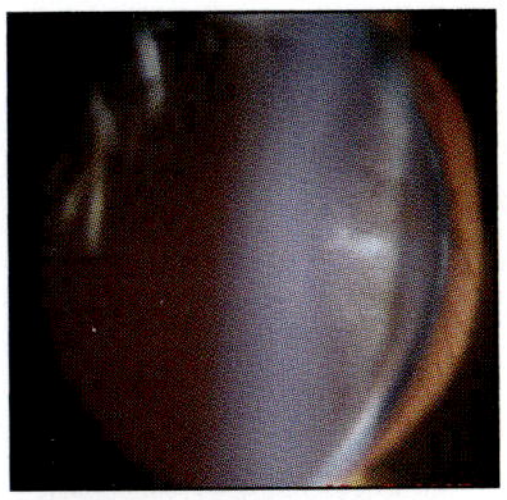

Figure 1. Although quiet, the patient's left eye has minor folds in Descemet's membrane and a capsular plaque.

RICHARD E. BRAUNSTEIN, MD

This patient has a presentation consistent with postoperative *P. acnes* endophthalmitis. Caused by *P. acnes*, a gram-positive anaerobic bacillus, this condition presents as a white intracapsular plaque in the setting of decreased vision, conjunctival injection, intraocular inflammation with or without hypopyon, and keratic precipitates. The positive culture from the anterior segment of this patient solidifies the diagnosis.

P. acnes endophthalmitis has traditionally been treated via a stepwise approach. Many patients are successfully managed with topical corticosteroids. This patient may benefit from a more frequent regimen of topical corticosteroids in conjunction with a topical NSAID. If topical therapy is ineffective at controlling her inflammation and improving her vision, the literature supports an intravitreal injection of vancomycin 1 mg/0.1 mL.[1,2] Reviews of treatment strategies for *P. acnes* endophthalmitis reported a 50% to 100% failure rate for an intraocular antibiotic injection as a primary treatment.[1,2] When intraocular antibiotics fail to control the inflammation, a pars plana vitrectomy and either a partial or a total capsulectomy with or without IOL exchange is indicated. Data from the aforementioned studies demonstrated a recurrence rate of 14% to 44% in patients treated with partial capsulectomy and a recurrence rate of zero in patients treated with total capsulectomy and IOL removal.

For this culture-positive patient, I would recommend an intravitreal injection of vancomycin combined with frequent topical anti-inflammatory therapy. If this therapy failed to resolve the inflammation, I would attempt a pars plana vitrectomy with subtotal posterior capsulectomy, irrigation of the capsular bag, and a repeat intravitreal injection of vancomycin prior to performing a total capsulectomy and removing the IOL.

NICK MAMALIS, MD

This patient's history of inflammation associated with slight pain and redness, photophobia, and a partial response to prednisolone drops is consistent with a case of delayed-onset or chronic endophthalmitis. On Figure 1, the white plaque in the periphery of the capsule is consistent with *P. acnes*, which was confirmed by the testing of an extract from the patient's aqueous.

Treating *P. acnes* chronic endophthalmitis can be challenging, because the organism may be sequestered within the capsular bag or between the implant and the capsular bag, where it is difficult for antibiotics to reach sufficiently high levels to eradicate the bacterium. Such can be the case even after a direct injection of an antibiotic into the lens capsular bag. Conservative treatment for *P. acnes* chronic endophthalmitis consists of the intravitreal injection of an antibiotic (vancomycin) combined with either pars plana vitrectomy or pars plana vitrectomy and partial posterior capsulectomy. Only approximately 50% of patients treated with this limited therapy, however, showed successful eradication of the infection. Two relatively large retrospective studies have confirmed these findings.[1,2] Aldave et al reported on the experience of treating *P. acnes* endophthalmitis at Wills Eye Hospital in Philadelphia,[2] and Clark et al reported similar results for the treatment of patients at the Bascom Palmer Eye Institute in Miami and at the Cleveland Clinic.[1] Both studies confirmed that the limited surgical interventions described earlier eradicated infection in approximately half of the patients. The infection recurred in the remaining 50% of patients, who required a more aggressive surgical intervention, including total capsulectomy with the removal of the IOL combined with an injection of intravitreal antibiotics and pars plana vitrectomy. The complete removal of the lens capsular bag with the IOL cured this condition in all patients treated in this manner.

Given the findings of the aforementioned studies, this patient should undergo initial management with a limited pars plana vitrectomy and posterior capsulectomy followed by intravitreal vancomycin as well as an injection of 1 mg of vancomycin directly into the remaining capsular bag. If the signs of infection recur following this treatment, then the patient will have to undergo a complete removal of the lens capsular bag and IOL with an exchange for either an ACIOL or a sutured PCIOL without the presence of the lens capsular bag. This treatment is usually definitive, even if the more conservative treatment initially fails.

ROBERT KAUFER, MD

Fortunately, the complication presented in this case is infrequent. This patient's endophthalmitis must be managed for the macular inflammation to decrease. Otherwise, her visual acuity will be compromised.

My approach would be to explant the IOL and the entire capsular bag and then inject vancomycin into the anterior chamber. If the capsular plaque were localized in one place (in this case, it occupies 360°), one could consider partially removing the capsule. If vitreous were present in the anterior chamber, a vitrectomy would be indicated.

After administering sub-Tenon's anesthesia, I would inject an ophthalmic viscosurgical device into the anterior chamber to permit maneuvering of the lens. I have found it difficult to fold a silicone lens in the anterior chamber. I would therefore remove the IOL from the bag and cut it into two pieces in order to extract it through a 3-mm incision. Next, I would remove the entire capsular bag while trying to preserve the hyaloid face and prevent vitreous from moving anteriorly. Once I had removed the lens and capsule, I would irrigate the anterior chamber thoroughly with vancomycin 1 mg/0.1 mL and instill a miotic agent.

Postoperatively, the posterior portion of the patient's eye should be tranquil. The macular inflammation should dissipate, and, with proper refractive correction, the patient's visual acuity should improve. I would wait 3 months for her refraction to stabilize, during which time the patient could use a contact lens. I would then proceed to implant an ACIOL. Another possibility would be to suture a PCIOL to the iris or sclera. Given the age of this patient, however, I would consider the ACIOL to be safer.

DANIEL M. MILLER, MD, PhD

The differential diagnosis in cases of delayed inflammation after cataract surgery includes noninfectious uveitis such as sarcoid- or HLA-B27-associated inflammation and infectious endophthalmitis. Causative organisms in delayed-onset endophthalmitis are *Staphylococcus epidermidis, Streptococcus viridans*, other coagulase-negative staphylococci, *P. acnes*, gram-negative rods, and—less commonly—*Candida* or *Aspergillus* in immunosuppressed or systemically ill patients.[3]

P. acnes is an anaerobic, gram-positive, pleomorphic bacillus that grows extremely slowly in anaerobic culture.[4] The association of this organism with acute endophthalmitis after cataract surgery was first reported in 1978.[5] Subsequently, *P. acnes* was shown to be a common cause of delayed-onset endophthalmitis after cataract surgery.[6,7] The key clinical feature of delayed-onset endophthalmitis caused by *P. acnes* is a white, intracapsular plaque composed of sequestered organisms in the relatively anaerobic peripheral capsular bag. The diagnosis can be established by anaerobic culture and by polymerase chain reaction.[4,5,8]

The management of *P. acnes* endophthalmitis is challenging. Intraocular inflammation can recur many months and years after a primary treatment modality, so clinicians should view with caution reports of successful intervention with relatively short follow-up periods. Topical and intraocular antibiotics alone typically do not eradicate the organism, because *P. acnes* may be encapsulated in the peripheral capsule.[1,2,7] Two series of *P. acnes* endophthalmitis following cataract surgery provided information on the relative effectiveness of a variety of therapeutic interventions,[1,2] as described in the comments of my coauthors.

The patient in this case has moderate-to-severe visual loss associated with her infection as well as a progressive course despite topical prednisolone. *P. acnes* endophthalmitis is likely to recur with less aggressive treatment, because the peripheral capsular plaque in 360° of the capsule eliminates the possibility that a focal capsulectomy would result in long-term success. Similarly, conservative measures such as irrigating the peripheral capsule with antibiotics and rotating/mobilizing the IOL within the capsule without capsulectomy are unlikely to treat all sequestered *P. acnes*. I would recommend a pars plana vitrectomy, a total capsulectomy, intravitreal vancomycin, and an IOL exchange in this case. ■

This article originally appeared in the August 2007 issue of CRSToday.

1. Clark WL, Kaiser PK, Flynn HW, et al. Treatment strategies and visual acuity outcomes in chronic postoperative *Propionibacterium acnes* endophthalmitis. *Ophthalmology.* 1999;106:1665-1670.
2. Aldave AJ, Stein JD, Deramo VA, et al. Treatment strategies for postoperative *Propionibacterium acnes* endophthalmitis. *Ophthalmology.* 1999;106:2395-2401.
3. Benz MS, Scott IU, Flynn HW, et al. Endophthalmitis isolates and antibiotic sensitivities: a 6 year review of culture proven cases. *Am J Ophthalmol.* 2004;137:38-42.
4. Hall GS, Pratt-Rippin K, Meisler DM, et al. Growth curve for *Proprionibacterium acnes. Curr Eye Res.* 1994;13:465-466.
5. Forster RK, Zachary IG, Cottingham A Jr, Norton EWD. Further observations in the diagnosis, etiology, and treatment of endophthalmitis. *Trans Am Ophthalmol Soc.* 1978;73:221-230.
6. Meisler DM, Palestine AG, Vastine DW, et al. Chronic *Proprionibacterium* endophthalmitis after extracapsular cataract extraction and intraocular lens implantation. *Am J Ophthalmol.* 1986;102:733-739.
7. Meisler DM, Mandelbaum S. *Proprionibacterium*-associated endophthalmitis after extracapsular cataract extraction. Review of reported cases. *Ophthalmology.* 1989;96:54-61.
8. Lai J, Chen K, Lin Y, et al. *Proprionibacterium acnes* DNA from an explanted intraocular lens detected by polymerase chain reaction in a case of chronic pseudophakic endophthalmitis. *J Cataract Refract Surg.* 2006;32:522-525.

CHAPTER 103

TASS: What Every Anterior Segment Surgeon Needs to Know

HENRY F. EDELHAUSER, PhD; AND DANIEL G. DAWSON, MD

A symposium held during the 2004 annual meeting of the AAO in New Orleans highlighted toxic anterior segment syndrome (TASS).[1] From the questions posed at the end of the session, it became apparent that most of the audience knew little about this postoperative complication, primarily because of a lack of information in the ophthalmic literature and partially because of differences in terminology. This article therefore reviews the etiology, treatment, and prevention of TASS.

DIFFERENTIAL DIAGNOSIS

Since 1980, several published articles have described a severe form of inflammation that appears in the anterior segment within 24 hours after intraocular surgery.[2-4] Called *TASS* since 2002,[5] this postoperative complication causes severe anterior segment inflammation, usually with hypopyon, and can result in varying degrees of long-term damage to anterior segment structures.[6,7] Although TASS was sometimes referred to as *sterile endophthalmitis*, the two conditions are different, because the former involves only the anterior segment of the eye, has a more acute onset (within 24 hours after surgery vs 3 to 7 days for endophthalmitis), always cultures negatively for bacteria, and responds to steroid treatment.

TASS can be triggered by the introduction of toxic substances into the anterior segment of the eye, which results in cellular death (ie, necrosis or apoptosis) and extracellular tissue damage to the corneal endothelium, trabecular meshwork, iris, or lens. The eye's innate immune system summons inflammatory cells to the anterior segment where they can attack the foreign toxins. Unfortunately, this acute immune response has advantages and disadvantages. Although it helps to remove toxic substances, dead tissue, and damaged extracellular matrices, the excessive intensity of the response further damages already compromised ocular tissue.

The degree of damage caused by TASS depends on many factors, including the type and amount of substance introduced into the eye, the duration of exposure, and how quickly treatment begins. An especially acute form of TASS, called *toxic endothelial cell destruction syndrome*, predominantly affects the corneal endothelium,[7] whereas toxic endophthalmitis or sterile endophthalmitis significantly affects the posterior segment.

Although some of the causes of TASS have been known for some time (eg, intraocular irrigating solutions, pH, osmolality, drug concentrations, or preservative levels outside the tolerable range for intraocular tissues to survive),[8] it was not until hospitals and surgery centers started reporting local endemic outbreaks that different etiologies of this condition began to emerge.[9-13] Most recent cases can be attributed to problems in the procedures used to clean and sterilize ophthalmic instruments. Specific contributing factors include the inadequate rinsing of heat-stable detergents from reusable intraocular instruments (particularly those with retained viscoelastic residue),[9-11] the formation of metal residues on reusable surgical instruments during cleaning with a gas sterilization system, or the deposit of a heat-stable bacterial endotoxin on intraocular instruments before or during steam autoclave sterilization. The heat-stable bacteria usually originate in the water reservoirs of ultrasonic cleaners or steam sterilizers.[13]

PREVENTING TASS

The primary treatment for TASS is topical steroids. Once toxic substances damage the eye, however, these drugs only suppress the secondary inflammatory response. The best way to manage TASS is to prevent it.

When performing cataract surgery, one must ensure that the whole surgical team (nurses, OR technicians, and physicians) knows what irrigating solutions and viscoelastics are appropriate for use in the eye and how to properly dilute drugs intended for intracameral use. One should keep the use of reusable intraocular instruments to a minimum and make sure that the OR technicians who clean and sterilize the reusable instruments follow the proper protocols. They should:

- rinse or flush all instruments with sterile deionized water thoroughly to remove residual detergents or enzymatic cleaners from their surfaces and lumens between each cleaning step;
- replace the water in ultrasonic cleaning baths every day. Rinse the baths with alcohol before refilling them to prevent the growth of gram-negative bacteria that have heat-stable lipopolysaccharide endotoxins in their membranes; and
- change the water reservoirs in steam sterilizers at least once a week.

Finally, one should ensure that all intraocular medications used during anterior segment surgery are free of preservatives,[5] diluted to the correct concentration for intraocular use, and have the proper pH and osmolality range for intraocular tissues. Also, only physiologic irrigating solutions such as BSS or BSS Plus (Alcon Laboratories, Inc., Fort Worth, TX) should be used during the procedure.

KNOWN SOURCES OF TASS-CAUSING TOXINS

- Preservatives in ocular medications; incompatible drug concentration, pH (6.5 to 8.5), or osmolality (200 to 400 m Osm)
- Endotoxins deposited on reusable or nonreusable surgical instruments not free of pyrogen by contaminated water sources
- Incomplete surgical solutions or irrigants that lack the necessary buffer and five-ion content
- Residual detergent on reusable surgical instruments
- Residual metal toxins on reusable cannulas after plasma gas sterilization

ISOLATING THE SOURCE

In case of an outbreak of TASS, the surgeon is responsible for notifying the surgical team and the surgery center's management. The surgery center should treat all cases of TASS as an environmental toxin and infection control breakdown. They may have to identify protocol changes that coincided with the timeframe of the outbreak.[14] The center should check if patients treated by other surgeons in different ORs developed similar cases of TASS. Useful strategies for identifying the source of TASS-causing toxins usually include appointing a staff member to coordinate the clinical review and making flow charts to track the changes or factors potentially responsible for the outbreak.

CONCLUSION

The recent review by Mamalis et al[14] is a useful source for those needing more information about TASS. All surgeons should know about TASS, particularly how to prevent it and how to differentiate this condition from endophthalmitis. It is also important to know that TASS, toxic endothelial cell destruction, and toxic endophthalmitis are all varying degrees of the same condition. ■

Supported in part by NIH grants R01 EY-00933 and T32-EY-7092.

This article originally appeared in the July 2006 issue of CRSToday.

1. TASS: what you don't know could be toxic. Symposium held during: The Annual Meeting of the American Academy of Ophthalmolog; October 25, 2004; New Orleans, LA.
2. Meltzer DW. Sterile hypopyon following intraocular lens surgery. *Arch Ophthalmol.* 1980;98:100-104.
3. Apple DJ, Mamalis N, Steinmetz RL, et al. Phacoanaphylactic endophthalmitis associated with extracapsular cataract extraction and posterior chamber intraocular lens. *Arch Ophthalmol.* 1984;102:1528-1532.
4. Abrahams IW. Diagnosis and surgical management of phacoanaphylactic uveitis following extracapsular cataract extraction with intraocular lens implantation. *Am Intraocular Implant Soc J.* 1985:11:444-447.
5. Jehan FS, Mamalis N, Spencer TS, et al. Postoperative sterile endophthalmitis (TASS) associated with the Memorylens. *J Cataract Refract Surg.* 2000:26:1773-1777.
6. Monson MC, Mamalis N, Olson RJ. Toxic anterior segment inflammation following cataract surgery. *J Cataract Refract Surg.* 1992;18:184-189.
7. Breebaart A, Nuyts R, Pels E, et al. Toxic endothelial cell destruction of the cornea after routine extracapsular cataract surgery. *Arch Ophthalmol.* 1990;108:1121-1125.
8. Parikh CH, Edelhauser HF. Ocular surgical pharmacology: corneal endothelial safety and toxicity. *Curr Opin Ophthalmol.* 2003;14:178-185.
9. Richburg F, Reidy J, Apple D, Olson R. Sterile hypopyon secondary to ultrasonic cleaning solution. *J Cataract Refract Surg.* 1986;12:248-251.
10. Worst JGF. A retrospective review on the sterilization of intraocular lenses and the incidence of sterile hypopyon. *Am Intraocular Implant Soc J.* 1980;6:10-12.
11. Kim JH. Intraocular inflammation of denatured viscoelastic substance in cases of cataract extraction and lens implantation. *J Cataract Refract Surg.* 1987;13:537-542.
12. Duffy R, Brown S, Caldwell K, et al. An epidemic of corneal destruction caused by plasma gas sterilization. The Toxic Endothelial Cell Destruction Syndrome Investigative Team. *Arch Ophthalmol.* 2000;118:1167-1176.
13. Whitby JL, Hitchins VM. Endotoxin levels in steam and reservoirs of tabletop steam sterilizers. *J Refract Surg.* 2002;18:51-57.
14. Mamalis N, Edelhauser HF, Dawson DG, et al. Toxic anterior segment syndrome. *J Cataract Refract Surg.* 2006;32:324-333.

CHAPTER 104

TASS Versus Endophthalmitis

RANDALL J. OLSON, MD

Imagine that you performed several uncomplicated surgeries yesterday. The first patient you see today with moderate pain, horrible vision, profound corneal edema, and unusual inflammation and hypopyon is enough to make your heart stop. When you realize that, of your eight postoperative patients, all have unusual inflammation and three cases are severe, you wonder if you ever want to practice medicine again. Such has been the story reported to me, including by one of my former fellows, who seriously considered giving up surgery. It is the horror of toxic anterior segment syndrome (TASS).

One problem is that TASS and endophthalmitis can appear exactly the same, but the treatment for each is different. TASS can improve in time without a special treatment, whereas a diagnosis of endophthalmitis must be made as soon as possible in order to potentially achieve a good result. Distinguishing between the two conditions is therefore an important factor in dealing with either disease determining a diagnosis is not an academic exercise as more ophthalmologists encounter TASS. In fact, I know my colleagues feel that this complication is dramatically underreported because many cases of unusual inflammation were probably TASS that resolved and thus remained undiagnosed.

I believe it is possible to tell the difference between the two types of inflammation most of the time. A few signs and symptoms can help ophthalmologists decide the best course of treatment when examining the patient.

CLINICAL FINDINGS

Timing of the Disease

Because TASS is a toxic insult, it virtually always shows up as an unusual inflammation on the day after surgery. Although endophthalmitis can manifest 1 day postoperatively, the Endophthalmitis Vitrectomy Study[1] has shown that most cases of endophthalmitis do not show up until later. Therefore, unusual changes on the day after surgery may indicate TASS, but alone this finding is not definitive.

Pain

Although both TASS and endophthalmitis can cause significant or no pain, it has been my and my colleagues' experience that pain more often indicates endophthalmitis. Unless the IOP is very high, TASS is associated with remarkably little pain but significant inflammation. Again, this is a differentiating point that is helpful but not definitive in regard to determining whether or not a patient has TASS.

Conjunctival and Lid Reaction

Because TASS represents a localized chemical or toxic reaction in the intraocular anterior segment, it is often surprising how little conjunctival or scleral injection is seen at presentation. Furthermore, lid swelling is uncommon. The presence of conjunctival or lid injection and swelling therefore suggest endophthalmitis.

Corneal Edema

It is exceedingly rare to have limbal-to-limbal, 360° corneal edema on the first postoperative day. Even corneal edema caused by complicated and difficult cataract surgery (eg, with Fuchs' corneal dystrophy) is generally sectorial and often most noticeable near the wound or centrally and opposite the wound where most of our surgery is performed. Ninety degrees away, surgeons can find patches of cornea without edema. With TASS, all of the endothelium functions poorly.

Limbus-to-limbus edema is thus a very important differentiating finding. If this symptom is present on the first postoperative day, you can feel at least 95% confident that the problem is TASS. Nonetheless, endophthalmitis should never be eliminated as a diagnosis until the therapeutic response is measured!

Iris Findings

In an eye with TASS, a fixed, dilated pupil—often with spotty or diffuse areas of iris atrophy—is not uncommon. That finding is unlikely in endophthalmitis. Be aware that iris damage associated with TASS only occurs in some cases, however.

IOP

TASS can have a profound impact on the trabecular meshwork. Depending upon the amount of inflammation, there may be some ciliary body shutdown and hypotony, but many eyes have severely elevated IOP, often as high as 50 to 60 mm Hg. Extremely high IOP early in the postoperative period is an unusual finding for endophthalmitis and points toward a diagnosis of TASS. The trabecular meshwork is one of the less sensitive structures. Surgeons may encounter many cases with profound corneal edema and a largely unresponsive pupil without damage to the trabecular meshwork.

Therapeutic Response

If you suspect TASS, then the patient's therapeutic response to topical steroids is the definitive test. Assume TASS with any eye that exhibits an unusual amount of inflammation and limbus-to-limbus corneal edema on the first postoperative day until proven otherwise. These patients should receive frequent (every 30 to 40 minutes) drops of topical steroids and remain in the office to be monitored during the day. Steroids can suppress inflammation from endophthalmitis for a short period of time. If the patient is no worse by the end of the day, however, you can assume TASS is the problem. If you sense that the patient's condition is worsening despite steroid treatment, then endophthalmitis is the likely diagnosis, and the patient should be treated promptly.

Regardless of how the patient responds to steroids during the day, he should be seen promptly the next day and monitored on a daily basis until a diagnosis is absolutely certain.

CONCLUSION

My colleagues and I feel quite comfortable distinguishing between the two conditions in regard to the initial treatment. Never take TASS lightly however. Until a therapeutic response to topical steroids is clearly present for several days, endophthalmitis should be a consideration. Fortunately, the clues outlined herein should facilitate the differential diagnosis. ■

This article originally appeared in the July 2006 issue of CRSToday.

1. Results of the Endophthalmitis Vitrectomy Study. A randomized trail of immediate vitrectomy and of intravenous antibiotics for the treatment of postoperative bacterial endophthalmitis. Endophthalmitis Vitrectomy Study Group. *Arch Ophthalmol.* 1995;113:1479-1496.

CHAPTER 105

TASS Outbreaks: What Should We Do?

NICK MAMALIS, MD

Toxic anterior segment syndrome (TASS) is an acute, sterile, postoperative anterior segment inflammation that may occur following any anterior segment surgery.[1] The hallmark of TASS is an inflammatory reaction in the anterior segment of the eye that starts within 12 to 48 hours after surgery. The most common clinical findings in these patients are diffuse, limbus-to-limbus corneal edema (Figure 1), increased inflammation in the anterior chamber with the possible formation of a hypopyon (Figure 2), and the deposition of fibrin.[2,3] The eye may also have a dilated pupil with an irregularity to the iris (Figure 3) and potential damage to the trabecular meshwork with subsequent secondary glaucoma. The inflammation is sterile and must be distinguished from an infectious endophthalmitis. This article summarizes the causes of, responses to, and prevention of TASS and provides information on the resources available to affected surgeons and centers.

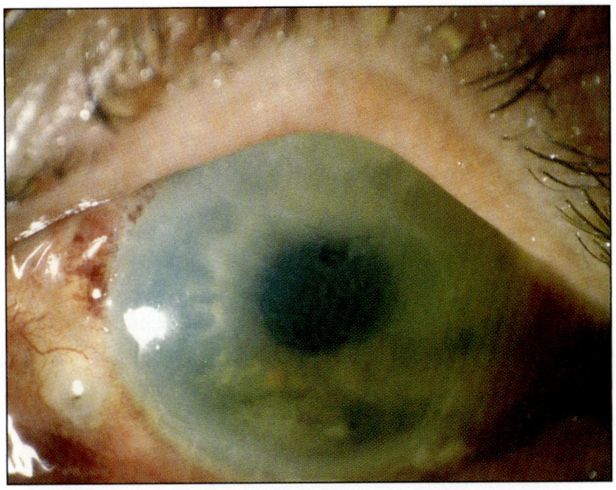

Figure 1. The eye exhibits diffuse, limbus-to-limbus corneal edema. (Reprinted with permission from Mamalis N, Edelhauser HF, Dawson DG, et al. Toxic anterior segment syndrome [review/update]. *J Cataract Refract Surg.* 2006;32:324-333.)

THE CAUSES OF TASS

Cases of TASS may occur singly or, more often, in groups or clusters. The potential factors in the etiology of the condition are widespread.[3-7] TASS may be due to problems with irrigating or

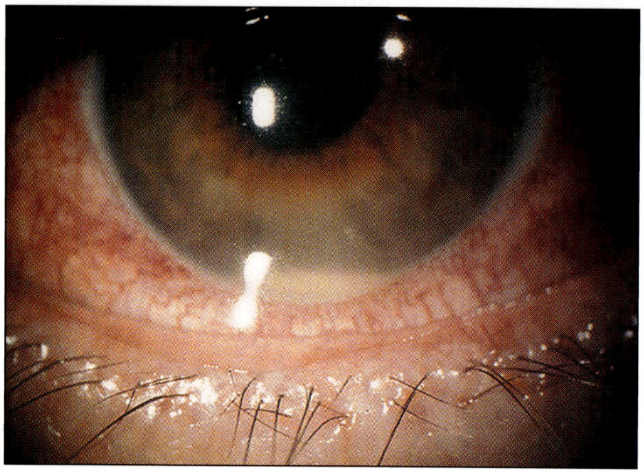

Figure 2. Marked anterior segment inflammation with hypopyon formation is evident. (Reprinted with permission from Mamalis N, Edelhauser HF, Dawson DG, et al. Toxic anterior segment syndrome [review/update]. *J Cataract Refract Surg.* 2006;32:324-333.)

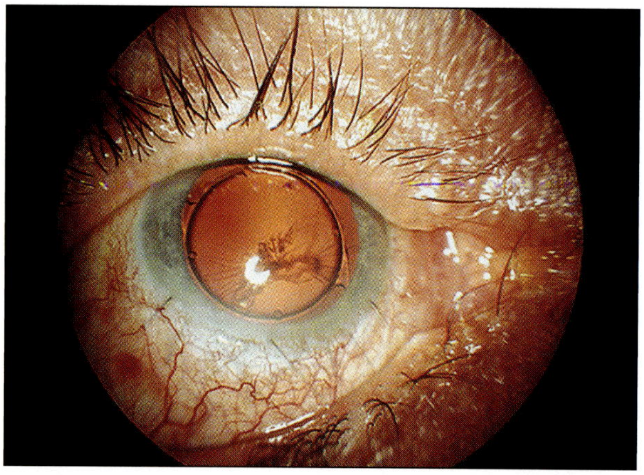

Figure 3. The eye has a dilated, irregular pupil secondary to iris damage. (Reprinted with permission from Mamalis N, Edelhauser HF, Dawson DG, et al. Toxic anterior segment syndrome [review/update]. *J Cataract Refract Surg.* 2006;32:324-333.)

balanced salt solutions or any medication, including antibiotics and analgesic agents that are injected into the eye during surgery. Topical drops or ointments that gain access to the anterior chamber may trigger an inflammatory reaction. In addition, any enzymes or detergents used to clean instruments or cannulas between cases are potential sources of postoperative inflammation. Contamination with a heat-stable endotoxin can occur from multiple different sources involved in the cleaning and sterilization of instruments and handpieces. Lastly, any residual material such as ophthalmic viscosurgical devices, cortex, or cleaning materials that remain in handpieces or cannulas can cause TASS.

AN ANALYSIS OF TASS

Once an outbreak of TASS has been recognized, it is important for all members of the surgical team to work together on its analysis. The effort should include not only the physicians involved but also the surgical nurses, OR technicians, and anyone participating in the preparation of the medications or solutions used in anterior segment surgery. In addition, staff members responsible for the cleaning and maintenance of autoclaves and ultrasound baths should participate.

The surgeons and representatives from the surgical center or hospital (including all involved nursing staff and personnel) should undertake a complete review of all OR protocols. They should carefully evaluate the procedures used in the sterilization and preparation of instruments in order to rule out any potential source of TASS. A complete analysis of all medications or fluids used during anterior segment surgery is also necessary. It is helpful to appoint a coordinator from the surgical center to oversee the review of the factors possibly involved in TASS.

It is beneficial to establish flowcharts and follow protocols to track changes or factors that could be responsible for the outbreak. Investigators should carefully evaluate any fluids, solutions, or medications used during the surgery and record all involved lot and batch numbers for potential etiologic agents.

THE PREVENTION OF TASS

Several steps can help prevent additional cases of TASS from occurring. All staff involved in the cleaning and sterilization of intraocular instruments should receive thorough instruction regarding the protocols for these processes. This effort can result in the elimination of residue that could accumulate on reusable instruments and cause a toxic reaction. The center should limit the use of such instruments and rely on disposable products, especially cannulas, when possible to eliminate a potential source of TASS. Instruments that need to be reused (eg, phaco and I/A handpieces) should be thoroughly rinsed at the conclusion of each case with at least 120 mL of sterile, deionized water through both their irrigation and aspiration ports. The staff should replace the fluid on a daily basis in any ultrasound or water baths used to clean instruments in order to limit the possible growth of gram-negative bacteria, which may lead to a buildup of heat-stable lipopolysaccaride endotoxins. In addition, the staff should regularly clean the inside of these baths thoroughly.

Changing the water reservoir of steam autoclave sterilizers, when applicable, on a weekly basis will prevent the buildup of gram-negative bacteria with lipopolysaccaride endotoxins. In addition, the staff should thoroughly clean the inside of the autoclave at least once a week in order to prevent the accumulation of any potentially toxic, residual material.

Other possible sources of TASS include medications or solutions used within the eye. The surgeon and staff should carefully review all of the medications that are used during routine anterior segment surgery. They must ensure that medications are indeed free of preservatives if they are supposed to be. It is important that the epinephrine in the irrigating solution be without bisulphate preservatives. Anesthetic medicines such as intracameral lidocaine should also be noted to be free of preservatives, because even low levels within the anterior chamber of the eye can trigger an inflammatory reaction. Lastly, the surgeon and staff should take great care to ensure that any antibiotics or similar medications, either in the irrigating solution or injected into the eye at the conclusion of the case, are in the proper doses.

THE RESOURCES AVAILABLE

Attempting to analyze the source of a potential TASS outbreak can be difficult for a surgeon or surgical center. Outside help is available to assist in the analysis of a potential occurrence of TASS. The ASCRS has helped to establish the Intermountain

Ocular Research Center, for which I am the director, at the University of Utah in Salt Lake City to evaluate the causes and prevention of TASS (see *Helping to Prevent TASS*). Protocols developed at the center can help guide this analysis, and ophthalmic research fellows are available to provide an on-site analysis of TASS outbreaks if necessary. Henry Edelhauser, PhD, has also established a response team at the Emory University Eye Center to provide assistance in the evaluation and prevention of outbreaks of TASS.

Both centers have worked with the Centers for Disease Control and Prevention as well as the FDA in the analysis of possible TASS outbreaks. Physicians and surgical centers may consider both of these centers as resources to help investigate incidents of TASS in order to track down the etiologic agents involved and help eliminate the potential sources of this sterile, postoperative inflammation. ■

This article originally appeared in the July 2006 issue of CRSToday.

1. Monson MC, Mamalis N, Olson RJ. Toxic anterior segment inflammation following cataract surgery. *J Cataract Refract Surg.* 1992;18:184-189.
2. Mamalis N. Toxic anterior segment syndrome (editorial). *J Cataract Refract Surg.* 2006;32:181-182.
3. Mamalis N, Edelhauser HF, Dawson DG, et al. Toxic anterior segment syndrome (review/update). *J Cataract Refract Surg.* 2006;32:324-333.
4. Kreisler KR, Martin SS, Young CW, et al. Postoperative inflammation following cataract extraction caused by bacterial contamination of the cleaning bath detergent. *J Cataract Refract Surg.* 1992;18:106-110.
5. Parikh CH, Edelhauser HF. Ocular surgical pharmacology: corneal and endothelial safety and toxicity. *Curr Opin Ophthalmol.* 2003;14:178-185.
6. Parikh C, Sippy BD, Martin DF, Edelhauser HF. Effects of enzymatic sterilization detergents on the corneal endothelium. *Arch Ophthalmol.* 2002;120:156-172.
7. Kim JH. Intraocular inflammation of denatured viscoelastic substance in cases of cataract extraction and lens implantation. *J Cataract Refract Surg.* 1987;13:537-542.

CHAPTER 106

Investigating a TASS Outbreak

THOMAS L. BEARDSLEY, MD

The occurrence of toxic anterior segment syndrome (TASS) is an unexpected and unsettling event that will disrupt an otherwise routine postoperative examination. Because the primary treatment of TASS is prevention, an immediate and comprehensive evaluation of the entire surgical procedure must occur. In addition to this month's cover series in *Cataract & Refractive Surgery Today*, all surgeons should be familiar with a recent, thorough review of TASS published in the *Journal of Cataract and Refractive Surgery*.[1] After a diagnosis of TASS, the entire surgical team must give input on every perioperative process during its review. In order to evaluate all potential sources of TASS completely, I would suggest that each surgery center designate its own team of CSIs (in this case, cataract surgery investigators).

EARLY DIAGNOSIS

The process begins with a timely and accurate diagnosis of TASS as opposed to normal postoperative inflammation or infectious endophthalmitis. I feel it is critical for the operating surgeon to perform the initial postoperative examinations within 24 hours. Only the surgeon has the knowledge of the patient and the details of the operation necessary to judge the appropriate amount of postoperative inflammation or edema.

Many ophthalmologists examine their patients at the slit lamp hours after surgery. Signs of TASS can appear within hours of the procedure, and the CSIs can be notified before the end of the day. The early postoperative examination may also reveal other problems such as an elevated IOP or a leaking wound.

Because there are numerous reported causes of TASS, it can be difficult to isolate a specific etiology in each outbreak. The frequency and pattern of observed cases can help lead the CSI team. Clusters of cases enable investigators to review commonalities between surgeries and perhaps identify a product or inconsistency common to the affected patients. It will be harder to determine a cause for sporadic or isolated cases after the fact. The postoperative examination is critical to differentiate between unique cases and clusters in which some of the patients' signs are subtle.

NOTIFICATION

After identifying TASS in the postoperative clinic, the surgeon should immediately communicate the finding to the surgery center's director, who should in turn notify the surgeons scheduled to use the ORs next. If the problem is widespread, further intraocular surgery should be canceled. With sporadic cases, the director must decide whether or not to maintain the surgical schedule with an emphasis on diligently following established OR procedures and policies until the problem is identified. The surgery center's director should notify all of the OR staff and convene the CSI team to begin an immediate re-evaluation of the previous day's operations. Of course, the affected patients should be fully informed of the unexpected complication. It may be appropriate to notify the major vendors of the center's surgical supplies, because these individuals may be helpful in identifying a more widespread outbreak.

DATA COLLECTION

The CSI team should re-evaluate all of the products used during the entire surgical schedule that day as quickly as possible. They should check every medication, fluid, and disposable product used pre- and intraoperatively and catalog these items by manufacturer, lot number, expiration date, appropriate concentration, and type of preservative, if any. This effort may entail dumpster diving for the trash bags if they are still available. Residual, unused product such as balanced salt solution or viscoelastic should be saved for chemical and biological analysis. Samples can be sent to the Centers for Disease Control and Prevention in Atlanta, the vendor, or an independent laboratory for analysis.

In their catalog, the CSI team should also include the OR pack, phaco pack, IOL, lens inserters, and every other disposable product used. The list should also identify which surgical instruments were used and, particularly, the method of sterilization for each case. The CSI team should note any variations in the surgery center's environment such as power outages; a malfunction of the heating, ventilation, or air conditioning; or a disruption of the water supply.

If cases of TASS continue to occur sporadically, the staff may begin the tedious task of recording all of these data preoperatively until the problem is identified. This detailed information may lead investigators toward a common cause not only at the center in question but elsewhere as well in cases caused by tainted products. Nick Mamalis, MD, at the Intermountain Ocular Research Center in Salt Lake City has developed a protocol for data collection in cases of postoperative inflammation, including TASS and endophthalmitis.

REVIEW OF OR PROTOCOL

The surgeon, the OR staff, and the investigating team should thoroughly review all aspects of the cataract operation. This process should include the sterile preparation of the patient, the staff's sterile technique, the setup of the phaco machine and intraocular irrigating fluid, the preparation of all intraocular medications, the storage and handling of injectable products, such as the IOL, and the cleaning of the surgical instruments on the back table prior to their sterilization.

It may be that staff turnover or stress from an increase in surgical volume and demands for more efficiency resulted in errors or deficiencies in the OR protocol. The surgical staff must remain diligent in the ordering, preparation, and use of every intraocular product. Staff members must avoid cutting corners or absentmindedly deviating from established policies and procedures. The center should institute checks and balances in all critical phases, including the drawing up of intraocular injections.

REVIEW OF CLEANING AND STERILIZING PROCEDURE

Many cases of TASS result from deficiencies in the cleaning and sterilization of the surgical instruments. Any substance used during the cleaning process can result in TASS if enough of it enters the eye. Detergents, enzymes, and residual metallic ions that are left on instruments by faulty cleaning have been implicated. In addition, heat-stable bacterial endotoxins in sterilizer reservoirs or water baths may contaminate instruments. Denatured viscoelastic trapped in surgical instruments and cannulas can also result in TASS.

Probably the most important area for review by your CSI team is the use and maintenance of the sterilizers. The investigators should sample the water reservoir, the water supply, or the steam generator for impurities. It is important to look for residual endotoxin and other heat-stable bacterial byproducts inside the units.

Everyone involved in the cleaning and sterilization process should be adequately knowledgeable about proper techniques. Someone should consult with the manufacturer to ensure the proper care, cleaning, and maintenance of the sterilizer. Moreover, the hospital or the American Society of Ophthalmic Registered Nurses can provide recommendations on the cleaning and care of instruments. The surgical staff should implement a frequent, vigorous, and thorough cleaning process for the sterilizers that may go beyond the recommended schedule of the vendor.

REPORTING CASES

It may not be possible to determine the cause of TASS in isolated instances, especially if the culprit was a single slipup in protocol during surgery. A local investigative team can and should address recurring cases due to internal problems with the use of a product, sterilization, medication, etc.

In the case of tainted products, a nationwide reporting system may help identify the potential source of the contamination. Physicians should inform their colleagues through meetings or Web-based chat rooms such as Eye-mail on the ASCRS' Web site. The ASCRS has set up a national registry for TASS and postoperative endophthalmitis at the University of Utah under the direction of Dr. Mamalis, as noted earlier. One may also contact Henry Edelhauser, PhD, at the Emory Eye Center in Atlanta. If necessary, surgeons may involve the Centers for Disease Control and Prevention through contact with the Emory Eye Center. ■

This article originally appeared in the July 2006 issue of CRSToday.

1. Mamalis N, Edelhauser HF, Dawson EG, et al. Toxic anterior segment syndrome. *J Cataract Refract Surg.* 2006;32:324-333.

CHAPTER 107

Autoclave Contamination and TASS

SIMON HOLLAND, MB, FRCSC; AND DOUGLAS MORCK, DVM, PhD

Endotoxin is a possible cause of toxic anterior segment syndrome (TASS).[1,2] Bacterial endotoxin or lipopolysaccharide (LPS) is produced by gram-negative bacteria and is a potent inflammatory mediator that causes septic shock syndrome. The Lipid A portion of the LPS molecule is thought to be responsible for this potent inflammatory effect. Endotoxin is heat stable and can readily survive short-cycle sterilization.[3] Endotoxins are also recognized as an important cause of diffuse lamellar keratitis (DLK) and have been identified in the steam distillate of the Statim sterilizers (Scican Inc., Pittsburgh, PA).[4] Thus, although bacteria such as *Pseudomonas* are killed by short-cycle sterilization (3.5 minutes at 180° C), their endotoxins are released from the cells' walls in the sterilizer. These endotoxins remain biologically active and can be deposited on instruments used in anterior segment cataract surgery.

Previous outbreaks of TASS have also been linked to the contamination of the ultrasonic baths with similar bacteria[5] and to the liquid detergent used in the cleaning bath.[1] Our recent experience with an outbreak showed an association between the contamination of an autoclave reservoir with gram-negative, endotoxin-producing bacteria and TASS.[6]

OUTBREAK INVESTIGATED

Our hospital experienced an outbreak of TASS that began with four cases occurring during a 3-week period. After it investigated the incident, the only suggestion to control the outbreak from the hospital's infection control department was for surgeons to switch

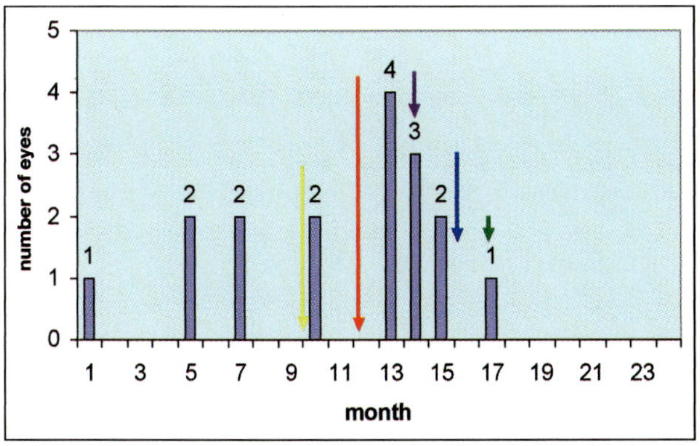

Figure 1. This graph shows the epidemiological curve of a TASS outbreak.

from multi- to single-use phaco tips. This change in protocol proved ineffective in preventing further cases of TASS (Figure 1). The method of sterilization ophthalmologists in the hospital used was a combination of a short cycle with the Statim sterilizers and a prolonged-cycle system with sterilizers from the hospital's central sterile department. Culturing of the Statim sterilizers showed a heavy growth of gram-negative bacteria (predominantly *Sphingomonas, Ralstonia,* and *Pseudomonas*), but no additional action was taken based on these results at that time.

Another cluster of 10 TASS cases occurred between months 13 and 17 of the reported outbreak. Surgeons limited their use of short-cycle sterilization and replaced reusable with disposable cannulas. Although these steps proved partially effective, the outbreak continued. Further bacterial cultures and biofilm sampling of the Statim sterilizer reservoirs showed the same bacteria and associated biofilms within the reservoirs (Figure 2).

Our hospital replaced its three Statim sterilizers and instituted a rigorous cleaning protocol for the new units that included emptying them daily, cleaning their reservoirs with a quaternary ammonium compound daily, and periodically replacing their inner tubing. The sterilizers had been in use for more than 8 years and had never been serviced or cleaned. Following these interventions, the outbreak ceased, and no further cases have been reported at the hospital in the 2 years since.

PROTOCOL FOR THE DURATION OF AN OUTBREAK

- Empty the sterilizer at the end of each surgical day.
- Fill with boiling tap water and drain. Repeat.
- Fill reservoir with distilled water and empty. Repeat.
- Leave 70% alcohol in reservoir overnight.
- Fill with boiling tap water and drain.
- Fill with distilled water and drain.
- Fill with distilled water and run two cycles.
  Note: Diluted hypochlorite may be substituted for 70% alcohol.
- The inner tubing of the sterilizer must be changed monthly at minimum.

This protocol is not approved by the FDA or the manufacturers of sterilizers.

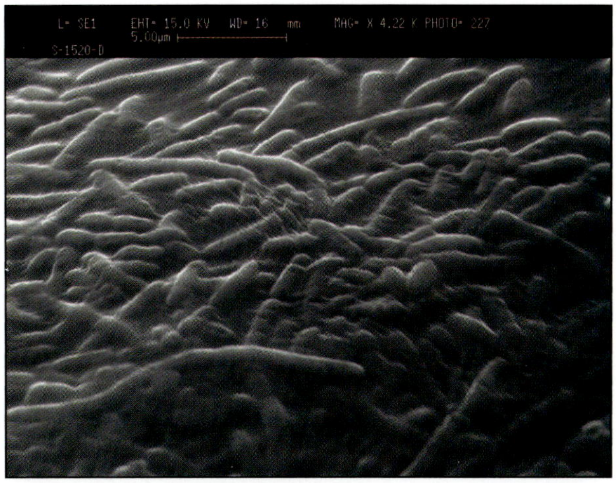

Figure 2. Bacterial biofilm coats the mesh of an in-line filtering system in a Statim sterilizer.

PROTOCOLS FOR THE MAINTENANCE OF A STERILIZER'S RESERVOIR

We have found the following protocols effective in controlling biofilm and the contamination of sterilizers' reservoirs with bacterial endotoxin. These procedures are not approved by the sterilizers' manufacturers or the FDA. Maintenance based on the endotoxin theory has thus far proven successful against outbreaks of both TASS and DLK.[3,6] We recommend appropriately cleaning reservoirs to clinics experiencing cases of TASS.

During periods without a case of TASS, a clinic's staff should perform routine maintenance of the sterilizer on each surgical day (see *Routine Maintenance for a Sterilizer*). The unit's inner tubing should be replaced monthly.

During an outbreak of TASS or DLK, the sterilizer may become contaminated (see *Protocol for the Duration of an Outbreak*). Modified protocols may be necessary based on the severity of the outbreak as well as the nature of the bacterial biofilm identified. Although most biofilm produced by bacteria is inactivated by 70% alcohol, we have found a difference in the substance's susceptibility to various biocides depending on the specific bacteria.[7] During confirmed outbreaks, household bleach (sodium hypochlorite) diluted in distilled water may be substituted for 70% alcohol. We recommend seeking further advice from those with experience such as ourselves before using hypochlorite 0.525% (ie, commercial household bleach 5.25% diluted 1:10 with water) due to the potential for damaging the sterilizer's lining and tubes. Our use of this solution in specific outbreaks was based on our assessment of the resistance of involved bacterial biofilm to the biocidal agents that are more easily employed (ie, 70% alcohol).

CONCLUSION

Short-cycle, steam-generating, tabletop sterilizers such as the Statim have proven to be efficient in high-volume cataract surgical centers due to their simplicity of use, rapid cycles, cassette-based system, reliability, and economy. Most units use a sterilization time of 3.5 minutes and a total sterilization cycle time of 6 minutes compared with the 45-minute cycles of standard sterilizers. Short-cycle sterilizers are not without their problems, however. One major disadvantage is their inability to deactivate bacterial endotoxin, which can be found in the steam distillate.[4] This drawback creates the potential for the toxic material to be deposited on "sterilized" instruments. Bacterial endotoxin (LPS) is a potent initiator of inflammation; very low levels can incite significant inflammation. Fortunately, relatively simple measures of sterilizer maintenance, although not approved by the manufacturers, have proven highly effective at reducing bacterial biofilm, the typical source of endotoxin in short-cycle sterilization systems.

Because TASS is multifactorial, it is often difficult to determine if one or more causes are involved. We have investigated two recent outbreaks in which autoclave contamination appeared to have an important role. Other factors such as the incomplete cleaning of ultrasonic baths[5] and inadequate rinsing of the lumens of reusable cannulas and phaco tips have a greater potential to incite TASS if short-cycle sterilizers are used because of their inability to deactivate endotoxins. ■

This article originally appeared in the July 2006 issue of CRSToday.

1. Kreisler KR, Martin SS, Young CW, et al. Postoperative inflammation following cataract extraction caused by bacterial contamination of the cleaning bath detergent. *J Cataract Refract Surg.* 1992;18:106-110.
2. Mamalis N, Edelhauser HF, Dawson DG, et al. Toxic anterior segment syndrome. Review/update. *J Cataract Refract Surg.* 2006;32:324-333.
3. Holland SP, Mathias RG, Morck DW, et al. Diffuse lamellar keratitis related to endotoxins released from sterilizer reservoir biofilms. *Ophthalmology.* 2000;107:1227-1233.
4. Whitby JL, Hitchins VM. Endotoxin levels in steam and reservoirs of table-top steam sterilizers. *J Cataract Refract Surg.* 2002;18:51-52.
5. Richburg FA, Reidy JJ, Apple DJ, Olson RJ. Sterile hypopyon secondary to ultrasonic cleaning solution. *J Cataract Refract Surg.* 1986;12:248-251.
6. Holland SP, Chavez G, Morck D, Mathias R. Toxic anterior segment syndrome (TASS) associated with short cycle sterilization and BSS. Paper presented at: The ASCRS/ASOA Symposium & Congress; March 19, 2006; San Francisco, CA.
7. Nguyen V, Ceri H, Stremick CA, et al. MBEC evaluation of biocides for Burkholderia pickettii isolated from a laser corneal surgery clinic. Abstract presented at: The Biofilms 2000 Meeting of the American Society of Microbiology; July 2000; Big Sky, MT.

CHAPTER 108

TASS and Intraocular Ointment

LILIANA WERNER, MD, PHD

Several studies have identified substances and toxins that cause toxic anterior segment syndrome (TASS) after phacoemulsification and the implantation of IOLs. This article shares a series of cases in which this inflammatory syndrome was associated with the postoperative use of ophthalmic ointment.

A REVIEW OF THE LITERATURE

The penetration of ointments after ocular surgery is a recognized complication. In 1973, Fraunfelder and Hanna[1] published the results of a survey sent to 400 randomly selected ophthalmologists. Of the 327 responses, 65 (20%) reported seeing ointment trapped in 95 anterior chambers after ocular surgery. Twenty-five of these patients had developed glaucoma or uveitis thought to be a result of the ointment.

In 1999, Garzozi et al[2] described a patient treated with ophthalmic ointment after RK who later presented with a bubble floating in his anterior chamber. They observed anterior uveitis and elevated IOP in this eye during the early postoperative period as well as at 41 and 61 months after the procedure.

In another case, Aralikatti et al[3] observed a white substance in the anterior segment of a patient's eye 1 day after he underwent phacoemulsification through an oblique, self-sealing, clear corneal incision. The researchers assumed the substance they saw overlying the patient's pupil was ointment that had entered the anterior chamber and adhered to the newly implanted IOL. More recently, Riedl et al[4] described ointment entering the anterior chamber after cataract surgery through a temporal corneal incision. In this case, the patient was noted to have vitreous and "pieces of cortex" in the anterior chamber 5 weeks after surgery, followed by inflammation and elevated IOP.

The aforementioned cases demonstrate that the penetration of ointment into the anterior chamber may cause toxic complications, a finding confirmed in an experimental study by Scheie et al.[5] When the investigators injected bases of common ophthalmic ointment into the anterior chambers of rabbits' eyes, they found that the amount of ointment instilled was a major predictor of the severity of the eye's intraocular reaction.

TASS OUTBREAK

Recently, my colleagues and I[6] analyzed eight cases of TASS that were associated with an oily substance in the anterior chambers of patients treated at the Department of Eye Medicine and Surgery of Hamilton Health Sciences in Hamilton, Ontario, Canada. The substance was later identified as an ointment instilled in the patients' eyes after uneventful phacoemulsification.

A single surgeon had implanted the same three-piece silicone IOL into the eyes of all patients through clear corneal incisions. The procedures took place between May and October 2003.

Solutions and agents used during the procedure included BSS (Alcon Laboratories, Inc., Fort Worth, TX), epinephrine, pilocarpine hydrochloride, Amvisc Plus (Bausch & Lomb, Rochester, NY), and vancomycin. Postoperative medications included combination gentamicin/betamethasone ophthalmic ointment (Garasone; Schering-Plough, Kenilworth, NJ) and pilocarpine gel. After he applied the ointment, the surgeon attached tight patches to each eye at the end of the procedures.

DETECTION AND TREATMENT

On the first postoperative day, four patients presented with diffuse corneal edema and elevated IOP. Upon examination, the surgeon observed a filmy coating on the corneal epithelium of the eyes within the anterior chambers (Figure 1A). The same material was observed in another eye's anterior chamber, but this patient did not develop corneal edema until the second postoperative week. The three remaining patients developed an oily bubble floating inside their anterior chambers (Figure 1B). The bubble was later found to be ointment coating the IOL.

Most of the affected patients needed more than one additional surgical procedure to resolve the complications resulting from TASS. These operations included penetrating keratoplasty, IOL explantation and exchange, aspiration of the oily bubble and polishing of the IOL, vitrectomy and washout of the anterior chamber, trabeculectomy for uncontrolled IOP, and Nd:YAG laser to remove the ointment from the IOL's surface. Table 1 lists the procedures performed on individual patients.

LABORATORY ANALYSIS

To rule out reusable ophthalmic instruments and other factors as the source of the contaminants that caused TASS in the patients from Hamilton Health Sciences, my colleagues and I analyzed the substance retrieved from the surface of six explanted IOLs. Gross examination and light microscopy of two IOLs confirmed there was an oily residue over large areas of the lens' optical surfaces (Figure 2).

Gas chromatography-mass spectrometry (GC-MS) of the remaining four explanted IOLs revealed that the implants' surfaces were covered with a mixed-chain hydrocarbon that was consistent with the topical antibiotic/steroid ointment that was applied to the eyes after surgery.

Under the same experimental conditions, we performed GC-MS on the silicone sleeves used to protect the phaco tips during the autoclaving process as well as on the lidocaine and pilocarpine gel used during or after cataract surgery. The substance did not match the material that we retrieved from the explanted IOLs. We concluded that the ointment applied after cataract surgery was the most likely cause of TASS in these cases.

CLEAR CORNEAL INCISIONS

The mechanism by which ophthalmic ointment entered the anterior chambers of the eight patients reviewed in our study may be related to how the surgeon bandaged their eyes after cataract surgery.

Experimental studies with cadaveric eyes demonstrated that the self-sealing properties of unsutured clear corneal wounds can be compromised by variations in IOP or the application of external pressure.[7] When IOP measurements were low, the edges of the corneal wound tended to gape. In a retrospective study, Shingleton et al[8] found that a significant percentage of eyes that underwent clear corneal phacoemulsification had an IOP of 5 mm Hg or lower 30 minutes after surgery. By patching the patients' eyes tightly after cataract surgery, the surgeon at Hamilton Health Sciences may have created a gaping wound through which the ointment gained access to the anterior chamber. Other postoperative factors, including changes in IOP as well as manipulation of the eye by blinking or rubbing, have also been implicated as compromisers of the clear corneal wound's integrity.

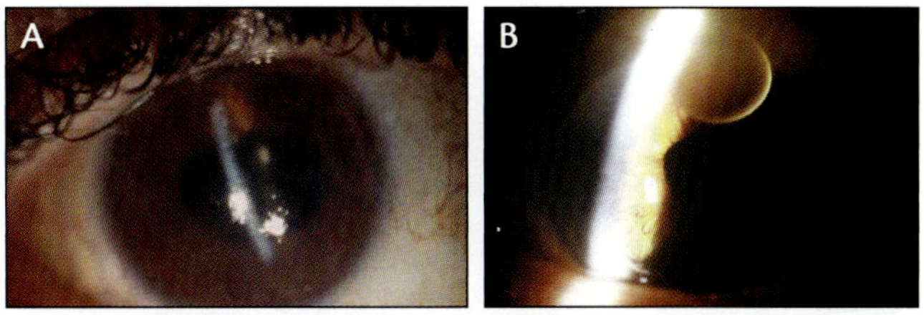

Figure 1. Pictured are slit-lamp clinical photographs taken during the first postoperative week from two of the eight TASS cases. The oily material coated the corneal endothelium and caused edema (A). The material can be seen as a large bubble floating in the anterior chamber (B). (Reprinted with permission from Werner L, Sher JH, Taylor JR, et al. Toxic anterior segment syndrome and possible association with ointment in the anterior chamber following cataract surgery. *J Cataract Refract Surg.* 2006;32:227-235.)

DELAYED ONSET OF TASS

Typically, TASS appears approximately 24 hours after surgery, but my colleagues and I recently analyzed a case in which a patient developed problems related to intraocular ointment much later in the postoperative period.[9] Eight months after uneventful, bilateral phacoemulsification followed by the implantation of three-piece silicone IOLs, the patient developed recurrent anterior chamber inflammation. At first, the physician suspected the patient's IOLs were unstable and performed two lens positioning procedures 11 and 13 months after the IOLs' initial implantation. Eighteen months after cataract removal (5 months after the last surgical procedure), the patient presented with a greasy film on his IOL. His doctor initiated anti-inflammatory and antibiotic treatment, but the patient's clinical outcome did not improve.

Twenty-seven months after the IOLs' initial implantation, the patient's silicone lenses were replaced with new lenses made of a hydrophilic acrylic material. GC-MS analysis of the explanted lens detected compounds that matched one of the ointments with which the patient was treated postoperatively.

Chen et al[10] reported similar findings in a case where they observed an oily material in a patient's anterior chamber 34 months after cataract surgery. Fourier transform infrared and confocal Raman microspectroscopy identified this material as ointment.

TABLE 1. INTRAOCULAR OINTMENT AFTER CATARACT SURGERY

Patients	Clinical Signs		Additional Surgical Procedures					
	Film in Anterior Chamber	Oily Bubble in Anterior Chamber	Penetrating Keratoplasty	IOL Explantation/ Exchange	Aspiration/ IOL Polishing	Vitrectomy/ Anterior Chamber Washout	Trabeculectomy	Nd:YAG on Intraocular Ointment
1	X		X	X				
2		X		X				
3	X		X	X		X		
4	X			X				X
5		X			X			
6	X		X	X				
7	X		X	X		X	X	
8		X			X			

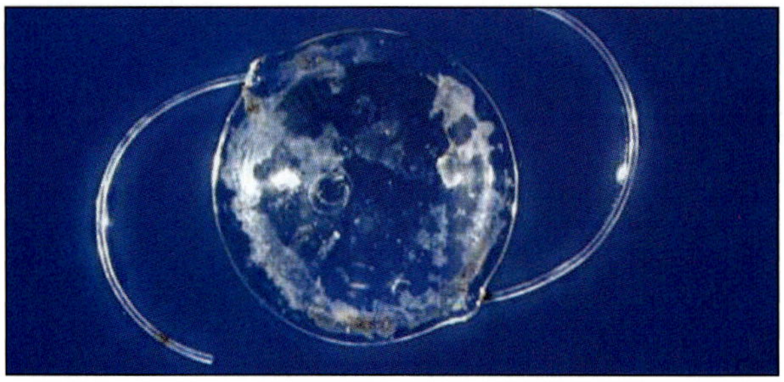

Figure 2. When this IOL was explanted from one of the patients with TASS, large areas of the lens' anterior and posterior surfaces were coated with an oily material.

CONCLUSION

To prevent topical ointments from entering the anterior chamber and causing TASS after cataract surgery, surgeons should be aware of the dynamics of self-sealing clear corneal incisions as well as of the associated risks of using postoperative ointments and eye patches. They also should anticipate the possibility of intraocular penetration when using any kind of ointment after other penetrating procedures.

Another potential cause of TASS is the introduction of oily materials into the eye by devices or equipment during cataract surgery. Any kind of lubricating material used during the sterilization of instruments, cannulas, or phaco tips should be considered a potential source of contamination, although this did not appear to contribute to the eight cases at Hamilton Health Sciences. Regardless, the surgeons at that facility did not see additional cases of TASS after replacing the ointment with topical drops after cataract surgery. ■

This article originally appeared in the July 2006 issue of CRSToday.

1. Fraunfelder FT, Hanna C. Ophthalmic ointment. *Trans Am Acad Ophthalmol Otolaryngol.* 1973;77:467-475.
2. Garzozi HJ, Muallem M, Harris A. Recurrent anterior uveitis and glaucoma associated with inadvertent entry of ointment into the anterior chamber after radial keratotomy. *J Cataract Refract Surg.* 1999;25:1685-1687.
3. Aralikatti AK, Needham AD, Lee MW, Prasad S. Entry of antibiotic ointment into the anterior chamber after uneventful phacoemulsification. *J Cataract Refract Surg.* 2003;29:595-597.
4. Reidl M, Maca S, Amon M, et al. Intraocular ointment after small-incision cataract surgery causing chronic uveitis and secondary glaucoma. *J Cataract Refract Surg.* 2003;29:1022-1025.
5. Scheie HG, Rubenstein RA, Katowitz JA. Ophthalmic ointment bases in the anterior chamber; clinical and experimental observations. *Arch Ophthalmol.* 1965;73:36-42.
6. Werner L, Sher JH, Taylor JR, et al. Toxic anterior segment syndrome and possible association with ointment in the anterior chamber following cataract surgery. *J Cataract Refract Surg.* 2006;32:227-235.
7. Sarayba MA, Taban M, Ignacio TS, et al. Inflow of ocular surface fluid through clear corneal cataract incisions: a laboratory model. *Am J Ophthalmol.* 2004;138:206-210.
8. Shingleton BJ, Wadhwani RA, O'Donoghue MW, et al. Evaluation of intraocular pressure in the immediate period after phacoemulsification. *J Cataract Refract Surg.* 2001;27:524-527.
9. Chew JJ, Werner L, Mackman G, Mamalis N. Late opacification of a silicone intraocular lens caused by ophthalmic ointment. *J Cataract Refract Surg.* 2006;32:341-346.
10. Chen KH, Lin SY, Li MJ, Cheng WT. Retained antibiotic ophthalmic ointment on an intraocular lens 34 months after sutureless cataract surgery. *Am J Ophthalmol.* 2005;139:743-745.

CHAPTER 109

IOLs and TASS

LUTHER L. FRY, MD

A small amount of postoperative inflammation is always associated with cataract surgery. Toxic anterior segment syndrome (TASS) represents an inordinate amount of inflammation, usually with hypopyon. The complication was called *sterile endophthalmitis* and *sterile hypopyon*[1-4] before being more appropriately named *TASS* by Monson et al[5] in 1992. Lens-induced TASS has likely occurred since Harold Ridley implanted the first IOLs in 1949, but only in the past 15 years has the problem been well recognized as a toxic syndrome.

DIFFERENTIAL DIAGNOSIS

It is difficult to distinguish TASS from infectious endophthalmitis, but the distinction is important, because the treatment of each complication is so different. Several clinical findings help to separate the two. The onset of TASS is generally earlier, 1 versus 4 to 7 days. With TASS, the vitreous is usually clear, and the heavy administration of topical steroids yields improvement. If performed, a vitreous tap and culture show no organisms in TASS. A confounder, unfortunately, is that the results of Gram staining and culturing may also not be positive with infectious endophthalmitis, depending on the care taken and method used.

A variant of TASS involves severe endothelial damage with limbus-to-limbus edema. This problem is usually not induced by the IOL but by a toxin such as detergent or sterile water that has entered the anterior chamber. Mamalis et al[6] published a review of TASS that is an excellent resource for ophthalmologists.

If the clinical appearance of the eye and the characteristics of the infection are suspicious for TASS rather than an infectious etiology, it seems reasonable to dose the patient heavily with topical steroids for 8 to12 hours and then reevaluate the eye before proceeding to vitrectomy and intraocular antibiotics.

ANECDOTAL CASES

The 1970s

Early uveitis-glaucoma-hyphema (UGH) syndrome with poorly manufactured ACIOLs was not strictly TASS, but the problem plagued ophthalmologists in the 1970s. The original Choyce Mark VIII anterior chamber lens (Rayner Intraocular Lenses Ltd., East Sussex, UK) was never associated with UGH syndrome. Unfortunately, the company's production capacity was limited and the lens in short supply. US manufacturers began to produce copies of the lens, but they were poorly made with rough edges. Also, the IOLs were injection molded rather than lathe cut. The injection-molded PMMA tended to warp over time in the eye. This warpage and the lens' rough edges led to iris chafing and UGH syndrome. Fortunately, the Choyce VIII lenses were easily exchanged. Closed-loop lenses were more difficult to remove and frequently required surgeons to cut the loops and leave portions in the angle.

When used with intracapsular surgery, metal looped, Binkhorst-style lenses were too heavy and caused fraying of the iris sphincter, UGH syndrome, and dislocation or subluxation of the IOL.

The initial Binkhorst and Worst Medallion IOLs (both manufactured by Dutch Medical Workshop) came in a glass tube filled with NaOH solution. The other side of the tube was filled with a neutralizing solution. After neutralizing the lenses, ophthalmologists washed them with 2L of normal saline solution to eliminate residual NaOH. Although I had no related complications, there were reports of severe damage to the anterior segment in cases where the NaOH was not fully neutralized and removed.

Interestingly, the lenses stored in this solution had a reputation for the least postoperative inflammation. The reason was probably that the NaOH dissolved and washed off residual contaminants, particularly polishing compound.

Morcher GmbH (Stuttgart, Germany) had a problem with TASS involving gamma-radiation–sterilized IOLs around 1970. Its exact cause was not determined.

Orcolon

The IOP is frequently high with TASS, due either to a clogging of the trabecular meshwork or a direct, toxic effect. One unusual variant occurred with Orcolon (polyacrylamide gel; Optical Radiation Corporation) around 1991.[7-9] This viscoelastic performed well in clinical trials. After its FDA approval, however, there were a number of cases in which the eye, after doing well initially, suddenly developed an IOP in the 50s along with pain but little inflammation. The increased pressure was minimally affected by aqueous suppressants and responded only to paracentesis and filtering surgery. It was as if the trabecular meshwork suddenly and totally shut down 1 week after surgery.

In my first case of a shutdown trabecular meshwork, I had no idea what had happened. I made some calls, and Randy Craven, MD, a glaucoma specialist in Denver, advised me of the Orcolon disaster. At that time, Optical Radiation Corporation had a particularly aggressive and effective sales representative covering the Denver area, and a number of the doctors there were using both Orcolon and the Memorylens (CIBA Vision, Duluth, GA). In retrospect, it was a terrible combination. As one of the few glaucoma specialists in Denver at that time, Dr. Craven rapidly accumulated a lot of experience with Orcolon-associated glaucoma.

Only a few eyes in which Orcolon was used developed this form of glaucoma. At that time, the pre-rolled Memorylens had just been approved. With the initial lenses, I waited for the IOL to unroll partially, which took a few minutes, and then aspirated the viscoelastic. Those eyes are the ones that developed the glaucoma. Apparently, the prolonged contact time with the viscoelastic allowed it to penetrate the trabecular meshwork and cause the problem.

It was a mystery why the complication was never encountered in the clinical trials. It turned out that, when Orcolon's production went from small to large lots, the glass bottles in which it was made were rinsed and autoclaved after each batch. Residual Orcolon on the glass containers' walls was polymerized by the autoclaving, and then microscopic particles flaked into the next batch. They were invisible to conventional microscopy and only observable by phase contrast microscopy. These particles apparently embedded in the trabecular meshwork and set off some type of inflammatory reaction that culminated in a complete shutdown of the meshwork. After the reaction was understood, ophthalmologists could see small, inflammatory precipitates on the surface of the trabecular meshwork by careful gonioscopy. Early, heavy dosing of topical steroids could rescue eyes developing Orcolon-related glaucoma.

Unfortunately, the rash of subsequent lawsuits derailed a full investigation of the problem's etiology, and few reported the condition in the literature. A useful animal model of glaucoma might have been found.

The Memorylens

My personal experience is fortunately fairly limited, but I think it might be instructive to share some of it. In 1999, a small number of eyes in which I had implanted a Memorylens developed what appeared to be infectious endophthalmitis postoperatively.[10] The first few I referred for vitrectomy and intraocular antibiotics. All did well, and none had any identifiable organism. I thought the results were due to inadequate culturing and Gram staining techniques by the vitreoretinal surgeons. After hearing about cases of sterile postoperative inflammation across the country, I realized that TASS was likely the culprit. A couple of cases thereafter were successfully treated with heavily dosed topical steroids alone. An investigation by CIBA Vision identified residual polishing compound as the apparent problem.

CONCLUSION

Although IOL-related TASS still occurs, it is fortunately increasingly rare. Manufacturers' awareness of the importance of removing polishing and cleaning compounds from the IOLs has vastly reduced the problem. Most cases now appear to derive from endotoxins in sterilizers' reservoirs, detergent in instruments' lumens, and other local issues. Vigilance continues to be necessary. ■

This article originally appeared in the July 2006 issue of CRSToday.

1. Meltzer DW. Sterile hypopyon following intraocular lens surgery. *Arch Ophthalmol.* 1980;98:100-104.
2. Richburg FA, Reidy JJ, Apple DJ, Olson RJ. Sterile hypopyon secondary to ultrasonic cleaning solution. *J Cataract Refract Surg.* 1986;12:248-251.
3. Kim JH. Intraocular inflammation of denatured viscoelastic substance in cases of cataract extraction and lens implantation. *J Cataract Refract Surg.* 1987;13:536-542.
4. Nelson DB, Donnenfeld ED, Perry HD. Sterile endophthalmitis after sutureless cataract surgery. *Ophthalmology.* 1992;99:1655-1657.
5. Monson MC, Mamalis N, Olson RJ. Toxic anterior segment inflammation following cataract surgery. *J Cataract Refract Surg.* 1992;18:184-189.
6. Mamalis N, Edelhauser HF, Dawson DG, et al. Toxic anterior segment syndrome. *J Cataract Refract Surg.* 2006;32:324-333.
7. Siegel MJ, Spiro JA, Miller JA, et al. Secondary glaucoma and uveitis associated with Orcolon. *Arch Ophthalmol.* 1991;109:1496-1498.
8. Herrington RG, Ball SF, Updegraff SA. Delayed sustained increase in intraocular pressure secondary to the use of polyacrylamide gel (Orcolon) in the anterior chamber. *Ophthalmic Surg.* 1993;24:658-662.
9. *Wall Street Journal.* May 27, 1992; B7.
10. Jehan FS, Mamalis N, Spencer TS, et al. Postoperative sterile endophthalmitis (TASS) associated with the MemoryLens. *J Cataract Refract Surg.* 2000;26:1773-1777.

CHAPTER 110

Balanced Salt Solution and TASS

STANLEY J. BERKE, MD; ROBERT B. NELSON, PA-C; AND LILLIAN ROTH PONTACOLONE, RN, CNOR

This article recounts our experience concerning the 2005 nationwide outbreak of toxic anterior segment syndrome (TASS) related to Endosol balanced salt solution (manufactured by Cytosol Ophthalmics, Lenoir, NC; distributed by Advanced Medical Optic, Inc., Santa Ana, CA). As part of this outbreak, we discovered our first nine cases of TASS on September 22, 2005. One surgeon in our center urgently reported these cases on the first postoperative day. He described a significant reaction in the anterior chamber in seven patients and fibrin in two patients. All nine patients were referred to a retina specialist, who performed a vitreous tap with intravitreal antibiotics in the two severe cases (fibrin) and suggested medical treatment and close monitoring for the other seven milder cases (significant anterior chamber reaction).

ACCOUNTING FOR PATIENTS' OUTBREAKS

The trending and tracking of patient information on our endophthalmitis investigation form began immediately after the discovery of our first cases of TASS. We also initiated a top-down staff review of all aseptic techniques, terminal cleaning of the ORs, and instrument processing protocols. Sterilization logs and spore tests for these specific cases were the first for us to review, and all were normal.

No common denominator was initially identified as the cause of the TASS outbreak. However, there was an onset of symptoms of TASS within 12 to 18 hours after surgery. We took more than 50 environmental cultures of our surgery center. Walls, machines, tables, mayo stands, air vents, etc, were all cultured and showed no growth. We began spore testing every instrument load that went into the autoclaves, and, again, all were normal. We did a top-down terminal cleanup of each OR and changed the cleaning solution. We scrupulously examined our course of cleaning and processing the instruments and made changes along the way. We thought that the problem might be related to an enzymatic cleaner used to decontaminate the instruments, but, after switching the agent, TASS cases still emerged. Next, we began to document the specific lot numbers of any product that went into an eye or onto its surface, including viscoelastics, medications, solutions, and lenses.

For 6 weeks, we continued to see isolated cases. In total, we discovered 37 occurrences out of 1,100 patients from September 22 to October 31, 2005. During that time, we initiated our own comprehensive internal investigation, through which we studied each reported case by looking for common threads and tracking the results on a spreadsheet.

IDENTIFYING THE CULPRIT

When we could identify no definitive cause, we contacted Nick Mamalis, MD, at the John A. Moran Eye Center in Salt Lake City. Dr. Mamalis received a grant from the ASCRS to study TASS outbreaks as well as endophthalmitis. At that time, we had 25 to 30 cases on our spreadsheet. We shared our findings with his team. At about the same time, we began to suspect that the balanced salt solution might be involved. Advanced Medical Optics, Inc., supplied 95% of our balanced salt solution. At first, we felt the solution was an unlikely cause, because the cases were sporadic. When we finally contacted the company by e-mail to ask if they had any reports of similar cases, we got a response from the corporate offices within 10 minutes. Executives from Advanced Medical Optics, Inc., disclosed that they were getting reports from other sites nationwide. They acknowledged probably 10 sites at that time with some 200 cases. Per its standard protocol, Advanced Medical Optics, Inc., immediately began coordinating with Cytosol, which conducted tests of samples received from suspected lots. After Cytosol's study results indicated no evidence of toxins, Advanced Medical Optics, Inc., began working with independent laboratories to define the breadth of the outbreak.

CASES OF TASS NATIONWIDE

The matter was discussed at our quarterly quality assurance meeting. Dr. Berke, Quality Assurance Chairperson, and David Nelson, MD, Medical Director, were actively involved. Dr. Berke posted a question on the American Glaucoma Society's and ASCRS' Web sites, and Mr. Nelson posted a similar question on our New York State ASC Society Web site. Soon enough, we began to hear of many more TASS cases and locations nationwide. We stayed in touch with Advanced Medical Optics, Inc., and introduced Dr. Mamalis to the company's clinical team that was investigating this outbreak. He then guided the company through the rest of the investigative process.

On November 1, 2005, we removed all of Cytosol's balanced salt solution from our shelves and switched to one manufactured by Baxter Healthcare Corporation (Vancouver, Canada). Advanced Medical Optics, Inc., also stopped shipping Endosol balanced salt solution and issued a safety alert on November 10 to eye surgeons and ORs nationally as well as to member lists at the AAO and ASCRS with a warning not to use the solution due to the TASS outbreak. On November 18, Advanced Medical Optics, Inc., issued a voluntary market withdrawal of all of its Endosol manufactured by Cytosol. We have had no cases of TASS reported since.

Following extensive testing and inspection of its manufacturing operations by the FDA, Cytosol initiated a recall on February 15, 2006, of all balanced salt solution manufactured at its Braintree, Massachusetts, facility.

The incidences we had of TASS responded well to high doses of steroids, and the patients have for the most part recovered well. Some of the more severely affected individuals have permanent visual and ocular problems. In the end, we understand that Advanced Medical Optics, Inc., identified approximately 25 sites and more than 500 cases of TASS related to the Endosol balanced salt solution manufactured by Cytosol.

FURTHER INVESTIGATION

During the time of the outbreak and since, we have remained in contact with Dr. Mamalis. Dr. Berke has received many reports of TASS from colleagues via the American Glaucoma Society's and ASCRS' chat rooms. We have fully cooperated with Cytosol/Advanced Medical Optics, Inc., by sharing our data and sending representative samples of the involved agent for the companies' testing.

In early December 2005, Preeta Kutty, MD, of the Centers for Disease Control and Prevention (CDC) in Atlanta contacted us. Dr. Kutty revealed that the CDC was actively involved in investigating this national outbreak of TASS. We sent the CDC samples of the balanced salt solution from Advanced Medical Optics, Inc., for analysis, have shared our case data with them, and have cooperated fully with their investigation.

When seven of the bottles involved in TASS cases at our ambulatory surgery unit were tested by the CDC for endotoxins, only one came back as positive with a level of 1.085 EU/mL (EU = endotoxin units, a measurement for endotoxin activity). The other six samples tested negative with endotoxin levels of less than 0.195 EU/mL.

FDA REGULATIONS

According to the FDA, water and sterile water for injection or irrigation have an allowable endotoxin limit of 0.25 EU/mL. However, bacteriostatic water for injection and sterile water for inhalation have been given a slightly higher bacterial endotoxin limit of 0.50 EU/mL.[1]

The endotoxin limits are defined by the route of administration, the dose or amount of product delivered, and the threshold pyrogenic response (5 EU/kg of body weight/hr).[1]

Unfortunately, there are no standards specifically for balanced salt solution or any other ocular irrigating solutions. We feel strongly that all ophthalmic surgical solutions should be completely free of endotoxins and that getting this standard revised immediately by the FDA should be a major objective of both the AAO and the ASCRS.

EMOTIONAL PERSPECTIVES

Dealing with an outbreak of TASS (or endophthalmitis) is an emotional time for surgeons, managers, and staff members at a surgicenter or hospital OR. There can be a sense of isolation and uncertainty as well as grave concern for patients' safety. Without the knowledge that an outbreak is widespread, identifying and eliminating the cause of TASS is a lonely struggle. Managers in particular face a debate over closing the facility with the associated loss of revenue, the dilution of confidence by attending surgeons, and the damage to the center's reputation in the local healthcare community after a cluster of cases. Those ramifications are difficult to measure.

The entire staff at our surgicenter worked as a fine-tuned machine to find the cause of TASS. It was incredible (and most rewarding) that we had implemented every change that Dr. Mamalis had recommended prior to receiving his advice. We are especially proud of how professionally the management team performed during a difficult time. The effort that went into identifying the cases and gathering the relevant data was extraordinary. Our attending staff members were notified of the problem and willingly reported their cases, thus allowing us the opportunity to see the trend develop. There is an impulse to downplay complications for fear of the potentially negative impact on the institution, but the emphasis should be on quality patient care. We are confident that this dilemma is now behind us, and we will continue to work with Dr. Mamalis and the CDC in supplying them with any and all additional information about our experiences with TASS. ■

This article originally appeared in the July 2006 issue of CRSToday.

1. ITG subject: bacterial endotoxins/pyrons. Department of Health, Education, and Welfare Public Service; Food and Drug Administration. March 20, 1985; No. 40. Available at http://www.fda.gov/ora/inspect_ref/itg/itg40.html. Accessed May 31, 2006.

CHAPTER 111

When TASS Strikes: A Nurse's Perspective

SUSAN CLOUSER, RN, MSN, CRNO

Toxic anterior segment syndrome (TASS) is a postoperative inflammation of the anterior chamber that is caused by a toxic substance's entering the eye during anterior segment surgery. The conditions in the OR are therefore suspect. For that reason, there may be no more ominous words from an ophthalmic surgeon to a surgery center's administrator or director of nursing than "My patients have TASS. What are you going to do about it?" Finding the cause of the problem can be a nerve-wracking and exhausting process.

A surgeon's report of TASS merits serious attention. Many times, the cases will be isolated, or they will occur in clusters with significant amounts of time between the groupings. There is a resultant tendency to put the investigation on a back burner as the pressures of everyday operation continue. Although an outbreak of TASS cannot be allowed to paralyze a surgery center, its source must be identified, or the problem is certain to recur. An incidence of TASS at a surgery center requires communication, education, investigation, and an initiation of change.

COMMUNICATION

When confronted by a case of TASS, it is a natural impulse to want to keep the bad news quiet. It is important, however, for the ophthalmologist to share the information with the medical director and other surgeons who use the ORs. Doing so may yield additional information for the investigation. Surgeons have often seen mild cases of TASS without recognizing them, and those cases therefore go unreported. Knowing that another surgeon in the facility has encountered a problem with TASS may cause them to remember instances of postoperative inflammation experienced by their own patients. This information may rule out some etiologies and thus narrow the list of possible causes.

It is also wise to alert the surgery center's staff to the situation. Not only will these individuals be able to participate in problem solving, but they will also understand why the ophthalmologist may be more anxious during subsequent surgeries until a cause has been identified and eliminated.

EDUCATION

OR Staff

Part of communicating with the surgery center's staff involves education. Without an understanding of the etiologies and consequences of TASS, the members of the surgical team cannot be effective problem solvers.

The first step is to prepare an in-service meeting for the surgery center's staff that provides a description of TASS and an example of how it differs from endophthalmitis. The discussion should emphasize that the outbreak is an issue of toxicity, not sterility. Once they understand the nature of TASS, staff members' awareness will be heightened for potential causes.

It is important to create an environment of inquiry and investigation, not of culpability and blame. The OR staff involved in the cases already feels guilty. It is important to make staff members understand that TASS is not the fault of someone but of something.

Surgeons

It may be necessary to educate other ophthalmic surgeons working in the facility who are not familiar with TASS to prevent them from panicking and taking their surgery elsewhere. They need reassurance that the situation is under serious investigation. Doctors familiar with TASS and its treatment can offer advice on managing patients, should that be required.

INVESTIGATION

A Task Force

The next step is to form a task force that includes the surgery center's administrator, director of nursing, medical director, and instrument technician as well as the surgeon and OR staff who were involved in the cases. Someone knowledgeable about the workings of the OR should lead the investigation and be given a free hand.

The first areas to investigate are those known to be common causes of TASS. They include the cleaning and sterilization of instruments, medications, and particulates.

Instruments

Of all the potential causes of TASS, the majority of cases involve the cleaning, processing, and sterilization of instruments. Policies and procedures should be established for each of these areas. The policy will state the chief standards, and the procedure will enumerate the steps for achieving these standards.

Manual cleaning is required for delicate ophthalmic microsurgical instruments. A soft bristle brush should be used to remove blood, tissue, and other residues such as viscoelastic from the instruments. If a detergent is used, it should be of neutral pH, and the instruments should undergo copious irrigation with deionized, distilled, or sterile water to ensure no residue remains that can later be introduced into an eye. These precautions are most important with cannulated items such as the phaco and I/A handpieces. The staff should use a compressed-air or medical-grade nitrogen flush to remove the remaining water. The difficulty in cleaning instruments with a fine bore such as cannulas precludes their reuse.

A procedure for cleaning instruments should address whether or not instruments should be put in a washer/sterilizer or ultrasonic cleaner; if used, the types of water, detergent, and cleaners; and the necessity of mechanical hand washing. Whoever writes the standard procedure for cleaning instruments should consult the manufacturers' guidelines for the instruments' care. A documented, standardized method for cleaning ophthalmic instruments that is adopted and used by all personnel greatly decreases the likelihood of TASS. It is important to ensure that all employees involved in the cleaning of instruments, particularly new staff, are properly oriented and that there are frequent procedural reviews.

Medications

Another common source of TASS is perioperative medications. A large number of cataract surgeons use topical anesthesia, which may be a misnomer, because this type of anesthesia frequently includes intracameral lidocaine. Topical anesthesia often begins with the instillation of proparacaine or tetracaine drops followed by the off-label use of lidocaine gel. Multidose bottles of topical anesthetic, whether in liquid or viscous form, contain a preservative such as benzalkonium chloride, and some lidocaine gels have preservatives as well. Irrigating these substances completely from the eye before the start of the procedure is imperative, or they may enter the anterior chamber on an instrument.

Intraocular medications (eg, anesthetics, epinephrine, or miotics) placed directly in the anterior chamber and those injected into a 500-mL bottle of balanced salt solution (eg, epinephrine 1:1000 or antibiotics) must also be free of preservatives. The medical director should work with the pharmacist and drug supplier to ensure that any substitutions due to back orders or discontinued items meet the center's preservative-free criterion.

Viscoelastics in their original form pose no threat to the eye. If these materials remain on instruments after surgery, however, they can combine with detergents and enzymatic cleaners or become denatured in the sterilization process and lead to TASS. As mentioned earlier, appropriate cleaning removes viscoelastics from the instruments.

Particulates

Particulate matter most commonly comes from the powder on surgical gloves and fibers from items in the pack such as towels and gowns. The use of powder-free gloves by all personnel eliminates the talc, and switching to low-linting draping material and gowns minimizes airborne particulate matter.

INITIATION OF CHANGE

Eliminating the common causes of TASS from the facility may eradicate TASS. If cases still occur, the task force should re-examine the center's procedures and look for other less familiar etiologies such as endotoxin contamination or water-supply variances. Whichever cause seems more likely should be eliminated to see if it is the culprit. It is important to avoid the shotgun approach (eg, changing multiple things simultaneously). Although the TASS outbreak may stop, its cause will remain unknown. Moreover, changes made without supporting data can increase the staff's workload and/or the facility's costs unnecessarily.

CONCLUSION

TASS has numerous possible causes, each of which must be investigated and eliminated from the ORs. Once the surgery center is again free of TASS, the surgeons and staff should remain vigilant for new potential causes and stop the problem before it starts. ■

This article originally appeared in the July 2006 issue of CRSToday.

CHAPTER 112

Avoiding Complications With Intraocular Medications

JAMES P. GILLS, MD

The delivery, type, and level of medications for cataract surgery continually evolve to meet the changing requirements of surgical technique. Ophthalmologists now intracamerally inject lidocaine to reduce patients' pain and discomfort during surgery, prophylactic antibiotics to prevent endophthalmitis, NSAIDs for mydriasis, and, more recently, triamcinolone acetonide to control postoperative inflammation. The proper combinations of drugs and dosage levels are critical for avoiding cystoid macular edema (CME), endophthalmitis, and corneal clouding.

LIDOCAINE

Although cataract surgeons now commonly use topical anesthesia, it does not eliminate all sensation of pressure or discomfort in every patient. My colleagues and I intracamerally inject unpreserved lidocaine to minimize the sensations that often accompany surgical maneuvers that manipulate the iris root and can cause the patient anxiety and discomfort.[1]

In rare instances, we have found that the intracameral injection of lidocaine can result in transient visual loss, as would occur during a retrobulbar block.[2] In the four cases in which we observed this phenomenon, the posterior capsule was not intact, which possibly allowed the lidocaine to migrate posteriorly into the vitreous. Visual recovery was complete within hours, and there was no retinal damage. Nevertheless, surgeons should thoroughly investigate any visual loss after topical anesthesia with lidocaine in order to rule out vascular occlusion or any other complication.

ANTIBIOTICS

My colleagues and I have used prophylactic antibiotics to prevent endophthalmitis since 1985.[3] At first, we added the antibiotics to the irrigating solution, but we now include them in the intracameral injection in order to achieve a consistent dose. We add ceftazidime 30 µg and vancomycin 50 µg to the postoperative injection. This regimen provides widespread coverage against endophthalmitis. In high doses, these two antibiotics would interact and precipitate out of the solution, but we have had no problems with the minute concentrations we use.

A study by Axer-Siegel et al[4] suggested that antibiotics in the irrigating solution may increase the occurrence of CME. We have had very low incidences of this complication, whether the antibiotic was delivered in the irrigating solution or by injection. In fact, our incidence of CME is lower than that of the control group cited in the study. Perhaps our low incidence is due to our postoperatively injecting NSAIDs into the anterior chamber and, until recently, postoperative steroids to reduce inflammation. We now use triamcinolone acetonide intracamerally.

TRIAMCINOLONE ACETONIDE

Technique

Investigators have shown that triamcinolone acetonide injected into the vitreous is well tolerated and causes minimal toxicity.[5] Intravitreally injected triamcinolone acetonide is known to enter the anterior chamber[6,7] and even deposit submacularly[8] without adverse effect. My colleagues and I hypothesized that very low doses of the agent injected directly into the anterior chamber, posterior capsule, and vitreous could adequately control inflammation after cataract surgery with few or no complications.

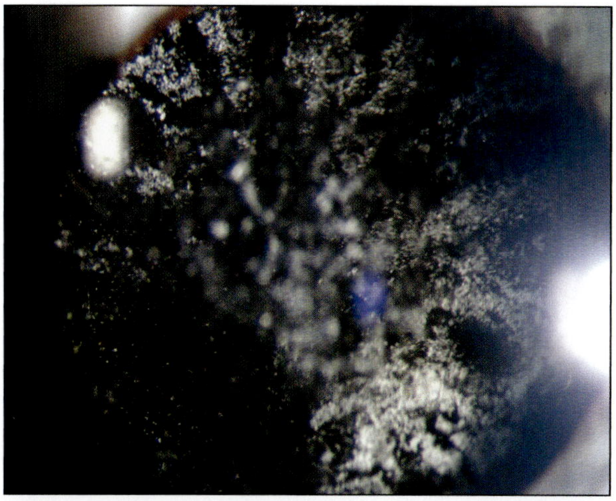

Figure 1. Slit-lamp examination reveals Kenalog in the posterior capsule and vitreous.

Because we already injected antibiotics and anti-inflammatories into the anterior chamber at the end of each case, we added triamcinolone acetonide to our anterior chamber solution. As we did not know the appropriate dosage for controlling inflammation after cataract surgery, we began conservatively with low dosages (0.25 mg) and gradually increased to between 3 and 4 mg for diabetic patients. The solution is injected through a 23-, 25-, or 27-gauge cannula, which is pointed in a posterior direction to facilitate flow through the zonules. Although we place as much of the solution as possible behind the posterior capsule in the vitreous to reduce the amount of medication against the endothelium, some of the solution migrates throughout the anterior chamber. Ideally, dilute triamcinolone acetonide is visible in the anterior chamber, capsular bag, and posterior chamber at the end of the case (Figure 1). After injecting all of the solution, we inject balanced saline soultion to firm the anterior chamber. We ask patients to look upward and sleep on their backs to help disperse the corticosteroid from the anterior chamber to the vitreous.

As we gradually increased the dosage of triamcinolone, fewer eyes required topical steroids postoperatively (from 45% at the lowest dose to only 2% at the 1.8- to 2.1-mg level). None of the eyes that received 2.8 mg or more required additional steroid treatment. Similarly, we saw a decrease in the rate of clinical CME as the dose of triamcinolone acetonide increased. At 1.8 mg or more, CME did not occur.

Concerns

High doses of triamcinolone acetonide on the endothelium will cause cloudiness of the cornea, an increase in corneal thickness, and endothelial cell loss. We have found that a dose of 1.5 mg or less inserted near the zonules, with balanced saline solution injected over the triamcinolone acetonide to fill the chamber and protect the endothelium, will safely eliminate the need for postoperative topical steroids in approximately 95% of cases.

Increased IOP has been noted within the first 3 months of intravitreally injecting triamcinolone acetonide.[9-11] We inject much lower doses of the agent into the anterior chamber and vitreous, and our incidence of IOP spikes has been lower with intracameral administration than postoperative drops. Low doses of the corticosteroid may reduce any trabeculitis that is present and may slightly lower IOP.

There is no uniformity in the way that the agent clears from the eye. Younger patients' eyes clear quickly, whereas older patients, glaucoma patients, and hyperopes retain the medicine for days, sometimes weeks. Thus, we administer a higher dose in long versus short eyes.

Crystals of triamcinolone acetonide spread throughout the eye, iris, wound sites, and capsular bag, and they enter the vitreous. In some cases, the agent may pool in the anterior chamber, where it resembles a hypopyon. Much of the drug may progress through the anterior chamber's different channels of access such as the trabecular meshwork or the iris itself. When we performed gonioscopy on some patients, however, especially early on in those with the pseudohypopyon, the examination revealed triamcinolone acetonide in the trabecular meshwork, largely inferiorly. That we observed so few particles at 1 week suggests either an embodiment of the corticosteroid in the ocular tissues or drainage through the trabecular meshwork or areas of pseudofacility of the aqueous outflow.

Although endophthalmitis has been a concern with intravitreal injections of the drug, we have had no absolute culture-proven incidence of endophthalmitis or other infection in more than 15,000 cases. Because intravitreal injections by retinal surgeons use a higher dosage of the agent and are administered by a different technique, they may cause the sterile endophthalmitis. Our prophylactic use of antibiotics and anti-inflammatories in the intracameral injection solution may help avoid infection.

TOXIC ANTERIOR SEGMENT SYNDROME

Toxic anterior segment syndrome (TASS) occurs when a noninfectious toxic agent enters the anterior segment during surgery and causes an inflammatory response.[12] The many agents identified as possible causes of TASS include contaminated balanced saline solution, injected antibiotics, endotoxins produced by bacteria, and residue on surgical instruments.

Often mistaken for infectious endophthalmitis, TASS has several distinguishing features. Unlike the former complication, TASS has an earlier onset, often the day of surgery or the following day. With TASS, the edema is usually more profound, iris atrophy is significant, and inflammation increases markedly, sometimes with a hypopyon. TASS often produces a fixed, dilated pupil and high IOP (Figure 2).

We experienced a cluster of TASS cases after we began using extra lidocaine 1% for hydrodissection, a practice based on a study by Vargas et al[13] that demonstrated reduced epithelialization on the capsule. We concluded that the lidocaine caused TASS because (1) the complication developed after we began using extra lidocaine, (2) TASS only occurred in patients who received topical anesthesia and intraocular lidocaine, and (3) one case involved the rotation of a toric lens, and lidocaine was the only fluid injected. We now inject 0.5mL of lidocaine 1% after making the cataract incision, and we no longer use additional lidocaine for hydrodissection. We have had no occurrences of TASS since making this change.

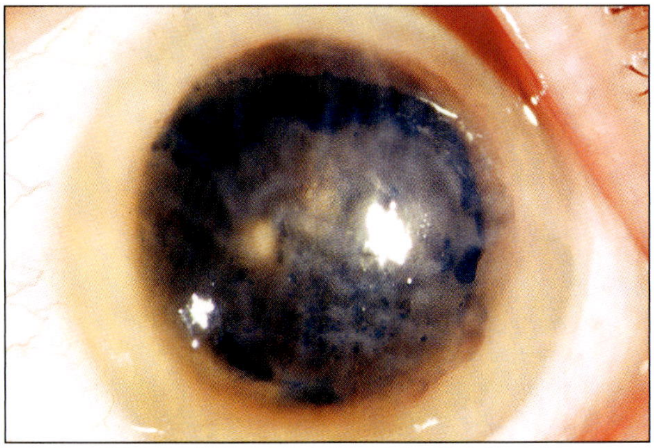

Figure 2. Acute corneal edema occurs after clear lens extraction.

SUMMARY

Although intracameral drugs have decreased the complications of cataract surgery by reducing endophthalmitis and CME, many of these agents can cause serious side effects. The key to avoiding complications is using the right combination of drugs and the lowest doses required for a beneficial effect. Our administration of anti-inflammatory agents reduces the inflammation, while the antibiotics reduce the potential for infection. ■

This article originally appeared in the April 2005 issue of CRSToday.

1. Gills JP, Cherchio M, Raanan MG. The use of intraoperative unpreserved lidocaine to control discomfort during IOL surgery under topical anesthesia. *J Cataract Refract Surg.* 1997;23:527-535.
2. Gills JP, Martin RG, Cherchio M. Topical anesthesia and intraocular lidocaine. In: Gills JP, ed. *Cataract Surgery: The State of the Art.* Thorofare, NJ: Slack, Inc.; 1998: 9-17.
3. Gills JP. Prevention of endophthalmitis by intraocular solution filtration and antibiotics. *J Am Intraocul Implant Soc.* 1985;11:185-186.
4. Axer-Siegel R, Stiebel-Kalish H, Rosenblatt I, et al. Cystoid macular edema after cataract surgery with vancomycin. *Ophthalmology.* 1999;106:1660-1664.
5. McCuen BW 2nd, Bessler M, Tano Y, et al. The lack of toxicity of intravitreally administered triamcinolone acetonide. *Am J Ophthalmol.* 1981;91:785-788.
6. Jonas JB. Concentration of intravitreally injected triamcinolone acetonide in aqueous humour. *Br J Ophthalmol.* 2002;86:1066.
7. Beer PM, Bakri SJ, Singh RJ, et al. Intraocular concentration and pharmacokinetics of triamcinolone acetonide after a single intravitreal injection. *Ophthalmology.* 2003;110:681-686.
8. Enaida H, Sakamoto T, Ueno A, et al. Submacular deposition of triamcinolone acetonide after triamcinolone-assisted vitrectomy. *Am J Ophthalmol.* 2003;135:243-246.
9. Bakri SJ, Beer PM. The effect of intravitreal triamcinolone acetonide on intraocular pressure. *Ophthalmic Surg Lasers Imaging.* 2003;34:386-390.
10. Wingate RJ, Beaumont PE. Intravitreal triamcinolone and elevated intraocular pressure. *Aust N Z J Ophthal.* 1999;27:6:431-434.
11. Jonas JB, Kreissig I, Degenring R: Intraocular pressure after intravitreal injection of triamcinolone acetonide. *Br J Ophthalmol.* 2003;87:24-27.
12. Rongé LJ. Toxic anterior segment syndrome: why sterile isn't clean enough. *EyeNet.* 2002 November/December. Available at: http://www.aao.org/aao/news/eyenet/cataract/cataract_nov.htm. Accessed March 10, 2005.
13. Vargas LG, Escobar-Gomez M, Apple DJ, et al. Pharmacologic prevention of posterior capsule opacification: in vitro effects of preservative-free lidocaine 1% on lens epithelial cells. *J Cataract Refract Surg.* 2004;29:1585-1592.

CHAPTER 113

Managing Retained Lens Fragments

JUDY E. KIM, MD, AND DENNIS P. HAN, MD

The posterior dislocation of lens fragments is an infrequent but well-known complication of cataract surgery.[1-5] Its incidence (reported at between 0.3% to 1.0%)[5,6] is higher with phacoemulsification than with extracapsular cataract surgery. The complication can be stressful to the surgeon, and it may result in significant inconvenience to and prolonged recovery for the patient. Additional surgery such as pars plana vitrectomy is frequently necessary. Retained lens fragments may lead to sight-threatening problems such as chronic uveitis, corneal edema, cystoid macular edema, increased IOP, and retinal detachment. Appropriate management, however, can minimize secondary complications and achieve a good visual prognosis in a majority of patients.

RISK FACTORS

The risk factors for dislocated lenticular material include the presence of a hard nucleus, a miotic pupil with difficult visualization, weakened zonules (due to pseudoexfoliation, Marfan's syndrome, or previous trauma), deep-set eyes, traumatic cataract, previous vitrectomy, the patient's movement during surgery, and the surgeon's inexperience with the phaco technique.[5] Capsular rupture, zonular dehiscence, and the posterior dislocation of lenticular fragments most commonly occur during emulsification of the lens and cortical clean-up. Preventing and recognizing capsular tears during these steps of cataract surgery are therefore paramount.

PREOPERATIVE MANAGEMENT

Patients usually expect an excellent visual outcome after cataract surgery. Informed consent that includes a discussion of the risk of dislocated lens material is important, not just for medicolegal reasons, but also because it may reduce pressure on the cataract surgeon to solve the problem during cataract surgery, an effort that may actually be counterproductive.

INTRAOPERATIVE MANAGEMENT

Most important is to minimize attempts at retrieving intravitreal lens fragments in order to avoid traction on the vitreous. Aggressive efforts at retrieval anteriorly without concomitant posterior vitrectomy can result in giant retinal tears and retinal detachments.[7-9] One should avoid irrigating posteriorly dislocated fragments into the pupillary space. Various techniques such as posterior-assisted levitation via the pars plana have been described, but they should be performed judiciously.[10,11]

One should minimize further extension of the capsular tear as well as forward movement of the vitreous. In the absence of anteriorly displaced vitreous, one may inject viscoelastic material into the anterior chamber to prevent further anterior migration of the vitreous. Inserting a second instrument behind the lens fragment can prevent posterior migration. Some have reported using a Sheet's glide to act as a barrier to aid with emulsification of residual lens material in the anterior chamber.[12] Other options include converting to extracapsular cataract extraction or removing lenticular material using toothed lens-fragment forceps.

If anterior migration of the vitreous has occurred, the surgeon should perform a careful and thorough anterior vitrectomy prior to removing the retained lens material. One should also pay attention to any cortical material that may have migrated into the anterior chamber and into the angle, because it can also cause significant postoperative inflammation.

It is important that the surgeon remain calm and resist the urge to chase after the dropped lens material. Instead, one should remove only the fragments that are readily retrievable and perform a thorough anterior vitrectomy as needed.

A posterior chamber IOL (PCIOL) is an option if a sufficient amount of lens capsule remains. Otherwise, one may consider inserting an anterior chamber IOL (ACIOL) or leaving the eye aphakic for future management with a sutured PCIOL or an ACIOL. A comparison of various IOL placements revealed no significant difference in patients' final visual outcomes.[1] It is acceptable to leave the patient aphakic if a rock-hard nucleus dislocates posteriorly; such cases may require the retina surgeon to deliver the lens fragment through a limbal incision, if fragmentation proves difficult. In the rare instance of a PCIOL's posterior dislocation during management, the surgeon should avoid inserting another IOL until a retina specialist has removed the first one.

Silicone IOLs should be avoided in eyes with dislocated lens fragments, because some patients may need posterior-segment surgery and possible repair of a retinal detachment, requiring air-fluid exchange or the use of silicone-oil tamponade. Moisture tends to condense on IOLs made of silicone during air-fluid exchange and reduce visualization during the posterior-segment surgery. Silicone oil may become irreversibly adherent to silicone IOLs and may necessitate the IOL's eventual removal.

It is wise to place a suture at the site of the corneal incision. Attempts to retrieve lenticular fragments may have violated the integrity of the wound's construction, and it may no longer be watertight, which will increase the risk of wound leak, hypotony, choroidal hemorrhage, and endophthalmitis. Furthermore, watertight incisions are easier to manage during work in the posterior segment.

POSTOPERATIVE MANAGEMENT

Inflammation

Frequent topical corticosteroids and cycloplegic agents should control postoperative inflammation. An antiglaucoma medication may be necessary, because more than one-half of these eyes may have elevated IOP prior to vitrectomy.[2-5,13] The surgeon should closely monitor corneal edema, high IOP, and the development of cystoid macular edema. In addition, one should keep in mind that, in rare instances, severe postoperative inflammation may be due to concomitant endophthalmitis, which should be detected and treated as soon as possible.[14]

The Timing of Vitrectomy

A 1994 survey of anterior segment surgeons found that they refer 77% of cases of retained lens fragments to vitreoretinal surgeons and manage 23% themselves.[6] If the retained lens fragment is small, it may be resorbed over time without surgical intervention. A prospective nonrandomized study by Rossetti and Doro, however, found that vitrectomy can yield faster visual rehabilitation and a better quality of vision when compared with nonvitrectomized eyes, but the procedure poses a risk of retinal detachment.[15] Cataract surgeons should obtain a retinal consultation as soon as possible in cases with a large fragment dropped posteriorly, poor visualization of the fundus, retinal detachment, significant inflammation, vitreous hemorrhage, or elevated IOP.

The optimal timing of vitrectomy for the removal of lenticular material has not been firmly established. Although larger studies did not show an association between the timing of vitrectomy and visual outcome, smaller studies have suggested a trend toward less inflammation and a possibly improved visual outcome with earlier vitrectomy.[1,13,16-18]

Vitrectomy may be performed on the same day, if a retina surgeon is readily available, in order to avoid a second surgery. Because same-day surgery is not possible in most settings and the best timing of surgery is undecided, the cataract surgeon should consider staged management.

Initial aggressive pharmacological therapy and delayed vitrectomy may permit time to improve corneal edema and acute postoperative inflammation as well as visualization during pars plana vitrectomy. Nevertheless, it would be prudent to seek a retinal consult early in order to rule out retinal tears and detachments and to manage secondary complications in a timely manner. In general, pars plana vitrectomy may be performed within 1 to 3 weeks, if there are no other significant secondary complications.

Visual Outcome

Excellent visual outcomes are possible for patients undergoing vitrectomy for retained lens fragments. In most reports, over one-half of patients achieved a final visual acuity of 20/40 or better.[1-5,19-21]

The causes of a poor visual outcome include cystoid macular edema, preexisting ocular disease, corneal edema and decompensation, retinal detachment (both before and after vitrectomy), and an epiretinal membrane.[20,21] In a series by Moore et al that included 343 patients, retinal detachment was observed prior to vitrectomy in 7.3% and occurred after vitrectomy in 5.5%, with an overall rate of 12.8%.[8] Complicated detachments with giant retinal tears occurred as well. Only 18% of the eyes with retinal detachment achieved a visual acuity of 20/40 or better. Poor visual acuity prior to pars plana vitrectomy and the presence of a retinal tear at the time of vitrectomy were associated with a higher rate of subsequent retinal detachment.[8,9]

Because the risk of retinal tears and detachment is correlated with vitreous manipulation, both during cataract surgery and pars plana vitrectomy, cataract and retina surgeons should minimize vitreous traction as much as possible. They should thoroughly inspect the peripheral retina in these patients. Long-term follow-up is recommended in eyes that had retained lens fragments in order to detect and manage the delayed onset of complications, such as cystoid macular edema, epiretinal membrane, or retinal detachment.[21]

In summary, the dislocation of lenticular material into the vitreous cavity during cataract surgery is a rare but potentially serious, sight-threatening complication. Pars plana vitrectomy is effective for removing retained lens fragments, lowering the IOP, and reducing inflammation. Ophthalmologists must take every care to reduce the possibility of retinal detachment, which is a major cause of poor visual outcomes. The majority of patients with retained lens fragments have a good visual prognosis, when the cataract and retina surgeons work as a team to minimize secondary complications through the appropriate and timely management of the case. ■

This article originally appeared in the August 2005 issue of CRSToday.

1. Kim JE, Flynn HW Jr, Smiddy WE, et al. Retained lens fragments after phacoemulsification. *Ophthalmology.* 1994;101:1827-1832.
2. Bourne MJ, Tasman W, Regillo C, et al. Outcomes of vitrectomy for retained lens fragments. *Ophthalmology.* 1996;103:971-976.
3. Margherio RR, Margherio AR, Pendergast SD, et al. Vitrectomy for retained lens fragments after phacoemulsification. *Ophthalmology.* 1997;104:1426-1432.
4. Hansson LJ, Larsson J. Vitrectomy for retained lens fragments in the vitreous after phacoemulsification. *J Cataract Refract Surg.* 2002;28:1007-1011.
5. Monshizadeh R, Samiy N, Haimovici R. Management of retained intravitreal lens fragments after cataract surgery. *Surv Ophthalmol.* 1999;43:397-404.
6. Leaming DV. Practice styles and preferences of ASCRS members—1994 survey. *J Cataract Refract Surg.* 1995;21:378-385.
7. Olsson RB, Ritland JS, Bjornsson OM, et al. A retrospective study of patients with retained nuclear fragments after cataract extraction. *Acta Ophthalmol Scand.* 200;78:677-679.
8. Moore JK, Scott IU, Flynn HW Jr, et al. Retinal detachment in eyes undergoing pars plana vitrectomy for removal of retained lens fragments. *Ophthalmology.* 2003;110:709-713.
9. Smiddy WE, Guererro JL, Pinto R, Feuer W. Retinal detachment rate after vitrectomy for retained lens material after phacoemulsification. *Am J Ophthalmol.* 2003;135:183-187.
10. Chang DF, Packard RB. Posterior assisted levitation for nucleus retrieval using Viscoat after posterior capsule rupture. *J Cataract Refract Surg.* 2003;29:1860-1865.
11. Lifshitz T, Levy J. Posterior assisted levitation: long-term follow-up data. *J Cataract Refract Surg.* 2005;31:499-502.
12. Frankel J. Managing retained intravitreal lens fragments after cataract surgery. *Surv Ophthalmol.* 2000;44:363-364.
13. Yeo LMW, Charteris DG, Bunce C, et al. Retained intravitreal lens fragments after phacoemulsification: a clinicopathological correlation. *Br J Ophthalmol.* 1999;83:1135-1138.
14. Kim JE, Flynn HW Jr, Rubsamen PE, et al. Endophthalmitis in patients with retained lens fragments after phacoemulsification. *Ophthalmology.* 1996;103:575-578.
15. Rossetti A, Doro D. Retained intravitreal lens fragments after phacoemulsification: complications and visual outcome in vitrectomized and nonvitrectomized eyes. *J Cataract Refract Surg.* 2002;28:310-315.
16. Wilkinson CP, Green WR. Vitrectomy for retained lens material after cataract extraction. The relationship between histopathologic findings and the time of vitreous surgery. *Ophthalmology.* 2001;108:1633-1637.
17. Kageyama T, Ayaki M, Ogasawara M, et al. Results of vitrectomy performed at the time of phacoemulsification complicated by intravitreal lens fragments. Br J Ophthalmol. 2001;85:1038-1040.
18. Stefaniotou M, Aspiotis M, Pappa C, et al. Timing of dislocated nuclear fragment management after cataract surgery. *J Cataract Refract Surg.* 2003;29:1985-1988.
19. Vilar NF, Flynn HW Jr, Smiddy WE, et al. Removal of retained lens fragments after phacoemulsification reverses secondary glaucoma and restores visual acuity. *Ophthalmology.* 1997;104:787-792.
20. Scott IU, Flynn HW Jr, Smiddy WE, et al. Clinical features and outcomes of pars plana vitrectomy in patients with retained lens fragments. *Ophthalmology.* 2003;110:567-572.
21. Greven C, Piccione K. Delayed visual loss after pars plana vitrectomy for retained lens fragments. *Retina.* 2004;24:363-367.

CHAPTER 114

Incidence of Retinal Detachment With Myopic Lens-Based Surgery

BARRY SEIBEL, MD

Laser vision correction has benefited countless myopes by reducing their dependence on glasses and correspondingly enhancing their quality of life. However, with increasing degrees of laser vision correction available, the postoperative quality of vision may possibly decrease for reasons such as severe flattening of the corneal curvature as well as induced spherical aberration, especially at the junction of the treated and untreated corneal tissues. Therefore, highly myopic patients, whose quality of life is poorest due to their absolute dependence on thick spectacles or contact lenses, are often not ideal candidates for corneal refractive surgery. For these individuals, lens-based surgery in the form of phakic IOLs or refractive lens exchange may offer hope for visual improvement. These types of surgeries may also benefit moderately myopic patients with cataracts as well as treat presbyopia and effectively reduce higher-order aberrations with proper IOL choice.

CHOOSING THE BEST PROCEDURE

Despite lens-based surgery's potentially superior visual outcomes compared with corneal procedures, the surgeon must examine its risk-benefit ratio in order to validate the appropriateness of the approach. An examination of the Ophthalmic Mutual Insurance Company's consent forms for the two procedures reveals their striking similarity regarding such risks as infection, corneal edema/scarring (which could possibly require a penetrating keratoplasty), possible equipment malfunction, retinal detachment, hemorrhage, retinal vein or artery occlusion, blindness, and the loss of the eye.[1] The two consent forms differ slightly in that LASIK's risks include an incorrect laser power setting and a patient's under- or overresponse. Refractive lens exchange includes the risk of a miscalculated IOL power, a poorly positioned IOL, and cystoid macular edema. Although the last is listed only with refractive lens exchange, its actual rate is extremely low.[2]

Although retinal detachment is a potential risk for both surgical modalities, a review of the literature reveals a potential disparity in relative risk, because there is considerable variability in findings regarding the incidence of retinal detachment in refractive lens exchange. Furthermore, the studies differ greatly with regard to their scopes, criteria, and follow-up durations. For example, Güell et al examined 44 eyes with a mean correction of -15.77 D for 4 years and found a 0% retinal detachment rate.[3] Fernandez-Vega et al examined 190 eyes with a 26- to 39-mm axial length for 5 years and found a 2.1% rate of retinal detachment.[4] Pucci examined 25 eyes with corrections of greater than -12.00 D for 43 months and found a 4% incidence of retinal detachment.[5] Arne studied 36 eyes with -17.00 D manifest refractions and 28-mm axial lengths for 4 years and found a 5.5% incidence of retinal detachment (in two eyes, both of which received PMMA IOLs and underwent a YAG posterior capsulotomy.[6] Fritch examined 481 eyes with axial lengths greater than 26 mm for 7 years and found only a 0.4% incidence of retinal detachment, one-tenth the rate of Pucci's study.[7] The highest rate of retinal detachment (8.1%) was found by Colin et al,[8] who examined 52 eyes that were treated for more than 12.00 D of myopia for 7 years.

SANDERS' ANALYSIS

In order to sort through this somewhat perplexing range of outcomes from differently designed studies, Sanders performed an extensive review of 14 studies of retinal lens exchange with a PCIOL.[2] These studies included a total of 1,372 myopic eyes (range, -6.00 to -33.75 D) of patients mostly in their 30s and 40s. All but 46 surgeries were performed with phacoemulsification, and the follow-up ranged from 15 to 45.9 months. Of all eyes, only 14 developed retinal detachments, an incidence of 1%. Sanders also examined the rate of cystoid macular edema in this review of the literature and found it to be only 0.1%. Although some of the studies were somewhat limited in their length of follow-up, Sanders' review is commendable for attempting to apply some homogeneity to this area of study.

Moreover, this review is significant for looking beyond the simple incidence of retinal detachment to the visual sequelae of this event. Sanders noted that retinal reattachment rates averaged 85%, with some series quoting success rates as high as 98%. However, the final BCVA after reattachment varied, with 60% of patients achieving 20/40 or better, 20% achieving 20/50 to 20/100, and 20% being worse than 20/100. By combining these visual outcomes data with the actual retinal detachment data from the 14 studies, Sanders determined an overall long-term incremental risk of moderate-to-severe vision loss with myopic refractive lens exchange of 4%.

Sanders' estimate was based on his compiled 1% incidence of retinal detachment with myopic refractive lens exchange. His estimate for visual loss would have been considerably worse had he used data from Colin et al, who showed an 8.1% rate of retinal detachment at 7 years.[8] These data are disturbing for several reasons. For example, comparing them with the 4.8% incidence of retinal detachment predicted by Perkins[9] at 7 years shows an incremental risk of this complication with refractive lens exchange of 3.3%. Moreover, the Colin study mirrored the Perkins study at 4 years with a 2% incidence (one eye in the Colin study). The three additional eyes with retinal detachment in the Colin study underwent a Nd:YAG posterior capsulotomy at 4 to 4.5 years postoperatively, and they all experienced retinal detachment within 2 years afterward. Arne's article also showed an association with Nd:YAG capsulotomy.[6]

MECHANISM OF RETINAL DETACHMENT WITH REFRACTIVE LENS EXCHANGE

The mechanism of YAG-induced retinal detachment is thought to be that the laser's energy and resultant shock waves destabilize the hyaluronic acid matrix that supports the vitreous-cortex structure and lead to an anomalous posterior vitreous detachment, which in turn produces a retinal detachment.[10] Another theory predicts that the YAG energy disrupts the anterior hyaloid face, decreases the concentration of hyaluronic acid, and leads to an anomalous posterior vitreous detachment, which in turn leads to retinal detachment.[11]

Even without a YAG laser capsulotomy, cataract surgery alone can conceivably induce a retinal detachment. For example, the anterior shifting of the vitreous can produce peripheral and posterior retinal traction that leads to breaks. Although this anterior shifting is reduced by a properly placed PCIOL with posterior angulated haptics, it can still occur intraoperatively prior to the IOL's placement. Retinal traction may also occur as a result of the inertial destabilization of vitreous intraoperatively, although this retinal traction is also likely reduced by a properly placed PCIOL with posterior angulated haptics. Prior to such stabilization by the IOL, variable anterior chamber pressures and turbulence may proportionately and adversely mobilize the vitreous; therefore, attention to phacodynamic settings and proper instrument manipulation may be helpful in reducing the vitreous' movement.[12] These vitreous dynamics could conceivable play a role in phakic IOL implantation in which anterior chamber pressures also vary with attendant changes in the anterior chamber's depth and potential retinal traction.

Additional considerations come into play when postulating the mechanism of retinal detachment in young myopes, in whom early vitreous liquefaction (synchesis) increases the chance for vitreous collapse (syneresis) and posterior vitreous detachment. The last produces an inertial destabilization of the vitreous that creates traction on the anteriorly attached retina, but these forces do not typically result in a retinal tear in a naturally occurring posterior vitreous detachment in an older patient due to the weaker vitreoretinal adhesions that produced this detachment initially. However, an anomalous posterior vitreous detachment occurs in young myopes prior to normal age-related vitreoretinal dehiscence; therefore, a break is more likely due to inertial vitreal traction's being more directly transmitted to the retina. Furthermore, the young myope will have synchesis as described earlier, which is more likely to dissect through a break as opposed to formed vitreous; this dissection typically results in retinal detachment.[13]

PRESENT AND FUTURE GUIDELINES

Given the potentially increased risk of retinal detachment in myopic refractive lens exchange, what should ophthalmologists do now and in the future? They should inform patients of the disparity in the literature. Some articles state an unchanged or even reduced risk of retinal detachment relative to a myope's natural history. They may also mention the most conservative estimates, with Sanders stating a 4% incremental risk of moderate-to-severe visual loss with retinal lens exchange and Colin et al suggesting a 3% incremental risk of retinal detachment. A retinal specialist should evaluate these patients preoperatively and consider retinal detachment prophylaxis such as laser or cryoretinopexy for suspicious areas. However, Goldberg found equivocal benefits of retinal detachment prophylaxis.[14] He noted retinal breaks in or away from areas of prophylactic treatment. Inflammation from treatment could also induce other sequelae such as an epiretinal membrane, posterior vitreous detachment, or retinal detachment.

Moving into the future with myopic refractive lens exchange, a new, large database of age-matched controls must be established for the natural history of myopia for varying levels of axial length and ametropia to verify the baseline incidence of retinal detachment. The Perkins data[9] are limited and 25 years old, and yet they form the benchmark for judging the incremental risk of retinal detachment. A large, prospective, multicenter study of refractive lens exchange should be organized with standardization of modern small-incision techniques and technology, notwithstanding the inevitable change in these factors with the rapid advances in this area of ophthalmology. The study should also span10 or more years, given the late occurrences of retinal detachment in the Colin study. Also for the future, more studies are needed to validate the role of retinal detachment prophylaxis preoperatively given the doubts cast by Goldberg.[14] Objective evaluative modalities of the vitreous should be developed as preoperative predictors of retinal detachment risk with myopic refractive lens exchange, such as dynamic light scattering or 3-D B-scan ultrasonography.[14] Further evaluation is also needed on the potential role of pharmacologic vitreolysis for prophylaxis against retinal detachment in the face of anomalous posterior vitreous detachments.

In summation, the literature has indicated a potentially increased risk of retinal detachment[14] with refractive lens exchange in myopia. With proper informed consent and meticulous attention to surgical technique (to minimize the disturbance of the vitreous and reduce the likelihood of posterior capsular opacification requiring Nd:YAG posterior capsulotomy), refractive lens exchange is a viable procedure that can significantly enhance the quality of life for these myopic patients. ■

This article originally appeared in the August 2005 issue of CRSToday.

1. Ophthalmic Mutual Insurance Company. Risk Management Forms. San Francisco, California.
2. Sanders, DR. Actual and theoretical risks for visual loss following use of the implantable contact lens for moderate to high myopia. *J Cataract Refractive Surg.* 2003;29:1323-1332.
3. Güell JL, Rodriguez-Arenas AF, Gris O, et al. Phacoemulsification of the crystalline lens and implantation of an intraocular lens for the correction of moderate and high myopia: four-year follow-up. *J Cataract Refract Surg.* 2003;29:34-38.
4. Fernandez-Vega L, Alfonso JF, Villacampa T. Clear lens extraction for the correction of high myopia. *Ophthalmology.* 2003;110:2349-2354.
5. Pucci V. Clear lens phacoemulsification for correction of high myopia. *J Cataract Refract Surg.* 2001;27:896-900.
6. Arne JL. Phakic intraocular lens implantation versus clear lens extraction in highly myopic eyes of 30- to 50-year-old patients. *J Cataract Refract Surg.* 2004;30:2092-2096.
7. Fritch CD. Risk of retinal detachment in myopic eyes after intraocular lens implantation: a 7-year study. *J Cataract Refract Surg.* 1998;24:1357-1360.
8. Colin J, Rabinet A, Cochener B. Retinal detachment after clear lens extraction for high myopia: seven-year follow-up. *Ophthalmology.* 1999;106:2281-2284.
9. Perkins ES. Morbidity from myopia. *Sight Saving Review.* 1979;49:11-19.
10. Michels R. Other causes of retinal detachment. In: Retinal Detachment, 2nd ed. St. Louis, MO: Mosby; 1996: 195-197.
11. Smith TR, Moscoso WE, Trokel S, Auran J. The barrier function in neodymium YAG laser capsulotomy. *Arch Ophthalmol.* 113:645.
12. Seibel BS. Logic of setting machine parameters. In: Phacodynamics. 4th ed. Thorofare, NJ: Slack, Inc.; 2005: 154-167.
13. Sebag J. Structure, Function, and Age-Related Changes of the Human Vitreous. In: Vitreous and Vitreo-Retinal Interface. Schepens C, Neetens A, eds. New York, NY: Springer-Verlag: 1987: 37-57.
14. Goldberg MF. Clear lens extraction for axial myopia. An appraisal. *Ophthalmology.* 1987;9:571-582.

CHAPTER 115

Best Practices for Cystoid Macular Edema Prophylaxis

JOHN R. WITTPENN, JR, MD

All surgeons recognize the risk factors for cystoid macular edema (CME) and will respond appropriately. Doctors have often told me, "When I have a high-risk patient, I often treat him with an NSAID to prevent CME." The question is, what about patients who you do not identify as high risk? What are the chances of those patients with no risk factors developing clinically significant or even subclinical CME that would affect their visual function? Is it important that we use prophylaxis in all cases?

I believe that all surgeons should prescribe a nonsteroidal anti-inflammatory drug (NSAID) for all cataract patients, not just high-risk ones. As the data discussed herein show, using at least ketorolac with a steroid produces a statistically significant improvement in visual outcomes.

DIFFERENT MECHANISMS OF ACTION

Some surgeons feel that NSAIDs are not necessary if they prescribe a steroid, because both of these agents block prostaglandin synthesis. The two work differently, however. Although steroids block the arachidonic acid cascade, the binding is not an irreversible blockage, but rather a reversible bond (ie, only a partial blockage). NSAIDs block cyclooxygenase COX-1 and COX-2 inhibitors in a nonreversible bond. In other words, once a COX-1 or COX-2 enzyme is blocked, it is out of the system. Therefore, prescribing steroids and NSAIDs together produces synergistic effects, as recent studies show.

TREATING NON–HIGH-RISK PATIENTS

Criteria

My colleagues and I conducted a large, multicenter, randomized, masked trial that examined the importance of adding ketorolac to steroids in 546 patients undergoing cataract surgery.[1] We specifically identified patients who had no risk factors for CME. The study criteria included (1) zero risk factors for CME, (2) complication-free surgery, and (3) an expected amount of inflammation on the first day after surgery. If patients experienced an unexpected amount of inflammation (eg, toxic anterior segment syndrome), they were eliminated from the study. Our goal was to study the patients who were most likely not to have CME and find out if there was still an advantage to adding ketorolac to their medication regimen. We found that there was, in fact, a benefit.

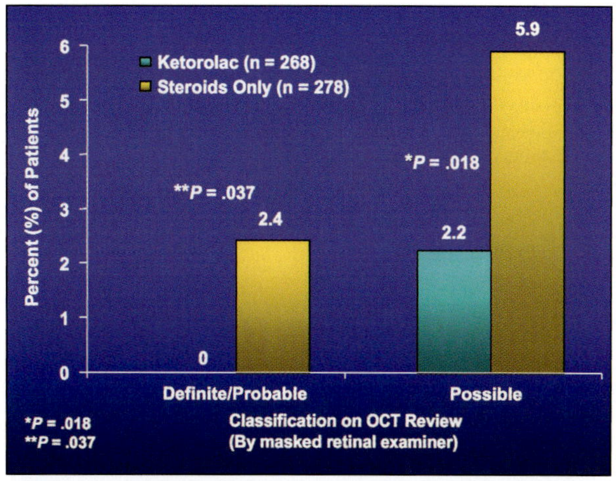

Figure 1. Incidence of CME on examination with ocular coherence tomography.

Outcomes

The patients' outcomes were evaluated by a masked retinal analyst who compared preoperative and 4-week postoperative optical coherence tomography (OCT). We found that the CME rate was statistically significant between the two treatment groups (Figure 1). The group that received only steroids had a 2.4% rate of definite or probable CME and a loss of visual acuity

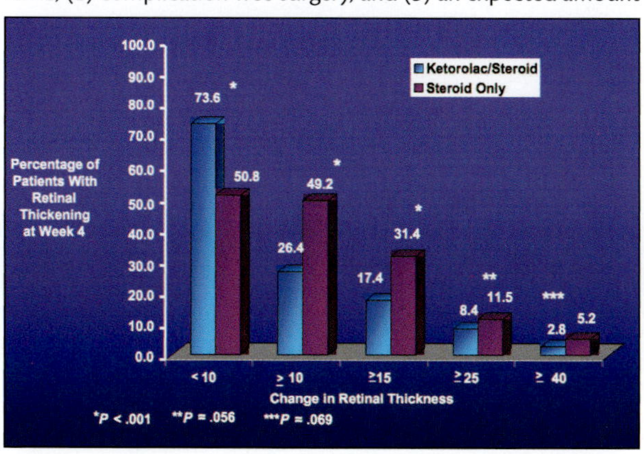

Figure 2. Incidence of retinal thickening between the two treatment groups.

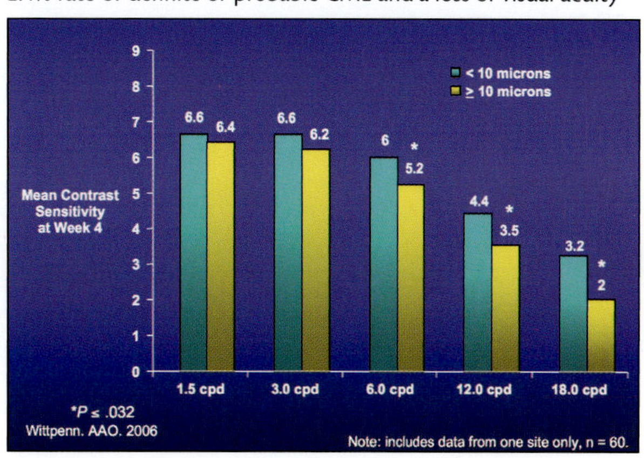

Figure 3. Limiting retinal thickening improves contrast sensitivity.

ranging from 20/30 to 20/100. The group of patients who received ketorolac plus steroid had no cases of definite or probable CME. Furthermore, when all patients of both groups were compared for retinal thickening, more than half of the steroid-only patients had macular thickening of greater than 10 µm, whereas only 25% of the ketorolac group had this degree of thickening, which was also statistically significant (Figure 2). Patients with less than 10 µm of thickening exhibited statistically significant better contrast sensitivity (Figure 3).

CME and Contrast Sensitivity

Unfortunately, one of my patients in the steroid-only group developed CME. At 4 weeks postoperatively, her BCVA was 20/40, and I treated her with the combination therapy. Two months later, her condition had improved to 20/20 BCVA. She has a cataract in her other eye, which is about 20/30- BCVA. To this day, she will not let me remove the cataract, because she insists this eye is her better eye. The reason is that the eye with CME has abnormal contrast sensitivity. Although she can read the letters on an eye chart easily and we consider her to be a cured patient, her final visual function is so poor that she still considers this eye her worse eye.

NSAID Dose Response Curve

In a smaller study of 100 patients reported by Eric Donnenfeld, MD, patients were grouped to receive ketorolac starting 3 days, 1 day, 1 hour, or not at all before cataract surgery. All patients except the last group received ketorolac and a steroid following cataract surgery. In comparing the four groups at 15 days, the group receiving ketorolac for 1 or 3 days preoperatively had less pain during and after surgery, faster surgery, and no cases of CME. The study highlighted the importance of beginning ketorolac at least 1 day before surgery.[2]

NSAIDS AND MULTIFOCAL IOLS

These studies emphasize the importance of using NSAIDs and steroids in combination for all cataract patients. Furthermore, to paraphrase Steven Dell, MD, this regimen is hypercritical when working with multifocal IOLs. Another study by Dr. Donnenfeld and Kerry Solomon, MD, presented at the ASCRS last year compared ketorolac plus steroid to steroid alone in multifocal IOL patients. They enrolled 26 patients undergoing bilateral multifocal IOL cataract surgery into the study. One eye of each patient was treated with steroids plus ketorolac, and the other eye with steroids only. They reported that the eyes receiving both ketorolac and steroid had better BCVA and statistically significant better contrast sensitivity. Subjectively, more patients preferred the ketorolac-plus-steroid eye when questioned.

DOSING RECOMMENDATIONS

Macular thickening is an issue for all cataract patients. They demand and we strive to give them the absolute best vision. CME or any degree of macular thickening is an unacceptable problem. As a result of these studies on ketorolac, I believe that the gold standard of care for all cataract surgery patients should include preoperative ketorolac for 1 to 3 days followed by a combination of a steroid and ketorolac postoperatively for 4 to 5 weeks. If the patient has high risk factors for CME, I initiate treatment for 1 week preoperatively and plan to continue the treatment for 8 to 12 weeks. Since the newer NSAIDs have been shown in studies to reduce inflammation following cataract surgery, many assume these agents will provide similar results with regard to macular thickening, although we still need to see studies confirming these assumptions. Finally, surgeons should note that these are off-label indications for all NSAIDs. ■

This article originally appeared in CRSToday*'s March 2008 Premium Cataract Surgery supplement.*

1. Wittpenn J Jr, Silverstein SM, Hunkeler JD, et al. A masked comparison of acular LS plus steroid vs. steroid alone for the prevention of macular leakage in cataract patients. Poster presented at: The AAO/APOA Annual Joint Meeting; November 12, 2006; Las Vegas, NV.
2. Donnenfeld ED, Perry HD, Wittpenn J Jr, et al. Preoperative ketorolac tromethamine 0.4% in phacoemulsification outcomes: pharmacokinetic-response curve. *J Cataract Refract Surg.* 2006;32:9:1474-1482.

CHAPTER 116

Improving Quality of Vision

MICHAEL B. RAIZMAN, MD

Nonsteroidal anti-inflammatory drugs (NSAIDs) are becoming more popular to use during cataract surgery. Ophthalmologists now seem to recognize the value of this class of drugs. There are four reasons why I advocate the use of topical NSAIDs during cataract surgery. First, these agents effectively reduce postoperative inflammation. Second, they probably prevent cystoid macular edema (CME).[1,2] The third reason is that NSAIDs maintain intraoperative meiosis (this was the first indication for these drugs during cataract surgery).[3] Finally, topical NSAIDs have been shown to improve comfort during and after surgery.[4-7] I routinely use topical anesthesia, and I believe that nonsteroidal drops assist in keeping my patients comfortable. This use of topical NSAIDs is equally important for comfort in refractive surgery.

EXPERIENCE

Several patients in the mid-1990s prompted me to investigate the role of topical NSAIDs in preventing CME. At Tufts University School of Medicine, some of my associates, including Carmen Puliafito, MD, and Joel Schuman, MD, were collaborating with engineers from the Massachusetts Institute of Technology on the first prototype of the device that performed optical coherence tomography (OCT). Some of my patients were complaining of poor vision after cataract surgery despite what I considered to be a good outcome. One of my patients saw 20/20 but complained of metamorphopsia. The Amsler grid was described as having wavy lines centrally. OCT revealed significant parafoveal edema despite a normal foveal pit and normal foveal thickness.

Another patient complained of distorted vision in one eye. The

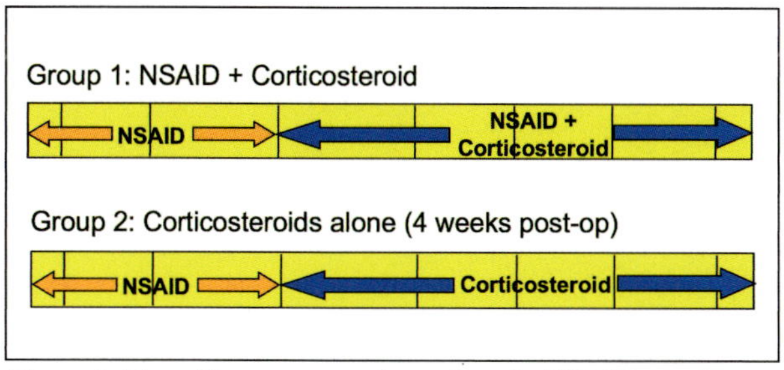

Figure 1. The efficacy comparison of topical NSAIDs and steroids in reducing the incidence of CME in patients undergoing cataract surgery (n = 60).

first eye had 20/20 vision after cataract surgery with a normal OCT. The second eye had 20/25 visual acuity, but the patient was quite upset with the difference between the vision in the two eyes. Although the foveal pit appeared normal in the eye with 20/25 acuity, the macular thickness was 50 µm greater than in the eye with 20/20 vision. This patient was treated with topical NSAID drops, and after several weeks, the acuity and the OCT returned to normal.

We now realize that our patients are more demanding with cataract surgery. They expect excellent visual outcomes. We have learned from our refractive surgery patients that the quality of vision is critical. We no longer depend solely on the Snellen visual acuity. Contract sensitivity is also important. Our patients also demand a rapid recovery of vision and minimal discomfort.

PREVALENCE

We recognize that CME can occur with perfect cataract surgery. Although endophthalmitis is of great concern, postoperative macular edema is far more common. A variety of studies indicate that CME may occur between 8% and 12% of the time in routine, uncomplicated clear cornea phaco surgery. Patients with diabetes may have a rate as high as 32%, even in the absence of diabetic retinopathy.[8] Patients with diabetic retinopathy may have an 80% chance of increased macular thickening with routine cataract surgery.

Although it is possible to treat CME after it develops, not all patients will respond to therapy, and some macular edema is permanent and can cause significant reduction in visual acuity. In my view, it is better to do our best to prevent CME rather than wait for its development.

Risk Factors

There are a number of factors that increase the risk of CME. The presence of uveitis or other pre-existing inflammation is a strong risk factor. Macular edema after surgery in the contralateral eye is another risk factor. Any macular disorders including epiretinal membranes, traction on the macula, retinal vascular abnormalities, retinitis pigmentosa, and previous surgery can all increase the risk of CME.

Regimen

The optimal regimen for topical NSAIDs around cataract surgery is not known. Cal Roberts, MD, showed that providing 3 days of nonsteroidal therapy before surgery reduces the amount of postoperative inflammation compared to 1 or 2 days of therapy. We do not know whether 3 days of preoperative therapy are required to prevent postoperative CME.[9] A shorter course of preoperative therapy is adequate to reduce discomfort and maintain pupil dilation during surgery. I have my patients use NSAID drops for 3 days before surgery. In some high-risk cases, I may use these drops for 1 week before surgery.[10]

After surgery, I regularly prescribe NSAID drops for 4 weeks in routine cases and at least 6 weeks in patients with high risk factors. Patients with diabetic retinopathy routinely receive 6 to 12 weeks of therapy. In all cases, I use topical NSAIDs in combination with topical corticosteroids after cataract surgery. Approximately 90% of patients may have complete control of inflammation with a NSAID drop alone. It is not possible to predict which patients fall into the 10% that are inadequately treated with topical NSAIDs. For this reason, I treat all patients with a combination of drops. I stop the steroid at 4 weeks and continue the NSAID drop if necessary.

In a small study that I performed in the late 1990s, I treated half of my patients with topical corticosteroids after routine cataract surgery.[1] The other half received topical corticosteroids in combination with topical NSAIDs for 4 weeks. The group that received the nonsteroid drops had no CME, as demonstrated on OCT. The group that received corticosteroids alone had a 12% rate of CME as demonstrated by OCT (Figure 1). Larger studies have corroborated my findings. Wittpenn and associates found a 12% rate of CME in patients who received prednisolone acetate alone.[11] In their study of patients who received prednisolone acetate and ketorolac, only 1% developed CME. Braunstein showed similar efficacy with nepefenac after routine cataract surgery.[12]

RECOMMENDATION

In summary, although CME may not be as devastating as endophthalmitis, it is far more common and deserves our attention. Even mild CME is clinically relevant, and our patients are demanding optimal outcomes. I strongly recommend the use of topical NSAIDs routinely in cataract surgery. ■

This article originally appeared in the February 2008 CRSToday *supplement.*

1. Samiy N, Foster CS. The role of nonsteroidal anti-inflammatory drugs in ocular inflammation. *Int Ophthalmol Clin.* 1996;36:1:195-206.
2. McColgin AZ, Raizman MB. Efficacy of topical diclofenac in reducing the incidence of postoperative cystoid macular edema. *Invest Ophthmol Vis Sci.* 1999;40(suppl):S289.
3. Flach, AJ. Topical nonsteroidal antiinflammatory drugs in ophthalmology. *Int Ophthalmol Clin.* 2002;42:1:1-11.
4. Yee RW, Ketorolac Radial Keratotomy Study Group. Analgesic efficacy and safety of nonpreserved ketorolac ophthalmic solution following radial keratotomy. *Am J Ophthalmol.* 1998;125:472-480.
5. Eiferman RA, Hoffman RS, Sher NA. Topical diclofenac reduced pain following photorefractive keratectomy. *Arch Ophthalmol.* 1993;111:1022.
6. Szerenyi K, Sorken K, Garbus JJ, et al. Decrease in normal human corneal sensitivity with topical diclofenac sodium. *Am J Ophthalmol.* 1994;118:312-315.
7. Price MO, Price FW. Efficacy of topical ketorolac tromethamine 0.4% for control of pain or discomfort associated with cataract surgery. *Curr Med Res Opin.* 2004;20:12:2015-2019.
8. Pollack A, Leiba H, Bukelman A, Oliver M. Cystoid macular edema following cataract extraction in patients with diabetes. *Br J Ophthalmol.* 1992;76:4:221-224.
9. Roberts C. Improving quality of vision with nonsteroidal agents. Paper presented at: The ASCRS Symposium on Cataract, IOL and Refractive Surgery; March 19, 2006; San Francisco, CA.
10. Heier, JS. Preventing Post-cataract extraction CME: early identification of patients at risk and prophylactic treatment may avert vision loss. *Ophthalmology Management.* 2004;39:63-72.
11. Wittpenn J Jr, Silverstein MD, Hunkeler JD, et al. A masked comparison of Acular LS plus steroid vs steroid alone for the prevention of macular leakage in cataract patients. Poster presented at: The AAO/APAO 2006 Joint Meeting; November 11, 2006; Las Vegas, NV.
12. Wolf EJ, Braunstein A, Shih CY, Braunstein RE. Incidence of visually significant pseudophakic macualr edema after uneventful phacoemulsification in patients treated with nepafenac. Paper presented at: The ASCRS Symposium on Cataract, IOL and Refractive Surgery; April 30, 2007; San Diego, CA.

CHAPTER 117

Pseudophakic Cystoid Macular Edema

TINA A. SCHEUFELE, MD, AND JEFFREY S. HEIER, MD

Cystoid macular edema (CME) is still the most frequent cause of decreased vision after cataract surgery, although its incidence has declined with advances in surgical techniques (most notably, the change from intracapsular to extracapsular cataract extraction [ECCE]). Clinical CME has historically been defined as a reduction in vision to 20/40 or less that is attributable to ophthalmoscopically or angiographically visible CME. The condition occurs in as many as 1% to 6% of patients after uncomplicated phaco surgery.[1,2]

Advances in technique, instrumentation, and pharmacology have increased expectations for surgical outcomes, from both the patient's and the surgeon's perspective. Less dramatic visual deficits than 20/40 may be considered clinically significant today. For example, a patient may be symptomatic with a visual acuity of 20/25 or 20/30 or subtle metamorphopsia. Angiographic CME, in which visual acuity is unaffected but CME is present on fluorescein angiography, is seen in up to 19% of these patients.[3] The incidence may be higher in patients with a greater degree of postoperative inflammation.[4] Pseudophakic CME classically presents 4 to 6 weeks after cataract surgery, but it has occurred as early as 3 weeks or as late as 6 months postoperatively.[5]

MECHANISM

Uveal stimulation or the release of lens epithelial cells during intraocular surgery promotes prostaglandin synthesis in the anterior chamber.[6] Prostaglandins disrupt the blood-aqueous barrier and thus permit cytokines and other inflammatory mediators to enter the anterior chamber.[6] The prostaglandins and inflammatory mediators are then believed to diffuse through the vitreous to the retina, where they result in a breakdown of the blood-retinal barrier that leads to CME. Older patients and those with various other ocular conditions (including diabetes mellitus, uveitis, and retinal vascular occlusions) may be more susceptible to a breakdown of the blood-retinal barrier.[6] The relative contributions of the inflammatory mediators and other predisposing factors are still unknown.

RISK FACTORS

Surgical

The risk of pseudophakic CME appears to be lower with phaco surgery than with either ECCE or intracapsular cataract extraction, perhaps because of reduced postoperative inflammation.[7] The amount of inflammation, and hence the risk of CME, is greater with higher phaco power (>1 J).[8]

Surgical complications dramatically increase the risk of CME. A ruptured posterior capsule is associated with an 11.5% to 20% incidence of clinical CME in patients undergoing phacoemulsification.[4,9] In those undergoing ECCE, the incidence may be as high as 30.8%.[10] Retained lens fragments further increase the risk of clinical CME to as much as 29% after phacoemulsification.[11] Immediate pars plana vitrectomy, although often not possible, may reduce this risk.[12]

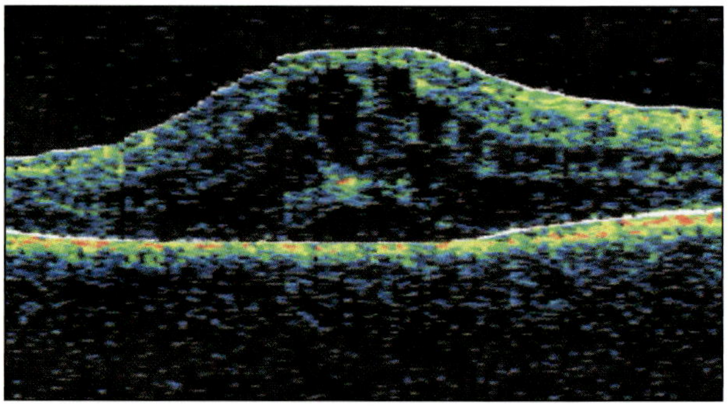

Figure 1. Optical coherence tomography (OCT) shows intraretinal cystic spaces and a small amount of subretinal fluid consistent with CME.

Chronic CME in the setting of complicated cataract surgery may be due to mechanical traction on the retina or persistent inflammation. The former may be caused by vitreous strands adherent to the cataract wound. In the past, chronic inflammation was often seen with rigid anterior chamber IOLs (ACIOLs) as a result of iris trauma. Today, the incidence of CME with a well-positioned, open-looped ACIOL is much lower, although certain patients may still do better with sutured-in posterior chamber IOLs (PCIOLs).[13]

Approximately 1% of patients may develop CME after Nd:YAG capsulotomy.[14] This complication often occurs 1 to 5 months later and is believed to be related to opening the posterior capsule rather than to the energy of the Nd:YAG laser.[15]

Retinal Pathology

Patients with diabetes are at an increased risk of both clinically significant diabetic macular edema and CME following cataract surgery. In individuals with diabetic retinopathy but no macular edema prior to ECCE, the incidence of clinical CME may be as high as 75%.[13] If no diabetic retinopathy is present prior to surgery, the incidence of clinical CME is much lower (11%).[16] CME is also more likely to persist longer in diabetics, whether or not retinopathy is present.[16] Specifically, chronic (> 6 months) postoperative CME is more likely in patients with systemic hypertension or diabetes, probably because of a greater permeability of the blood-retinal barrier.[17]

Other underlying retinal pathology may cause CME. A recent study reported a 17% incidence of CME in pseudophakic patients after pars plana vitrectomy for retinal detachment.[18] In the investigators' personal experience (ongoing study), patients who have previously undergone repair of retinal detachment are at a higher risk of CME after cataract extraction. This risk is present independent of whether the patient developed CME after the previous retinal surgery. The investigators have also observed an increased risk of CME in eyes that have had previous retinal venous occlusions (regardless of past macular edema) and in patients whose fellow eye had CME. Epiretinal membranes and idiopathic juxtafoveal

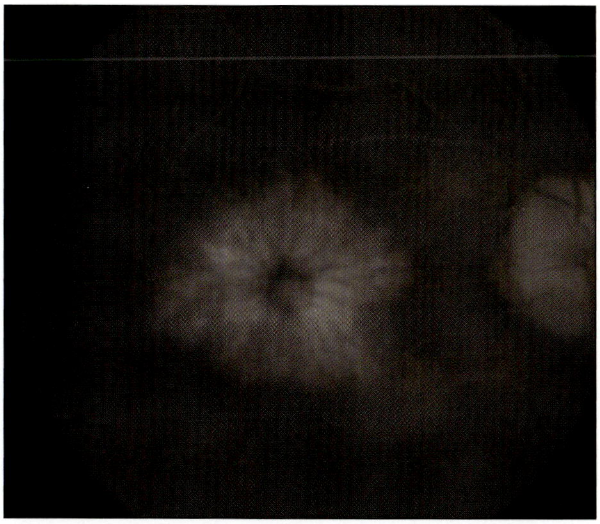

Figure 2. This fluorescein angiogram of an eye with CME shows the typical petaloid pattern of late leakage in the fovea.

telangiectasia may also cause CME, which often will not respond to pharmacotherapy.

In patients with a history of uveitis, CME is an important cause of poor vision postoperatively. The incidence of CME in pars planitis may be as high as 50% after phacoemulsification with the implantation of a PCIOL.[19] The condition is often refractory to topical therapy alone in these patients and may require peri- or intraocular steroid injections.

Medication

The perioperative use of antiglaucoma eye drops such as epinephrine, dipivefrin, and the prostaglandin analogues has been shown to increase the risk of CME.[8,20] Recently, the preservative benzalkonium chloride, which is found in many other ocular medications as well, has been independently associated with an increased incidence of CME, an effect attributed to the release of prostaglandins and other inflammatory mediators.[20] The relative contributions of these medications and their preservatives are not fully understood.

PROPHYLAXIS

Topical steroids alone do not suppress the synthesis of inflammatory mediators, such as the prostaglandins.[21] Topical NSAIDs, by suppressing the cyclooxygenase pathway responsible for prostaglandin production, have been shown to reduce aqueous flare and the development of CME when used after cataract surgery.[21] Starting a topical NSAID such as ketorolac (Acular; Allergan, Inc., Irvine, CA) or diclofenac (Voltaren; Novartis Pharmaceuticals Corporation, East Hanover, NJ) q.i.d. for 3 days prior to cataract surgery and maintaining the patient on the NSAID for a minimum of 1 month postoperatively may be the best routine prophylaxis against CME.[22]

If possible, one should halt prostaglandin analogues perioperatively, because endogenous prostaglandins have been implicated in the mechanism of CME.[6] A recent study in the United Kingdom found that 40% of the 519 ophthalmologists surveyed stopped these agents in at least some of their patients prior to cataract surgery.[23] Most stopped the drug less than 1 week before surgery and did not resume it until 30 to 60 days after surgery.[23]

For uveitic patients, most important is maximum control of their intraocular inflammation with topical or oral steroids or with systemic immunosuppressants, if necessary. One may manage patients with refractory or recurrent uveitis or pars planitis with oral prednisolone (0.5 mg/kg) initiated 2 weeks prior to surgery and tapered gradually postoperatively.[24] This regimen has been shown to decrease aqueous flare and inflammation.[24]

Postoperatively, patients at high risk for CME should be treated prophylactically with topical NSAIDs for at least 6 to 12 weeks.

DIAGNOSIS

OCT of CME shows intraretinal cystic spaces and occasionally a small amount of subretinal fluid (Figure 1). OCT may be sufficient for diagnosis in patients whose presentation is classic. In diabetics or patients with an atypical presentation, however, fluorescein angiography assists the diagnosis by ruling out other causes of macular edema such as diabetic retinopathy, venous occlusive disease, choroidal neovascularization, or idiopathic juxtafoveal retinal telangiectasia.

In CME, the fluorescein angiogram shows a petaloid pattern of late leakage in the fovea (Figure 2). Hyperfluorescence of the optic disc is typically present in pseudophakic CME, but this clinical sign is often absent in other etiologies, including clinically significant diabetic macular edema, epiretinal membrane, or age-related macular degeneration.

It is important to consider other conditions that may mimic CME but will not respond to topical treatment. Cataract extraction may worsen diabetic macular edema. Patients with diabetes or with a history of prior retinal detachment or retinal vascular occlusion may develop an epiretinal membrane, often best appreciated on OCT. This technology is also helpful in diagnosing vitreomacular traction. Finally, choroidal neovascular membranes and juxtafoveal telangiectasia may cause intraretinal edema, both of which are best evaluated by fluorescein angiography.

TREATMENT

Initial Approach

After a confirmed diagnosis of pseudophakic CME, OCT is an objective and relatively sensitive method of monitoring the patient's response to treatment. We initiate topical therapy consisting of prednisolone acetate and an NSAID q.i.d. for at least 6 weeks in all patients with pseudophakic CME. If we observe a treatment response, the patient continues therapy until the edema resolves, which may take several months. Once the swelling abates, we taper the drops by one drop per week.[25] Acular and Voltaren appear to be equally effective NSAIDs.[26] Acular LS (0.4%; Allergan, Inc.) is generally preferred over Acular 0.5% because it causes less ocular irritation.

It is still not known whether topical NSAIDs alone are as effective as the combination of topical NSAIDs and steroids. A recent small study found no statistically significant difference in the response of pseudophakic CME to ketorolac alone versus ketorolac and prednisolone.[27] An earlier study, however, found a statistical benefit with the combination of topical steroids and NSAIDs.[25] It is possible that these drugs may act synergistically to restore the blood-retinal barrier by blocking prostaglandin synthesis (NSAIDs) and decreasing intraocular inflammation (steroids).

The FDA recently approved a new twice-daily topical NSAID (bromfenac 0.09% [Xibrom; Ista Pharmaceuticals, Inc., Irvine, CA]) for controlling inflammation after cataract surgery.[28] Its effectiveness for the treatment of CME has not been studied. If effective, it may increase patients' compliance.

CME in patients on prostaglandin analogues usually responds favorably to the cessation of the prostaglandin drug and the initiation of therapy with a topical NSAID.

If Topical Therapy Fails

Topical therapy alone is usually effective in treating routine pseudophakic CME, but it may fail in patients who have other risk factors. If no improvement occurs after 6 weeks of strict compliance, one may consider periocular or intravitreal steroids. For refractory pseudophakic CME, intravitreal Kenalog (Bristol-Myers Squibb Company, New York, NY) may reduce macular edema and improve vision, but this effect may only last 2 to 4 months.[29]

Pars plana vitrectomy may be indicated when macular edema is associated with epiretinal membranes, suspected retained lens fragments, or pars planitis that is unresponsive to maximum medical therapy. Even in the absence of vitreoretinal abnormalities or the aforementioned surgical indications, research has shown that pars plana vitrectomy resolves chronic CME in some patients.[30] ■

This article originally appeared in the August 2005 issue of CRSToday.

1. Ray S, D'Amico DJ. Pseudophakic cystoid macular edema. *Semin Ophthalmol.* 2002;17:167-180.
2. Powe NR, Schein OD, Gieser SC, et al. Synthesis of the literature on visual acuity and complications following cataract extraction with intraocular lens implantation. *Arch Ophthalmol.* 1994;112:239-252.
3. Ursell PG, Spalton DJ, Whitcup SM, Nussenblatt RB. Cystoid macular edema after phacoemulsification: relationship to blood-aqueous barrier damage and visual acuity. *J Cataract Refract Surg.* 1999;25:1492-1497.
4. Collins JF, Krol WF, Kirk GF, Gaster RN; VA Cooperative Cataract Study Group. The effect of vitreous presentation during extracapsular cataract surgery on the postoperative visual acuity at one year. *Am J Ophthalmol.* 2004;138:536-542.
5. Nikica G, Ljerka HP, Jelena P. Cystoid macular edema in anterior chamber lens implantation following posterior capsule rupture. *Doc Ophthalmol.* 1992;81:309-315.
6. Miyake K, Ibaraki N. Prostaglandins and cystoid macular edema. *Surv Ophthalmol.* 2002;47(suppl):S203-S218.
7. Pande MV, Spalton DJ, Kerr-Muir MG, Marshall J. Postoperative inflammatory response to phacoemulsification and extracapsular cataract surgery: aqueous flare and cells. *J Cataract Refract Surg.* 1996;22(suppl 1):770-774.
8. Ferrari TM, Cavallo M, Durante G, et al. Macular edema induced by phacoemulsification. *Doc Ophthalmol.* 1999;97:325-327.
9. Frost NA, Sparrow JM, Strong NP, et al. Vitreous loss in planned extracapsular cataract extraction does lead to a poorer visual outcome. *Eye.* 1995;9:446-451.
10. Ah-Fat FG, Sharma MK, Majid MA, Yang YC. Vitreous loss during conversion from conventional extracapsular cataract extraction to phacoemulsification. *J Cataract Refract Surg.* 1993;24:801-805.
11. Scott IU, Flynn HW Jr, Smiddy WE, et al. Clinical features and outcomes of pars plana vitrectomy in patients with retained lens fragments. *Ophthalmology.* 2003;110:1567-1572.
12. Lai TY, Kwok AK, Yeung YS. Immediate pars plana vitrectomy for dislocated intravitreal lens fragments during cataract surgery. *Eye.* E-publication ahead of print.
13. Evereklioglu C, Er H, Bekir NA, et al. Comparison of secondary implantation of flexible open-loop anterior chamber and scleral-fixated posterior chamber intraocular lenses. *J Cataract Refract Surg.* 2003;29:301-308.
14. Steinert RF, Puliafito CA, Kumar SR, et al. Cystoid macular edema, retinal detachment, and glaucoma after Nd:YAG laser posterior capsulotomy. *Am J Ophthalmol.* 1991;112:373-380.
15. Winslow RL, Taylor BC. Retinal complications following YAG laser capsulotomy. *Ophthalmology.* 1985;92:785-789.
16. Pollack A, Leiba H, Bukelman A, Oliver M. Cystoid macular oedema following cataract extraction in patients with diabetes. *Br J Ophthalmol.* 1992;76:221-224.
17. Dick II JSB, Jampol LM, Haller JA. Macular edema. In: Ryan SJ, ed. *Retina.* St. Louis, MO: Mosby; 2001: 967-981.
18. Campo RV, Sipperley JO, Sneed SR, et al. Pars plana vitrectomy without scleral buckle for pseudophakic retinal detachments. *Ophthalmology.* 1999;106:1811-1815.
19. Ganesh SK, Babu K, Biswas J. Phacoemulsification with intraocular lens implantation in cases of pars planitis. *J Cataract Refract Surg.* 2004;30:2072-2076.
20. Miyake K, Ibaraki N, Goto Y. ESCRS Binkhorst lecture 2002: pseudophakic preservative maculopathy. *J Cataract Refract Surg.* 2003;29:1800-1810.
21. Arcieri ES, Santana A, Rocha FN, et al. Blood-aqueous barrier changes after the use of prostaglandin analogues in patients with pseudophakia and aphakia: a 6-month randomized trial. *Arch Ophthalmol.* 2005;123:186-192.
22. Guttman C. NSAIDs vital tool for optimized cataract outcomes. *Ophthalmology Times.* 2005 April;30:8:1,42.
23. Ahad MA, McKee HDR. Stopping prostaglandin analogues in uneventful cataract surgery. *J Cataract Refract Surg.* 2004:30;2644-2645.
24. Rahman I, Jones NP. Long-term results of cataract extraction with intraocular lens implantation in patients with uveitis. *Eye.* 2005;19:191-197.
25. Heier JS, Topping TM, Baumann W, et al. Ketorolac versus prednisolone versus combination therapy in the treatment of acute pseudophakic cystoid macular edema. *Ophthalmology.* 2000;107:2034-2039.
26. Rho DS. Treatment of acute pseudophakic cystoid macular edema: diclofenac versus ketorolac. *J Cataract Refract Surg.* 2003;29:2378-2384.
27. Singal N, Hopkins J. Pseudophakic cystoid macular edema: ketorolac alone vs ketorolac plus prednisolone. *Can J Ophthalmol.* 2004;39:245-250.
28. Guttman C. Twice-daily NSAID relieves post-cataract inflammation. *Ophthalmology Times.* 2005 May;30:9:1,8.
29. Benhamou N, Massin P, Haouchine B. Intravitreal triamcinolone for refractory pseudophakic macular edema. *Am J Ophthalmol.* 2003;135:246-249.
30. Pendergast SD, Margherio RR, Williams GA, Cox MS Jr. Vitrectomy for chronic pseudophakic cystoid macular edema. *Am J Ophthalmol.* 1999;128:317-23.

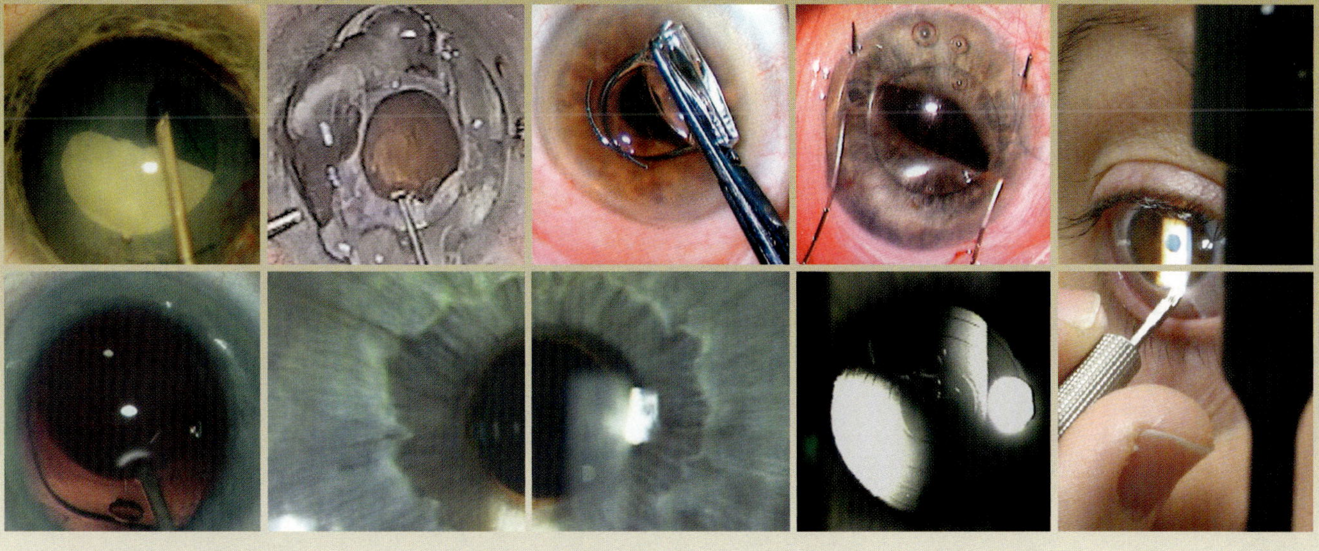

INTRAOCULAR LENSES

ASPHERIC IOLS

COMPLICATIONS OF IOLS

ASTIGMATISM MANAGEMENT

REFRACTIVE IOLS

COMPLICATIONS OF PREMIUM IOLS

CHAPTER 118

Highly Accurate IOL Calculations

WARREN E. HILL, MD

Accurate IOL calculations begin with identifying the patient's visual goals. No one needs to explain this concept to a LASIK surgeon, but cataract surgeons all too often overlook this basic starting point. With patients' expectations continuing to increase, it is becoming more important to follow the lead of our refractive colleagues and take the time to agree upon a refractive goal with each patient prior to cataract surgery. It may come as a surprise that your patients will often give you an answer other than emmetropia. For example, a patient of mine is a well-known chef who told me that his world exists mainly at arm's length. We agreed before surgery that -1.50 D would be our refractive target. Conversely, for a pilot, the refractive goal would undoubtedly be plano. Ascertaining individual preferences, especially if a specific occupational concern is important, can convert those patients who clearly know what they want into a small army of ambassadors for your practice.

THE COMPONENTS OF ACCURATE CALCULATIONS

For normal eyes, using the best aspects of today's technology makes it possible to consistently achieve highly accurate postoperative results. As always, however, the devil is in the details, meaning that we have to execute all components of the exercise correctly. Patient selection, accurate keratometry, the method of biometry, the IOL power formula selected, and even the surgical technique all play important roles. To concentrate all of our attention on biometry is to miss the point. For example, if the keratometry is off by 0.75 D, then the final postoperative refraction will be off by that same amount. Using the SRK/T formula in the setting of high-axial hyperopia will probably produce a hyperopic result. If the capsulorhexis is much larger than the optic of the IOL, a myopic shift may occur following the contraction of the capsular bag. Finally, knowing when to repeat a measurement that does not fall within an established set of validation criteria is as important as knowing how to carry out the measurement correctly in the first place. Highly accurate IOL power calculations are the result of a collection of many nuances, all linked together and each needing optimization.

AN EXCITING TIME

Refractive surprises have occurred ever since Sir Harold Ridley implanted the first IOL in 1949. With steady technological advances, the overall accuracy of our refractive outcomes has generally doubled every 5 to 10 years. With the introduction of the IOLMaster (Carl Zeiss Meditec Inc., Dublin, CA) in North America in 2000, refractive outcomes within 0.25 D of the targeted refraction became a reality for the first time. This milestone allows us to set our sights on far more sophisticated endeavors, such as allowing our patients to fully enjoy the correction of spherical aberration. We are clearly entering a very exciting time in the history of IOL power calculations.

There are several patient groups for whom it is not always possible to deliver a highly accurate refractive result, however. At present, consistently accurate refractive outcomes remain elusive for those with prior keratorefractive surgery, keratoconus, extreme axial myopia with posterior staphyloma, nanophthalmic eyes, or eyes with silicone oil.

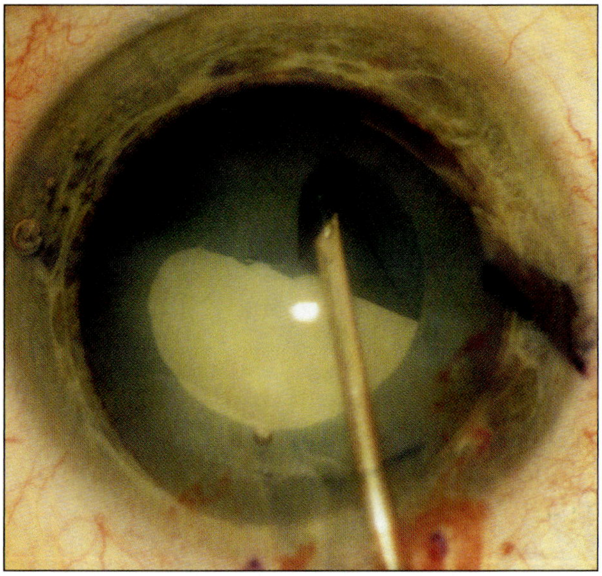

Figure 1. In terms of highly accurate refractive outcomes, the proper construction of the capsulorhexis is the defining portion of the surgical procedure.

BASIC KERATOMETRY

When was the last time you calibrated all of the keratometers in your office? If your office has more than one keratometer, or employs several different methods of corneal power measurement (eg, simulated keratometry, automated keratometry, and manual keratometry), multiple instruments will introduce another variable into the process. I strongly recommend assigning a single instrument that was recently calibrated against a set of standard calibration spheres to the task of all pre- and postoperative keratometry.

It is also helpful for each office to establish a set of keratometry validation guidelines. In my office, if the Ks are very flat (less than 40.00 D) or very steep (greater than 48.00 D), a second person double-checks the measurements and signs the chart. If the total keratometric power between eyes is greater than1.50 D, a second staff member repeats the measurements. If the mires are distorted, or the total astigmatism for either eye is greater than 4.00 D, we will typically obtain a topographic axial map to screen for keratoconus. Lastly, if there are any difficulties in obtaining the measurements that cannot be resolved, we ask the patient to return for repeat keratometry on another day.

BIOMETRY

There are currently four methods available for ophthalmic biometry: applanation A-scan; immersion A-scan; immersion A/B-scan; and optical coherence biometry using the IOLMaster.

Surgeons interested in highly accurate outcomes have mostly abandoned applanation biometry, which yields a falsely short axial length due to variable amounts of corneal compression. It is also highly operator dependent and often leads to corneal irritation. Of the ultrasound-based biometric methods, immersion biometry is a much better choice. Although it has the same 10-MHz resolution as the applanation method, it is much more consistent because there is no corneal compression and the measurement displayed is closer to the true axial length. Contrary to popular belief, the immersion technique is actually quite simple to perform, especially when used in conjunction with the Prager shell. Moreover, because immersion biometry is far more consistent than applanation biometry, it often takes less time.

The main limitation to accuracy with 10-MHz A-scan ultrasound is that it uses a relatively broad, low-resolution sound wave to measure the distance from the corneal vertex to the vitreoretinal interface. Moreover, the region surrounding the fovea has a variable retinal thickness, with the foveal center being thinner than the area immediately adjacent to it. Typically, both of these areas are included in an A-scan biometric measurement.

The most sophisticated form of ultrasound-based biometry is a combined immersion vector A/B-scan. By this technique, familiar to our retinal colleagues, a horizontal immersion B-scan is carried out with a simultaneous vector A-scan that can be manually positioned to measure from the center of the corneal vertex to the location of the fovea.[1] The disadvantages of A/B biometry are that the equipment is generally somewhat expensive and a higher level of operator skill is required. In my office, if we are not able to use the IOLMaster due to the presence of a dense axial opacity, immersion A/B biometry is our method of choice.

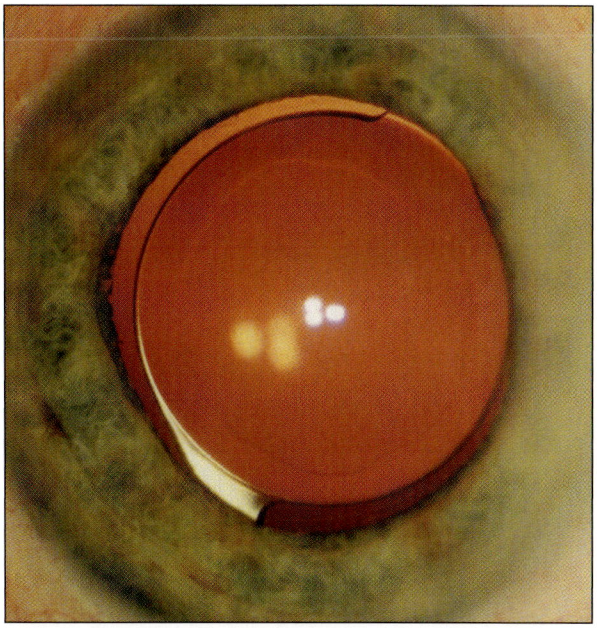

Figure 2. The capsulorhexis should be round, centered, and smaller than the optic of the IOL.

THE IOLMASTER

In my opinion, the IOLMaster represents the single most important advance in IOL power calculations since the introduction of ultrasound biometry 3 decades ago. Interestingly, the technological foundation of this instrument is based on principles laid down during the 19th century by the German-American physicist Albert Michelson.[2] More than 100 years after its invention, the Michelson interferometer was introduced to ophthalmology via our colleagues in astronomy and physics. It is likely that, in the future, similar technological advancements will come to us from other unrelated disciplines and will have an equally important impact.

One of several reasons why the IOLMaster has a much higher resolution than ultrasound is that the axial-length measurement is based on a very short 780-nm light wave, rather than a much longer 10-MHz sound wave. By optical coherence biometry, the IOLMaster measures the distance from the corneal vertex to the retinal pigment epithelium (not affected by variations in retinal thickness) and then subtracts the foveal thickness. This approximation to an axial length by immersion ultrasound is based on a comparison to the exquisitely accurate Grieshaber Biometric System (Alcon Grieshaber AG, Schaffhausen, Switzerland), an ultra-high–resolution ultrasound biometer that employs four 40-MHz counters and is capable of an astonishing accuracy of 20μm.[3] In essence, the IOLMaster is the equivalent of an upright, noncontact, immersion A-scan but with a fivefold increase in resolution.[4]

There are four situations in which the IOLMaster is best suited for accurate biometry: (1) nanophthalmia or extreme axial hyperopia, because small errors in axial length are important; (2) extreme axial myopia, especially in the presence of a peripapillary posterior staphyloma; (3) prior retinal detachment with silicone oil; and (4) pseudophakia, polypseudophakia, and phakic IOLs. Ophthalmologists are now starting to measure eyes that develop cataracts after phakic IOL implantation, and the IOLMaster can measure straight through the phakic IOL on the phakic setting with excellent results.[5]

When the IOLMaster debuted, it was presented mostly as a point-and-shoot device with which the axial-length display with the highest signal-to-noise ratio was considered the best choice. Unfortunately, it is not quite that simple. Using the IOLMaster requires the correct interpretation of the axial-length display, with the signal-to-noise ratio being helpful but not the most important determiner of the overall quality of the axial length measurement. Ideally, the axial-length display should have tall and slender primary maxima, with a thin and well-defined termination, much like the familiar silhouette of the Chrysler building in New York City.[4] Careful attention to the axial-length display will avoid double peaks and other problems that could lead to potentially inaccurate measurements.

VALIDATION GUIDELINES FOR AXIAL LENGTH

If the preoperative refraction and keratometry are equal between both eyes, but one eye measures 28mm and the other eye measures 26 mm, something is obviously wrong. A 27-mm axial length displayed for a patient with a +4.00 D refractive error suggests an error. As originally suggested by Holladay,[6] it is important to follow a set of axial-length validation guidelines as the basis of a protocol to double-check any measurements that may not correlate with the overall clinical picture. In my office, if the difference between eyes is greater than 0.33 mm, a second person independently verifies the results. If the axial length is less than 22 mm or greater than 26 mm, a second person reviews or repeats the measurements. We do likewise if the axial length correlates poorly with the refractive data or if there is any difficulty in obtaining consistent measurements.

IOL FORMULAE

In North America, the three commonly used, theoretical IOL power calculation formulas (Hoffer Q, Holladay 1, and SRK/T) are derived from the same mathematical backbone. The main difference between these third-generation, two-variable formulas is the way in which they calculate the final position of the IOL, commonly known as the *effective thin-lens position.*[7]

Limitations of all third-generation, theoretical, two-variable formulas are that they work best near schematic eye parameters, apply a number of broad assumptions to all eyes, and, apart from the lens constant, predict the final position of the optic of the IOL based solely on central corneal power and axial length. For example, some formulae assume that the anterior and posterior segments of the eye are mostly proportional, or that there is always the same relationship between central corneal power and the effective lens position, which is not always true, especially in axial hyperopia.[7,8]

By the late 1980s, the Holladay 1 formula was available, which works well for eyes with normal and long axial lengths. This formula was followed in 1990 by the SRK/T formula, which works well for normal-to-moderately long axial lengths. Several years later, the Hoffer Q formula was added, which works well for eyes with short and normal axial lengths. Presently, regression formulae such as Binkhorst II, SRK I, and SRK II are now mostly of historical interest only. Interestingly, SRK II is still widely used by many in spite of its obvious limitations.

In 1991, Wolfgang Haigis, MS, PhD, the head of the Biometry Department of the University of Würzburg Eye Hospital in Germany, published the Haigis formula. Using the same mathematical backbone as other theoretic formulas, the Haigis formula approaches the problem of IOL power accuracy with three constants (a0, a1, and a2) and adds a measured anterior chamber depth for a third required variable. With the a0 constant optimized in a manner similar to SRK/T, and the a1 and a2 constants based on schematic eye parameters, the formula performs as if it were a very good third-generation two-variable formula. When all three constants are optimized by regression analysis based on surgeon-specific IOL data, however, the range of the Haigis formula can be extended greatly to cover both high-axial hyperopia and high-axial myopia. The main limitations to using the Haigis formula for all axial lengths are that only Dr. Haigis and I presently carry out the required regression analysis and a patient database of approximately 200 cases containing a wide range of axial lengths is required.

The Holladay 2 formula, available since 1998, is considered by many to be the most accurate of the theoretic formulas currently offered. The formula is easy to optimize and works well across a wide range of axial lengths. Its main limitations are that it requires the manual input of seven variables and it is relatively expensive to purchase. Surgical practices serious about their refractive outcomes will typically use the Holladay 2 formula.

Because most biometric equipment already comes with several theoretic formulas, a simple rule to follow is to use the Holladay 1 formula for normal-to-long eyes and the Hoffer Q formula for normal-to-short eyes. However, it should eventually be the goal of every surgical practice to use a more modern formula such as Haigis or Holladay 2.

What are useful IOL power calculation validation guidelines? Of course, both eyes should be measured at the same time to serve as a basis for comparison. If the IOL power difference between eyes is greater than 1.00 D, or if there is any question about the accuracy of the axial length or keratometry, the results should be double-checked. Also, if the calculated IOL power does not match what you expected to see, such as a +28.00-D IOL recommended for an axial myope, repeating the measurements is mandatory.

SURGICAL TECHNIQUE

For highly accurate refractive outcomes, the capsulorhexis should be considered the defining portion of the surgical procedure (Figure 1). Ideally, the capsulorhexis should be round, smaller than the optic, and centered. If carried out correctly, the optic of the lens implant should remain at the plane of the zonules. If the capsulorhexis is much larger than the optic, the forces of capsular bag contraction may shift the optic anteriorly, inducing a myopic shift late in the postoperative course. Also, at the conclusion of the case, the optic of the IOL should be centered directly beneath the capsulorhexis so that the capsular bag can uniformly shrink-wrap around it (Figure 2). This approach is another important step for ensuring consistent refractive outcomes. A failure to pay close attention to the capsulorhexis can impact on the refractive outcome more than ultrasound-based biometry or keratometry.

SUMMARY

Understand the current limitations of technology. There are some patients to whom you cannot promise a highly accurate outcome. Assign a single instrument for the task of keratometry for added consistency. Use the IOLMaster or immersion biometry rather than an applanation technique. Develop a set of validation criteria for each part of the measurement process and have a second person carefully review and/or repeat any part that falls outside of these guidelines. Consider switching to one of the newer IOL power calculation formulae for improved accuracy. Optimize your surgical technique by making the capsulorhexis round, smaller than the optic, and centered. By embracing current technology and paying careful attention to details, every ophthalmologist can achieve highly accurate refractive outcomes. ■

This article originally appeared in the March 2006 issue of CRSToday.

1. Hill WE, Byrne SF. Complex axial length measurements & unusual IOL power calculations. In: *Focal Points: Clinical Modules for Ophthalmologists.* San Francisco: American Academy of Ophthalmology; 2004;22:9.

2. Hill WE. The IOLMaster. *Techniques in Ophthalmology.* 2003;1:1:62.

3. Haigis W, Lege B, Miller N, Schneider B. Comparison of immersion ultrasound biometry and partial coherence interferometry for intraocular lens calculation according to Haigis. *Graefes Arch Clin Exp Ophthalmol.* 2000;238:765-773.

4. Vogel A, Dick B, Krummenauer F. Reproducibility of optical biometry using partial coherence interferometry. Intraobserver and interobserver reliability. *J Cataract Refract Surg.* 2001;27:1961-1968.

5. Salz JJ, Neuhann T, Trindade F, et al. Consultation section: cataract surgical problem. *J Cataract Refract Surg.* 2003;29:1058-1063.

6. Holladay JT, Prager TC, Chandler TY, et al. A three part system for refining intraocular lens power calculations. *J Cataract Refract Surg.* 1988;14:17-24.

7. Holladay JT. Standardizing constants for ultrasonic biometry, keratometry, and intraocular lens power calculations. *J Cataract Refract Surg.* 1997;23:1356-1370.

8. Holladay JT, Gills JP, Leidlen J, Cherchio M. Achieving emmetropia in extremely short eyes with two piggyback posterior chamber intraocular lenses. *Ophthalmology.* 1996;103:1118-1123.

CHAPTER 119

Spherical Aberration 101

LISA MARTÉN, MD; TRACY SWARTZ, OD; AND MING WANG, MD, PHD

Spherical aberration is an imperfection in an image that is due to the spherical shape of the lens or mirror used to create that image. There is an intrinsic defect in spherical mirrors that prohibits the mirror from focusing light toward a single point. Light rays that strike the outer edges of the mirror focus at a different point than those rays that strike the inner portions of the mirror, and the result is a blurry image. The image of a point formed by a lens with a spherical aberration is usually a bright dot surrounded by a halo of light. Spherical aberration softens the contrast and blurs the details of images[1] as if looking through a fog. This article provides a short, basic review of spherical aberration.

The quantity and sign of spherical aberrations relies on the wavelength of light. A spherical aberration depends upon the focal length, aperture, shape, and distance of an object from the visual axis. The resulting amount of aberrant light, or image blur, is relative to the diameter and inversely proportional to the focal length of the lens/mirror. Spherical aberration is responsible for the blurred form at negative distances and a smoother appearance at positive distances.[2] Off-axis rays of light are focused closer to the lens than the paraxial rays. In simple terms, as one moves away from the center of the lens, the refractive (light-bending) power of the lens increases. When a light bundle strikes at a lens position farther from the lens' center, it will be bent more than when the light bundle strikes at a lens position closer to the center. Hence, along the radial direction, the farther away the point on the lens at which a light bundle strikes, the more powerful refractively the lens becomes. Depending on the focal point at which someone is looking, the center of the image will be clearly focused, while the edges of the field appear fuzzy and dim.

HOW TO DECREASE SPHERICAL ABERRATION

Because rays of light spread across several points on the z plane along its axis, the intensity of the light as well as its lateral and axial resolution are decreased. As someone views an image through different points along the focal axis, the image can lose detail and become distorted.[3]

Spherical aberration is important to the clarity of images produced through photography, microscopes, telescopes, and the human eye. Various methods can minimize spherical aberration and improve an image's quality. Corrective factors are employed, for example, in the Hubble telescope. Mathematical formulae are used to calculate an appropriate series of lenses that will reduce spherical aberration. Scientists can apply the Coddington shape and position factors to minimize the bending of light into its best form, thereby reducing spherical aberration.

Spherical mirrors cause most spherical aberrations and are commonly corrected with a parabolic mirror. Parabolic optics correct the aberration, because their outer edges have a different curvature than the center, resulting in sharp, clear images. In microscopy, common methods used to minimize spherical aberration include decreasing the size of the aperture and using collared water or oil immersion. The system must be adjusted, however, for different focal planes. Newer, self-adjusting programs have been developed for microscopy to automatically set the optics to minimize spherical aberration.[3]

SPHERICAL ABERRATION OF THE HUMAN EYE

Corneal asphericity (Q-value) has a value of -0.50 in an ideal visual system. This value is indicative of a prolate shape and results in zero spherical aberration. Unfortunately, a zero Q-value is not anatomically possible due to the necessary framework of the junction between the cornea and the sclera. Instead the human Q-value averages -0.26 due to the limbal transition. The human visual system therefore suffers from a small amount of spherical aberration, which rises as the pupil's size increases.

The natural curvature of the cornea induces positive spherical aberration, although the relaxed natural lens induces negative spherical aberration.[2,4] The spherical aberration of the posterior corneal surface is negative when a person is young and becomes positive with age, thus making the posterior corneal measurement important for calculating the total spherical aberration of the entire eye.[2]

The anterior surface of the cornea, internal optics of the posterior

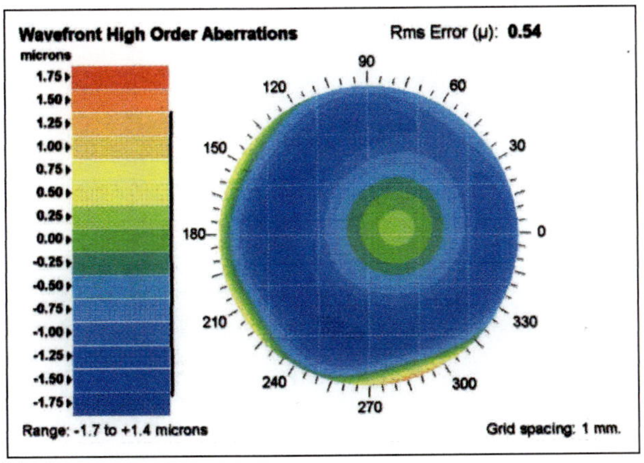

Figure 1. Pictured is a wavefront aberrometry map of a patient after myopic LASIK.

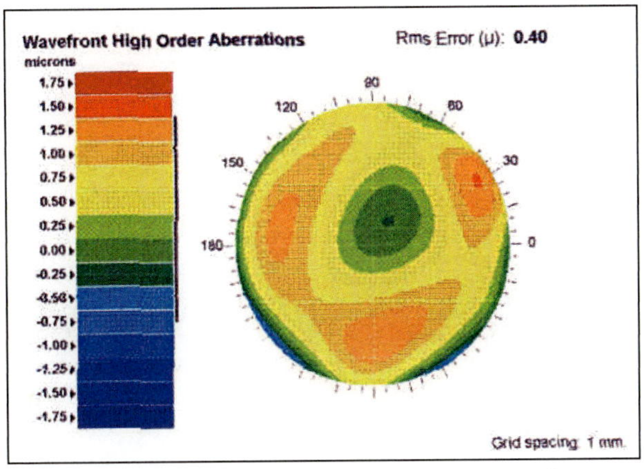

Figure 2. Pictured is a wavefront aberrometry map of a patient after hyperopic LASIK.

cornea, and crystalline lens all contribute to the aberration of a wavefront passing through the eye.[5] It is possible to measure the lower and higher optical aberrations with a wavefront aberrometer. By shining a small spot of light onto the retina and observing the amount that is reflected from within the eye, one can quantify the amount of lower-order aberrations (eg, astigmatism, myopia, hyperopia) and higher-order aberrations (eg, coma, spherical aberration). The Hartmann-Shack sensor, which was originally developed for measuring the aberrations of optical instruments and general refracting surfaces in astronomical telescopes, is now used to measure aberrations of the human eye. The Hartmann-Shack sensor sends information to a computer software program, which decomposes wavefront aberrations into a set of Zernike polynomials.[6] Other techniques include ray tracing and instruments based on the Tscherning principle.

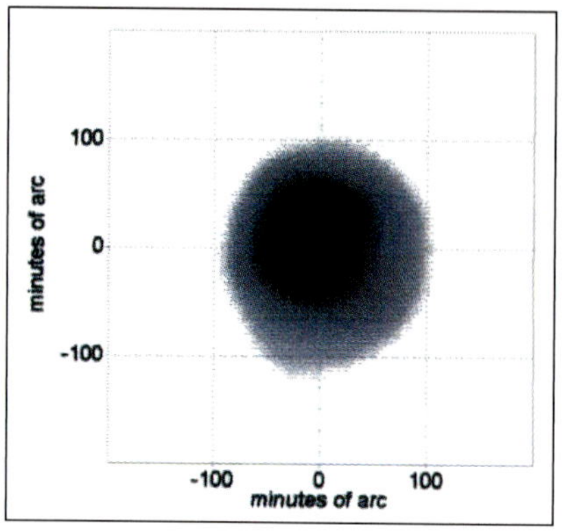

Figure 3. Pictured is a simulated image of a point of light as seen by a patient with increased spherical aberration.

In the human eye, it is difficult to insert lenses of different sizes and powers to minimize spherical aberration. Given the dynamic change of spherical aberration, many would argue against such a procedure. Contact lenses can be easily changed and are one option for correction. The design of regular soft contact lenses of high negative or positive power should aim to produce -0.07 D/mm of spherical aberration. Patients can usually tolerate an interval between -0.15 and +0.01 D/mm of spherical aberration for a 6-mm pupil.[7,8] After cataract surgery, specially designed aspheric contact lenses can compensate for the cornea's positive spherical aberration that tends to increase with age.

Wavefront aberrometry may identify patients who have significant amounts of spherical aberration prior to elective keratorefractive surgery, and wavefront systems to program computerized ablation may prevent an increase in visual symptoms related to corneal properties. Spherical aberration may result from large changes in the corneal curvature such as that induced by myopic or hyperopic LASIK. Note the effect of the flattening of the central cornea with myopic treatments (Figure 1) and that of a hyperopic treatment (Figure 2). The aberrations are in opposite directions. The effect of spherical aberration can be simulated using Snellen E representation as well as in the point of light as shown in Figure 3.

Advances in keratorefractive and IOL technology have incorporated the reduction of spherical aberration into the optical correction. IOLs with negative spherical aberration can negate or offset the positive spherical aberration of the cornea.[9] Future technologies will increasingly consider both the lens' and cornea's aberration, to yield optimal overall optical performance.

IN SUMMARY

Understanding spherical aberration in the human eye is important in modern-day refractive surgery procedures. It is present in the cornea as well as the crystalline lens in their native states. Furthermore, spherical aberrations can be created iatrogenically by keratorefractive or lenticular surgeries. The pupil's size, the lens' shape, and the cornea's curvature and shape all influence spherical aberration. New technologies, including wavefront imaging, have ushered in a new era of understanding the human eye's higher-order aberrations. Technologies such as wavefront-driven or corneal topography-based treatments are being developed to minimize the spherical aberration created by surgeons. ■

This article originally appeared in the November/December 2006 issue of CRSToday.

1. Smith WJ. Modern optical engineering. 3rd ed. New York, NY: McGraw-Hill; 2000.
2. Sicam VA, Dubbelman M, van der Heijde RG. Spherical aberration of the anterior and posterior surfaces of the human cornea. *J Opt Soc Am A Opt Image Sci Vis.* 2006;23:544-549.
3. Monks C. Optical spherical aberration correction. *GIT Imaging and Microscopy.* March 2004;2-3.
4. Smith G, Cox MJ, Calver R, Garner LF. The spherical aberration of the crystalline lens of the human eye. *Vision Res.* 2001;41:235-243.
5. Kelly JE, Mihashi T, Howland HC. Compensation of corneal horizontal/vertical astigmatism, lateral coma, and spherical aberration by internal optics of the eye. *J Vis.* 2004;4:262-271.
6. Carvalho LA, Castro JC, Carvalho LA. Measuring higher order optical aberrations of the human eye: techniques and applications. *Braz J Med Biol Res.* 2002;35:1395-1406.
7. Legras R, Chateau N, Charman WN. Assessment of just-noticeable differences for refractive errors and spherical aberration using visual simulation. *Optom Vis Sci.* 2004;81:718-728.
8. Dietze HH, Cox MJ. Correcting ocular spherical aberration with soft contact lenses. *J Opt Soc Am A Opt Image Sci Vis.* 2004;21:473-485.
9. Holladay JT, Piers PA, Kozanyi G, et al. A new intraocular lens designed to reduce spherical aberration of pseudophakic eyes. *J Refract Surg.* 2002;18:683-701.

CHAPTER 120

Maximizing Optical Quality

MARK PACKER, MD; I. HOWARD FINE, MD; AND RICHARD S. HOFFMAN, MD

The youthful, accommodating, emmetropic, and minimally aberrated eye is the standard by which the results of cataract and refractive surgery are evaluated.[1] The erosion of accommodation and the decline in functional vision that occur with age[2] are linked to changes in the crystalline lens.[3,4] Cataract and refractive lens exchange surgery offer an intuitive avenue for correcting presbyopia as well as for reversing increased lenticular spherical aberration. Because the optical wavefront of the cornea remains essentially stable throughout life,[5] refractive lens exchange represents a permanent solution to the challenges of restoring accommodation and achieving a youthful quality of vision.

The positive spherical aberration of a spherical pseudophakic IOL tends to increase total optical aberrations, a problem that has led to the development of aspheric IOLs.[6] These designs may reduce or eliminate ocular spherical aberration and improve functional vision compared with a spherical pseudophakic implant.

Three aspheric IOL designs are currently marketed in the US: the Tecnis Z9000 IOL (Advanced Medical Optics, Inc., Santa Ana, CA); the Acrysof IQ IOL (Alcon Laboratories, Inc., Fort Worth, TX); and the Sofport AO IOL (Bausch & Lomb, Rochester, NY).

ASPHERIC IOLS

Tecnis IOL

The Tecnis IOL was designed with a modified prolate anterior surface to compensate for the average corneal spherical aberration found in the adult eye. This lens introduces -0.27 μm of spherical aberration into the eye. The results for clinical studies of the Tecnis IOL, which were submitted to the FDA, showed that the IOL eliminated patients' mean spherical aberration and significantly improved their functional vision compared with a standard spherical IOL.[7]

Acrysof IQ IOL

The Acrysof IQ IOL incorporates both the ultraviolet- and blue-light–filtering chromophores found in the single-piece acrylic Acrysof Natural IOL (Alcon Laboratories, Inc). The Acrysof IQ lens, however, has a posterior, aspheric surface designed to compensate for spherical aberration by addressing the effects of overrefraction at the periphery. It adds -0.20 μm of spherical aberration to the eye.

Sofport AO IOL

The Sofport AO IOL is an aspheric IOL that has been specifically designed with zero spherical aberration so that it will not contribute to any preexisting higher-order aberrations. This lens' silicone, sharp-edged optic design incorporates haptics with zero angulation to permit atraumatic placement in the capsular bag.

STUDIES COMPARING DIFFERENT ASPHERIC IOLS

According to the literature, the Tecnis IOL has demonstrably reduced spherical aberration and provided superior contrast sensitivity and contrast acuity in comparison to a variety of spherical IOLs (as of press time, there were no peer-reviewed publications evaluating the clinical results with either of the other two aspheric IOLs available in the US).[8-15] Data show that the mean spherical aberration in the eyes implanted with the Tecnis IOL is, as stated by executives from the FDA, "not different from zero."[16] Subjects in the FDA-monitored night driving simulation study of the Tecnis IOL performed functionally better in 20 of 24 driving conditions (and statistically better in 10 conditions) when using BSCVA with the eye implanted with the Tecnis IOL compared to BSCVA with the eye implanted with the Acrysof IQ.[6] These findings represent the basis for the FDA labeling indicating that the Tecnis IOL improves functional vision and enhances highway safety "for elderly drivers and those with whom they share the road."[6] Optical laboratory studies' results nevertheless have cast doubt on the efficacy of IOLs with negative spherical aberration (eg, the Tecnis and Acrysof IQ) due to the range of tilt and decentration of pseudophakic lenses in general[17,18].

MULTIFOCAL IOLS

Array Lens

From 1997 until 2005, the only FDA-approved multifocal IOL available was the Array IOL (Advanced Medical Optics, Inc.) This zonal progressive lens has five concentric zones on its anterior surface. Zones one, three, and five are distance dominant, whereas zones two and four are near dominant. The lens has an aspheric component whereby each zone repeats the entire refractive sequence corresponding to distance, intermediate, and near foci. This configuration provides patients with vision over a range of distances.

The lens uses 100% of the incoming available light and is weighted for optimum light distribution. With typically sized pupils, approximately half of the light is distributed for distance, one third for near vision, and the remainder for intermediate vision. Because the lens utilizes a continuous surface construction, there is no loss of light through diffraction and no degradation of image quality as a result of surface discontinuities.[19] The lens has a foldable silicone optic that is 6mm in diameter, PMMA haptics, and an overall diameter of 13mm. It can be inserted through a clear corneal incision that is 2.8mm wide by means of the Unfolder injector system (Advanced Medical Optics, Inc.).

Rezoom Lens

In 2005, the FDA approved two new multifocal designs, the Rezoom IOL (Advanced Medical Optics, Inc.) and the Acrysof Restor IOL (Alcon Laboratories, Inc.). The former represents new engineering of the Array platform, including a hydrophobic acrylic material and a shift of the zonal progression. Zones one, three, and five are all distance dominant, whereas zones two and four are near dominant. The large, distance-dominant, central zone one is designed to provide vision in bright light (eg, for daytime driving). The Rezoom IOL's expanded zone three facilitates distance vision in moderate-to-low light when the pupil is more fully dilated, and zone five is designed to supply distance vision in low light (eg, for nighttime driving). Zone two, the large zone immediately peripheral to zone one, is intended to give near vision in moderate-to-low light. Zone four serves to provide near vision for lower-light situations. Aspheric transitions between the zones offer intermediate vision. The near-dominant zones provide +3.50 D of add power at the IOL's plane for near vision, yielding approximately +2.57 D of add power in the spectacle plane. This power addition translates to a near point of vision of 39cm or 16 inches.

Optiedge technology (Advanced Medical Optics, Inc.) inhibits the migration of lens epithelial cells without causing visual disturbances or glare (sata on file with Advanced Medical Optics, Inc.). Buehl et al[20] demonstrated low rates of posterior capsular opacification (PCO) in cataract patients implanted with an IOL that has a modified, sharp, posterior optic edge design.

The Rezoom IOL reduces the amount of light that goes to the near foci in low-light conditions (ie, larger pupils) and reallocates it to the distance foci. The intermediate power of this lens allows the formation of images on the retina, even if the distance and near powers form slightly out-of-focus images. The intermediate power should theoretically reduce the unfocused light on the retina, leading to fewer halos and less glare. Reduced photic phenomena (such as internal reflections and edge glares) and minimized PCO are the goals of the IOL's Optiedge design.

Acrysof Restor Lens

The Acrysof Restor IOL employs a central apodized diffractive area surrounded by a purely refractive outer zone. This lens has a central 3.6-mm diffractive optic region. Twelve concentric diffractive zones on the anterior surface of the lens divide the light into two diffractive orders to create two lens powers. A region that has no diffractive structure over the remainder of the 6.0-mm–diameter lens surrounds the central 3.6-mm zone. The near correction is calculated at +4.00 D at the lens' plane, resulting in approximately +3.20 D at the spectacle plane. This add power provides a defocus curve of 6.00 D of pseudoaccommodation at the 20/40 level.

The apodized diffractive structure of the Acrysof Restor IOL provides a gradual centrifugal decrease in step height of 12 diffractive circular structures. This design creates a transition of light between the foci and theoretically reduces disturbing optical phenomena like glare and halos. The results of a current study of the Acrysof Restor IOL show excellent near visual acuity and no compromise of subjects' distance vision, with approximately 80% not needing spectacles for near, distance, or intermediate vision.[21]

With the Acrysof Restor lens, the logic of placing the diffractive element centrally depends upon the near synkinesis of convergence, accommodation, and miosis. As the pupil constricts, the focal dominance of the lens shifts from almost purely distance to equal parts distance and near. This approach conserves efficiency for mesopic activities when the pupil is larger (eg, nighttime driving) but reduces near vision under mesopic conditions (eg, reading a menu by candlelight).

Comparative Studies

Many investigators have evaluated both the objective and subjective qualities of contrast sensitivity, stereoacuity, glare, and photic phenomena following the implantation of multifocal IOLs. Refractive multifocal IOLs such as the Array are better than diffractive multifocal IOLs in terms of contrast sensitivity and glare.[22] Recent reports comparing refractive and diffractive IOLs, however, revealed similar distance-vision qualities evaluated by modulation transfer functions but better near vision for the diffractive lens.

In terms of contrast sensitivity testing, the Array produces a small loss of contrast sensitivity that is equivalent to one line of visual acuity at the 11% contrast level using Regan contrast sensitivity charts.[23] This loss of contrast sensitivity at low levels of contrast is only present when the Array is implanted monocularly. It is not seen in patients with bilateral implants and binocular testing.[24] Regan testing, however, is not as sensitive as sine wave grating tests that evaluate a broader range of spatial frequencies. With the latter approach, reduced contrast sensitivity occurred in eyes implanted with the Array in the lower spatial frequencies compared with monofocal lenses when a halogen glare source was absent. When a moderate glare source was introduced, no significant difference in contrast sensitivity between the multifocal or monofocal lenses was observed.[25]

Practitioners implanting the Array have noted a period of neural adaptation in patients.[26] Similarly, researchers have shown that contrast sensitivity normalizes over a 6-month period.[27]

According to recent reports, there is a reduction in tritan color contrast sensitivity function in refractive multifocal IOLs compared with monofocal lenses under conditions of glare. These differences were significant for distance vision in the lower spatial frequencies and for near vision in the low and middle spatial frequencies.[28] A newer aspheric multifocal IOL, the Progress 3 (Domilens Laboratories, Lyon, France; not available in the US), also significantly lowers mean contrast sensitivity with the Pelli-Robson chart when compared to monofocal IOLs.[29]

Ultimately, these contrast sensitivity tests reveal that, in order to deliver multiple foci to the retina, there is always some loss of efficiency with multifocal IOLs when compared with monofocal IOLs. Contrast sensitivity loss, random-dot stereopsis, and aniseikonia improve, however, when multifocal IOLs are placed bilaterally versus unilaterally.[30] A recent publication evaluating a three-zone refractive multifocal IOL showed an improvement in stereopsis, less aniseikonia, and a greater likelihood of spectacle independence with bilateral versus unilateral implantation.[31] There is also evidence that contrast sensitivity with multifocal IOLs improves over time, approximating the levels found with spherical monofocal lenses by 6 months postoperatively.[25]

Disadvantages

One of the persistent drawbacks of multifocal lens technology has been the potential for patients to see glare or halos around point sources of light at night in the early weeks and months following surgery.[32,33] A meta-analysis of the peer-reviewed literature on multifocal IOLs shows a greater incidence of glare and halos with the multifocal than monofocal IOLs.[34] According to a clinical investigation of the Acrysof Restor IOL, 23.2% of subjects implanted bilaterally complained of moderate halos at night, although 7.2% complained of severe halos, versus 1.9% and 1.3%, respectively, of subjects implanted bilaterally with a control monofocal IOL.[35] Severe halos were reported by 15.3% of subjects bilaterally implanted with the Array IOL, the Rezoom IOL's precedecessor.[36] Fortunately, most people learn to disregard halos with time, and bilateral implantation appears to improve these subjective symptoms.[37]

ASPHERIC MULTIFOCAL IOL

The Tecnis Multifocal IOL (Advanced Medical Optics, Inc.) is a wavefront-designed, diffractive, foldable IOL with a modified prolate anterior surface. It has received CE Marking for the treatment of presbyopia, and clinical trials in the United States are ongoing. Optical bench studies reveal a superior modulation transfer function at both distance and near compared with standard monofocal IOLs with a 5-mm pupil and equivalence to standard monofocal IOLs with a 4-mm pupil. When compared to the Array multifocal IOL, the Tecnis Multifocal IOL performed better in the presence of a 2-mm pupil at near and a 5-mm pupil at distance and near. From these laboratory studies, it appears that combining diffractive multifocal optics with an aspheric, prolate design may enhance the functional vision of pseudophakic patients.[38]

Huetz et al[39] performed a prospective, randomized study comparing three bilaterally implanted multifocal IOLs: the Array; the Acrysof Restor; and the Tecnis Multifocal. They found faster uncorrected and best distance-corrected reading speeds among patients with the Tecnis Multifocal than the other lenses under both photopic and mesopic conditions. The reading speed with the Tecnis Multifocal was significantly faster with near correction under photopic conditions, and it was significantly better than in patients with the Acrysof Restor (but not the Array) under mesopic conditions. The latter finding probably reflects the fact that the larger pupil under mesopic conditions benefits near vision with the zonal progressive Array but reduces near vision with the apodized diffractive Acrysof Restor. Anecdotally, our patients, after receiving refractive multifocal lenses (Array and Rezoom), have remarked that they read more easily in dim versus bright light.

ONE SIZE DOES NOT FIT ALL

The availability of presbyopia-correcting IOLs, refractive lens exchange, and customized aspheric IOLs is changing ophthalmic practice. Informed consent takes on a new meaning when the surgeon and the patient decide together which IOL technology best fits his lifestyle and visual demands. Customizing the selection of IOLs is now essential to the practice of refractive lenticular surgery. ■

This article originally appeared in the November/December 2006 issue of CRSToday.

1. Schallhorn SC. Deciphering wavefront higher-order aberrations. *Cataract & Refractive Surgery Today.* 2002;2:1:47-48.

2. Rohaly AM, Owsley C. Modeling the contrast-sensitivity functions of older adults. *J Opt Soc Am A.* 1993;10:1591-1599.
3. Artal P, Berrio E, Guirao A, Piers P. Contribution of the cornea and internal surfaces to the change of ocular aberrations with age. *J Opt Soc Am A.* 2002;19:137-143.
4. Glasser A, Campbell MC. Biometric, optical and physical changes in the isolated human crystalline lens with age in relation to presbyopia. *Vision Res.* 1999;39:1991-2015.
5. Wang L, Dai E, Koch DD, Nathoo A. Optical aberrations of the human anterior cornea. *J Cataract Refract Surg.* 2003;29:1514-1521.
6. Holladay JT, Piers PA, Koranyi G, et al. A new intraocular lens design to reduce spherical aberration of pseudophakic eyes. *J Refract Surg.* 2002;18:683-691.
7. Tecnis Foldable Ultraviolet Light-Absorbing Posterior Chamber IOL [package insert]. Santa Ana, CA: Advanced Medical Optics, Inc.; 2005.
8. Packer M, Fine IH, Hoffman RS, Piers PA. Initial clinical experience with an anterior surface modified prolate intraocular lens. *J Refract Surg.* 2002;18:692-696.
9. Mester U, Dillinger P, Anterist N. Impact of a modified optic design on visual function: clinical comparative study. *J Cataract Refract Surg.* 2003;29:652-660.
10. Packer M, Fine IH, Hoffman RS, Piers PA. Improved functional vision with a modified prolate intraocular lens. *J Cataract Refract Surg.* 2004;30:986-992.
11. Bellucci R, Scialdone A, Buratto L, et al. Visual acuity and contrast sensitivity comparison between Tecnis and AcrySof SA60AT intraocular lenses: a multicenter randomized study. *J Cataract Refract Surg.* 2005;31:712-717.
12. Kennis H, Huygens M, Callebaut F. Comparing the contrast sensitivity of a modified prolate anterior surface IOL and of two spherical IOLs. *Bull Soc Belge Ophtalmol.* 2004;294:49-58.
13. Kershner RM. Retinal image contrast and functional visual performance with aspheric, silicone, and acrylic intraocular lenses: prospective evaluation. *J Cataract Refract Surg.* 2003;29:1684-1694.
14. Ricci F, Scuderi G, Missiroli F, et al. Low contrast visual acuity in pseudophakic patients implanted with an anterior surface modified prolate intraocular lens. *Acta Ophthalmol Scand.* 2004;82:718-722.
15. Martinez Palmer A, Palacin Miranda B, Castilla Cespedes M, et al. Spherical aberration influence in visual function after cataract surgery: prospective randomized trial [in Spanish]. *Arch Soc Esp Oftalmol.* 2005;80:71-77.
16. Tecnis Foldable Ultraviolet Light-Absorbing Posterior Chamber IOL [package insert]. Santa Ana, CA: Advanced Medical Optics, Inc.; 2005.
17. Dietze HH, Cox MJ. Limitations of correcting spherical aberration with aspheric intraocular lenses. *J Refract Surg.* 2005;21(suppl):541-546.
18. Altmann GE, Nichamin LD, Lane SS, Pepose JS. Optical performance of 3 intraocular lens designs in the presence of decentration. *J Cataract Refract Surg.* 2005;31:574-585.
19. Fine IH. Design and early clinical studies of the AMO Array multifocal IOL. In: Maxwell A, Nordan LT, eds. *Current Concepts of Multifocal Intraocular Lenses.* Thorofare, NJ: Slack, Inc.; 1991:105-115.
20. Buehl W, Findl O, Menapace B, et al. Effect of an acrylic intraocular lens with a sharp posterior optic edge on posterior capsule opacification. *J Cataract Refract Surg.* 2002;28:1105-1111.
21. AcrySof ReSTOR Apodized Diffractive Optic Posterior Chamber Intraocular Lenses. Premarket Approval Application (PMA) P040020. Available at: http://www.fda.gov/cdrh/pdf4/p040020b.pdf. Accessed on December 22, 2005.
22. Pieh S, Weghaupt H, Skorpik C. Contrast sensitivity and glare disability with diffractive and refractive multifocal intraocular lenses. *J Cataract Refract Surg.* 1998;24:659-662.
23. Steinert RF, Post CT, Brint SF et al: A progressive, randomized, double-masked comparison of a zonal-progressive multifocal intraocular lens and a monofocal intraocular lens. *Ophthalmology.* 1992;99:853-861.
24. Arens B, Freudenthaler N, Quentin CD. Binocular function after bilateral implantation of monofocal and refractive multifocal intraocular lenses. *J Cataract Refract Surg.* 1999;25:399-404.
25. Schmitz S, Dick HB, Krummenauer F, et al. Contrast sensitivity and glare disability by halogen light after monofocal and multifocal lens implantation. *Br J Ophthalmol.* 2000;84:1109-1112.
26. Presbyopic lens exchange improves patients' quality of life. *Ophthalmology Times.* July 15, 2002. Available at: http://www.ophthalmologytimes.com/ophthalmologytimes/article/articleDetail.jsp?id=24614. Accessed October 18, 2005.
27. Montés-Micó R, Alió JL. Distance and near contrast sensitivity function after multifocal intraocular lens implantation. *J Cataract Refract Surg.* 2003;29:703-711.
28. Pieh S, Hanselmayer G, Lackner B, et al. Tritan colour contrast sensitivity function in refractive multifocal intraocular lenses. *Br J Ophthalmol.* 2001;85:811-815.
29. Kamlesh S, Dadeya S, Kaushik S. Contrast sensitivity and depth of focus with aspheric multifocal versus conventional monofocal intraocular lens. *Can J Ophthalmol.* 2001;36:197-201.
30. Haring G, Gronemeyer A, Hedderich J, et al. Stereoacuity and aniseikonia after unilateral and bilateral implantation of the Array refractive multifocal intraocular lens. *J Cataract Refract Surg.* 1999;25:1151-1156.
31. Shoji N, Shimizu K. Binocular function of the patient with the refractive multifocal intraocular lens. *J Cataract Refract Surg.* 2002;28:1012-1017.
32. Haring G, Dick HB, Krummenauer F, et al. Subjective photic phenomena with refractive multifocal and monofocal intraocular lenses. Results of a multicenter questionnaire. *J Cataract Refract Surg.* 2001;27:245-249.
33. Sen HN, Sarikkola AU, Uusitalo RJ, Laatikainen L. Quality of vision after AMO Array multifocal intraocular lens implantation. *J Cataract Refract Surg.* 2004;30:2483-2493.
34. Leyland M, Zinicola E. Multifocal versus monofocal intraocular lenses in cataract surgery: a systematic review. *Ophthalmology.* 2003;110:1789-1798.
35. AcrySof ReSTOR Apodized Diffractive Optic Posterior Chamber Intraocular Lenses. Premarket Approval Application (PMA) P040020. Available at: http://www.fda.gov/cdrh/pdf4/p040020b.pdf. Accessed on: October 19, 2005.
36. ReZoom Acrylic Multifocal Posterior Chamber Intraocular Lenses [package insert]. Santa Ana, CA: Advanced Medical Optics, Inc.; 2005.
37. Hoffman RS, Fine IH, Packer M. Refractive lens exchange with a multifocal IOL. *Curr Opin Ophthalmol.* 2003;14:24-30.
38. Packer M, Fine IH, Hoffman RS. The Tecnis Multifocal IOL. In: Fine IH, Packer M, Hoffman RS, eds. *Refractive Lens Surgery.* Heidelberg, Berlin: Springer-Verlag; 2005:147.
39. Huetz WW, Grolmus R, Eckhardt B. Reading acuity and reading speed with different types of multifocal IOLs. Paper presented at: the XXIII Congress of the ESCRS; September 10, 2005; Lisbon, Portugal.

CHAPTER 121

Spherical Aberration: The Next Frontier

JACK T. HOLLADAY, MD, MSEE

Spherical aberration is the property of a single spherical surface to refract rays too strongly as one moves from the center of the pupil peripherally compared with the paraxial (central) focus (Figure 1). The image formed when spherical aberration is present causes a halo (or blur) around the paraxial image (Figure 2). The terminology is the same in an optical system with multiple surfaces such as the human eye, which has four refracting surfaces (the anterior/posterior cornea and the anterior/posterior crystalline lens). If the system has more optical power away from the optical axis, toward the periphery, there is *positive* spherical aberration. If the opposite is true, then it is *negative*. Spherical aberration is radially symmetric, meaning that all semimeridians are identical and have the same ray-tracing diagram as if it were the only aberration in the system.

This article analyzes spherical aberration mathematically in order to identify the optimal amount to target for the human eye.

THE MATHEMATICS OF ASPHERIC SURFACES AND SPHERICAL ABERRATION: THE ANTERIOR CORNEA

Biological single surfaces are rarely spherical. More often they are aspheric, as are the surfaces of the cornea and crystalline lens. Some of the simplest aspheric surfaces are referred to as *conic sections*, because they can be created by taking a section of a cone. If we allow these surfaces to have a toric apex (astigmatism), then the resulting surfaces are hyperboloid, paraboloid, prolate ellipsoid, spheroid, and oblate ellipsoid. Each of these surfaces can be determined by three variables: horizontal and vertical apical radii (R_{xz} and R_{yz}) and an asphericity quotient (Q-value) in a three-dimensional Cartesian coordinate system (X, Y, and Z).

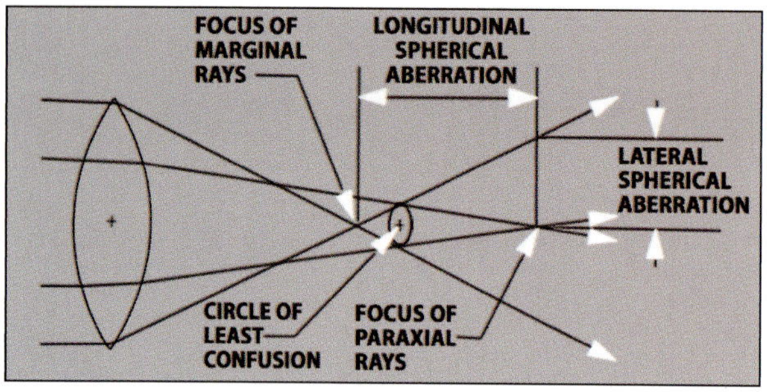

Figure 1. This diagram of positive spherical aberration illustrates longitudinal and lateral spherical aberration.

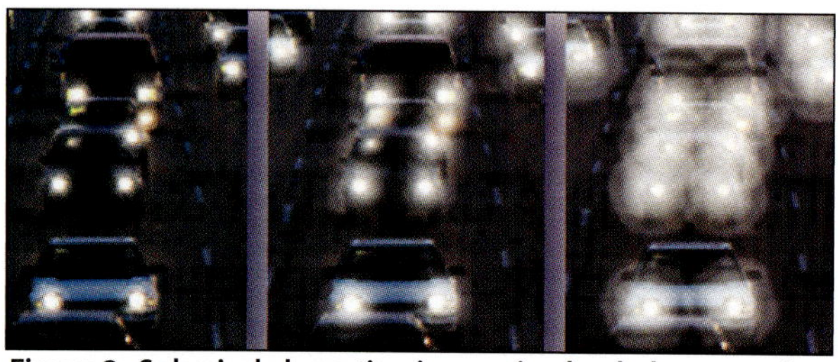

Figure 2. Spherical aberration is perceived as halos around lights that cause the symptoms of glare. Increasing amounts of spherical aberration create larger halos.

Equation 1.

$$Z = c \mp c^* \sqrt{(1 - \frac{X^2}{R_{xz}c} - \frac{Y^2}{R_{yz}c})}$$

where Equation 2.

$$R_{SEQ} = \frac{2R_{xz}R_{yz}}{R_{xz} + R_{yz}} \quad \& \quad c = \frac{R_{SEQ}}{(1 + Q_{SEQ})}$$

Table 1 shows the values of Q and their corresponding surfaces. Figure 3 provides a cross-section (two-dimensional plot) of these surfaces.

Figure 4 illustrates a colored ray tracing of a spherical surface. The *longitudinal spherical aberration* (LSA') is the difference between the marginal focus (L'_m) and the paraxial focus (L'_p) along the optical axis. *Transverse spherical aberration* (TSA') is the height of the marginal ray at the paraxial focal plane.

Written as formulas, it is

Equation 3a. $LSA' = L'_m - L'_p$

Equation 3b. $TSA' = H' = (LSA')\tan U'_m$

where U'_m is the slope of the marginal ray after refraction. When the marginal ray intercept is anterior to the paraxial focus, the spherical aberration is positive. If posterior to the paraxial focus, it is negative.

The longitudinal spherical aberration can also be expressed as a series

Equation 4. $LSA' = a\,Y^2 + b\,Y^4 + c\,Y^6 + \ldots$

where the first term is referred to as *third-order LSA*, the second term as *fifth-order LSA*, etc., and the *a* is the coefficient of the third-order term, the *b* is the coefficient of the fifth-order term, etc. In most simple optical systems, including the normal human eye, it is rare to have more than third-order LSA, so the first term is all that is used clinically. In optical design, the term *zonal* SA_z is used. Instead of the marginal ray, it is customary to use a ray of height that is 0.707 of the marginal ray (Y_m) such that the areas inside and outside this diameter are equal. The resulting equations for third-order LSA are

Equation 5a. *Marginal Third-Order*

$$LSA'_m = aY_m^2$$

Equation 5b. *Zonal Third-Order*

$$LSA'_z = a\frac{Y_m^2}{2}$$

where

$$a = \frac{LSA'_m}{Y_m^2}$$

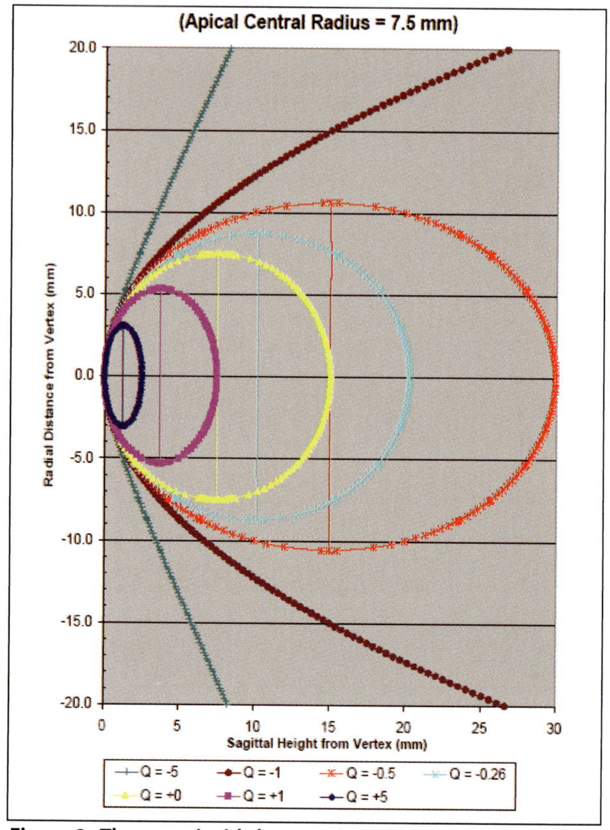

Figure 3. These conicoids have various Q-values. Blue (Q = +5) is an oblate ellipsoid, magenta (Q = +1) is an oblate ellipsoid, yellow (Q = 0) is a sphere, aqua (Q = -0.26, mean human cornea) is a prolate ellipsoid, red (Q = -0.50) is a prolate ellipsoid, brown (Q = -1) is a paraboloid, and green (Q = -5) is a hyperboloid.

When only third-order spherical aberration is present, the "best" focus (circle of least confusion) is midway between the paraxial focus and marginal focus (one half of LSA_m). If third- and fifth-order spherical aberration are present, then the best focus moves to three quarters of LSA_m.

The spherical aberration may also be described using wave aberration form, which expresses the aberration of the wave at the refracting surface.

Equation 6.

$$W = w_4Y^4 + w_6Y^6 + w_8Y^8 + \ldots$$

Similar to Equation 4, the wave aberration for third-order spher-

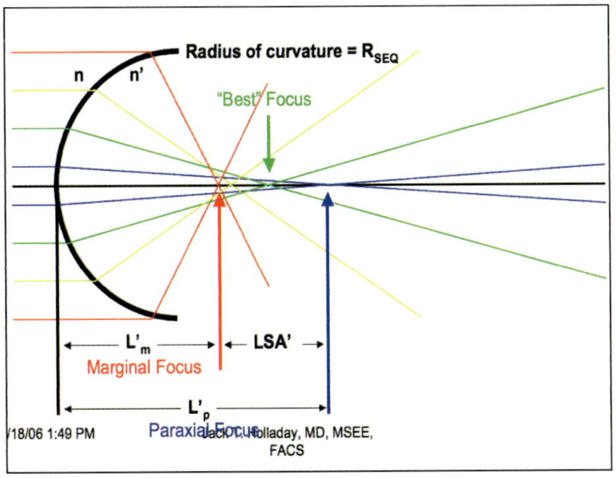

Figure 4. This diagram of positive spherical aberration shows marginal focus (L'_m), paraxial focus (L'_p), and longitudinal spherical aberration (LSA'). When only primary (third-order spherical aberration) is present, the best focus is midway between the marginal and paraxial foci.

ical aberration is the first term, fifth-order spherical aberration is the second term, etc. For an aspheric surface, the primary spherical aberration (third-order) may be determined with the following equation[1]:

Equation 7.

$$w_4 = \frac{\frac{n'}{L'_m}\left(\frac{1}{L'_m}-\frac{1}{R_{SEQ}}\right)^2 - \frac{n}{L}\left(-\frac{1}{L}+\frac{1}{R_{SEQ}}\right)^2}{8} + \frac{Q_{SEQ}(n'-n)}{8R_{SEQ}^3}$$

where n is the index of refraction of the media of the object, n' is the index of refraction of the media of the image, L is the distance to the object, and L' is the distance to the image from the vertex of the surface for the marginal ray.

A number of observations can be made when looking at this equation. The first term (divided by eight) is the spherical aberration of a spherical surface, and the second term (after the plus sign) is the additional term necessary to describe the primary spherical aberration of an aspheric surface with a Q-value of Q_{SEQ}. In this equation, the primary spherical aberration coefficient is a proportional Q-value (as Q becomes more positive, the spherical aberration increases) and inversely related to the apical radius (as the apical radius decreases or K-reading increases, the spherical aberration increases). For any single object and apical spheroequivalent radius, there is a spheroequivalent Q-value that will give zero primary spherical aberration (note: this is only true for a single object at a given distance, not for an object at any other distance).

TABLE 1. Q-VALUES AND THEIR CORRESPONDING SURFACES

Q-Value	Surface
$Q < -1$	Hyperboloid
$Q = -1$	Paraboloid
$-1 < Q < 0$	Prolate ellipsoid
$Q = 0$	Spheroid
$Q > 0$	Oblate ellipsoid

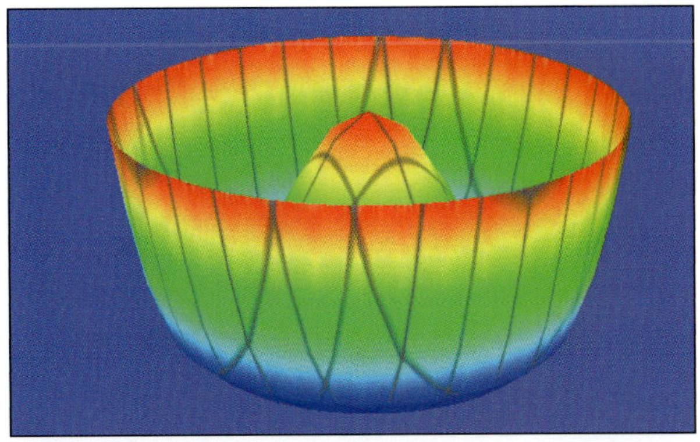

Figure 5. The surface of the Z(4,0) Zernike term for primary (third-order) spherical aberration is shown.

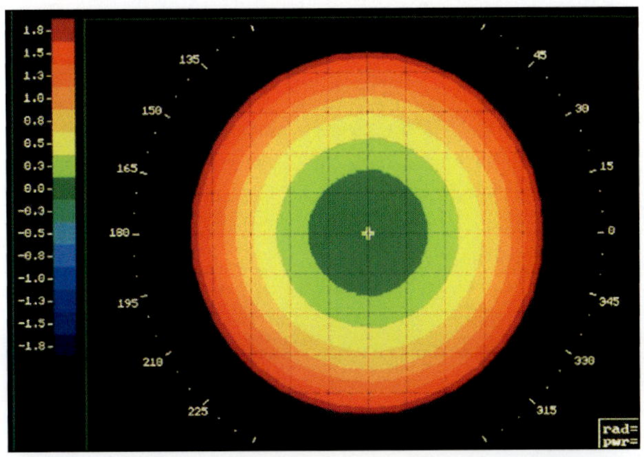

Figure 6. Shown is a refractive power map of the anterior surface of the corneal aspheric model with a central radius of 7.695 mm (K-reading = 43.86D), a Q-value of -0.26, and a stromal index of refraction of 1.376. The increase in refractive power is shown by warmer colors. At 3 mm from the center, the additional refractive power equals +1.00 D.

If we want to find the surface that has no spherical aberration for any object and image, the optical path difference must be the same for any rays traced through the system at height Y and must satisfy the following two-dimensional equation (Y and Z as defined in Equation 1 with X = 0):

Equation 8.

$$n'\sqrt{Y^2+(L'-Z)^2} + n\sqrt{Y^2+(Z-L)^2} = n'L'-nL$$

Equation 8 is a form of the famous Descartes equation. Unfortunately, for all objects at any distance, the aspheric surface is not a conic section, so none of the aforementioned conic surfaces (Equation 2) can eliminate spherical aberration for *any* object at *any* finite distance. If the object is at infinity, then the formula reduces to the simple equation

Equation 9.

$$Q = -\frac{n^2}{n'^2}$$

This equation shows that, for an object at infinity, the negative of the ratio of the anterior index of refraction and squared divided by the posterior index of refraction squared is the perfect Q-value

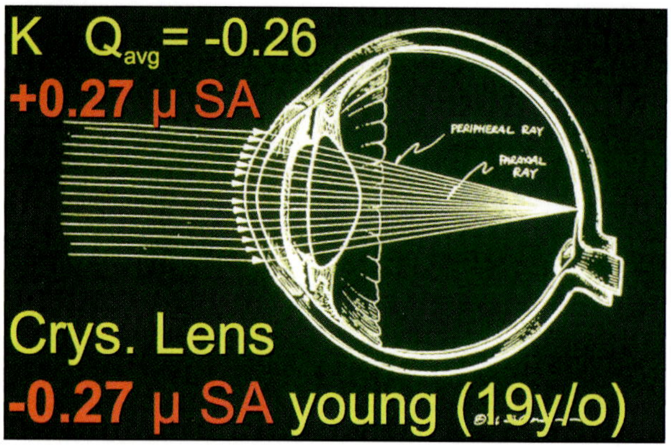

Figure 7. The ocular spherical aberration (entire eye) is nearly zero young in life (approximately 19 years of age), because the negative spherical aberration of the crystalline lens is almost equal and opposite to the positive spherical aberration of the cornea.

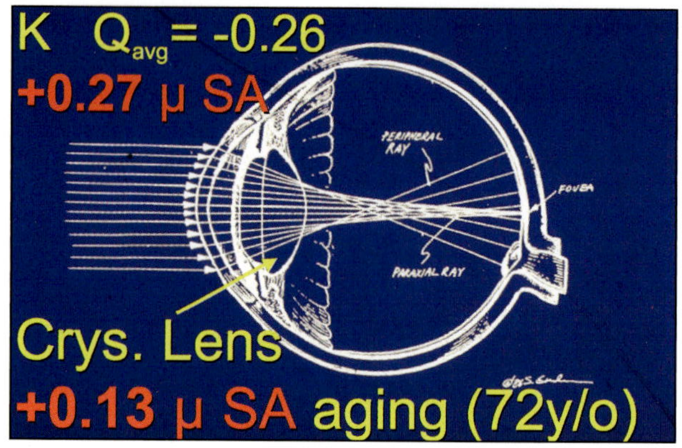

Figure 8. The human cornea and crystalline lens both have positive spherical aberration later in life due to the progressive increase in spherical aberration of the crystalline lens with age.

(conic surface) to eliminate spherical aberration. For the cornea, the index of refraction is 1.376, and the anterior medium is air. The ideal asphericity for the anterior surface of the cornea to eliminate spherical aberration for a distant object would therefore be a prolate ellipsoid with

Equation 10. *Q= - (1.0002/1.3762) = -0.528.*

Several investigators have shown that the mean Q-value of the anterior cornea over a 6-mm zone is -0.260 (0.00 to -0.50) with a wide variance.[2] The normal human cornea with a Q-value of -0.260 has less positive spherical aberration than a sphere (Q = 0), but it is rarely free of spherical aberration (Q = -0.53). An important clinical point is that, even if the anterior cornea did have a Q-value of -0.528, it would only be free of spherical aberration for an object at infinity. An object at any distance other than infinity will result in spherical aberration.

Another common method of describing a wavefront aberration over a circular pupil with radius ρ is the Zernike polynomials. They are easily related to the classical aberrations, but two terms are required for aberrations that are not rotationally symmetric such as astigmatism and coma. Such terms are decomposed into an x and a y component, but they can be easily combined into one term with a single magnitude and orientation.

The term for primary (third-order) spherical aberration is given by the following Zernike polynomial:

Equation 11.

$$Z(4,0) = 5^{1/2}(6\rho^4 - 6\rho^2 + 1)$$

All of the Zernike terms above Z(0,0) have an average value of zero, and all terms are orthogonal and therefore mutually exclusive. Because each term has an average value of zero over the entire surface, the reference plane of zero (Figure 5 where zero is green) is not the paraxial focus but the best focus (circle of least confusion), as seen in Figure 4. For positive spherical aberration, the paraxial focus would be hyperopic (posterior to the best focus), and the marginal focus would be myopic (anterior to the best focus).

If we use the mean keratometric power of the human cornea (43.86 D, yielding a radius of curvature of 7.695 mm [keratometric index of refraction = 1.3375]), the mean human Q-value of -0.26, and the corneal stromal index of refraction of 1.376, the calculated primary spherical aberration using the Zernike transform Z(4,0) is +0.189 µm for a 6-mm–diameter zone on a virgin cornea. We can also look at the spherical aberration as the change in refractive power on the cornea, which is much more familiar to the clinician.

Figure 6 is the topographic refractive power map of the conic anterior surface of the average human cornea with a central radius of 7.695mm (K-reading = 43.86 D) and a Q-value of -0.26 with a stromal index of refraction of 1.376. The increase in refractive power is shown by warmer colors. At a 3-mm radius from the center (6-mm diameter), the additional refractive power equals +1.00 D or +1.00 D of marginal spherical aberration. The paraxial focus (L'_p) in media 1.376 is 28.1604 mm, the marginal focus at 3 mm (L'_m) is 27.5741, and the difference (LSA') is +0.586 mm (+586 µm). We see that, for the average anterior aspheric surface of the human cornea, the spherical aberration has a wavefront Z(4.0) of +0.189 µm, a refractive power spherical aberration of +1.00 D, and a longitudinal spherical aberration of +586 µm—three different ways of describing the same amount of spherical aberration.

Unfortunately, using the actual topographic height data, these values are approximately 30% less than the actual measured, average, virgin, human, anterior corneal spherical aberration Z(4,0), which has been shown to be +0.270 µm.[3,4] The refractive power spherical aberration is +1.42D, and the longitudinal spherical aberration is +837 µm.

Recent studies explain the cause of this disparity and demonstrate that the conic with apical radii and Q-values (Equations 1 and 2) do not exactly reflect the true shape of the cornea, especially after corneal refractive surgery.[5-8] As a result, the K-reading and Q-value should never be used to determine the spherical aberration Z(4,0) term, because significant errors will occur.

Topographers such as the OPD Scan (Nidek, Inc., Fremont, CA) and the Pentacam (Oculus Optikgeräte GmbH, Wetzlar, Germany) calculate the Zernike terms for the topographic examination and display a report of these values. Most topographers do not have this feature in their software and require separate software programs such as VOL-CT (Sarver and Associates, Inc., Carbondale, IL) that take exported examinations from the topographers, import the information into VOL-CT, and then compute all of the Zernike terms and many other parameters. Unfortunately, this is the only accurate method available to clinicians today for most topographers that allows the exact calculation of the spherical aberration for choosing the correct aspheric IOL after cataract surgery.

With newer instruments such as the Pentacam and Visante OCT (Carl Zeiss Meditec, Inc., Dublin, CA) that are not Placido ring based, the central zone of the cornea is no longer a scotoma, and data are measured all the way to the center. These instruments have shown that the normal cornea is flatter in the central 2 mm, becomes steeper from 2 to 4 mm, and then begins to flatten beyond 4 mm. To accurately represent the true corneal shape measured with these newer instruments, the simple ellipsoid is not adequate, and we must use a figured ellipsoid. It differs from the standard ellipsoid given in Equations 2 and 3 in that the Q-value is not a constant but an equation that varies as one moves radially from the center of the cornea. If we compute the apical radii and keep them constant, the Q-value usually gets more negative from the normal cornea's center to its periphery. A simple second-order polynomial is sufficient to describe this change.

Equation 7. $Q=a+b\rho+c\rho 2$, *where* $\rho 2 = X2 + Y2$ and ρ is the radial distance from the center (apex). To use the figured ellipsoid, we would therefore need five variables (R_{xz}, R_{yz}, a, b, and c): two principal apical radii for astigmatism and three coefficients for the Q-value as a function of the radial distance from the center, compared with only three for the standard conic surface. An excellent measure of the quality of the fit of any surface to the actual height data is the root mean square (RMS) error of the fit. The difference in the actual height data from the cornea and the height of the model surface is determined at each point. The difference at each point is then squared, the mean value of the sum of all of the squares is determined, and the square root of this value is calculated. A fit with an RMS error of < 0.5µm is excellent and represents a true fit.

OCULAR SPHERICAL ABERRATION: THE ENTIRE EYE

Studies measuring ocular (entire eye) spherical aberration agree on two findings. First, there is a great deal of variation in ocular spherical aberration at any age. Second, the average ocular spherical aberration is nearer to zero when people are around 15 to 20 years of age than when older. The *ocular spherical aberration* is the sum of the spherical aberration from the four refracting surfaces of the eye (the anterior/posterior cornea and the anterior/posterior crystalline lens).

Studies have demonstrated that the cornea has a stable shape throughout life in the absence of anterior corneal disease such as dry eye or anterior membrane dystrophy.[9] As mentioned earlier, the average spherical aberration of the anterior cornea is +0.270 µm over a 6-mm zone. Glasser and Campbell have shown in vitro that the spherical aberration of the crystalline lens increases (from negative to positive) as a function of age.[10] Two more recent in vivo studies[11,12] have shown that the ocular spherical aberration is lowest in people aged 15 to 20. The variation is wide, however, and the trends of spherical aberration versus age only explain between 5% and 12% of the data. These statistics are similar to refractive error, color vision, contrast sensitivity, etc.

The best performance is around 19 years of age rather than older, but, even at that age, most people have spherical aberration that will likely become more positive as they grow older. Figure 7 is a ray-traced diagram with the ocular spherical aberration (entire eye) nearly zero at around 19 years of age, because the negative spherical aberration of the crystalline lens is almost equal and opposite to the positive spherical aberration of the cornea. Figure 8 depicts the spherical aberration in the aging human eye, where the cornea and crystalline lens both have positive spherical aberration.

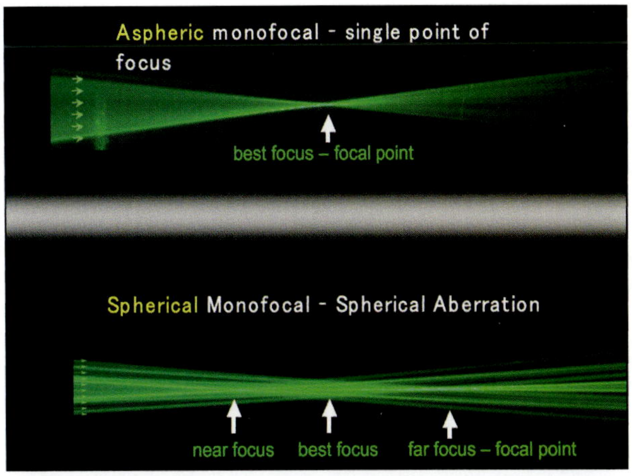

Figure 9. The light's path through different IOLs is visualized by projecting a monofocal, green (550-nm) light bundle through a lens positioned in water.

IDEAL SPHERICAL ABERRATION IN THE HUMAN EYE

Knowing that the ocular spherical aberration is nearly zero when the eye is at its peak performance does not necessarily prove that zero is the ideal target, especially as people age. Some proposed concepts about spherical aberration are erroneous. Two fallacies are that the depth of focus increases with positive spherical aberration and that these changes naturally and beneficially reduce the effects of presbyopia on the quality of near vision.

First, the term is *spherical aberration.* By definition, an *aberration* reduces the quality of the ocular image. It is true that some aberrations are worse than others. For example, Huber[13] demonstrated better distance vision with similar amounts of with- versus against-the-rule astigmatism, and Sawusch and Guyton[14] demonstrated that against-the-rule astigmatism was better for near vision. The observations are true and relate to the Arabic alphabet. There are more vertical than horizontal strokes in the 26 letters of the English alphabet. Leaving the vertical line of the Conoid of Sturm on the retina therefore allows people to recognize more letters and explains the seemingly paradoxical results from Huber and Sawusch and Guyton.

Several researchers have demonstrated with image simulation how, together, certain higher-order aberrations can provide clearer images than lower amounts of other aberrations.[15-19] Additionally, McClellan et al have shown that we do not perceive chromatic aberration (rainbows of at least 1.50 D around white light), because they are balanced by achromatic higher-order aberrations in the eye.[20] All of these observations and explanations are true and underscore the complex interplay of parameters in the eye that result in our excellent vision.

Spherical aberration does not increase depth of focus. Figure 9 depicts the pencil (fan) of rays passing through a 6-mm aperture, coming into focus, and then passing out of focus. Of note, the aspheric IOL (no spherical aberration in the system) brings rays into a single point of focus, whereas the spherical IOL with spherical aberration does not (forms a blurred circle of least confusion). The only difference between these two lenses is at the best focus, where the aspheric surface comes to a single point and the spherical lens does not. At ±0.50D and beyond, the pencil of light is the same diameter in both the spherical and aspheric IOLs with corresponding, equally blurred circles. There is no difference in the depth of focus, only the clarity of best focus.

The same comparison can be made between a +20.00 D conoid aspheric indirect ophthalmoscopic lens and a spherical +20.00 D lens from the trial lens set. The aspheric indirect lens creates a much clearer image than the spherical trial lens, because it eliminates spherical aberration. If there were any increased depth of focus due to the spherical aberration of the spherical lens or any other perceived improvement, we would all be using the $5 spherical trial lens and not the $300 aspheric conoid lens.

In fact, plus or minus spherical aberration yields a blurred halo around the image, and no spherical aberration yields the best possible image. In presbyopia or pseudophakia with an aspheric monofocal IOL, it may actually be desirable to have negative spherical aberration (rays in the periphery bend less than paraxial rays, thus resulting in more power centrally than peripherally). The reason is the synkinetic reflex when viewing an object at near. When an object is brought close to the eye, the synkinetic reflex includes convergence, accommodation, and miosis of the pupil. If negative ocular spherical aberration is present, then the power of the eye increases and makes the near image clearer when the pupil constricts. The negative spherical aberration when the pupil constricts still creates a halo, but the near vision with presbyopia is better. With positive spherical aberration, when the pupil constricts, the power centrally is weaker and actually reduces the quality of the image at near.

Suggestions that residual positive spherical aberration when the pupil constricts is beneficial refer to population-based studies or Top Gun pilots who have an average of +0.1μm. Referring to these studies is misleading, because the average age of the subjects is between 35 and 45 years.[21] These individuals have excellent vision, but the quality of their vision was better when they were 19 years old and their spherical aberration was nearer to zero. Also, if the RMS value rather than the coefficient of the spherical aberration is used, it is always positive and only relates to the magnitude and not the sign (positive or negative) of the aberration. The target of zero still provides the best result.

Also, we must carefully consider clinical studies comparing spherical aberration and the quality of contrast sensitivity function, macular threshold testing, etc. If other higher-order aberrations are present in the cornea, then any conclusions about spherical aberration and quality of vision are suspect, unless the other aberrations are also analyzed independently.[13-18]

In addition, if pseudophakic patients are left slightly myopic (-0.25 D), uncorrected contrast sensitivity function or macular threshold studies may actually show better results with slightly positive spherical aberration. In mesopic or photopic conditions, the average size of the pupil is between 3 and 4 mm, and the central part of the aperture is slightly hyperopic, balancing the mild myopia. If the patient's minimal myopic refraction is corrected, zero spherical aberration will always give the best results, provided there are no other higher-order aberrations present to confuse the issue. If all parameters of testing are controlled properly, zero will always yield the best quality of vision. If the magnitude of the positive and negative spherical aberration is equal, they will also perform the same. The only difference will be improved near vision with negative spherical aberration due to the constriction of the pupil as described earlier. Pablo Artal, PhD, has confirmed these findings clinically in his laboratory.[22]

Excimer laser surgery has also confirmed these findings. Standard hyperopic treatments induce negative spherical aberration versus positive spherical aberration with myopic treatments. If patients are emmetropic with presbyopia, the hyperopes with negative spherical aberration will have better near vision than their myopic counterparts with positive spherical aberration. The negative value is also the basis of presbyopic LASIK and Near Vision CK (Refractec, Inc., Irvine, CA), which produces an exaggeratedly prolate cornea with negative spherical aberration.

What is the optimal ocular spherical aberration we should target with aspheric IOLs and corneal ablation? From the material already presented in this article, it should be clear that we should target zero spherical aberration in the young individuals with no presbyopia who are scheduled for LASIK or PRK. Because they can accommodate, they will derive no benefit from the introduction of negative spherical aberration. In the presbyope or pseudophake with little or no accommodation, negative spherical aberration may be beneficial if they want to depend less on readers. If they are not bothered by using reading glasses, then zero spherical aberration is still the best target.

Several clinical studies have demonstrated improved quality with reduced ocular spherical aberration for aspheric IOLs after cataract surgery.[23-33] They have determined the improvement in contrast sensitivity to be approximately 0.3 log units (3dB) or 40% to 50% improved retinal image contrast. These results are predictable because modern small-incision cataract surgery introduces minimal new corneal aberrations and the optical qualities of IOLs' surfaces far surpass those of the cornea. Measuring the corneal spherical aberration over a 6-mm zone and matching this value with the aspheric IOL with the closest negative spherical aberration is the correct approach. If the surgeon cannot make an exact match, leaving the patient slightly negative is the best choice.

Unlike cataract surgery, unfortunately, modern corneal refractive surgery often introduces aberrations into the optical system when changing the refractive properties of the eye (primarily sphere and cylinder). The causes include nonhomogeneity of the excimer beam, reduced tension of the corneal collagen fibers in the LASIK flap, biomechanical changes of the cornea, and epithelial healing and remodeling. Although these factors are much harder to control and predict than cataract surgery, further research will realize the full benefits of ocular and topographic wavefront-guided treatments and result in the improvement of all aberrations, not just sphere and cylinder.

Another consideration that we cannot ignore, when looking at outcome measures such as visual acuity and contrast sensitivity function, is that our visual system includes an optical, sensory, and computer processor. The last of these compares the retinal image to stored images and also enhances the quality of the image. This neural adaptation has both a rapid and a long-term phase. The latter extends from 3 months to 1 year and is present whether the optical changes improve or degrade the retinal image.

Multifocal IOLs, which reduce the contrast of the image by 30% and are associated with halos, show that fewer than 1% of patients notice or are bothered by these effects by 1 year postoperatively. The same is true when the optical system is improved. In the original studies of the Tecnis aspheric IOL, Mester et al[30] and others[34] showed that the contrast sensitivity function continued to improve from 3 months to 1 year as the brain adjusted to the improved image. The point is that studies performed before the 1-year mark, when the optical system has been altered, do not necessarily reflect the patient's final outcome.

CONCLUSION

Our refractive surgical goal should be to eliminate or at least reduce all of the optical aberrations of the eye, including spherical aberration. We should remember, however, that it may take 6 to 12 months of neural adaptation for the patient to fully appreciate and exhibit improvement in subjective measures such as visual acuity and contrast sensitivity function. Older presbyopic patients may benefit from a small amount of residual negative spherical aberration in order to achieve better unaided near vision and depend less on readers—a similar compromise as with modern diffractive and refractive multifocal IOLs. Finally, there is no benefit to leaving any positive spherical aberration in the optical system, because it degrades the image and reduces patients' near vision as their pupils constrict. ■

This article originally appeared in the November/December 2006 issue of CRSToday.

1. Smith G, Atchison DA. *The Eye and Visual Optical Instruments.* New York: Cambridge University Press; 1997.
2. Kiely PM, Smith G, Carney LG. The mean shape of the human cornea. *Opt Acta.* 1982;29:1027-1040.
3. Holladay JT, Piers PA, Koranyi G, et al. A new intraocular lens design to reduce spherical aberration of pseudophakic eyes. *J Refract Surg.* 2002;18:683-691.
4. Wang L, Dai E, Koch DD, Nathoo A. Optical aberrations of the human anterior cornea. *J Cataract Refract Surg.* 2003;29:1514-1521.
5. Tuan KM, Chernyak D. Corneal asphericity and visual function after wavefront-guided LASIK. *Optom Vis Sci.* 2006;83:605-610.
6. Kanellopoulos AJ. Topography-guided custom retreatments in 27 symptomatic eyes. *J Refract Surg.* 2005;21:S513-S518.
7. Somani S, Tuan KA, Chernyak D. Corneal asphericity and retinal image quality: a case study and simulations. *J Refract Surg.* 2004;20:S581-S585.
8. Roberts C. Characterization of the inherent error in a spherically-biased corneal topography system in mapping a radially aspheric surface. *J Refract Corneal Surg.* 1994;10:103-111; discussion 112-116.
9. Guirao A, Gonzales C, Redondo M, et al. Average performance of the human eye as a function of age in the normal population. *Invest Ophthalmol Vis Science.* 1999;40:203-213.
10. Glasser A, Campbell MCW. Presbyopia and the optical changes in the human crystalline lens with age. *Vision Res.* 1998;38:209-229.
11. Wang L, Santaella RM, Booth M, Koch DD. Higher-order aberrations from the internal optics of the eye. *J Cataract Refract Surg.* 2005;31:1512-1519.
12. Holzer MP, Goebels S, Aufarth GU. Total, corneal and internal aberrations of the human eye. Paper presented at: The DOC; May 27, 2006; Nuremburg, Germany.
13. Huber C. Planned myopic astigmatism as a substitute for accommodation in pseudophakia. *J Am Intraocul Implant Soc.* 1981;7:244-249.
14. Sawusch MR, Guyton DL. Optimal astigmatism to enhance depth of focus after cataract surgery. *Ophthalmology.* 1991;98:1025-1029.
15. Charman WN. The Charles F. Prentice Award Lecture 2005: optics of the human eye: progress and problems. *Optom Vis Sci.* 2006;83:335-345.
16. Chen L, Singer B, Guirao A, et al. Image metrics for predicting subjective image quality. *Optom Vis Sci.* 2005;82:358-369.
17. Marsack JD, Thibos LN, Applegate RA. Metrics of optical quality derived from wave aberrations predict visual performance. *J Vis.* 2004;4:322-328.
18. Cheng X, Bradley A, Thibos LN. Predicting subjective judgment of best focus with objective image quality metrics. *J Vis.* 2004;4:310-321.
19. Cheng X, Thibos LN, Bradley A. Estimating visual quality from wavefront aberration measurements. *J Refract Surg.* 2003;19:S579-S584.
20. McClellan JS, Marcos S, Prieto PM, Burns SA. Imperfect optics may be the eye's defence against chromatic blur. *Nature.* 2002;417:174-176.
21. Levy Y, Segal O, Avni I, Zadok D. Ocular higher-order aberrations in eyes with supernormal vision. *Am J Ophthalmol.* 2005;139:225-228.
22. Artal P. Visual performance with varying amounts of spherical aberration. Paper presented at: The ARVO Annual Meeting; May 6, 2006; Fort Lauderdale, FL.
23. Bellucci R, Scialdone A, Buratto L, et al. Visual acuity and contrast sensitivity comparison between Tecnis and AcrySof SA60AT intraocular lenses: a multicenter study. *J Cataract Refract Surg.* 2005:31:712-717.
24. Denoyer A, Roger F, Majzoub S, Pisella PJ. Quality of vision after cataract surgery in patients with prolate aspherical lens. *J Fr Ophtalmol.* 2006;29:157-163.
25. Franchini A. Comparative assessment of contrast with spherical and aspherical intraocular lenses. *J Cataract Refract Surg.* 2006;32:1307-1319.
26. Kennis H, Huygens M, Callebaut F. Comparing the contrast sensitivity of a modified prolate anterior surface IOL and of two spherical IOLs. *Bull Soc Belge Ophtalmol.* 2004;294:49-58.
27. Kershner RM. Retinal image contrast and functional visual performance with aspheric, silicone, and acrylic intraocular lenses. Prospective evaluation. *J Cataract Refract Surg.* 2003;29:1684-1694.
28. Lanzagorta-Aresti A, Palacios-Pozo E, Taboada-Esteve JF, et al. Contrast sensitivity to intraocular lens Tecnis Z-9000. *Arch Soc Esp Oftalmo.* 2005;80:651-658.
29. Martinez PA, Palacin MB, Castilla CM, et al. Spherical aberration influence in visual function after cataract surgery: prospective randomized trial. *Arch Soc Esp Oftalmo.* 2005;80:71-78.
30. Mester U, Dillinger P, Anterist N. Impact of a modified optic design on visual function: clinical comparative study. *J Cataract Refract Surg.* 2003;29:652-660.
31. Munoz G, Albarran-Diego C, Montes-Mico R, et al. Spherical aberration and contrast sensitivity after cataract surgery with the Tecnis Z9000 intraocular lens. *J Cataract Refract Surg.* 2006;32:1320-1327.
32. Packer M, Fine IH, Hoffman RS, Piers PA. Prospective randomized trial of an anterior surface modified prolate intraocular lens. *J Refract Surg.* 2002;18:692-696.
33. Packer M, Fine IH, Hoffman RS, Piers PA. Improved functional vision with a modified prolate intraocular lens. *J Cataract Refract Surg.* 2004;30:986-992.
34. Artal P, Chen L, Fernandez EJ, et al. Neural compensation for the eye's optical aberrations. *J Vis.* 2004;4:281-287.

CHAPTER 122

Aspheric IOLs Are Predicted to Reduce the Frequency of Car Accidents

DOUGLAS D. KOCH, MD

As surgeons, we can tell patients that aspheric IOLs offer a quality of vision that is superior to that provided by standard monofocal IOLs. Furthermore, aspheric implants perform better in difficult visual situations, such as night driving.[1,2] IOLs with a negative spherical aberration (such as the Tecnis IOL [Advanced Medical Optics, Inc., Santa Ana, CA]) are designed to counteract the mean amount of positive anterior corneal spherical aberration found in the general population of patients with cataracts. By reducing ocular spherical aberration, these IOLs have been shown to improve patients' functional vision and their visual performance in simulated night driving conditions.[3]

SOCIOECONOMIC NOTE

At least two IOLs with negative asphericity have been granted New-Technology IOL status,[4] which increased the amount of reimbursement to ASCs by $50 per lens. Assuming 2.5 million cataract procedures are performed per year and a 50% market penetration, the annual cost of this surgery to the United States government (taxpayers) and other third-party payers is roughly $62 million. In the long run, however, IOLs with negative asphericity will likely save patients and the government money—and lives. According to a study by the Potomac Institute for Policy Studies, located in Arlington, Virginia, the enhanced vision of patients who receive aspheric IOLs will result in a decrease in the rate of automobile accidents.[2]

IMPROVED DRIVING RESPONSE TIMES

In the study by the Potomac group of braking response time, 60 eyes of 30 patients underwent cataract surgery and were randomly assigned to receive either the Tecnis lens or a standard IOL. The investigators measured subjects' visual acuity, spherical aberration, and contrast sensitivity. Across all ages and pupillary sizes, the average amount of spherical aberration was significantly lower in the eyes that received the Tecnis IOL.

Ninety days after surgery, the investigators tested the patients' ability to drive at night at a modern driving simulation facility. The lighting was adjusted to approximate the conditions of rural or city driving. The former involved a straight, level road and a constant vehicular speed of 55 miles per hour. The road for city driving was similar, but the simulation included lights, cars, and storefront illumination in the forward view. The experiment tested patients' ability to detect and recognize highway signs and adult pedestrians. Patients signaled their identification of objects and people by pressing a button.

The investigators reported that patients who received the Tecnis IOL identified pedestrians, roadways' hash lines, and other objects more quickly than those who received a standard monofocal lens. The Tecnis group had an average 45-foot advantage in terms of braking/stopping sooner, which translated as a 0.5-second improvement in response time. Of interest, the superior braking reaction in the Tecnis group exceeded the benefits of other technological advances in automotive safety and lighting (eg, rear center, high-mounted brake lights).

How does improved reaction time increase driving safety? Using three different methodologies, the Potomac Institute study estimated that aspheric IOLs would result in a 10% reduction in accidents among those who received this lens. The anticipated savings could exceed $1 billion per year, with a prevention of more than 70,000 personal injuries annually.

IN SUMMARY

To my knowledge, the driving simulation and theoretical studies from the Potomac Institute are the best indicators that, by enhancing quality of vision, aspheric IOLs can have a major impact in improving driver safety. Greater safety on the roads will cost society less in terms of automobile accidents (not to mention the prevention of death or injury), despite the initial cost of the IOL. ■

This article originally appeared in October 2008 issue of CRSToday.

1. McBride DK, Matson W. Assessing the significance of optically produced reduction in braking response time: possible impacts on automotive safety among the elderly. Arlington, VA: *Potomac Institute for Policy Studies*; April 2003.
2. McBride DK, Matson W. Assessing the significance of optically produced reduction in automobile crashes in an aging American population: possible economic impacts. Arlington, VA: *Potomac Institute for Policy Studies*; July 2004.
3. The Tecnis 1-Piece IOL [package insert]. Santa Ana, CA: *Advanced Medical Optics*, Inc.; 2007.
4. Centers for Medicare & Medicaid Services Press Release. CMS announces approval of New Technology Intraocular Lens. January 26, 2006. http://www.cms.hhs.gov/apps/media/press/release.asp?Counter=1762. Accessed July 21, 2008.

CHAPTER 123

Customizing the Correction of Spherical Aberration

GEORGE BEIKO, BM, BCh, FRCSC

Until recently, the goal of cataract surgery has been to restore a patient's Snellen visual acuity to its greatest potential. Surgeons have emphasized minimizing sphere and cylinder and helping patients obtain emmetropic results. Now, the goal of cataract surgery is to restore patients' youthful contrast sensitivity and accommodative potential. This article investigates how aspheric IOLs may help us achieve this ideal.

QUANTIFYING SPHERICAL ABERRATION

From the wavefront analysis of the optical system, we know that aberrations other than sphere and cylinder significantly affect visual function. We can characterize these aberrations with Zernike transformations.

Research has shown an inverse association between the Zernike coefficient for spherical aberration and contrast sensitivity. In other words, spherical aberration increases as contrast sensitivity decreases.[1-4] The best contrast sensitivity has been measured in people between 20 and 30 years of age.

In the phakic eye, the anterior corneal surface, posterior corneal surface, crystalline lens, and retina all contribute to the total number of higher-order aberrations. In the aphakic eye, however, 98.2% of the aberrations arise from the anterior corneal surface.[5] For the purposes of this discussion, corneal higher-order aberrations will represent those of the entire eye in cataract patients.

Zernike coefficients of the eye's higher-order aberrations can be derived from corneal topographic data.[1,5-8] Because studies have shown that small-incision cataract surgery does not significantly affect postoperative corneal topography,[4-9] we can use measurements of higher-order aberrations obtained preoperatively to manipulate the outcome of cataract surgery. If our goal is to achieve optimal spherical aberration and maximal contrast sensitivity, we can implant an aspheric IOL that will neutralize the patient's preoperative spherical aberration.

ASPHERIC IOLS AND VISUAL QUALITY

The cornea has a positive spherical aberration of approximately 0.27 µm[10-12] for a 6.0-mm diameter, a measurement that does not vary significantly with aging. The implantation of an aspheric IOL such as the Tecnis Z9000 (Advanced Medical Optics, Inc., Santa Ana, CA), which possesses a spherical aberration of -0.27 µm, can reportedly improve image quality and contrast sensitivity under mesopic and photopic conditions versus the implantation of a

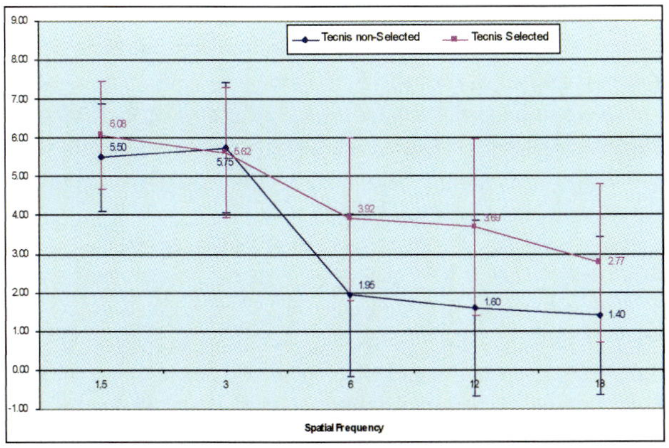

Figure 1. Patients targeted for 0.10 µm of residual spherical aberration (Tecnis selected) had better postoperative contrast sensitivity in photopic conditions versus patients targeted for zero spherical aberration (Tecnis nonselected).

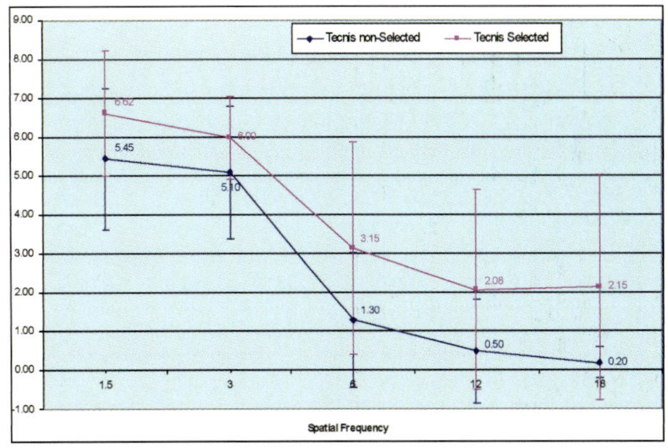

Figure 2. Patients targeted for 0.10 µm of residual spherical aberration (Tecnis selected) had better postoperative contrast sensitivity in mesopic conditions versus patients targeted for zero spherical aberration (Tecnis nonselected).

standard IOL. The spherical aberration of standard spherical IOLs tends to increase with the lens' power.[13-15]

Simulated night driving tests showed that patients who received the Tecnis IOL identified a pedestrian 45 feet or 0.5 seconds sooner at 55 mph than those implanted with a spherical IOL.[16] These results suggest that the correction of spherical aberration not only improves vision but also increases patients' safety. It is important to remember, however, that these previously mentioned studies compared patients who had no residual spherical aberration with the Tecnis lens with those who had 0.30 to 0.40 µm of postoperative spherical aberration with spherical IOLs.

Currently, the FDA has approved three IOLs for the correction of spherical aberration: the Tecnis; the Sofport AO (Bausch & Lomb, Rochester, NY); and the Acrysof IQ (Alcon Laboratories, Inc., Fort Worth, TX). The three lenses use different strategies to correct spherical aberration. Because the Sofport AO lens has no spherical aberration, it does not affect this characteristic of the eye. The Acrysof IQ has a negative spherical aberration of 0.20 µm and thus targets a mean postoperative spherical aberration of 0.10µm. The Tecnis lens (spherical aberration = -0.27 µm) targets the full correction of corneal spherical aberration.

IDENTIFYING THE OPTIMAL TARGET

Several studies have shown a potential correlation between spherical aberration and natural super vision (defined as 20/15 or better). Levy et al[17] measured the total spherical aberration in 70 eyes of 30 subjects (mean age = 24.3 ±7.7 years) with natural super vision. All measurements were made with the Nidek OPD scan wavefront aberrometer (Nidek Co., Ltd., Gamagori, Japan) across a naturally dilated, 6-mm pupil. The investigators found that the mean total spherical aberration in this population was +0.110 ±0.077 µm.[17]

Another study showed a correlation between some positive spherical aberration and better-than-average visual acuity and contrast sensitivity among student naval pilots.[18]

Based on these data, and considering an average corneal spherical aberration of +0.27 µm, I hypothesized that patients with a residual mean spherical aberration of approximately +0.10 µm after the implantation of a Tecnis lens would have better contrast sensitivity than those who had no residual spherical aberration. In an unpublished study, I compared 13 patients who had an average

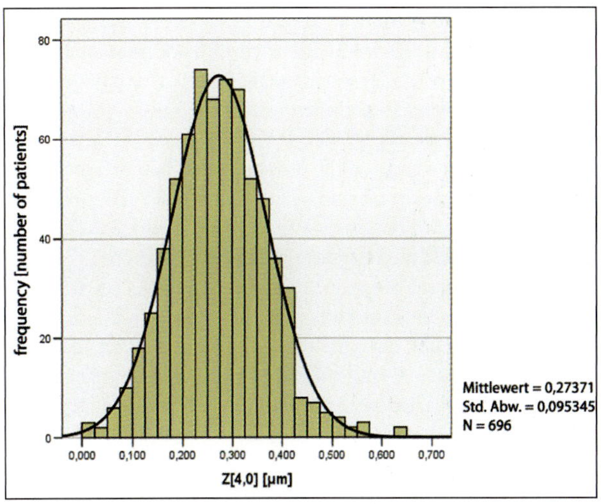

Figure 3. A normal Gaussian distribution of spherical aberration in 696 eyes shows a large standard deviation (±0.095) from the mean of 0.274 µm (Z [4,0]).

preoperative spherical aberration of +0.37 µm with 20 patients who had an average preoperative spherical aberration close to that found in the studies by Holladay et al[11] and by Beiko et al.[19]

Because the Tecnis' fixed spherical aberration is -0.27 µm, its implantation would leave the patients in the first group (Tecnis selected) with +0.10 µm of spherical aberration versus zero in the second group (Tecnis nonselected).

Postoperatively, I detected statistically significant differences between the groups for spatial frequencies of 12 cycles per degree under photopic conditions (Figure 1), and for six, 12, and 18 cycles per degree under mesopic conditions (Figure 2). In addition, the intergroup differences for spatial frequencies of six and 18 cycles per degree under photopic conditions (P=.0570 and P=.0585, respectively) were almost significant. Unlike in other studies that compared the Tecnis with hydrophobic acrylic IOLs,[13-15] the differences in contrast sensitivity between the two groups in this present study cannot be attributed their material and optical characteristics. My unpublished study confirmed that patients who had 0.10 µm of residual spherical aberration had better postoperative contrast sensitivity than those that had zero postoperative spherical aberration.

TABLE 1. LENS SELECTIONS FOR MINIMIZING POSTOPERATIVE SPHERICAL ABERRATION	
IOL Design	Preoperative Spherical Aberration (μm)
Clariflex,* Sofport AO,† Akreos AO†‡	Zero to 0.15
Acrysof IQ§	0.16 to 0.33
Tecnis Z9000*	> 0.33
Spherical IOLs	< Zero

*Advanced Medical Optics, Inc., Santa Ana, CA.
†Bausch & Lomb, Rochester, NY.
‡Not available in the US.
§Alcon Laboratories, Inc., Fort Worth, TX.

In an unpublished follow-up study, unselected patients whose corneal spherical aberration was similar to that of the general population (0.27 μm) were implanted with either the Acrysof IQ or the Sofport AO lens. The Acrysof IQ lens' performance was almost identical to that of the Tecnis in patients targeted for 0.10 μm of postoperative spherical aberration in the previous study. Under the same conditions, the Sofport AO performed similarly to the Tecnis nonselected group in the previous study. In terms of contrast sensitivity testing, targeting a mean spherical aberration of zero (as in the Tecnis nonselected group) or 0.27 μm (as in the Sofport AO group) was inferior to targeting 0.10 μm.

Based on the results of contrast sensitivity testing, I currently advocate personalizing cataract patients' postoperative outcomes by targeting for +0.10 μm of residual spherical aberration. Ideally, we would be able to choose from a range of powers on different IOL platforms. Because only a few aspheric IOLs are currently available, I measure patients' preoperative corneal spherical aberration and select an IOL as outlined in Table 1.

If it is not possible to measure spherical aberration directly in patients who have undergone refractive surgery, we may follow some general guidelines. Myopic laser ablation tends to increase the eye's spherical aberration, so an IOL with highly negative spherical aberration such as the Tecnis is probably appropriate. Conversely, hyperopic ablation tends to decrease the eye's spherical aberration, sometimes making it negative, so we might consider implanting a standard IOL with positive spherical aberration.

CAN WE BUY THE HYPE?

The manufacturers of aspheric IOLs have proposed that their implantation as part of a targeted strategy will give all cataract patients super vision. For this premise to be true, we would have to assume that patients' spherical aberrations cluster tightly around the mean and that each strategy targets the optimal value.

In order to investigate the manufacturers' proposals adequately, it is it is essential to know the distribution of corneal spherical aberration in the general population. A small standard deviation relative to the mean would support the idea that a few aspheric IOLs can provide optimal outcomes, whereas a larger value would suggest that surgeons need a wider range of IOLs to correct different degrees of spherical aberration.

In a recent study, my colleagues and I measured 0.274 ±0.095 μm of spherical aberration among 696 eyes and concluded that the large standard deviation of the Gaussian distribution does not support the manufacturers' assertions[19] (Figure 3).

CONCLUSION

The strategies for providing customized correction after cataract surgery are constantly evolving. For example, Yoon et al[20] reported that refractive surgery patients with +0.10 μm of preoperative spherical aberration achieve the best results when their myopia is undercorrected by 0.25 D. Although similar results have not been reported among cataract patients, the investigators' findings suggest that these individuals may benefit from a comparable strategy.

As we learn more about how higher-order aberrations affect visual quality, we may need to revise our preferred targets for minimizing postoperative spherical aberration. ■

This article originally appeared in the November/December 2006 issue of CRSToday.

1. Guirao A, Artal P. Corneal wave aberration from videokeratography: accuracy and limitations of the procedure. *J Opt Soc Am A Opt Image Sci Vis.* 2000;17:955-965.
2. Glasser A, Campbell MC. Biometric, optical and physical changes in the isolated human crystalline lens with age in relation to presbyopia. *Vision Res.* 1999;39:1991-2015.
3. Glasser A, Campbell MC. Presbyopia and the optical changes in the human crystalline lens with age. *Vision Res.* 1998;38:209-229.
4. Valois RL, Valois KK. Spatial Vision. Oxford, England: Oxford University Press; 1988.
5. Barbero S, Marcos S, Merayo-Lloves L, Moreno-Barriuso E. Validation of the estimation of corneal aberrations from videokeratography in keratoconus. *J Refract Surg.* 2002;18:263-270.
6. Rabinowitz YS, McDonnell PJ. Computer assisted corneal topography in keratoconus. *Refract Corneal Surg.* 1989;5:400-408.
7. Schweigerling J, Greivenkamp JE. Using corneal height maps and polynomial decompensation to determine corneal aberration. *Optom Vis Sci.* 1997;74:906-916.
8. Gobbe M, Guillan M, Marissa C. Measurement repeatability of corneal aberration. *J Refract Surg.* 2002;18:S567-S571.
9. Guirao A, Tejedor J, Artal P. Corneal aberrations before and after small-incision cataract surgery. *Invest Ophthalmol Vis Sci.* 2004;45:4312-4319.
10. Wang I, Dai E, Koch D, Nathoo A. Optical aberrations of the human anterior cornea. *J Cataract Refract Surg.* 2003;29:1514-1521.
11. Holladay JT, Piers PA, Koranyi G. A new intraocular lens design to reduce spherical aberration of pseudophakic eyes. *J Refract Surg.* 2002;18:683-691.
12. Beiko, G. Measurement of the wavefront aberrations using the Oculus Easygraph Topographic System. Paper presented at: The ASCRS/ASOA Symposium and Congress; May 2, 2004; San Diego, CA.
13. Kershner RM. Retinal image contrast and functional visual performance with aspheric, silicone, and acrylic intraocular lenses. Prospective evaluation. *J Cataract Refract Surg.* 2003;29:1684-1694.
14. Packer M, Fine IH, Hoffman RS, Piers PA. Initial clinical experience with an anterior surface modified prolate intraocular lens. *J Refract Surg.* 2002;18:692-696.
15. Barbero S, Marcos S, Jimenez-Alfaro I. Optical aberrations of intraocular lenses measured in vivo and in vitro. *J Opt Soc Am A Opt Image Sci Vis.* 2003;20:1841-1851.
16. Tecnis IOL [package insert]. Santa Ana, California; Advanced Medical Optics, Inc.; 2006.
17. Levy Y, Segal O, Avni I, Zadok D. Ocular higher-order aberrations in eyes with supernormal vision. *Am J Ophthalmol.* 2005;139:225-228.
18. Grimson JM, Schallhorn SC, Kaupp SE. Contrast sensitivity: establishing normative data for use in screening prospective naval pilots. *Aviat Space Environ Med.* 2002;73:28-35.
19. Beiko GHH, Haigis W, Steinmueller A. Distribution of the corneal spherical aberration in a comprehensive ophthalmology practice, and can keratometry be predictive of the value of the corneal spherical aberration? *J Cataract Refract Surg.* In press.
20. Yoon G, Subbaram M, MacRae S. The impact of correcting spherical aberration on hyperopic overcorrection after wavefront guided myopic refractive surgery. Paper presented at: The ARVO Annual Meeting; April 30, 2006; Fort Lauderdale, FL.

CHAPTER 124

At What Pupillary Size Does an Aspheric Matter?

THOMAS KOHNEN, MD, AND THOMAS KASPER, MD

Studies evaluating spherical-like aberrations in phakic eyes have shown rising values with increasing pupillary diameter.[1,2] This fact is also important in pseudophakic eyes, especially for the implantation of aspheric IOLs. These lenses were designed to compensate for corneal, primary spherical aberration (Z[4,0]), and they should restore the pseudophakic eye to the Z(4,0) values of young phakic eyes. Because earlier clinical research did not take different pupillary sizes into account, we designed a study protocol to evaluate higher-order aberrations as a function of the pupil's diameter.[3]

SUBJECTS AND METHODS

Patients

We included the eyes of 21 patients who needed IOL implantation because of cataract. They randomly received an aspheric Tecnis IOL (Z9000; Advanced Medical Optics, Inc., Santa Ana, CA) in one eye and a spherical Sensar IOL (AR40e; Advanced Medical Optics, Inc.) in their contralateral eye. No subject had eye disease other than cataract. The study population reflected a normal cataract population with a mean age of 71 years (range, 59 to 82 years). Professor Kohnen performed all of the surgeries, and no intra- or postoperative complications occurred.

Wavefront Measurement and Analysis

One month after cataract surgery, we used a Hartmann-Shack sensor (Zywave; Bausch & Lomb, Rochester, NY) to perform wavefront measurements of the whole eye under maximal pharmacological mydriasis. Using VOLPro software (Sarver and Associates, Inc., Carbondale, IL), we calculated higher-order aberrations, including Z(4,0), for virtual pupillary diameters of 3 to 6 mm, and we performed intraindividual comparisons.

To exclude influences on the whole eye's measurement from differences in corneal Z(4,0), we performed corneal topographic measurements (Orbscan IIz; Bausch & Lomb) and calculated the Z(4,0) of the central 6-mm zone.

Measurement of Pupillary Size

To evaluate the physiological pupillary size of the study population under different lighting conditions, we measured the pupil's size with a digital infrared pupillometer (Procyon P2000SA Pupillometer; Procyon Instruments Ltd., Grosmont, England). All measurements were performed without pharmacological treatment for luminance levels of 6.61 lux (highly mesopic), 0.88 lux (mesopic), and 0.07 lux (low mesopic).

RESULTS

Higher-Order Aberrations of the Whole Eye as a Function of Pupillary Diameter

We found rising values for all of the evaluated wavefront errors with the virtual pupil's increasing diameter regardless of the IOL implanted.

The most interesting wavefront error after the implantation of aspheric IOLs is Z(4,0). For the Tecnis IOL, we found statistically significantly lower values for all calculated pupillary diameters (3 to 6 mm). The absolute amount of the differences for small pupils (3 and 4 mm) was minor, but it rose as the pupil's size grew (5 and 6 mm). It is remarkable that some of the eyes with aspheric IOLs even reached negative values.

For total higher-order aberrations (third- to fifth-order RMS), we found statistically significant differences with lower values in the aspheric group only with a pupillary diameter of 6 mm. Coma-like aberrations such as third- and fifth-order RMS did not show any statistically significant differences between the study groups at any calculated pupillary diameter.

Z(4,0) of the Cornea

We did not find a statistically significant difference for Z(4,0) of the central 6-mm cornea between the study groups. We therefore concluded that all calculated differences in Z(4,0) of the whole eye were the consequence of the implantation of different types of IOLs.

Physiological Pupillary Sizes Under Mesopic Conditions

The median pupillary sizes under highly mesopic luminance were 3.25 mm (Tecnis group) and 3.20 mm (Sensar group). The pupil's size increased under mesopic illumination to as great as 4.04 and 4.05 mm, respectively. Under low mesopic luminance (0.07 lux), the median pupillary diameters were 4.90 and 5.03 mm in the Tecnis and Sensar groups, respectively. Inspecting the absolute values of pupillary size, we found that only one patient reached a 5-mm pupillary diameter under mesopic conditions. For low mesopic conditions, 23 of the 42 eyes (55%) attained a 5-mm pupil. We did not find any statistically significant differences between the groups.

DISCUSSION

Spherical aberrations, mainly Z(4,0), affect optical quality by reducing image contrast. A recognition of this problem led to the design of new IOLs such as the Tecnis to reduce Z(4,0) and thus increase contrast sensitivity after cataract surgery. Aspheric lenses should reduce the level of Z(4,0) to that of young eyes. Of interest is whether every cataract patient can profit from the implantation of this type of IOL.

To answer this question, we focused on pupillary diameter. It is commonly understood that the elderly have smaller pupils than the young. In our study, for example, just 55% of subjects attained a pupillary size of 5mm, and they did so only under nearly scotopic lighting conditions of 0.07 lux. For mesopic conditions, only one of 21 patients reached this pupillary size.

Why do we think 5mm is an important margin? Our calculations of Z(4,0) of the whole eye also yielded statistically lower values for 3- and 4-mm pupils. Nevertheless, these statistical differences were based on small differences of the absolute values. Clear differences were only present for 5- and 6-mm pupils. Moreover, Z(4,0) did not affect optical quality alone. A statistically significant difference for total higher-order aberrations (third- to fifth-order RMS) could only be calculated at the 6-mm pupillary diameter. Higher-order aberration values, however, are only one element of optical quality. It is not known what difference in Z(4,0) or total higher-order aberrations must be reached to obtain a clinical relevance with better contrast sensitivity.

It is our conclusion that patients with larger pupils can derive a greater benefit from aspheric IOLs than people with smaller pupils. These theoretical considerations must be proven by clinical testing of contrast sensitivity. In a subsequent investigation, we tested our study population with the observer-independent Frankfurt-Freiburg Contrast and Acuity Test System under different mesopic luminance conditions. We did not find any statistically significant difference between the Tecnis and Sensar IOLs.[4]

These results support our theory that patients with larger pupils than ours had could profit more from aspheric IOLs. This idea can only be proven, however, by new studies that compare contrast sensitivity after the implantation of aspheric IOLs in eyes with pupils that are larger or smaller than 5mm. ■

This article originally appeared in the November/December 2006 issue of CRSToday.

1. Castejon-Mochon JF, Lopez-Gil N, Benito A, Artal P. Ocular wave-front aberration statistics in a normal young population. *Vision Res.* 2002;42:1611-1617.
2. Wang Y, Zhao K, Jin Y, et al. Changes of higher order aberration with various pupil sizes in the myopic eye. *J Refract Surg.* 2003;19(2 suppl):S270-S274.
3. Kasper T, Bühren J, Kohnen T. Intraindividual comparison of higher-order aberrations after implantation of aspherical and spherical intraocular lenses as a function of pupil diameter. *J Cataract Refract Surg.* 2006;32:78-84.
4. Kasper T, Bühren J, Kohnen T. Visual performance of aspheric and spherical intraocular lenses: intraindividual comparison of visual acuity, contrast sensitivity and higher-order aberrations. *J Cataract Refract Surg.* In press.

CHAPTER 125

The Effect of Decentration on Higher-Order Aberrations

EDWIN J. SARVER, PhD; LI WANG, MD, PhD; AND DOUGLAS D. KOCH, MD

The average human cornea contains a certain amount of positive spherical aberration.[1,2] Because spherical IOLs also have positive spherical aberration, implanting them in the eye increases the degree of this higher-order aberration in the optical system. This fact suggests that implanting IOLs with one or more negatively aspheric surfaces (aspheric IOLs)[3-8] will benefit patients by neutralizing the natural spherical aberrations of their corneas. At minimum, aspheric IOLs should not induce additional

TABLE 1. CORNEAL SHAPES OPTIMIZED FOR MODEL IOLs WITH NEGATIVE, ZERO, AND POSITIVE SPHERICAL ABERRATION

Model Cornea	Optimized for IOL	Corneal K-Value	Spherical Aberration (µm)
Cornea with negative spherical aberration	IOL with positive spherical aberration	-0.967061	-0.2374
Cornea with zero spherical aberration	IOL with zero spherical aberration	-0.632661	-0.0446
Cornea with positive spherical aberration	IOL with negative spherical aberration	-0.140545	0.2701

TABLE 2. SPHERICAL ABERRATIONS INDUCED IN MODEL CORNEAS BY DECENTERED IOLs

Model Cornea	IOL With Positive Spherical Aberration			IOL With Zero Spherical Aberration			IOL With Negative Spherical Aberration		
	Decentration (mm)			Decentration (mm)			Decentration (mm)		
	Zero	0.5	1.0	Zero	0.5	1.0	Zero	0.5	1.0
Cornea with negative spherical aberration	0.0001 µm	0.0032 µm	0.0131 µm	-0.0941 µm	-0.0933 µm	-0.0910 µm	-0.2462 µm	-0.2496 µm	-0.2602 µm
Cornea with zero spherical aberration	0.0934 µm	0.0965 µm	0.1061 µm	Zero	0.0008 µm	0.0031 µm	-0.1503 µm	-0.1536 µm	-0.1636 µm
Cornea with positive spherical aberration	0.2400 µm	0.2429 µm	0.2522 µm	0.1477 µm	0.1485 µm	0.1508 µm	Zero	-0.0030 µm	-0.0120 µm

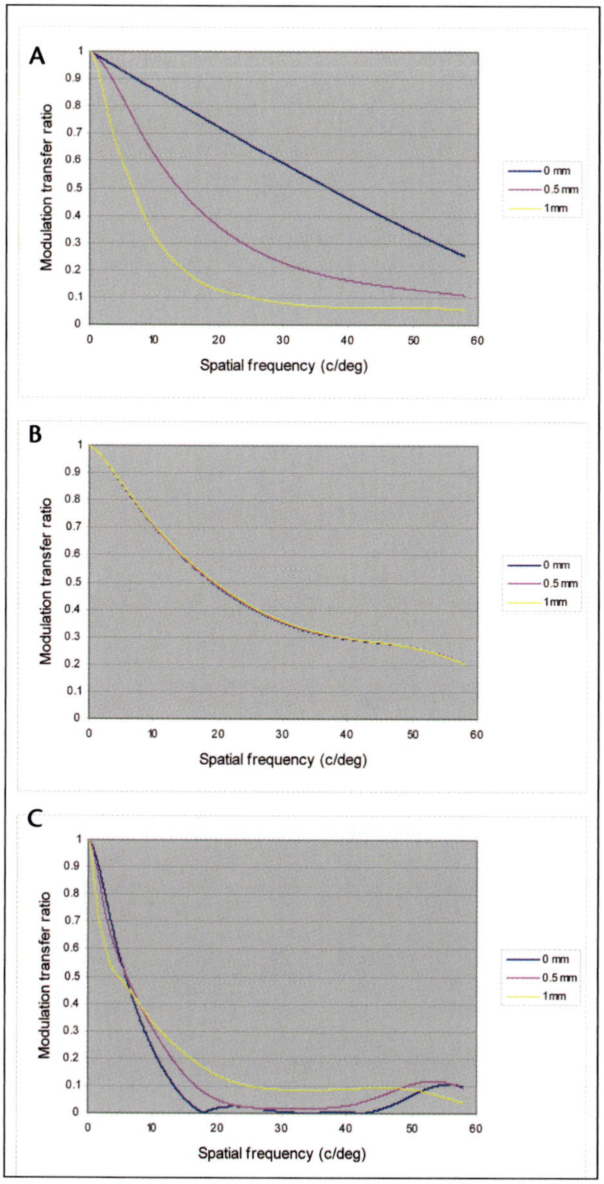

Figure 1. These graphs show the modulation transfer functions for the Soflex spherical IOL (A), the Sofport AO aspheric IOL (B), and the Tecnis aspheric IOL (C) imposed on a cornea with negative spherical aberration. Each IOL is decentered by zero, 0.5, and 1.0mm.

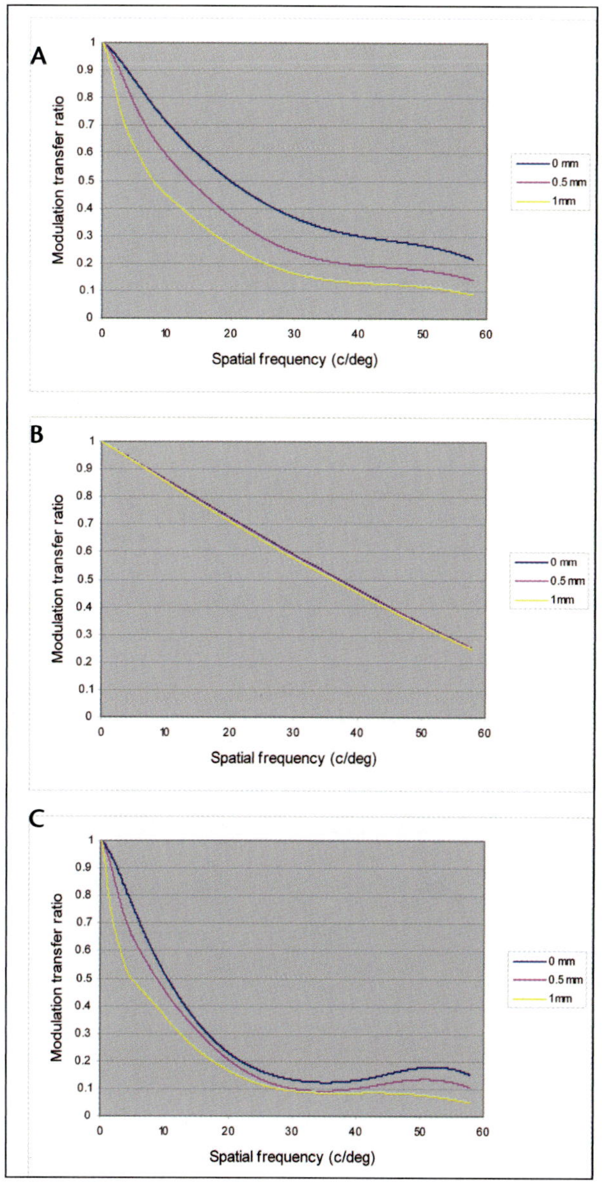

Figure 2. These graphs show the modulation transfer functions for the Soflex spherical IOL (A), the Sofport AO aspheric IOL (B), and the Tecnis aspheric IOL (C) imposed on a cornea with zero spherical aberration. Each IOL is decentered by zero, 0.5, and 1.0mm.

positive spherical aberration. The decentration of an implanted aspheric IOL, however, may overshadow the lens' apparent benefits by inducing coma or reducing modulation transfer.[1,3,9]

This article presents the results of a study in which we measured the effect of decentration on the performance of aspheric IOLs.

METHOD

We used a commercial optical engineering program from Zemax Development Corporation (Bellevue, WA) to perform optical ray tracing and analysis of aspheric schematic eye models and IOL models based on the parameters described by Altmann et al.[3]

The schematic eye model was fixed to 5mm, which is the midrange of the pupil's diameter for 60-year-old subjects over various lighting conditions. The 22.00-D IOL models had positive, negative, and zero spherical aberration, and the decentration values used in the study were zero (on axis), 0.5, and 1.0 mm.

For each of the three IOL models, we determined the corneal asphericity (K-value) needed to optimize the eye model and produced three corneal shapes that matched the IOLs' apical radii of curvature. Table 1 lists the optimized corneal models and their corresponding spherical aberrations. It is unlikely that a natural cornea would have -0.2374 μm^2 of spherical aberration, but the model was useful for the present analysis.

For each of the three corneal shapes, we substituted one of the IOL models (on axis) and optimized the distance to the retina for best focus. We then obtained the modulation transfer functions and Zernike aberrations for the three values of decentration using 512 X 512 rays.

TABLE 3. ASTIGMATISM INDUCED BY DECENTERED IOLs

Model Cornea	IOL With Positive Spherical Aberration			IOL With Zero Spherical Aberration			IOL With Negative Spherical Aberration		
	Decentration (mm)			Decentration (mm)			Decentration (mm)		
	Zero	0.5	1.0	Zero	0.5	1.0	Zero	0.5	1.0
Cornea with negative spherical aberration	Zero	-0.0505 µm	-0.2074 µm	Zero	-0.0094 µm	0.0076 µm	Zero	0.0998 µm	0.4086 µm
Cornea with zero spherical aberration	Zero	-0.0503 µm	-0.2066 µm	Zero	0.0021 µm	0.0077 µm	Zero	0.0993 µm	0.4064 µm
Cornea with positive spherical aberration	Zero	-0.0500 µm	-0.2054 µm	Zero	0.0021 µm	0.0078 µm	Zero	0.0985 µm	0.4031 µm

TABLE 4. COMA INDUCED BY DECENTERED IOLs

Model Cornea	IOL With Positive Spherical Aberration			IOL With Zero Spherical Aberration			IOL With Negative Spherical Aberration		
	Decentration (mm)			Decentration (mm)			Decentration (mm)		
	Zero	0.5	1.0	Zero	0.5	1.0	Zero	0.5	1.0
Cornea with negative spherical aberration	Zero	-0.1459 µm	-0.3028 µm	Zero	-0.0094 µm	-0.0210 µm	Zero	0.2269 µm	0.4679 µm
Cornea with zero spherical aberration	Zero	-0.1451 µm	-0.3012 µm	Zero	-0.0096 µm	-0.0214 µm	Zero	0.2243 µm	0.4626 µm
Cornea with positive spherical aberration	Zero	-0.1439 µm	-0.2988 µm	Zero	-0.0099 µm	-0.0220 µm	Zero	0.2203 µm	0.4543 µm

RESULTS

Figures 1, 2, and 3 show the modulation transfer functions for the decentration values of zero, 0.5, and 1.0 mm imposed on model corneas with negative, positive, and zero spherical aberration, respectively.

The Zernike aberrations for spherical aberration (Z[4,0]), astigmatism (Z[2,2]), and coma (Z[-1,3]) are listed in Tables 2, 3 and 4. Because the decentration of the IOLs was performed only in the y direction, the other terms for astigmatism and coma were zero.

DISCUSSION

We can make several observations about the optical performance of the IOLs as a function of the corneal shape and the amount of decentration of the IOL. Maintaining minimal decentration (less than 0.5 mm) and matching the IOL to the amount of corneal spherical aberration will provide the best optical performance. For misalignments of 0.5 mm or more, the IOL with zero spherical aberration (Sofport AO; Bausch & Lomb, Rochester, NY) provides better visual quality than the spherical (Soflex; Bausch & Lomb) or the aspheric (Tecnis; Advanced Medical Optics, Santa Ana, CA) IOL.

All three IOLs appear to perform about the same in terms of ocular spherical aberration as a function of decentration (Table 2). The IOLs produce approximately the same level of ocular spherical aberration in the resulting eye model when each of them is decentered. The IOL with zero spherical aberration appears to cause slightly less total ocular spherical aberration only because it is optimized for the central range of the corneas under consideration. Surprisingly, the astigmatism and coma induced due to decentration is relatively independent of the corneal shape (Tables 3 and 4).

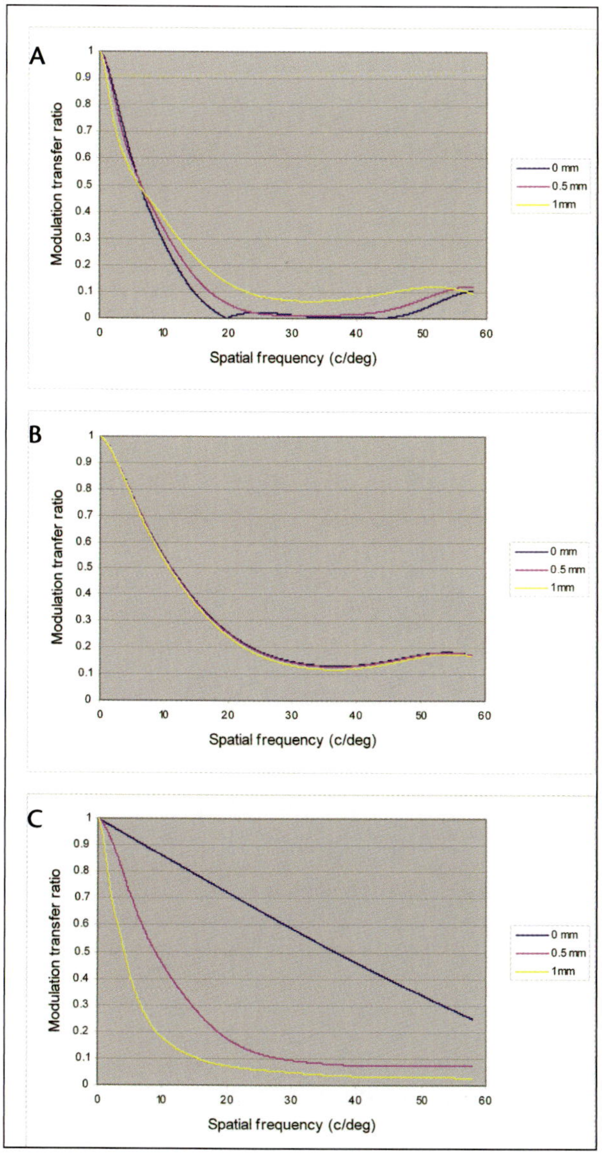

Figure 3. These graphs show the modulation transfer functions for the Soflex spherical IOL (A), the Sofport AO aspheric IOL (B), and the Tecnis aspheric IOL (C) imposed on a cornea with positive spherical aberration. Each IOL is decentered by zero, 0.5, and 1.0 mm.

Spherical IOLs decentered by 0.5 and 1.0 mm induced 14 to 25 times more coma and astigmatism than similarly decentered IOLs with zero spherical aberration. IOLs with negative spherical aberration induced even higher degrees of coma and astigmatism versus IOLs with zero spherical aberration (23 to 50 times as much) when both were decentered by 0.5 and 1.0 mm.

Although a more thorough optical analysis of the IOLs' decentration would include the effects of tilt, defocus, and polychromatic changes, we can draw the following generalizations from our study.

First, IOLs should be selected as a function of the corneal spherical aberration and anticipated decentration for best performance. Second, the modulation transfer function of IOLs with zero spherical aberration is not affected by zero to 1.0 mm of decentration. Third, the modulation transfer function of spherical and aspheric IOLs is adversely affected by 0.5 to 1.0 mm of decentration. Finally, IOLs with zero spherical aberration induce less coma and astigmatism if they decenter than IOLs with positive and negative spherical aberration.

CONCLUSION

Our study shows how the decentration of an aspheric IOL causes ocular aberrations and demonstrates that the magnitude of the induced aberrations is a function of the aspheric IOL. ■

This article originally appeared in the November/December 2006 issue of CRSToday.

1. Krueger RR, MacRae SM, Applegate RA. The future of customization. In: Kreuger RR, Applegate RA, MacRae SM, eds. *Wavefront Customized Visual Correction. The Quest for Super Vision II.* Thorofare, NJ; Slack Incorporated; 2004:363-373.
2. Wang L, Dai E, Koch DD, Nathoo A. Optical aberrations of the human anterior cornea. *J Cataract Refract Surg.* 2003;29:1514-1521.
3. Altmann GE, Nichamin LD, Lane SS, Pepose JS. Optical performance of 3 intraocular lens designs in the presence of decentration. *J Cataract Refract Surg.* 2005;31:574-585.
4. Bellucci R, Morselli S, Piers P. Comparison of wavefront aberrations and optical quality of eyes implanted with five different intraocular lenses. *J Refract Surg.* 2004;20:297-306.
5. Packer M, Fine IH, Hoffman RS, Piers PA. Improved functional vision with a modified prolate intraocular lens. *J Cataract Refract Surg.* 2004;30:986-992.
6. Kershner RM. Retinal image contrast and functional visual performance with aspheric, silicone, and acrylic intraocular lenses. Prospective evaluation. *J Cataract Refract Surg.* 2003;29:1684-1694.
7. Mester U, Dillinger P, Anterist N. Impact of a modified optic design on visual function: clinical comparative study. *J Cataract Refract Surg.* 2003;29:652-660.
8. Holladay JT, Piers PA, Koranyi G, et al. A new intraocular lens design to reduce spherical aberration of pseudophakic eyes. *J Refract Surg.* 2002;18:683-691.
9. Wang L, Koch DD. Effect of decentration of wavefront-corrected intraocular lenses on the higher-order aberrations of the eye. *Arch Ophthalmol.* 2005;123:1226-1230.
10. Atchison DA, Smith G, eds. The aging eye. In: *Optics of the Human Eye.* Edinburgh, UK: Butterworth Heinemann; 2000:221-229.

CHAPTER 126

Do Aspheric IOLs Worsen Pseudoaccommodation?

PABLO ARTAL, PhD, AND JUAN TABERNERO, MSc

Recent studies[1,2] on the location of aberrations in the normal eye have suggested that the young crystalline lens partially compensates for positive corneal aberrations by virtue of its negative spherical aberration but that this effect is lost with age.[3] In contrast, the cornea changes little with age. The manufacturers of ophthalmic lenses have therefore developed aspheric designs to correct for the spherical aberration of the cornea.[4,5] Laboratory studies using adaptive optics[6] and clinical studies have demonstrated the visual benefit of these IOLs.[7]

Correcting the corneal spherical aberration improves the contrast of the retinal image. A question is whether that strategy also reduces depth of focus and therefore renders the pseudophakic eye more vulnerable to errors in defocus. Another important issue is the impact of a misaligned IOL on optical and visual performance. In some cases, the benefit of correcting spherical aberration could be reduced or even negated by the introduction of off-axis aberrations due to the lens' misalignment.

We developed ray-tracing modeling using actual data and have found it to be an extremely useful tool for predicting the optical performance of different types of IOLs after cataract surgery.[8] As this article describes, our results were not what one might expect.

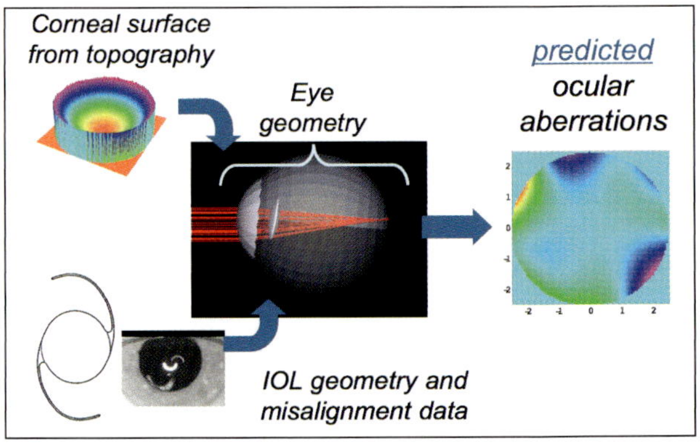

Figure 1. A schematic diagram of the customized ray-tracing modeling is provided. The authors obtained the predicted aberrations from actual data on the cornea, IOL, and eye.

VIRTUAL CATARACT SURGERY

We combined data on the measured corneal topography; the IOL's tilt, decentration, and geometry; and the eye's geometry to predict—through computational ray tracing—the optical performance of eyes implanted with two different types of IOLs. We called this procedure *virtual cataract surgery*. We estimated the wavefront aberration of the cornea from corneal elevations at a sample of points obtained with a Placido-based corneal topographer (Atlas; Carl Zeiss Meditec, Inc., Dublin, CA). To estimate the IOL's tilt and decentration, we developed an instrument based on recording the Purkinje images of a semicircular ring of infrared LEDs for several, well-defined fixations. For each patient, we obtained measurements of axial length and the IOL's axial position.

All of these data were incorporated into the computer ray-tracing model, developed using optical software (Zemax Development Corp., San Diego, CA). The corneal surface was decentered relative to the pupillary center by those values obtained from the corneal topographer. We measured the degree of the IOL's tilt and decentration for each subject postoperatively with our Purkinje-meter system and then incorporated the information into our calculations together with the IOL's axial position, the ocular axial length, and the geometrical details. The specifics of the IOLs' geometry and refractive indices were provided by their manufacturer, Advanced Medical Optics, Inc. (Santa Ana, CA), and we incorporated the information into the model. We compared the company's Tecnis TM Z9000 and Ceeon 911A lenses. Both are foldable, silicone IOLs with a high refractive index (1.458) and a 6-mm optical zone. The Ceeon model is a biconvex lens with spherical surfaces, whereas the Tecnis is an aspheric IOL designed to correct for the average value of corneal spherical aberration.

We incorporated experimental data from a series of cataract patients into the computer model to predict the virtual postoperative ocular aberrations for a variety of conditions and the two types of lenses. Figure 1 provides a schematic view of the complete customized procedure with real aberrations for one patient. We measured the ocular wavefront aberration using our own research-based, prototypic, nearly infrared, Hartmann-Shack wavefront sensor adapted to the clinical environment. This system consists of a microlens array, conjugate with the eye's pupil, and a camera placed at its focal plane. The comparison of the predicted and measured aberrations in several real patients validated our modeling approach.

DEPTH OF FOCUS WITH ASPHERIC AND SPHERICAL IOLs

We studied the depth of focus (pseudoaccommodation) provided to real eyes by both the conventional Ceeon lens and the aspheric Tecnis. We predicted the retinal image quality in 24 patients with the lenses for different values of defocus. As an optical quality metric, we calculated the modulation transfer function at six cycles per degree. Figure 2 shows the average value for all patients as a function of defocus for both IOLs. At best focus, visual performance was better with the aspheric lens, as one would expect. For different values of defocus, however, the Tecnis lens performed better or similarly to the spherical lens. This finding indicates that the aspheric Tecnis IOL generally improves retinal contrast at best focus and also for small values of defocus. In other words, actual pseudoaccommodation is not compromised.

Our results may seem counterintuitive. In a simple, rotationally symmetric eye model for which defocus and spherical aberration are the only variables, removing spherical aberration does indeed

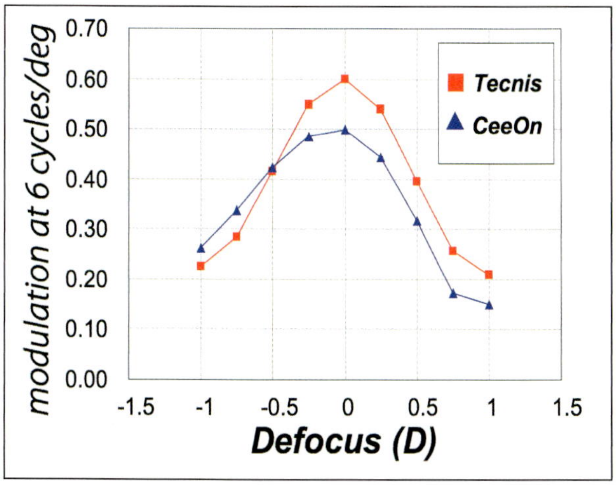

Figure 2. The average values of the modulation at six cycles per degree for different values of defocus are shown in red for the Tecnis lens and in blue for the Ceeon lens. The authors obtained these results with their customized ray-tracing modeling in a group of real patients.

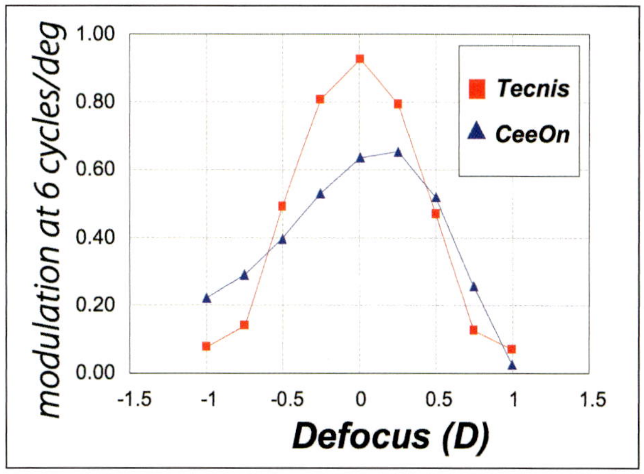

Figure 3. Again, the average values of the modulation at six cycles per degree for different values of defocus are shown in red for the Tecnis IOL and in blue for the Ceeon lens. To obtain these results, the authors used an overly simple approach that took only spherical aberration and defocus into account. This unrealistic prediction suggests that aspheric IOLs reduce depth of focus.

reduce the depth of focus. Figure 3 shows that type of calculation with our modeling when only symmetrical terms were considered. In such an unrealistic case, the Tecnis IOL would perform best at best focus, but the Ceeon lens would be superior for certain degrees of defocus. The eyes of real cataract patients are not affected by spherical aberration alone, however. In the presence of the other higher-order aberrations, correcting spherical aberration improves visual quality at best focus and also for a small refractive error that may occur intraoperatively (Figure 2). Aspheric IOLs therefore do not compromise patients' depth of focus. ■

This article originally appeared in the November/December 2006 issue of CRSToday.

1. Artal P, Guirao A, Berrio E, Williams DR. Compensation of corneal aberrations by the internal optics in the human eye. *J Vis.* 2001;1:1-8.
2. Artal P, Benito A, Tabernero J. The human eye is an example of robust optical design. *J Vis.* 2006;6:1-7.
3. Artal P, Berrio E, Guirao A, Piers P. Contribution of the cornea and internal surfaces to the change of ocular aberrations with age. *J Opt Soc Am A Opt Image Sci Vis.* 2002; 19:137-143.
4. Guirao A, Redondo M, Geraghty E, et al. Corneal optical aberrations and retinal image quality in patients in whom monofocal intraocular lenses were implanted. *Arch Ophthalmol.* 2002;120:1143-1151.
5. Holladay JT, Piers PA, Koranyi G, et al. A new intraocular lens design to reduce spherical aberration of pseudophakic eyes. *J Refract Surg.* 2002;18:683-691.
6. Piers PA, Fernandez EJ, Manzanera S, et al. Adaptive optics simulation of intraocular lenses with modified spherical aberration. *Invest Ophthalmol Vis Sci.* 2004;45:4601-4610.
7. Mester U, Dillinger P, Anterist N. Impact of a modified optic design on visual function: clinical comparative study. *J Cataract Refract Surg.* 2003;29:652-660.
8. Tabernero J, Piers P, Benito A, et al. Predicting the optical performance of eyes implanted with IOLs to correct spherical aberration. *Invest Ophthalmol Vis Sci.* 2006;47:4651-4658.

CHAPTER 127

Akreos IOLs

ROSA BRAGA-MELE, MED, MD, FRCSC

An increasing number of technologies in cataract surgery are launched internationally before making their way to the US market. One such example is the Akreos family of lenses (Adapt AO, Adapt AO with Violet Shield, and the Micro-Incision sub–2-mm Adapt AO lens; all from Bausch & Lomb, Rochester, NY). These lenses are aberration-free, aspheric, hydrophilic acrylic IOLs with a unique 360° square edge. Combining Sofport AO's (Bausch & Lomb) aberration-free aspheric design for reduced dysphotopsia, low posterior capsular opacification, and high patient satisfaction with four square haptics and a steep anterior surface to minimize glare, the Akreos offers a versatile acrylic platform. This article provides an overview on this family of IOLs.

ADAPTABILITY

The Akreos Adapt AO and Sofport AO IOLs have aspheric anterior and posterior surfaces that induce no spherical aberration, because they distribute power uniformly from their center to their edge. Like the Sofport AO lens, the Akreos IOL is neutral to the cornea and therefore suitable for patients regardless of their corneal shape; even patients with preexisting corneal aberration, previous LASIK treatment, or keratoconus are candidates for this lens. The Akreos' even distribution of power allows the IOL to work independently from the imperfect alignment of the natural eye, and it is therefore less affected by decentration—thus providing more predictable refractive and visual outcomes, even in patients with zonular weakness or eccentric pupils.[1] The Akreos IOL has four contact points in three dimensions to fit the capsular bag. It is the first lens to adapt automatically to differently sized eyes. The lens offers other unique design elements, including a steep anterior surface and moderate refractive index of 1.458 (hydrated), to minimize glare. It has four haptics for an anterior/posterior square edge, which offers a 360° posterior barrier, including the haptic/optic junction.

HYDROPHILIC ACRYLIC MATERIAL

Akreos lenses are made of hydrophilic acrylic materials that offer incredible elasticity and allow the lenses to be folded before insertion. The folding method is easy for doctors and nurses, and the lenses may be implanted through small wound assists, which expedite healing times. The Akreos Adapt AO lens may be inserted through a 2.2-mm incision with wound assist, while the Akreos Micro-Incision lens can be inserted through a 1.5-mm incision. The lenses' copolymer composition was developed to provide advanced optical performance without compromising patients' comfort.

KEY BENEFITS

The Akreos IOLs have not been associated with glistenings or observable microvacuoles (data on file with Bausch & Lomb). In addition, the unique hydrophilic acrylic material used in these IOLs makes them much more resistant to damage during YAG procedures than hydrophobic acrylic and silicone lenses.[2] There have been no reports of brown deposits on the acrylic Akreos IOLs in uveitic eyes. The incidence is about 38.5 times more likely to occur with hydrophobic acrylics (such as the Acrysof MA60BM [Alcon Laboratories, Inc., Fort Worth, TX] and the Sensar AR40 [Advanced Medical Optics, Inc., Santa Ana, CA]) when compared to hydrophilic acrylics (Akreos or hydrophobic silicone IOLs).[3] One reason for this difference may be that the acrylic is highly biocompatible; it is therefore frequently used successfully in patients with inflammatory conditions.[4] The Akreos IOLs may also be less susceptible to biocontamination and have lower rates of endophthalmitis due to their lower ratio of early adhesion and bacterial density compared with hydrophobic products.[5] Compared with IOLs that have higher refractive indices (lenses made of silicone and hydrophobic acrylic), the Akreos IOLs induce less dysphotopsia, because their water content helps to minimize glare as well as external and internal reflections.[6-9]

AKREOS AND THE US MARKET

More than 1.5 million Akreos lenses have been implanted in Europe during the last 3 years. The IOLs' success in the US depends on whether surgeons appreciate the benefits of the IOLs' hydrophilic acrylic material. The Akreos Adapt, and its next-generation Micro-Incision lens for sub–2-mm microincisional surgery, are safe, reliable, and predictable in terms of their insertion and ocular stability.[10] The 30 patients in whom I have implanted the lens to date, all have shown excellent ocular stability and visual outcomes. The Akreos Adapt AO IOL is expected to enter the US market this year, pending FDA approval. The Akreos AO Micro-Incision sub–2-mm lens is currently expected to debut in the US in 2008. ■

This article originally appeared in the February 2007 issue of CRSToday.

1. Haustermans A. The Akreos advanced optics IOL: no additional spherical aberration. *Cataract & Refractive Surgery Today Europe.*2006;1;1:55.
2. Trinavarat A, Atchaneeyasakul L, Udompunturak S. Neodymium:YAG laser damage threshold of foldable intraocular lenses. *J Cataract Refract Surg.*2001;27:775-780.
3. Manuchehri K, Mohamed S, Cheung D, et al. Brown deposits in the optic of foldable intraocular lenses in patients with uveitis. *Eye.* 2004;18:54-58.
4. Abela-Formanek C, Amom M, Schauersberger J, et al. Uveal and capsular biocompatibility of 2 foldable acrylic intraocular lenses in patients with uveitis or pseudoexfoliation syndrome: comparison to a control group. *J Cataract Refract Surg.*2002;28:1160-1172.
5. Schauersberger J, Amon M, Aichinger D, Georgopoulos A. Bacterial adhesion to rigid and foldable posterior chamber intraocular lenses: in vitro study. *J Cataract Refract Surg.* 2003;29:361-366.
6. Davison JA. Positive and negative dysphotopsia in patients with acrylic intraocular lenses. *J Cataract Refract Surg.* 2000;26:1346-1355.
7. Farbowitz, MA, Zabriskie NA, Crandall AS, et. al. Visual complaints associated with the AcrySof acrylic intraocular lens. *J Cataract Refract Surg.* 2000;26;1339-1345.
8. Holladay JT, Lang A, Portney V. Analysis of edge glare phenomena in intraocular lens edge designs. *J Cataract Refract Surg.* 1999;25:748-752.
9. Erie JC, Bandhauer MH, McLaren JW. Analysis of postoperative glare and intraocular lens design. *J Cataract Refract Surg.* 2001;27:614-621.
10. Spath U, Liekfeld A, Hartmann C, Pham DT. Evaluation of posterior capsule opacification after implantation of the Akreos Disc and Akreos Fit acrylic intraocular lenses. *Klin Monatsbl Augenheilkd.* 2003;220:695-698.

CHAPTER 128

Analyzing Explanted IOLs

LILIANA WERNER, MD, PhD

Every week, the John A. Moran Eye Center at the University of Utah in Salt Lake City receives discolored or opacified IOLs explanted from cataract patients. As of 2006, my colleagues and I at the Berlin Eye Research Institute in Germany have also received explanted ocular devices from institutions all over the world, especially from Europe. Our sample from both sites contains a wide range of designs and materials, including some not currently available in the United States (Figure 1).

First-line treatments for decreased vision after cataract surgery may include Nd:YAG laser capsulotomy or vitrectomy, depending on the underlying cause. These interventions are not effective, however, if the problem is caused by an opacified or discolored IOL. The only way to improve vision in these situations may be to replace the opacified device.

This article summarizes our analyses of explanted IOLs and discusses the pathologic processes underlying the opacification of these lenses.

TRACKING CAUSE AND EFFECT

To better understand the pathologic processes that affect the clarity of IOLs, my colleagues and I examined opacified lenses with gross and light microscopy, scanning electron microscopy, energy dispersive x-ray spectroscopy, gas chromatography-mass spectroscopy, and other methods.[1] Our analyses revealed several factors that can compromise an IOL's optical clarity, some of which may be prevented (see *Strategies for Preventing Some Causes of IOL Opacification*).

Depending on the underlying process, IOLs can become opacified or discolored at any time during or after surgery. We described two cases in which single-piece hydrophobic acrylic SA60AT IOLs (Alcon Laboratories, Inc., Fort Worth, TX) were explanted because fragments of the ophthalmic viscosurgical device (OVD) used to load the lenses into the injectors crystallized intraoperatively on their surfaces.[2]

An analysis of three-piece silicone IOLs explanted from six patients who developed cloudy vision a few hours after cataract surgery showed that the environment in which lenses are stored preoperatively could affect their behavior in the eye. Investigators determined that the chemicals used to clean a storage facility caused the IOLs' normally hydrophobic surfaces to become more hydrophilic. After the silicone lenses were implanted, they absorbed excessive water and became opaque.[3,4]

The high-water content (73%) of an explanted Acqua hydrophilic acrylic IOL (Mediphacos, Belo Horizonte, Brazil, [not available in the US]) appeared to contribute to the len's uptake of trypan blue during cataract surgery.[5] Compared with other hydrophilic acrylic IOLs, which contain less water and are stored in balanced salt solution or distilled water prior to their insertion, the Acqua IOL is implanted in a dry state. Consequently, the lens reaches its full size only after it absorbs additional fluid from the capsular bag. The use of capsular dyes is contraindicated with the Acqua IOL because it will absorb any dye left in the eye following surgery.

In some cases, lenticular opacification affects only visual acuity, whereas in others the underlying cause has potentially serious consequences. In the July 2006 issue of *Cataract & Refractive Surgery Today*, I described eight cases of Toxic Anterior Segment Syndrome that were associated with an oily substance in the anterior chambers of cataract patients treated at the Department of Eye Medicine and Surgery of Hamilton Health Sciences in Hamilton, Ontario.[6,7] The substance was identified as an ointment instilled in the patients' eyes that had entered the anterior chamber through the clear corneal incision. To prevent this complication, surgeons should construct corneal wounds appropriately, ensure the wound's integrity postoperatively, and avoid patching the operated eye tightly after applying ophthalmic ointment. Surgeons should also consider replacing ointment with antibiotic drops.

LONG-TERM COMPLICATIONS

The analyses of explanted IOLs has identified pathological processes that seem to target specific materials and cause complications

STRATEGIES FOR PREVENTING SOME CAUSES OF IOL OPACIFICATION

- Follow the manufacturer's recommendations for loading IOLs into injectors and storing OVD. Surgeons should take special care to minimize the period of contact between the OVD and the lens before its injection into the eye.
- Store IOLs in a clean, dry environment, and avoid exposing them to chemicals that could alter their surface properties.
- Avoid using capsular dyes with IOLs that have a very high water content.
- Construct clear corneal incisions properly, ensure the wound's integrity at the end of the procedure, and avoid patching eyes tightly after instilling ophthalmic ointment.
- Do not implant silicone IOLs in patients who are likely to need retinal surgery in the future, because silicone IOLs interact with silicone oil.
- Remove all residual cortex from the capsular bag before implanting piggybacked IOLs. Either insert both lenses into the capsular bag through a capsulorhexis with a relatively large diameter or implant the anterior IOL in the sulcus and the posterior IOL in the bag through a small capsulorhexis.

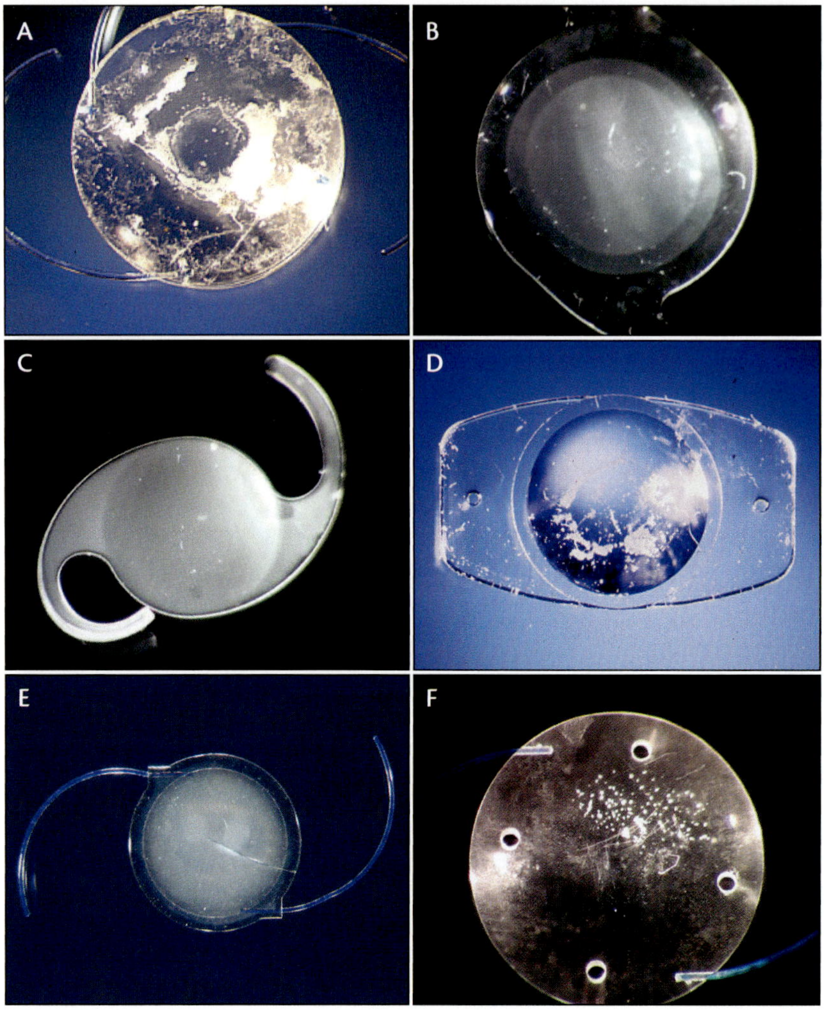

Figure 1. Examples of IOLs explanted in different countries and analyzed at the John A. Moran Eye Center at the University of Utah in Salt Lake City or the Berlin Eye Research Institute in Germany. The lenses were manufactured from different biomaterials and exhibit opacification of their optics due to conditions such as interlenticular opacification (A), calcification (B to D), contamination by exogenous molecules (E), or incipient snowflake degeneration (F). All these conditions were discussed in: Werner L. Causes of intraocular lens opacification or discoloration. *J Cataract Refract Surg*. 2007;33:713-726.

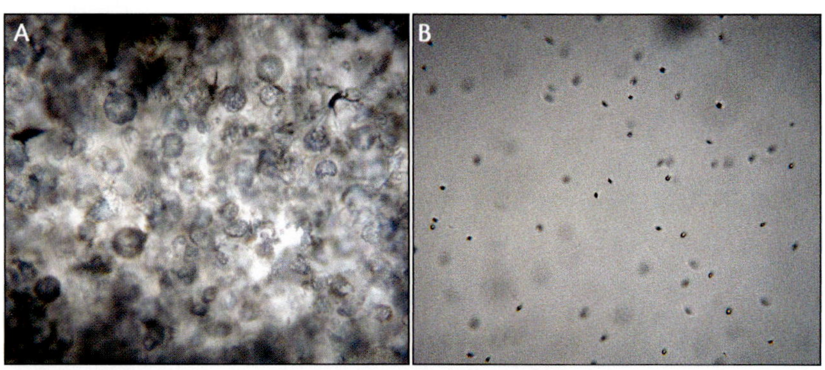

Figure 2. Light microscopic photographs showing the aspect of the dry lesions in the snowflake degeneration of a PMMA IOL (A) and of the fluid-filled vacuoles, known as glistenings, within a hydrophobic acrylic lens (B).

that appear several months to years after the IOL's implantation.

Surgeons should note that because silicone oils used during retinal surgery adhere to silicone IOLs, they should avoid using this type of lens in patients who might need treatment for severe vitreoretinal disease in the future.[1] The literature also describes a few cases in which patients with asteroid hyalosis developed calcified deposits on their silicone IOLs.[8,9]

Since 1999, my colleagues and I have identified several factors that contributed to the deposition of calcium and phosphate on or within hydrophilic acrylic IOLs, including a change in the polishing process (MemoryLens; Ciba Vision, Duluth, GA)[10] and contamination from silicone compounds used in packaging materials (Hydroview; Bausch & Lomb, Rochester, NY; Aqua-Sense; Ophthalmic Innovations International, Ontario, CA).[11,12] We also observed calcification of another hydrophilic acrylic IOL (SC60B-OUV IOL; Medical Developmental Research, Inc., Clearwater, FL),[13] which some researchers[14] have attributed to premature aging of its UV-blocking agent.

Although interlenticular opacification, a process in which residual cortex adheres to the opposing surfaces of piggybacked IOLs, does not cause the lenses themselves to become cloudy, it can be associated with the explantation of pairs of hydrophobic acrylic IOLs.[15]

All the cases of interlenticular opacification that my colleagues and I have analyzed to date occurred when two posterior chamber hydrophobic acrylic IOLs were implanted in the capsular bag through a small capsulorhexis. In every instance, the capsulorhexis' margins overlapped the anterior IOL's optic edge for 360°.

Because the pathogenesis of interlenticular opacification is similar to pearl-like posterior capsular opacification, surgeons should always perform careful cortical cleanup before implanting piggybacked IOLs. They can also reduce the risk of this complication by implanting both IOLs in the capsular bag through a relatively large capsulorhexis or by placing the anterior IOL in the sulcus and the posterior IOL into the capsule through a small capsulorhexis.

PMMA lenses may be associated

with a form of opacification known as *snowflake degeneration*.[16,17] This pathological process first appears as scattered white-brown spots within the IOL's substance that can increase in intensity and number over time and eventually affect visual acuity. Snowflake lesions tend to form in the central anterior area of PMMA IOLs' optics, which suggests an association with long-term exposure to UV radiation. Manufacturing variations in some PMMA IOLs fabricated in the 1980s to early 1990s may be responsible for the lens' progressive degeneration. Snowflake lesions are dry and thus differ from glistenings because the latter are fluid-filled vacuoles that can be observed with any IOL material. Glistenings are largely described in association with hydrophobic acrylic lenses, however, and are generally stated to be clinically insignificant[18] (Figure 2).

CONCLUSION

My colleagues and I hope that our research will help surgeons identify the cause of an IOL's opacification, decide if and when explantation is necessary, and reduce the risk that patients will undergo unnecessary capsulotomy or vitrectomy. ■

I would like to thank my colleagues at the University of Utah, Nick Mamalis, MD, and the many research fellows who have been involved in these studies throughout the past years. I also thank my colleagues at the Berlin Eye Research Institute, Manfred Tetz, MD, Mona Tawfik, MD, and Matthias Mueller, Dipl-Ing, for their support and collaboration in this project.

Analyses of explanted IOLs at the John A. Moran Eye Center have been supported in part by the Research to Prevent Blindness Olga Keith Wiess Scholar Award (to Liliana Werner, MD, PhD). Dr. Werner also has received an ESCRS Research Grant for the project "Analyses of Intraocular Lenses and Other Ocular Implants Explanted in Europe Because of Different Complications," performed at the Berlin Eye Research Institute.

This article originally appeared in the September 2007 issue of CRSToday.

1. Werner L. Causes of intraocular opacification or discoloration. *J Cataract Refract Surg.* 2007;33:713-726.
2. Hickman MS, Werner L, Mamalis N, et al. Intraoperative explantation of two single-piece hydrophobic acrylic intraocular lenses due to surface deposits. *Eye.* 2006;20:1054-1060.
3. Hilgert CR, Hilgert A, Höfling-Lima AL, et al. Early opacification of SI-40NB silicone intraocular lenses. *J Cataract Refract Surg.* 2004;30:2225-2229.
4. Werner L, Dornelles F, Hilgert CR, et al. Early opacification of silicone intraocular lenses: laboratory analysis of 6 explants. *J Cataract Refract Surg.* 2006;499-504.
5. Werner L, Apple DJ, Crema AS, et al. Permanent blue discoloration of a hydrogel intraocular lens by intraoperative trypan blue. *J Cataract Refract Surg.* 2002;28:1278-1286.
6. Werner L. TASS and intraocular ointment. *Cataract & Refractive Surgery Today.* 2006;6:7:62-64.
7. Werner L, Sher JH, Taylor JR, et al. Toxic anterior segment syndrome and possible association with ointment in the anterior chamber following cataract surgery. *J Cataract Refract Surg.* 2006;32:227-235.
8. Foot L, Werner L, Gills JP, et al. Surface calcification of silicone plate intraocular lenses in patients with asteroid hyalosis. *Am J Ophthalmol.* 2004;137:979-987.
9. Werner L, Kollarits CR, Mamalis N, Olson RJ. Surface calcification of a 3-piece silicone IOL in a patient with asteroid hyalosis: a clinicopathologic case report. *Ophthalmology.* 2005;139:734-735.
10. Neuhann IM, Werner L, Izak AM, et al. Late postoperative opacification of a hydrophilic acrylic (hydrogel) intraocular lens: a clinicopathological analysis of 106 explants. *Ophthalmology.* 2004;111:2094-2101.
11. Werner L, Apple DJ, Escobar-Gomez M, et al. Postoperative deposition of calcium on the surfaces of a hydrogel intraocular lens. *Ophthalmology.* 2000;107:2179-2185.
12. Werner L, Hunter B, Stevens S, et al. Role of silicone contamination on calcification of hydrophilic acrylic intraocular lenses. *Am J Ophthalmol.* 2006;141:45-43.
13. Werner L, Apple DJ, Kaskaloglu M, Pandey SK. Dense opacification of the optical component of a hydrophilic acrylic intraocular lens: a clinicopathological analysis of 9 explanted lenses. *J Cataract Refract Surg.* 2001;27:1485-1492.
14. Frohn A, Dick B, Augustin AJ, Grus FH. Late opacification of the foldable hydrophilic acrylic lens SC60B-OUV. *Ophthalmology.* 2001;108:1999-2004.
15. Werner L, Apple DJ, Pandey SK, et al. Analysis of elements of interlenticular opacification. *Am J Ophthalmol.* 2002;133:320-326.
16. Apple DJ, Werner L. Complications of cataract and refractive surgery: a clinicopathological documentation. *Trans Am Ophthalmol Soc.* 2001;99:95-109.
17. Dahle N, Werner L, Fry L, Mamalis N. Localized, central optic snowflake degeneration of a PMMA intraocular lens: Clinical report with pathological correlation. *Arch Ophthalmol.* 2006;124:1350-1353.
18. Tognetto D, Toto L, Sanguinetti G, Ravalico G. Glistenings in foldable intraocular lenses. *J Cataract Refract Surg.* 2002;28:1211-1216.

CHAPTER 129

IOL Selection for the Weakened Capsular Bag

DAVID F. CHANG, MD

Devices designed to help stabilize the loosened capsular bag during phacoemulsification include (1) capsular tension rings (CTRs; Morcher GmbH, Stuttgart, Germany [distributed in the United States by FCI Ophthalmics, Inc., Marshfield Hills, MA], and OPHTEC, Groningen, the Netherlands), (2) the Ahmed capsular tension segment (Morcher GmbH), and (3) capsule retractors such as the Mackool Cataract Support System (Duckworth & Kent Ltd., Hertfordshire, England, and Impex, Staten Island, NY). Thanks to these devices and to techniques such as phaco chop, surgeons are frequently able to preserve the capsular bag despite the multiple challenges posed by weakened zonules. The surgeon, however, is then faced with a new set of decisions. Is the capsular bag suitable for the long-term support of an IOL? Which IOL should be used? Is a CTR or other implantable device, such as a Cionni modified CTR (Morcher GmbH), necessary? The same questions must be considered for all eyes with pseudoexfoliation (PXF) in light of the increasing incidence of late, spontaneous dislocation of the capsular bag.[1-4]

SPONTANEOUS DISLOCATION OF THE CAPSULAR BAG

At the 2000 Annual Meeting of the AAO, Mamalis et al[1] reported their initial series of nine patients with PXF who presented with late, spontaneous dislocation of the capsular bag. These dislocations occurred between 5 and 10 years after the original surgery. The investigators' case series comprised eight PMMA IOLs and one plate haptic silicone IOL, and it was published in *Ophthalmology*

1 year later.[2] I reported on two cases of spontaneous dislocation in PXF patients with three-piece silicone IOLs.[3] At the 2002 AAO Annual Meeting Spotlight on Cataracts Symposium, Alan Crandall, MD, of Salt Lake City updated his series, which numbered 19 patients at that time.[4]

I was impressed by the contraction of the capsulorhexis in the four patients whom I have managed with this complication. I was the primary surgeon for three of them (Figure 1). Exaggerated contraction of the capsulorhexis is usually an indication of weak zonules.[5-7] It also seems likely, however, that capsulophimosis and extensive anterior capsular fibrosis exerted excessive centripetal strain on the already weakened zonules in these eyes.

Given that the capsulorhexis technique was not widely adopted until the early 1990s, and considering the 5- to 10-year latency for this complication, it makes sense that we surgeons are seeing an increasing frequency and growing awareness of this complication during the past few years. In assessing the risk of delayed spontaneous bag dislocation in PXF, however, what is not known is the denominator. Complicating any evaluation of preventive measures is the fact that dislocation may take more than 10 years to occur. Nonetheless, I believe it is possible to make rational choices based upon our current knowledge of IOL design and materials.

CTRS AND PXF

Does every patient with PXF require a CTR? This decision is controversial, and the extent of zonular deficiency should be a determinant. Significant zonular weakness would certainly be a reasonable indication for a CTR. Many PXF patients, however, exhibit no intraoperative evidence of zonular laxity, and I do not think that a CTR is necessary in such cases. Nevertheless, there are several surgical and IOL design objectives that make sense for any patient with PXF.

Thorough cortical cleanup is especially important in PXF eyes. Although the circumferential anterior capsular overlap of the optic edge is desirable, an excessively small-diameter capsulorhexis must be avoided in these patients. IOLs with optic diameters smaller than 6 mm should be avoided for this reason. Following IOL implantation, a small capsulorhexis can be secondarily enlarged if necessary. After obliquely cutting one edge with a long Vannas scissors, I re-tear the opening under viscoelastic.

Because hydrophobic acrylic IOLs are associated with less anterior capsular fibrosis when compared with silicone lenses,[8,9] I believe that the former material is preferable for PXF eyes. Three-piece lens designs with broad, stiff PMMA haptics are able to exert the maximum centrifugal tension against the capsular fornices. They are preferable to the soft, floppy single-piece haptics for this reason. At the most recent AAO Annual Meeting, Da Reitz Pereira et al[10] reported on a large retrospective study comparing the single-piece and three-piece AcrySof IOLs (Alcon Laboratories, Inc., Fort Worth, TX). With a single surgeon and identical capsulorhexis sizing, the single-piece AcrySof group demonstrated a significantly higher incidence of capsular contraction syndrome. Three percent of the single-piece AcrySof group required a YAG anterior capsulotomy for this condition versus none of the three-piece group. One should probably avoid silicone plate haptic IOLs in PXF eyes, because of these lenses' haptic design and higher tendency for anterior capsular fibrosis.

Finally, one should specifically examine the anterior capsular reaction at the final 1-month postoperative visit in patients with PXF. If there already are signs of early contracture and fibrosis, prophylactic YAG relaxing cuts in the capsulorhexis edge should be considered.

In any eye in which the surgeon notes intraoperative signs of zonular laxity, the placement of a CTR is prudent. The goals would be to (1) prevent capsulophimosis, (2) reduce centripetal zonular stress by resisting capsulorhexis contraction, and (3) avoid IOL decentration caused by asymmetric capsular fibrosis. There are numerous situations, however, where a CTR alone might not afford sufficient long-term capsular support. Such cases include eyes with a large zonular dialysis or severe, diffuse circumferential weakness. It is for these eyes that the Cionni modified CTR or the Ahmed capsular tension segment were designed. Unfortunately, neither device is currently FDA-approved in the US.

If a CTR is not available, there are other options to consider. As an alternative to enlarging a small-diameter capsulorhexis, one could make relaxing incisions in the capsulorhexis edge after placing the IOL in the bag. With a temporal incision, I would orient the haptics along the horizontal axis (3- to 9-o'clock position) and make two opposing cuts in the capsulorhexis edge superiorly and inferiorly (12- and 6-o'clock positions). The cuts should not extend too far peripherally, because they merely need to prevent the sphincter-like contraction of the capsulorhexis margin.

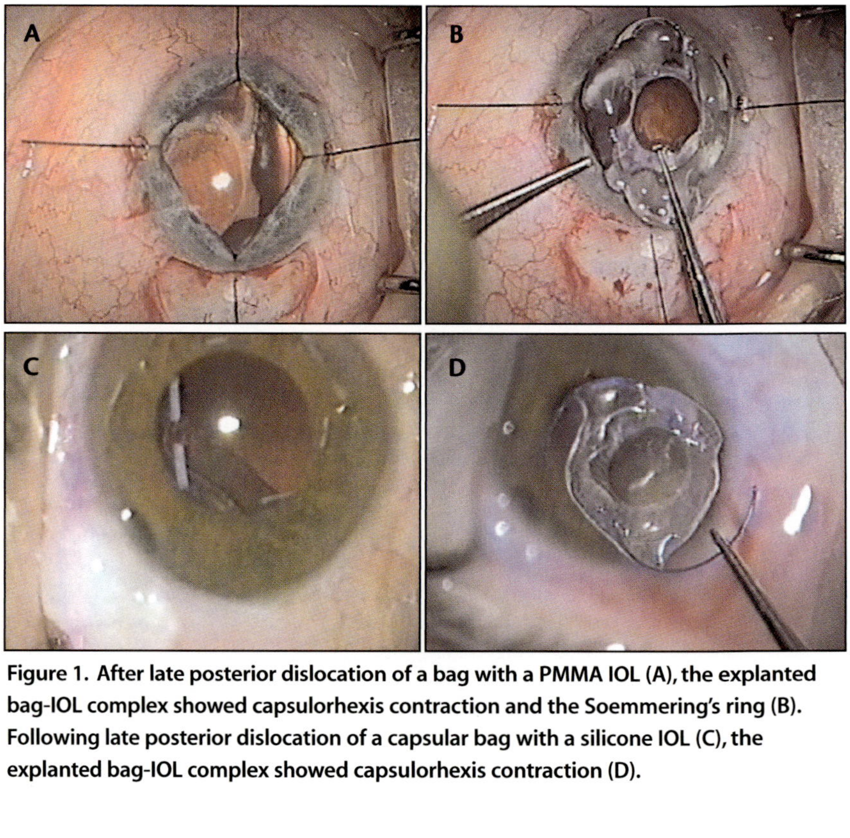

Figure 1. After late posterior dislocation of a bag with a PMMA IOL (A), the explanted bag-IOL complex showed capsulorhexis contraction and the Soemmering's ring (B). Following late posterior dislocation of a capsular bag with a silicone IOL (C), the explanted bag-IOL complex showed capsulorhexis contraction (D).

Finally, one could place the IOL in the sulcus (Figure 2). The sulcus diameter can be estimated by adding 1.5 mm to the white-to-white horizontal corneal diameter. Thus, the typical foldable IOL of 13 mm in overall length is too short for a corneal diameter of 12 mm or greater. STAAR Surgical Company (Monrovia, CA) makes a 13.5-mm foldable silicone IOL (model AQ 2010 V) that is my preference for sulcus placement. The IOL power should be reduced by 0.50 to 1.00 D from that calculated for capsular bag placement.[11] The single-piece AcrySof is not only too short for sulcus placement, but it has thicker, sharp-edged haptics that can cause pigment dispersion. If sulcus placement is elected because of a severe zonular dialysis, one should consider making multiple relaxing cuts in the capsulorhexis edge to avoid extensive and asymmetric bag contracture with avulsion of the remaining hemisphere of weak zonules.

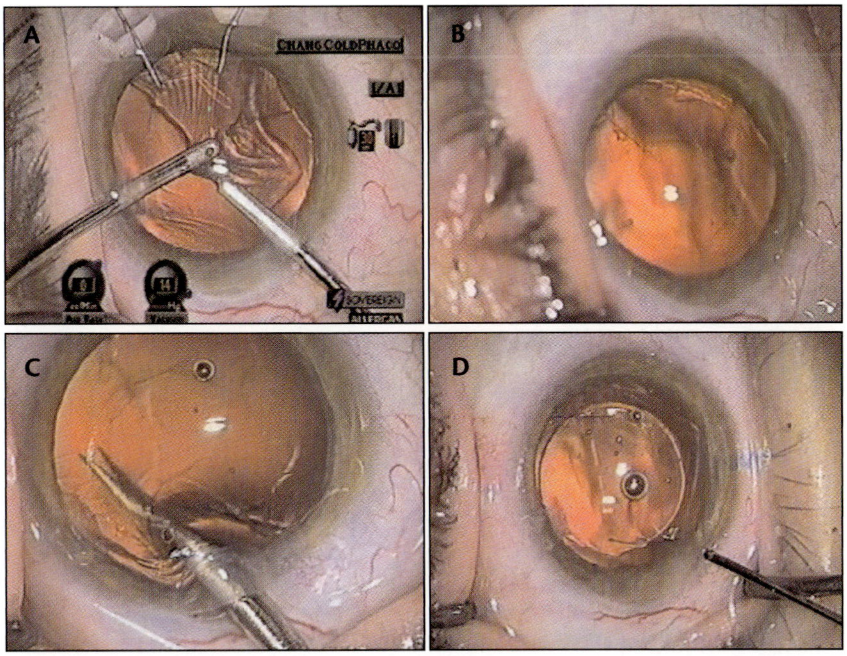

Figure 2. Mackool capsule retractors supported a nasal area of large zonular dialysis during bimanual cortical irrigation and aspiration (A). Despite the preservation of the capsular bag, a large nasal zonular dialysis was visible after the removal of the capsule retractors (B). The surgeon used long Vannas scissors to make multiple radial cuts in the nasal capsulorhexis edge (C). The surgeon placed a 13.5-mm-long, foldable silicone IOL in the sulcus, with the haptic axis oriented 90° from the zonular defect (D).

CONCLUSION

Whereas excellent results may be obtained with a wide range of IOL materials and designs in routine cases, eyes with weak zonules are at greater risk for delayed IOL subluxation, dislocation, and capsulophimosis. Surgeons should strive to minimize anterior capsular fibrosis and capsulorhexis contraction through a combination of surgical technique and IOL selection. ■

This article originally appeared in the May 2004 issue of CRSToday.

1. Mamalis N, Jehan FS, Crandall AS. Spontaneous late dislocation of intraocular lens within capsular bag in pseudoexfoliation patients. Paper presented at: The AAO Annual Meeting; October 24, 2000; Dallas, TX.
2. Jahan FS, Mamalis N, Crandall AS. Spontaneous late dislocation of intraocular lens within the capsular bag in pseudoexfoliation patients. *Ophthalmology.* 2001;108:1727-1731.
3. Chang DF. Prevention of bag-fixated IOL dislocation in pseudoexfoliation. *Ophthalmology.* 2002;109:5-6.
4. Crandall A. Late bag dislocation in pseudoexfoliation. Paper presented at: The AAO Annual Meeting; October 21, 2002; Orlando, FL.
5. Hansen SO, Crandall AS, Olson RJ. Progressive constriction of the anterior capsular opening following intact capsulorhexis. *J Cataract Refract Surg.* 1993;19:77-82.
6. Davison JA. Capsule contraction syndrome. *J Cataract Refract Surg.* 1993;19:582-589.
7. Hayashi H, Hayashi K, Nakao F, Hayashi F. Anterior capsule contraction and intraocular lens dislocation in eyes with pseudoexfoliation syndrome. *Br J Ophthalmol.* 1998;82:1429-1432.
8. Hayashi H, Hayashi K, Nakao F, Hayashi F. Reduction in the area of the anterior capsule opening after polymethylmethacrylate, silicone, and soft acrylic intraocular lens implantation. *Am J Ophthalmol.* 1997;123:441-447.
9. Werner L, Pandey SK, Apple DJ, et al. Anterior capsule opacification. *Ophthalmology.* 2001;108:1675-1681.
10. Da Reitz Pereira C, Rauser ME, LaBree L. Anterior capsule contraction syndrome with the AcrySof SA60AT acrylic lens. Paper presented at: The AAO Annual Meeting; November 18, 2003; Anaheim, CA.
11. Suto C, Hori S, Fukuyama E, Akura J. Adjusting intraocular lens power for sulcus fixation. *J Cataract Refract Surg.* 2003;29:1913-1917.

CHAPTER 130

Radial Rhexis Tear or Sulcus Implantation

LISA BROTHERS ARBISSER, MD

The goal of cataract surgery is to achieve 100% capsular bag placement of the IOL in the setting of an intact continuous curvilinear capsulorhexis (CCC) and posterior capsule. Although a laudable aim, cataract surgeons sometimes fall short. Knowing how to compensate for complications related to suboptimal surgical anatomy is essential to providing our patients with optimal outcomes.

CCC TEARS

My lens of choice for routine cataract surgery is a one-piece, acrylic, truncated-edge, blue-blocking implant (SN60 AT; Alcon Laboratories, Inc., Fort Worth, TX). This lens' attributes include maximum capsular biocompatibility, acceptable uveal biocompatibility, maximum refractive stability and predictability of effective lens position (ELP), reduced capsular opacification, ease of insertion, and theoretically maximized macular protection. Many of these traits make this lens ideal for cases in which the anterior CCC tears.

In the complicated setting of a CCC tear, one salient reason to use a one-piece acrylic IOL in the bag is the lack of pent-up energy the lens disperses as it unfolds within the eye, thus allowing a controlled placement during insertion. Silicone IOLs generally release more energy during folder ejection than do acrylic implants. The force of an explosively unfolding lens extends to the capsule's edge and can result in a radial tear that often extends through the equator. Three-piece lenses are tricky to place without applying some pressure on the capsule. A two-handed technique that uses a "Y" hook through the paracentesis incision to support the trailing haptic near the haptic-optic junction reduces these insertion forces compared with dialing or one-handed pronation of PMMA haptics. Surgeons should never consider inserting a plate-haptic lens without an intact capsule.

To place the AcrySof one-piece IOL, the surgeon folds the acrylic haptics onto the optic, inserts the implant into the loading cartridge, implants the entire body of the lens into the viscoelastic-expanded bag, and gently floats the implant into position. As long as the trailing optic-haptic junction clears the rhexis' edge, no force is transmitted to the capsule's edge upon lens insertion or unfolding, and the tear does not extend.

The second reason to choose a one-piece acrylic IOL is its immediate and long-term force distribution. Hydrophobic acrylic causes the least capsular fibrosis, and, because of its tackiness, firmly bonds to the capsule. Third-generation silicone is quite biocompatible with the uvea but less so with the capsule. When unbalanced, due to fibrosis in the presence of a tear, the shrinking capsule can cause postoperative movement of the three-piece lens as it applies asymmetric forces to the bag. In a small eye, PMMA haptics may have a sufficient diameter to cause a Maddox rod effect on the posterior capsule with axial striae. These same forces translate to the anterior capsular edge. In the presence of CCC discontinuity, asymmetric forces may increase over time and lead to lens decentration. If the surgeon must place a three-piece lens inside a capsular bag that has a single radial tear, Howard Gimbel, MD, of Loma Linda, California, has recommended intentionally creating a small radial incision 180° away from the tear,[1] a technique that may help distribute the forces over time. I find this maneuver unnecessary for one-piece acrylic IOLs, because the haptics distribute forces evenly to the bag and do not lose their memory; this IOL design produces predictable centration even in this compromised situation.

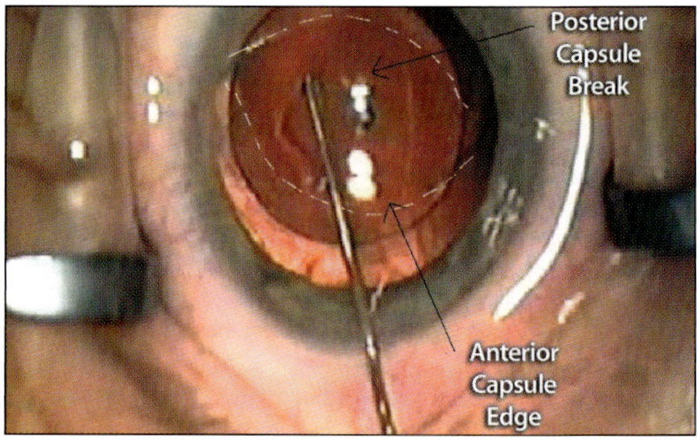

Figure 1. A three-piece acrylic lens with its haptics in the sulcus and its optic captured through the CCC in the bag tamponades the posterior capsular break and ensures lens centration.

TORN POSTERIOR CAPSULE

Although some physicians advocate using a one-piece acrylic lens in the capsular bag in the case of a torn posterior capsule, I limit in-the-bag implantation to eyes in which the posterior capsular tear is converted to a true posterior CCC. Even limited or round posterior tears are undependable intraoperatively and postoperatively. For an unconverted posterior capsular tear with an intact anterior capsulorhexis, I choose any three-piece IOL for sulcus implantation with optic capture, as first described by Neuhann.[2] The diameter of the CCC must be at least 1 mm smaller than the optic's diameter and centered (my goal in every case).

For a torn posterior capsule with an intact CCC, I implant the lens initially in the sulcus. Then, I apply gentle posterior pressure to the surface of the optic, 90° away from the optic-haptic junctions. I use a sweep or lens manipulator, first near the distal edge and then the proximal edge, to push the optic under the CCC edge. Thus, the optic sinks into the bag, thus causing the CCC to ovalize (Figure 1). This maneuver firmly fixates the optic-haptic junctions at the apex of the oval, a situation that provides ideal stability. Because the implantation does not depend on the relationship between the haptic diameter and the sulcus length for centration, any three-piece foldable lens is acceptable. If the CCC is centered, the optic will remain centered forever. Because the optic is drawn backward toward the plane of the anterior capsule, it minimally changes the ELP so that the lens power need not be modified for lower IOL powers. For IOLs exceeding 23.00 D, the altered lens position warrants a 0.50-D decrease in the power of the lens implanted. Pigment dispersion, sometimes seen in pure sulcus implantation, is absent because the optic is drawn back and the edges are covered by the anterior capsule. Optic capture also prevents an undesirable fusion of the anterior and posterior capsules' leaves, a situation that can lead to early capsular opacity that requires a capsulotomy.

In an eye for which in-the-bag or optic-capture options are impossible, the surgeon must plan the sulcus location of both the haptic and the optic. We know that the diameter of the sulcus is roughly the white-to-white measurement plus 2 mm. There must be capsular support 180° apart on opposite sides of the sulcus for haptic placement as well as reasonable zonular stability in order for lens placement to depend solely on the sulcus for fixation. The main concerns with this approach are centration and uveal biocompatibility. One-piece acrylic lenses do not belong in the sulcus; they are too short, thick, and tacky, and they lack angulation. Most three-piece IOLs measure 13 mm or less from haptic to haptic and are too small for some eyes. The ideal lens features angulated haptics with excellent memory, a large haptic diameter of 13.5 to 14.0 mm, a third-generation silicone composition, a 6.5-mm optic for optimal uveal biocompatibility and greater coverage in case of minor decentration, and round edges to reduce chaffing of the iris pigment epithelium. The IOL's profile must be slim, especially in the case of a secondary piggyback lens, where one IOL is already in the bag. No lens precisely fits this description.

My lens of choice for the sulcus component of a piggyback strategy is the AQ series three-piece silicone lens (STAAR Surgical Company, Monrovia, CA) with large, stiff elastimide haptics and a thin profile. I consider an MA50 three-piece acrylic lens (Alcon Laboratories, Inc.) with its larger 6.5-mm optic as my backup for primary sulcus use when neither capsular leaf is intact. It is worth remembering that sulcus fixation results in a more anterior ELP than bag fixation, which is assumed by our current power calculation formulas. Therefore, I reduce the anterior chamber depth and surgeon's factor components of the formula by 0.30 mm and the A-constant by approximately 0.50 D. In practical use, the higher the lens power is, the more effect the positional change will exert.

CALCULATING LENS POWER

When the calculated lens power is between 15.00 and 23.00 D, I reduce the power of the sulcus lens by 1.00 D. A lens of under 15.00 D I reduce by 0.50 D, and one greater than 23.00 D I reduce by 1.50 D to approximate the equivalency of my refractive aim.

When in doubt about the security of sulcus fixation, I prefer iris fixation with a 10–0 PROLENE (Ethicon, Inc., Somerville, NJ) suture to avoid IOL subluxation or dislocation in the future. The growing number of reports on excellent long-term results with modern, open-looped, four-point–fixation anterior chamber lenses make this alternative extremely viable as well.[3] ■

This article originally appeared in the May 2004 issue of CRSToday.

1. Gimbel HV, DeBroth BM. Intaocular lens optic capture. *J Cataract Refract Surg.* 2004;30:200-206.
2. Petternel V, Menapace, R, Findl O, et al. Effect of optic edge design and haptic angulation on postoperative intraocular lens position change. *J Cataract Refract Surg.* 2004;30:52-57.
3. Holladay JT. International intraocular lens and implant registry 2004. *J Cataract Refract Surg.* 2004;30:207-229.

CHAPTER 131

CCC, PCCC, or Membrane Capture

HOWARD V. GIMBEL, MD, MPH, FRCSC

The objectives of IOL implantation are (1) a centered lens, (2) capsular fixation, and (3) a barrier to vitreous migration. In the absence of bag fixation, these objectives may be achieved by optic capture using either anterior continuous curvilinear capsulorhexis (CCC) capture, posterior CCC (PCCC) capture, or capsular membrane capture.

An absence of bag fixation can occur at any stage of primary cataract surgery (Table 1) and is almost certain to occur in secondary IOL surgery, such as during removal and replacement, repositioning, or secondary IOL placement after extracapsular cataract extraction (Table 2). The surgeon usually cannot reopen a fused capsular bag for bag fixation of an IOL. He may remove a defective IOL from a fused capsular bag by sliding the loops out of the membrane; if this is not possible, he may cut off the loops and leave them in the membrane. He may use a similar removal technique for an eccentric IOL with only one loop in the bag.

The surgeon may easily remove from but not reposition into the capsular bag a mobile sulcus IOL, which may cause uveitis, glaucoma, or hypema (UGH) syndrome. In some cases, he may form a new CCC peripheral to the original one (which is fused to the posterior capsule) to create a bag sulcus for the IOL loops, but this option is rarely possible.

TABLE 1. ABSENCE OF CAPSULAR BAG FIXATION OF IOLs DURING CATARACT AND IOL SURGERY

Complication	Type
Traumatic capsular tear	• Anterior • Anterior and posterior • Equatorial
Iatrogenic capsular tear	• Anterior • Posterior • Anterior and posterior • Equatorial

Aphakia after extracapsular cataract extraction usually provides a capsular membrane for sulcus IOL placement but not bag placement. These surgical challenges lend themselves to secondary surgical

TABLE 2. ABSENCE OF IOL CAPSULAR BAG FIXATION DURING SECONDARY IOL SURGERY

Procedure	Complication
Removal and replacement	• IOL material degradation • Nd:YAG-pitted IOLs
Repositioning	• Subluxated sulcus IOL • Eccentric IOLs (one loop out of the bag) • Mobile sulcus IOLs causing UGH syndrome
Secondary IOL placement	• Aphakia after extracapsular cataract extraction

techniques that utilize membrane IOL capture. This article discusses surgical alternatives for optic capture that maximize the potential for capsular bag IOL fixation in primary and secondary surgery (Table 3).

CCC IOL FIXATION

Various capsule and membrane optic capture techniques have been described in detail in the literature.[1] Surgeons may perform the capsulorhexis fixation method of optic capture when an intact anterior capsulorhexis opening is present and the capsular bag's integrity is compromised. Most often, the surgeon performs anterior capsulorhexis IOL fixation when a large posterior capsular tear—although it has not extended around the equator of the capsule to the CCC—is too large to convert to a PCCC or to safely receive an IOL. If vitreous prolapse has occurred, the surgeon should perform an anterior vitrectomy, while taking care to avoid extending the posterior capsular tear and violating the anterior capsular edge with the vitrectomy handpiece. Once he has removed all of the prolapsed vitreous, the surgeon may place viscoelastic into the anterior chamber and ciliary sulcus before inserting the IOL into the ciliary sulcus. If he deems the anterior capsulorhexis opening to be reasonably centered and smaller than the IOL's optic, he may place the optic through the capsulorhexis using gentle pressure on first one side and then the other of the IOL's anterior surface, 90° away from the haptic-optic junctions. The haptics remain in the ciliary sulcus while the surgeon captures the IOL's optic posteriorly through the capsulorhexis opening.

SULCUS-PLACED HAPTICS AND OPTIC CAPTURE THROUGH THE PCCC

The surgeon may consider this technique as an alternative to sulcus IOL placement in cases in which the anterior CCC has more than one large tear to the equator of the capsule that compromises the secure placement of the haptics into the capsular bag. In addition, an intact PCCC must be present, either as a result of a primary PCCC or a small posterior tear that is converted into a PCCC.[2] In this situation, the surgeon may position the IOL in the ciliary sulcus and capture the optic posteriorly through the anterior and posterior capsulorhexis openings. This approach maintains centration of the IOL and prevents Elshnig pearl formation posterior to the IOL. I recommend that surgeons use a highly viscous viscoelastic material during the capture to avoid extending an anterior capsular leaflet tear to the PCCC.

HAPTICS IN THE CAPSULAR BAG AND OPTIC CAPTURE THROUGH THE PCCC

The surgeon performs a posterior capture of the IOL optic under an ocular viscoelastic device. He applies gentle pressure to one half of the IOL's optic, 90° from the haptic-optic junction, and then exerts slow and gentle pressure on the second half of the optic through the capsulorhexis opening. The physician should perform an anterior vitrectomy if vitreous herniates through the posterior capsulorhexis opening.

The technique of posterior capsulorhexis with optic capture has been used to prevent secondary opacification of the visual axis in children, but it may also be appropriate in adults.[3] In localities where access to Nd:YAG lasers is limited, or if the patient is unable to sit up or cooperate for an Nd:YAG capsulotomy, this technique may be considered as a method to eliminate the need for surgical discission of the opacified posterior capsule. Also, the technique of optic capture has the advantage of preventing vitreous herniation that may occur if the surgeon performs a primary posterior capsulotomy in the absence of optic capture.

HAPTICS IN THE CAPSULAR BAG AND OPTIC CAPTURE THROUGH A CCC

Bringing the IOL's optic anteriorly through the CCC effectively achieves a reverse capsulorhexis fixation. This technique is useful

TABLE 3. OPTIC CAPTURE OPTIONS

Position of Haptics	Optic Capture Procedure
Haptics in sulcus	• CCC optic capture • PCCC optic capture—CCC torn
Haptics in capsular bag	• CCC optic capture after posterior capsular tear too extensive for conversion to a PCCC • CCC optic capture for anterior piggyback IOL • PCCC optic capture *Pediatric* - without anterior vitrectomy - after anterior vitrectomy *Adult* - disability, ie, ankylosing spondylitis - dementia - geographic limitations
Haptics in sulcus, anterior to capsular membrane	• Membrane optic capture
Haptics posterior to capsular membrane (dislocated)	• Membrane optic capture

when a large posterior capsular tear occurs or a small tear extends after the surgeon places an IOL in the capsular bag, thus making stable IOL fixation uncertain. The surgeon may also use this technique if, while he performs a PCCC under an in-the-bag IOL's optic, a radial tear of the PCCC occurs that renders the IOL unstable within the capsular bag. The surgeon may then bring the IOL's optic forward and capture it through the anterior CCC, thus creating IOL stability and ensuring lens centration. Another use of this technique is to bring the optic of a piggyback IOL out of the capsular bag while leaving the haptics in the bag. This approach may reduce the incidence of pearl accumulation in the interface between the two IOLs while maintaining capsular fixation of the second IOL.

HAPTICS IN THE SULCUS AND IOL CAPTURE THROUGH A MEMBRANE OPENING

This technique is useful for secondary procedures such as repositioning decentered IOLs or fixating replacement IOLs (when in-the-bag lenses must be replaced for reasons such as optical degradation from Nd:YAG pits, calcification or crystallization). Decentration of the IOL may occur because of poor initial positioning, such as one haptic in the sulcus and one in the bag. This problem may also occur because of asymmetric contraction of the capsular bag. The surgeon may bring the IOL into the sulcus or perform an IOL replacement by placing the haptics in the sulcus and capturing the optic through the capsular membrane opening. The surgeon may use a vitrector to enlarge a membrane opening that is too small or eccentric. If no opening is present, he may use a PCCC or the anterior vitrectomy handpiece to make an opening slightly smaller than the size of the optic through which to perform the optic capture. Capsular membrane openings that are enlarged or made with the vitrector usually resist tearing and extension because of the fibrosis located between the capsules or on the capsule around the previous opening. Capturing the IOL's optic through the membrane opening achieves better long-term centration of the IOL and avoids, or at least minimizes, the chaffing of uveal tissues.

This technique is particularly useful if the IOL being repositioned (1) has an overall length that may be appropriate for the capsular bag but not long enough for the sulcus or (2) has haptics that are crimped and no longer suitable for sulcus placement. Capturing the IOL through the membrane opening can achieve IOL stability, eliminate IOL movement, and minimize the risk of late displacement. Another benefit of IOL capture through a membrane opening is that it creates a tight barrier between the anterior and posterior segments. This barrier can eliminate the possibility of the vitreous' moving forward into the anterior chamber, a situation that may result in vitreous traction. The barrier can also decrease the risk of vitreous factors' diffusing to the anterior segment and imparting possible toxic effects to the trabecular meshwork.

PARS PLANA IOL REPOSITIONING WITH OPTIC CAPTURE

This technique is useful in the presence of a non–plate-haptic posterior chamber IOL that has subluxated or completely dislocated posteriorly into the vitreous. A circumstance such as this can occur after an Nd:YAG capsulotomy.

A posterior segment surgeon performs pars plana IOL repositioning with optic capture from behind the capsular membrane after completing the vitrectomy. He leaves the haptics posterior to the capsular membrane and pushes the IOL's optic anteriorly through the opening in the membrane. If the capsular opening is too small or the membrane has become fibrotic, scarred, and too stiff to capture the IOL's optic, he may be able to fashion an appropriately sized opening in the membrane remnant with the vitrector. This opening, at least in one meridian, needs to be slightly smaller (approximately 1 mm) than the diameter of the optic to be able to capture the optic and provide adequate support.

SUMMARY

These capture techniques provide alternatives to simple sulcus placement, sutured sulcus placement, iris suturing, iris fixation, or IOL placement in the anterior chamber. By considering these alternatives, the surgeon extends the possibilities of capsular fixation of the IOL in either primary or secondary surgical scenarios and reduces the risk of UGH syndrome and other complications from IOL/tissue contact and interaction. ■

This article originally appeared in the May 2004 issue of CRSToday.

1. Gimbel HV, Debroff BM. Intraocular lens optic capture. *J Cataract Refract Surg.* 2004;30:1:200-206.
2. Gimbel HV. Posterior capsule tears using phaco-emulsification: Cause, prevention and management. *Eur J Implant Ref Surg.* 1990;2:63-69.
3. Gimbel HV, DeBroff BM. Posterior capsulorhexis with optic capture: Maintaining a clear visual axis after pediatric cataract surgery. *J Cataract Refract Surg.* 1994;20:658-664.

CHAPTER 132

Sclerally Sutured PCIOLs: Part I

ELIZABETH A. DAVIS, MD

Most cataract surgery performed today in the United States is extracapsular cataract extraction with phacoemulsification and the implantation of a posterior chamber IOL (PCIOL). When an intact posterior capsule is present, almost all surgeons favor in-the-bag placement of a PCIOL. In the absence of capsular support, however, the choice of lens type and the technique used to secure it in the eye is much more controversial.

Anterior chamber intraocular lenses (ACIOLs) are easier to insert than PCIOLs (particularly sutured PCIOLs), but they have been associated with various complications, including pseudophakic bullous keratopathy, iris atrophy, glaucoma, and the uveitis-glaucoma-hyphema syndrome.[1-4] Although the newer Kelman-Multiflex–style open-loop ACIOLs offer a significant improvement over the previous closed-loop lenses, these lenses cannot be implanted in the absence of adequate iris support or when there is significant angle pathology.

Unlike ACIOLs, sutured PCIOLs are located away from the corneal endothelium and anterior chamber angle and closer to the nodal point of the eye. They are therefore less likely to cause endothelial cell loss, peripheral anterior synechiae, or secondary angle-closure glaucoma.[5] Unfortunately, suturing a PCIOL is much more difficult technically. In the case of transsclerally sutured IOLs, multiple loops of the suture can become entangled or twisted. An inability to directly visualize the sulcus means that the surgeon essentially must perform the procedure blind. A lack of symmetry in suture placement for each of the haptics can lead to lens tilt or decentration. Furthermore, a more anteriorly placed lens can produce a myopic outcome, whereas a more posteriorly placed lens can result in postoperative hyperopia.

MY TECHNIQUE

Prior to suturing a PCIOL transsclerally, it is important to perform a thorough vitrectomy, which prevents vitreous from displacing the IOL or prolapsing around the edges of the optic. I retract the iris during the vitrectomy in order to remove any vitreous from the sulcus, where the sutures will emerge. I do not want to incarcerate vitreous with the sutures, because this situation can cause traction on the retina and potentially lead to a retinal detachment.

I prefer to use a large optic, which I find to be slightly more forgiving of any decentration than a smaller one. I personally use a Storz P366UV PMMA PCIOL (Bausch & Lomb, Rochester, NY). It has a 6.5-mm optic and an overall length of 13.4 mm. Each of the haptics has an eyelet through which I pass a double-armed, 10–0 PROLENE suture (polypropylene; Ethicon, Inc., Somerville, NJ), which exits from the sclera. This technique results in four-point fixation of the PCIOL—the most stable fixation, in my opinion. I also believe there is less risk of lens tilt with this technique. Generally, I try to have the sutures emerge at the 7- to 8-o'clock and 1- to 2-o'clock positions. I avoid the 3- and 9-o'clock positions because of the risk of encountering the ciliary arteries.

When I combine suturing a PCIOL with a corneal transplant, then the procedure is done open-sky. Otherwise, I make a 6.5-mm scleral tunnel. With the open-sky technique, I prefer the needles of the PROLENE suture to be short (Ethicon CS140-6; 6.2-mm needle). If I am using a scleral tunnel, then the needles that I use for the distal haptic are long (Sharpoint 2xSSL15, Surgical Specialties Corporation, Reading, PA; 14.99-mm needle), and the needles that I use for the proximal haptic are short and curved (Ethicon CS140-6; 6.2-mm needle). I bury the knots of the exiting sutures beneath either a scleral or conjunctival flap.

RESULTS AND COMPLICATIONS

Although excellent results have been achieved with transsclerally sutured PCIOLs, complications are not rare. For instance, the sutures may erode through the scleral flaps and cause irritation. They may also loosen or break and cause either tilting or dislocation of the optic. In addition, a persistent suture extending between intraocular and extraocular environments may provide a track for bacteria to enter the eye and establish endophthalmitis. A choroidal hemorrhage and detachment can occur from inadvertent injury to the ciliary body. Moreover, traction on the peripheral retina or vitreous during suture placement in the sulcus may increase the risk of retinal detachment.[6]

Interestingly, despite the uncomplicated placement of the polypropylene sutures through the sulcus, histopathologic studies[7] have shown that the distal haptics probably lie outside the ciliary sulcus. This situation may relate to the surgeon's difficulty observing the sulcus intraoperatively during suture placement, even when limbal indentation is performed. Furthermore, fibrosis of the haptic to the ciliary body does not universally occur. As a result, the sutures provide the primary support for the lens, thereby preventing dislocation into the vitreous. Nevertheless, several cases of suture removal from transsclerally fixated PCIOLs without lens dislocation have been reported.[8-10]

Late cases of sutured IOL dislocations have occurred. After more than 15 years at Minnesota Eye Consultants, my colleagues Richard Lindstrom, MD, and David Hardten, MD, and I are aware of eight patients who have experienced suture erosion and the dislocation of implants that were transsclerally sutured an average of 10 years earlier. All of the patients required surgical repair, which was quite challenging in certain instances. Reports and experiences such as these have prompted some surgeons to advocate the use of 9–0, rather than 10–0, polypropylene or even 8–0 GoreTex sutures (W. L. Gore and Associates, Milpitas, CA), as mentioned to me by Randall Olson, MD (written communication, February 2004).

CONCLUSION

Despite rare but significant late complications, I feel that the transscleral suturing of PCIOLs plays a role in cases of capsular compromise. These lenses are preferred to ACIOLs when the cornea shows signs of compromise (eg, guttata), if the anterior chamber is shallow, or if the patient has glaucoma or angle pathology. They are also preferred over iris-fixated IOLs in cases of iris atrophy. Each case is unique, however, and must be individualized. ■

This article originally appeared in the May 2004 issue of CRSToday.

1. Insler MS, Kook MS, Kaufman HE. Penetrating keratoplasty for pseudophakic bullous keratopathy associated with semiflexible, closed-loop anterior-chamber lenses. *Am J Ophthalmol.* 1989;107:252-256.
2. Smith PW, Wong SK, Stark WJ, et al. Complications of semi-flexible closed loop anterior chamber lenses. *Arch Ophthalmol.* 1987;105:52-57.
3. Lim ES, Apple DJ, Tsai JC, et al. An analysis of flexible anterior chamber lenses with special reference to the normalized rate of lens explantation. *Ophthalmology.* 1991;98:243-246.
4. Speaker MG, Lugo M, Laibson PR, et al. Penetrating keratoplasty for pseudophakic bullous keratopathy. *Ophthalmology.* 1988;95:1260-1268.
5. Soong HK, Musch DC, Kowal V, et al. Implantation of posterior chamber intraocular lenses in the absence of lens capsule during penetrating keratoplasty. *Arch Ophthalmol.* 1990;107:660-665.
6. Rajpal RK, Carney MD, Weinberg RS, et al. Complications of transscleral sutured posterior chamber intraocular lenses. *Ophthalmology.* 1991;98(suppl):144.
7. Lubniewski AJ, Holland EJ, Van Meter WS, et al. Histologic study of eyes with transsclerally sutured posterior chamber intraocular lenses. *Am J Ophthalmol.* 1990;110:237-243.
8. Johnson SM. Results of exchanging anterior chamber lenses with sulcus fixated posterior chamber IOLs without capsular support in penetrating keratoplasty. *Ophthalmic Surg.* 1989;20:465-468.
9. Lindquist TD, Agapitos PJ, Lindstrom RL, et al. Transscleral fixation of posterior chamber intraocular lenses in the absence of capsular support. *Ophthalmic Surg.* 1989;20:769-775.
10. Davis RM, Best D, Gilbert GE. Comparison of intraocular lens fixation techniques performed during penetrating keratoplasty. *Am J Ophthalmol.* 1991;111:743-749.

CHAPTER 133

Sclerally Sutured PCIOLs: Part II

ROGER F. STEINERT, MD

Three primary options exist for IOL fixation in the absence of capsular support: a transsclerally sutured posterior chamber IOL (PCIOL), a peripheral iris-sutured PCIOL, and a flexible open-loop anterior chamber IOL. If both the posterior capsule and the iris are disrupted or absent, then sutured transscleral PCIOLs are the only lens option. This article describes the techniques for transscleral suture fixation of a PCIOL.

SURGICAL PEARLS

Many different techniques for the placement of transsclerally sutured PCIOLs have been presented in the literature.[1] Sclerally sutured lenses can be sutured from the inside out (ab interno) or by passing the needles from the outside of the eye inward (ab externo). A combination of scleral and iris sutures has also been described.[2] Transscleral sutures may be oriented vertically, obliquely, or horizontally, although direct 3- and 9-o'clock horizontal fixation is inadvisable because of the danger of suturing through the long ciliary arteries and nerves at these locations. It is important to perform an extensive anterior vitrectomy in most cases before placing a sutured PCIOL in order to avoid vitreous incarceration and subsequent retinal traction and detachment.

A common error with sclerally sutured PCIOLs is placing the haptics too far posteriorly. The goal is to have the haptics rest in the ciliary sulcus. Anatomical studies[3] have shown that the ciliary sulcus is only 0.83 mm posterior to the limbus in the vertical meridian and just 0.46 mm posterior to the limbus in the horizontal meridian. The surgeon can detect when he is passing a needle too anteriorly by iris movement that occurs as the needle penetrates the peripheral iris stroma near the angle. In order to determine the correct location for the needle to penetrate the external sclera, the surgeon must be mindful that the aforementioned anatomical studies are based on a strict perpendicularity of the needle relative to the scleral wall. If the surgeon passes the needle through the scleral wall at an oblique angle (usually tilted toward the iris plane), then the external scleral point will need to be located more posteriorly in order for the interior scleral point to be at the level of the ciliary sulcus.

The surgeon has the option of creating scleral flaps so that the polypropylene suture knot is buried, thereby avoiding exposed suture ends. Cautery is recommended to retract exposed barbs, should they occur postoperatively, in order to eliminate a possible entry track for microorganisms or the epithelium. If the suture knot is rotated, as in the technique of Stephen Lane, MD, of St. Paul, Minnesota, then no scleral flap is needed.

PCIOLs made specifically for suturing to the sclera feature eyelets on their haptics to aid suture fixation, and they have large-diameter optics (7 mm) to compensate for possible decentration. Some commonly used models of sclerally sutured IOLs include the CZ70BD (Alcon Laboratories, Inc., Fort Worth, TX) and the C540MC (CIBA Vision, Duluth, GA).

The ab interno technique for the transscleral suture fixation of a PCIOL typically utilizes polypropylene suture material. A long needle is required for the pass across the anterior chamber; the Ethicon CIF-4 and Ethicon STC-6 (Ethicon Inc., Somerville, NJ) are common choices. The surgeon passes the needles under the iris and aims for the ciliary sulcus. A girth hitch may be used to attach the polypropylene suture loop to the IOL haptic (Figure 1). Alternatively, the surgeon may tie the sutures to the haptic, to the haptic's eyelets, or proximal to one of the haptic's eyelets. The needles exit the eye under the previously dissected scleral flaps, and the sutures are tied. Alternatively, to avoid dissecting the scleral flaps and avoid the potential for later erosion of the flap and conjunctiva (with resultant exposure of the suture ends), the surgeon may pass the suture through the positioning hole in the haptic and rotate the knot below the scleral surface (Figure 2). The ab interno technique is adaptable to foldable IOL implantation as well, which allows suture fixation of the IOL while retaining a small incision. Minimizing the incision size is particularly important if capsular support is lost during primary cataract surgery through a small, clear corneal incision.

The principal advantages of the ab interno, inside-to-outside approach are that it is more straightforward and possibly faster

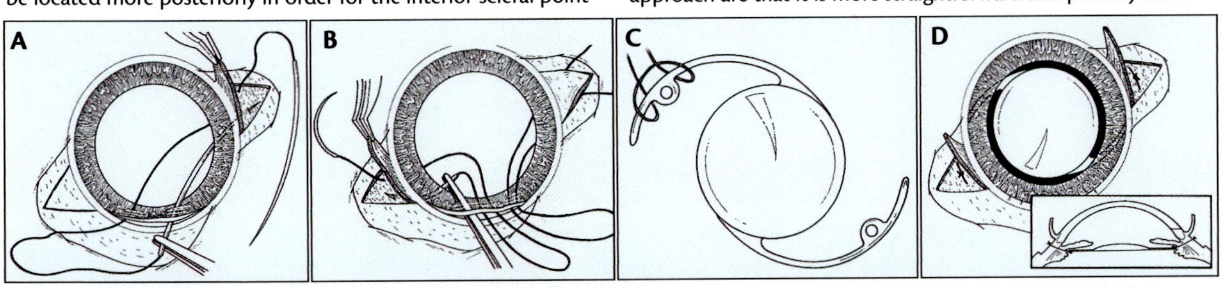

Figure 1. The ab interno technique with four-point fixation requires scleral flaps. The first double-armed suture on the long Ethicon CIF-4 needle is placed first (A). The second double-armed suture on the CS 160 or equivalent needle is placed 180° away. This maneuver requires the surgeon to place the needle holder's tip inside the anterior chamber, while taking care to avoid causing endothelial trauma (B). The suture is placed around the haptic hole with a girth hitch loop (C). The surgeon places the IOL in the eye, cuts the sutures, and ties them tightly. He then replaces the scleral flap and sutures the conjunctiva closed (D). (Reprinted with permission from Steinert RF, Arkin MS. Secondary intraocular lenses. In: Steinert RF, ed. *Cataract Surgery: Techniques, Complications, and Management*. 2nd ed. Philadelphia: WB Saunders; 2004.)

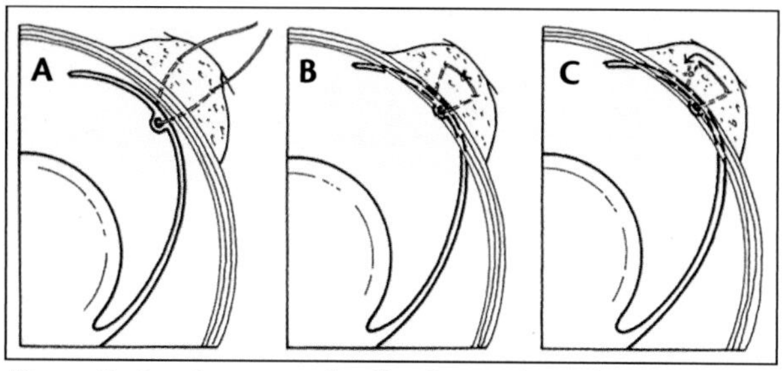

Figure 2. For the two-point fixation variant, the suture placement is identical to that in Figure 3, except that the surgeon passes the second needle of each double-armed suture through the haptic's positioning hole before passing it through the sclera 1.5 to 2.0 mm lateral to the first needle penetration site (A). The knot is tied tightly; four single throws utilizing a slip-knot technique are advisable to achieve a low-profile knot that will also be secure (B). Rotating the knot below the scleral surface leaves only a smooth loop of suture on the scleral surface that is then covered with conjunctiva (C). (Reprinted with permission from Steinert RF, Arkin MS. Secondary intraocular lenses. In: Steinert RF, ed. *Cataract Surgery: Techniques, Complications, and Management*. 2nd ed. Philadelphia: WB Saunders; 2004.)

than the ab externo, outside-to-inside technique. The ab interno approach is also easier to perform in conjunction with penetrating keratoplasty. The disadvantages of this technique include the fact that the surgeon must pass the needle under the iris without direct visualization and that he must rely on the indentation of the iris, with visualization of the pressure of the needle from behind the iris, to ensure the correct placement of the suture in the ciliary sulcus.

Lewis[4] first described the ab externo technique of passing the scleral needles from the outside inward (Figure 3). The sutures used for the procedure are 10–0 polypropylene, with a long straight needle such as the Ethicon STC-6 (Ethicon Inc.). Alcon Laboratories, Inc., produces the Pair Pack Fixation Suture, which is a hybrid combining an SC-5 straight needle on one end and an AUM-5 corneal needle on the other. This suture is specifically designed for the outside-to-inside technique of sclerally sutured PCIOLs. The surgeon passes the long, straight needle perpendicularly through the sclera (usually under partial-thickness scleral flaps), approximately 0.75 mm posterior to the limbus. Inside the eye, the needle should penetrate at the ciliary sulcus. The needle is then "docked" inside the tip of a 25-, 27-, or 28-gauge hollow needle, which the surgeon has passed through the ciliary sulcus on the opposite side, also with an outside-to-inside technique. After the long straight needle with the 10–0 polypropylene is docked within the hollow needle, the latter needle is withdrawn with the solid needle inside of it. In this way, the surgeon pulls the polypropylene suture across the eye. He then uses a hook to pull the suture out through a superior limbal wound. The suture is cut, and each end is tied to a haptic of the IOL. After placing the IOL into position, the surgeon secures the scleral sutures to the sclera.

This procedure can be performed with two sutures per haptic if the surgeon desires four-point fixation to ensure stability (Figure 4A and B). The surgeon ties the sutures to the haptics and buries the external knot under a scleral flap. The alternative procedure, illustrated in Figure 4C, allows the rotation of the knot in order to avoid the necessity for scleral flaps and the potential of late exposure of the suture ends; the anti-rotational stability of true four-point fixation is not achieved, however.

The advantage of the outside-to-inside approach is a greater assurance of the location of internal scleral penetration at the ciliary sulcus. Taking precise measurements and avoiding the highly vascularized pars plicata can minimize bleeding. In addition, the anterior chamber remains closed during the needle passes, thereby decreasing the duration of ocular hypotony. The disadvantages of the ab externo approach are that it takes longer than the ab interno approach and that it is not applicable with the open-sky situation of penetrating keratoplasty. In addition, if the surgeon performs more than one suture pass, it may be confusing to keep track of the origins and courses of the various suture ends.

IOL tilting is a serious but avoidable complication of sclerally sutured PCIOLs.[5] If the surgeon elects a double-suture technique with knot rotation, he must be meticulous in achieving a suture orientation that permits easy rotation of the knot (Figure 5A and B) and in avoiding suture configurations that will resist the rotation of the knot (Figure 5C through H). Furthermore, the surgeon should orient the suture pass through the opposite haptics in a direction that will resist the rotation of the IOL out of the iris plane (Figure 5I), rather than allow rotation (Figure 5J).

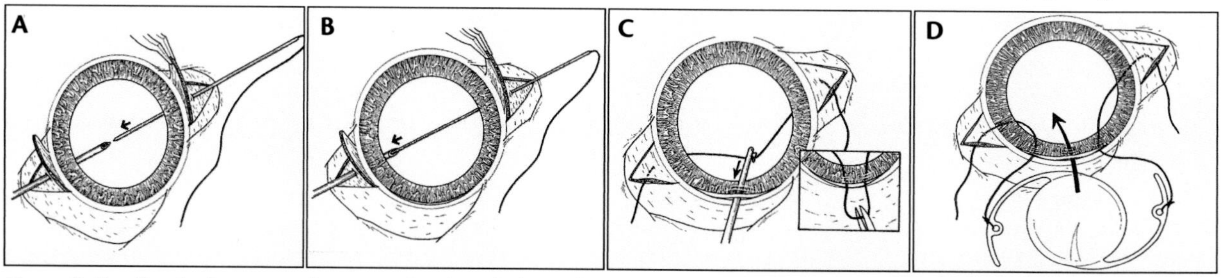

Figure 3. For the single-suture, ab externo Lewis technique, the surgeon passes a straight needle with a suture under scleral flaps from one side while a hypodermic needle enters the eye 180° away (A). The solid needle is "docked" into the hollow needles, and the two needles are withdrawn to the left so that the suture then traverses the anterior chamber (B). A Kuglen or similar hook draws the suture out of the main incision (C). After cutting and tying the suture to the IOL's haptic, the surgeon inserts the lens in the eye and secures each end of the suture to the sclera by making a midscleral pass and then tying the suture to itself (D). (Reprinted with permission from Steinert RF, Arkin MS. Secondary intraocular lenses. In: Steinert RF, ed. *Cataract Surgery: Techniques, Complications, and Management*. 2nd ed. Philadelphia: WB Saunders; 2004.)

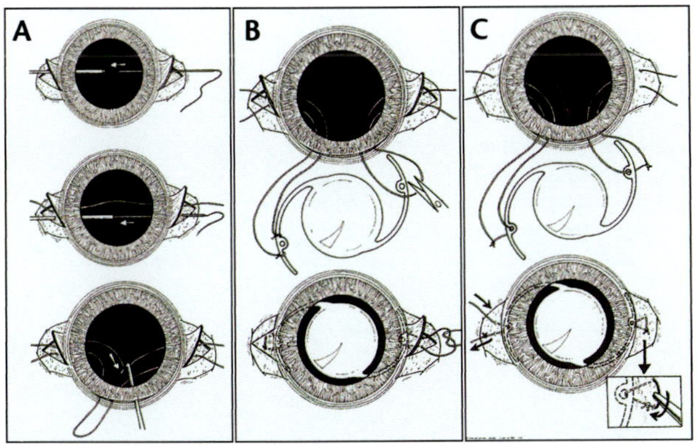

Figure 4. The double-suture variant of the Lewis ab externo technique begins similarly to the single-suture technique, except that the suture's entry point under the scleral flap is displaced to one side (top). The second suture is passed parallel to the first, with 1.0 to 1.5 mm between the two sutures (middle). Care must be taken to keep the sutures taut and thereby avoid crossing them or confusing which suture originates from each scleral site; a Kuglen hook or similar instrument simultaneously withdraws the suture loop through the previously prepared principal incision (bottom) (A). To achieve four-point stable fixation, the surgeon ties the cut sutures to the haptic on either side of the eyelet (top). The surgeon then places the IOL in the posterior chamber while keeping the sutures taut to avoid entanglement. The ends are then tied under the scleral flaps, and the conjunctiva is closed over the flaps (bottom) (B). In this variant of the double-suture ab externo technique, the goal is to achieve a loop of suture where the knot can be rotated beneath the sclera, thus avoiding the necessity of a scleral flap and the potential for late erosion of the knot or suture ends. The cut ends of each suture are passed through the haptic positioning hole and tied (top). As the IOL is positioned in the posterior chamber, one end of the suture on each side is pulled so that the knot passes through the sclera to the external eye, where it is cut off (bottom). The surgeon then ties together the remaining suture ends and rotates the knot beneath the sclera (inset) (C). (Reprinted with permission from Steinert RF, Arkin MS. Secondary intraocular lenses. In: Steinert RF, ed. *Cataract Surgery: Techniques, Complications, and Management*. 2nd ed. Philadelphia: WB Saunders; 2004.)

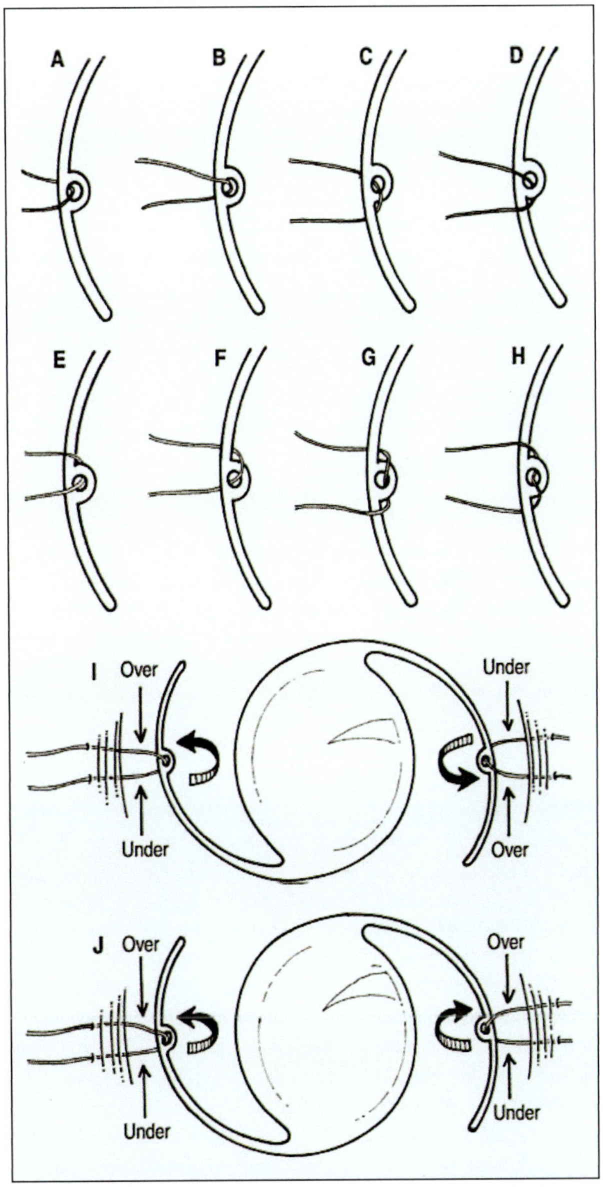

Figure 5. A suture passed through the positioning hole may wrap around the haptic in eight basic configurations. Unless the appropriate pathways are used (A and B), the surgeon's ability to rotate the suture will be impaired or fully prevented by the circuitous route taken by the suture (C through H). Because there are two haptics, a total of 16 configurations are therefore possible. The surgeon should take care to use configuration A on one haptic, and the opposite configuration B on the other haptic. In that manner, the torque of the IOL is resisted; as one haptic starts to rotate in the direction not resisted by the suture loop, the other haptic meets more resistance (arrows) (I). When both suture loops have the same configuration, the suture does not resist the torque of the IOL (arrows) (J). (Reprinted with permission from Steinert RF, Arkin MS. Secondary intraocular lenses. In: Steinert RF, ed. *Cataract Surgery: Techniques, Complications, and Management*. 2nd ed. Philadelphia: WB Saunders; 2004.)

CONCLUSIONS

Little debate exists that the placement of a standard PCIOL is the method of choice for a secondary IOL in the presence of sufficient capsular support. In cases without capsular support, the decision is more difficult. It is impossible to reach firm conclusions regarding sutured PCIOLs with presently available information. It seems clear that some surgeons have prematurely disregarded modern anterior chamber IOLs, which provide a valuable alternative to sutured PCIOLs for many patients. The visual results for most patients with sclerally sutured lenses are comparable to those with other lens types.

On the other hand, a properly performed scleral suture IOL fixation yields the most anatomically correct alternative in the absence of an intact lens capsule support system. A meticulous surgical technique will reward the surgeon who pursues this approach. ■

Portions of this article are adapted with permission from Steinert RF, Arkin MS. Secondary intraocular lenses. In: Steinert RF, ed. Cataract Surgery: Techniques, Complications, and Management. *2nd ed. Philadelphia: WB Saunders; 2004.*

This article originally appeared in the May 2044 issue of CRSToday.

1. Steinert RF, Arkin MS. Secondary Intraocular Lenses. In: Steinert RF, ed. *Cataract Surgery: Techniques, Complications, and Management.* 2nd ed. Philadelphia: WB Saunders; 2004: 429-441.
2. Stark WJ, Gottsch JD, Goodman DF, et al. Posterior chamber intraocular lens implantation in the absence of capsular support. *Arch Ophthalmol.* 1989;107:1078-1083.
3. Duffey RJ, Holland EJ, Agapitos PJ, Lindstrom RL. Anatomic study of transsclerally sutured intraocular lens implantation. *Am J Ophthalmol.* 1989;108:300-309.
4. Lewis JS. Ab externo sulcus fixation. *Ophthalmic Surg.* 1991;22:692-695.
5. Hayashi K, Hayashi H, Nakao F, Hayashi F. Intraocular lens tilt and decentration, anterior chamber depth, and refractive error after transscleral suture fixation surgery. *Ophthalmology.* 1999;106:878-882.

CHAPTER 134

Iris-Sutured PCIOLs

GARY P. CONDON, MD

Patients who are longstanding aphakes or who have significantly compromised capsular support at the time of cataract extraction are challenging cases for IOL implantation. Today, surgeons may choose from three available options: (1) an anterior chamber IOL (ACIOL); (2) a posterior chamber IOL (PCIOL); and (3) an iris-sutured PCIOL. Each lens type has its own advantages and disadvantages.

OPTIONS FOR IOL FIXATION

ACIOLs

New-generation ACIOLs are easy to insert and fairly safe, but they require a large corneal incision for implantation. These lenses also carry the long-term risk of inflammation, pigment dispersion, increased IOP, and possible adverse effects on corneal clarity.[1,2]

Scleral-Sutured PCIOLs

Surgeons enthusiastically embraced the concept of suturing a PCIOL to the sclera in the late 1980s, but many surgeons have since found it to be a complicated procedure requiring much manipulation of the eye and possible bleeding as they pass the suture needle through choroidal tissue without direct visualization.[3] Long-term problems now becoming evident include a substantial possibility of the sutures' eventually breaking, thus leading to IOL dislocation. Another potential complication is that the buried sutures may become exposed, thereby opening a pathway for infectious agents to enter the eye and potentially cause late endophthalmitis.[4,5]

Iris-Sutured PCIOLs

The concept of iris-sutured PCIOLs dates back to 1976 and the work of Malcolm McCannel, MD, of Edina, Minnesota, who proposed the idea of a retrievable suture that the surgeon could pass through anterior segment tissues.[6] The ends of the sutures could be grasped through a small corneal stab wound and tied. Surgeons could employ this technique for recentering previously implanted IOLs that had become dislocated.

A Comparison

Schein et al conducted a prospective study of IOL fixation during penetrating keratoplasty and concluded that iris suturing resulted in fewer complications than scleral suturing or anterior chamber placement.[7] A recent extensive review of the literature on IOL fixation in the absence of capsular support, however, failed to determine clear differences among the visual outcomes

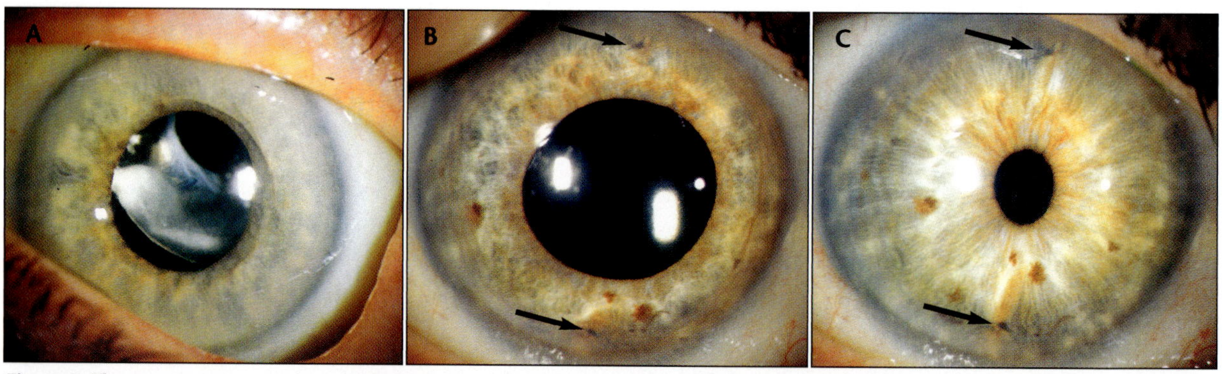

Figure 1. The surgeon may use the modified McCannel suture to reposition and fixate a dislocated IOL. Preoperatively, the significant dislocation of this IOL can clearly be seen through the dilated pupil. The lens is actually still inside the capsular bag, which became detached as a result of pseudoexfoliation. Because this lens was not amenable to simple refixation, the author removed and exchanged it for an iris-sutured IOL (A). After fixation with sutures placed through the peripheral iris (arrows), the IOL optic is well centered, as seen on the dilated view (B). Because the sutures are located in the peripheral, nondynamic area of the iris, little if any displacement occurs from the dilated to the photopic pupil. This situation minimizes the long-term physical stress on the sutures (C).

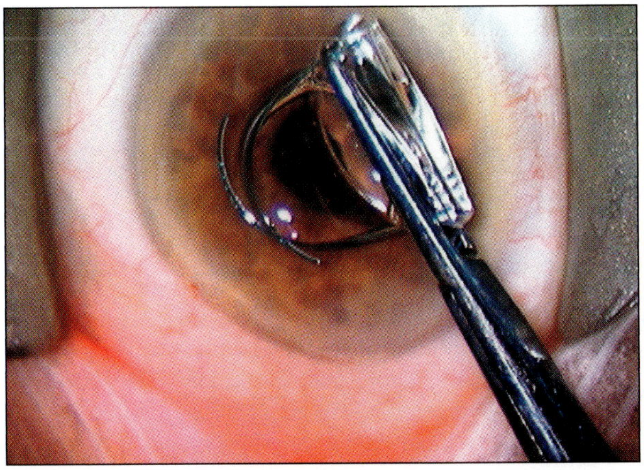

Figure 2. The author folds the AcrySof MA60AC multipiece acrylic IOL across the 3- to 9-o'clock meridian and grasps the lens in the Fine Inserter II.

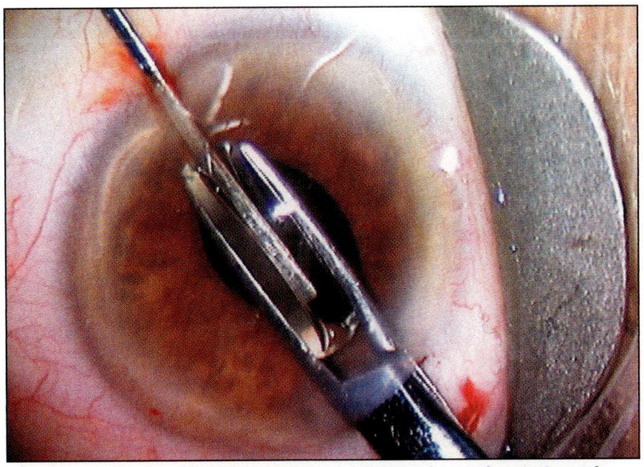

Figure 3. The leading haptic is compressed gently against the edge of the optic as the IOL enters the incision. Once the IOL is inside the anterior chamber, the author directs both haptics downward through the pupil while holding the optic just above the iris plane. The author relaxes the optic slightly within the inserter, passes a Cleasby iris spatula through the paracentesis, and gently places the spatula within the fold of the optic.

or complication rates of these three fixation methods.[8]

I had used the McCannel technique to fixate dislocated IOLs—with sutures placed in the peripheral iris—and had found it to be reliable and safe. One of the technique's advantages is that it does not leave patients with the large corneal incision that is required when exchanging a PCIOL for an ACIOL. Although a dislocated PCIOL could also be repositioned with scleral-suture fixation, I believe the potential risk of suture erosion and late endophthalmitis is unacceptable. Iris fixation keeps the sutures entirely within the eye. The peripheral iris is also a nondynamic location where less long-term stress will be placed on the sutures (Figure 1).

One question remained: How could this approach be used in patients who did not already have an IOL behind the iris? The answer came with the introduction of the three-piece AcrySof lens (Alcon Laboratories, Inc., Fort Worth, TX), which I found to unfold inside the eye in a slow, controlled fashion. By allowing the lens to unfold over a spatula, I was able to place the haptics behind the iris while keeping the optic in the anterior chamber. The temporary optic capture holds the lens in position while I place modified McCannel sutures in the peripheral iris to fixate the haptics. The final step is to prolapse the optic through the pupil.

Although this technique is well suited to acrylic lenses such as the AcrySof, I would not recommend trying it with a silicone lens. The rapid unfolding and more slippery surface of silicone lens optics might make it difficult to control and maneuver them with the spatula.

I and others now prefer an iris-suturing technique using the foldable multipiece AcrySof lens in cases of primary or secondary IOL implantation in the absence of capsular support.[9,10]

SURGICAL TECHNIQUE

To achieve pupil constriction and topical anesthesia, I apply topical pilocarpine 4% to the eye 30 minutes preoperatively, followed by intravenous sedation and topical tetracaine 1%. With a 3.0-mm disposable keratome, I create a 3.5-mm clear corneal tunnel incision temporally, while taking care to avoid the prior incision site in secondary implant cases. Preservative-free lidocaine 1.5% and acetylcholine are placed in the anterior chamber. I deepen the chamber slightly with Provisc (sodium hyaluronate 1.0%; Alcon Laboratories, Inc.) while avoiding posterior iris displacement and pupillary expansion. A 1-mm peripheral paracentesis stab incision is made opposite the corneal incision.

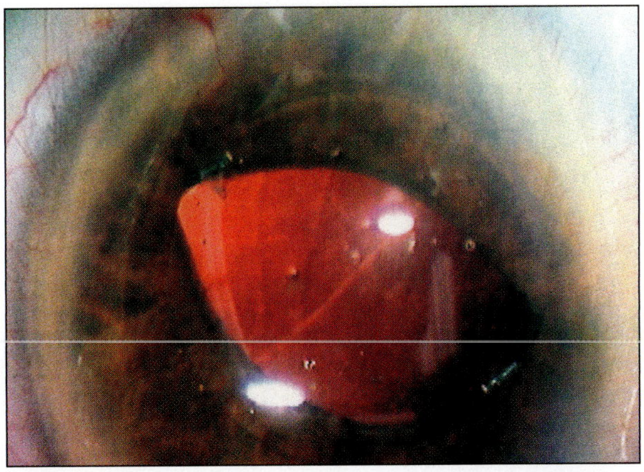

Figure 4. After the author positions and stabilizes the optic with the spatula, the haptics lie behind the iris, and pupillary capture immobilizes the optic in the anterior chamber.

I used to reduce the power of the multipiece AcrySof model MA60AC IOL (Alcon Laboratories, Inc.) by 1.00 D from the value calculated for in-the-bag placement.[9] Currently, I usually do not reduce the calculated power at all, because most patients receiving an iris-sutured IOL have a very deep anterior chamber postoperatively. In none of my current cases is the lens power reduced by more than 0.50 D.

I fold the lens across the 3- to 9-o'clock meridian, thereby creating a "bucket handle" or slight "mustache" haptic configuration. I hold the IOL in a Fine Inserter II instrument (05-2339-R; Rhein Medical Inc., Tampa, FL) (Figure 2).

While taking care to avoid kinking the haptic, I gently compress the leading haptic against the edge of the optic as the IOL enters the incision. Once the IOL is in the anterior chamber, both haptics are directed downward through the pupil while the optic is held

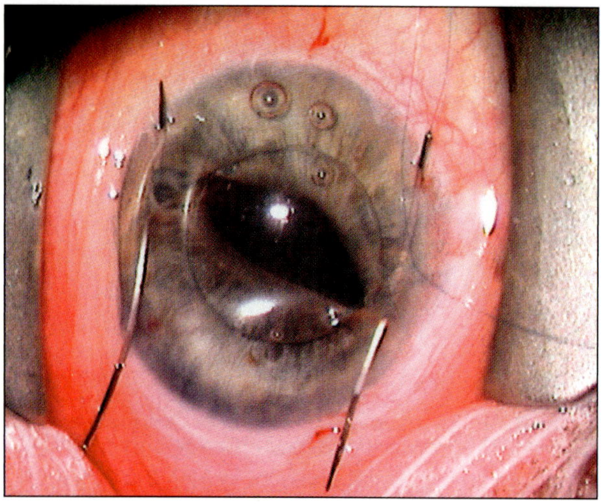

Figure 5. Each IOL haptic is fixated with a 10–0 polypropylene suture passed through a paracentesis, then through peripheral iris, behind the haptic, back through the iris, and out through peripheral cornea. The surgeon will retrieve the suture ends through paracenteses made directly over each peripheral haptic.

just above the iris plane. After slightly relaxing the optic within the inserter, I pass a Cleasby iris spatula (Storz E 0485-C; Bausch & Lomb, Rochester, NY) through the paracentesis and gently place it within the fold of the optic (Figure 3). The IOL slowly unfolds, which results in the haptics' extending behind the posterior iris surface. The spatula supports the optic above the iris plane during unfolding so that the optic is completely captured by the pupil and stabilized (Figure 4). I then remove the spatula.

To fixate the haptic to the peripheral iris, I make an additional paracentesis (located slightly oblique to the meridian of the IOL's haptic) so that the needle can enter the anterior chamber without distorting the soft globe. A 10–0 polypropylene suture on an Ethicon CIF-4 (Ethicon Inc., Somerville, NJ) or an Alcon PC-7 needle passes through the paracentesis perpendicular to the haptic orientation. The needle tip is advanced down through the peripheral iris, behind the haptic, and back out through iris and peripheral cornea, approximately 4 clock hours from the initial entry.

Creating another additional paracentesis directly over the haptic allows the retrieval of both ends of the suture. The knot is initiated with a triple throw, and gentle traction is applied as the haptic is pulled toward the iris and the knot is secured. In most of my cases, I have used a Siepser sliding knot[11] through the entry paracentesis, a technique that I feel provides more security for the haptic. I secure the second haptic in the same manner (Figure 5) and trim the sutures.

Next, I use a lens manipulator to prolapse the optic into the posterior chamber. Gentle manual or automated irrigation removes the viscoelastic. All incisions should be checked to ensure that they are watertight and free of any vitreous strands. Postoperative medications include a topical steroid/antibiotic combination and a topical ophthalmic nonsteroidal anti-inflammatory tapered over approximately 8 weeks, depending upon the patient's postoperative status.

RESULTS

At the 2003 ASCRS meeting, I reported on a review of 30 cases in which investigators (including myself) implanted AcrySof IOLs using the modified McCannel suture for iris fixation.[12] Most of the patients were aphakes, but the other cases involved IOL exchange or a dislocated crystalline lens. The mean follow-up period was approximately 1 year, and we saw no cases of significant IOL decentration or tilt, uveitis, or CME. A few eyes experienced transient pigment dispersion, but there were no new cases of glaucoma and no eyes with pre-existing glaucoma requiring an increase in medication. In one case, an iris tear occurred intraoperatively.

I have personally performed more than 35 cases with the modified McCannel technique during the past 4 years. The results continue to be excellent. My co-investigators and I have encountered one late IOL subluxation and one lens that dislocated because the haptic became disinserted from the lens optic. The latter case was easily corrected using a new lens implanted by the same method, and that patient is doing well today. Based on the accumulating experience, I recommend this technique to other surgeons confronting similar cases where capsular support is absent. ■

This article originally appeared in the May 2004 issue of CRSToday.

1. Amino K, Yamakawa R. Long-term results of out-of-the-bag intraocular lens implantation. *J Cataract Refract Surg.* 2000;26:266-270.
2. Drolsum L. Long-term follow-up of secondary flexible, open-loop, anterior chamber intraocular lenses. *J Cataract Refract Surg.* 2003;29:498-503.
3. Evereklioglu C, Er H, Bekir NA, et al. Comparison of secondary implantation of flexible open-loop anterior chamber and scleral-fixated posterior chamber intraocular lenses. *J Cataract Refract Surg.* 2003;29:301-308.
4. Schechter RJ. Suture-wick endophthalmitis with sutured posterior chamber intraocular lenses. *J Cataract Refract Surg.* 1990;16:755-756.
5. Solomon K, Gussler JR, Gussler C, Van Meter WS. Incidence and management of complications of transsclerally sutured posterior chamber lenses. *J Cataract Refract Surg.* 1993;19:488-493.
6. McCannel MA. A retrievable suture idea for anterior uveal problems. *Ophthalmic Surg.* 1976;7:2:98-103.
7. Schein OD, Kenyon KR, Steinert RF, et al. A randomized trial of intraocular lens fixation techniques with penetrating keratoplasty. *Ophthalmology.* 1993;100:1437-1443.
8. Wagoner MD, Cox TA, Ariyasu RG, et al. Intraocular lens implantation in the absence of capsular support: a report by the American Academy of Ophthalmology. *Ophthalmology.* 2003;110:840-859.
9. Condon GP. Simplified small-incision peripheral iris fixation of an AcrySof intraocular lens in the absence of capsule support. *J Cataract Refract Surg.* 2003;29:1663-1667.
10. Stutzman RD, Stark WJ. Surgical technique for suture fixation of an acrylic intraocular lens in the absence of capsule support. *J Cataract Refract Surg.* 2003;29:1658-1662.
11. Siepser SB. The closed chamber slipping suture technique for iris repair. *Ann Ophthalmol.* 1994;26:71-72.
12. Condon GP, Ahmed IK, Masket S, et al. Iris fixation of foldable PC IOLs with modified McCannel slip-knot suture. Paper presented at: The ASCRS/ASOA Symposium on Cataract, IOL and Refractive Surgery; April 14, 2003; San Francisco, CA.

CHAPTER 135

Suture Fixation of the Capsular Bag

ROBERT J. CIONNI, MD

Weakened or missing zonules present a serious challenge to the cataract surgeon. Fortunately, the use of a capsular tension ring (CTR) in these cases has been shown to decrease the risk of complications.[1-4] Nevertheless, although a CTR can be helpful in patients who have a moderate loss of zonular support, eyes with profound zonular compromise (or lens subluxation) may not obtain adequate stabilization or centration despite CTR placement. In 1997, Robert Osher, MD, of Cincinnati demonstrated the idea of *synthetic zonules* by suturing the CTR to the scleral wall with a 10–0 PROLENE suture (Ethicon Inc., Somerville, NJ).[5] Vladimir Pfeifer, MD, of Ljubljana, Slovenia, preferred to fashion a small peripheral capsulorhexis through which a similar suture passage could be made.[6] Although both techniques provide a solution for eyes with severe zonular insufficiency, they violate the integrity of the peripheral capsular bag and thereby risk its rupture. The modified CTR (Morcher GmbH, Stuttgart, Germany) differs from the CTR in that the former has a fixation hook that loops anteriorly into a second plane, wraps around the capsulorhexis edge, and thereby allows scleral fixation without violating the integrity of the capsular bag (Figures 1 through 3).[7]

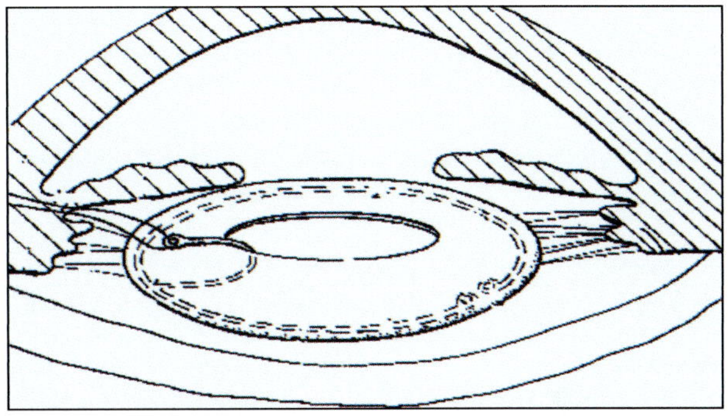

Figure 1. The modified CTR model 1-L can be sutured through the ciliary sulcus to the scleral wall without violating the integrity of the capsular bag.

MODIFIED CTR TECHNIQUE

The Capsulorhexis

I usually work through a near-clear corneal incision and place a generous amount of a dispersive viscoelastic over the area of zonular dialysis to tamponade vitreous. Next, placing a cohesive viscoelastic over the crystalline lens provides a deep, noncollapsing anterior chamber. I then initiate the capsulorhexis in an area remote from the dialysis in order to make use of the stronger remaining zonules for countertraction. The capsulotomy should be large enough to allow for easy nucleus manipulation. It may be necessary to stabilize the capsular bag with a dull second instrument or with an iris retractor to complete the capsulorhexis.

The Modified CTR

Although the modified CTR may be inserted into the capsular bag at any point after the creation of the capsulorhexis, a bulky nucleus can make visualization and the placement of the device difficult. I prefer to remove the nucleus and as much cortex as possible before placing the ring. It is often necessary to stabilize the bag during phacoemulsification with iris retractors.[8] The capsular tension segment (Morcher GmbH) designed by Ike Ahmed, MD, of Toronto can provide a broader area of temporary stabilization. Hydrodissection maximally frees the nucleus and thereby decreases zonular stress during manipulation of the nucleus. Moreover, hydrodissecting the nucleus completely into the anterior chamber greatly simplifies nuclear removal and helps eliminate zonular stress during phacoemulsification.

Slow-motion phacoemulsification using low vacuum and aspiration settings to minimize the infusion reduces the risk of vitreous prolapse or of further stress to the zonules.[9] Viscoelastic injected between the nuclear quadrants and peripheral capsular bag lifts the nuclear fragments while expanding and stabilizing the bag during phacoemulsification.[10] Injecting viscoelastic against the residual anterior capsular rim and peripheral capsular bag separates the cortex from its adhesions to the capsule for easier aspiration.

Before inserting the modified CTR, I preload a double-armed 9–0 PROLENE or 8–0 GoreTex suture (W. L. Gore and Associates, Milpitas, CA) through the eyelet of the fixation hook. Alternatively, the suture can be single-armed, and the free end of the suture may be tied to the fixation hook's eyelet. Next, I place viscoelastic just under the surface of the residual anterior capsular rim to dissect any residual cortex away from the peripheral capsule, thereby making cortical entrapment less likely. Fully expanding the capsular bag with viscoelastic allows the modified CTR to glide around the bag's equator more easily. Using a smooth forceps, I insert the device through the main incision and dial it into the capsular bag. If the fixation hook does not "capture" anterior to the capsulorhexis edge, I manipulate it anteriorly with the Osher Y-Hook (Duckworth & Kent Ltd., Hertfordshire, England) or a Sinskey hook and use a second dull instrument to retract the capsulorhexis edge. The fixation hook is "dialed" until its eyelet is centered at the site of zonular weakness.

Next, I displace the fixation hook to the scleral wall to be certain that the chosen location will result in bag centration. After fashioning a scleral flap at this site, I direct the needles to exit through the ciliary sulcus while remaining anterior to the anterior capsule at all times. The needles should exit the scleral wall approximately 1.5 mm apart and 1.5 mm posterior to the corneal-scleral junction to prevent postoperative iris chaffing. I then cinch the sutures to achieve centration and tie them. If a single-armed suture is used, the needle is passed through partial-thickness sclera beneath the scleral flap and then tied to itself. After suture fixation of the modified CTR, any remaining cortex may be aspirated. I then reinflate the capsular bag with viscoelastic in preparation for IOL implantation. I prefer the single-piece AcrySof posterior chamber IOL (Alcon Laboratories, Inc., Fort Worth, TX) in these cases for its ease of insertion, low

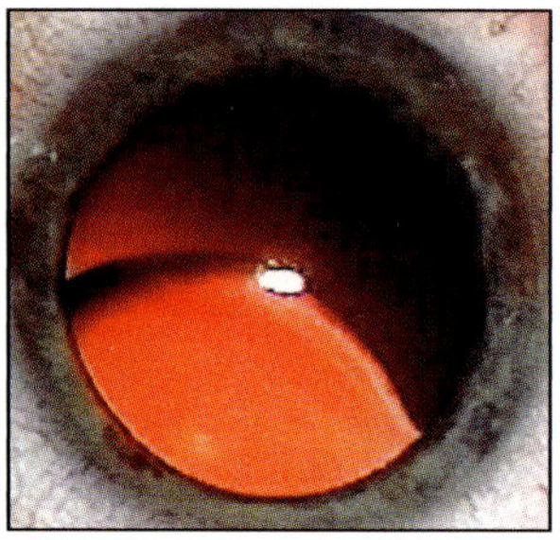

Figure 2. Preoperatively, this eye exhibited congenital lens subluxation due to Marfan's syndrome.

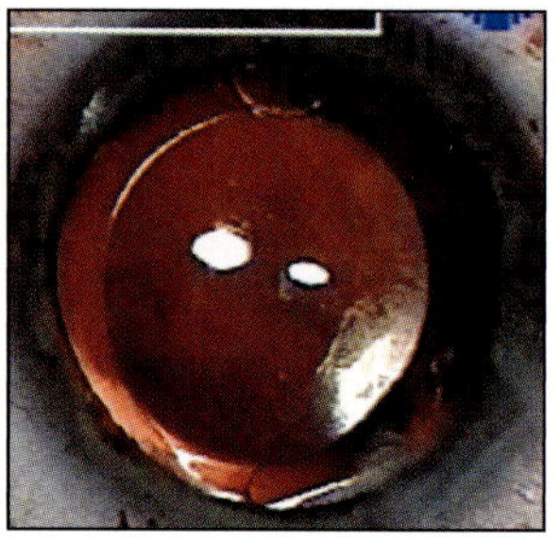

Figure 3. After placement of a modified CTR, the surgeon centers a posterior chamber IOL in the bag.

rate of posterior capsular opacification, and ability to stay well centered.

I manually remove viscoelastic either through the sideport incision or with an automated I/A handpiece. Instilling Miochol (CIBA Vision, Duluth, GA) ensures that the pupil becomes round. After re-approximating conjunctiva over the scleral flap, I hydrate the corneal incision and ensure that it is watertight.

CONCLUSION

CTRs and modified CTRs of any model should not be used if a complete continuous capsulorhexis is not attained or if a posterior capsular tear occurs, because the expansile forces may cause the capsular bag to rupture. Surgical options in such cases include either suturing the IOL to the iris or to the scleral wall or implanting an anterior chamber IOL.

At present, only Morcher's CTR (distributed in the United States by FCI Ophthalmics, Inc., Marshfield Hills, MA) has been approved for use in the US. Although the modified CTR can improve the surgical management of eyes with significant zonular weakness, it is important that the surgeon be familiar with advanced surgical techniques, because these cases represent some of the most difficult procedures that we ophthalmologists encounter. ■

This article originally appeared in the May 2004 issue of CRSToday.

1. Cionni RJ, Osher RH. Management of zonular dialysis with the endocapsular ring. *J Cataract Refract Surg.* 1995;21:245-249.
2. Cionni RJ, Osher RH. Management of profound zonular dialysis or weakness with a new endocapsular ring designed for scleral fixation. *J Cataract Refract Surg.* 1998;24:1299-1306.
3. Hara T, Hara T, Yamada Y. "Equator ring" for maintenance of the completely circular contour of the capsular bag equator after cataract removal. *Ophthalmic Surg.* 1991;22:358-359.
4. Legler U, Witschel B, et al. The capsular tension ring: a new device for complicated cataract surgery. Paper presented at: The ASCRS/ASOA Symposium on Cataract, IOL and Refractive Surgery; May 1993; Seattle, WA.
5. Osher RH. Synthetic zonules. *Video Journal of Cataract and Refractive Surgery.* 1997;8;(1).
6. Pfeifer V. Suturing the CTR. *Video Journal of Cataract and Refractive Surgery.* 1998;14(4).
7. Cionni RJ, Osher RH, Marques DM, et al. Modified capsular tension ring for patients with congenital loss of zonular support. *J Cataract Refract Surg.* 2003;29:1668-1673.
8. Merriam J, Zheng L. Iris hooks for phacoemulsification of the subluxated lens. *J Cataract Refract Surg.* 1997;23:1295.
9. Osher RH. Slow motion phacoemulsification approach. *J Cataract Refract Surg.* 1993;19:667.
10. Cionni RJ, Osher RH. Complications of phacoemulsification. In: Weinstock FJ, ed. *Management and Care of the Cataract Patient.* Cambridge, MA: Blackwell Scientific Publications Inc.; 1992: 209-210.

CHAPTER 136

Anterior Chamber IOLs

MANUS C. KRAFF, MD

After Danheim's and Barraquer's initial problems with anterior chamber IOLs (ACIOLs) in the 1950s, Peter Choyce, MD, developed eight iterations of the ACIOL in England over the course of the next decade. Dr. Choyce's lens was relatively successful in Europe by the 1970s, and the manufacture of ACIOLs began in the United States during the middle of that decade. Poor manufacturing techniques, lens warping, and rough edges resulted in problems associated with the American ACIOLs such as uveitis, glaucoma, and hyphema (dubbed *UGH syndrome*) as well as painful, inflamed, and uncomfortable eyes. The fact lost on surgeons was that these complications occurred mainly with lenses manufactured in the US.

The second era of problems with ACIOLs occurred from 1979 to 1982. Small, tubular haptics implanted in the angle caused chronic inflammation and an overgrowth of iris tissue that resulted in UGH syndrome as well as chronic CME. Concern over implicated ACIOLs such as the Azar, Leiske, Sheppard, Hesburg, and Stableflex obscured the fact that well-manufactured lenses, including the Rayner's Choyce Mark VIII, Precision Cosmet, and, later, the flexible Kelman Tripod and Quadraflex, did not produce the chronic inflammation leading to UGH syndrome and iris distortion.

All ACIOLs were lumped together as inferior lens products that should not be used. Surgeons developed myriad techniques (many of which were supremely difficult technically and caused trauma to the eye) that allowed them to avoid using ACIOLs. They began suturing posterior chamber IOLs (PCIOLs) to the sclera or iris from the posterior chamber. This article addresses ACIOLs' place in surgical practice and shares my results with this lens type.

ADVANTAGES OF AN ACIOL

These lenses are useful as secondary IOLs after intracapsular cataract extraction (ICCE). They are also appropriate for eyes in which there is insufficient capsular support for a PCIOL due to intraoperative traumatic capsular rupture. ACIOLs are indicated in cases of major zonular dehiscence and/or subluxation of the crystalline lens as well as after the removal of a subluxated PCIOL.

In the last three surgical scenarios just described, implanting an ACIOL is technically much easier, far less traumatic to the eye, and much more time efficient when compared with a sutured PCIOL. ACIOLs are the preferred lens type after a successfully performed ICCE with or without vitreous loss. In certain cases of severely compromised zonules, this surgical approach may be associated with a decreased incidence of posterior dislocation of the crystalline lens compared with phacoemulsification. In such cases, the implantation of an ACIOL after a planned ICCE avoids the risk of dropped lenticular fragments, as can occur if phacoemulsification

TABLE 1. VISUAL ACUITY AFTER ACIOL IMPLANTATION	
BSCVA	Percentage of Patients
20/15	4%
20/20	19%
20/25	34%
20/30	9%
20/40	6%
20/50	8%
20/60	11%
<20/60	9%

is attempted. Moreover, because an ACIOL is in contact with mesodermal tissue (eg, anterior iris), this lens type poses less risk of pigmentary glaucoma, uveitis, hyphema, and CME than does a PCIOL, which is in contact with the iris pigment (eg, neural ectoderm). Because a PCIOL's haptics are not in the bag, they may cause friction and erosion of iris pigment and vascular tissue upon pupillary movement, thereby resulting in intermittent bleeding (posterior or anterior) and/or pigmentary glaucoma.

FIVE-YEAR DATA

A review of my own surgical data from the past 5 years revealed the use of ACIOLs in 53 eyes (approximately 1.5%). The Kelman Quadriflex lens was used exclusively in this study, and my follow-up data range from 6 months to 5 years. Of the ACIOLs implanted, 31 were secondary IOLs, 12 were placed in cases of a subluxated crystalline lens, eight replaced subluxated PCIOLs that I had removed, and two were placed after intraoperative capsular rupture and in the absence of sufficient capsular support for a PCIOL. The median age of the patients who received an ACIOL was 59 years (range, 26 to 92 years).

Table 1 shows the postoperative visual acuities for the study patients. Seventy-two percent achieved a postoperative BSCVA of 20/40 or better, and 79% saw 20/50 or better after ACIOL implantation. Only 9% had a BSCVA worse than 20/60. When analyzed by patient's age, 84% of patients younger than 70 years and 68% of those 70 years of age or older achieved a BSCVA of 20/40 or better.

CONCLUSION

A definite, although small, need for ACIOLs exists today. This type of lens and the surgery involved are far less traumatic to the eye and easier for the ophthalmologist to implant/perform. ■

This article originally appeared in the May 2004 issue of CRSToday.

CHAPTER 137

Managing Dislocated IOLs

GREGG T. KOKAME, MD

The dislocation or subluxation of IOLs has been an uncommon but recurrent complication throughout the history of their implantation. If the IOL is subluxated but still stable within the anterior segment, the surgeon may use an anterior approach to fixate the implant. If the IOL is unstable or dislocated posteriorly into the vitreous cavity, he should approach and retrieve the IOL via the posterior segment or pars plana vitrectomy and then reposition, exchange, or remove the lens.[1-7]

THE APPROACH

With IOLs that are unstable or posteriorly dislocated into the vitreous cavity, the advantages of a pars plana surgical approach include (1) a closed system with continuous infusion that allows precise maneuvers in a controlled surgical environment, (2) the clear visualization of surgical maneuvers through an undistorted cornea, and (3) bimanual manipulation of the unstable, dislocated implant. In addition, the surgeon can support the dislocated IOL from a posterior-to-anterior direction by passing instruments through the pars plana (Figure 1) as opposed to using a limbal or clear corneal approach, which requires passing instruments in an anterior-to-posterior direction to manipulate the dislocated IOL. Although improved techniques and instrumentation have greatly facilitated the management of these cases, new IOL designs and presentations such as in-the-bag IOL dislocations (where the IOL is encased within the capsular bag and dislocated due to zonular dehiscence[8,9]) present new challenges in management.

HOW TO PROCEED

The decision to remove, exchange, or reposition the IOL depends on the clinical situation. It is advisable to remove the lens in eyes with a poor visual prognosis, associated complicated retinal pathology such as retinal detachment, or damaged IOLs.[1-3] Exchanging the IOL for either a flexible-loop ACIOL or a sclerally fixated PCIOL is a reasonable management option, but it has the disadvantage of creating a large wound in the anterior segment for the removal of the dislocated IOL and the implantation of a new one.[1-3,7]

Repositioning the dislocated IOL reuses the original IOL, the refractive power of which provided functional vision prior to dislocation, and avoids the need for a large wound in the anterior segment.[1-7] Difficulties in manipulating the unstable dislocated IOL and trying to loop sutures around it have led some surgeons to abandon repositioning procedures, however. Moreover, a comparative, multisurgeon series found no difference in visual outcomes after the repositioning of the dislocated IOL versus its exchange for an ACIOL.[7]

REPOSITIONING DISLOCATED IOLS

Background

Manipulating an unstable, dislocated IOL in the vitreous cavity is technically difficult. For that reason, surgeons have developed many techniques to reposition and, if necessary, sclerally fixate a PCIOL's haptics.[1-6] Ideally, there is an intact rim of peripheral

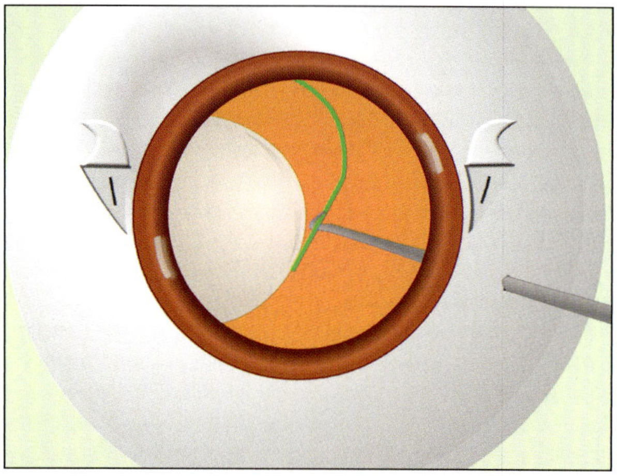

Figure 1. From the surgeon's view, the dislocated IOL is stabilized and supported with an instrument through a pars plana sclerotomy from a posterior-to-anterior direction. (Reprinted with permission from Kokame GT, Yamamoto I, Mandel H. Scleral fixation of dislocated posterior chamber intraocular lenses: temporary haptic externalization through a clear corneal incision. *J Cataract Refract Surg*. 2004;30:1049-1056.)

capsule over which the surgeon can reposition the IOL and its supporting haptics, thus minimizing surgical trauma and allowing the quickest recovery of vision. If the dislocation occurs many years after the IOL's initial implantation even if there is a residual capsular rim, however, I have found that either the capsular-zonular support system has become incapable of supporting the IOL's haptics long-term, or the original IOL's haptics are too flexible or are inadequate to prevent repeat dislocation over time. In cases of late, recurrent dislocation, the surgeon should place at least one scleral-fixation suture.

If the capsular support for the haptics is inadequate, the surgeon may reposition dislocated PCIOLs with scleral-fixation sutures. With adequate capsular support for one haptic (at least 5 clock hours), he may use scleral fixation for one haptic and the residual capsule for the other haptic.[4,5] If there is inadequate capsular support for one haptic, then I prefer to remove the residual capsule during the pars plana vitrectomy and sclerally fixate both haptics. In order to evaluate and plan for the surgical procedure, it is important to conduct a careful, tangential, slit-lamp examination for residual capsular support during the preoperative examination.

Creating the Suture Loop for Scleral Fixation

There are several techniques for looping a suture around the haptic of a dislocated IOL in eyes with inadequate residual capsular support.[1-6] Internal looping techniques are too numerous to describe in depth in this article, but they include multiple passes of the needle around the haptic through sclerotomies or paracentesis sites, looping the haptic with a threaded needle or a loop passed through a needle, holding a suture loop with a forceps, or lassoing the haptic with a pretied loop or slipknot.[1-3] These techniques work well if the IOL is relatively stable in a position posterior to the pupil so that it does not fall posteriorly during looping maneuvers. These intraocular maneuvers can be cumbersome and frustrating, however, when the dislocated IOL is unstable and mobile in the vitreous cavity, especially following pars plana vitrectomy.

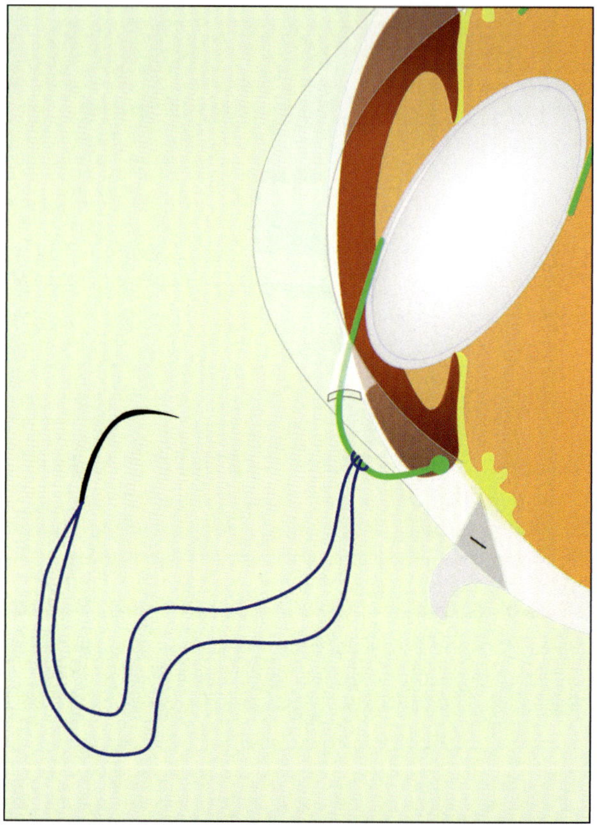

Figure 2. In this cross-sectional, sagittal view, the surgeon brings the implant up into the anterior chamber and externalizes the haptic through a clear corneal incision. He has tightened the suture loop around the haptic and cauterized the tip of the haptic to create a bulb to prevent slippage. (Reprinted with permission from Kokame GT, Yamamoto I, Mandel H. Scleral fixation of dislocated posterior chamber intraocular lenses: temporary haptic externalization through a clear corneal incision. *J Cataract Refract Surg*. 2004;30:1049-1056.)

Haptic Externalization

A technique called *haptic externalization* allows the surgeon to securely place the scleral-fixation suture prior to reimplantating an IOL into the eye. It also stabilizes the previously unstable IOL and thus makes further manipulation safer and more controlled.[4-6] Clement Chan, MD, first described haptic externalization through a pars plicata fixation sclerotomy.[6] Once the surgeon externalizes the haptic, he tightens the suture loop down around the haptic and reimplants it.

In order to stabilize dislocated IOLs, I developed a technique of bringing the dislocated PCIOL back into the anterior chamber and then externalizing the haptic through a clear corneal incision (Figure 2). After I fixate the suture to the haptic outside the eye, I pass the suture posteriorly through the clear corneal incision, through the pupil, and posterior to the iris, where I retrieve it through a fixation sclerotomy, 1.25 mm posterior to the limbus (Figure 3). The implant is then in its usual position, and I can reimplant it in a controlled fashion. The clear corneal externalization allows me direct visualization of the haptic externalization and thus minimizes the risk of damage to the haptic during externalization.

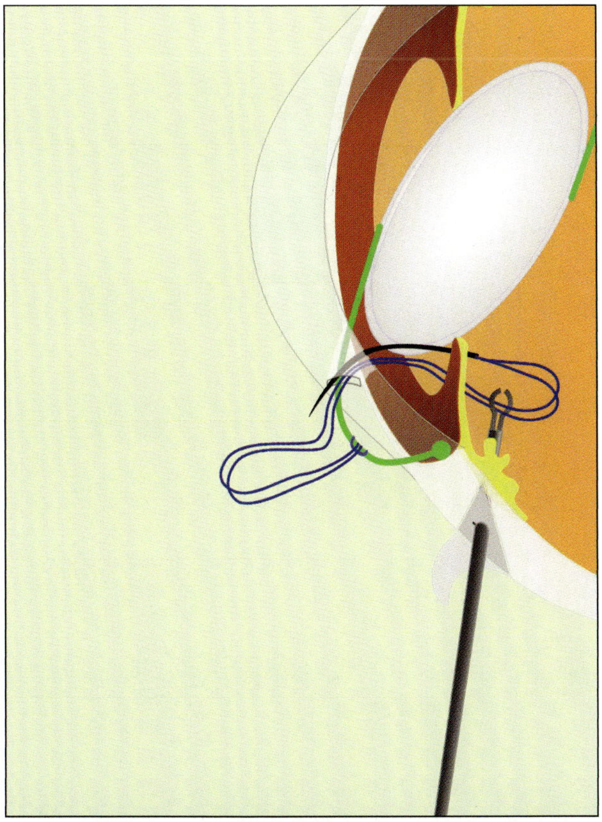

Figure 3. In this cross-sectional, sagittal view, the surgeon passes the long, curved needle backward through the clear corneal incision, through the pupil, and posterior to the iris, where he retrieves the suture through a pars plicata fixation sclerotomy, 1.25 mm posterior to the limbus. The surgeon will then reimplant the IOL and tie the sutures around the haptic to a separate scleral-fixation suture underneath the scleral flap. (Reprinted with permission from Kokame GT, Yamamoto I, Mandel H. Scleral fixation of dislocated posterior chamber intraocular lenses: temporary haptic externalization through a clear corneal incision. *J Cataract Refract Surg*. 2004;30:1049-1056.)

One important hint for performing an externalization technique is to grasp the tip of the haptic and to follow its curve during externalization to prevent breaking or bending the haptic.

In-the-Bag IOL Dislocations

Managing in-the-bag dislocation of an IOL is especially challenging, because the haptics are enmeshed within the residual capsule and lens debris. Although the highest incidence of this complication has been reported with pseudoexfoliation,[8,9] it can also occur with uveitis and trauma or without an identifiable cause.[9] If the complex is still relatively stable within the anterior segment, the surgeon may grasp and remove the entire complex through an anterior segment wound. In addition, some surgeons have found posterior-assisted levitation[10] with viscoelastic to be a useful approach that floats the complex anteriorly in order to allow its removal from this direction. Suturing through the capsular bag is another alternative for achieving scleral fixation. "Cheesewiring" the suture loop through the residual capsule as well as inadequate long-term stability of the suture loops around the haptics through the capsule may be a risk for future redislocation, however.[11]

Presently, if an IOL in the bag dislocates into the vitreous cavity, I prefer to (1) use a posterior segment approach with vitrectomy, (2) stabilize the IOL-capsular bag complex with a forceps, and (3) dissect the residual capsule and lens debris off the haptics and possibly the optic of the dislocated IOL. I may then externalize and fixate the haptics to the sclera by tightening the suture loops directly onto the haptic in order to minimize the IOL's future redislocation.[9,11] ■

This article originally appeared in the August 2005 issue of CRSToday.

1. Mello MO, Scott IU, Smiddy WE, et al. Surgical management and outcomes of dislocated intraocular lenses. *Ophthalmology*. 2000;107:62-67.
2. Chan CK, Agarwal A, Agarwal S, Agarwal A. Management of dislocated intraocular implants. *Ophthalmol Clin North Am*. 2001;14:681-693.
3. Smiddy WE, Ibanez GV, Alfonso E, Flynn HW Jr. Surgical management of dislocated intraocular lenses. *J Cataract Refract Surg*. 1995;21:64-69.
4. Kokame GT, Yamamoto I, Mandel H. Scleral fixation of dislocated posterior chamber intraocular lenses. Temporary haptic externalization through a clear corneal incision. *J Cataract Refract Surg*. 2004;30:1049-1056.
5. Kokame GT, Atebara NH, Bennett MD. Modified technique of haptic externalization for scleral fixation of posterior chamber implants. *Am J Ophthalmol*. 2001;131:129-131.
6. Chan CK. An improved technique for management of dislocated posterior chamber implants. *Ophthalmology*. 1992;99:51-57.
7. Sarrafizadeh R, Ruby AJ, Hassan TS, et al. A comparison of visual results and complications in eyes with posterior chamber intraocular lens dislocation treated with pars plana vitrectomy and lens repositioning or lens exchange. *Ophthalmology*. 2001;108:82-89.
8. Jehan FS, Mamalis N, Crandall AS. Spontaneous late dislocation of intraocular lens within the capsular bag in pseudoexfoliation patients. *Ophthalmology*. 2001;108:1727-1731.
9. Gross JG, Kokame GT, Weinberg DV. The Dislocated In-The-Bag Intraocular Lens Study Group. In-the-bag intraocular lens dislocation. *Am J Ophthalmol*. 2004;137:630-635.
10. Chang DF. Viscoelastic levitation of posteriorly dislocated intraocular lenses from the anterior vitreous. *J Cataract Refract Surg*. 2002;28:1515-1519.
11. Kokame GT, Gross JG, Weinberg DV. The Dislocated In-the-Bag Intraocular Lens Study Group. In-the-bag intraocular lens dislocation. Author Reply. *Am J Ophthalmol*. 2005;139:953-954.

CHAPTER 138

Managing Cylinder Intraoperatively

STEVEN J. DELL, MD

Approximately 30% of patients have more than 1.00 D of preexisting astigmatism, but how many of us are addressing astigmatism when we remove a cataract or perform a refractive lens exchange? While surveys indicate many surgeons state that they correct astigmatism, I suspect that a high percentage of them do not do so. If you talk to field representatives from the companies that manufacture IOLs, I think they would estimate that 80% of cataract surgeons do not correct astigmatism when they remove a cataract. In my opinion, the correction of astigmatism is an integral component of modern cataract surgery, and it can be safely and conveniently performed at the time of the cataract removal.

WHY CORRECT ASTIGMATISM?

We surgeons go to great lengths in our IOL calculations. We use equipment like the IOLMaster (Carl Zeiss Meditec, Inc., Dublin, CA) to measure the axial length, we are careful about keratometry (K), and we analyze our outcomes. These measures only address the spherical component of the postoperative refractive error. We need to correct astigmatism as well. Many patients, however, expect emmetropia after standard, traditional cataract surgery. If you perform refractive lens exchange or implant premium IOLs, addressing astigmatism is essential.

Small-incision cataract surgery predictably introduces a relatively small amount of astigmatism. Existing software tools such as http://www.LRIcalculator.com (Advanced Medical Optics, Inc., Santa Ana, CA) and http://www.acrysoftoriccalculator.com (Alcon Laboratories, Inc., Fort Worth, TX) on the Web enable you to modify your limbal relaxing incision (LRI) nomogram or your toric IOL calculations, based upon the anticipated flattening of the cornea after cataract surgery. Thus, many cases of cylinder can be addressed intraoperatively.

POSTPONING THE CORRECTION

The most precise method for addressing astigmatism is laser vision correction after healing has occurred from the cataract surgery, but it is also the most expensive technique and requires two surgical events. Nonetheless, patients achieve refractive stability more quickly after cataract surgery without LRIs. In addition, delaying astigmatic correction for a separate procedure allows you to address any residual spherical refractive error.

For these reasons, some surgeons plan to perform laser vision correction after cataract surgery, especially for cases of high astigmatism or when the chances of a refractive miss are high, as might be the case with extremes in axial length.

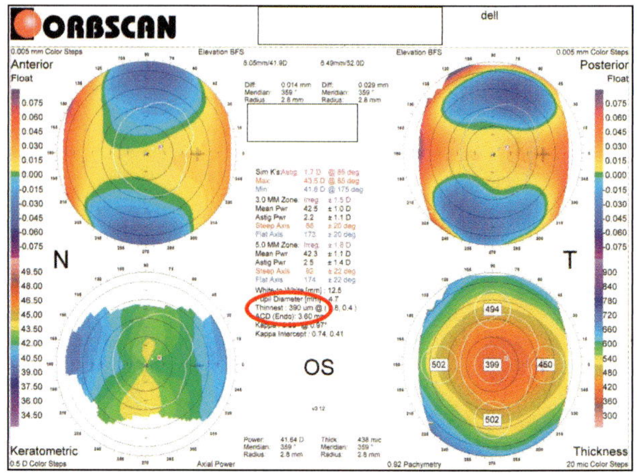

Figure 1. An abnormally thin (390 µm) cornea has a relatively normal surfact topography.

EXCLUDING ECTATIC AND/OR IRREGULAR CORNEAS

Irregular corneas or those with ectasia should not receive treatment of their astigmatism. Figure 1 demonstrates a topography that is relatively normal on the surface, but this unadulterated cornea is 390 µm thick at its thinnest point. Figure 2 shows another cornea that has a normal range of automated Ks but clearly has an abnormal topography. Figure 3 shows an eye that has mild infe-

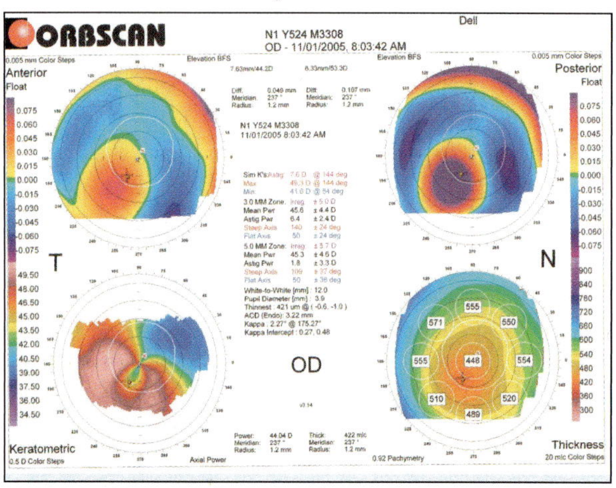

Figure 2. This cornea has normal K readings but abnormal topography.

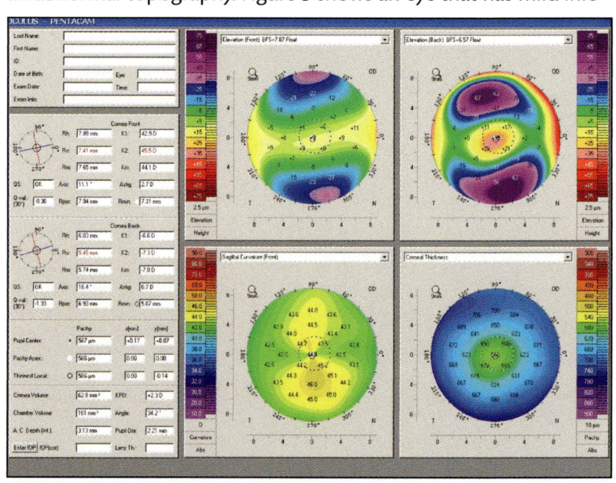

Figure 3. This cornea has mild inferior steepening and an abnormal posterior float.

rior steepening but a very abnormal posterior float. Corneas such as these have an elevated risk of ectasia with LASIK or LRIs and should be identified preoperatively.

NOMOGRAMS BASED ON ARC VERSUS CORD LENGTH

The effect of an arcuate incision on the cornea relates to its distance and length from the center of the cornea. In a small eye, because the incision is closer to the cornea than in a large eye, any given cord length of an incision will achieve more effect. On the other hand, the degree of arc-based nomograms (eg, 30° or 45°) automatically correct for this phenomenon, because the length of the incision subtending a certain number degrees of arc shortens as it moves closer to the center of the cornea. One drawback for LRIs based on degree of arc is that their nomograms tend to be complicated.

Nomograms based on cord length have the advantage of relative simplicity, but care must be exercised in small eyes to avoid over-corrections. Once again, this is because a 6-mm cord-length incision in a small eye would subtend a much larger angle than it would in a large eye. You can, however, get very good results with nomograms based on cord length.

TORIC IOLS

The advantage of toric IOLs is that they can correct cylinder and sphere simultaneously, potentially with greater accuracy than an LRI. You do not have to make any extra corneal incisions, and you can avoid the neurotrophia potentially associated with long corneal incisions. The lenses approved in the US, however, are available in a limited range of powers. Furthermore, a misalignment of the astigmatic axis of a toric IOL will reduce the effect.

I would recommend against toric IOLs in eyes with zonular dehiscence, weak zonules, and pseudoexfoliation because of the high risk of the lens' dislocation.

CONCLUSION

Astigmatic management will play an increasing role in cataract surgery as patients come to expect independence from glasses postoperatively. With premium IOL surgery, the need to address astigmatism is even more important. Familiarity with these techniques will help us meet the rising expectations of our patients. ■

This article originally appeared in the February 2008 issue of CRSToday.

CHAPTER 139

Corneal Correction of Astigmatism During Cataract Surgery

UDAY DEVGAN, MD

In the age of refractive cataract surgery, addressing the patient's preexisting corneal astigmatism at the time of surgery is important to delivering postoperative emmetropia and satisfaction. Minimizing postoperative astigmatism (no more than 0.50 to 0.75 D) is particularly important for achieving optimal results with multifocal IOLs (Figure 1).

Treating astigmatism with an excimer laser in pseudophakic patients is precise, but many cataract surgeons may not have access to this modality. Toric IOLs are an alternative, but they do not correct presbyopia. Another viable option is to treat the astigmatism via corneal incisions—a relatively safe and easy method with a minimal learning curve.

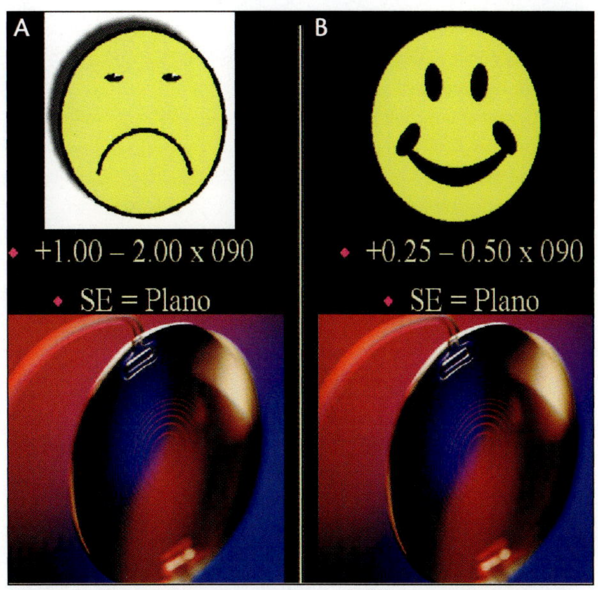

Figure 1. Pictured is a comparison of differences between patients with identical postoperative spherical equivalents, but markedly differently astigmatism. The patient with a multifocal IOL with 2.00 D of cylinder will probably be unhappy (A), whereas the patient with the same IOL and only 0.50 D of cylinder likely will be happy (B).

BASIC CONCEPTS

Understanding the basics of corneal incisions is an important first step. There are five primary concepts:

1. The corneal coupling effect explains why making a relaxing incision in the cornea flattens that meridian and steepens the cornea 90° away. For peripheral relaxing incisions, like limbal relaxing incisions (LRIs), this coupling ratio is 1:1. No change in the IOL power is needed because the cornea's spherical equivalent has not changed.
2. The larger the corneal incision is, the more it will flatten that meridian, and the more steepening it will cause 90° away.
3. The more central an incision is, the more flattening it will cause at that meridian. Peripheral incisions, like LRIs, have less

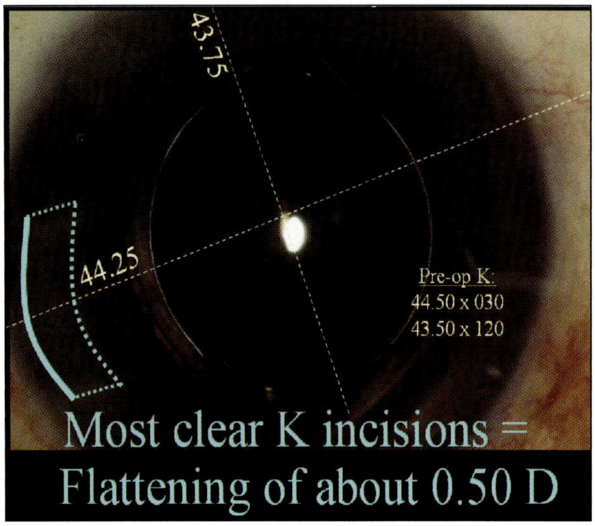

Figure 2. Most clear corneal phaco incisions cause a net flattening of about 0.50 D.

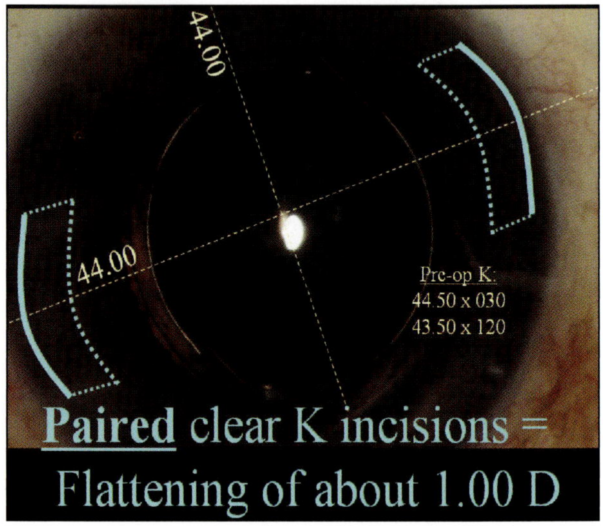

Figure 3. Making two paired clear corneal phaco incisions 180° apart can increase the net flattening.

effect but are more forgiving and less likely to induce irregular astigmatism. Central incisions such as astigmatic keratotomies (AKs) are significantly stronger in their effect, but they are also more likely to cause irregular astigmatism.

4. With penetrating incisions, short tunnels cause more flattening than long ones. For example, with the clear corneal incisions used during cataract surgery, the shorter the tunnel length, the more the flattening effect at that meridian and the steeper the effect 90° away. The long, square corneal incisions seal well and have little effect on astigmatism. The short tunnels are better able to reduce the astigmatism in their meridian, but they are more likely to leak at the end of the surgery.

5. With nonpenetrating incisions such as LRIs and AKs, the deeper the cuts, the more the flattening effect. Most LRIs are performed with set depths of 500, 550, or 600 µm, whereas AKs are usually performed at a depth that is a percentage of the total corneal thickness at that site. Although surgeons are less likely to cause an unintentional corneal perforation with the shallower incisions, they have less ability to modulate the astigmatism.

A FIRST STEP

It is important for cataract surgeons to know the effect of their incisions. Most temporal clear corneal incisions of 2.6 to 3.0mm cause about 0.25 to 0.75 D (with an average of about 0.50 D) of flattening at that meridian.[1] In order to determine the effect of your incisions,

Intralimbal Relaxing Incision
Nomogram for Modern Phaco Surgery
Empiric blade-depth setting of 600µm
Louis D. "Skip" Nichamin, MD ~ Laurel Eye Clinic, Brookville, PA

SPHERICAL
(up to +0.75 X 90 or +0.50 X 180)
Incision Design — **"Neutral" temporal clear corneal incision (ie, 3.5mm. or less, single plane, just anterior to vascular arcade)**

AGAINST-THE-RULE
(Steep Axis 0-44°/136°-180°)

PREOPERATIVE CYLINDER	Paired Incisions in Degrees of Arc* 30-40 yrs old	41-50 yrs old	51-60 yrs old	61-70 yrs old	71-80 yrs old	81-90 yrs old	91+ yrs old
+0.75 to +1.25	Nasal limbal arc only*					35°	
	55°	50°	45°	40°	35°		
+1.50 to +2.00	70°	65°	60°	55°	45°	40°	35°
+2.25 to +2.75	90°	80°	70°	60°	50°	45°	40°
+3.00 to +3.75	90° o.z = 8mm	90° o.z. = 9mm	85°	70°	60°	50°	45°

Incision Design — The temporal incision, if greater than 40° of arc, is made by first creating a two-plane, grooved phaco incision (600 µ depth), which is then extended to the appropriate arc length at the conclusion of surgery.

WITH-THE-RULE
(Steep Axis 45°-135°)

PREOPERATIVE CYLINDER	Paired Incisions in Degrees of Arc 30-40 yrs old	41-50 yrs old	51-60 yrs old	61-70 yrs old	71-80 yrs old	81-90 yrs old	91+ yrs old
+1.00 to +1.50	50°	45°	40°	35°	30°		
+1.75 to +2.25	60°	55°	50°	45°	40°	35°	30°
+2.50 to +3.00	70°	65°	60°	55°	50°	45°	40°
+3.25 to +3.75	80°	75°	70°	65°	60°	55°	45°

Incision Design — "Neutral" temporal clear corneal along with the following peripheral arcuate incisions

When placing intralimbal relaxing incisions following or concomitant with radial relaxing incisions, total arc length is decreased by 50%

(Courtesy of Louis "Skip" D. Nichamin, MD.)

Figure 4. Skip Nichamin, MD, has developed an accurate nomogram for the treatment of corneal astigmatism at the time of cataract surgery. He uses an empiric blade depth of 600µm, and his nomogram depends on the age of the patient as well as the amount of preoperative corneal astigmatism.

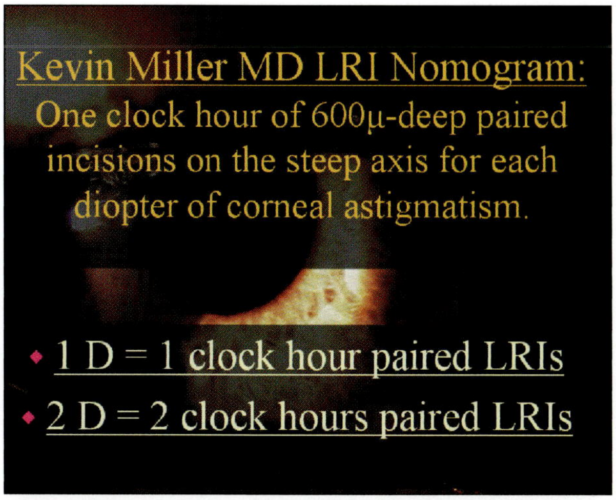

(Courtesy of Kevin Miller, MD.)

Figure 5. The simplest of all nomograms comes from Kevin Miller, MD, who has found no significant differences between depths of 450 μm and 600 μm. His nomogram is easy to remember, as it is just 1 clock hour of paired incisions for each diopter of symmetrical corneal astigmatism.

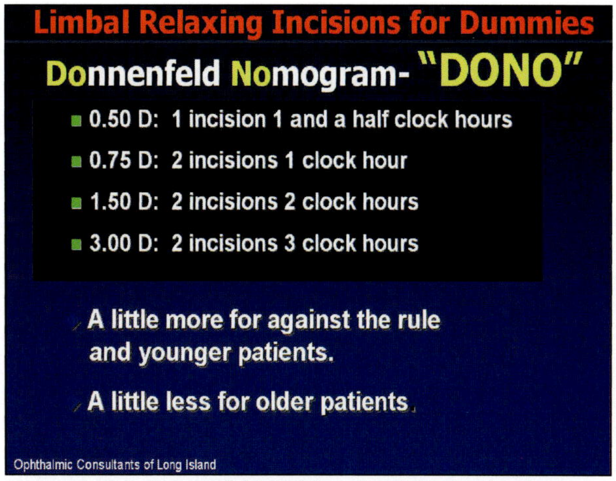

(Courtesy of Eric D. Donnenfeld, MD.)

Figure 6. Eric Donnenfeld, MD, has developed a simple nomogram for his LRI procedures. Note that he uses a blade depth of 600 μm and makes a mild correction for age as well.

carefully measure the pre- and postoperative keratometry and calculate the difference. Surgeons can place the corneal incision on the steep axis in order to induce an intentional astigmatic reduction of about 0.50 D[2] (Figure 2).

The surgeon can even make a second, full-thickness, perforating, clear corneal incision 180° away from the main incision in order to further increase the astigmatic effect.[3] I would suggest making this second clear corneal incision at the end of the case, while the anterior chamber is still inflated with viscoelastic. This technique for managing astigmatism does not require the purchase of any additional instruments (Figure 3).

LRIs can provide ophthalmologists with additional control in effectively managing astigmatism during cataract surgery. Nomograms guide the extent and location of these incisions.

Among the pioneers of LRIs at the time of cataract surgery are Louis D. "Skip" Nichamin, MD;[4] James Gills, MD[5]; and Douglas Koch, MD.[6] Each has developed and published his own nomogram that yields excellent results (Figure 4).

A SIMPLER STEP

Some of the simplest nomograms for astigmatic incisions come from Kevin Miller, MD, and Eric Donnenfeld, MD (Figures 5 and 6). Both nomograms are based upon the clock hours of treatment. Dr. Miller's nomogram can be summed up as follows: perform 1 clock hour of paired incisions at 600 μm on the steep axis for each diopter of corneal astigmatism. Dr. Donnenfeld's nomogram is so easy that he calls it *LRIs for dummies*.

TIPS AND TRICKS

Double even triple check that you are making the incisions on the correct axis. The most common mistake is making the incision 90° off, thereby doubling the patient's astigmatism.

Preoperative corneal topography allows surgeons to understand the extent and location of the corneal astigmatism and to screen out patients who may have subclinical keratoconus.

Do not overcorrect the astigmatism, as this will flip the axis and give the patient astigmatism to which he is not accustomed. Overcorrection of with-the-rule astigmatism will result in new against-the-rule astigmatism and an unhappy patient. It is far better to leave the patient a little undercorrected.

Apply a thin coating of a dispersive viscoelastic to the external cornea prior to performing the LRI. Doing so will help the blade glide smoothly and prevent roughing up the epithelium.

Mark the 90° position with a surgical marking pen while the patient is seated upright and before injecting anesthetics (topical drops are fine). This technique will ensure that any cyclotorsion of the eye does not cause a misplacement of the incisions.

I feel that the best instruments for making corneal relaxing incisions are diamond knives, which are available in preset or adjustable depths from many manufacturers. In particular, Accutome Inc. (Malvern, PA) makes diamond LRI knives for less than $500.

CONCLUSION

The arena of multifocal IOLs, premium IOLs, and refractive lens surgery, requires the surgeons be able to reduce or eliminate corneal astigmatism at the time of lenticular surgery. With a minimal investment of instruments and time, most can begin with the simple nomograms presented herein, track their results, and then hone their technique. Managing corneal astigmatism is an important part of refractive cataract surgery that I teach to all of my residents and regularly perform in my own private practice. ■

This article originally appeared in the January 2007 issue of CRSToday.

1. Borasio E, Mehta JS, Maurino V. Torque and flattening effects of clear corneal temporal and on-axis incisions for phacoemulsification. *J Cataract Refract Surg.* 2006;32:2030-2038.
2. Kaufmann C, Peter J, Ooi K, et al. Limbal relaxing incisions versus on-axis incisions to reduce corneal astigmatism at the time of cataract surgery. *J Cataract Refract Surg.* 2005;31:2261-2265.
3. Khokhar S Lohiya P, Murugiesan V, Panda A. Corneal astigmatism correction with opposite clear corneal incisions or single clear corneal incision: comparative analysis. *J Cataract Refract Surg.* 2006;9:1432-1437.
4. Nichamin LD. Nomogram for limbal relaxing incisions. *J Cataract Refract Surg.* 2006;32:1408.
5. Gills JP. Treating astigmatism at the time of cataract surgery. *Curr Opin Ophthalmol.* 2002;13:2-6.
6. Wang L, Misra M, Koch DD. Peripheral corneal relaxing incisions combined with cataract surgery. *J Cataract Refract Surg.* 2003;29:712-722.

CHAPTER 140

Where Is the Axis?

R. BRUCE WALLACE III, MD

A growing interest in presbyopia-correcting IOLs has helped to renew ophthalmologists' attention to preoperative biometry in order to maximize the accuracy of their IOL power calculations. Additionally, the surgical correction of astigmatism is becoming more common. For those surgeons who plan to use only monofocal IOLs, toric IOLs such as the ones from STAAR Surgical Company (Monrovia, CA) and Alcon Laboratories, Inc. (Fort Worth, TX) can provide an answer to their cylinder-correction needs. However, toricity is not yet available on a presbyopia-correcting IOL platform. For now, surgeons must couple corneal refractive procedures with presbyopia-correcting IOLs of the appropriate spherical power to achieve the desired result.

SURGERY TO REDUCE POSTOPERATIVE ASTIGMATISM

Central corneal surgery such as PRK, Epi-LASIK, and LASIK can reduce unwanted postoperative astigmatism, but these procedures are relatively expensive alternatives to incisional, peripheral, corneal surgery such as limbal relaxing incisions (LRIs). Excimer laser ablation also means another surgical event for patients, and some of these patients may have other ocular conditions such as dry eye, which might adversely affect their postoperative outcome. Most surgeons have found that LRIs provide a safe and effective means of correcting unwanted cylinder with remarkable postoperative stability. For these reasons, LRIs have become a popular method to reduce astigmatism.

FINDING THE AXIS

Astigmatic procedures require the surgeon to select the proper axis of astigmatism. With toric IOLs and LRIs, the plus axis is the reference point. With corneal laser correction, the minus axis is the reference point.

What are surgeons' choices to measure and determine where the axis is? Most depend on keratometry because the refractive cylinder may be influenced by lenticular astigmatism, which will be eliminated after the lens is removed. Many cataract surgeons like manual keratometry instead of automated methods because visualizing the regularity and sharpness of the corneal mires can help determine the quality of the manual reading. In addition, more cataract practices have been investing in corneal topography to determine the pattern of the astigmatism as well as its amount and location.

AXIS LOCATION STUDY

My colleagues and I performed a study to decipher the best way to locate the proper axis for astigmatic correction.[1] We found a surprising variance between refractive, keratometric, and corneal topographic axis locations among patients with 2.00 D or less of measurable cylinder. However, for eyes with more than 2.50 D, we began to see a stronger correlation of the axis' location with all methods used to measure corneal cylinder.

Most of our patients needing astigmatic correction with lenticular procedures will have less than 2.50 D of cylinder. Therefore, the surgeon must "guesstimate" the axis' position using the current methods to measure corneal curvature. Fortunately, astigmatic correction is usually more forgiving than spherical correction, especially for patients with 0.50 to 2.00 D of cylinder.

Most of my patients in need of astigmatic correction benefit from LRIs. When planning the incisions, I pay most attention to the axis' location and cylindrical pattern as displayed by the corneal topographic map. If I find a significant disparity between corneal topography and keratometry (ie, more than 30°), I may elect to postpone the LRI until after the lens' replacement and usually will offer any needed astigmatic correction for this eye in tandem with lens surgery on the fellow eye.

CONCLUSION

All methods to surgically correct astigmatism during (and after) lens replacement depend on choosing the correct axis of the corneal cylindrical power. Because this axis can be difficult to locate, especially with astigmatism of less than 2.00D, the surgeon will need to make a judgment call as to the placement of the astigmatic correction. If unsuccessful, the ophthalmologist can still fine-tune eyes with problematic levels of astigmatism. Fortunately, because astigmatic surgery is relatively forgiving, most of these patients will be satisfied with their UCVA after their initial astigmatic procedure. ■

This article originally appeared in the May 2006 issue of CRSToday.

1. Wallace RB. On-axis cataract incisions: where is the axis? In: *1995 ASCRS Symposium of Cataract, IOL and Refractive Surgery Best Papers of Sessions.* ASCRS: Fairfax, Virginia; 1995; 67-72.

CHAPTER 141

Corneal Relaxing Incisions

LOUIS "SKIP" D. NICHAMIN, MD

The need to manage preexisting astigmatism has become a requisite of modern phaco surgery. Ophthalmologists' experience with keratorefractive surgery has proven that astigmatism of as little as 0.75 D may leave a patient symptomatic with visual blur, ghosting, and halos. To fully embrace the notion of refractive cataract surgery, the dedicated surgeon must aspire to a level of accuracy equated with corneal-based refractive surgery. The most popular approach to achieve this goal is the use of corneal incisions—specifically, limbal relaxing incisions (LRIs).

HISTORY

The modern era of cataract and astigmatic surgery began in the mid-1980s, when Robert Osher, MD, and other pioneering surgeons first suggested that astigmatic keratotomy might be combined with cataract and implant surgery.[1,2] In time, the benefit of moving these incisions to a more peripheral limbal location became evident.[3-5]

LRIs hold several advantages compared with astigmatic keratotomy incisions placed at a more central optical zone. They include a lesser tendency to cause a shift in the resultant axis of cylinder and a lower likelihood of inducing irregular astigmatism. LRIs are also easier to create and are more forgiving overall. Another advantage involves the coupling ratio, which describes the amount of flattening that occurs in the incised meridian relative to the amount of steepening that results 90° away. Because paired LRIs (when kept at or under 90° of arc length) exhibit a consistent 1:1 ratio, they elicit little change in spheroequivalence and obviate the need to change the IOL's power.

MEASUREMENTS

Perhaps the most challenging aspect of astigmatic surgery involves determining the quantity and exact location of the cylinder to be corrected. Unfortunately, preoperative measurements—keratometry, refraction, and corneal topography—do not always correlate. Lenticular astigmatism may account for some of this disparity, particularly in cases where there is a wide variance between the refraction and corneal measurements. Some discrepancies, however, are likely due to the inherent shortcomings of the traditional measurements of astigmatism. Standard keratometry, for example, measures only two points in each meridian at a single optical zone of approximately 3mm.

When faced with confounding measurements, one solution is to compromise and average the disparate readings. For example, if the refraction shows 2.00 D of astigmatism and keratometry reveals only 1.00 D, it would be reasonable to correct for 1.50 D. Alternatively, if the preoperative calculations vary widely, one may defer placing the relaxing incisions until the patient's refraction stabilizes after cataract surgery. The LRIs may be safely performed in the office in an appropriate treatment-room setting.

Corneal topography can also be helpful when the refraction and keratometry do not agree. It is also useful for detecting subtle corneal pathology such as forme fruste keratoconus, which would likely contraindicate the use of LRIs, or subtle irregular astigmatism such as that caused by epithelial basement membrane dystrophy.

POTENTIAL PROBLEMS

- Infection
- Weakening of the globe
- Perforation
- Decreased corneal sensation
- Induced irregular astigmatism
- Misalignment/axis shift
- Wound gape and discomfort
- Operating upon the wrong (opposite) axis!

Reprinted with permission from Gills J, ed. A Complete Surgical Guide for Correcting Astigmatism: an Ophthalmic Manifesto. *Thorofare, NJ: Slack, Inc.; 2003.*

NOMOGRAMS

After calculating the amount of astigmatism to correct, one must consult a nomogram[6] to determine the appropriate arc length of the incisions. My nomogram of choice originated with the work of Stephen Hollis, MD, and incorporates concepts (particularly age modifiers) taught by Spencer Thornton, MD.[7] Astigmatism is considered to be with the rule if the steep axis (plus cylinder) is between 45° and 135° (Table 1). Against-the-rule astigmatism falls between 0° to 44° and 136° to 180°. One aligns the patient's age with the amount of preoperative cylinder to be corrected and finds the suggested arc length that the incisions should subtend.

Cataract surgeons commonly set the blade's depth (typically at 600µm) empirically when performing LRIs. In the setting of refractive lens exchange surgery or when employing presbyopia-correcting IOLs—when ultimate precision is required—I prefer to perform pachymetry and adjust the blade's depth. One may perform pachymetry either preoperatively or at the time of surgery. Readings are taken over the entire arc length of the intended incision, and an adjustable micrometer diamond blade is then set to approximately 90% of the thinnest reading obtained. Refinements to the blade's depth setting as well as nomogram adjustments may be necessary depending upon individual surgical technique, the instruments used, and the style of the blade.

In eyes that have previously undergone RK, the surgeon should reduce the length of the incisions by approximately 50%. It may be best to avoid relaxing incisions in favor of a toric IOL in eyes that have undergone significant prior keratotomy surgery.

SURGICAL PEARLS

When

Generally, one places the relaxing incisions at the outset of surgery in order to minimize epithelial disruption. The one exception is when the phaco incision intersects or is encompassed within an LRI of greater than 40° of arc. Extending the incision to its full arc length at the start of surgery may produce significant gaping and edema secondary to the intraoperative manipulation of the wound. In this setting, one first makes the phaco incision by creating a shortened LRI, the arc length of which corresponds to the

TABLE 1. THE "NAPA" NOMOGRAM

WITH THE RULE (Steep Axis 45° to 135°)

PREOPERATIVE CYLINDER (Diopters)	Paired Incisions in Degrees of Arc 20 to 30 years old	31 to 40 years old	41 to 50 years old	51 to 60 years old	61 to 70 years old	71 to 80 years old
0.75	40	35	35	30	30	
1.00	45	40	40	35	35	30
1.25	55	50	45	40	35	35
1.50	60	55	50	45	40	40
1.75	65	60	55	50	45	45
2.00	70	65	60	55	50	45
2.25	75	70	65	60	55	50
2.50	80	75	70	65	60	55
2.75	85	80	75	70	65	60
3.00	90	90	85	80	70	65

AGAINST THE RULE (Steep Axis 0° to 44°/136° to 180°)

PREOPERATIVE CYLINDER (Diopters)	Paired Incisions in Degrees of Arc 20 to 30 years old	31 to 40 years old	41 to 50 years old	51 to 60 years old	61 to 70 years old	71 to 80 years old
0.75	45	40	40	35	35	30
1.00	50	45	45	40	40	35
1.25	55	55	50	45	40	35
1.50	60	60	55	50	45	40
1.75	65	65	60	55	50	45
2.00	70	70	65	60	55	50
2.25	75	75	70	65	60	55
2.50	80	80	75	70	65	60
2.75	85	85	80	75	70	65
3.00	90	90	85	80	75	70

Blade's depth setting is at 90% of the thinnest pachymetry.

Reprinted with permission from Gills J, ed. A Complete Surgical Guide for Correcting Astigmatism: an Ophthalmic Manifesto. *Thorofare, NJ: Slack, Inc.; 2003.*

width of the phaco and IOL incision. It is essentially a two-planed, grooved phaco incision with a depth of 600 µm (or as determined by pachymetry).

After implanting the IOL but before removing the viscoelastic, while the globe is still firm, the surgeon extends the relaxing incision to its full arc length as dictated by the nomogram. When the LRI is superimposed upon the phaco tunnel, one creates the phaco incision by pressing the bottom surface of the keratome blade downward upon the outer or posterior edge of the LRI. The keratome is then advanced into the LRI at a plane parallel to the iris. This angulation will promote a dissection at midstromal depth, which will help ensure an adequately long tunnel and a self-sealing closure.

Where

Properly centering the incisions over the steep corneal meridian is of the utmost importance. According to Euler's theorem, an axis deviation of 5°, 10°, or 15° will result in a 17%, 33%, or 50% reduction in effect, respectively.[8] This decrease holds true for both relaxing incisions and toric IOLs. Also, growing evidence supports the notion that significant cyclotorsion may occur when the patient assumes a supine position.[9] For this reason, most surgeons advocate placing an orientation mark at the 12:00- or 6:00-o'clock position on the limbus while the patient is upright. Doing so is particularly important when administering anesthesia by injection, which may result in unpredictable ocular rotation.

An additional tip for centering the relaxing incisions is to identify the steep meridian (plus cylinder axis) intraoperatively with some form of keratoscopy. The steep meridian over which the incisions are to be placed corresponds to the shorter axis of the reflected corneal mire. To mark the steep meridian, surgeons often use a Mendez ring or similar degree gauge, which is aligned with the previously placed limbal orientation mark, and then locate the axis of cylinder on the 360° gauge.

One should place the LRI at the most peripheral extent of clear corneal tissue, just inside the true surgical limbus—even in the presence of pannus. One may ignore bleeding if it occurs, because it will cease spontaneously. Placing the incisions farther out at the true surgical limbus will likely reduce their effect significantly due to both increased thickness of the tissue and a variation in its composition. LRIs are, therefore, really *intralimbal* in nature.

How

It is important to hold the knife perpendicular to the corneal surface in order to achieve a consistent depth and effect and to avoid gaping of the incision. Adequate support of the hand and wrist is important, and one ought to hold the blade as if throwing a dart. In other words, one should be able to rotate the instrument between one's thumb and index finger as it advances. Typically, surgeons create the incisions on the right side of the globe with their right hand, and they use their left hand for incisions on the left side of the globe. In most cases, it is more efficient to pull the blade toward (versus away from) oneself.

COMPLICATIONS

Even though LRIs are a safe and effective way of managing astigmatism at the time of cataract surgery, any surgical technique has potential complications (see *Potential Problems*). The most likely error involves incisions placed on the wrong axis, usually a 90° error with positioning upon the opposite, flat meridian. The error increases (likely doubles) the patient's preexisting cylinder. I recommend employing safety checks (eg, a written plan showing the proper orientation that is posted in the OR) to prevent this frustrating complication. Incisions are always placed upon the plus-cylinder axis and opposite to the minus-cylinder axis.

Although rare, corneal perforation is possible, potentially due to the blade's improper depth or as a result of a defect in the micrometer's mechanism. The latter problem may arise after repeated autoclaving and many sterilizing runs. Periodic inspection and calibration are warranted, even with preset single-depth knives. Unlike radial microperforations, circumferential punctures will rarely self-seal and will likely require the placement of temporary sutures.

SUMMARY

The refinement of the refractive outcome may be the single most pressing challenge faced by today's cataract surgeons. Astigmatic relaxing incisions are the most common method used to address preexisting cylinder. Moving these incisions to an intralimbal location greatly reduces the incidence of complications and difficulties compared with astigmatic keratotomy. ■

This article originally appeared in the May 2006 issue of CRSToday.

1. Osher RH. Combining phacoemulsification with corneal relaxing incisions for reduction of preexisting astigmatism. Paper presented at: The Annual Meeting of the American Intra-Ocular Implant Society; 1984; Los Angeles, CA.
2. Maloney WF. Refractive cataract replacement: a comprehensive approach to maximize the refractive benefits of cataract extraction. Paper presented at: The ASCRS Annual Meeting; 1986; Los Angeles, CA.
3. Budak K, Friedman NF, Koch DD. Limbal relaxing incisions with cataract surgery. *J Cataract Refract Surg.* 1998;24:503-508.
4. Muller-Jensen K, Fischer P, Siepe U. Limbal relaxing incisions to correct astigmatism in clear corneal cataract surgery. *J Refract Surg.* 1999;15:586-589.
5. Nichamin LD. Changing approach to astigmatism management during phacoemulsification: peripheral arcuate astigmatic relaxing incisions. Paper presented at: The ASCRS/ASOA Symposium & Congress; May 20, 2000; Boston, MA.
6. Gills JP. A *Complete Guide to Astigmatism Management.* Thorofare, NJ: Slack, Inc.; 2003.
7. Thornton SP. *Radial and Astigmatic Keratotomy: the American System of Precise, Predictable Refractive Surgery.* Thorofare, NJ: Slack, Inc.; 1994.
8. Abrams D. Ophthalmic optics and refraction. In: Duke-Elder SS, ed. *System of Ophthalmology.* St. Louis, MO: Mosby; 1970: 671-674.
9. Swami AU, Steinert RF, Osborne WE, et al. Rotational malposition during laser in situ keratomileusis. *Am J Ophthalmol.* 2002;133:561-562.

CHAPTER 142

The Importance of LRIs

ERIC D. DONNENFELD, MD

The single most important component of providing good surgical outcomes for patients with refractive IOLs is the treatment of residual corneal astigmatism. Astigmatism decreases visual acuity through meridional blur; one axis of the cornea is steeper than the other, causing the cornea to distort images. As little as small as 0.50 D of astigmatism may result in glare, symptomatic blur, ghosting, and halos. If we want to provide our refractive IOL patients with successful surgical outcomes, we need to treat their residual postoperative astigmatism. Although ophthalmologists can accomplish this goal with excimer photoablation and conductive keratoplasty, they should not dismiss limbal relaxing incisions (LRIs) as a valid alternative. Furthermore, reducing corneal astigmatism with LRIs is more cost effective and convenient than other techniques. Here is why I think all refractive IOL surgeons should know how to perform this simple and effective procedure.

ZERO TOLERANCE POLICY

A common belief about refractive surgery is that patients who receive presbyopia-correcting IOLs willingly tolerate small refractive errors after cataract surgery. In fact, nothing could be further from the truth. These individuals are incredibly sensitive to even minor refractive errors, including astigmatism. I have found that most patients can tolerate postoperative astigmatism of 0.50 D or less. If their preoperative topography suggests they will have between 0.50 and 1.50 D of residual cylinder, I plan to perform LRIs. I do not treat such a small degree of astigmatism with excimer photoablation, because I believe this procedure exposes patients to unnecessary expenses and potential postoperative

TABLE 1. THE DONNENFELD NOMOGRAM (DONO) FOR LRIs

Preoperative Astigmatism	Number of Incisions*	Length of Incisions, Clock Hours†
0.50 D	1	1.5
0.75 D	2	1
1.50 D	2	2
3.00 D‡	2	3

**All incisions are placed 0.5 mm from the limbus in the correct axis.*

†Patients who have against-the-rule astigmatism or who are less than 45 years old may benefit from slightly longer incisions. Shorter incisions may be indicated for patients older than 65 years.

‡I will use LRIs to correct up to 3.00 D of astigmatism if a laser correction is contraindicated for financial or medical reasons.

complications. I reserve laser treatment for patients who have more than 1.50 D of postoperative astigmatism.

PATIENTS WILL NOT PAY

It is true that most insurance plans, including Medicare, do not reimburse surgeons for correcting preexisting corneal astigmatism during cataract surgery. Patients, therefore, must pay out of pocket for this service. I have found, however, that most patients are happy to pay for markedly improved uncorrected vision, which is why I usually bundle the cost of LRIs with any additional charges for multifocal or accommodating IOLs.

NOMOGRAMS ARE TOO COMPLEX

Notable surgeons such as Louis "Skip" D. Nichamin, MD[1]; Douglas Koch, MD[2]; and James Gills, MD,[3] have proposed different nomograms for correcting small amounts of cylinder with LRIs. Although these formulae are meant to simplify the placement of the incisions, their specific adjustments for age and cylinder can give the impression that the procedure is overly complex, precise, and unforgiving. Instead, I believe that LRIs are as much an art as a science.

CORRECTING ASTIGMATISM

In order to provide refractive IOL patients with successful surgical outcomes, we need to treat their preexisting, surgically induced, and residual postoperative astigmatism. Although excimer photoablation is extremely effective, we should consider limbal relaxing incisions (LRIs) as an alternative.

THE INCISION'S LOCATION

Before performing LRIs, we first need to ask ourselves a very simple question: Where are we going to place them?

Surgeons should refer to a printout of the patient's preoperative corneal topography or keratometry to determine the incision's location. I advise that surgeons never base their incision on the refractive axis during cataract surgery, because lenticular astigmatism may be a factor, which will be absent following surgery. The one exception to this rule is after toric IOL implantation when keratometry is meaningless and the refraction is the correct axis for the incision. Although both keratometry and topography are useful, I prefer the latter. An important point is that the biggest mistake I see doctors make when performing LRIs is that they plot their incisions at their keratometric or topographic axis preoperatively and do not consider the surgically induced cylinder.

INDUCING CYLINDER

When placing LRIs, it is important to consider how the cataract incision will affect the patient's existing astigmatism. A simple way to determine the effect of the cataract incision on astigmatism is to place the incision exactly in the steep or flat corneal axis. The difference between the pre- and postoperative cylinder is induced by the incision. If the cylinder is at 90°, for example, and a surgeon places the incision at 90° and starts with 1.00 D of cylinder, he will end up with 0.50 D of cylinder. In other words, the incision created 0.50 D of cylinder. That is not what happens most of the time, however. Usually the incision is placed off axis and the two vector forces of preexisting cylinder and surgically induced cylinder are calculated with vector analysis.

NOMOGRAMS

When determining how much cylinder an incision will create, a nomogram from Warren Hill, MD, is helpful and available at http://www.drhill.com. Most doctors produce a little less than 0.50 D of cylinder, depending on where they

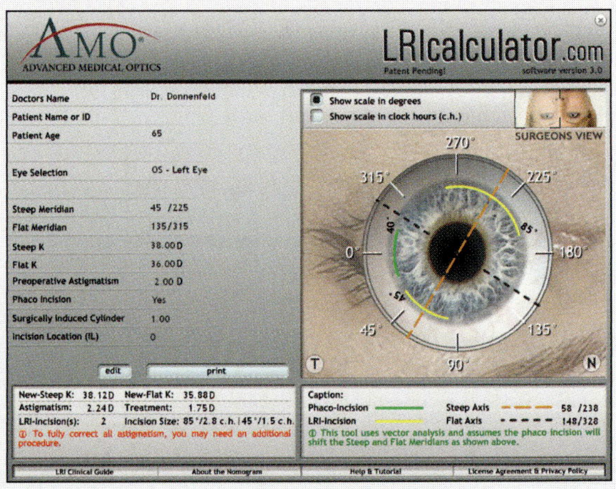

Figure 1. LRI calculator print output page.

place the incision.

Surgeons can also use a vector analysis of the preexisting cylinder and the cylinder induced by the incision to determine the location and length of the LRI. For most surgeons, however, this is not practical. Instead of learning vector analysis, surgeons can visit http://www.LRICalculator.com, a Web site created by Advanced Medical Optics, Inc. (Santa Ana, CA), that will instruct them where to place incisions. The Web site includes my Donnenfeld nomogram. Users of the Web site get a surgeon's view of the eye, which illustrates where the steep axis is located based on topography or keratometry. Users then enter the steep and flat keratometry readings. The Web site will use a green line to indicate where the incision should be made. The yellow line signifies the preoperative keratometry, and the black line represents the flat axis. Surgeons can print out the diagram to bring to the OR, or the office, to use as a template (Figure 1).

CONCLUSION

Patients who receive presbyopia-correcting IOLs will not tolerate a small refractive error. I routinely treat 0.50 D of cylinder in a symptomatic patient. When a surgeon transitions from cataract to refractive IOL surgery, it is important to pay attention to details. One of the most important concepts is to treat small residual refractive errors. Learning to perform LRIs is a major step that many surgeons will take to become excellent refractive cataract surgeons, and the good news is that it is an easy change to make. ■

In general, it is best for surgeons to practice the basic techniques for placing LRIs and eventually develop their own nomograms to achieve consistent results. This is how I developed the simple nomogram (the Donnenfeld nomogram or DONO) that I use in my practice (Table 1).

THE DONNENFELD NOMOGRAM

For surgeons new to LRIs, I suggest beginning by performing the procedure in the OR in conjunction with routine cataract surgery. I recommend adding peribulbar anesthesia to the operative regimen.

I place LRIs at the beginning of cataract surgery, because I prefer to work with a firm, well-hydrated eye. The cornea tends to become thinner as it dehydrates under the operating microscope. I determine where to place the corneal incisions by referring to a printout of the patient's preoperative corneal topography. I hold the map upside down to orient the patient's position on the operating table. Next, I grasp the episclera at the limbus with a 0.12-caliber forceps approximately 180° away from the incision's intended site. To place the incision, I apply a diamond blade (usually preset to 0.6 mm) to the eye and hold it in place for a second to ascertain that I have achieved the full depth before extending the cut to the length required to correct the targeted amount of astigmatism.

When placing LRIs, it is important to consider how the surgically induced cylinder will affect the patient's existing astigmatism. For example, because I make superior incisions, I will include an additional 0.50 D of against-the-rule cylinder to an LRI intended to treat a 0.50 D of preexisting against-the-rule cylinder. On the other hand, I know that my surgical technique will correct 0.50 D of cylinder in a patient who has with-the-rule astigmatism. Surgeons who prefer an oblique approach or are who treating a patient with oblique astigmatism can use a vector analysis of the preexisting cylinder and the cylinder induced by the incision to determine the location and length of the LRI. A new Web site, www.lricalculator.com, provides a vector analysis of the preexisting corneal astigmatism and the surgically induced cylinder. The Web site then calculates the new cylinder to be treated as well as the axis and creates a surgical diagram and plan, which can be copied and brought to the OR.

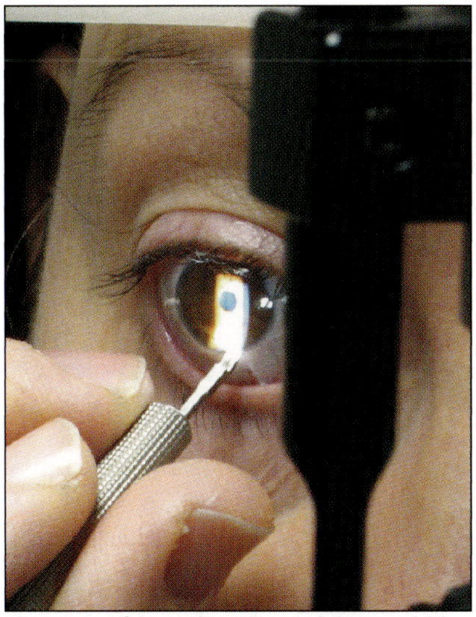

Figure 1. This patient is receiving an LRI to correct with-the-rule astigmatism.

INADEQUATE EQUIPMENT

Another inaccurate assumption about why surgeons hesitate to perform LRIs is that they are not comfortable with this technique. Instead, I think that surgeons do not perform LRIs as often as they could because they do not have access to operating microscopes in their offices. A simple solution in this situation is to perform LRIs at the slit lamp (Figure 1).

I prepare patients for in-office LRIs by anesthetizing their eye with lidocaine gel. When I am satisfied that the patient's head is positioned correctly on the chin rest, I look at his eye through the phoropter and use a diamond blade to create a small LRI, just as I would under an operating microscope. One small incision will correct 0.50 to 0.75 D of cylinder. The whole procedure takes approximately 30 seconds, and the patient's vision improves immediately. To prevent postoperative inflammation and infection, I prescribe prednisolone acetate 1% and gatifloxacin 0.3% q.i.d. for 5 days.

CONCLUSION

I believe that LRIs are underutilized for correcting residual astigmatism after the implantation of presbyopia- correcting IOLs. Ophthalmologists who successfully transition from cataract to refractive IOL surgery do so, because they pay attention to the details that improve their patients' visual outcomes. For many of these surgeons, this means learning to perform LRIs. ■

This article originally appeared in the February 2008 issue of CRSToday.

1. Nichamin LD. Nomogram for limbal relaxing incisions. *J Cataract Refract Surg.* 2006;32:1048.
2. Wang L, Misra M, Koch DD. Peripheral corneal relaxing incisions combined with cataract surgery. *J Cataract Refract Surg.* 2003;29:712-722.
3. Gills JP. Treating astigmatism at the time of cataract surgery. *Curr Opinion Ophthalmol.* 2002;13:2-6.

CHAPTER 143

The Shortcomings of LRIs

JOHN F. DOANE, MD

Interest in limbal relaxing incisions (LRIs) is increasing, as more surgeons start implanting presbyopia-correcting IOLs. The reduction of corneal astigmatism to 0.50 D or less is felt by most surgeons to be a necessity for patients to achieve acceptable UCVA with either accommodating or multifocal IOLs. From a surgical standpoint, LRIs compete with laser vision correction for addressing corneal astigmatism. The "red tape" associated with laser vision correction can be a tremendous hassle for the IOL surgeon who does not perform laser procedures. This form of correction is expensive and requires a second surgical setting. LRIs, however, are inadequate in certain instances.

IRRATIONAL EXUBERANCE

As with RK, surgeons can push the use of LRIs too far (Figure 1). Although some ophthalmologists assert that these incisions can correct up to 4.00 D of astigmatism or even higher when

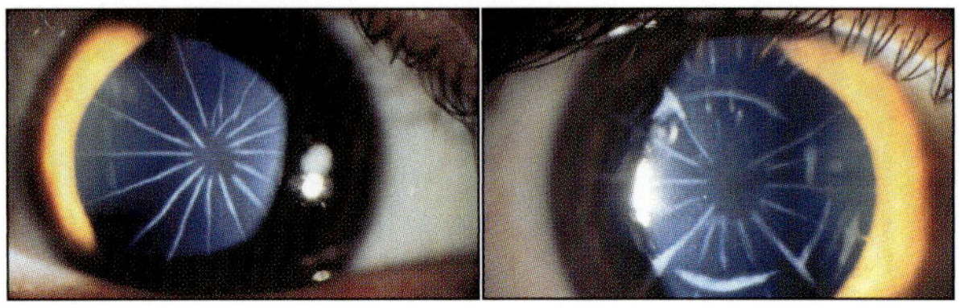

Figure 1. The surgeon pushed the limits of LRIs in these two eyes to their detriment. Most ophthalmologists believe that LRIs can treat 3.00 D of corneal astigmatism at most.

combined with more central (7- to 8-mm optical zone) astigmatic keratotomy, most surgeons feel 2.50 to 3.00 D is the upper limit of correction for LRIs. PRK or LASIK is probably more predictable for treating higher amounts of corneal astigmatism.

MISPLACEMENT OF THE LRI'S AXIAL MERIDIAN

If a surgeon loses the proper meridional alignment under the operating microscope, very complex astigmatic refractions may occur such as nonorthogonal astigmatism. A more typical error is when a surgeon performs the astigmatic correction 90° away from where it should be placed, which will usually double the amount of astigmatism in the original axis.

OVER- AND UNDERCORRECTIONS

With LRIs, a reasonable goal is to reduce the corneal cylinder to 0.50 D or less. In my opinion, it is probably better to under- versus overcorrect an astigmatic error. The causes of overcorrection include incisions that are too deep, too central, or too long. The causes of undercorrection include incisions that are too shallow, too short, or, more commonly, too peripheral to have an effect. *Undercorrections* are defined as residual astigmatism magnitude in the original meridian, and *overcorrections* typically are defined as residual astigmatism 90° away from the original merdian. With a flipped astigmatic axis, it is advisable not to chase one's tail by performing LRIs in the new meridian (Figure 1). I recommend that surgeons wait for the refraction to stabilize and then reduce the astigmatism with excimer laser ablation.

HOW LRIS WORK

The mechanism of action for LRIs is to increase the arc length in the steep or short axis of the cornea.

In my experience, the steep meridian of the astigmatism usually determines the success of the LRI procedure. Treating with-the-rule astigmatism (steep vertical meridian) is more predictable and stable than against-the-rule astigmatism (steepest horizontal meridian), in which the LRIs tend to gape for a much longer period than those oriented across the vertical meridian of the cornea. In my experience, postoperative dry eye symptoms are more common with against-the-rule versus with-the-rule LRIs of the same length. This finding is likely analogous to severing the horizontal nerve plexi with a superior hinge versus only severing one horizontal plexus for a nasal hinge in LASIK.

There are a few nuances regarding patients requiring LRIs that are worth reviewing. I advise surgeons to be cautious with the hyperopic patient who needs against-the-rule LRIs. The placement of the main cataract entry wound superiorly in a clear corneal fashion can induce significant astigmatism, because a small corneal diameter is common in hyperopic eyes. If a hyperopic patient with a small corneal diameter presents needing an LRI to treat against-the-rule astigmatism, I recommend a scleral tunnel incision either temporally or superiorly so the entry into the anterior chamber is as peripheral as possible. The scleral tunnel incision will make the main incision as astigmatically neutral as possible. The smaller the optical zone, the greater the impact on the induction of astigmatism than a larger optical zone. Therefore, a temporal clear corneal incision will induce less astigmatism than a superior clear corneal incision, because the point of entry into the anterior chamber is farther out with a temporal approach than a superior approach. Surgeons can expect that, with a temporal clear corneal incision one will flatten the meridian about 0.50 D or conversely steepen the vertical meridian an additional 0.50 D. Due to this effect, if a patient has greater than 0.50 D of with-the-rule astigmatism preoperatively, I will perform LRIs. If the patient has 0.75 D or less of against-the-rule astigmatism preoperatively, performing a temporal clear corneal incision should correct it.

Surgeons must double-check their comparisons of the steep axis on keratometry versus topography. In addition, it can be helpful to draw a picture of where they plan to make the LRIs. This drawing should be available for viewing in the OR when the surgeon is sitting at the 12-o'clock position so that he does not lose proper anatomic orientation. He can invert the topography at the time of surgery in order to confirm the orientation is correct.

PACHYMETRY

Corneal pachymetry is an important variable. I find that a 600-µm blade works well for most LRIs. I recommend that surgeons use an adjustable blade, however, if the central cornea is thinner than 500 µm or thicker than 600 µm or if the peripheral cornea has age-related thinning.

An eye with a central corneal thickness of 650 µm and a normal endothelium probably has a peripheral cornea that is much thicker than in the average eye. In this instance, a 600-µm LRI may produce little-to-no astigmatic effect, although an adjustable-depth incision on the order of 650 µm may give a nearly perfect result. Conversely, if the cornea is normal on topography but the central pachymetry is 500 µm, a 550-µm setting on the LRI blade will likely achieve excellent results, whereas a 600-µm setting may lead to an overcorrection.

CONCLUSION

Incisional keratotomy is a learned skill. I recommend adhering to one type of system, starting conservatively, mastering the system, and then refining the technique. Most surgeons have found that LRIs are most predictable for less than 3.00 D of corneal astigmatism, with success achieved more often with with-the-rule, oblique, and then against-the-rule astigmatism. I advise the enhancement of LRIs, if needed, with an excimer laser. Finally, the basic goal of an LRI (for the patient, surgical staff, and surgeon) is to leave the patient with 0.50 D or less of astigmatism. It is best to undercorrect the patient's vision rather than flip the axis. ■

This article originally appeared in the February 2008 issue of CRSToday.

CHAPTER 144

Clinical Pearls for Success With the AcrySof Toric IOL

ROBERT J. CIONNI, MD

For years, we surgeons have relied on astigmatic keratotomy or limbal relaxing incisions (LRIs) to reduce corneal astigmatism at the time of cataract surgery. With the advent of the single-piece acrylic toric IOL, we now have an option that is more predictable and stable. The FDA study for the AcrySof Toric IOL (Alcon Laboratories, Inc., Fort Worth, TX) demonstrated that 97% of patients who had at least 1.00 D of astigmatism preoperatively no longer wore glasses for tasks at distance after the lens' bilateral implantation.[1] Based on my own clinical experience, these IOLs satisfy patients more than ignoring their preoperative astigmatism or attempting to correct it with LRIs. The AcrySof Toric IOL's accuracy and its ease of use make it a good choice for those surgeons who are reluctant to perform LRIs at the time of cataract surgery. Additionally, ophthalmologists who have yet to enter the refractive IOL market may agree that the high degree of patients' satisfaction with these IOLs makes them an ideal introductory technology. The following pearls offer readers guidance on adding the AcrySof Toric IOL to their surgical armamentarium.

PATIENT SELECTION

Almost any patient who has 1.00 D or more of regular corneal astigmatism and who wishes to be less dependent on glasses is a good candidate for a toric IOL. Of course, the surgeon must consider the refractive state of the patient's fellow eye. Even individuals with more than 3.00 D of cylinder will appreciate the reduction in astigmatism that these IOLs can offer.

PREOPERATIVE EDUCATION

I strongly recommend providing patients who receive a cataract evaluation or re-evaluation with a pamphlet describing what astigmatism is and what IOL options are available. When patients discover that they can eliminate their distance glasses with these IOLs, they are eager to find out whether or not they are candidates for this option. Before I began using such a pamphlet, I would spend an inordinate amount of time explaining astigmatism to patients. Now, I simply say that, for the best quality of vision and the greatest chance of limiting their need for glasses after surgery, the AcrySof Toric IOL is their best option.

PREOPERATIVE TESTING

I rely on manual keratometry (K) readings for my toric IOL calculations. One must be certain, however, that the testing is accurate and reliable. I always confirm the manual K readings with those from the IOLMaster (Carl Zeiss Meditec, Inc., Dublin, CA) and corneal topography. Additionally, I like to see that these values make sense compared with the patient's refraction and past glasses prescriptions. If they do not match, I look for a reason why such as dry eye or irregular astigmatism. The reason for the difference may be lenticular astigmatism, but this is not always the case. Occasionally, the offsetting cylinder is not in the lens but somewhere else in the visual system. In these instances, placing a toric IOL may actually make the astigmatism worse. If the numbers do not make sense, I caution the patient that implanting a toric IOL may not produce the desired result, and we may then make a joint decision to forego the technology.

PREOPERATIVE CALCULATIONS

After determining the desired spherical power using a new-generation formula such as the Holladay II, it is time to figure out the toric power and the IOL's axial orientation to achieve the desired astigmatic result. The AcrySof Toric IOL Calculator is available at http://www.acrysoftoriccalculator.com. The surgeon enters data including K readings, IOL power, intended axis for the cataract incision, and the estimated effect of his cataract incision. For instance, my 2.2-mm temporal incision induces approximately 0.25 D of astigmatism 90° from where I make it. The calculator determines which toric power to use and the best axis for the lens' orientation. The printout includes a colored diagram of the eye showing the incision and the IOL's axis. I strongly recommend hanging the AcrySof Toric IOL Calculator printout in the OR so that it accords with the surgeon's view. I find it helps me to remain oriented during the IOL's implantation.

SURGERY

Prior to surgery, I mark the patient's eye while he is upright to identify the horizontal and vertical meridians. If this step is performed while the patient is lying down on the stretcher, the marks could be off by up to 30° due to cyclotorsion that can occur while the patient is in a supine position. This step can be performed freehand with a marking pen or one of the commercially available premarkers.

Next, I use an axis marker to stain the incisional axis and the intended axis for the IOL's orientation. Of the several instruments now available, I have found the Mastel marker (Mastel Precision Inc., Rapid City, SD) the easiest to use and the most accurate for aligning the marks through the center of the corneal apex.

Surgery is routine up until the IOL's implantation, which requires a little consideration. After injecting the lens into the capsular bag, the surgeon rotates it clockwise until the astigmatic markings on the optic are about 10° shy of the final intended axis. The goal here is not to allow the IOL to rotate past the end-point axis during removal of the viscoelastic. After evacuating the viscoelastic, the surgeon rotates the implant the last few degrees with the I/A tip or with a second instrument while irrigating with the I/A tip. Alternatively, one can perform the final rotation with an irrigating cannula through the sideport incision.

CONCLUSION

The AcrySof Toric IOL provides patients with a high chance of decreased dependence on spectacles. Its ease of use, predictability, and stability make it ideal for astigmatic correction during cataract surgery. As patients' satisfaction is almost certain with this IOL, it is a great point of entry into the premium IOL market for those surgeons who have yet to take the plunge. ■

This article originally appeared in the February 2008 issue of CRSToday.

1. AcrySof Toric Posterior Chamber IOL – P900014/S015. Available at http://www.fda.gov/cdrh/pdf/p930014s015.html. Accessed January 28, 2008.

CHAPTER 145

The Surgically Induced Astigmatism Calculator

WARREN E. HILL, MD

Since the introduction of phacoemulsification, improvements in the safety and predictability of cataract surgery combined with an astonishing array of technical advances, have raised the expectations of both patients and surgeons alike. A focus on meeting the individual refractive goal for each patient has become the norm while the occasional refractive surprise of only a few years ago has become unacceptable.

As a result, cataract surgeons are now also refractive surgeons, and they must constantly work to achieve the best possible outcome for each patient. Eliminating, or at least reducing, corneal astigmatism is particularly important with patients receiving premium IOLs. To manage corneal astigmatism with the greatest degree of accuracy and predictability, surgeons must understand the impact of the cataract incision. The Surgically Induced Astigmatism Calculator was developed to give surgeons a useful tool to better understand and individually determine this important value.

NEED

The Surgically Induced Astigmatism Calculator uses vector analysis to calculate the change in corneal astigmatism resulting from the cataract procedure. The calculator allows surgeons to generate several different types of reports that summarize individual case information by the type, size, and location of the corneal incision. Like all of the tools on my Web site, the calculater made available to the ophthalmic community free of charge.

Although temporal clear corneal incisions induce less astigmatism than those of similar size placed elsewhere on the eye, no incision is truly astigmatically neutral. The cataract incision's vector (having both a magnitude and a direction) invariably changes the vector of the preoperative corneal astigmatism, depending on the incision's location, size, and architecture. The two are added together to create a new vector, representing the postoperative corneal astigmatism. If this second influencing vector (the cataract incision) is not taken into account, the resulting change in both the axis and the magnitude of the postoperative astigmatism will typically result in an undercorrection of the corneal astigmatism by a toric IOL.

It is helpful to keep in mind that the astigmatism induced by the cataract incision can vary widely among surgeons based on factors such as the incision's location, size, and architecture; whether the ophthalmologist is right- or left-handed; and any stretching of the incision during the insertion of the IOL. The Surgically Induced Astigmatism Calculator accounts for these factors.

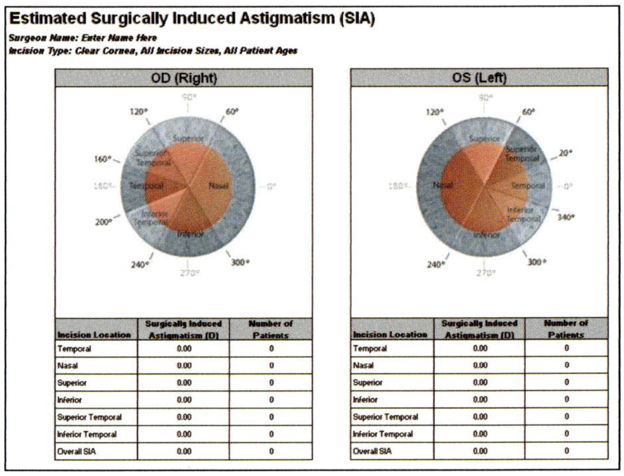

Figure 1. The Surgically Induced Astigmatism Calculator uses vector analysis to determine the amount of surgically induced astigmatism created during the cataract procedure. Surgeons can generate reports that sort their surgical data by the incision's type, size, and location.

Once surgeons know a baseline amount of astigmatism normally induced by their incision, they can use it to manage their patients' postoperative corneal astigmatism more effectively. Surgeons can change the incision's size and location relative to the steep meridian in order to achieve different effects. They can also plan to use adjunctive astigmatic treatment when the amount of preoperative astigmatism is too great to be sufficiently reduced by the cataract incision alone.

HOW TO USE THE SURGICALLY INDUCED ASTIGMATISM CALCULATOR

Surgeons can download the Surgically Induced Astigmatism Calculator free of charge from the physician download area at my Web site at http://www.doctor-hill.com in a Microsoft Excel format (Microsoft Office 2000 [Microsoft Corp., Redmond, WA] or later for personal computers and Office 2001 [Microsoft Corp.] or in the future for Macs [Apple Computer, Inc., Cupertino, CA]) (Figure 1).

The user enters the following information for sequential cataract surgery cases:

- Date of the surgery;
- Chart or case number;

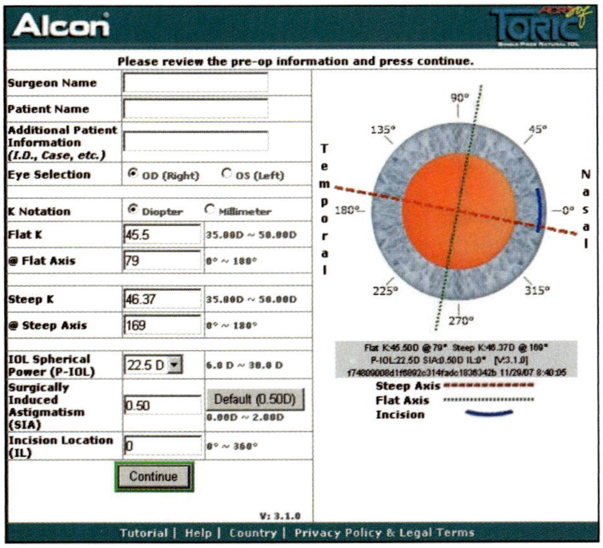

Figure 2. Surgeons implanting the AcrySof Toric IOL can use the Surgically Induced Astigmatism Calculator to generate a personalized value for surgically induced astigmatism. That value can replace the 0.50 D default value used with the AcrySof Toric IOL calculator. The latter calculator, pictured here, can then determine with more precision the most effective toric IOL power and axis of implantation.

- Patient's date of birth;
- Operative eye (OD/OS);
- Whether or not the patient has had previous corneal surgery;
- The incision's location, description, size, and type;
- Preoperative steep keratometry (K) reading, flat K, steep meridian, and flat meridian; and
- Postoperative steep K, flat K, steep meridian, and flat meridian.

A pull-down menu facilitates certain data entry. Based on the operative eye and the location of the incision, the calculator will determine if the incision was temporal, nasal, superior, or inferior, and this cell will be automatically filled.

After surgeons enters a minimum of 10 cases, they can click *create report* to obtain the magnitude (in diopters) of their surgically induced astigmatism. The results are sorted by the incision's type, size, and location. As desired by the operator, the data can be further sorted by the patient's age.

When preparing to use the calculator, surgeons should keep the following points in mind. Surgeons should make the location of the incision and its architecture as consistent as possible. They should obtain postoperative K values at the last postoperative visit or whenever they seem stable. Surgeons should use the same instrument for all preoperative and postoperative corneal power measurements. We as surgeon should take care not to mistakenly flip the pre- and postoperative meridians. Postoperatively, the axis for the steep preoperative principal meridian should shift by between 5° and 20°. A postoperative change in the power of the steep axis of the cornea should not be greater than 1.00 D unless the cataract incision is very large. Double-check K values that are very steep or very flat. The axes of the steep and flat meridians should be 90° apart. If not, they should differ by no more than ±5° from a 90° separation. Values outside this range may indicate irregular astigmatism and should be evaluated by topography. Additional instructions and tips are included with the calculator.

Surgeons implanting the AcrySof Toric IOL (Alcon Laboratories, Inc., Fort Worth, TX) can enter their calculated, individualized value for surgically induced astigmatism generated by the Surgically Induced Astigmatism Calculator into the AcrySof Toric IOL calculator at http://www.acrysoftoriccalculator.com to determine the most effective toric IOL power and the final axis of implantation as calculated by vector analysis (Figure 2). The AcrySof Toric IOL calculator also determines the amount of anticipated residual refractive astigmatism so the surgeon can decide whether or not it would be useful to adjust the location of the cataract incision to optimize this correction.

SUBMIT YOUR DATA

I ask all surgeons who use the Surgically Induced Astigmatism Calculator to contribute their information to a HIPAA-compliant database for further analysis. The goal of this effort is to study the magnitude of surgically induced astigmatism as a function of the incision's location, type, architecture, and size. To date, little has been published in this area.

Surgeons may send their data to me once they enter a minimum of 20 cases into the Surgically Induced Astigmatism Calculator, but 50 to 100 cases are preferable. Instructions for submitting data are included with the download of the Surgically Induced Astigmatism Calculator.

CONCLUSION

By using the new Surgically Induced Astigmatism Calculator, cataract surgeons can now more precisely manage their patients' corneal astigmatism and improve their outcomes by knowing how much their cataract incision affects preexisting corneal astigmatism. A value for surgically induced astigmatism can be generated using as few as 10 cases, but this value will be more meaningful using data from 50 to 100 cases. ■

This article originally appeared in the February 2008 issue of CRSToday.

CHAPTER 146

The STAAR Toric IOL

STEPHEN BYLSMA, MD

In the aphakic state, the cornea alone determines the magnitude and axis of refractive astigmatism. In today's efforts to achieve pseudophakic emmetropia, it is critical to reduce higher magnitudes of natural corneal astigmatism.[1] The alternative of correcting astigmatism with an IOL has distinct advantages compared with treatments directed at corneal tissue involving incisions[2-16] or laser ablation.[17-20] Implanting a toric IOL is a single-step, reliable, small-incision approach with a result that is independent of the postoperative corneal healing response. Toric IOLs can also correct higher degrees of cylinder than can corneal procedures.[21-24]

The Acrysof Toric IOL (Alcon Laboratories, Inc., Fort Worth, TX) has a single-piece design similar to that of the STAAR Toric IOL (STAAR Surgical Company, Monrovia, CA), but the former features compressible haptics made of acrylic rather than silicone. The Acrysof Toric IOL's recent approval by the FDA makes it worthwhile to review the results with the STAAR Toric IOL, the lens that has been the standard of care.

A HISTORICAL PERSPECTIVE

Investigations in the early 1990s used spherical (nontoric) IOLs to evaluate the rotational stability of various IOL designs.[22,25,26] Three-piece lenses using polypropylene haptics showed significant counterclockwise rotation.[22] Later studies demonstrated similarly frequent rotation within 2 weeks of implantation with loop- and plate-haptic designs but also showed that only the plate-haptic IOL was stable long term.[27] The latter design also demonstrated significantly less decentration when compared to a three-piece lens.[28]

The first study of a toric IOL (STAAR 4203T; STAAR Surgical Company) in the United States showed this plate-haptic design to undergo rotations of more than 30° in fewer than 5% of cases.[29] Results from the phase 1 FDA trial showed that, in 95% of cases, the toric IOL was within 30° of the intended axis, with a mean achieved reduction in refractive cylinder of 1.25 D.[30]

These early data indicated that, although rotations occasionally occurred in the early postoperative period, the plate-haptic design remained stable in the long term. The STAAR Toric IOL's AA4203-TF model (10.8-mm length) underwent a full FDA clinical trial that led to its approval in 1998. The longer (11.2-mm) AA4203-TL model was later created for use in larger myopic eyes.

THE STAAR TORIC IOL'S DESIGN

The foldable STAAR Toric lens is a plate-haptic PCIOL (Figure 1) made of first-generation silicone and is implanted through a 3-mm incision. The TF model is available in spherical equivalent powers of 21.50 to 28.50 D versus 9.50 to 23.50 D for the TL model. The TL model's lower power range increases its stability against off-axis rotation in the large capsules of myopic eyes. Both versions of the lens have two 1.5-mm fenestration holes in the haptics to encourage capsular fibrosis, which promotes long-term rotational stability of the IOL and prevents its posterior displacement after an Nd:YAG capsulotomy.

Manufactured as a plus-cylinder lens, the STAAR Toric IOL features two hash marks at the peripheral optic junction that designate the axis of the toric power and should be aligned along the steep keratometric axis. The anterior-posterior orientation of this lens is important. It is packaged with the toric power facing upward, and the manufacturer's labeling calls for the anterior, toric surface to be implanted facing the anterior capsule. Alternatively, the STAAR Toric IOL may be implanted in a reverse configuration to promote rotational stability.[31,32]

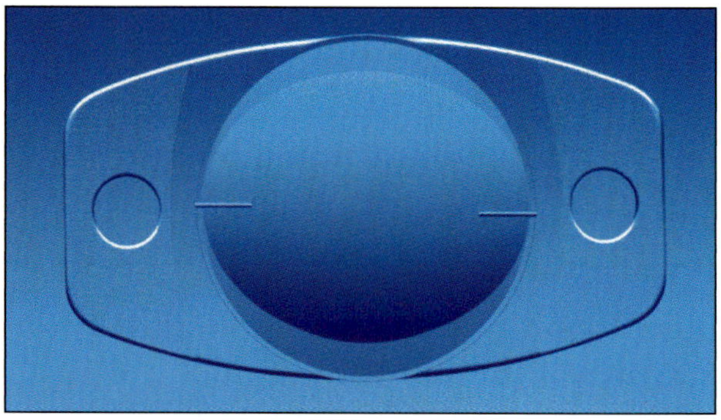

Figure 1. The STAAR Toric IOL.

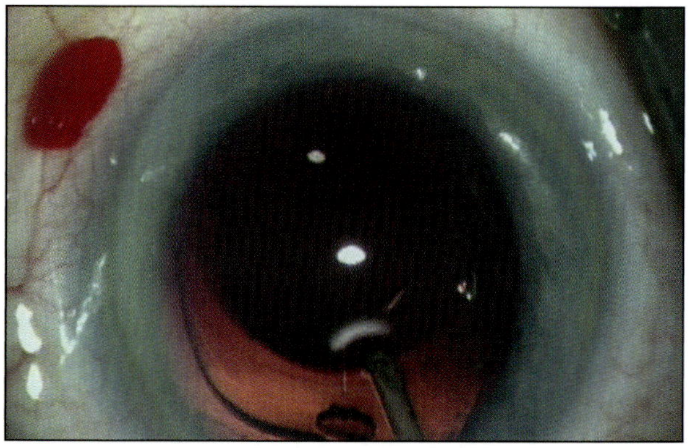

Figure 2. The author places the trailing haptic.

MODERN-DAY CLINICAL RESULTS

The TF and TL models both predictably improve UCVA, although the incidence of early off-axis rotation with them varies.[30-39] In sum, the studies show that the STAAR Toric IOL is more effective than limbal relaxing incisions (LRIs)[33,34] and that it is reliable in reducing postoperative refractive astigmatism, is consistent in producing a UCVA of 20/40 or better, has a low incidence of early positional problems, and shows long-term stability.[34-38] The longer TL model is more stable than the TF model.[39] Other clinical studies have used the STAAR Toric IOL to correct excessive astigmatism by combining the lens with LRIs or using multiple STAAR Toric IOLs in a piggyback fashion.[40-42]

As a group, these studies clearly demonstrate that the STAAR Toric IOL produces a predictable and beneficial clinical reduction in preoperative refractive cylinder but also that it has a tendency toward occasional, early, off-axis rotation, the incidence and severity of which vary. The differences in these studies are likely due to many factors, including (1) the availability of only the shorter TF model in early studies, (2) variability between surgeons in their removal of viscoelastic posterior to the IOL, (3) torsional rotations that may occur when the patient is recumbent versus upright or due to unintentional misalignments, (4) implantation on the improper axis, (5) large capsules due to myopia, old age, or mature, brunescent cataracts, or (6) rubbing of the eye by the patient during the early postoperative period.

Recent advances have decreased the frequency of early misalignment with the STAAR Toric IOL. Foremost is the availability of the longer TL model for use in myopic eyes.[39] Another is the reversed positioning in which the optic's toric surface faces the posterior rather than the anterior capsule.[31,32] This implantation technique improves UCVA and increases the refractive effect, despite a theoretical 8% reduction of toric power that occurs when the toric surface resides closer to the nodal point. The more precise rotational alignment was more important than the mild theoretical reduction of toric power. The IOL's reverse positioning is now recommended and widely practiced in the US.

Fortunately, the infrequent misalignments can be fully corrected. Because these rotations occur in the early postoperative period, before capsular fibrosis or contraction has begun, repositioning the implant will restore its beneficial effect. Other IOL designs that rotate months after capsular fibrosis and contraction are very difficult to reposition. The optimal time for repositioning the STAAR Toric IOL is 2 weeks postoperatively. If manipulated earlier, the problem may recur. In contrast, later repositioning is difficult due to capsular fibrosis.

PERIOPERATIVE MANAGEMENT

Surgeons may use IOL formulae and nomograms as for any other IOL to determine which spherical equivalent power of the STAAR Toric lens to implant. They should then choose the +2.00 or +3.50 D version depending on the degree of keratometric cylinder. The manufacturer states that the +2.00 D IOL should be used in eyes with 1.40 to 2.30 D of corneal astigmatism and that the +3.50 lens is indicated for corneal astigmatism greater than 2.30D. In my experience, it is best to choose the toric power based on the modified, "reverse" nomogram. For keratometric asymmetry of 1.20 to 2.10 D, I use the +2.00 D toric power in the reverse position. For corneal astigmatism above 2.20 D, I use the +3.50 D IOL in the reverse position. Eyes with less than 1.20 D of corneal cylinder should not receive the STAAR Toric IOL, because a flip in the refractive astigmatic axis may result.

Like any plus-cylinder lens, the STAAR Toric IOL should be oriented to neutralize the keratometric astigmatism. The surgeon determines the intended axis of implantation preoperatively based on keratometric data. Topography and other imaging can help verify that the astigmatism is regular (irregular corneal astigmatism will not be appropriately corrected by the STAAR Toric IOL) and determine the steep corneal axis. Alternatively, the intended axis for implantation may be identified intraoperatively by qualitative keratometry.

As with all plate-haptic IOLs, the STAAR Toric lens should only be implanted with an intact capsule and a complete, continuous curvilinear capsulorhexis. Using the current cartridge, surgeons may deliver the IOL through a 3-mm clear corneal incision. The cartridge's tip does not need to enter entirely into the anterior chamber, but it does need to pass fully through the corneal incision. Surgeons must retract the plunger several times as the IOL is pushed down the cartridge to ensure no overriding of the plunger that could tear the trailing haptic. The leading haptic is inserted into a capsule filled with viscoelastic, and the trailing haptic is placed with a second instrument, as with other plate-haptic IOLs (Figure 2).

Surgeons may use the I/A tip, cystotome, or another second instrument to orient the IOL to the desired axis. The careful removal of viscoelastic from between the posterior capsule and the lens is important to help avert the early rotation of the IOL. This step occurs prior to the lens' final orientation along the desired axis. Some surgeons prefer to leave the eye slightly soft to encourage early contact between the capsule and the lens.

Although some eyes may require an Nd:YAG capsulotomy for posterior capsular opacification, there have been no reports of subsequent off-axis deviation of the IOL.

CONCLUSION

Although many cataract and refractive surgeons have gladly relied on the STAAR Toric IOL, others have avoided the technology for reasons such as its construction from first-generation silicone, its plate-haptic design, concerns about early off-axis rotations, and significant economic benefits from LRIs. With the availability of the Acrysof Toric IOL, US surgeons have a choice of toric IOLs for the first time. As our experience accumulates with the new lens, we may evaluate any improvements it offers in light of the extensive data and experience with the STAAR Toric IOL. Particular areas meriting comparison include ease of implantation, the frequency of early and late off-axis deviations, the facility of correcting such problems if they do occur, and long-term refractive stability. ■

This article originally appeared in the May 2006 issue of CRSToday.

1. Fine IH, Hoffman RS. Refractive aspects of cataract surgery. *Curr Opin Ophthalmol.* 1996;7:21-25.
2. Grabow HB. Intraocular correction of refractive errors. In: Kershner RM, ed. *Refractive Keratotomy for Cataract Surgery and the Correction of Astigmatism.* Thorofare, NJ: Slack, Inc.; 1994: 79-115.
3. Maloney WF, Sanders DR, Pearcy DE. Astigmatic keratotomy to correct preexisting astigmatism in cataract patients. *J Cataract Refract Surg.* 1990;16:297-304.
4. Osher RH. Transverse astigmatic keratotomy combined with cataract surgery. In: Thompson K, Waring G, eds. *Contemporary Refractive Surgery—Ophthalmology Clinics of North America.* Philadelphia: W.B. Saunders; 1992: 717-725.
5. Price FW, Grene RB, Marks RG, et al. Astigmatism reduction clinical trial: a multicenter prospective evaluation of the predictability of arcuate keratotomy. *Arch Ophthalmol.* 1995;113:277-282.
6. Kershner RM. Keratolenticuloplasty: arcuate keratotomy for cataract surgery and astigmatism. *J Cataract Refract Surg.* 1995;21:274-277.
7. Buzard KA, Laranjeira E, Fundingsland BR. Clinical results of arcuate incisions to correct astigmatism. *J Cataract Refract Surg.* 1996;22:436-440.
8. Troutman RC, Swinger C. Relaxing incision for control of postoperative astigmatism following keratoplasty. *Ophthalmology.* 1980;11:117-120.
9. Gills JP, Fenzl RE. Analysis of astigmatic keratotomy with a 5.0mm optical clear zone. *Am J Ophthalmol.* 1996;121:731-732.
10. Budak K, Friedman NJ, Kock DD. Limbal relaxing incisions with cataract surgery. *J Cataract Refract Surg.* 1998;24:503-508.
11. Muller-Jensen K, Fischer P, Siepe U. Limbal relaxing incisions to correct astigmatism in clear corneal cataract surgery. *J Refract Surg.* 1999;15:586-589.
12. Nichamin LD, Wallace RB. Reducing astigmatism. In: Wallace R, ed. *Refractive Cataract Surgery and Multifocal IOLs.* Thorofare, NJ: Slack, Inc.; 2001: 167-172.
13. Budak K, Yilmaz G, Aslan BS, Duman S. Limbal relaxing incisions in congenital astigmatism: 6 month follow-up. *J Cataract Refract Surg.* 2001;27:715-719.
14. Shepherd JR. Correction of preexisting astigmatism at the time of small incision cataract surgery. *J Cataract Refract Surg.* 1989;15:55-57.
15. Lever J, Dahan E. Opposite clear corneal incisions to correct preexisting astigmatism in cataract surgery. *J Cataract Refract Surg.* 2000;26:803-805.
16. Kohnen T, Koch DD. Methods to control astigmatism in cataract surgery. *Curr Opin Ophthalmol.* 1996;7:75-80.
17. Ayala M, Perez-Santonja JJ, Artola A, et al. Laser in situ keratomileusis to correct residual myopia after cataract surgery. *J Refract Surg.* 2001;17:12-16.
18. Nichamin LD. Bioptics for the pseudophakic patient. In: Gills JP, ed. *A Complete Guide to Astigmatism Management.* Thorofare, NJ: Slack, Inc.; 2003: 37-39.
19. McDonnell PJ, Moreira H, Garbus J, et al. Photorefractive keratectomy to create toric ablations for correction of astigmatism. *Arch Ophthalmol.* 1991;109:710-713.
20. Artola A, Ayala M, Claramonte P, et al. Photorefractive keratectomy for residual myopia after cataract surgery. *J Cataract Refract Surg.* 1999;25:1456-1460.
21. Frohn A, Dick HB, Thiel HJ. Implantation of a toric poly(methyl methacrylate) intraocular lens to correct high astigmatism. *J Cataract Refract Surg.* 1999;25:1675-1678.
22. Shimizu K, Misawa A, Suzuki Y. Toric intraocular lenses: correcting astigmatism while controlling axis shift. *J Cataract Refract Surg.* 1994;20:523-526.
23. Schwartz DM, Jethmalani JM, Sandstedt CA, et al. Post implantation adjustable intraocular lenses. *Ophthalmol Clin North Am.* 2001;14:339-345.
24. Tehrani M, Stoffelns B, Dick B. Implantation of a custom intraocular lens with a 30-diopter torus for the correction of high astigmatism after penetrating keratoplasty. *J Cataract*

Refract Surg. 2003;29:2444-2447.
25. Sanders DR, Grabow HB, Shepherd J. The toric IOL. In: Grills JP, Martin RG, Sanders DR, eds. *Sutureless Cataract Surgery.* Thorofare, NJ: Slack, Inc.; 1992: 183-197.
26. Grabow HB, Martin RG. STAAR AA-4203 one-piece plate-haptic silicone IOL. In: Martin RG, Gills JP, Sanders DR, eds. *Foldable Intraocular Lens.* Thorofare, NJ: Slack, Inc.; 1993: 237-250.
27. Patel CK, Ormonde S, Rosen PH, Bron AJ. Postoperative intraocular lens rotation: a randomized comparison of plate and loop haptic implants. *Ophthalmology.* 1999;106:2190-2195; discussion: 2196.
28. Hwang IP, Clinch TE, Moshifar M, et al. Decentration of 3 piece versus plate-haptic silicone intraocular lenses. *J Cataract Refract Surg.* 1998;24:1505-1508.
29. Grabow HB. Early results with foldable toric IOL implantation. *Eur J Implant Refract Surg.* 1994;6:177-178.
30. Grabow HB. Toric intraocular lens report. *Ann Ophthalmol Glauc.* 1997;29:161-163.
31. Bylsma S. Toric intraocular lenses. In: Roy FH, Arzabe CW, eds. *Master Techniques in Cataract and Refractive Surgery.* Thorofare, NJ: Slack, Inc.; 2004: 165-170.
32. Bylsma S. STAAR Toric IOL. In: Fine IH, Packer M, Hoffman RS, eds. *Refractive Lens Surgery.* New York: Springer; 2005: 59-69.
33. Sun XY, Vicary D, Montgomery P, Griffiths M, Toric intraocular lenses for correcting astigmatism in 130 eyes. *Ophthalmology.* 2000;107:1776-1781.
34. Kershner RM. Toric intraocular lenses for correcting astigmatism in 130 eyes (discussion). *Ophthalmology.* 2000;107:1781-1782.
35. Rushwurm I, Scholz U, Zehetmayer M, et al. Astigmatism correction with a foldable toric intraocular lens in cataract patients. *J Cataract Refract Surg.* 2000;26:1022-1027.
36. Leyland M, Zinicola E, Bloom P, Lee N. Prospective evaluation of a plate haptic toric intraocular lens. *Eye.* 2001;15(Pt 2):202-205.
37. Nguyen TM, Miller KM. Digital overlay technique for documenting toric intraocular lens axis orientation. *J Cataract Refract Surg.* 2000;26:1496-1504.
38. Till JS, Yoder PR, Wilcox TK, et al. Toric intraocular lens implantation: 100 consecutive cases. *J Cataract Refract Surg.* 2002;28:295-301.
39. Chang DF. Early rotational stability of the longer Staar toric intraocular lens: fifty consecutive cases. *J Cataract Refract Surg.* 2003;29:935-940.
40. Gills J, Van der Karr M, Cherchio M. Combined toric intraocular lens implantation and relaxing incisions to reduce high preexisting astigmatism. *J Cataract Refract Surg.* 2002;28:1585-1588.
41. Gills JP. Sutured piggyback toric intraocular lenses to correct high astigmatism. *J Cataract Refract Surg.* 2003;29:402-404.
42. Gills JP, Van Der Karr MA. Correcting high astigmatism with piggy back toric intraocular lens implantation. *J Cataract Refract Surg.* 2002;28:547-549.

CHAPTER 147

Comparing the STAAR and AcrySof Toric IOLs

DAVID F. CHANG, MD

The STAAR Toric IOL (STAAR Surgical Company, Monrovia, CA) was approved by the FDA in November 1998, and it was the only toric IOL on the US market until recently. The 10.8-mm long TF model lens was the design studied in the FDA clinical trials. In an effort to decrease malrotation of the lens, the company released the longer 11.2-mm TL model in 1999.

Early postoperative rotation of the smaller TF IOL was a significant problem. In the FDA-monitored clinical study, 24% of the IOLs ended up more than 10° off axis (12% were more than 20° off, 8% were more than 30° off, and 5% were more than 45° off axis). Subsequently, a number of clinical studies of the STAAR toric IOL were published confirming a significant incidence of rotation greater than 10° to 15° postoperatively with the TF model[1-4] (Table 1).

I undertook my own study of the rotational stability of the longer TL model when it became available.[5] My evaluation of 90 consecutive toric IOL implantations included 80 TL IOLs and 10 TF IOLs (the TL model is not available in powers greater than 24.00 D). Of the TL toric implants, 73% were within 5°, 89% were within 10°, and 96% were within 15° of the targeted axis. My repositioning rate was 2.5% (two of 80) with the TL IOL and 3.3% overall (one of 10 TF IOLs was repositioned). Until my study, all of the published articles looking at the STAAR Toric IOL had reported on the only available model at the time, the TF. With respect to the TL model, the published literature on rotational stability was therefore misleading.

The recently approved AcrySof Toric IOL (Alcon Laboratories, Inc., Fort Worth, TX) has demonstrated excellent rotational stability in the FDA-monitored clinical study with an average of less than 4° postoperative rotation. The rotational stability of my first 20 AcrySof Toric IOLs confirms these results at 1-month minimum follow-up; 85% of the IOLs were within 5° of the targeted axis, and 100% were within 10° of the targeted axis.

The widespread adoption of the STAAR Toric IOL was hampered by surgeons' misperception that the TL model also exhibited poor rotational stability and their general reluctance to use silicone plate haptic lenses. Having a single-piece hydrophobic acrylic toric IOL available is therefore a welcome option. ■

TABLE 1. EARLY POSTOPERATIVE ROTATION IN STUDIES OF THE STAAR TORIC TF IOL

Study	Reported Rotation*
FDA clinical trial	12% > 20° (1%)
Sun et al[1]	25% > 20° (1%)
Ruhswurm et al[2]	19% > 10° (11%)
Leyland et al[3]	18% > 30° (1%)
Till et al[4]	14% > 15° [37% TL]† (3%)

**All of the studies shown except for that by Till et al[4] exclusively used the shorter TF model. Comparative results from Chang[5,6] using the longer TL model appear in parentheses.*
†In this study, 37% of the IOLs used were the TL model.

This article originally appeared in the May 2007 issue of CRSToday.

1. Sun XY, Vicary D, Montgomery P, Griffiths, M. Toric intraocular lenses for correcting astigmatism in 130 eyes. *Ophthalmology.* 2000;107:1776-1781; discussion:1781-1782.
2. Ruhswurm I, Scholz U, Zehetmayer M, et al. Astigmatism correction with foldable toric intraocular lens in cataract patients. *J Cataract Refract Surg.* 2000;26:1022-1027.
3. Leyland M, Zinicola P, Bloom P, Lee N. Prospective evaluation of a plate haptic toric intraocular lens. *Eye.* 2001;15:202-205.
4. Till JS, Yoder PR, Wilcox TK, Spielman JL. Toric intraocular lens implantation: 100 consecutive cases. *J Cataract Refract Surg.* 2002;28:295-301.
5. Chang DF. Early rotational stability of the longer STAAR Toric IOL—50 consecutive (TL) IOLs. *J Cataract Refract Surg.* 2003;29:935-940.
6. Chang DF. Early rotational stability of the longer STAAR Toric IOL: 70 consecutive cases. Paper presented at: The ASCRS/ASOA Symposium on Cataract, IOL and Refractive Surgery; April 14, 2003; San Francisco, CA.

CHAPTER 148

Toric IOLs Versus LRIs Versus Bioptics

KEVIN M. MILLER, MD

Every method for correcting astigmatism at the time of cataract or refractive lens exchange surgery has advantages and disadvantages. The ideal approach, if there is one, corrects all astigmatism with one procedure and does not require a secondary intervention. In most cases, limbal relaxing incisions (LRIs) or toric IOLs can correct astigmatism. Individuals who have residual cylinder after surgery or those whose cylinder is too great to correct by either of these methods alone or in combination may achieve the best result from postoperative keratorefractive surgery (bioptics).

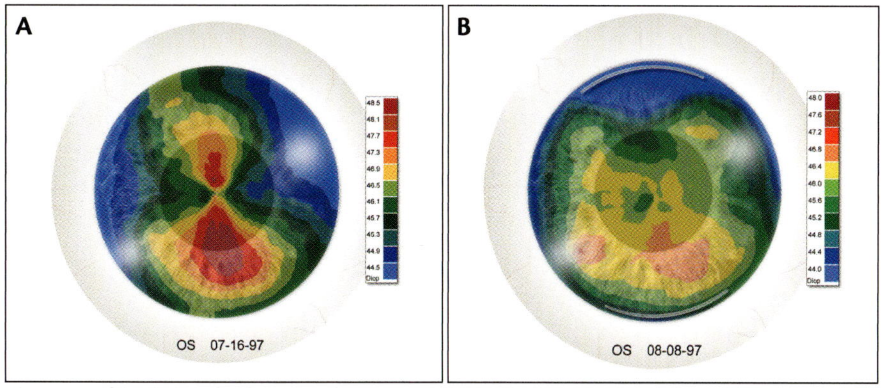

Figure 1. This patient had 2.00D of symmetric bowtie corneal astigmatism (A). Note the change in topography after the placement of paired 2–clock-hour LRIs in the steep meridian (B).

LRIS

The name of this procedure is somewhat misleading, because LRIs are usually placed on the peripheral cornea just inside the limbus, rather than on the limbus itself. The technique is easy to learn and perform, thanks in part to the availability of many nomograms, all of which produce approximately the same result.

Whereas toric IOLs are placed behind the cornea and may induce distortion, LRIs offer the advantage of correcting astigmatism at the source, the cornea. They predictably correct up to 3.00D of cylinder and will not rotate, as an IOL may.

Moreover, LRIs can correct symmetric and asymmetric bowtie corneal astigmatism (Figures 1 and 2). For example, the technique can address astigmatism that is steeper on one side of the cornea than the other as well as floppy bowties where the axis changes continuously across the entrance pupil.

On the con side, LRIs are often longer and thus less predictable than simple cataract incisions, because wound healing is more of a factor. Additionally, large LRIs may gape and be difficult to hydrate after phacoemulsification.

TORIC IOLS

Because toric lenses can be implanted through a standard phaco incision, patients recover more quickly than after LRIs, and the wound architecture may be more resilient to ocular trauma. Unlike astigmatic keratotomies, toric IOLs do not induce irregular astigmatism, and they can correct high amounts of astigmatism at the IOL plane. Currently, the highest power of toric IOL available is 3.50D (STAAR Toric IOL; STAAR Surgical Company, Monrovia, CA).

A major drawback of the STAAR Toric IOL is its tendency to rotate off axis. This problem was more common (up to 10%) in the shorter TF model and is less likely with the longer TL model.

According to unpublished clinical trials, the Acrysof Toric IOL (Alcon Laboratories, Inc., Fort Worth, TX) is rotationally stable in the eye and will only be off axis if placed so during surgery.

As mentioned earlier, correcting astigmatism with lenses at the IOL plane versus the cornea produces distortion. If the lens is not placed precisely on the axis of postoperative cylinder, the resulting astigmatism will have a new, usually oblique angle. Patients may have trouble adapting to the new refractive error, especially if they require spectacle correction. Finally, unlike LRIs, toric IOLs are not effective at correcting asymmetric bowtie corneal astigmatism.

BIOPTICS

The term *bioptics* refers to the combination of two surgical approaches to correcting astigmatism. For instance, one may perform keratorefractive surgery (LASIK, LASEK, PRK) several weeks after implanting a toric IOL for high astigmatism. This particular combination, however, is not my first choice, because most patients prefer to undergo one rather than two surgeries. LRIs or a toric lens can successfully address up to 3.00 D of cylinder. For astigmatism of up to 5.00 D, I favor the technique popularized by James Gills, MD, of Tarpon Springs, Florida. He combines the implantation of a toric IOL with the placement of LRIs. Bioptics may be the most reasonable strategy for patients who have more than 5.00 D of corneal astigmatism.

With bioptics, it is advisable to leave a residual myopic spherical equivalent refractive error, because LASIK, LASEK, and PRK are most successful for the treatment of compound myopic astigmatism rather than mixed astigmatism. Surgeons should make every attempt to maximize the cylindrical correction with a toric IOL before the subsequent excimer laser procedure.

Alcon Laboratories, Inc., plans to introduce toric IOLs with powers as great as 5.00 D soon. The availability of these new lenses should significantly reduce the need for excimer laser procedures after astigmatic cataract surgery.

MY APPROACH

I tend to be practical about correcting corneal astigmatism at the time of cataract surgery and have always treated up to 1.50 D of corneal astigmatism with LRIs. If Alcon Laboratories, Inc., successfully obtains premium pricing for the Acrysof Toric IOL and ophthalmologists are allowed to apply a refractive surcharge for the additional work associated with its implantation, then this lens may be an economically sound option for correcting low levels of astigmatism.

For up to 3.00 D of corneal astigmatism, I implant a toric IOL. I combine LRIs and toric IOLs for higher amounts of corneal astigmatism. I reserve bioptics for eyes with more than 5.00 D of astigmatism, but I plan to abandon this technique when higher-powered toric IOLs become commercially available.

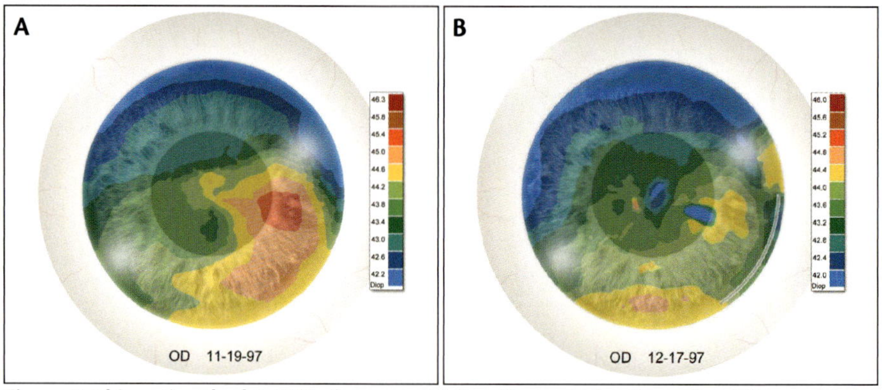

Figure 2. This patient had 1.00 D of asymmetric bowtie corneal astigmatism (A). Postoperative topography shows improvement after a single 2–clock-hour LRI was placed in the steep meridian (B).

FINAL THOUGHTS

The introduction of presbyopia-correcting IOLs radically changed the landscape of cataract surgery. Now, it is incumbent on cataract surgeons to achieve excellent postoperative refractive results. In essence, performing precise biometry and neutralizing astigmatism are paramount to satisfying patients and helping them attain independence from spectacles.

Ophthalmologists who have not given much consideration to the surgical correction of astigmatism in the past will be increasingly called upon to do so in the future. ■

This article originally appeared in the May 2006 issue of CRSToday.

CHAPTER 149

Correcting High Astigmatism During Cataract Surgery

ROBERT H. OSHER, MD; ROGER F. STEINERT, MD; LOUIS "SKIP" D. NICHAMIN, MD; AND KEVIN L. WALTZ, OD, MD

CASE PRESENTATION

A 60-year-old symptomatic patient presents with bilateral cataracts as well as 4.00 D of against-the-rule astigmatism in each eye. What would your strategy be for reducing the astigmatism in the initial eye undergoing surgery?

ROBERT H. OSHER, MD

A European surgeon who has access to high-powered toric lenses would manage this case differently. My approach, however, would be similar to that presented in a recent edition of the *Video Journal of Cataract and Refractive Surgery.*[1] After performing microcoaxial phacoemulsification through a 2.2-mm incision, which is astigmatically neutral, I would implant an AcrySof Toric lens (model T5; Alcon Laboratories, Inc., Fort Worth, TX) into the capsular bag and leave the IOL oriented as close to the steepest meridian as possible. If the placement were precise, this lens would correct 2.00 D of astigmatism in the corneal plane. I would treat the remaining 2.00 D with astigmatic keratotomy (AK).

Since 1983, I have used corneal relaxing incisions to reduce preexisting astigmatism. Although these incisions have a greater effect than limbal relaxing incisions (LRIs), the results are variable and highly dependent upon the incisions' depth and length, the size of the optical zone relative to the corneal diameter, the patient's age, and the type of astigmatism. AK is an acquired art in contrast to toric lenses, which are becoming a more precise science. Inaccuracy in identifying and marking the steepest meridian, however, remains a problem that must be improved. Nevertheless, the combined approach I described offers a satisfactory method for managing the cataract surgery patient with high astigmatism.

ROGER F. STEINERT, MD

Ophthalmologists have three effective modalities for dealing with astigmatism at cataract surgery: LRIs; toric IOLs; and LASIK/surface ablation. The disadvantages of excimer laser-based correction are its cost and the need for a separate procedure. Of the three options, however, it is the only one proven to be highly accurate.

In this case, the age of the patient and his high level of astigmatism make excimer laser refractive surgery the optimal choice based on its accuracy and optical superiority. Its added cost compared with a toric IOL is modest for most practices.

LOUIS "SKIP" D. NICHAMIN, MD

The decision whether to use corneal relaxing incisions or a toric IOL to reduce preexisting astigmatism at the time of cataract surgery is determined by the surgeon's level of comfort and experience with each modality as well as specific characteristics of a given patient. I am fortunate to have learned incisional keratotomy and astigmatic theory from pioneers such as Spencer Thornton, MD. I began correcting astigmatism at the time of cataract surgery in the late 1980s, as first described by Dr. Osher[2,3] and later by William Maloney, MD.[4] In the early 1990s, I became familiar with LRIs through my good friend David Dillman, MD, who first observed Stephen Hollis, MD, as he performed this important variation of AK. I have gradually modified Dr. Hollis' nomogram[5] and have achieved superb results with stable outcomes during the past 10 years.[6]

Using the current NAPA (*N*ichamin *a*ge- and *p*achymetry-*a*djusted) nomogram along with pachymetry-guided adjustable depth settings of the diamond blade, I can typically correct up to 2.00 to 3.00 D of astigmatism based upon the patient's age.[7]

In the presented case, the first factor in my decision would be the patient's desire for a premium multifocal or accommodating IOL versus a standard monofocal implant. If he chose a presbyopia-correcting lens, I would perform LRIs at the time of cataract/IOL surgery followed by a planned bioptics laser enhancement for the expected residual cylinder (again, LRIs are only capable of correcting up to 3.00 D of cylinder) and any remaining spherical error. If the patient were not interested in a presbyopia-correcting IOL, I would either combine LRIs with a toric lens or perform LRIs at the time of the implant surgery with the expectation of a planned bioptics enhancement. Because the toric lenses currently available in the United States only correct up to 3.00 D of astigmatism at the corneal plane, some type of combined procedure would be necessary for this particular patient. I still strongly prefer LRIs to "conventional" corneal AK based on the former's more forgiving nature, at least in my experience.

KEVIN L. WALTZ, OD, MD

The STAAR Toric IOL (STAAR Surgical Company, Monrovia, CA) combined with opposing full-thickness corneal incisions on the steep corneal axis would be the most effective and efficient way to treat 4.00 D of preexisting corneal astigmatism at the time of cataract surgery. The STAAR Toric IOL is available with 2.00 or 3.50 D of astigmatic power. The higher-powered lens with a single, on-axis incision would effectively treat the 4.00 D of corneal cylinder. Alternatively, two opposing full-thickness incisions on the steep axis of the cornea would treat approximately 2.00 D of the corneal cylinder, and the remainder could be treated with the lower-powered STAAR Toric IOL. Treating more of the corneal astigmatism would eliminate it, not just compensate for it. Varying the incision's width and distance from the visual axis would allow the surgeon to fine-tune the refractive effect. Ideally, he would use one of the incisions for the cataract's extraction and the lens' insertion, but it is not mandatory. ■

This article originally appeared in the February 2008 issue of CRSToday.

1. Osher RH. Correcting high astigmatism with combined toric lens and astigmatic keratotomy. *Video Journal of Cataract and Refractive Surgery.* 2007;23(3).
2. Osher RH. Astigmatic keratotomy: a new approach to reducing preexisting astigmatism at the time of cataract surgery. Paper presented at: Welsh Cataract Congress; 1984; Houston, TX.
3. Osher RH. Combining phacoemulsification with corneal relaxing incisions for reduction of preexisting astigmatism. Paper presented at: The Annual Meeting of the American Intraocular Implant Society; 1984; Los Angeles, CA.
4. Maloney WF. Refractive cataract replacement: a comprehensive approach to maximize refractive benefits of cataract extraction. Paper presented at: The Annual Meeting of the American Society of Cataract and Refractive Surgery; 1986; Los Angeles, CA.
5. Nichamin LD. Management of astigmatism in conjunction with lens surgery. In: Tasman W, Jaeger EA, eds. *Duane's Ophthalmology on CD-ROM.* Philadelphia, PA: Lippincott, Williams & Wilkins; 2006.
6. Nichamin LD. Changing approach to astigmatism management during phacoemulsification: peripheral arcuate astigmatic relaxing incisions. Paper presented at: The ASCRS Symposium on Cataract, IOL and Refractive Surgery; May 20, 2000; Boston, MA.
7. Nichamin LD. Astigmatism control. *Ophthalmol Clin North Am.* 2006;19:485-493.

CHAPTER 150

LASIK Bioptics

Y. RALPH CHU, MD

The evolution of cataract surgery techniques and advancements in IOLs have blurred the line between refractive and cataract surgery. Improved technologies as well as patients' higher expectations have heightened the importance of treating postoperative residual refractive error, which can be the cause of increased night vision complaints. Patients receiving presbyopia-correcting IOLs can be very sensitive to small amounts of astigmatism (≥ 0.75 D). They may experience more significant degradation in their quality of vision and be more likely to notice a decrease in their ability to read without correction than patients without residual astigmatism.

A surgical technique that can precisely treat this type of residual refractive error is essential. A planned bioptics procedure with LASIK or advanced surface ablation is an excellent way to maximize patients' outcomes.

HISTORY OF BIOPTICS

The concept of bioptics was first described by Roberto Zaldivar, MD,[1] when he performed LASIK to correct residual refractive error in eyes that had received phakic IOLs. Dr. Zaldivar found that the bioptics procedure was an effective and predictable method for correcting residual error in patients who had extreme preoperative myopia of up to -35.00 D. In 1994, José Güell, MD, described his concept of adjustable refractive surgery[2]; he performed LASIK to correct residual ametropia after different types of intraocular surgeries, including implantation surgeries for IOLs and phakic IOLs, penetrating keratoplasties, and corneal refractive surgeries such as PRK and radial and arcuate keratotomy.[3] Currently, ophthalmologists use the term *bioptics* when techniques for IOL implantation are followed by a procedure involving excimer laser corneal ablation such as LASIK,

Epi-LASIK, or PRK.[4-9] The advantage of placing the IOL first is the improvement in the patient's quality of vision. Using corneal refractive surgical techniques, such as LASIK, as a secondary enhancement tool improves the accuracy of the final refractive outcome.

REASONS FOR BIOPTICS

Potential candidates for a planned bioptics procedure include patients who wish to minimize their dependence on corrective eyewear after lens surgery. If a patient desires a presbyopia-correcting IOL and has more than 0.75 D of residual postoperative astigmatism with a healthy cornea, he may be a good candidate for a planned bioptics procedure. Most available excimer lasers can effectively treat up to 5.00 D of astigmatism. For higher levels, the surgeon may use a combination of limbal relaxing incisions with bioptics to effectively fine-tune the refractive outcome.

PATIENT ASSESSMENT

Surgeons should first confirm the health of the cornea and ocular surface with a complete anterior segment examination, including corneal topography, corneal pachymetry, and Schirmer's testing. Other tests such as tear breakup time and Lissamine Green staining (Accutome, Inc., Malvern, PA) can also be considered to assess the quality of the ocular surface.

Many patients undergoing cataract surgery and lens implantation are more than 50 years of age and thus have a higher risk of dry eye after a corneal ablative procedure. A surgeon can manage the ocular surface prior to considering further corneal surgery. Artificial tears, Restasis (Allergan, Inc. Irvine, CA), and punctal plugs are options. If a patient's Schirmer's test is significantly low, advanced surface ablation such as Epi-LASIK can help minimize the risk of severe dry eye postoperatively. Eyes with asymmetric topography may also do better with advanced surface ablation as opposed to LASIK due to the risk of potential ectasia.

Pupillometry is essential, especially if a patient is considering choosing a presbyopia-correcting IOL with a bioptics procedure. Although many patients with astigmatism have grown accustomed to dealing with moderate-to-severe amounts of glare and halo, a thorough discussion of these phenomena before surgery can help manage patients' expectations.

TECHNIQUE FOR BIOPTICS

Timing of Flap Creation

One of the biggest questions when performing a planned LASIK bioptics procedure is when to create the LASIK flap. One may cut the flap 1 to 2 weeks in advance or at the time of the intraocular surgery.[2,3] Cutting the flap prior to placing the IOL avoids the possible risks related to a microkeratome use in eyes that contain an IOL. The major potential risk of using a microkeratome in an eye with an IOL is corneal endothelial damage.

Creating the flap before the intraocular procedure allows the earlier correction of residual ametropia (4 to 6 weeks after the intraocular surgery). The surgeon can simply lift the LASIK flap instead of risking potential complications due to the increased IOP secondary to placing a microkeratome suction ring on these eyes. A potential disadvantage of creating the flap before the intraocular procedure is the increased risk of epithelial ingrowth after lifting the flap for the enhancement procedure.

Another technique is to perform the bioptics procedure in a sequential fashion. After the IOL surgery, the eye is allowed to heal, and the refraction is permitted to stabilize for at least 3 months prior to the LASIK enhancement.[1,4-6] The advantage of this approach is that it avoids having to lift the flap on the eye, thus minimizing the incidence of epithelial ingrowth and other potential flap-related complications, such as diffuse lamellar keratitis, for these patients. There is a difference between cutting a new flap after the intraocular procedure and lifting a previously created flap in terms of the risk of epithelial ingrowth. This risk is higher with a relifted versus freshly cut flap. This sequential method is the only option for patients awaiting advanced surface ablation.

Type of LASIK Correction

Surgeons must also decide whether to use conventional or wavefront-guided laser ablation. My colleagues and I found that this choice depends on the type of lens implant. Currently, it is difficult to obtain accurate wavefront measurements consistently in eyes that have multifocal IOLs. Using a conventional laser treatment technique based on a patient's preoperative manifest refraction seems to provide the most accurate results. Wavefront-guided corrections are an option in patients who have received monofocal IOLs. Further study is needed concerning combining wavefront-driven ablations with newer IOLs such as toric and aspheric lenses.

CONCLUSION

Planned LASIK bioptics, limbal relaxing incisions, and toric IOLs are essential tools for treating postoperative residual astigmatism. For patients with extreme degrees of astigmatism, combining all three modalities may be necessary.[9]

Bioptics offers several advantages over IOL implantation or LASIK surgery alone. The theoretical benefits of the combined technique include maximization of the optical zone's size and improved predictability of the refractive outcome.[1] Moreover, bioptics allows patients with degrees of astigmatism and refractive error outside the limits of each individual procedure to obtain satisfactory results.

The biggest concern associated with a bioptics procedure is that it carries the risks of two procedures. The patient has to accept the risks of IOL surgery (endophthalmitis and bleeding) as well as those of corneal refractive surgery, which include irregular astigmatism, dry eye, and keratectasia as well as subjective complaints of halos, glare, and ghost images.[10,11] ■

This article originally appeared in the May 2006 issue of CRSToday.

1. Zaldivar R, Davidorf JM, Oscherow S, et al. Combined posterior chamber phakic intraocular lens and laser in situ keratomileusis: bioptics for extreme myopia. *J Refract Surg.* 1999;15:299-308.
2. Güell JL. The adjustable refractive surgery concept. *J Refract Surg.* 1998;14:271.
3. Güell JL, Gris O, Muller A, et al. LASIK for the correction of residual refractive errors from previous surgical procedures. *Ophthalmic Surg Lasers.* 1999;30:341-349.
4. Pershin KB, Pashinova NF. Fine tuning excimer laser correction after intraocular lens implantation and corneal transplantation. *J Refract Surg.* 2000;16(suppl):S257-S260.
5. Pershin KB, Pashinova NF, Miovich O. LASIK over pseudophakia - bioptics. *J Refract Surg.* 2001;17(suppl):S270.
6. Velarde JI, Anton PG, Valentin-Gamazo L. Intraocular lens implantation and laser in situ keratomileusis (bioptics) to correct high myopia and hyperopia with astigmatism. *J Refract Surg.* 2001;17(suppl):S234-S237.
7. Zaldivar R, Oscherow S, Piezzi V. Bioptics in phakic and pseudophakic intraocular lens with the Nidek EC-5000 excimer laser. *J Refract Surg.* 2002;18(suppl):S336-S339.
8. Güell JL. When and how to use bioptics. *Review of Ophthalmology.* Available at: http://www.revophth.com/index.asp?page=1_53.htm. Accessed April 7, 2006.
9. Nichamin L. How to get the best from bioptics. *Review of Ophthalmology.* Available at: http://www.revophth.com/index.asp?page=1_289.htm. Accessed April 7, 2006.
10. El Danasoury MA. Prospective bilateral study of night glare after laser in situ keratomileusis with single zone and transition zone ablation. *J Refract Surg.* 1998;14:512-516.
11. Pallikaris IG. Quality of vision in refractive surgery. *J Refract Surg.* 1998;14:551-558.

CHAPTER 151

Reducing Astigmatism With Conductive Keratoplasty

ELIZABETH A. DAVIS, MD

Conductive keratoplasty (CK; Refractec, Inc., Irvine, CA) is the application of radiofrequency energy to the peripheral cornea to reshape its curvature. Using a combination of various spot patterns, CK is able to correct between 0.50 and 2.00 D of hyperopia, presbyopia, and astigmatism. The safety of CK is also to be noted.1 Because the procedure does not remove corneal tissue, it does not weaken the cornea structurally. A loss of BCVA did not occur in CK's FDA clinical trials, and, if the complication has ever occurred since then, it is tremendously rare.1 Furthermore, because CK does not sever corneal nerve fibers, dry eye is not a complication.

CK can be titrated. In the case of an undercorrection, the surgeon can place additional spots at a later time. Because the procedure is so quick and easy to perform, it is best to start conservatively with few spots and a large optical zone (7 to 8 mm). Depending on the outcome, enhancements may involve placing more spots in the same or next smaller zone for a greater effect.

Nearly one third of patients undergoing cataract surgery have more than 1.00 D of astigmatism. Given that most surgeons actually worsen or induce astigmatism unless they perform on-axis incisions, about half of these operated eyes have more than 1.00 D of astigmatism postoperatively—a degree of cylinder that is incompatible with 20/20 vision. Only 1.00 D of residual astigmatism will reduce UCVA to 20/30, although 1.50 D of residual astigmatism reduces it to 20/50. There is no effect on spherical equivalent. Surgeons should continue to aim for emmetropia with lens calculations as they would with astigmatic keratotomy.

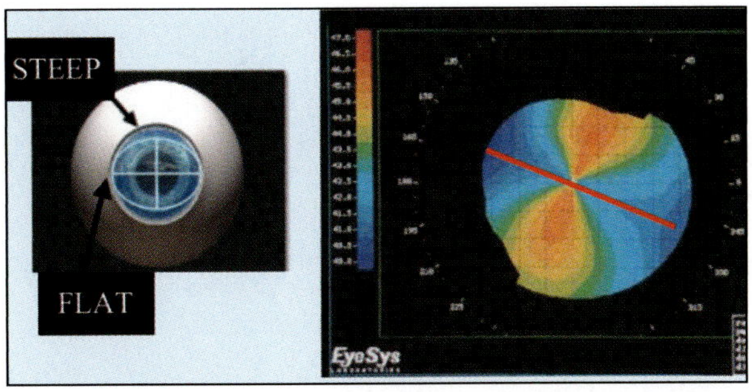

Figure 1. The author marked the flat axis with an RK marker.

In the current era of refractive cataract surgery, especially with the new technology presbyopia-correcting IOLs, our postoperative refractive goal should be 0.50 D or less of cylinder. Performing CK for astigmatism at the time of cataract surgery is a simple and effective method of achieving such results.

MY EXPERIENCE

Currently, I use CK to treat eyes with more than 1.25 D but less than 3.25 D of astigmatism. In an ongoing study, my colleague and partner, Richard L. Lindstrom, MD, and I have treated nine eyes. The median age of patients was 63 years. Our results are presented in Table 1. There have been no complications, no induction of

TABLE 1. CK FOR ASTIGMATISM PRIOR TO CATARACT SURGERY

	Preoperatively	2 Weeks Postoperatively	1 Month Postoperatively
UCVA	N/A	20/30	20/30
BCVA	20/50	20/20	20/20
Spherical Equivalent	-1.71 D (range, -7.00 to 2.50 D)	-0.29 D	-0.50 D
Mean Cylinder (preoperatively) and Reduction in Cylinder (postoperatively)	Manifest 1.41 D (range, 0.75 to 2.50 D) Keratometric 1.56 D (range, 1.25 to 2.13 D) Topographic 1.84 D (range, 1.12 to 3.00 D)	Manifest 0.75 D reduction Keratometric 1.02 D reduction Topographic 0.87 D reduction	Manifest 0.75 D reduction Keratometric 0.78 D reduction Topographic 1.12 D reduction

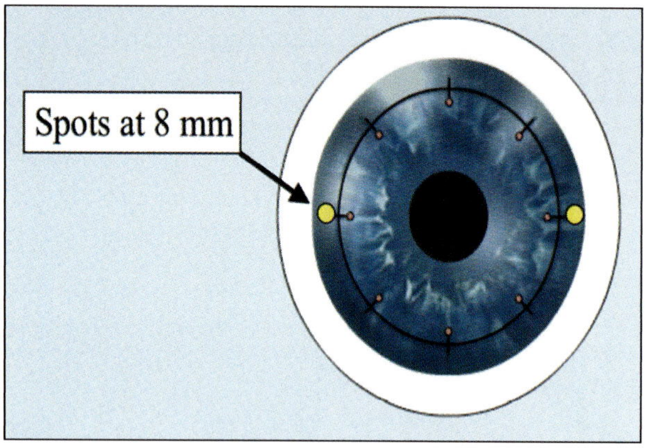

Figure 2. Using a CK marker,the author highlighted the 6-,7-,and 8-mm optical zones.

astigmatism, and no loss of BCVA. Follow-up examinations are ongoing, and we have performed additional procedures.

TECHNICAL PEARLS

I prefer to perform CK for astigmatism prior to making any incisions for the cataract surgery. I apply an anesthetic of topical proparacaine to the cornea and then administer a povidone-iodine swab of the eyelids. I then place the Viewpoint lid speculum (Refractec, Inc.) on the eye. Next, I mark the cornea under the operating microscope; I use an RK marker to indicate the flat axis (Figure 1) and a CK marker to denote the 6-, 7-, and 8- mm optical zones (Figure 2). Using moderate-to-light pressure of the CK probe, I place one spot on either side of the flat meridian (minus cylinder axis) at the 8-mm optical zone for a total of two spots.

The CK for astigmatism procedure takes only 3 minutes. Afterward, the speculum is removed, and the patient is prepped and draped with a standard sterile technique. I reglove and proceed with cataract surgery.

CONCLUSION

Dr. Lindstrom and I estimate that 90% of astigmatic treatments during and after cataract surgery could be achieved with CK alone. If a greater effect than can be achieved with CK were needed, astigmatic keratotomy or excimer laser correction could be performed. In my opinion, CK for astigmatism is an ideal solution for the refractive cataract surgeon who wants to offer patients greater spectacle independence. It is safe, easy to perform, quick, and effective. ■

This article originally appeared in the March 2007 issue of CRSToday.

1. McDonald MB, Durrie D, Asbell P, et al. Treatment of presbyopia with conductive keratoplasty: six-month results of the 1-year United States FDA clinical trial. *Cornea.* 2004;23:661-668.

CHAPTER 152

Top 10 Pearls for a Successful IOL Practice

ERIC D. DONNENFELD, MD

In addition to providing superb surgery with excellent clinical outcomes, one of the most valuable skills a surgeon and his staff can develop in the interest of building a successful refractive IOL practice is the ability to educate patients about the benefits of this surgery. At the third annual Refractive IOL Symposium recently held in Las Vegas, Nevada, leading experts in the field of refractive and lenticular surgery disclosed their practice management pearls that can help all surgeons gain more success in this field. Following is a synopsis of their insights.

1. **The surgeon and staff must communicate to the patient that they care about him and believe in refractive IOLs.** It is extraordinarily important that you offer patients what they want and need rather than try to sell them something. You must have faith in refractive IOL technology and a solid understanding of its benefit. Patients can easily sense doubt when a physician does not truly believe what he is telling them, and they will not be convinced of the merits of the technology. More importantly, surgeons should not recommend a technology that they do not believe in. They should feel comfortable implanting refractive IOLs in their family members' eyes before offering these lenses to their patients.

2. **All patients are candidates for premium refractive IOLs until they tell us they are not.** Monocular patients with macular degeneration and glaucoma should be informed about multifocal IOLs, although they may not be good candidates. There are several reasons for this strategy. First, telling patients about alternative choices for their surgical treatment is part of the informed consent process, even if they are not ideal candidates for those procedures. More importantly, a patient should be told why he is not a good candidate for a procedure so that he understands that you are considering his best interests. Additionally, patients whom you implant with a monofocal lens instead will still tell their relatives and friends about alternative treatments that you explained to them.

3. **What else do you own that you use every single day and does not devalue over time?** This message should be relayed to each patient considering premium refractive IOLs. The ability to improve one's lifestyle and quality of vision is something that does not degrade over time. Refractive IOLs are an investment in future happiness for many patients—something they should consider when seeking a refractive IOL consultation. It is important that we surgeons convey the value of this investment.

4. **Your staff's participation in patient education is important to the success of your refractive IOL business.** It is not good enough for just the surgeon to believe in refractive IOLs; the staff must acknowledge their importance as well. Only once the staff is convinced of the value of these lenses can they improve efficiency in patient care by becoming better communicators of the value of this technology. Often, ophthalmologists return from a meeting with new ideas for the practice, and the staff listens to the ideas and waits for the physician to return to his old habits. You must convince your staff that the changes are going to be permanent and then solicit their help in implementing these changes so that integrating refractive IOLs into your practice is seamless.

5. **You must set reasonable expectations for the surgery, bond with patients, and help them understand that their surgery is a process.** Two tenets of successful patient communication are to form a relationship with the patient and listen to him. Once you understand the patient's needs, it is much easier to recommend appropriate treatments for him. Also, you must explain to all refractive IOL patients that the treatment is a process and that additional surgeries, medications, and therapies may be necessary for them to achieve the full potential of their IOLs. Set this expectation preoperatively and discuss the possibility of postoperative limbal relaxing incisions, excimer laser photoablation, Nd:YAG capsulotomy, and topical medications to improve the tear film.

6. **Supply educational handouts, especially before the consultation.** It is very helpful for a patient to come into the office with an understanding of what he is going to be told by the ophthalmologist. It is a little overwhelming for a layperson to absorb all of the information that we provide in a short time. Handouts help the patient understand the different options available as well as the risks and benefits of each. Handouts should be provided to patients as early as possible in the consultative process; my staff and I prefer to mail them when the initial consultation is scheduled. Providing this information before their first visit helps patients develop some expectations for the appointment and perhaps a list of questions for the surgeon that they otherwise would not know to ask.

7. **Bring family members into the consultation whenever possible.** This is an extraordinarily important pearl for all refractive IOL surgeons. Family members are supportive, they ask important questions, and very commonly, they will help the patient make a good informed decision. It is very difficult for a patient to absorb all of the information about refractive IOL surgery on his own, and relatives can help in the educational process. Incidentally, family members will often convince a patient that he deserves the benefit of a premium refractive IOL. It is extremely heartwarming to hear a family member say that this is a gift that he wants to give the patient.

8. **Set up a good phone contact system so potential patients are not turned away.** Too often, the person answering the phone

at a physician's office is the least trained and lowest-paid person in the office. Because an individual's initial phone call is the first contact he has with an office, the person answering the phone should be positive and reflect the inviting atmosphere in your practice—a preview of what his experience in the practice will be like. In addition to helping to grow a practice, a receptionist with good phone skills can also be influential in setting callers' expectations for their first visit as well as in bringing in patients who need more immediate attention.

9. Give your staff a reward system based on your success. It is advantageous for staff members to benefit from the physician's success. Employees who are well rewarded for their hard work generally continue to perform better than staff members who are on a fixed salary. My administrators and I reward our staff members because we feel that they are an integral part of our success.

10. Improve scheduling and add dedicated times for refractive patients. One of the most difficult concepts for ophthalmologists to understand is that when they introduce new technology and a new patient population to the practice, something else must be given up in its place. The only way to be successful at offering premium refractive IOLs is to dedicate significant time and effort to this area, which requires giving up another part of the practice. The sacrificed service may be glaucoma or general ophthalmology, but success with refractive IOLs demands some type of change in the physician's schedule. I send my postoperative patients who have stable refractions to an associate ophthalmologist or optometrist for routine eye care. However, I make sure that the patient knows that he may always return to me for any ocular problems or additional procedures if necessary.

These 10 pearls for developing a refractive IOL practice are amassed from contributions by the entire faculty of the annual Refractive IOL Symposium run by *Cataract & Refractive Surgery Today*. I believe they represent valid and important concepts for success that practices will want to adopt in the coming years, as refractive IOLs become a more integral part of our routine practices. ■

This article originally appeared in the November 2007 issue of CRSToday.

CHAPTER 153

The Patient Experience in a Successful Refractive IOL Practice

JOHN F. DOANE, MD

Some patients consider the symptoms of presbyopia to be the worst experience that has ever happened in their lives. I consider having to explain presbyopia to patients or laypeople as the worst experience that I have had to endure in my clinical practice. Frequently, when the discussion starts, the patient and significant other are confused; by the time it ends, they are overwhelmed. These discussions with patients undergoing laser vision correction have troubled me for more than a decade and have motivated me to effectively communicate the concepts, natural progression, and prognosis of presbyopic symptoms to patients. Importantly, this talk is a catalyst to discussing which surgical option makes the most sense for an individual patient.

KEEP IT SIMPLE

My first goal in the initial consultation is to very simply draw the optical mechanics of the eye (Figure 1). I explain to the patient that the cornea and lens focus light into the eye, and the retina is like the "film" in a 35-mm camera. I tell him that the cornea is a fixed optic, but the lens can change in order to focus up close. Now for the first bombshell: I tell the patient that at age 40 and beyond, his focusing ability will decrease (Figure 2). For me, it has been helpful, if not relationship-saving, to tell each patient that everyone will experience this process after age 40. No one is immune to this progression.

FOCAL POINTS

The next step in the refractive preoperative workup that needs to be addressed is the patient's focal-point needs after surgery. This conversation sets the foundation for the patient to recognize and decide what optical aides, if any, he is willing to live with for the rest of his life. Patients must understand that there are three basic focal-point ranges used on a daily basis. Although this is an obvious concept, I believe an educated and informed patient is an asset to both himself and the surgeon postoperatively. I describe distance (driving vision) as the ability to view from 8 feet to infinity, intermediate (dashboard, computer screen, cell phone, PDA) as viewing ability from 8 feet to 2 feet, and near (reading documents) as 2 feet and closer (Figure 3).

I then describe historically what standard distance monofocal IOL surgery has provided patients. I try to illustrate the vision that the patient will obtain both uni- and bilaterally, depending on which IOL we select based on the end-target refraction. If we treat the right and left eyes for plano, we can show the patient that he will have both eyes for distance vision (Figure 4). The monofocal pseudophakic patient will need glasses for near tasks, and his need for correction may be unpredictable for intermediate tasks. I handle the issue of intermediate vision case by case, depending on the unique optics of a patient's eye.

TOLERATING MONOVISION

The first opportunity to suggest something other than creating iatrogenic presbyopia (ie, implanting monofocal IOLs with plano sphere refraction), is the discussion of monovision. In my experience, approximately 50% of patients will tolerate monovision happily. In this dialogue, using the distance, intermediate, and near plot (Figure 5), I again explain that if we select the right eye for plano and the left for -2.00 D, that the right eye will provide distance focus, the left will provide near focus, and the combination of the two will provide intermediate. With this choice, I make it very clear that at least 15% of patients will require glasses when driving at night, some may want reading glasses on occasion to "feel more balanced," and roughly 1% of patients will not like monovision and will require both eyes to be set for a plano sphere refraction.

At this point, I have presented the same information to the patient as I did before presbyopic IOLs became available. If I stopped here and did not give the presbyopic IOL talk, I will have shortchanged the patient and not provided him with all available options. If presbyopic IOLs are not discussed or at least described even briefly, this omission may later create distrust in the physician-patient relationship.

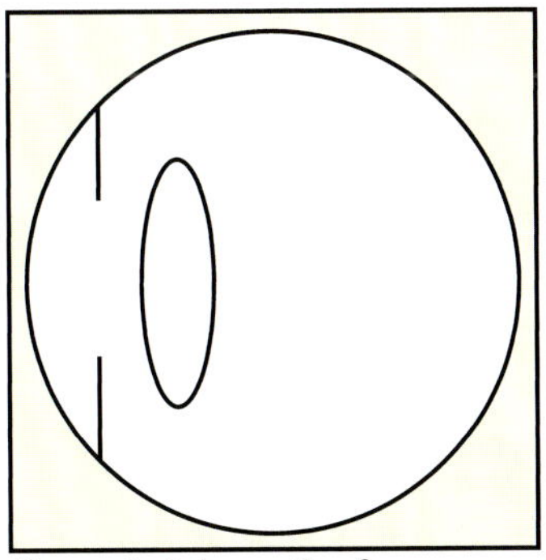

Figure 1. Schematic of an eye with the cornea and lens to the left and the retina to the right.

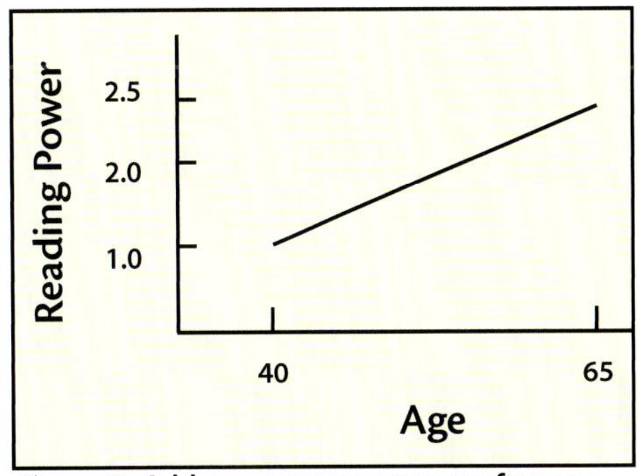

Figure 2. Add power to see at near after age 40: x-axis = age; y-axis = add power required.

Distance		8 feet to ⟶ the horizon
Intermediate	2 feet ⟷ 8 feet	(1.00 to 1.75 D good for life)
Near ⟵	2 feet	

Figure 3. Descriptor of three focal points: distance = 8 feet to the horizon, intermediate = 2 to 8 feet, and near = 2 feet.

THE GOAL

I show patients the ideal goal for presbyopic IOLs (Figure 6). In this scenario, we want both eyes to see at distance, intermediate, and near equally and at a very high level. I firmly believe patients want and expect near-perfect vision (at least 20/20) at distance, intermediate, and near with essentially no or minimal unwanted subjective visual phenomenon. At present, there is not an individual presbyopic IOL that will provide this type of vision every time for every patient, but there are techniques to maximize overall visual function. Accommodative IOLs such as the Crystalens (Eyeonics, Inc., Aliso Viejo, CA) involve targeting plano sphere in one eye and slight monovision (-0.50 to -1.00 D) in the other eye. For multifocal IOLs, either mixing the Acrysof Restor IOL (Alcon Laboratories, Inc., Fort Worth, TX) and the Crystalens or the Acrysof Restor and the Rezoom IOL (Advanced Medical Optics, Inc., Santa Ana, CA) can compensate for the weakness of one lens with the strength of the other.

POSSIBLE CONCERNS

Finally, I tell the patient there are two issues that may arise despite a perfect surgery. I tell him there is a 20% chance that I will perform YAG laser capsulotomy in the first year to improve his vision at distance, near, or both. I also emphasize that the best results occur in most cases when the final refraction is plano sphere from target with optimal refraction postoperatively and that he may require laser vision correction to perfect the unaided vision. For me, the chance for this correction is about 20% per eye.

IN SUMMARY

The information in this article may seem somewhat tedious, but it is complete, and I have found it to be essential for a healthy physician-patient relationship. At the conclusion of my discussion with the patient, I date and sign the document and place it in his chart. It is not uncommon for patients to ask for a copy of this sheet to review with their spouse. Until we have a lens that with 99% certainty can provide 20/20 or better unaided vision for distance, intermediate, and near in each eye (separately and with little-to-no unwanted subjective symptoms), surgeons and their staff should educate all pseudophakic IOL patients using the guidelines in this article, because they can minimize patient misunderstandings. I have elected to overeducate before surgery, as I find it much easier to deal with a patient and situation postoperatively if we have reviewed as many outcomes as possible in advance. ■

This article originally appeared in the November 2007 issue of CRSToday.

D	R & L
I	??????
N	Glasses

Figure 4. Descriptor that both the right (R) and left (L) eyes will be for distance (D), that near (N) will require glasses, and intermediate (I) is patient dependent (question marks).

D	R
I	R L
N	L (-2.00 D)

Figure 5. Descriptor showing the right eye (R) for distance (D) and the left eye (L) with a -2.00 D refractive error will provide near (N) focus, and both eyes (R and L) will provide intermediate (I) vision.

D	R L
I	R L
N	R L

Figure 6. Descriptor showing that both the right (R) and left (L) eyes will provide distance (D), intermediate (I), and near (N) focal points either independently or simultaneously.

CHAPTER 154

Patient Selection for Refractive IOLs

KERRY D. SOLOMON, MD

Patient selection for refractive IOLs is probably the single most important determinant of success for you and your practice as well as for patients' satisfaction. The entire staff of a practice needs to understand the significance of patients' having a choice of technology. Of paramount consequence is how patients learn about the different available refractive IOLs. In addition, staff members must ensure that they receive the proper education and informed consent.

An ophthalmologist who wants to implement refractive IOL technology into his practice needs first to spend time with his entire staff (from the receptionist to the schedulers to the technical staff) to make sure everyone understands his commitment to and belief in this treatment modality. It is comforting for patients to receive answers to their questions from staff members who have a great deal of refractive IOL knowledge. A well-informed counselor certainly provides assurance and confidence to patients as they explore their lens-related surgerical options.

My colleagues and I try to explain to patients that they have choices in IOLs. Most of them are interested in learning more about their options. We provide educational material in the form of brochures, DVD, and VHS tapes. Additionally, we invite our patients to ask questions of our staff members and physicians until they are satisfied with the answers.

PATIENT SELECTION

The ideal candidate for a refractive IOL is one who understands the technology's abilities and limitations. Furthermore, patients with minimal astigmatism and an otherwise healthy ocular surface, retina, macula, and optic nerve are preferable candidates for refractive IOL implantation.

Ideally, physicians want IOL patients to have less than 1.00 D of astigmatism. Managing cylinder in these patients is crucial. I have had great success with limbal relaxing incisions for patients with 1.50 D or less of astigmatism. If patients have more than this amount of pre-existing, regular, symmetric astigmatism, I perform bioptics, where I cut LASIK flaps 1 to 2 weeks before proceeding with the cataract surgery. When the refraction is stable postoperatively, 3 to 6 weeks after surgery, I lift the flaps and perform LASIK in order to treat the preexisting refractive astigmatism or any residual sphere.

ADDITIONAL EVALUATION

Anatomically, the ocular surface needs to be healthy for IOL implantation. I always note the status of the meibomian gland orifices and lid hygiene. I pay attention to the ocular tear film to make sure that the cornea stays moist and that the wetting ability of the tears is satisfactory for good ocular health. It is important to stain the ocular surface with Lissamine Green dye (Accutome Inc., Malvern, PA) and to look for any evidence of dryness. Punctal occlusion, topical lubricants, and Restasis (Allergan, Inc., Irvine, CA) are often prescribed preoperatively to optimize the ocular surface before proceeding with refractive lens exchange or cataract surgery.

Furthermore, I perform a thorough retinal examination with pupillary dilation to ensure the health of the retina. I pay attention to the macula to ensure minimal, if any, changes in retinal pigment epithelium or the presence of drusen. My staff and I perform preoperative analysis with optical coherence tomography on all patients to rule out the presence of fine epiretinal membranes, which may be too subtle to detect by retinal examination. If this analysis indicates any such membranes, I exclude the patient from refractive IOL technology because of the high possibility of cystoid macular edema and ocular and visual distortion.

ASSESSING PATIENTS' VISUAL GOALS

An equally important part of patient selection with IOLs is to gain a general feeling of the patient's visual goals and expectations; they need to be realistic in order for the patient to experience success with refractive lens technologies. I prefer patients to be somewhat flexible and compromising in terms of their visual outcomes. In fact, I often describe what these lenses can deliver as a compromise to the visual system. If they are interested in superb vision for distance and near, then I would recommend a monofocal lens. An aspheric monofocal IOL would be the lens of choice for all patients who desire the best quality of vision possible. For patients who are willing to make a visual compromise for the convenience of being less dependent on glasses, then presbyopia-correcting or refractive IOLs would be an excellent option.

DISCUSSION TOPICS

My staff and I give a general discussion of the compromises that exist with refractive lenses, such as those with which reading vision is optimal and less optimal. We explain the need for finding the "sweet spot" with any refractive lens technology. We talk about possible adjustments in their personal life, such as adjusting their lighting situations and the location of their computers based on refractive lens technologies. We also broach nighttime vision, because all of the refractive lens technologies are associated with scotopic visual symptoms. Fortunately, these symptoms, including halos, typically do not affect nighttime driving activities. I provide patients with statistics about the incidence of night vision symptoms; I believe there is roughly a 5% to 7% chance that these phenomena could be severe and possibly limit daily activities. I encourage patients to keep me well informed as to how they are doing. If they feel they have severe night vision symptoms, I may attempt an IOL exchange.

My staff and I also raise the topic of surgical touch-ups after patients' IOL surgery in the form of astigmatic treatments and fine-tuning their distance and near vision. We talk about the possibility of needing lens exchanges, piggyback lenses, and/or subsequent laser vision correction.

Finally, I remind patients that, although refractive lens technology is quite successful (90% of patients in my practice do not use glasses), approximately 10% still use spectacles. Most patients need them in low-light settings or occasionally for intermediate vision. Although this number of those that use eyeglasses is small, I think it is important for prospective IOL patients to understand the risk preoperatively. I tell our patients that some still use reading glasses for almost all of their daily activities. However, although not a guarantee, the success of these new lens technologies is quite high. ■

This article originally appeared in the July 2006 issue of CRSToday.

CHAPTER 155

Screening and Evaluating Presbyopic Patients

STEVEN J. DELL, MD

Consultations for cataract and refractive lens exchange surgery have become significantly more complicated. Ten years ago, I would diagnose a cataract and discuss the risks and benefits of as well as the alternatives for surgery with the patient. That was about it. The most complex question I would encounter was the occasional request for monovision. The type of IOL was rarely a topic for discussion. Overall, patients were happy to achieve good uncorrected distance vision, with readers needed for close vision. They were delighted to avoid the week of bed rest and aphakic spectacles they had seen their parents endure after cataract surgery in the 1960s and 1970s.

Today, consultations range from discussions similar to the aforementioned to explanations of the nuanced advantages of aspheric IOLs, descriptions of accommodating and multifocal IOLs, and the possibility of laser vision correction as an enhancement procedure. Recent decisions by the Centers for Medicare & Medicaid Services have introduced into the equation the possibility of large financial contributions by patients for New Technology IOLs. Moreover, people sometimes perform exhaustive research on the Internet before choosing a surgeon. In fact, I can assure you that some future potential patients will read this article. A strength and weakness of the Internet is that the information is completely unfiltered, and patients may present with demands for a technology that is completely inappropriate for them. Sometimes, I yearn for the serenity of a LASIK consultation with an obsessive-compulsive optical engineer.

Discussions with patients about cataract and refractive lens exchange surgery were taking a long time, and some people left confused, resulting in additional follow-up consultations. Still, I realized the importance of clearly conveying the complexities of the various IOL options to patients. As the volume of these consultations threatened to overwhelm my clinic, I instituted some changes.

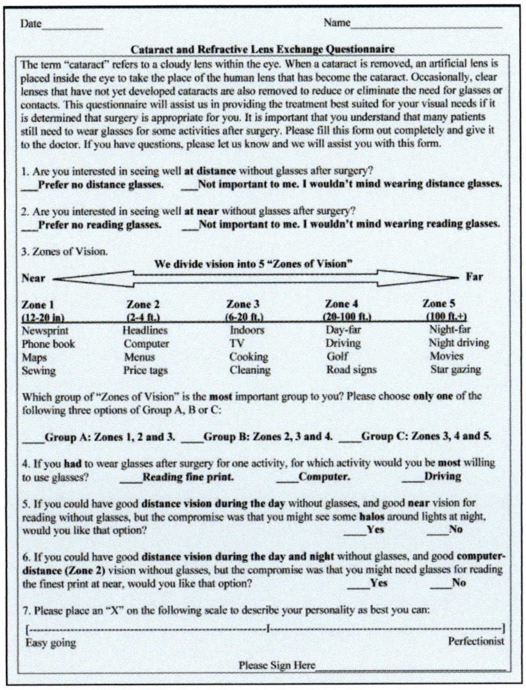

Date__________ Name______________________

Cataract and Refractive Lens Exchange Questionnaire

The term "cataract" refers to a cloudy lens within the eye. When a cataract is removed, an artificial lens is placed inside the eye to take the place of the human lens that has become the cataract. Occasionally, clear lenses that have not yet developed cataracts are also removed to reduce or eliminate the need for glasses or contacts. This questionnaire will assist us in providing the treatment best suited for your visual needs if it is determined that surgery is appropriate for you. It is important that you understand that many patients still need to wear glasses for some activities after surgery. Please fill this form out completely and give it to the doctor. If you have questions, please let us know and we will assist you with this form.

1. Are you interested in seeing well **at distance** without glasses after surgery?
___**Prefer no distance glasses.** ___**Not important to me. I wouldn't mind wearing distance glasses.**

2. Are you interested in seeing well **at near** without glasses after surgery?
___**Prefer no reading glasses.** ___**Not important to me. I wouldn't mind wearing reading glasses.**

3. Zones of Vision.

We divide vision into 5 "Zones of Vision"

Near ⟷ **Far**

Zone 1 (12-20 in)	**Zone 2 (2-4 ft.)**	**Zone 3 (6-20 ft.)**	**Zone 4 (20-100 ft.)**	**Zone 5 (100 ft.+)**
Newsprint	Headlines	Indoors	Day-far	Night-far
Phone book	Computer	TV	Driving	Night driving
Maps	Menus	Cooking	Golf	Movies
Sewing	Price tags	Cleaning	Road signs	Star gazing

Which group of "Zones of Vision" is the **most** important group to you? Please choose **only one** of the following three options of Group A, B or C:

___**Group A: Zones 1, 2 and 3.** ___**Group B: Zones 2, 3 and 4.** ___**Group C: Zones 3, 4 and 5.**

4. If you **had** to wear glasses after surgery for one activity, for which activity would you be **most** willing to use glasses? ___**Reading fine print.** ___**Computer.** ___**Driving**

5. If you could have good **distance vision during the day** without glasses, and good **near** vision for reading without glasses, but the compromise was that you might see some **halos** around lights at night, would you like that option? ___**Yes** ___**No**

6. If you could have good **distance vision during the day and night** without glasses, and good **computer-distance (Zone 2)** vision without glasses, but the compromise was that you might need glasses for reading the finest print at near, would you like that option? ___**Yes** ___**No**

7. Please place an "X" on the following scale to describe your personality as best you can:

[--|--]
Easy going Perfectionist

Please Sign Here______________________

Figure 1. Dr. Dell's questionnaire for patients.

GATHERING INFORMATION

During the workup process, individuals considering cataract or refractive IOL surgery watch a video introducing the concept of a presbyopia-correcting IOL. Next, they complete a questionnaire (Figure 1) that clarifies their postoperative visual goals. Although the survey provides a wealth of information, I have learned that, perhaps most importantly, it alters patients' perceptions of the surgery. The very nature of the questions lets them know that compromises are inherent in any surgical option. The final question asks patients to rate their personalities from easygoing to perfectionist. The technician working the patient up also rates the patient on this scale, and I do the same after my consultation.

COUNSELING PATIENTS

With the survey results in hand, my consultation becomes relatively straightforward. Typically, I will direct cataract surgery patients who are interested in good uncorrected distance vision and have corneal astigmatism toward a limbal relaxing incision or a toric IOL. Both options involve an out-of-pocket expense for patients. If they also want good uncorrected near vision, the discussion focuses on presbyopia-correcting IOLs or monovision. Because all of the presbyopia-correcting IOLs can produce successful results, a definitive recommendation from the surgeon is important. This advice should be based upon the technologies with which the surgeon is most comfortable. The patient deserves a statement such as "Based upon what I see today and what you have told me, I believe the best technology for you is X." Meandering, circular discussions of every possible combination of IOLs serve the interests of no one.

I typically tell patients interested in presbyopia- correcting IOLs that spectacles of some variety are in their future, but I explain that my goal is to reduce their need for glasses to a bare minimum. This is an important psychological milestone for patients. If they balk at this statement, I may reconsider their candidacy for these IOLs.

I also tell these patients that the treatment plan sometimes involves a second procedure to touch up the results of the first surgery. I stipulate that I will gladly perform the enhancement at a discount but that I am unable to do it for free. You may wish to actuarially bundle the costs of these enhancements into the price of your surgical procedure. Regardless, the patient will appreciate knowing this policy in advance.

If your patients undergo surgery with an expectation of perfection, you will be severely faulted if you do not deliver. Many fail to grasp the concept of variable human responses to surgery despite being told about it several times. Educating patients so they truly understand the possible outcomes of their surgery will make you both happier.

FOLLOWING UP

I often survey patients postoperatively to see how they rate their vision. Although, in general, those with the best objective vision are subjectively the happiest, it is amazing to observe the occasional total lack of correlation between these metrics. Some patients seem eternally happy no matter what I do, and some are clearly unhappy before, during, and after their surgical experience. It would be nice if these two types of patients would identify themselves upon their initial presentation to the clinic. Based upon the results of the postoperative surveys, I continue to make subtle refinements in my surgical strategies.

CONCLUSION

New IOL technologies have made the surgeon's job more interesting and complex. The stakes are higher now that patients are paying out of their own pockets for certain lenses and/or astigmatic correction. It is important to identify what they desire to achieve with surgery quickly and accurately, to set their expectations appropriately, and to recognize that their psychological makeup may affect their perception of the surgical outcome. ■

The Dell questionnaire is available at http://www.crstoday.com/Pages/DellIndex.doc.

This article originally appeared in the March 2007 issue of CRSToday.

CHAPTER 156

Mastering Preoperative Interviews

FRANK A. BUCCI JR, MD

The typical large-volume cataract practice is usually efficient at educating patients about what to expect during cataract surgery. Surgical counselors distribute informative brochures and videos and talk to patients about their upcoming surgery in an effort to decrease their anxiety and, by extension, the doctor's chair time. Combining high-quality cataract surgery with efficient patient flow in both the clinic and ambulatory surgical center has traditionally resulted in excellent outcomes, high patient satisfaction, and economic prosperity for the practice.

THE NEW PARADIGM

The landscape of cataract surgery is changing, however. The reimbursement ruling by the Centers for Medicare and Medicaid in 2005 introduced new treatment options for cataract surgeons to offer their patients: multifocal or presbyopia-correcting IOLs (also called *premium refractive IOLs*). Every cataract patient may now upgrade to a premium refractive IOL that can reduce or eliminate his need for reading glasses if he is willing to pay out of pocket for it. High-volume cataract surgeons are experiencing greater chair time yet disappointing conversion rates with cataract patients when discussing premium refractive IOLs. Typically, these efficient, successful cataract practices respond to this problem by doing more of what they do well. They assume that their patients need more and higher-quality information about these treatment options in order to make definitive decisions quicker, so they provide new and greater quantities of information about presbyopic IOLs "so the patient can decide."

What results from intensifying the transfer of information from the practice to the patient? Frustration. The conversion rates to premium refractive IOLs remain poor. Giving patients more information only serves to confuse them further, thus increasing the number of questions they have and lengthening their surgeon's chair time. In addition, surgeons are surprised when the extra chair time fails to prevent excessive complaining by premium refractive IOL patients about issues that were discussed, such as halos.

What accounts for these challenges of premium refractive IOLs that are frustrating physicians? This treatment category introduces a new paradigm in cataract surgery—one of elective surgery. Within this new doctor/patient relationship, the pathology/cataract model fails. In the paradigm of elective IOL surgery, the quality of the surgeon's preoperative decision making is directly related to and depends on the amount of valuable information moving not from the practice to the patient, but from the patient to the doctor.

IMPROVING INTERACTION

The surgeon can only glean valuable information from his patient if he improves the quality of the doctor/patient relationship. He must educate himself as to who the patient really is and what this person wants to achieve. There are two important first steps toward acquiring the information necessary for engaging in proper patient selection. The first is asking patients open-ended questions that elicit spontaneous responses, and the second step is improving one's listening and observational skills. The patient will give you all the information you need to know—if you will let him. Combine this information with a thorough preoperative examination, and then make a definitive treatment recommendation to the patient that will lead to the highest levels of success based on your professional opinion. Do not ask the patient to decide about the details of his treatment; instead, lead him to the best alternatives based on the history he has revealed about himself in the preoperative consultation and examination.

FINER POINTS OF THE PREOPERATIVE INTERVIEW

Important Questions to Ask

Some of the obvious characteristics patients divulge in their preoperative interviews include their visual expectations (personality), visual demands (lifestyle), visual function, refractive status, and economic status. The two most interesting and revealing questions, however, are the patient's lens status (a cataractous vs clear lens) and his "purpose for the consultation."

Lenticular status frequently divides potential refractive IOL patients into subcategories based on age and culture (Table 1).

TABLE 1. CHARACTERISTICS OF POTENTIAL PATIENTS

Cataract	Lensectomy
• Late 60s, 70s, 80s	• 40s, 50s, and early 60s
• "Brokaw cataract" WWII	• "Boomer cataract" & clear lens
• Accepting by culture	• Demanding by culture
• Poor corrected preop VA	• Excellent corrected preop VA
• Reasonable expectations	• High expectations
• Pay less - expect less	• Pay more - expect more
• Less litigious	• More litigious
• Less computer	• More computer

Lensectomy and younger cataract patients (baby boomers) are generally more demanding. They will compare their postimplantation vision with their excellent preoperative corrected vision. The inherent visual improvement that comes with all cataract surgery makes the entire process more forgiving when cataracts are removed in elderly individuals. These older patients are more accepting by culture, have paid less for the procedure, perform less demanding visual tasks, and in general, are less exacting and less litigious.

The "purpose for the consultation" may be the most revealing answer a surgical candidate can give. We need simply to ask why the patient is seeking an evaluation. Is he pursuing a diagnosis and treatment for pathology (cataract), or is he seeking spectacle independence? Even if the prospective patients were identical twins with identical examinations upon presentation, any difference in their reason for consulting a surgeon causes a significant divergence in the course of the preoperative examination.

Patients seeking treatment for a possible cataract have little or no awareness of refractive options. Those seeking spectacle independence are usually very educated by the media, seminars, the Internet, word of mouth, or optometric consultations regarding their refractive options. If the patient who is concerned about having a cataract is told that no cataract is present, he is delighted and returns home telling his family that he does not need "that growth" removed from his eye. If the patient seeking spectacle independence is told he does not have a cataract, he is extremely upset that he has "missed out" on the potentially large discount for a presbyopia-correcting IOL.

If Cataract Is Present

If the pathology-minded patient is told that he has a cataract, it may be initially difficult to efficiently and effectively present all the refractive options and economic realities. With these patients, I implement what I call the *three core questions*. The answers to these questions are either "yes" or "no" and quickly elevate you, the surgeon, to a new level of awareness about the patient.

1. Do you have any interest in achieving spectacle independence?
2. Would you be willing to tolerate some light phenomena while driving at night to achieve this freedom?
3. Would you be willing to pay an amount out of pocket to achieve this increased freedom from glasses?

If the answer to the first question is "no," then I will likely implant the patient with a monofocal IOL (with or without monovision) that is covered by insurance. If the sequence of answers is yes-yes-no, then we offer what I call *the opportunity*. We inform the patient that many presbyopes who wear bifocals but do not have cataracts pay in excess of $4,000 per eye to be free of their glasses. Because the patient has cataracts, however, he will pay less than $2,000 per eye to achieve the same outcome. We are careful not to directly compare the cost of upgrading to a premium IOL to the "free" IOL that comes with his health insurance. If the candidate's sequence of answers is yes-yes-yes, he will eventually choose a premium IOL.

If Cataract Is Not Present

If the patient seeking spectacle independence does not have a cataract, we then need to distinguish the emmetropes from the nonemmetropes. *If the patient is not an emmetrope, will he undergo LASIK or a refractive lensectomy?* I begin the differentiating process with the one fundamental question: "*If we use customized LASIK to give you excellent distance vision, and all you need is reading glasses after surgery, will that make you happy?*" If I receive a strong "yes," I perform LASIK. If I receive a strong "no," I discuss the essential aspects of refractive lens exchange with the patient and often end up performing that procedure. If I hear a weak "yes" or weak "no," I begin to discuss the pros and cons of each procedure in a balanced fashion. I watch and listen to the responses. Patients will lead you to an awareness of which procedure is best for them. Do not quickly manipulate the patient into having a particular procedure—you will get burned. I advocate a respectful exchange with patients by offering information, listening to their responses, and seeking to perceive the "truth" about their needs. *Who is this individual and what does he really want to achieve?* With practice, the quality of your decision making will escalate. When you decide that you have enough valuable information and you are aware of which treatment option is best for the patient, then proceed to lead him in a balanced manner to the procedure that you have determined will best satisfy him.

Strategy With Emmetropic Presbyopes

If the patient is an emmetropic presbyope, my approach changes significantly. Because these patients already have relatively good uncorrected distance acuity, they are more difficult to please. I strongly "counsel down" their expectations. I tell them that I am very respectful and cautious about performing intraocular surgery in patients with 20/20 uncorrected distance vision. I explain that if they can fully appreciate the high-risk profile of this surgery, I might offer them a presbyopia-correcting IOL in their nondominant eye, and I will likely require a significant period (months) of neuroadaptation after their first implantation before even considering surgery in their second eye. I discuss every possible complication. After offering the procedure in one eye, I then begin to withdraw this offer. I closely observe the patient's reaction, which will reveal his true desire for spectacle independence. In my opinion, a strong, sincere desire for spectacle independence has the greatest correlation with postoperative success when implanting multifocal IOLs than any other patient characteristic.

CONCLUSION

The new paradigm of elective implant surgery demands that surgeons facilitate a genuine doctor/patient relationship. The *three core questions, the opportunity*, and the *one fundamental question* are only tools I use for stimulating patients so I can then observe, listen to, and learn from their elicited response. The basic underlying principle of my approach is that if you choose to listen to your patients, they will give you the answers. ■

This article originally appeared in the November 2007 issue of CRSToday.

CHAPTER 157

The Mindset of Presbyopic Refractive Patients

ERIC D. DONNENFELD, MD

The mindset of the presbyopic refractive patient is unique and differs greatly from that of most pre-presbyopic refractive patients. Presbyopic patients no longer accept the loss of near vision as an unavoidable complication of growing older. Instead, older patients consider any loss of form or function as a sign of aging, something to be avoided at all costs. This mindset is particularly common among baby boomers, who, as a generation, associate aging with weakness. Evidence of this attitude abounds in forms such as medication for erectile dysfunction (a market that generated sales of $1.5 billion in 2005 and may exceed $6 billion by 2010) and hair transplants (increasing annually at a rate of 25%).[1]

The presbyopic baby boomer considers presbyopia and cataracts to be the defining moments of middle and old age, respectively. How many patients in their 50s or 60s have visited your office with cataracts and said, "I thought cataracts only happened to old people"? To help refractive surgeons manage these challenging patients, this article lays to rest several myths about presbyopes.

DISPELLING THE MYTHS

No. 1: Patients with monovision are truly happy.

In fact, presbyopes are never happy. They are the grumpiest, most demanding patients I know, and I speak from experience, as a presbyope myself. Although monovision may make these patients less unhappy, their distance vision is never as clear as when they had binocular distance vision, and their reading vision is never as good as it was with a decent pair of reading glasses. At best, monovision makes presbyopic patients slightly happier, but it never provides the vision that they truly want.

No. 2: Presbyopic low myopes are happy if their vision is corrected to plano.

This assumption is obviously false. Presbyopic low myopes will never forgive you for correcting them to plano. They do not always fully understand that they cannot put away their glasses after refractive surgery and that they can never regain the perfect reading vision they once had. As bad as correcting low myopic presbyopes to plano may be, however, the ultimate disaster is a hyperopic overcorrection in a patient who was previously a low myope. These people are extraordinarily unhappy, because their near point is even worse than it was previously with glasses. I therefore strongly recommend a contact lens trial before considering refractive surgery on any low myope who is entertaining the option of a full-distance correction.

No. 3: Presbyopic patients understand that, after refractive surgery, their reading vision will still worsen as they age.

When you correct presbyopic patients to plano and their reading vision worsens with age, they will blame you and regard their loss of vision as a complication of the surgery. They will also want an enhancement for better reading vision but will be unhappy with their loss of distance vision. Finally, despite the informed consent and however many hours spent discussing the issue with them, these patients will never fully agree that you explained this issue to them or that they understood prior to surgery that their reading vision would worsen as they grew older.

No. 4: The inadvertently undercorrected presbyopic patient will be happy with an enhancement to plano.

I frequently see patients who were inadvertently left slightly myopic following refractive surgery (eg, the -5.00 D myope or the +3.00 D hyperope who is left -0.50 D). These patients will want to have their vision corrected to plano to improve their distance vision. They should always have a contact lens trial to see if they will truly be happy with a full distance correction, however. After an enhancement (despite your best efforts to warn them), they almost uniformly want to revert to the minimal undercorrection. Many of them do not understand how much they will miss the slight near vision they had before their enhancement.

No. 5: Conductive keratoplasty can provide blended vision, and the patient will not lose quality distance vision with the return of his near vision.

Although conductive keratoplasty (CK; Refractec, Inc., Irvine, CA) can be very useful, particularly for improving the near vision of hyperopic, astigmatic, multifocal IOL patients, the procedure almost always causes a loss of Snellen visual acuity or contrast sensitivity at distance and a loss of visual quality. I perform CK, but I always tell patients that it yields monovision, not blended vision.

No. 6: Presbyopic IOL patients will tolerate small refractive errors.

This idea is just wrong. Presbyopic IOL patients are incredibly sensitive to small refractive errors. If you are considering adding presbyopia-correcting IOLs to your surgical armamentarium, then you must, as a refractive cataract surgeon, use precise biometry and create astigmatically reproducible cataract incisions. In addition, you must be willing and able to treat postoperative refractive errors with a variety of different techniques, including the excimer laser (LASIK and PRK), limbal relaxing incisions, an IOL exchange, and possibly CK.

MANAGING PRESBYOPIC PATIENTS

When managing presbyopes, it is important to address their most common concerns preoperatively. When I speak with patients regarding refractive IOLs particularly, I always mention that they may have a slight blur at distance, their reading distance may be fixed, and they might not have the full range of reading vision that they had previously. In addition, I explain that they may see ghost images and halos at night. Although these compromises may seem significant, most patients tolerate them very well and view them as a small price to pay for excellent near vision.

The best presbyopic refractive candidates are hyperopes, patients with cataracts who have had a loss of BCVA, individuals with greater than -4.00 D of myopia who are accustomed to wearing bifocals or separate reading glasses, and patients who are willing to undergo enhancements for astigmatism or residual refractive errors. These are the patients to treat early in your learning curve with refractive cataract and excimer laser surgery. They are more likely than others to be happy with any improvement in their vision, because they had such poor visual quality originally.

CONCLUSION

Today, there are 90 million presbyopes in the US. The ultimate form of presbyopia is monofocal pseudophakia, and 3 million patients develop cataracts every year. The presbyopic refractive patient is the most demanding to visit our cataract and refractive practices on a daily basis. Nevertheless, those with successful visual outcomes whose expectations have been met are also the most grateful patients in our practices, and they represent an enormous opportunity for all of ophthalmology. ■

This article originally appeared in the March 2006 issue of CRSToday.

1. American Society of Plastic Surgeons. Available at: http://www.plasticsurgery.org. Accessed: February 1, 2006.

CHAPTER 158

Communicating IOLs' Value

KERRY ASSIL, MD

Recent developments within ophthalmology have led us to approach cataract and presbyopic patients differently than in the past. New lens technologies are available such as the Rezoom (Advanced Medical Optics, Inc., Santa Ana, CA), Acrysof Restor (Alcon Laboratories, Inc., Fort Worth, TX), and Crystalens (Eyeonics, Inc., Aliso Viejo, CA). In addition, the Centers for Medicare & Medicaid Services ruled last year that patients may pay a premium to receive presbyopia-correcting IOLs.

These changes combined with many middle-aged and older individuals' desire to enhance their quality of life as they age has prompted my colleagues and me to adjust how we present information to patients. This article offers tips on tailoring discussions to the patient's perspective and visual needs.

CATARACT PATIENTS

Keep conversations simple with cataract surgery patients. For example, I ask them if, after the surgery, they would like to see without glasses. If a patient demonstrates little enthusiasm, I drop the subject and schedule him for cataract surgery.

However, if a patient shows an interest in being free of glasses postoperatively, I discuss with him the availability of multifocal lenses and accommodating IOLs and how they can provide binocular vision. Additionally, I explain that the patient will see some halos, but not many patients are dissuaded by that fact.

It is important not to refer to a presbyopia-correcting IOL as a better lens. Patients who cannot afford a new-technology IOL or who choose a standard monofocal lens should not feel that their decision was wrong or that paying the premium would have gotten them better surgery. Instead, try to focus your conversation on lifestyle improvements. This idea also helps patients understand premium surgery. Medicare patients are not used to paying out of pocket for medical benefits, but they are increasingly familiar with spending money to better their lives.

PRESBYOPES

Conversations with ametropic and presbyopic patients differ from those with cataract patients. First, you need to educate presbyopic patients about the loss of accommodation associated with age. Second, discuss cataracts with these patients, because they typically are already experiencing some early lenticular changes. In my practice, I use the analogy of a dirty windshield to explain how the crystalline lens becomes opaque with time.

Many patients are already familiar with the excimer laser treatment, but you still need to explain that excimer laser correction will not fix the source of their problem, which is the growing inflexibility of their crystalline lens. Discuss how their natural lens can be replaced with a new one that can provide binocular vision. Further explain that, if they have LASIK, they will quite possibly require cataract extraction in the future. A conversation about postoperative halos is always necessary before implanting multifocal IOLs. Although the halos often diminish with time, they may be noted for 1 year or longer. Once the second eye is treated, the halos may lessen more rapidly.

Last, although I am cautious in recommending refractive lens exchange to presbyopic myopes, I will consider the procedure for patients with early cataracts, provided a retinal specialist has conducted a meticulous examination of the peripheral retina and ruled out an unacceptably high risk of retinal detachment.

PRACTICE DEVELOPMENT

We need to reestablish our traditional roles when dealing with privately paid procedures. First of all, patients need to understand that any clinical recommendation is based on their eye health, visual needs, and lifestyle—not how much money they have. I recommend not discussing money with patients at all. Instead, make them aware of the in-practice counselors who are available to discuss financial matters.

Surgeons need to be closely involved in patient care pre- and postoperatively, because older patients are used to having a relationship with their physicians. These patients will not tolerate not meeting their surgeons, especially when they are paying a premium for the procedure.

Surgeons implanting presbyopia-correcting IOLs must strive for excellent outcomes. Careful preoperative screenings are a must, meaning that no patient should have macular disease or other ocular pathology, and lens subtypes (Rezoom, Acrysof Restor, or Crystalens) should be selected to match the patient's physiology and lifestyle. Moreover, the surgeon should disqualify candidates who seem prone to unrealistic expectations or who have an underachieving personality. Tight surgical protocols should ensure the implantation of the correct lens for a specific patient's dioptric range. In addition, the ophthalmologist should have access to an excimer laser and be prepared to perform a refractive enhancement via LASIK or Epi-LASIK, a lens exchange, a piggyback IOL, an Nd:YAG capsulotomy, etc.

CONCLUSION

Prudent patient selection, coupled with proper care and communication, will help ensure that patients receiving presbyopia-correcting IOLs are happy with their visual results postoperatively. Good news spreads quickly from the mouths of satisfied patients. Although we have not been implanting this types of lens for very long, my colleagues and I have already had patients refer their friends to us. ■

This article originally appeared in the March 2006 issue of CRSToday.

CHAPTER 159

Managing Cataract Patients' Refractive Expectations

JAMES A. DAVISON, MD

Cataract patients have always been refractive surgery patients, and those with 20/20 UCVA postoperatively have always been the happiest. It was somewhat embarrassing to accept their praise, because we surgeons knew that we really just got lucky with their results. Patients accepted that astigmatism and variable measurements only allowed a lucky few to see well uncorrected, and they were generally happy to receive a prescription for glasses that provided them with good distance and near vision. Patients and surgeons were happy, because both had their expectations met.

Today's patients expect 20/20 UCVA after surgery. Those who pay a premium to receive a multifocal or accommodating IOL expect to see well at distance and near without glasses. The tough part is that all of the patients not paying out of pocket for a new-technology IOL also now expect to have a plano result, see at least 20/20 at distance without correction, and only wear reading glasses for near work. Surgeons' attitudes have likewise changed. Managing these refractive expectations involves six areas.

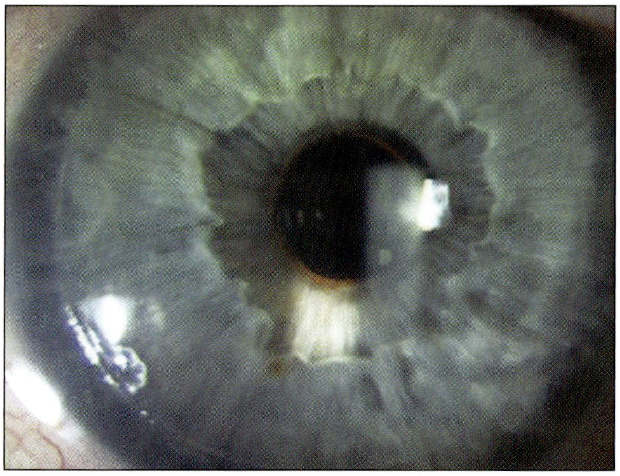

Figure 1. At 81 years of age, this patient was the oldest in the author's practice to undergo excimer laser surgery. Seven weeks after receiving an Acrysof Restor IOL, she underwent flap creation with the Intralase FS laser followed by LASIK. The procedure adjusted her final refraction and degree of astigmatism.

NO. 1: PATIENT SELECTION

Individuals who do not mind wearing glasses or who will not consider paying a premium are not candidates for a multifocal lens. I also feel that patients who have a lifelong history of glare, minimal nuclear cataract, and lots of complaints are poor candidates, and they may have an increased chance for glare after the implantation of any IOL. I rule out patients who have extraordinary expectations for perfection and who are intolerant of possible imperfection or the need for extra steps toward recovery. I also disqualify patients with any noteworthy compromise of their visual system (eg, significant macular pathology, corneal dystrophy, amblyopia).

Patients who previously underwent keratorefractive surgery are not the best candidates for multifocal IOLs. Although they are extremely motivated, achieving a plano result can be difficult, and a keratorefractive enhancement may not be possible. These individuals also may have higher-order aberrations that will diminish their quality of vision even under the best circumstances. Their expectations are usually very high, and they may view multifocal IOLs as the final step in their quest for perfect vision.

Finally, although patients who receive a multifocal IOL unilaterally may be satisfied, those who undergo bilateral implantation always have better results. Special discussion is therefore necessary with the former group.

NO. 2: REALISTIC EXPECTATIONS

I tell patients that no surgical procedure yields perfect results every time and that complications such as infection, hemorrhage, and retinal swelling can occur. The best results for a multifocal IOL were reported in the Acrysof Restor IOL's (Alcon Laboratories, Inc., Fort Worth, TX) FDA trials: 80% of patients never wore glasses; 85% had uncorrected 20/25 and J2 visual acuities; only 25% had at least moderate rings, halos, and glare; and 94% said they were happy and would have the procedure again or recommend it to a relative. Nevertheless, I emphasize the percentage of patients who

TABLE 1. RATES AND DEMOGRAPHICS OF ENHANCEMENTS				
ASTIGMATISM	1.00 D OR LESS	MORE THAN 1.00 D		
		No LRI	LRI	Total
Cases	90	10	19	29
Enhanced	1 (LASIK)	1 (LASIK)	4 (1 LASIK, 3 PRK)	5 (2 LASIK, 3 PRK)
Percentage	1%	10%	21%	17%

These statistics refer to the six of 119 cases that required secondary keratorefractive intervention after the implantation of an Acrysof Restor IOL.

did not achieve those results and stress that prospective cataract surgery patients could be among that group.

For the Acrysof Restor IOL, I explain that patients may need glasses for intermediate vision, such as for viewing a computer monitor, but that they may also require slight correction for their best possible distance and near vision. With the Rezoom IOL and Crystalens accommodating IOL (Eyeonics, Inc., Aliso Viejo, CA), I explain that patients may need some additional correction to see comfortably at near for long periods of time. I remark that halos and glare have not been a huge problem for my patients with the Acrysof Restor IOL. Finally, I note that reducing the residual refractive error is the key to success with all pseudophakic technology, especially multifocal and accommodating IOLs, and that some may require additional refractive surgery in order to achieve good results.

Subjects in the Acrysof Restor IOL's FDA clinical trials had 1.00 D of keratometric astigmatism or less. If my cataract patients have significant astigmatism, I impress upon them that their surgery should include concurrent limbal relaxing incisions (LRIs) but that astigmatism can rarely be eliminated. For those reasons, I say, there is approximately a 20% chance of their needing a subsequent refractive procedure.

I also warn patients that they may require an IOL exchange. Of my first 119 Acrysof Restor IOL implants, I had to exchange two, one for positive dysphotopsia and the other for blurred BCVA. I explain the concept of cortical adaptation and advise patients that their brain may not adapt quickly to or fully appreciate the new IOL technology.

NO. 3: BIOMETRY AND CALCULATIONS

Residual spherical equivalent ametropia reduces the effectiveness of a multifocal IOL, and a refractive error greater than 0.50 D is probably going to be significant. One must recognize that optimizing refractive outcomes entails striving for perfection in all components of preoperative measurements and IOL calculations. For my staff and me, the adoption and disciplined, consistent use of biometric technologies and calculation formulae are an ongoing process. We began with what we could best afford and control—contact A-scan, manual keratometry, and two-variable formulae.

Although the technicians with whom I work are very experienced with contact A-scan and manual keratometry, manual methods of measurement require higher degrees of human skill and are therefore subject to higher mean absolute error, even when perfectly calibrated. Multiple clinics and the use of numerous technicians and machines can further increase the variability. With these manual methods and two-variable formulae, my patients have an average residual spherical equivalent refractive error of +0.04 ±0.42 D. This standard deviation means that, 32% of the time, the residual refractive error will be beyond that range.

We have committed to reducing that standard deviation through the following actions. First, we have converted to immersion A-scans for all patients and have ordered six IOLMasters (Carl Zeiss Meditec Inc., Dublin, CA) for our main clinics, which should improve the consistency of our measurements. Additionally, we are scheduling trials of other technologies for automated keratometry.

Historically, we have used the third-generation, two-variable SRK-T formula for eyes of average length and the Hoffer Q for shorter eyes. We are converting to the Holladay 2, a multiple-variable formula that includes the axial length, keratometry, anterior chamber depth, lens' thickness, vertex distance, white-to-white measurement, and manifest refraction.

We are hoping that making this financial and scientific investment in these technologies and formulae will improve our refractive results.

NO. 4: SURGICAL EXCELLENCE

The standard, temporal, clear corneal 2.8-mm incision should induce no more than approximately 0.25 D of with-the-rule astigmatism overall. The IOL's optic should be perfectly centered and overlapped 360° by 0.25 to 0.40 mm of anterior capsule to ensure the consistent positioning of the lens and prevent posterior capsular opacification.

NO. 5: RESIDUAL REFRACTIVE ERROR

Residual refractive cylinder reduces the effectiveness of the optical system, and greater than 0.75 D will probably be significant. Preoperative keratometric astigmatism is a useful, although imperfect, predictor of postoperative pseudophakic refractive cylinder. Patients with greater than 1.00 D of keratometric astigmatism will usually require LRIs, which, in my hands, are effective in up to 80% of cases (Table 1). Six (5%) of my first 119 cases with the Acrysof Restor IOL required subsequent corneal refractive enhancements. Only 1% of those cases with ≤ 1.00 D of preoperative keratometric astigmatism required an enhancement versus 17% of those with > 1.00 D.

I was wary of performing LASIK with femtosecond flap creation (Intralase FS laser; Intralase Corp., Irvine, CA) at 7 weeks after surgery that included LRIs, so I opted for PRK in my first three eyes receiving an Acrysof Restor IOL. I have since performed the Intralase/LASIK procedure in two such patients without incident and will use this approach in the future (Figure 1). For preoperative keratometric astigmatism of greater than 2.50 D, a bioptics approach makes sense.

NO. 6: COMMITMENT AND REASSURANCE

Almost all patients will be very happy with their final surgical outcome. Some may need to wear glasses occasionally or undergo a refractive enhancement procedure. Others may require an IOL exchange if they cannot function adequately with their new multifocal vision system. It may take months for them to experience significant cortical adaptation. Throughout this process and during those many days, surgeons and their staffs should reassure patients that they are committed to achieving a satisfactory visual outcome.

Some patients will not wait months for improvement. Two of my patients waited only 2 months after undergoing implantation of the Acrysof Restor IOL before I had to exchange the lens for a monofocal IOL. These patients could not see well and refused to proceed with surgery on their second eye. One suffered significant positive dysphotopsia, which was only partially improved by the IOL exchange. The other had blurry BCVA at distance and near that the IOL exchange resolved. These patients required numerous surgical visits and additional surgery but were ultimately very satisfied with my staff and me because of our committment and the guidance, reassurance, and treatment they received to get them to the best possible vision they could recover. ■

This article originally appeared in the March 2006 issue of CRSToday.

CHAPTER 160

Pearls for Success With Presbyopia-Correcting IOLs

WILLIAM TRATTLER, MD, AND CARLOS BUZNEGO, MD

In 2005, US ophthalmologists anxiously awaited the release of the latest generation of multifocal IOLs to treat patients with presbyopia. Some surgeons achieved excellent results, whereas others did not. The varying levels of success are intriguing. In our practice, eight surgeons perform cataract surgery. For the first 6 months of 2007, four of the surgeons implanted presbyopia-correcting IOLs in 25% or more of their patients (range, 25% to 37%). In contrast, three other surgeons used presbyopia-correcting lenses in less than 7% (range, 0 to 7%) of their patients. We believe that the aforementioned differences in the level of success can be traced to pre-, intra-, and postoperative management and the setting of realistic postoperative expectations.

PREOPERATIVE PREPARATION AND TESTING

Education

Patients must understand that although current presbyopia-correcting lenses provide an unprecedented range of vision, they are not perfect. Informing patients that they may require glasses in specific situations is important, because surgeons cannot guarantee that patients will be 100% spectacle free after receiving a presbyopia-correcting IOL. Furthermore, patients should know that their reading vision in dim illumination may be less than satisfactory.

Besides these functional issues, patients should also understand that each type of presbyopia-correcting IOL would have different issues that patients need to be made aware of. For example, multifocal IOLs are more often associated with glare, flare, halos, and ghosting than monofocal or accommodating lenses.

Image Quality

Succeeding with multifocal IOLs entails understanding how they work. Essentially, these lenses provide multifocality by splitting light rays into near and distance foci. This diversion of some light rays maximizes the importance of ensuring that the rest of the visual pathway helps provide a high-quality image. Any compromises in image quality on the retina (defocus or opacity) will degrade the quality of vision. Deterioration of the visual processing system (eg, due to irregular corneal astigmatism, macular dysfunction, or optic nerve disease) will compound the reduction of contrast sensitivity from the multifocal optics. Patients with any significant compromise to macular or optic nerve function may be poor candidates for these IOLs.

Corneal Topography

Corneal topography can detect irregular astigmatism, frank and forme fruste keratoconus, and early and frank pellucid marginal degeneration. Because these patients' irregularly shaped corneas will reduce their BCVA, they are less than ideal candidates for presbyopia-correcting IOLs.

Recognizing Macular Dysfunction

Macular dysfunction, whether pre-existing or induced by intraocular surgery, can be a common reason for patient dissatisfaction following the implantation of a presbyopia-correcting IOL. Although some types of macular pathology are visible upon preoperative examination, a number of conditions are subtle and difficult to visualize in the presence of a visually significant cataract. Optical coherence tomography (OCT) of the macula, however, can help identify epiretinal membranes, vitreomacular traction syndrome, and early macular holes. Affected patients need to be educated about their preoperative condition and how it may affect their vision postoperatively.

INTRA- AND POSTOPERATIVE CONSIDERATIONS

Refractive Errors

Residual refractive errors (sphere and cylinder) are among the most obvious contributors to patients' dissatisfaction. Surgeon-specific A-constants, careful measurements of preoperative axial length and the breadth of corneal power, and accurate IOL calculations are critical. Astigmatism significantly degrades visual image quality, especially with multifocal IOLs, which can lead to complaints of poor quality of vision. For this reason, it is important to treat preexisting astigmatism of 0.75 D or more. Performing limbal relaxing incisions (LRIs) at the time of surgery can safely and effectively help these patients. For a large degree of preoperative astigmatism or residual refractive error postoperatively despite the placement of LRIs, surgeons should consider laser vision correction, conductive keratoplasty, or a piggyback IOL.

Cystoid Macular Edema

Small reductions in visual quality are magnified in patients with presbyopia-correcting IOLs, and cystoid macular edema (CME) is one of the most common and visually important causes. Surgeons should make every effort to reduce the risk of macular swelling, which jeopardizes patients' quick and full visual recovery from IOL surgery. A meticulous surgical technique will help to avoid trauma to the iris and capsular rupture, thus minimizing inflammation. Even a technically perfect surgery will liberate prostaglandins, which can induce macular thickening and CME.

NSAIDs

Many cataract surgeons routinely use steroids but not topical NSAIDs. A recent clinical study supports the synergistic effect of ketorolac 0.4% with prednisolone acetate 1% following cataract procedures.[1] In this large multicenter trial of healthy patients with healthy maculas, there was a statistically significant reduction in CME in cataract surgery patients treated with the combination of prednisolone acetate 1% and ketorolac 0.4% versus prednisolone acetate 1% only. The combination group also achieved better contrast sensitivity, particularly important with multifocal IOLs, which—as mentioned—reduce contrast sensitivity.

Dry Eye

Patients who report fluctuating vision may have dry eyes. An examination of their eyelids and ocular surface can reveal signs of dry eye, which can be worse following cataract surgery. The condition is exacerbated by LRIs, which can sever corneal nerves. The options for treatment include anti-inflammatory drops (topical cyclosporine and/or short-term use of a low-dose topical steroid), punctal plugs, and artificial tears.

Follow-Up

Inevitably, some patients will be disappointed with their visual results. In these cases, it is critical to repeat OCT to ensure that their maculas have remained healthy. A careful re-examination of the posterior capsule is also indicated, because mild posterior capsular opacification (which would not affect the vision of a monofocal patient) can reduce these individuals' contrast sensitivity and quality of vision. A YAG capsulotomy can improve their visual acuity and satisfaction.

CONCLUSION

The proper selection and counseling of patients are important to the success of presbyopia-correcting IOLs. Preoperative testing (corneal topography and OCT) will help to ensure that patients' eyes are healthy. The use of pre- and postoperative topical NSAIDs in conjunction with prednisolone acetate 1% can help optimize their quality of vision postoperatively. When patients are dissatisfied postoperatively, it is important to conduct careful evaluations for early posterior capsular opacification and dry eye, because the treatment of these conditions can help improve their visual results. ■

This article originally appeared in the September 2007 issue of CRSToday.

1. Wittpenn J, Silverstein S, Hunkeler J, et al. A masked comparison of Acular LS plus steroid versus steroid alone for the prevention of macular leakage in cataract patients. Presented at: The AAO Annual Meeting; November 12, 2006; Las Vegas, NV.

CHAPTER 161

IOL Power Calculations for Multifocal Lenses

JACK T. HOLLADAY, MD, MSEE

Ophthalmic surgical patients' expectations of multifocal IOLs are high, because they have been promised little-to-no dependence on spectacles or contact lenses postoperatively. Attaining this goal requires eliminating astigmatism and achieving a precise postoperative plano refraction within ±0.25 D. This article describes techniques for determining the proper IOL power for multifocal IOLs.

The accuracy of predicting the necessary power for an IOL is directly related to the accuracy of several measurements.[1,2] They include central corneal refractive power (keratometry readings), axial length (biometry), horizontal corneal diameter (horizontal white-to-white), anterior chamber depth, lenticular thickness, preoperative refraction, and the age of the patient.

UNDERSTANDING EFFECTIVE LENS POSITION

The term *effective lens position* was recommended to the FDA in 1995 to describe the position of an IOL in the eye (Figure 1), because the term *anterior chamber depth* is not anatomically accurate for lenses in the posterior chamber and can confuse the clinician.[3] Ophthalmologists' ability to predict the effective lens position has evolved in accuracy over the years, due both to advancements in formulas and to the technical skills of surgeons who consistently implant IOLs in the capsular bag. We now know that a 20.00 D IOL that is axially displaced by 0.5 mm from the predicted effective lens position will result in approximately 1.00 D of error in the patient's stabilized postoperative refraction. For piggyback lenses totaling 60.00 D, however, a 0.5-mm axial displacement will cause a 3.00 D refractive surprise; the error is directly proportional to the power of the implanted lens. This direct relationship to the power of the lens is why the problem is much less evident in extremely long eyes, because the power of the implanted IOL is so small to achieve emmetropia after cataract extraction.

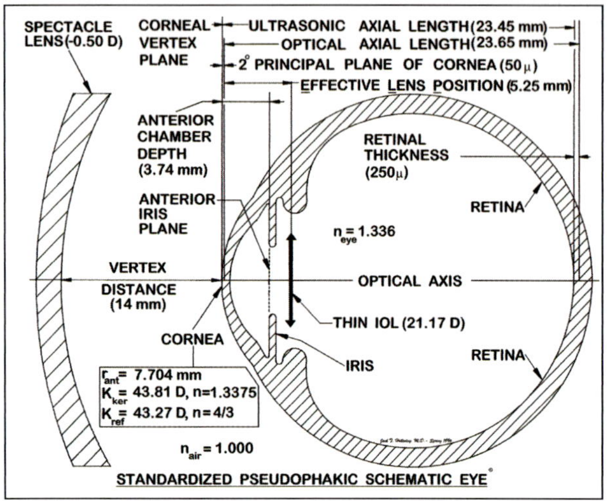

Figure 1. The effective lens position is measured from the corneal vertex plane to the plane of the thin IOL.

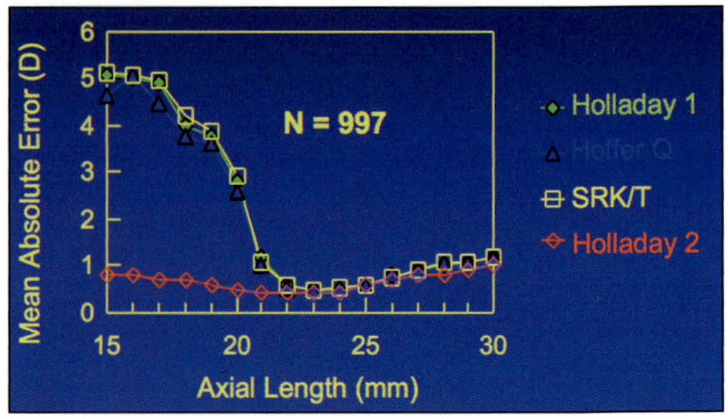

Figure 2. This graph compares the mean absolute predictive error (diopters) of the Holladay 1, Hoffer Q, and SRK/T formulas (two-variable predictors of effective lens position using measurements of keratometry and axial length) with the Holladay 2 formula (seven-variable predictor of effective lens position using measurements of keratometry, white-to-white, anterior chamber depth, lenticular thickness, age, and refraction).

The Holladay 2 formula (Holladay Consulting, Inc., Bellaire, TX) provides more predictable results in normal and unusual eyes than other recent formulas due to its application of seven preoperative variables that my colleagues and I found to be useful for significantly improving the prediction of the effective lens position in eyes ranging from 15 to 35 mm (Figure 2). Once these additional measurements become routine for clinicians, I expect that a new flurry of prediction formulas using seven or more variables will emerge, similar to the activity following our two-variable prediction formula in 1988.[2] The standard of care will reach a new level of predictive accuracy for extremely unusual eyes, just as it has for normal eyes. Calculations on patients with axial lengths of between 22 and 25 mm with corneal powers of between 42.00 and 46.00 D will do well with current third-generation formulas (the Holladay 1,[2] SRK/T,[4] and Hoffer Q[5]). For cases outside this range, the Holladay 2 should be used to ensure accuracy.

PRIMARY CATARACT SURGERY OR REFRACTIVE LENS EXCHANGE

The intraocular power calculations for refractive lens exchange are no different than those for cataract surgery. Refractive lens exchange is usually reserved for patients who are outside the range of other forms of refractive surgery. Consequently, the measurements of axial length, keratometry, and so forth are usually quite different from those in typical cataract surgery patients because of the exceptionally large refractive error and younger age of patients undergoing refractive lens exchange. In most highly myopic eyes, the axial lengths are extremely long (> 26 mm), whereas highly hyperopic eyes have very short axial lengths (< 21 mm).

In eyes with myopia exceeding -20.00 D, removing the crystalline lens often results in postoperative refractions near emmetropia with no IOL. The exact result depends on the power of the cornea and the axial length. The recommended lens powers range from -10.00 to +10.00 D in the majority of these cases. The correct axial length measurement is very difficult to obtain because of the abnormal anatomy of the posterior pole. Staphylomas are frequently present in these eyes, and the macula is often not at the location in the posterior pole where the A-scan measures the axial length[6] (Figure 3).

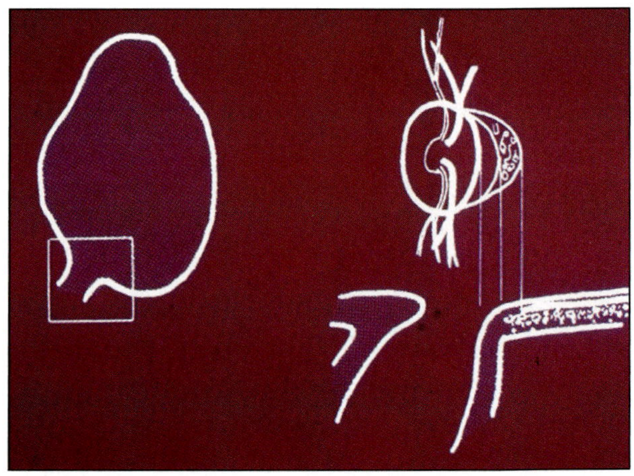

Figure 3. An eye with an axial length of more than 26 mm has a posterior staphyloma, resulting in the anatomic axial length measured from the anterior to posterior poles that is much different than the optical axial length from the corneal vertex to the fovea. (Reprinted with permission from Slack Incorporated. Holladay JT. *Quality of Vision: Essential Optics for the Cataract and Refractive Surgeon*. Thorofare, NJ: Slack Incorporated; 2007:54.)

It is especially important to measure the axial length of highly myopic eyes with optical coherence tomography (IOLMaster; Carl Zeiss Meditec, Inc., Dublin, CA) to ensure a measurement from the macula (fovea) to the corneal vertex. I have personally seen refractive surprises of 3.00 to 4.00 D, because the macula was on the edge of the staphyloma and the A-scan measured to the deepest part of the staphyloma. Such an error results in a hyperopic surprise, because the distance to the macula is much shorter than the distance to the center of the staphyloma. The third-generation theoretical formulas yield excellent results if the axial length measurement is accurate and stable.

In eyes shorter than 21 mm, it is equally important to use optical coherence tomography, because the measurements must be more precise than in normal eyes to achieve the same accuracy in the postoperative refraction.

PIGGYBACKING IOLS TO ACHIEVE POWERS ABOVE 34.00 D

For patients with axial lengths shorter than 21 mm, I recommend performing IOL power calculations with the Holladay 2 formula. In these eyes, the size of the anterior segment is unrelated to the axial length in 80% of cases.[7] Oftentimes, the anterior segment is of normal size, and only the posterior segment is abnormally short. In a few individuals (<20%), however, the anterior segment is proportionately small compared with the axial length (nanophthalmos). The differences in the size of the anterior segment in these cases can cause an average hyperopic error of 5.00 D with third-generation formulas, because they predict that the anterior chamber will be very shallow. Using the newer Holladay 2 formula can reduce the predictive error in these eyes to less than 1.00 D.

Accurate measurements of axial length and corneal power are especially important with piggyback lenses, because any error will be magnified by the extreme dioptric powers of the IOLs. With foldable IOLs, the surgeon places one implant in the bag and the other in the sulcus to avoid interlenticular membranes and posterior capsular opacification. When piggybacking a multifocal IOL, the surgeon may place the lens in front of or behind the monofocal IOL to achieve the best results, although the stronger-powered IOL is usually placed in the bag and the weaker IOL in the sulcus. One should never piggyback two multifocal IOLs, or the near power will be double what was intended. Choosing a monofocal IOL with a lens constant that is equal to the multifocal IOL's reduces the variability in the piggyback calculation.

CHOOSING THE POSTOPERATIVE REFRACTIVE TARGET

Determining the desired postoperative refractive target for multifocal IOLs is slightly different than for monofocal IOLs, where a slight amount of myopia may be beneficial. With the refractive ReZoom multifocal IOL (Advanced Medical Optics, Inc., Santa Ana, CA) and the diffractive AcrySof Restor multifocal IOL (Alcon Laboratories, Inc., Fort Worth, TX), the target should be exactly zero (plano) or the nearest hyperopic choice to zero. Patients' near vision with each of these lenses is excellent, but slight myopia moves the near point too close for comfortable reading.

For the Crystalens accommodating IOL (Eyeonics, Inc., Aliso Viejo, CA), the refractive target may be slightly myopic (-0.50 D) for the patient's "reading eye" to achieve slightly better near vision. This choice must be discussed with patients, however, especially if they may compare their two eyes for distance. They should understand the possibility of a slight sacrifice in depth perception to have near vision in one eye.

PERSONALIZED LENS CONSTANT

Every surgeon who offers premium IOLs (aspheric and multifocal) must personalize his IOL constants for these lenses. Although the design of the IOL is the primary factor in the constant, variations in surgical technique such as the placement of the IOL, the location and design of the incision, and differences in the calibration and design of axiometers and keratometers also affect the personalized lens constant. Most surgeons must perform 20 to 40 cases in order to personalize their lens constant. This process is the only way to achieve superior results with these IOLs and accuracy to within ±0.25 D for 95% of patients.[2,3]

SUMMARY

Optimal refractive outcomes with multifocal IOLs can only be achieved through the selection of appropriate patients, precise measurements with keratometry/topography and axiometry (preferably with the IOLMaster), and the employment of the other five variables discussed herein to ensure the correct sizing of the anterior segment and the accurate prediction of the effective lens position. Personalizing the lens constant is critical to eliminating the systematic variations that are present in all ophthalmic instruments and surgical techniques. Using these techniques will make excellent results and happy patients the rule with multifocal lenses. ■

This article originally appeared in the August 2007 issue of CRSToday.

1. Holladay JT, Prager TC, Ruiz RS, Lewis JW. Improving the predictability of intraocular lens calculations. *Arch Ophthalmol.* 1986;104:539-541.
2. Holladay JT, Prager TC, Chandler TY. A three-part system for refining intraocular lens power calculations. *J Cataract Refract Surg.* 1988;13:17-24.
3. Holladay JT. Standardizing constants for ultrasonic biometry, keratometry and intraocular lens power calculations. *J Cataract Refract Surg.* 1997;23:1356-1370.
4. Retzlaff JA, Sanders DR, Kraff MC. Development of the SRK/T intraocular lens implant power calculation formula. *J Cataract Refract Surg.* 1990;16:333-340.
5. Hoffer KJ. The Hoffer Q formula: a comparison of theoretic and regression formulas. *J Cataract Refract Surg.* 1993;19:700-712.
6. Zaldiver R, Shultz MC, Davidorf JM, Holladay JT. Intraocular lens power calculations in patients with extreme myopia. *J Cataract Refract Surg.* 2000;26:668-674.
7. Holladay JT, Gills JP, Leidlein J, Cherchio M. Achieving emmetropia in extremely short eyes with two piggy-back posterior chamber intraocular lenses. *Ophthalmology.* 1996;103:1118-1123.

CHAPTER 162

Clinical Pearls for Using the Restor

DAVID ALLEN, BSc, FRCS, FRCOphth

European surgeons such as myself have considerable experience with the Acrysof Restor apodized diffractive implant (Alcon Laboratories, Inc., Fort Worth, TX), because the lens received CE Marking that allowed its clinical use in the summer of 2003. Remarkably, the clinical results with the implant have been at least as good as those obtained during the formal studies performed for regulatory approval. I ascribe this success to three factors: the implant's performance, the careful selection of patients, and the surgical technique of the ophthalmologists implanting the IOL.

PATIENT SELECTION

Hyperopes Versus Myopes

Although this IOL provides better reading vision with fewer unwanted visual effects than other bifocal/multifocal IOLs currently on the market (based on data submitted to the FDA in support of approval for the Restor, Array [Advanced Medical Optics, Inc., Santa Ana, CA], and the Crystalens [Eyeonics, Inc., Aliso Viejo, CA]), the careful selection of patients is still important. Candidates must truly wish to be free from spectacles.

Patients who have age-related cataracts and who are hyperopic are the best candidates, because they will be delighted with their postoperative unaided distance vision. Having unaided near vision as well will prompt them to rave about their results to friends and family. I recommend that surgeons first implant the Restor in this subset of patients before working with more challenging patients such as low myopes, who always had unaided near vision until they developed cataracts.

Surgeons should reject patients whom they cannot guarantee a low level of postoperative astigmatism. The clinical studies required less than 1.00 D of preoperative keratometric astigmatism for all subjects. The company now recommends that surgeons use the Restor only when they can reasonably expect to achieve less than 1.00 D of astigmatism postoperatively.

Ophthalmologists may want to consider the Restor for refractive lens exchange, although the FDA has not approved the IOL for this indication. Again, it would be advisable to begin with hyperopes, because this lens will significantly improve their distance vision, even if their final refractive outcome is slightly off target. Myopes without significant astigmatism, however, will have clear, unaided vision at some relatively near distance despite their presbyopia. To satisfy these individuals, the surgeon must obtain an excellent refractive outcome.

Reading Vision

The Restor lens features a 4.00 D add at the IOL plane (around 3.20 D at the spectacle plane). One reason for this relatively large add is that it increases the spatial separation of the two images and therefore decreases the influence of the out-of-focus image on the focused one. As a result, patients' reading distance is best at approximately 31 to 32 cm.

Cataract patients over the age of 60 years have become accustomed to absolute presbyopia and a fixed reading distance of approximately 36cm (with a typical 2.50 or 2.75 D spectacle reading add). Developing presbyopes, on the other hand, have gradually increased their reading distance to compensate for their growing loss of accommodative amplitude and may have become used to a reading distance of arm's length or greater. Practitioners therefore must carefully prepare early presbyopic patients for a dramatic reduction in their best reading distance. In my clinical experience, however, patients' reading distance gradually extends a little and, after a few months, is probably nearer to 34 or 35 cm. The reason for this change is unclear.

SURGICAL CONSIDERATIONS

Binocularity

The binocular implantation of this IOL is recommended by the manufacturer. Most measures of visual function improve when measured binocularly, and patients are generally more comfortable when both of their eyes have broadly similar function. With the Restor, my colleagues and I have found that patients' binocular distance and reading performance is approximately one line better than the best uniocular result. Uniocular implantation in binocular patients is not absolutely contraindicated, but the surgeon and patient need to be aware that the results will not be quite as good.

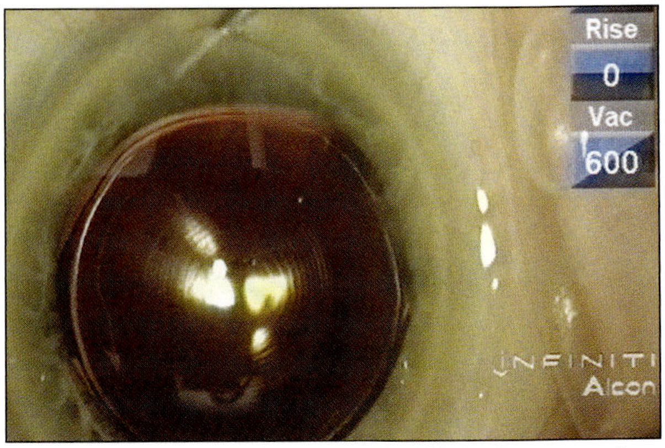

Figure 1. The diffractive grating just visible in the center of the IOL aids in its centration at the end of the procedure.

Planning

Ophthalmologists wishing to use the Restor implant should already have a consistent surgical technique, be familiar with using the Acrysof SA60 platform (Alcon Laboratories, Inc.), and be sure that they and their surgical team can routinely achieve the predicted refractive outcome. If the goal is to leave the patient independent of spectacles, then surgeons must be confident that they normally free patients from glasses for distance vision.

Using the correct A-constant is important. The company recommends an A-constant of 118.4 for ultrasound biometry with the standard SA60 lens but one of 118.2 for the Restor. Surgeons should similarly adjust their individualized A-constants or the one that they employ with the IOLMaster (Carl Zeiss Meditec Inc., Dublin, CA). This change is needed partly because the posterior surface of the IOL was made aspheric to improve the quality of the optical image.

Targeting a postoperative refraction that is slightly hyperopic (0 to +0.50 D) tends to increase patients' reading distance without compromising their unaided distance vision. This technique also reduces the incidence of unwanted nighttime visual phenomena, because the near image is more out of focus.

Technique

The surgical technique is the same as that for implanting a standard SA60 IOL. The capsulorhexis should be centered, round, and 5.0 to 5.5 mm in diameter so that the anterior capsule overlaps the IOL's anterior edge and thus reduces the incidence of posterior capsular opacification. It is best to insert the Restor lens with a cartridge, preferably the Monarch II IOL Delivery System with a B cartridge (Alcon Laboratories, Inc.). When removing the IOL from its packaging and transferring it to the cartridge, the surgeon should be careful to grasp the haptic or, if necessary, the optic close to its edge so as to avoid any possible damage to the diffractive grating, which occupies the central 3.6-mm diameter of the lens' anterior surface. This cartridge will fit snugly into the entrance of a 2.75-mm corneal incision.

It is, of course, important to ensure that the IOL sits securely within the capsule and that all viscoelastic material has been removed. With a strongly cohesive viscoelastic, directly aspirating behind the IOL optic is not necessary if the surgeon rocks and nudges the lens when aspirating the viscoelastic. If using a retentive substance such as Viscoat (Alcon Laboratories, Inc.), then one should directly aspirate the material from behind the optic. Once the haptics have fully returned to their preinsertion configuration, the ophthalmologist should ensure that the IOL's optic is centered, because the position of the lens will not change postoperatively (Figure 1). Regarding the lens' ability to provide two good-quality images, a decentration of up to 1 mm does not degrade optical function, but, in general terms, it is important to ensure the centration of the IOL's optic.

CONCLUSION

Although bifocal and multifocal IOLs have been available in different markets for almost 20 years, they have never had a major impact in terms of the proportion of patients receiving such lens technology. The combination of diffractive optics with apodization present in the Acrysof Restor IOL provided excellent unaided vision and freedom from spectacles for 85% of subjects who received the lens during the FDA clinical trial. This IOL should significantly affect the future of cataract surgery, but it still requires carefully selected patients and a meticulous surgical technique. ■

This article originally appeared in the June 2005 issue of CRSToday.

CHAPTER 163

Deciphering Diffraction

JAMES A. DAVISON, MD

Although light travels in a straight line, when it encounters the edge of an obstruction, it slows and spreads out slightly. This effect is called *diffraction*. It cannot be adequately explained with a ray-tracing model, because ray tracing should only be applied to smooth and continuous optical surfaces. Rays are normally perpendicular to a wavefront at every point, but, if the wavefront encounters an edge, simple ray tracing gives misleading results, because diffractive effects become dominant.

The Acrysof Restor refractive-diffractive IOL (Alcon Laboratories, Inc., Fort Worth, TX) uses a set of circular zones to focus light at two foci. The far focus is at the foveola, and the near focus is approximately 1mm in front of the foveola. There are a number of discontinuities, also known as *diffractive steps* or *zone boundaries*. There are zones between the discontinuities, but these do not act like the zones of a refractive multifocal IOL. That is, they do not alternate far-near-far-near. Instead, the diffractive effects created by the geometry of the steps combine with the refractive lens properties to create a unique design.

THE DESIGN IN DETAIL

The Restor's construction is inherently difficult to represent in a simple fashion for two reasons. First, there are the distractions of too much detail, such as the thickness of the optic, the range of wavelengths for visible light, the refractive indices of the media, and the anatomy of the fovea. Second, there is a huge number of light waves involved. Ignoring those distractions, Figure 1 schematically represents the distance from the lens to the foveola (19 mm) and the distance from the lens to the point of near focus (18 mm) in an emmetropic model eye.

The distances can be measured in wavelengths of light as well. Using green light as an example, there are approximately 46,000 wavelengths of 550-nm light in the vitreous from the lens to the foveola (the far image) and about 44,000 wavelengths from the lens to the add-power focus (the near image), which is approximately 1mm in front of the foveola. Starting at the first diffractive step of the Restor lens and moving radially outward, the location of the second zone boundary is where the difference of the distances between the two foci changes by just one wavelength on the IOL's optic. The other 11 zone boundaries are placed at additional, increasingly peripheral locations of one wavelength of change. As it turns out, in order to keep the same two points of focus (far and near) as zones are added, zone boundaries become progressively closer together peripherally. If the add power were lower, the second focus would move closer to the foveola (eg, it would be at 18.5 mm for a 2.00 D add), and the family of zones would move outward on the lens to maintain the one-wavelength requirement.

The magnitude of these numbers seems incredible, but changes in the optical path length of one wavelength of relating points that

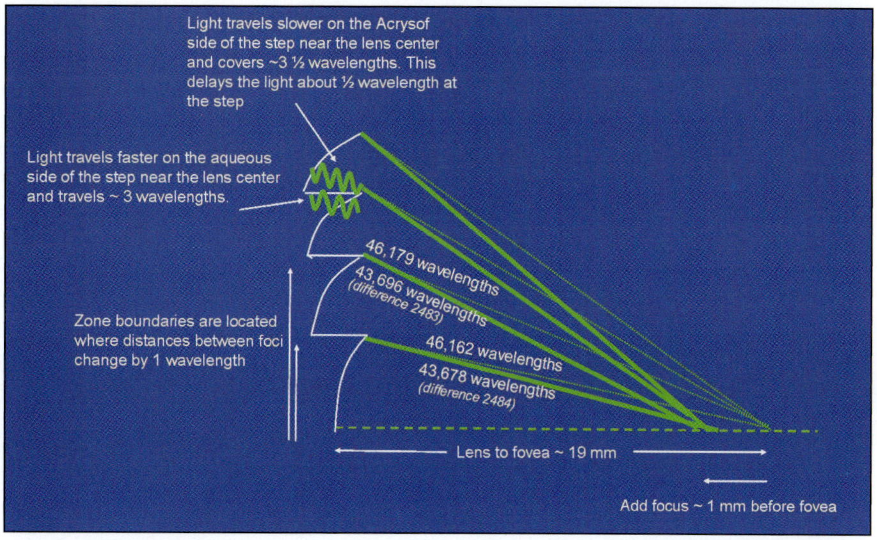

Figure 1. Due to a difference in the speed at which light passes through the plastic side of the step near the lens versus through aqueous, a phase delay creates two points of focus, one for distance and one for near.

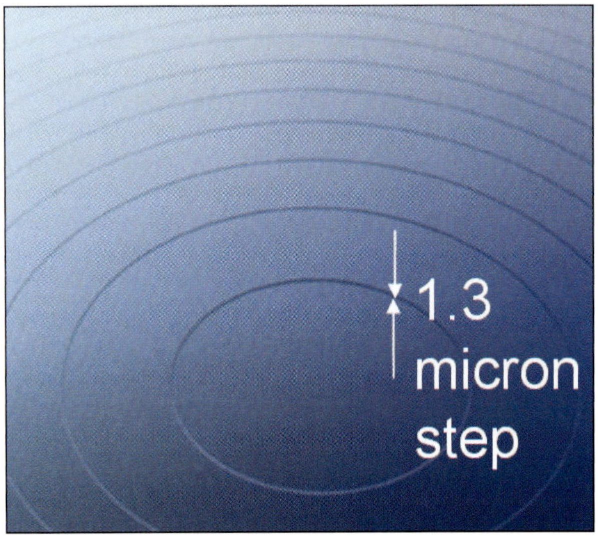

Figure 2. On the apodized diffractive anterior surface, the steps become progressively shorter, from 1.3 to 0.2 µm.

are thousands of wavelengths away specify the widths of the optical zones that lie within the zone boundaries. The engineering of the IOL with regard to these numbers is equally fascinating. That is, the company had to develop a cast-molding process that can reliably produce plastic lenses out of foldable Acrysof lens (Alcon Laboratories, Inc.) material that have step heights of approximately 1.3 µm and gradually decrease in a stepwise fashion to 0.2 µm peripherally. As 1.3 µm equals 1,300 nm, this is little more than two wavelengths of green light in air, or about three wavelengths in aqueous. Two-tenths of a micron is 200 nm or one-half a wavelength of blue light in air.

DIFFRACTIVE STEPS

The diffractive steps introduce phase delays for light at the zone boundaries. The height of the step is a measure of the phase delay, although the entire zone surface changes if the step height is altered. The reason is that, although the optical zones themselves have generally spherical surfaces, they are each composed of individually different curvatures that also differ from the underlying optical base curve of the lens. The characteristics of a diffractive IOL can be seen in the Restor lens' surface (Figure 2). The shape of the surface profile of each zone determines the predominant direction of light passing through the zone, while tiny steps at the zone boundaries adjust the phase of the light. The combination of the zone boundary's placement, the zone's surface profile, and the phase delay at the steps creates the overall optical properties.

The step height can be used as a simple descriptor of the overall optical properties of the Restor IOL. If there were no steps at the zone boundaries, for example, it would be a monofocal lens, and all the light would go to its base power. If the step heights all increased the optical path by one wavelength, then the lens would be monofocal, with all the light going to the add power; in this case, the curvatures of the individual zones would all be identical and similar to those of a refractive lens.

Something that is less obvious is that, if the step heights all increased the optical path by half a wavelength, then approximately 41% of the light would go to each of the two primary lens powers. This is theoretically and practically the best division of light that can be achieved by diffraction alone for two lens powers, and it results from the complex interaction between the zone boundaries'

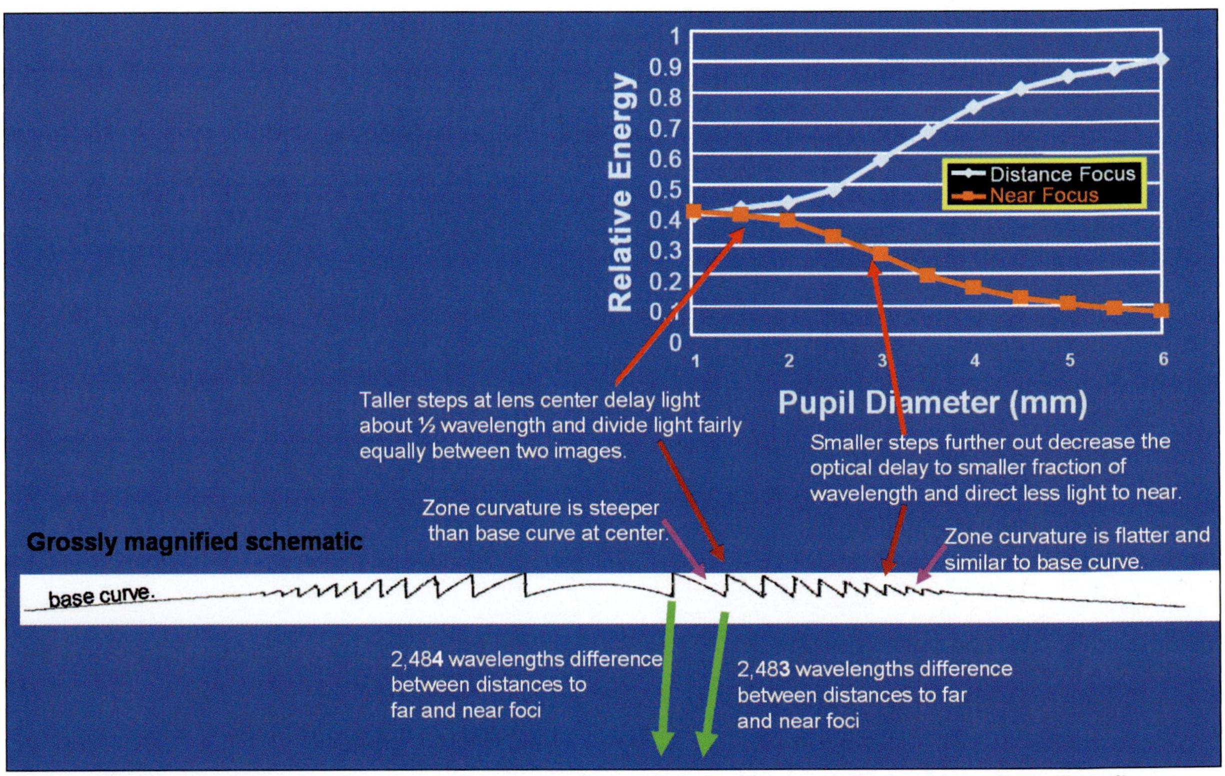

Figure 3. The Restor's apodization virtually equalizes the portions of light for distance and near with small pupillary diameters and increases the contribution for distance vision as the pupil becomes larger and more of the peripheral optic is utilized.

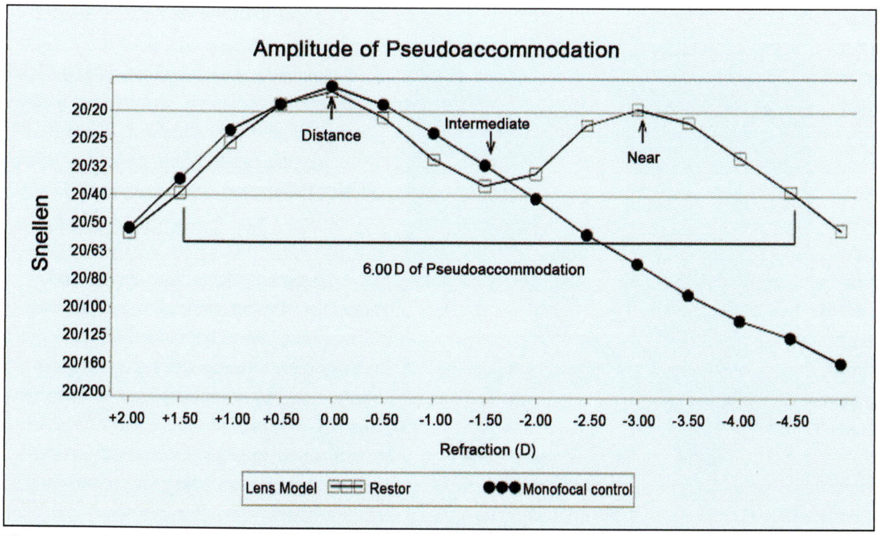

Figure 4. The monofocal IOL's peak performance is with zero diopters in the phoropter. The Restor IOL has two performance peaks, one with zero diopters and the other with -3.00 D dialed into the phoropter, because the lens possesses a plano correction and a +3.00 D correction. The Restor lens has a pseudoaccommodative range of 6.00 D versus 3.50 D for the monofocal IOL.

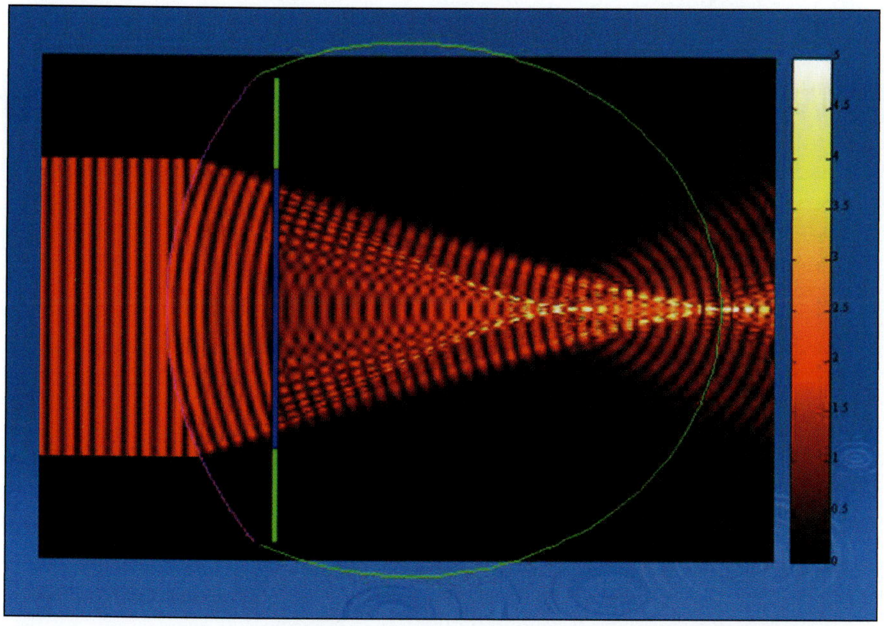

Figure 5. An eye with a 3-mm pupil sees a distant object through the Restor. Half of the light is projected to the foveola, and half is focused at a point 1 mm anterior to the fovea. The latter projection is so far forward that the patient cannot perceive a near image.

locations and the zonal structure. The step height essentially determines how much light goes to each image and provides control over energy balance. The additional light energy goes into other lens powers of -4.00, +8.00, -8.00, and +12.00 D, powers that are related to other image distances that geometrically have integral multiples of optical path distance (three wavelengths, five wavelengths, etc.). The images are not perceived, because they are extremely defocused and their energy is very low.

APODIZATION

Apodization refers to the change of a property across the optical surface from the center to periphery. The term could apply to a filter that is clear in the center and becomes increasingly opaque toward the periphery. In the case of the Restor's optic, the diffractive structure is apodized in order to control light energy's contribution to the two distant and near foci. This concept is illustrated in Figure 3, which compares the exaggerated surface with the approximate energy balance between the two images. Previous diffractive lenses have used the same step height for all the zone boundaries, a design that also makes all the zone curvatures similar to each other. For the Restor lens, with small pupils, the phase delay at the central steps is approximately half a wavelength, which divides the light energy fairly equally between the base and add powers. As pupils become larger, additional zones are used, with the step heights becoming progressively shorter and the zones less steeply curved. The phase delay at the steps is less, because the step heights get shorter, which results in less light's going to the add power and correspondingly more light's being used for far vision. The step heights actually straddle the base curve so that the calculation of the zone boundary's location is not affected by changes in step height.

Two factors are complementary when considering the design: the situations where near vision is used and the visibility of photic phenomena. In general, near vision is important primarily when the pupil is smaller because of normal high illumination levels for near work and the accommodative reflex. Photic phenomena due to the second image are more likely at night when the pupil is larger. The apodization profile for the Restor lens equally distributes energy between the two primary images for smaller pupils, but more light goes to the far lens power as the pupil becomes larger.

The peripherally decreasing step heights reduce the net contribution of energy to near and simultaneously increase the net contribution of energy to distance. In other words, depending on the pupillary diameter, the cumulative effect of the exposed zone surfaces and the step heights at the zone boundaries determines how much light goes to each of the two primary images.

The horizontal pattern of zone boundaries determines the 4.00 D add power in the optic plane (3.20 D in the spectacle plane). The fact that the space between boundaries gets progressively smaller from the optic's center to the periphery of the diffractive, 3.6-mm diameter is necessary to define the two focal points consistently across the optic. Put another way, the pattern of decreasing step widths is the necessary diffractive pattern to maintain the two focal points, both foveal and 1mm anterior to the fovea.

RANGE OF FOCUS

An increased depth of field can yield a pseudoaccommodative visual performance. The Restor lens has two fixed primary powers where retinal focus is sharpest and best acuity can be achieved. It also provides good visual acuity for two ranges of object distances. The midpoint of each range is each of the primary best-focusing distances. Figure 4 shows defocus curves measured in the phoropter that compare the Restor lens to a monofocal control. Far vision ranges are comparable for both lenses, but the Restor lens provides an additional range of vision around the best near focus of 32cm. Both primary lens powers of the Restor lens contribute to intermediate distance vision. With the Restor, the expanded performance of near and intermediate depths of field improves patients' vision of everything within arm's length.

The change in the intensity of defocused light varies with the type of object and other parameters. For a point source, the light from the second power has less than 1% of the intensity of the focused spot. For a line or other object, it may be 2% to 3%. The human visual system is designed to pick out structure in a scene and to ignore other optical phenomena, which arise normally in the phakic eye due to corneal tear film effects, dryness, and swelling; floaters; and other phenomena. Faint, secondary, defocused light is rarely noticeable, although it is more likely to be visible at night, when there are bright point sources against a dark background.

Restor patients do not report a loss of light, although the energy's focus is split between the two images. Human vision is very tolerant of the continual changes in light energy upon fluctuations in pupillary diameter and in illumination. The eye seeks details of interest and ignores modest changes in intensity. Objects are visible under luminance changes of more than a factor of 1 million, from a lighted office to outdoor sunshine. An intensity change of a factor of 2 is not normally noticeable.

ANALOGIES

Two analogies can describe diffraction. The first is sound waves traveling down a hall, encountering a corner, and then slowing and spreading out so that the sound wave travels around the corner and is heard 90° from the wave's original direction. The second analogy is not exactly correct but may be used to conceptualize light in its particulate form as photons and to compare it to atmospheric gas molecules as air. An air-vent diffuser in an automobile dashboard that directs air straight outward without deflection is analogous to distance vision, where the light is directed to the distance focal point at the fovea. The diffusers can be aimed downward to deflect the air stream in that direction, similar to if most of the light were deflected toward the shorter near focal point 1mm in front of the fovea. The diffuser can be placed in an in-between position so that half of the air is directed straight outward and half of it is deflected toward the near lower point. The Restor's refractive-apodized diffractive optic accomplishes the same objective in its most central zones by dividing the light wavefront so that half of it goes to the distance foveal focus point and half of it goes to the near point 1mm in front of it (Figure 5).

CONCLUSION

The Restor IOL represents a revolutionary integration of apodized diffractive structure on a platform with which ophthalmologists are familiar. Combined with the consistent centration of the Acrysof single-piece IOL, this new technology offers surgeons the opportunity to dramatically and almost immediately improve the quality of most patients' distance, near, and intermediate vision through lens replacement surgery. ■

This article originally appeared in the June 2005 issue of CRSToday.

CHAPTER 164

Centration and Diffractive Multifocal IOLs

JACK T. HOLLADAY, MD, MSEE

The Acrysof Restor (Alcon Laboratories, Inc., Fort Worth, TX) and Tecnis Multifocal (Advanced Medical Optics, Inc., Santa Ana, CA; not FDA approved) IOLs both use diffractive optics, as do other multifocal lenses available internationally. It is crucial to center on the pupil (rather than the center of the bag) all IOLs using this optic design.

REFRACTIVE VERSUS DIFFRACTIVE OPTICS

Lenses such as the Rezoom (Advanced Medical Optics, Inc.) use aspheric refractive zones and all of the available light to create multifocality. The Rezoom lens in particular was designed to provide patients with vision at all distances, with a balance that slightly favors distance and intermediate vision.

Diffractive multifocal lenses use higher-order optics to create two focal points, one at distance and one at near. The Acrysof Restor lens provides approximately a 3.00 D add (working distance of 33.00 cm or 13.13 inches) at the spectacle plane. The design emphasizes distance and near and provides a lesser visual performance at intermediate distances. The Rezoom lens provides approximately 2.70 D (working distance of 37.00 cm or 14.58 inches). The design emphasizes distance and intermediate vision. Diffractive IOLs generally use 40% of the available light for distance and 40% for a second focal point. The remaining 20% is lost to destructive interference.

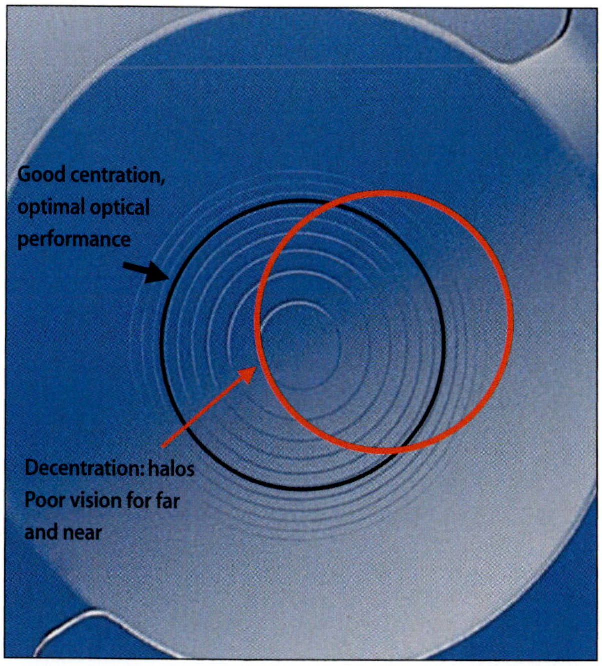

Figure 1. Good centration of the IOL with respect to the pupil (black arrow and circle) optimizes the lens' performance. Decentration (red arrow and circle) results in halos and poor vision at far and near.

The spacing and height of the rings that create the images for the bifocal IOLs determine the location of the focal points and the balance of light between them. Because tilting and decentration affect the rings' effective spacing and height to a much greater extent than refraction, the slight decentration or tilting of the IOL has a more significant effect on visual outcomes with diffractive versus refractive multifocal lenses. It is therefore imperative that the former be centered on the pupil.

CENTRATION

Paolo Vinciguerra, MD, first presented the issue of decentered diffractive multifocal IOLs in 2005.[1] He shared three cases of patients with these lenses whose visual performance was problematic due to the IOLs' decentration with respect to the pupil (Figures 1 and 2). In addition, he demonstrated simple techniques for recentering the lenses during the primary surgery and in the early postoperative period.

The Nidek OPD Scan (Nidek, Inc., Fremont, CA), unlike Hartmann-Shack or Tscherning wavefront analyzers, can measure the eye's wavefront optical performance using skiascopy reflexes, similar to retinoscopy. Using the Nidek OPD Scan, Dr. Vinciguerra could confirm the significant reduction in optical performance with a decentered diffractive multifocal lens and the subsequent improvement after the IOL's recentration on the pupil. In addition, he showed that the patients' visual acuity improved and their symptoms resolved. Marie Jose Tassignon of Antwerp, Belgium, also confirmed the problem with centration using the Tracey Wavefront System (Tracey Technologies, Houston, TX).[2]

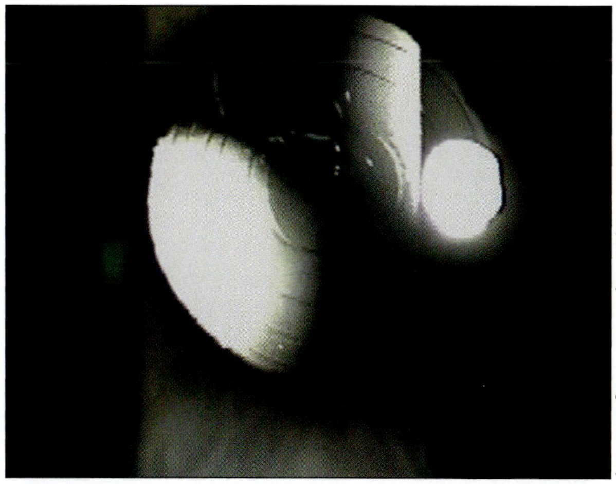

(Courtesy of Paolo Vinciguerra, MD.)

Figure 2. The IOL's diffractive rings are perfectly concentric with the pupil.

TECHNIQUE

The slight decentration of an IOL with respect to the pupil is common, because the pupillary center is nasal to the optical center of the eye (the geometric center of the cornea, crystalline lens, and bag after nuclear and cortical removal). A lens placed and centered in the capsular bag will almost always be temporal to the center of the pupil (0.3 mm on average).

Dr. Vinciguerra recommends that surgeons implanting diffractive multifocal IOLs place the haptics vertically at the 12- and 6-o'clock positions so that the lens can be slightly decentered nasally in the bag. Placing the haptics horizontally causes the IOL to return to the geometrically horizontal center. At the end of surgery, the lens optic will be slightly nasal in the bag when the diffractive rings are concentric with the pupil. Dr. Vinciguerra has shown that this technique eliminates problems with the lenses' optical performance. If he notes that the IOL is slightly decentered during the first postoperative week and the patient's visual performance is compromised, he will push the lens nasally to the center of the pupil while the patient is at the slit lamp.

CONCLUSION

Centering diffractive multifocal IOLs on the pupil is critical to their optimal performance. Although they are less sensitive to decentration, refractive multifocal IOLs should also be centered on the pupil, because severe cases of decentration can increase the lens' effective power and induce astigmatism and coma. ■

This article originally appeared in the April 2006 issue of CRSToday.

1. Vinciguerra P, Epstein D. Correction of presbyopia in cataract surgery. Paper presented at: The Refractive On-Line Symposium; September 15, 2005; Milan, Italy.
2. Tassignon MJ. Centration of multifocal IOLs. Paper presented at: World Ophthalmology Congress; February 23, 2006; São Paulo, Brazil.

CHAPTER 165

Experience With the Rezoom IOL

H. BURKHARD DICK, MD

Newly approved by the FDA, the Rezoom hydrophobic acrylic multifocal IOL (Advanced Medical Optics, Inc., Santa Ana, CA) has a 6-mm optic featuring five zones optimized and proportioned to provide good visual function across a range of distances. After implanting more than 40 of these IOLs, I have found the lens to be an improvement on the Array multifocal IOL (Advanced Medical Optics, Inc.).

LENS DESIGN

The five concentric, refractive zones provide true multifocal vision: zones 1, 3, and 5 are distance dominant; zones 2 and 4 are near dominant; and an aspheric transition between zones provides balanced intermediate vision. The second optical zone provides a sufficiently large near add. The IOL's Balanced View Optics Technology provides expanded distance-dominant zones and light distribution for good vision under a broad range of lighting conditions. The Rezoom IOL works satisfactorily at intermediate distance and under dim lighting conditions, an especially important capability for computer work.

I prefer an optic edge design that provides an uninterrupted 360° barrier against lens epithelial cell migration and is designed to minimize edge glare.[1,2] The Optiedge design (Advanced Medical Optics, Inc.), which has been incorporated into the Rezoom IOL, decreases the intensity of reflected images tremendously compared with square-edge designs.[3]

Surgeons already familiar with the Sensar three-piece monofocal IOL (Advanced Medical Optics, Inc.) should find the Rezoom lens easy to use, because the two IOLs' A-constants are the same and they unfold in the eye similarly. Additionally, the Unfolder Emerald injector system (Advanced Medical Optics, Inc.) allows the Rezoom to be implanted through a 2.7-mm incision. I have found that this IOL centers perfectly. In a rare case of capsular rupture with vitreous loss, the lens may be fixated in the sulcus.

Capsular fibrosis with this hydrophobic acrylic lens material was very low.[1,4] Moreover, with a low rate of posterior capsular opacification, the near portion of the lens' optic is not obscured by fibrosis. As a result, patients' reading capability should last longer compared with the silicone optic of the Array lens.[4] Rezoom patients' near visual acuity should remain stable for a long time.

STUDY RESULTS

I conducted a prospective, randomized, masked clinical trial to compare the Rezoom (n = 24) and the first-generation Array (n = 18) IOLs. Outcomes with the former proved superior in several regards.

The mean defocus acuity curves for both IOLs were similar; they demonstrated acceptable near vision and excellent intermediate vision, which is not achieved with current diffractive multifocal IOL designs. Patients who received the Rezoom lens reported that they saw comfortably without glasses at distance (100%), intermediate distance (95%), and near (71%). Sixty-seven percent of my Rezoom patients never wore glasses at 6 months postoperatively. All Rezoom patients reported driving easily, and they expressed great satisfaction with their depth and color perception, neither of which deteriorated during 6 months of follow-up.

Regarding distance-corrected near visual acuity, 83.3% of Rezoom patients saw 20/40 or better. The group's mean binocular distance UCVA was 20/20, and the mean binocular distance BCVA was 20/17. These patients' mean near UCVA at 40cm was 20/42, and their distance-corrected visual acuity at 40cm was 20/35. All Rezoom eyes had a binocular distance BCVA of 20/25 or better.

Compared to the Array IOL, the Rezoom IOL produced fewer photic phenomena. Specifically, the incidence of halos with the Rezoom was one-third that with the Array lens. The former was also associated with distinctly fewer incidences of starbursts. No Rezoom patient complained of severe halos, double vision, blurred near or far vision, or starbursts. Only one reported moderate starbursts for one eye.

CONCLUSION

Photic phenomena were less of a problem with the Rezoom IOL versus the first-generation multifocal Array lens. The latter is one of the few IOLs investigated thoroughly enough to provide practitioners with an excellent understanding of its functionality. I do not doubt that the Rezoom lens will be of benefit to my patients. ■

This article originally appeared in the June 2005 issue of CRSToday.

1. Buehl W, Findl O, Menapace R, et al. Effect of an acrylic intraocular lens with a sharp posterior optic edge on posterior capsule opacification. *J Cataract Refract Surg.* 2002;28:1105-1111.
2. Ellis MF. Sharp-edged intraocular lens design as a cause of permanent glare. *J Cataract Refract Surg.* 2001;27:1061-1064.
3. Franchini A, Gallarti BZ, Vaccari E. Computerized analysis of the effects of intraocular lens edge design on the quality of vision in pseudophakic patients. *J Cataract Refract Surg.* 2003;29:342-347.
4. Sacu S, Menapace R, Buehl W, et al. Effect of intraocular lens optic edge design and material on fibrotic capsule opacification and capsulorhexis contraction. *J Cataract Refract Surg.* 2004;30:1875-1882.

CHAPTER 166

The Tecnis Multifocal IOL

MANFRED R. TETZ, MD

The Tecnis Multifocal lens (not currently approved by the FDA; Advanced Medical Optics, Inc., Santa Ana, CA) has enhanced ophthalmologists' IOL options. Not only does this lens perform as a foldable, diffractive, multifocal IOL with an improved near addition, its optic also incorporates "intelligent asphericity" to counteract most corneal spherical aberrations. I now have more than 1 year's clinical experience with this lens.

DESIGN

The Tecnis Multifocal IOL is based on the aspheric optic design of the Tecnis IOL (Advanced Medical Optics, Inc.), which was engineered to reduce the spherical aberration of an average cornea. Based on a principle of diffraction—as is the Acrysof Restor IOL (Alcon Laboratories, Inc., Fort Worth, TX)—the Tecnis Multifocal IOL features diffractive rings on its posterior surface. The lens provides patients with a near and a distant focus, each of which is distinct. The rings start very close to the optic's center and then continue out toward the periphery, usually with an increasing distance between the rings. As a result, the multifocal effect's dependence on the pupil is limited. Even in the presence of relatively small pupils, this IOL provides excellent near vision.

INNOVATIVE TECHNOLOGY

The best innovation of the Tecnis Multifocal IOL lies in its combination of two optical principles: multifocality and an "intelligent" prolate, anterior, optical surface. Whereas multifocal IOLs have been known for reducing patients' contrast sensitivity (a loss inherent in the optical principle of multifocality), the Tecnis IOL improves contrast by reducing higher-order aberrations compared with a normal monofocal optic. Investigators are conducting tests of this lens with simulations of driving during the day and night[1] (Figure 1). One can therefore anticipate that the multifocal version of this lens will also offer benefits with regard to contrast sensitivity.

The amount of near addition that can be incorporated into either a refractive or diffractive lens appears to be limited. A refractive multifocal lens such as the Rezoom (Advanced Medical Optics, Inc.) has 3.50 D at the lens level, approximately 2.80 D on the corneal plane, and about 2.40 D on the spectacle plane. Diffractive lenses such as the Acrysof Restor and the Tecnis Multifocal are 4.00 D on the IOL plane, an amount that is equivalent to 3.00 D at the spectacle plane. Both IOLs therefore provide a superior near focus to that of refractive multifocal lenses; even if the final IOL power is a little off (eg, +0.25 or even +0.50 D), these diffractive multifocal IOLs still work efficiently.

The injectors for silicone IOLs from Advanced Medical Optics, Inc., work perfectly with the Tecnis line of IOLs, and the company's three versions of Healon may all be used.

CLINICAL RESULTS

A series of clinical studies[2-4] has demonstrated the excellent performance of the Tecnis monofocal IOL under mesopic and scotopic lighting conditions.

My results with the Tecnis Multifocal IOL during the past year have shown the lens to be especially effective in emmetropic and hyperopic presbyopes, because their corneas seem to be closer to the average corneal asphericity incorporated into the design of the lens. These patients' reading capabilities are excellent.

As for optical aberrations, every lens with more than one focus will be associated with some degree of glare or halos, because one image is laid over another. It may be that patients who receive the Tecnis Multifocal and whose corneas fit the parameters considered typical by the designers of the aspheric Tecnis platform will be less affected by halos. Regardless, this multifocal lens should be an excellent option for patients with hyperopic or emmetropic presbyopia who are undergoing cataract surgery or refractive lens exchange. ■

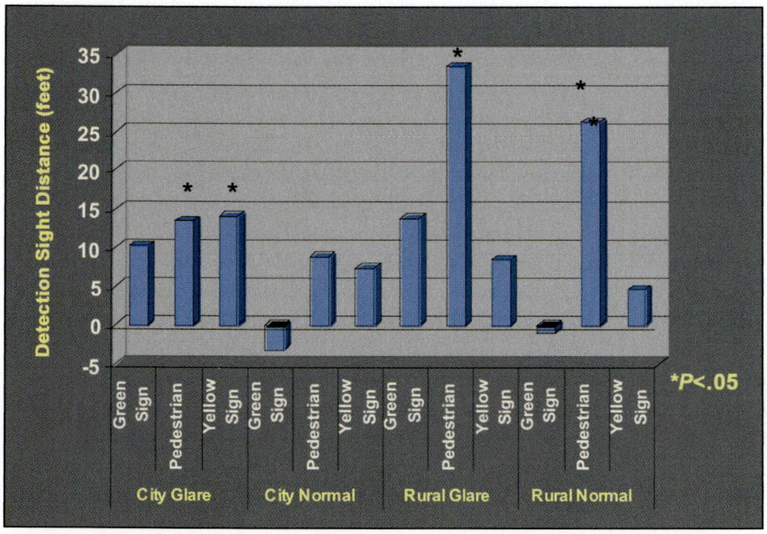

Figure 1. This graph shows the difference in patients' detection of objects using the wavefront-corrected Tecnis IOL versus a standard IOL. Positive bars indicate subjects' earlier detection of a target with the Tecnis versus the standard IOL.

This article originally appeared in the June 2005 issue of CRSToday.

1. Javitt J. Wavefront-corrected IOL (Tecnis Z9000) is associated with improved driving safety. Paper presented at: The 18th Congress of German Ophthalmic Surgeons (DOG); June 25, 2004; Nürnberg, Germany.
2. Mester U, Dillinger P, Anterist N. Impact of a modified optic design on visual function: clinical comparative study. *J Cataract Refract Surg.* 2003;29:652-660.
3. Chierego C, Scialdone A, Belluci R, Buratto L. Contrast sensitivity with Tecnis and with conventional IOL. Paper presented at: The XX Congress of the ESCRS; September 10, 2002; Nice, France.
4. Packer M, Fine IH, Hoffman RS, Piers PA. Improved functional vision with a modified prolate intraocular lens. *J Cataract Refract Surg.* 2004;30:986-992.

CHAPTER 167

Neural Adaptation to Aberrations

PABLO ARTAL, PhD

In healthy individuals, the visual system provides clear images of viewed objects despite optical aberrations that blur the retinal image.[1,2] Every eye is affected by specific aberrations that produce a particular light pattern on the retina of an object point: the point spread function. If the brain adjusts for a given eye's aberrations, the individual's vision should be clearest when looking through his usual aberrations rather than through unfamiliar optics. If this theory is correct, it has important implications for ophthalmology, especially with regard to procedures that modify the eye's optical properties such as refractive and cataract surgeries.

BACKGROUND

Neural adaptation and plasticity play a major role in many important visual tasks, and clinicians have capitalized on these properties for centuries. Many patients' complaints about unwanted visual phenomena disappear without any apparent reason except the passage of time. Common circumstances in which the visual system adjusts include the mechanisms of blur adaptation[3] and the adaptation to color or to distortions in the visual field. Similarly, a popular treatment for presbyopia is progressive addition lenses. Initially, most subjects notice the evident distortions in the retinal image caused by the lenses' optical surfaces.[4] After several days, these problems tend to disappear, and many patients are satisfied with this corrective modality.

RESEARCH

Several years ago, my colleagues and I sought to determine whether the visual system actually adapted to the eye's optical aberrations. We employed adaptive optics in our controlled, collaborative experiment with David Williams, PhD, at the University of Rochester in New York.[5] In addition to high-resolution retinal imaging, adaptive optics for vision can produce controlled patterns of aberration in the eye of a subject.

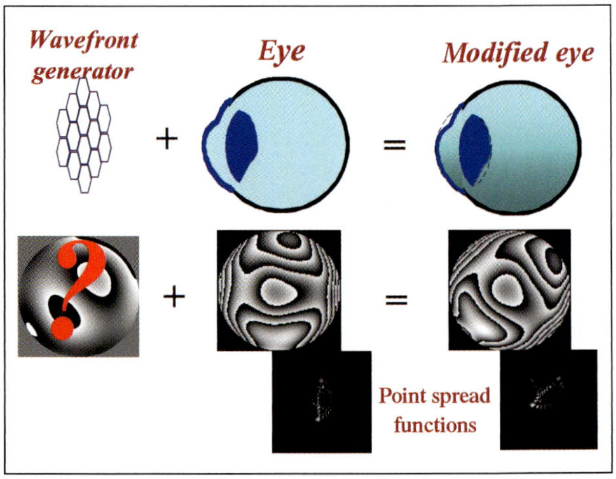

Figure 1. Aberrations and the point spread function are rotated using adaptive optics.

In our experiment, we conducted subjective blur matching with normal and rotated aberrations. The adaptive optics system consisted of a real-time wavefront sensor to measure the eye's aberrations and a deformable mirror to modify the aberrations. A visual channel presented a stimulus to the subject. With this instrument, we were able to rotate the aberrations (and the point spread functions) of the subject by maintaining their magnitude (Figure 1). We asked subjects to view a binary noise stimulus through the system, either with their natural aberrations or with a rotated version of their aberrations. They viewed the stimulus alternately for 500 milliseconds with both the normal and the rotated point spread function. The subjects' task was to adjust the magnitude of the aberrations to match the subjective blur of the stimulus to that seen when the wave aberration was in its normal orientation.

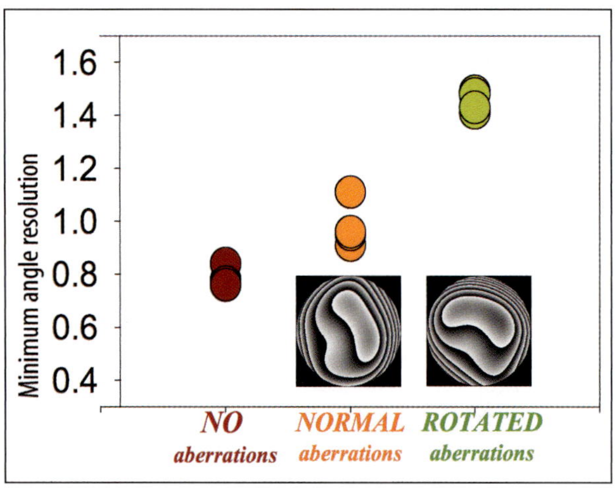

Figure 2. The visual acuity (expressed in minutes of arc) of the author's right eye is measured for corrected (brown), normal (orange), and rotated aberrations (green).

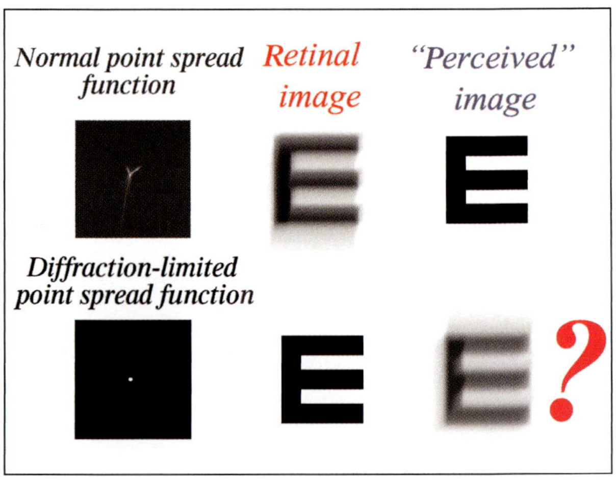

Figure 3. This cartoonish schematic diagram shows the possible effect of neural adaptation on the retinal images before and after their ideal correction.

In all subjects, the wavefront error of the rotated wave aberration required to match the blur with the normal wave aberration was less than in the normally oriented aberration case. This finding indicates that the subjective blur for the stimulus increased significantly when the point spread function was rotated.

We also measured visual acuity for different aberration profiles. Figure 2 shows, as an example, one subject's visual acuity expressed as a minimum angle of resolution in minutes of arc without any aberration, with the normal aberrations, and with the rotated aberrations. The subject's performance was lowest with the rotated version of the aberrations.

CONCLUSION

It is important to note the role of time in neural adaptation. Moreover, although it is obvious that the visual system cannot deal with a very large amount of aberrations, it is also relevant to understand the amount of aberrations that is required to induce the adaptation.

In the area of wavefront-guided, customized refractive surgery, neural adaptation to aberrations will reduce the immediate benefit to the patient of attempts to surgically produce diffraction-limited eyes. The reason is that the brain has adapted to a particular pattern of aberrations. After surgery, the neural compensation will still be acting for the previous pattern. Figure 3 simulates the possible effect. If the brain restores the degraded image, it will also initially degrade a perfect retinal image. Again, the importance of this action in practical terms depends on the time required to reverse the previous adaptation and to allow the visual system to adapt to the newly induced aberrations.

With IOLs, ophthalmologists are currently deeply interested in mixing and matching lenses in patients' eyes to increase their overall depth of focus. The role of neural adaptation in this approach is probably very important but related to binocular vision. The scenario is complex, involving both monocular aberrations and binocular interactions. More experiments are required, for example, to provide a better understanding of binocular performance as a function of individual or binocular aberrations. The use of adaptive optics extended to binocular applications can answer many questions. This exciting area of research should ultimately help clinicians provide patients with a superior quality of vision. ■

This article originally appeared in the August 2007 issue of CRSToday.

1. Artal P, Guirao A, Berrio E, Williams DR. Compensation of corneal aberrations by the internal optics in the human eye. *J Vis.* 2001;1:1-8.
2. Artal P, Benito A, Tabernero J. The human eye is an example of robust optical design. *J Vis.* 2006;6:1-7.
3. Webster MA, Georgeson MA, Webster SM. Neural adjustments to image blur. *Nat Neurosci.* 2002;5:839-849.
4. Villegas EA, Artal P. Comparison of aberrations in different types of progressive power lenses. *Ophthalmic Physiol Opt.* 2004;24:419-426.
5. Artal P, Chen L, Fernández EJ, et al. Neural compensation for the eye's optical aberrations. *J Vis.* 2004;4:281-287.

CHAPTER 168

Seven Tips for Successfully Implanting the Crystalens

D. MICHAEL COLVARD, MD

The Crystalens (Bausch & Lomb, Rochester, NY) can provide cataract surgery patients with a full and improved range of visual function without reducing the quality of their vision. Patients need not endure a period of neuroadaptation postoperatively, and their dependence on spectacles generally decreases after the IOL's implantation.

Achieving optimal results with the Crystalens HD or Five-O, however, requires you to pay greater attention to detail than is customary with monofocal lenses. IOL surgery for presbyopic correction is intrinsically a refractive procedure. The level of patients' satisfaction with the Crystalens depends on your ability to achieve a desired refractive outcome. To give patients the highest level of spectacle independence, you must manage their astigmatism effectively and provide them with their best possible UCVA. Here are several tips I have found helpful in achieving this goal.

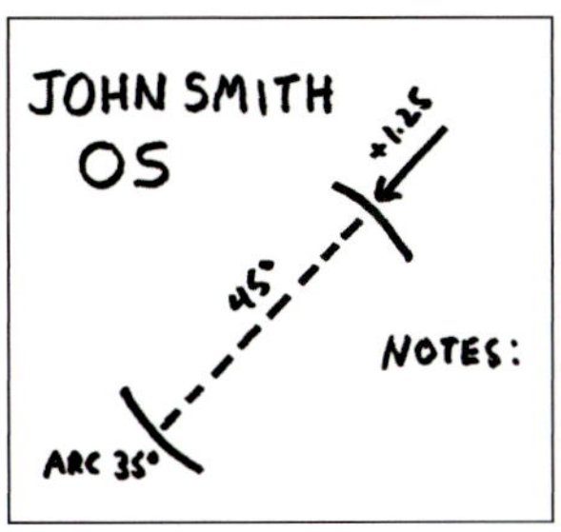

Figure 1. Create a diagram of the planned location of the primary incision and of the location and size of LRIs.

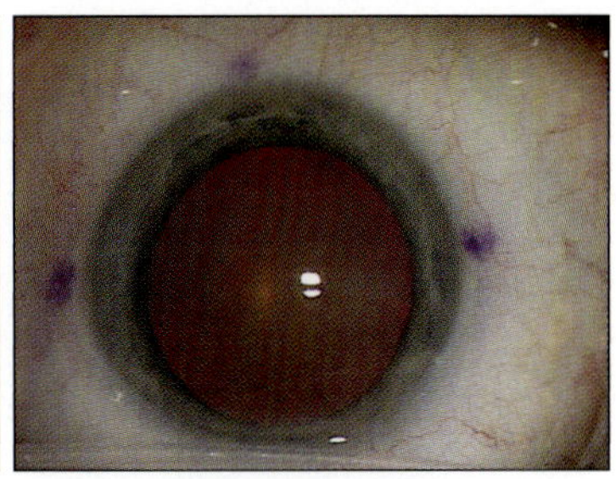

Figure 2. Mark the 0°, 180°, and 270° axes while the patient is upright.

TIP No. 1. MAKE A DETAILED DIAGRAM OF YOUR PLAN FOR MANAGING ASTIGMATISM

There is a general perception among ophthalmologists that limbal relaxing incisions (LRIs) are forgiving and therefore do not have to be very precise. Only the first part of this statement is true. LRIs are maximally effective only if they are placed in the proper location(s) and subtend the correct arc(s). It is useful to make a diagram based on keratometric and topographic findings that exactly describes your plan for surgically managing astigmatism (Figure 1). This drawing should describe the planned location of your primary incision and the size and exact location of the LRIs. I tape the diagram to the microscope or on the wall next to the patient before

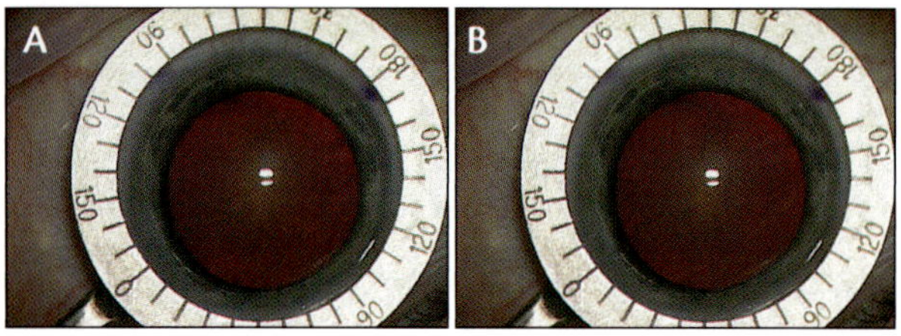

Figure 3. Using the horizontal and vertical markings to position the axis indicator (A), establish the location of the steep axis and LRIs under the microscope (B).

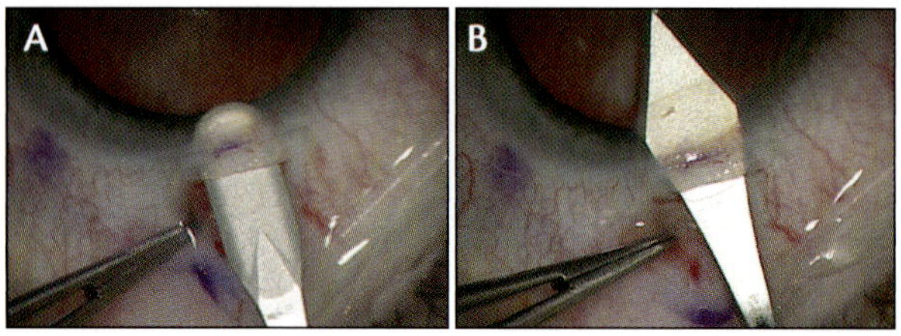

Figure 4. Use a scleral tunnel or a sutured corneal incision to ensure absolute stability of the anterior chamber. A well-constructed scleral tunnel incision started 1 to 2 mm posterior to the limbus (A) and carried at least 1.5 mm into clear cornea (B) usually does not require a suture.

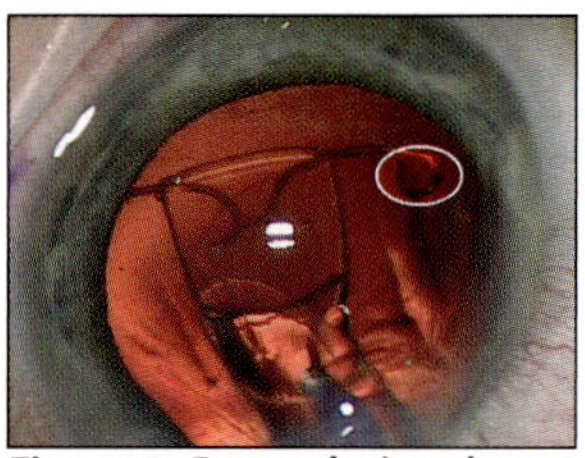

Figure 5. Pause during the Crystalens' insertion to inspect its distal polyamide haptics in order not to insert the IOL upside down. The round tip should always be on the right.

each case so that I know precisely what I need to do once I sit down. If you prefer to operate on the steep axis whenever possible (as I do), the diagram also helps the nurses to orient the microscope correctly before you enter the room.

TIP No. 2. MARK THE HORIZONTAL AND VERTICAL AXES PREOPERATIVELY WHILE THE PATIENT IS IN A SEATED POSITION

It is important to establish precisely the primary horizontal and vertical axes before the patient lies down. One approach is simply to touch the sclera with a surgical marking pen at the limbus at 0°, 180°, and 270° while the patient is sitting upright outside the OR (Figure 2). Once you begin to mark these axes preoperatively, you will quickly realize that cyclotorsion is not inconsequential. For a majority of patients in the supine position, the eye experiences a downward temporal rotation of approximately 20°. Failure to take cyclotorsion into account guarantees that you will place your LRIs in the wrong axis and that their effectiveness will be reduced.

TIP No. 3. MARK THE LOCATION OF THE STEEP AXIS AND THE LOCATION AND EXTENT OF LRIs UNDER THE MICROSCOPE

Once the patient has lain down and is in position under the microscope, use the horizontal and vertical markings you made preoperatively to position the axis indicator (Figure 3). If you prefer to operate on the steep axis, mark its location for the primary incision and the location and size of the LRI(s). If you always prefer to operate temporally, mark only the location and extent of the LRIs. It should be understood that, when placed off axis, even a small, relatively astigmatically neutral temporal incision may produce vectors of force that can influence the final postoperative astigmatic outcome. It is for this reason that I prefer to operate on the steep axis whenever doing so is feasible.

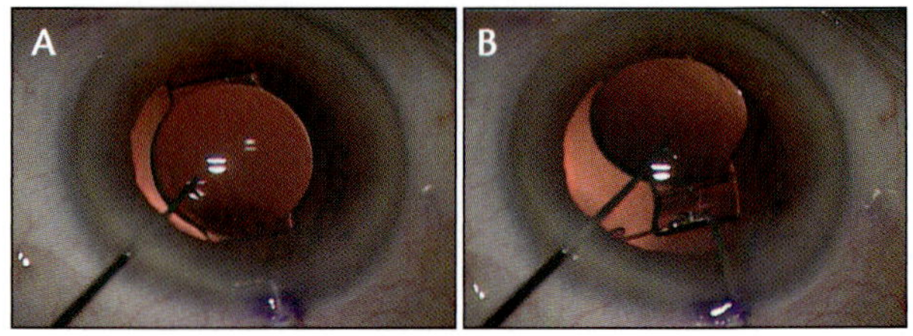

Figure 6. For capsular placement of the IOL, inject the distal haptics into the bag and "park" the proximal haptics in the anterior chamber on the anterior surface of the iris (A). Then, lift the optic with an instrument through the sideport, fold the proximal haptic inferiorly, and gently drop the IOL into the bag (B).

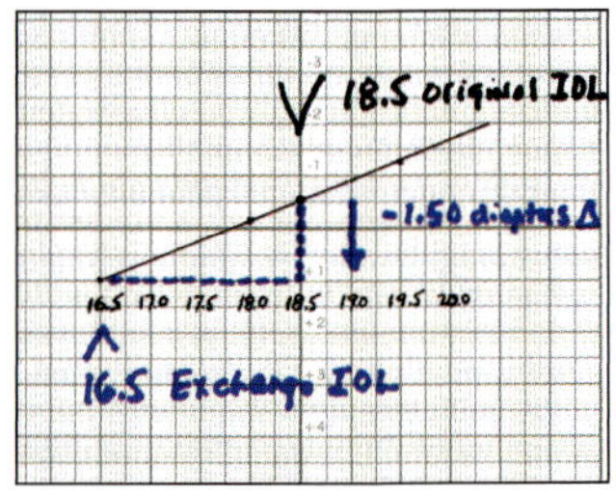

Figure 7. Use a dioptric power graph to select the proper IOL for exchange. Plot the preoperative biometric data by placing the range of dioptric powers on the abscissa and the range of predicted refractive outcomes on the ordinate. Decide the amount of refractive change you desire and select the new IOL power by dropping down the ordinate to correct a myopic error or moving up the ordinate to correct a hyperopic error.

TIP No. 4. CONSTRUCT A WATERTIGHT INCISION

The slightest bit of shallowing of the anterior chamber postoperatively can result in a forward vaulting of the Crystalens and the induction of myopia. The primary incision must be watertight, and sideport incisions must be beveled and well hydrated at the conclusion of the case to prevent a loss of chamber volume. Corneal incisions should be sutured, but a well-constructed scleral tunnel incision with an internal corneal flap of 1.5 mm or more usually does not require a suture (Figure 4). The scleral tunnel incision may seem a little "retro," but, in general, I prefer it for eyes receiving the Crystalens. I tell patients that they will notice a little red spot on the surface of their eye postoperatively that will go away in a week. I find this explanation simpler than telling them they will have a suture in their eye that will require removal. Patients seem to find a red spot easier to accept. It requires less explanation and no additional intervention.

TIP No. 5. PAUSE DURING INJECTION TO CHECK THE IOL's ORIENTATION

It is possible to implant the Crystalens upside down if you are not careful. This error can occur if the IOL is improperly loaded in the inserter or if the lens rotates excessively in the inserter during injection. You can easily verify the IOL's correct orientation by pausing during injection to inspect the flat circular knobs at the ends of the polyamide haptics as they exit the inserter. The lens is designed so that, when its proper side is up, the knob to the right is always rounded (round on right) and the knob to the left is oval

(Figure 5). If you see that the knob on the right is oval, rotate the injector 180° before the optic of the IOL leaves the inserter. You may then easily insert the Crystalens so that it is correctly oriented.

TIP No. 6. LIFT AND FOLD THE PROXIMAL HAPTIC INTO THE CAPSULAR BAG DURING THE IOL's INSERTION

There are many ways to place the Crystalens in the capsular bag. I find that the lift-and-fold technique is the easiest and most reliable and that it places a minimal amount of stress on the zonules (Figure 6). Using this approach, you inject the IOL so that the distal haptics are in the bag and the proximal haptics are "parked" inside the anterior chamber on the anterior surface of the iris. You then lift the optic with any spatula-like instrument introduced though the side-port incision. Next, using any hook that you may have or a chopper, introduced through the primary incision, fold the proximal haptic downward and gently drop the haptic into the capsular bag.

TIP No. 7. USE A DIOPTRIC POWER GRAPH TO SELECT THE PROPER IOL FOR EXCHANGE

Inevitably, a refractive outcome will occasionally be less than optimal. Even with precise biometry and the meticulous management of astigmatism, a small number of patients require additional attention in order to achieve a desired refractive endpoint. Options include IOL exchange, piggyback IOLs, and keratorefractive procedures. IOL exchanges should be carried out within the first several weeks after the initial surgery, because the polyamide haptics become fibrosed to the capsule after a few weeks, thus making the lens' removal more difficult.

The key to optimizing the refractive outcome is selecting the correct dioptric power for the replacement IOL. Doing so is easy. On a Cartesian graph, using the preoperative biometric data, simply plot the range of dioptric powers close to emmetropia on the abscissa and the range of predicted refractive outcomes on the ordinate (Figure 7). Then, decide the amount of refractive change required. Select the new IOL power by dropping down the ordinate the desired amount for myopic dioptric changes or by moving up the ordinate the desired amount for hyperopic corrections. ■

This article originally appeared in the August 2008 issue of CRSToday.

CHAPTER 169

Tips for Successfully Implanting the Crystalens

OMAR F. ALMALLAH, MD

All ophthalmic surgeons have heard the cliché *underpromise and overdeliver*. This was and remains good advice for the treatment of surgical pathologies. I do not believe the approach is appropriate, however, for a modern refractive cataract practice and presbyopic correction. Patients are now asked to pay out of pocket for the uncovered upgrades of presbyopia-correcting IOLs. Their expectations are therefore justifiably greater than those of patients undergoing conventional cataract surgery. If presbyopic correction is for what patients paid, that is what they receive, and it has to work reliably for them, barring a significant surgical complication. Imagine a commercial airline that promised, "Fly with us. We will get you there—maybe." I do not think it would be a successful slogan. We surgeons have adopted this attitude of underpromising in ophthalmology. I therefore was not surprised when my fellow audience members and I reported that anywhere from zero to 20% of our patients were choosing presbyopia-correcting IOLs during an informal poll, conducted at a session on presbyopic correction during the ASCRS Symposium on Cataract, IOL and Refractive Surgery in April 2007. I have no doubt that, similarly, air travel would lose its popularity if airlines could not reliably get people to their destinations.

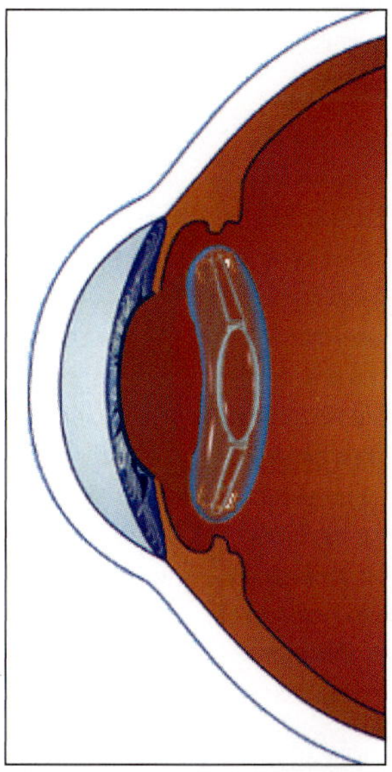

Figure 1. The surgeon properly orients the Crystalens in the bag with its optic showing acutely angulated haptics and the loop arch haptic lengths (or segments) seated in the bag so that there are no capsular striae.

Fully correcting a patient's vision is a noble goal and is our objective for all patients who undergo cataract surgery. We cannot provide this degree of correction to every patient, however; some have macular pathology or lack the financial resources to pay for the uncovered presbyopia-correcting IOL, for example. If no barriers to costs exist, spectacle-free vision is a logical choice for patients. I do not know anyone who loves presbyopia. I think it is time to present the option to every suitable candidate.

This article provides my recommendations for improving presbyopes' vision with the implantation of a Crystalens accommodating IOL (Eyeonics, Inc., Aliso Viejo, CA) and maintaining the lens' proper positioning within the capsular bag for successful postoperative outcomes.

AN IOL's POSITION

Success with presbyopia-correcting IOLs depends heavily on refractive predictability. We ophthalmologists understand the importance of accurate biometry and keratometry, surgeon-specific A-constants, and the appropriate choice of IOL power calculation formulae.[1] We sometimes pay too little attention to making sure the IOL remains in the proper position within the capsular bag after its implantation (Figure 1). Subtle changes in an IOL's location can result in significant refractive changes and are often an unrecognized reason for refractive surprises and even poor accommodative results.

The position of the Crystalens accommodating IOL is particularly important. This thin, flexible implant can lose its precise position in the capsular bag if the anterior chamber becomes shallow at any time intraoperatively (Figure 2A). The displacement can occur when the surgeon removes the viscoelastic from the anterior chamber and takes out the I/A instrument's tip. Subsequent deepening of the anterior chamber may not restore the IOL's original seating.

The Crystalens' haptics may move out of position from the deepest recesses of the fornix of the capsular bag, and they may not return to their original position upon the reformation of the anterior chamber with balanced salt solution. Another reason for the haptics' dislocation is that, after the viscoelastic's removal from the eye, the capsular bag will not expand like it did before. Finally, the haptics may be captured in a position that is eccentric and different from the original implantation site, which causes a subtle asymmetry to the IOL within the bag (Figure 2B). Striae in the posterior capsule are a clue that the IOL has shifted. Further pressurizing the anterior chamber may temporarily eliminate capsular striae, but they are frequently visible the next day at the slit lamp due to the improper fixation of the implant in the bag.

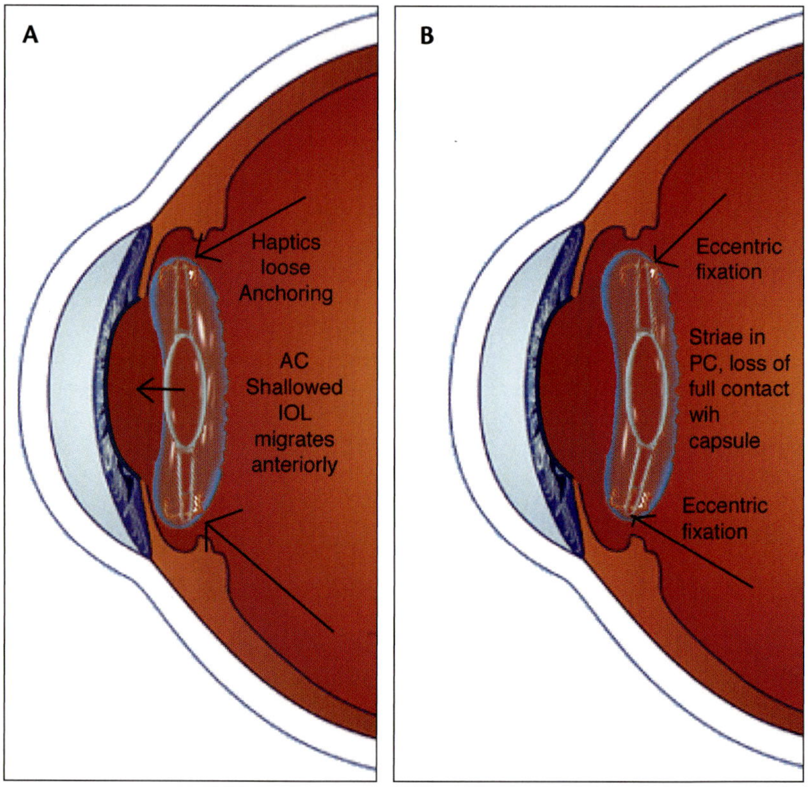

Figure 2. The anterior chamber becomes shallow after the Crystalens' optic, haptics, and loop arch haptic lengths lose their proper anchoring (A). After the author reforms the anterior chamber, the Crystalens may not be properly seated, because the loop arch haptic lengths could get caught in a loose bag. As a result, full contact of the IOL and haptics with the bag may be lost, which will degrade accommodation and/or present a myopic surprise (B).

The most common intracapsular dislocation is anterior, which explains why nearly all of the refractive surprises in the absence of miscalculated IOL powers with the Crystalens are myopic. The other significant complication of intracapsular dislocation is the patient's loss of accommodative function, which depends on the transmission of forces of the ciliary muscle from the capsular bag to the flexible Crystalens implant. If the capsular bag does not have unhindered contact with the full plate and loop arch lengths of the Crystalens' haptics, the degradation or loss of accommodative function is likely. This phenomenon may also play a role in refractive surprises following the implantation of a multifocal IOL. Surgeons therefore must adopt a strategy to avoid the shallowing of the anterior chamber after an IOL's implantation. Implementing the smallest possible incision is a priority. I use a 2.8-mm trapezoidal clear corneal incision for implanting the Crystalens with the STAAR plate haptic injector and the MTC-60c cartridge (both from STAAR Surgical Company, Monrovia, CA).

THE PREVENTION OF SUBLUXATION

Preventing the anterior chamber from becoming shallow once the Crystalens is seated is key to a successful result. I recommend surgeons reduce or, if possible, eliminate the sideport incision, which in my experience is a major source of leaky wounds. If elimination is not an option for bimanual surgery, then I suggest a proper square or nearly square clear corneal sideport design. In such cases, I favor square or nearly square clear corneal incisions with either the Williamson or Langerman modification of Fine's design.[2] Before removing the viscoeleastic from the anterior chamber, I perform stromal hydration of the sideport incisions (if applicable), the lateral walls of the clear corneal incision, and, most importantly, the roof of the clear corneal incision. Next, I preplace a suture to close the wound, but I leave it untied. Lastly, I proceed with I/A to remove the viscoelastic.

I have found that following the aforementioned steps prior to performing I/A maintains a deep anterior chamber and prevents the subluxation of the Crystalens. The hydrated clear corneal incision acts as a one-way valve, allowing the I/A instrument's tip into the anterior chamber but not permitting the aqueous to exit when the tip is removed.

A hydrated clear corneal incision is critical. No striae should appear in the posterior capsule, but the sharp angulations of the hinge should be visible while the patient is on the operating table. If any striae are present, simply deepening the chamber or repositioning the IOL is inadequate. If necessary, surgeons should inject a viscoelastic to reinflate the bag and remove all capsular folds—particularly in the deep fornices of the capsule—before repositioning the IOL. This process ensures proper fixation before the conclusion of the case. Ensuring that the Crystalens is properly positioned until wound healing secures the location of its haptics will decrease patients' loss of accommodation. By preplacing the suture, surgeons avoid having to manipulate the wound, which may lead to a shallow chamber at the end of the case. I feel it is very important to use a suture when implanting the Crystalens.

LATE COMPLICATIONS

Properly preparing the capsular bag prior to implanting the IOL can reduce the incidence of enduring complications. Surgeons should thoroughly vacuum the interior of the capsule to remove lens epithelial cells and polish the posterior capsule regardless of how clean it appears. It is also worth noting that, because a round capsulorhexis is more likely to fibrose in a symmetric fashion and is therefore less likely to exert asymmetric forces on the implant, its use reduces the risk of Z-syndrome or late subluxation.[3]

Occasional refractive surprises are inevitable, and they are easily addressed with keratorefractive surgery and/or piggyback lens implants.

CONCLUSION

Only with proper implantation will patients achieve accommodative function with the Crystalens. The techniques described herein allow me to deliver excellent results with this IOL consistently.

Because 1.50 D of accommodation is not adequate for many of my patients, I target their nondominant eye for -0.75 D and their dominant eye for emmetropia. I do not consider this approach to be monovision, because a -0.75 D eye will see 20/30 or better uncorrected at distance. I perform limbal relaxing incisions for astigmatism of 0.50 D or more, and I postoperatively employ customized ablation to eliminate any residual ametropia or aberrations that are clinically significant. Sometimes, a result that is 0.25 D off is sufficient reason for further surgical intervention. This much precision requires a great deal of commitment, but the rewards to patients and myself are commensurately great. ■

This article originally appeared in the July 2007 issue of CRSToday.

1. Holladay JT. Standardizing constants for ultrasonic biometry, keratometry, and intraocular lens power calculations. *J Cataract Refract Surg.* 1997:23:1356-1370.
2. Masket S, Belani S. Proper wound construction to prevent short-term ocular hypotony after clear corneal incision cataract surgery. *J Cataract Refract Surg.* 2007;33:383-386.
3. Gimbel HV, Neuhann T. Development, advantages and methods of the continuous circular capsulorhexis technique. *J Cataract Refract Surg.* 1990;16:1631-1637.

CHAPTER 170

A Systematic Approach to Selecting a Premium IOL

ERNST NICOLITZ, MD; DAVID MILLS, MD; LENKA CHAMPION, MD; AND LOUIS CATANIA, OD

One of the strongest factors in the successful use of premium IOLs is determining which model is the most appropriate for a given patient. Accurate choices require a brief preoperative interview to evaluate the patient's visual needs and preferences and to measure the refractive error and pupillary size. To facilitate this process, we created a chart (Table 1) that summarizes what we consider to be the optimal IOL selections based on the aforementioned criteria. The recommended lenses may represent a mixed or a matched approach. This article presents the rationale behind our chart and selections.

DISTANCE VISION

Ophthalmologists have long considered monofocal optics to be the optimal means for correcting distance vision. Whether the physiologic pupil is small or large, a monofocal optic will provide the best-quality distance vision. For that reason, the monofocal Crystalens Five-O and HD accommodating IOLs (Bausch & Lomb, Rochester, NY) are our premium lenses of choice in the category of distance vision. Distance-oriented patients will always have some degree of near and intermediate visual needs as well. The Crystalens should perform adequately in these areas by providing moderate levels of accommodation through translational movements in the preoperative emmetrope or hyperope[1] plus accommodative arching in the preoperative emmetrope, hyperope, and higher myope.[2]

Patients seeking distance correction who are emmetropic or hyperopic with small pupils preoperatively may also be well served by the ReZoom multifocal IOL (Advanced Medical Optics, Inc., Santa Ana, CA). Their small pupils will maximize the benefit of the lens' dominant (central) distance optic. Unlike other patients, presbyopic hyperopes and emmetropes will be more tolerant of the positive spherical aberrations created by the ReZoom IOL's transitional zones. These individuals generally have clinically significant preoperative levels of positive spherical aberration[3] to which they have cortically adapted as they have aged. We have therefore found that they require less postoperative adaptation to multifocal lenses.

NEAR VISION

The AcrySof Restor IOL (Alcon Laboratories, Inc., Fort Worth, TX) is the only near-dominant premium lens. In a preoperative emmetrope or hyperope with a large pupillary diameter (approximately 4 to 6 mm or greater when dilated), the IOL's peripheral refractive portion (beyond a 3.6-mm diameter) provides effective distance power. For near vision, the central near refractive power aligns well with the constricted pupil. We find that any positive spherical aberration created by the multifocality and diffractive (apodized) portion of this IOL is significantly less with the AcrySof Restor Aspheric IOL (Alcon Laboratories, Inc.) and is thus well tolerated by preoperative emmetropes or hyperopes with positive spherical aberrations.

TABLE 1. PREMIUM IOL SELECTIONS				
Patient's Visual Needs and Preference	**Preoperative Pupillary Size and Refraction**			
	Pupillary Size (constricted to dilated) 2 to 5 mm or less		**Pupillary Size (constricted to dilated) 3 to 6 mm or greater**	
	Myopia (>3.00 D)	**Emmetropia or hyperopia**	**Myopia (>3.00 D)**	**Emmetropia or hyperopia**
Distance	Crystalens	Crystalens or ReZoom	Crystalens	Crystalens
Near	*Mixed Optics* Acrysof Restor[a] and Crystalens	*Mixed Optics* Acrysof Restor Aspheric[a] and Crystalens	*Mixed Optics* Acrysof Restor[a] and Crystalens	Acrysof Restor Aspheric
Equal distance and near	Crystalens	*Mixed Optics* Crystalens[a] and Acrysof Restor Aspheric	Crystalens	*Mixed Optics* Crystalens[a] and Acrysof Restor Aspheric

[a]*Indicates dominant eye.*

The AcrySof Restor IOL's limitations include a lack of intermediate visual power and a compromise in distance vision with smaller pupillary diameters (less than 4 mm). Owing to the lens' dominant near power, however, this IOL is often the ideal choice to mix with the Crystalens. Through a combination of the optical characteristics of each lens, patients with near visual needs/preferences and small pupils benefit from quality near vision with the AcrySof Restor Aspheric IOL (for emmetropes or hyperopes) or the AcrySof Restor IOL (for myopes) in their dominant eye and the Crystalens in their nondominant eye for intermediate and distance vision.

EQUAL DISTANCE AND NEAR VISION

Most commonly, patients being screened for premium IOLs state their need and interest in distance and near vision. None of the currently available premium IOLs provides the highest quality vision at both ranges.

In most patients, the Crystalens provides sharp distance and intermediate vision and adequate near vision through transitional movement and accommodative arching. Individuals with 3.00 D or more of myopia may obtain the best range of intermediate and near power with this IOL.[4] The lower-powered silicone optic (in myopes) has a thinner center than the higher, plus-powered optic (in emmetropes and hyperopes). The thin center allows greater arching of the lens, which results in additional plus power. Translational movement requires millimeters of anterior shifting to induce plus power. In contrast, mere microns of bending or accommodative arching of the curvature of the IOL's optic provide the potential for far greater amounts of induced plus power than translational movement can produce. The Crystalens may also be a better choice for high myopes than a multifocal IOL, because these patients tend to have negative spherical aberrations. This group has never been happy with the positive spherical aberrations introduced by multifocal optics.

Patients who desire strong vision at distance and near may be well suited to a combination of the Crystalens and either the AcrySof Restor Aspheric IOL (for emmetropes or hyperopes) or the AcrySof Restor lens (for myopes). Implanting a Crystalens in the patient's dominant eye and the AcrySof Restor lens in his nondominant eye should provide optimal distance, intermediate, and near vision while maintaining uncompromised binocular distance vision (as opposed to a standard monovision approach).

CONCLUSION

Surgeons can select the proper premium IOLs for successful outcomes by taking into account patients' visual needs and preferences, assessing their preoperative refractive error and pupillary size, and analyzing the available IOLs' optics, strengths, and weaknesses. This process of lens selection can lead to greater efficiency, more accurate matching of IOLs and patients, and optimal visual results. It can also minimize patients' need for cortical adaptation while maximizing their satisfaction. ■

This article originally appeared in the August 2008 issue of CRSToday.

1. Hunter J, Campbell M, Geraghty E. Optical analysis of an accommodating intraocular lens. *J Cataract Refract Surg.* 2006;32(2):269-278.
2. Waltz KL. Understanding accommodation with the crystalens (accommodative arching). *Cataract & Refractive Surgery Today.* February 2006;6(2)(suppl):13-15.
3. Alio JL, Schimchak P, Negri HP, Montes-Mico R. Crystalline lens optical dysfunction through aging. *Ophthalmology.* 2005;112(11):2022-2029.
4. Kim JH, Park CS, Chung TY, Chung ES. Clinical evaluation of accommodative intraocular lens implantation in high myopic eyes. *Korean J Ophthalmol.* 2008;22(2):81-86.

CHAPTER 171

Mixing IOLs: What Are the Options?

ELIZABETH A. DAVIS, MD, AND RICHARD L. LINDSTROM, MD

The ideal IOL would provide perfect vision and seamless accommodation from distance to near without aberrations, a loss of contrast sensitivity, dysphotopsia, posterior capsular opacification, or a loss of function with time. Because every currently available lens has benefits and disadvantages, combining different IOLs in a single patient may enhance his outcome by maximizing his vision while reducing unwanted side effects.

At present, there are three main categories of IOLs: monofocal (spherical, aspheric, and toric); accommodating; and multifocal. This article focuses on the five basic possible combinations.

COMBINATION No. 1

One option is to combine two monofocal IOLs with different focal points to achieve monovision. This approach can be very successful, particularly in patients who have worn such a correction in contact lenses. Surgeons can choose the exact focal point of the near eye to suit the patient's needs. Targeting myopia of 1.00 to 1.75 D allows for functional intermediate vision, whereas a target of 2.00 to 2.50 D provides true near vision. The monovision approach requires neuroadaption, with suppression of the near eye when the subject gazes at distant objects and suppression of the distance eye when he focuses up close. The greater the disparity is between his eyes, the more difficult it is for the patient to neuroadapt. Nevertheless, there is the benefit of maintaining a high quality of vision with monofocal optics. Pseudophakic monovision is a good option in patients who are at risk of developing eye diseases that will impact their contrast sensitivity (eg, glaucoma, macular degeneration, diabetic retinopathy). It is also appropriate for patients who have undergone keratorefractive surgery (eg, excimer laser ablation, incisional keratotomy), because corneal irregularities may already impact their contrast acuity and visual quality.

COMBINATION No. 2

Another alternative is to mix a monofocal with an accommodating IOL. Patients should attain excellent distance and intermediate vision and fairly good near vision (J3). Targeting some myopia in the eye with the accommodating IOL can achieve a stronger near point, albeit with some sacrifice of distance acuity in that eye. This combination of IOLs may be particularly useful when the patient has undergone prior IOL surgery in one eye, which has a monofocal lens, and desires enhanced near vision in his second eye without sacrificing visual quality. The approach maintains a high quality of vision with monofocal optics. Like the previous combination, this option is appropriate for patients at risk for eye diseases and for those who have previously undergone corneal refractive surgery.

COMBINATION No. 3

Combining a monofocal with a multifocal IOL allows both of the patient's eyes to achieve excellent distance vision with the added benefit of some pseudoaccommodation in his multifocal eye. The ReZoom multifocal IOL (Advanced Medical Optics, Inc., Santa Ana, CA) provides excellent intermediate vision and good near vision, whereas the AcrySof Restor IOL (Alcon Laboratories, Inc., Fort Worth, TX) provides excellent near vision but minimal intermediate vision. With any multifocal IOL, patients may experience glare, halos, and reduced contrast acuity. Most find that these symptoms diminish with time. When unwanted visual phenomena do occur, their presence in only one eye may have a mitigating effect.

COMBINATION No. 4

Surgeons may mix an accommodating with a multifocal IOL. This combination produces a quality of vision similar to mixing a monofocal and a multifocal lens, but patients' intermediate vision should be superior. An accommodating IOL can be an appropriate choice for the second eye of patients who achieved good unaided visual acuity with a multifocal lens in their first eye but are struggling with glare and halos.

COMBINATION No. 5

Lastly, one can mix two multifocal IOLs of differing types. Many surgeons find this combination useful when a patient seems to be comfortable with and adaptable to multifocal optics but has a strong desire to improve both his uncorrected intermediate and near vision. Mixing a ReZoom and an AcrySof Restor IOL can achieve this result.

TIPS FOR SUCCESS

With any of the combinations described, it is imperative to treat preexisting conditions that may impair the patient's vision. For example, ophthalmologists should treat or manage malpositioned eyelids, blepharitis, dry eye, and anterior basement dystrophy before surgery. As always, counseling patients preoperatively is critical. The surgeon should understand the patient's needs and preferences. Additionally, the patient should understand the limitations of each combination and its potential compromises and side effects. He should be informed of the potential need for enhancement surgeries and the associated costs and risks.

Intraoperatively, surgeons must pay special attention to the centration and positioning of the IOL, particularly with toric, accommodating, and multifocal designs. Improper positioning may not only reduce these lenses' effectiveness, but it may also impair the patient's visual outcome. Reducing the incidence of posterior capsular opacification and capsular phimosis (for instance, through adequate capsulorhexis size, symmetric capsular shape, meticulous cortical cleanup, and capsule/optic overlap) is also important. In addition, having patients use NSAID drops for several weeks postoperatively may prevent cystoid macular edema, which even in subtle forms can impair contrast acuity. A plan to treat corneal astigmatism of 0.75 D or greater is often required. If a toric IOL is not used, then the surgeon should consider incisional keratotomies, laser excimer ablation, or conductive keratoplasty.

CONCLUSION

Mixing IOLs is a known and a successful strategy for many patients. The authors have achieved excellent outcomes with all of the combinations described in this article. The choice of which IOLs to implant depends upon the patient's lifestyle, preference, and personality. Until the perfect IOL is developed, mixing lens designs will remain a useful strategy for correcting patients' vision. ■

This article originally appeared in the August 2007 issue of CRSToday.

CHAPTER 172

Mixing the ReZoom and AcrySof Restor IOLs

FRANK A. BUCCI JR, MD

I began mixing the ReZoom IOL (Advanced Medical Optics, Inc., Santa Ana, CA) and AcrySof Restor IOL (Alcon Laboratories, Inc., Fort Worth, TX), because my patients were highly dissatisfied with the bilateral implantation of the latter. Most other US surgeons did not share my initial experience. What accounts for these differences in results?

CATARACT SURGERY VERSUS REFRACTIVE LENS EXCHANGE

The typical US surgeon using the AcrySof Restor lens treats more patients with cataract surgery than refractive lens exchange (a ratio greater than 20:1). These patient groups' expectations for their postoperative vision are extremely different (Table 1). The AcrySof Restor FDA study enrolled only cataract surgery patients who paid nothing for the bilateral implantation of the lens.[1] The criteria for success with a 75-year-old patient with a dense, nuclear sclerotic cataract versus a 50-year-old baby boomer undergoing refractive lens exchange are very dissimilar. The AcrySof Restor FDA study thus revealed little about how that IOL would perform in the 40- to 60-year-old refractive lens exchange patient.

ELECTIVE REFRACTIVE SURGERY AND PATIENTS' EXPECTATIONS

Patients Want What They Pay for

The original targeted market for these presbyopia-correcting IOLs was not cataract surgery patients but precataract presbyopes, but all patients are paying out of pocket for these lenses. Now these procedures are officially considered refractive surgeries, and an 80% success rate for any form of refractive surgery is unacceptable. Imagine telling LASIK patients that they have an 80% chance of functioning without glasses after a procedure that costs $3,000 to $5,000. The perception of visual improvement achieved by cataract patients averaging 70 years of age is dominated by the results associated with the extraction of the cataract, irrespective of the type of IOL implanted.

My Experience With the AcrySof Restor IOL

After hearing many positive presentations on the AcrySof Restor lens at the 2004 ESCRS meeting in Paris, I began wait-listing my multifocal IOL patients until the this IOL became available in the US on June 1, 2005. I quickly established a cohort of 55 bilateral AcrySof Restor recipients in a 3-month period.[2] Sixty-three percent underwent elective refractive lens exchange surgeries.

Seventeen of my 55 AcrySof Restor patients complained of a lack of intermediate vision, and one in three of my refractive lens exchange patients voicing this disappointment. It became apparent to me that baby boomers and younger cataract surgery patients would not tolerate the absence of functional intermediate vision.

During the same time period, I evaluated several patients who had received a unilateral Array lens (Advanced Medical Optics, Inc., Santa Ana, CA) and desired an IOL in their fellow eye in hopes of achieving sharper reading vision without additional halos. I implanted the AcrySof Restor lens in the fellow eyes of five such patients, and they were extremely happy and completely free of spectacles postoperatively. I therefore decided to explore combining the ReZoom and AcrySof Restor IOLs, because the former represents an upgrade of the Array lens.

MIXING THE REZOOM WITH THE ACRYSOF RESTOR

The first 110 patients in whom I implanted the combination of ReZoom and AcrySof Restor lenses achieved statistically and clinically better intermediate vision than those in whom I had bilaterally implanted the AcrySof Restor lens. The ReZoom/AcrySof Restor patients achieved J2.44 versus J3.60 for the bilateral AcrySof Restor patients, and none of the former group spontaneously complained about his intermediate vision. Moreover, my ReZoom/AcrySof Restor patients seemed to have the "wow" factor that is frequently observed in LASIK patients. In comparison, even my successful bilateral AcrySof Restor patients often seemed relatively "underwhelmed."

There were no statistically significant differences with regard to bilateral near vision between the two groups. The ReZoom/AcrySof Restor patients, however, frequently reported a more comfortable reading distance compared with the bilateral AcrySof Restor patients, who often thought their near point of focus was too close. Additionally, as Akaishi and Fabri[3] reported at the World Cornea Congress last year, I have observed subtle but significant losses in patients' BCVA and uncorrected distance visual acuity with the AcrySof Restor lens.

WAXY VISION

I recently reported on a group of patients[4] with a severe form of waxy vision, which I call *Vaseline vision dysphotopsia* (Vaseline; Unilever, PLC, London, United Kingdom). I diagnosed the problem in 13 of 300 eyes (4.33%) in which I implanted the AcrySof Restor lens, nine of which required explantation. The symptoms of Vaseline vision dysphotopsia are unique in that they (1) present almost immediately after the IOL's implantation, (2) are constant rather than intermittent, (3) are not dependent on a point source of light, (4) do not decrease with neuroadaptation, (5) appear to be psychologically draining as much as visually dysfunctional, and (6) are only relieved by the lens' explantation.

Nevertheless, my experience with multifocal IOLs has led me to two core conclusions. The first is that mixing a refractive with a diffractive multifocal IOL will greatly satisfy patients and produce a high level of spectacle independence. The second is that the AcrySof Restor IOL is not the optimal diffractive lens for the refractive IOL/diffractive IOL combination.

CONCLUSION

High levels of success with presbyopia-correcting IOLs entail selecting the proper patients and effectively setting their expec-

TABLE 1. A COMPARISON OF TWO PATIENT GROUPS

Traditional Cataract Surgery Patients	Refractive Lens Exchange Patients (Baby Boomers)
• Late 60s, 70s, and 80s	• 40s, 50s, and early 60s
• Accepting by culture	• Demanding by culture
• Poor corrected preoperative visual acuity	• Excellent corrected preoperative visual acuity
• Lower cost, lower expectations	• Higher costs, higher expectations
• Less litigious	• More litigious
• Less computer use	• More computer use

tations before surgery. The preoperative examination should confirm that they have full visual potential, with special attention paid to the cornea and the retina. Surgeons should also continually upgrade their skills at phacoemulsification and the correction of residual refractive errors such as corneal astigmatism. Although optimal IOL selection is a critical element, it is still only one of many essential building blocks (see *The 10 Ps*) necessary for producing a patient satisfied with presbyopia-correcting IOLs.

Akaishi and Fabri[3] reported superior reading speeds, greater pupillary independence, better-quality distance vision, and a lesser incidence of halos and glare with a combination of the ReZoom lens and the aspheric Tecnis Multifocal IOL (not approved in the US; Advanced Medical Optics, Inc.) compared with the ReZoom/AcrySof Restor combination. The diffractive rings of the Tecnis Multifocal IOL are spread throughout the lens' entire optic, whereas all of the rings are located within the central 3.6 mm of the AcrySof Restor lens' optic. It may be that the centralization of the rings produces the waxy vision and Vaseline vision dysphotopsia associated with the latter IOL. There have been no reports of waxy vision with the Tecnis Multifocal IOL. I therefore believe that combining the ReZoom and Tecnis Multifocal IOLs will be the optimal approach to presbyopic correction among patients undergoing cataract surgery and refractive lens exchange once the latter lens is approved by the FDA. ■

This article originally appeared in the August 2007 issue of CRSToday.

1. Acrysof ReSTOR apodized diffractive optic posterior chamber intraocular lenses, models MA60D3 and SA60D3 – P04002. Available at: http://www.fda.gov/cdrh/pdf4/p040020.html. Accessed July 24, 2007.
2. Bucci F. Bilateral multifocal cataract and lensectomy patients receiving ReZoom/ReSTOR – long term follow-up. Poster presented at: ARVO; May 8, 2007; Fort Lauderdale, FL.
3. Akaishi L, Fabri PP. PC IOLs mix and match technologies: Brazilian experience. Paper presented at: The World Ophthalmology Congress; February 2006; São Paolo, Brazil.
4. Bucci F. Vaseline vision dysphotopsia and explantation of the ReSTOR multifocal implant. Poster presented at: ARVO; May 8, 2007; Fort Lauderdale, FL.

THE 10 Ps

These points are important to consider when implanting presbyopia-correcting IOLs:

1. **P**ersonality: establish a relationship with the patient, who is more similar to someone undergoing LASIK than cataract surgery
2. **P**atient selection
3. **P**reoperative counseling to manage patients' postoperative expectations
4. **P**reoperative examination (especially of the cornea and retina) to assess patients' postoperative visual potential
5. **P**resbyopia-correcting IOL selection (target distance, intermediate, and near vision)
6. **P**rostaglandins' inhibition (use topical NSAIDs pre- and postoperatively)
7. **P**hacoemulsification and IOL implantation (be efficient and accurate)
8. **P**lano ± target (do not give away distance vision; treat residual refractive error)
9. **P**osterior capsular opacification (treat patients who have already lost contrast sensitivity)
10. **P**sychophysiology (continue to help patients neuroadapt to their lenses)

CHAPTER 173

Mixing Multifocal IOLs

JONATHAN D. CHRISTENBURY, MD

I underwent successful LASIK about 10 years ago for a -4.00 D refractive error. I enjoyed spectacle-free vision for a number of years until I developed the visual symptoms of presbyopia. I admit that I am a refractive surgery patient. I enjoyed being independent of spectacles. As my presbyopia increased, however, I became dependent on reading glasses for almost every near task, including computer work. I am very familiar with multifocal IOLs, because I have implanted a combination of the AcrySof Natural Restor IOL (Alcon Laboratories, Inc., Fort Worth, TX) and the ReZoom IOL (Advanced Medical Optics, Inc., Santa Ana, CA) in more than 4,000 patients since May 2005. Over time, I became envious of their good postoperative vision (95% of them are free of spectacles), and I finally decided to undergo refractive lens exchange. My positive experience has inspired confidence among my patients who are interested in this surgical option, and it has motivated me to offer the procedure to a wider population. As a surgeon who implants multifocal IOLs, I have learned that these lenses provide the best reading vision and that they only produce glare for the first couple of months postoperatively. If patients are told that these phenomena are transient and part of a normal healing process, very few of them, in my experience, comment about their night vision after 3- to 6-months postoperatively. I also observed that patients who receive a different multifocal lens in each eye seemed to have better intermediate vision and better reading vision in dim light than those who receive the same lens in both eyes. In my experience, multifocal and monofocal lenses appear to provide comparable visual acuity at distance.

Patients who have other combinations of lenses also report satisfactory postoperative vision, including those who have a ReZoom lens in one eye and an AcrySof Natural Restor IOL in the other. Although the lenses are tinted differently, none of my patients complained that combined IOLs affected their color perception.

Based on the aforementioned observations, I chose to undergo refractive lens exchange with the ReZoom and AcrySof Natural Restor IOLs. I was comfortable selecting this procedure after prior LASIK, because many of my patients have achieved good BSCVAs with the same treatment.

MY MIXED MULTIFOCAL IOL ROUTE

About 1.5 years ago, I decided to undergo multifocal IOL implantation in both eyes with the AcrySof Natural Restor lens in my left eye and the ReZoom IOL in my right, dominant eye.

I chose Stephen Slade, MD, of Houston to implant the lenses because I have known him for more than 15 years. Furthermore, he trained me to perform refractive surgical procedures, including astigmatic keratotomy, RK, and automated lamellar keratoplasty, and we were co-investigators for a number of FDA clinical trials of PRK and LASIK. Dr. Slade and I have also observed each other operating a number of times, both inside and outside the United States. Under Dr. Slade's tutelage, I learned a meticulous and conservative approach to surgery that I still follow today.

Preoperatively, I did my own biometric calculations, and I brought my own lenses to Dr. Slade's practice. Of course, he performed his own IOL calculations, testing, and full examinations, but he did agree with my choice of lens for each eye. I used the By-Pass K Method for calculating the power of my IOLs, because I have found it to be accurate in patients with a history of prior cornea refractive surgery in my own practice. Dr. Slade said I was one of the most cooperative ophthalmologists, or ophthalmologists' family members, he has treated.

My preoperative UCVA measured 20/20 OU, which allowed me to read some of the letters on the 20/15 Snellen line. In contrast, my unaided near vision was approximately 20/80. Without reading glasses, I was not able to read newsprint. I had 20/20 BCVA up close and had no significant distance refractive error because of having undergone LASIK. I had approximately 0.75 D of astigmatism in my left eye, which did not bother me.

Dr. Slade implanted the AcrySof Natural Restor IOL in my left eye on a Thursday. Due to my workload at that time, I had to wait a few weeks before Dr. Slade could place the ReZoom IOL in my right eye. Before I underwent the second procedure, my vision felt very unbalanced, a phenomenon that many patients had described to me after I had implanted their first multifocal IOL. Despite this effect, I returned to work the following Monday and resumed my regular clinical and surgical schedule. Interestingly, I quickly neuroadapted to my uneven vision and began to read with both eyes equally. I only used reading glasses intermittently between my first and second procedures.

I returned to work several days after Dr. Slade implanted the ReZoom lens in my right eye. I immediately noticed that my sense of being visually unbalanced had resolved and that I no longer needed glasses for reading. My near vision cleared first, then my distance vision. I had some mild fluctuation in my vision at first, but it did not interfere with my overall function. I was also interested to observe that my binocular intermediate and near vision was so much better than my monocular, intermediate, and near vision.

Over the next several months, my vision improved as I neuroadapted to the lens implants. At 3 months postoperatively, however, I began to notice that shiny objects and glossy pages were causing glare and that my vision was becoming hazy. Soon thereafter, I was diagnosed with mild capsular haze, and I consulted a local colleague who performed my bilateral YAG laser capsulotomy. My vision improved significantly the next day.

In the past, I have not hesitated to perform YAG laser capsulotomy on patients who developed similar complaints with their near vision after the implantation of multifocal IOLs. Mild posterior capsular opacification can significantly affect the quality of near vision provided by these lenses.

POSTOPERATIVE OUTCOMES

Since I underwent refractive lens exchange, I do not need glasses for driving, using the computer, or reading. I occasionally use magnifiers to minimize the visual effects from a lid lesion. I previously wore reading glasses while I positioned the IntraLase FS laser's suction ring (Advanced Medical Optics, Inc.) on my patients' corneas, but I rarely need them now.

Before the implantation of my ReZoom/AcrySof Natural Restor IOLs, I had difficulty picking up a collagen punctal plug in a dim examination room. I can do this now without difficulty. I did experience glare and halos for approximately 6 weeks postoperatively, but these problems have resolved. My experience has helped me be more empathetic with my own multifocal IOL patients. Because I experienced the common early nighttime visual symptoms, which resolved, I can offer positive reinforcement to my own patients as they progress through their own healing process.

I currently see 20/20 at distance and J1+ at near. In my office, I can sit in front of a computer monitor until my nose is approximately 8 inches away, and then I can roll slowly backward and have continuous vision of the computer screen until I am 3 or 4 feet away. I do not seem to have a gap in my vision.

I did experience some low contrast sensitivity before I underwent the YAG laser capsulotomy. Since then, my vision is so good that I have not bothered to test my contrast sensitivity.

TODAY'S PRACTICE

Many patients who are curious about cataract surgery or refractive correction will research multifocal IOL technology on the Internet, which I think helps them become more educated. Cataract surgery patients seem to be extremely satisfied with multifocal lens technology. Having their vision restored and becoming independent of spectacles are wonderful experiences for the active cataract patient population. One of my patients told me she "younged up!" Currently, my colleagues and I implant multifocal IOLs in 60% to 70% of our cataract procedures.

Many patients are still confused about the types of presbyopia-correcting IOLs available, however, and can be easily overwhelmed by the potential combinations. I try to keep the discussion as simple as possible by telling patients immediately whether or not they are good candidates for multifocal IOLs. If I think they are eligible for a combination of lenses, I tell them that I chose the ReZoom/AcrySof Natural Restor mix, because I have observed that it provides the best intermediate and near vision. Once they hear that I have undergone the procedure and learn about my results, they ultimately understand that it is a safe procedure, similar to LASIK, which many of their friends have undergone.

Although I have not performed the procedure on any of my staff members (they are all too young), I have implanted the AcrySof Natural Restor and ReZoom IOLs in a number of their family members. In some cases, I have performed refractive lens exchange with the AcrySof Restor and ReZoom IOLs off label in younger patients who are not candidates for LASIK or the Visian ICL (STAAR Surgical Company, Monrovia, CA). I do perform bilateral ReZoom implantation in patients who have mild amblyopia and advise them they are more likely to wear reading glasses for prolonged reading. I estimate that 95% of my patients with combined multifocal IOLs do not wear spectacles—including those who underwent LASIK for residual refractive error. When I am choosing a multifocal IOL for a patient who has significant corneal toricity, I target a predicted postoperative spherical equivalent of zero, because their perceived and functional vision will be better until LASIK or PRK is performed. This seems to be the easiest experience for astigmatic patients, even if some may require temporary astigmatic spectacles, and our excimer lasers are accurate when correcting mixed astigmatism. I think it is important to discourage patients from using reading glasses immediately after the implantation of a multifocal IOL, because the spectacles seem to slow neuroadaptation significantly.

TAKE-HOME POINTS

I have learned that managing expectations in refractive surgery in general is critical to having a happy refractive surgery patient. Many presbyopes, even if they are advised that their intermediate vision will not be adequate, are not happy patients. People require intermediate vision for many tasks, and the majority of us use computers for work. Also, presbyopic patients want clear distance vision in both eyes, just like they had with whatever optical correction they were using before presbyopia-correcting IOL surgery. The patients who are happiest with these lenses are those who rarely need spectacles to achieve functional reading, intermediate, and distance vision. To get there, the doctor and patient need to accept nighttime vision glare or halos for a couple of months. The best presbyopic correction I have experienced is the ReZoom/AcrySof Natural Restor IOL combination. Because of my personal experience, I know that night vision and quality of vision improves after a number of months because of neuroadaptation. ■

This article originally appeared in the October 2008 issue of CRSToday.

CHAPTER 174

Mixing Versus Matching IOLs

JAY S. PEPOSE, MD, PhD

The availability of three FDA-approved IOLs for the treatment of presbyopia allows surgeons to customize patients' binocular vision. Recently, my colleagues and I completed a prospective, nonrandomized, five-arm comparative trial of bilaterally implanted ReZoom zonal refractive multifocal IOLs (Advanced Medical Optics, Inc., Santa Ana, CA), bilaterally implanted AcrySof Restor apodized diffractive multifocal IOLs (Alcon Laboratories, Inc., Fort Worth, TX), bilaterally implanted Crystalens accommodating IOLs (Eyeonics, Inc., Aliso Viejo, CA), and combinations of the Crystalens/ReZoom IOLs and the Crystalens/AcrySof Restor IOLs, with the Crystalens implanted in the patient's dominant eye.[1] This article shares the outcomes of our study and discusses the possibilities of customizing IOLs to meet each patient's individual needs and lifestyle.

OUR RESULTS

The monocular results paralleled the binocular findings and are summarized in *Visual Outcomes in Patients With Various Combinations of Accommodating and Multifocal IOLs*. In brief, there were no statistically significant differences in uncorrected distance

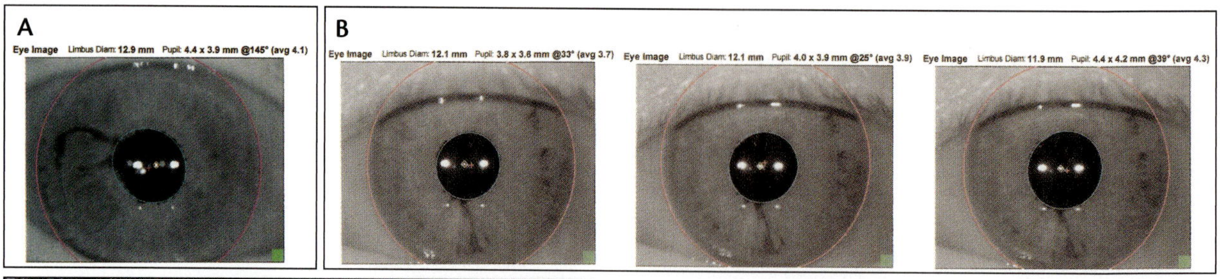

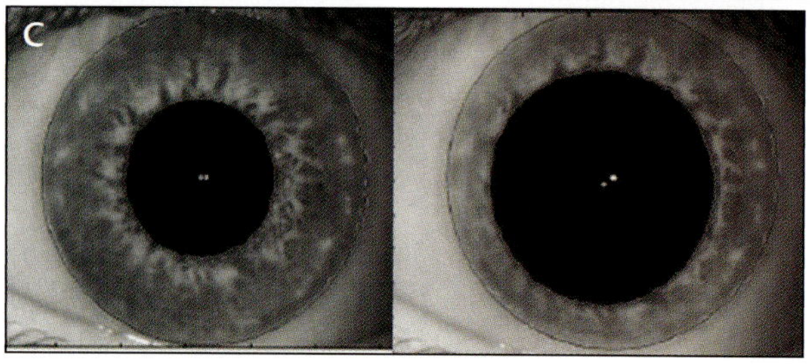

Figure 1. The pupil's shape (A), dynamics (B), and size (C) influence the optical performance of multifocal IOLs and their distribution of light energy at near, intermediate distance, and distance.

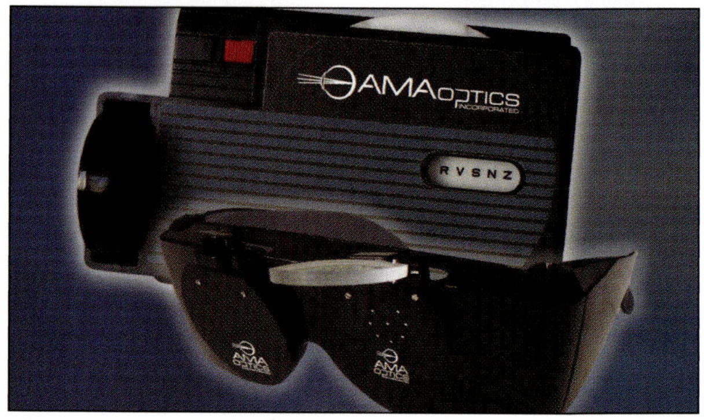

Figure 2. Testing a patient's potential acuity with devices such as the AMA Optics retinal acuity meter may help to preoperatively identify patients with concomitant retinal or optic nerve disorders that could compromise their visual outcomes.

vision between the five groups.

Contrast sensitivity testing was reduced at a number of spatial frequencies in patients with a multifocal IOL in one or both eyes, and photic complaints were more prevalent among these individuals compared with those who received the Crystalens bilaterally. Patients with a Crystalens in their dominant eye and an AcrySof Restor IOL in their nondominant eye achieved the best overall distance, intermediate, and near binocular vision. According to our quality-of-life surveys, however, they complained more of nighttime glare than those who received the Crystalens bilaterally.

The Art of Customization

True customization of these IOLs is an acquired art with some foundation in science. Despite flawless surgery, some patients may be highly dissatisfied with certain premium IOL channels, whereas others are ecstatic with the same combination of IOLs. The discrepancy may be the combined result of patients' preoperative expectations, pre- and postoperative refractions, degree of lenticular opacity, neural processing capabilities, foveal status together with the density and spacing of their cones, and personalities. Direct and open-ended questions can identify patients' special needs, such as a devotion to sewing or fly fishing or other tasks requiring a very short focal point. Patients who work in low-contrast situations, such as a radiology technician or a truck driver, may not be suitable candidates for multifocality. Those with macular

VISUAL OUTCOMES OF PATIENTS WITH VARIOUS COMBINATIONS OF ACCOMMODATING AND MULTIFOCAL IOLs

Monocular testing

- Crystalens eyes had statistically better best-corrected distance, uncorrected intermediate, distance-corrected intermediate, and best-corrected near vision than eyes with the AcrySof Restor (Alcon Laboratories, Inc., Fort Worth, TX) or ReZoom lens (Advanced Medical Optics, Inc., Santa Ana, CA), but they required the greatest reading add.
- ReZoom eyes had statistically better uncorrected intermediate and distance-corrected intermediate than the AcrySof Restor eyes.
- AcrySof Restor eyes had statistically better uncorrected near vision and required the lowest reading compared with eyes with the Crystalens or ReZoom IOL, but they had statistically worse uncorrected intermediate and distance-corrected intermediate vision than eyes with the Crystalens or ReZoom IOL.

Binocular testing

- A Crystalens in one or both eyes was better for intermediate vision with either multifocal IOL.
- An AcrySof Restor lens in one or both eyes was better for near vision than bilateral Crystalenses, bilateral ReZoom IOLs, or a combination of a Crystalens with the ReZoom lens.
- The Crystalens/AcrySof Restor combination provided the best mean intermediate and near visual acuities overall.

dysfunction or forms of optic neuropathy are also best counseled not to have a multifocal IOL. Patients who spend extended time on computers, cell phones, or iPods (Apple Inc., Cupertino, CA) require fairly strong intermediate vision, which was statistically better in our study with the bilaterally implanted Crystalens and ReZoom IOLs than the AcrySof Restor IOL in eyes targeted for emmetropia.

Because multifocal lenses split light differently at dissimilar pupillary diameters, surgeons must evaluate each patient's pupillary size, shape, and dynamics to predict how a given lens will perform in that person's eyes. In my experience, a patient with a relatively small or irregularly shaped scotopic or mesopic pupil may not obtain excellent near vision with the ReZoom lens, which is dominant for distance centrally (Figure 1A). A patient who has little dynamic range in pupillary size (Figure 1B) may obtain superior near vision with the AcrySof Restor IOL. He may be more likely to have dysphotopsia and nighttime complaints, however, although instilling a mydriatic drop and ensuring excellent centration of the IOL can lessen the problem. The Crystalens or monovision with an aspheric monofocal IOL is better suited to patients with large pupils (Figure 1C) who demonstrate a pupil-center shift under mesopic or scotopic conditions. Those with midsized pupils generally do well with the Crystalens or ReZoom IOL at most ranges of vision.

THE UNKNOWNS

A number of variables that cannot be anticipated may affect the outcome of cataract surgery. Besides an intraoperative complication, they include postoperative changes in the corneal wavefront; the IOL's final position, tilt, and decentration; residual defocus and astigmatism; the pattern of higher-order aberrations and phase reversals; and neural adaptive capability. Compared with accommodating IOLs, multifocal lenses generally introduce more higher-order aberrations, thus often making patients less tolerant of residual second-order aberrations (ie, defocus and astigmatism) and more likely to require a postoperative laser vision enhancement.

As a contingency plan, the preoperative workup for all premium-IOL candidates should include an initial evaluation for LASIK or laser surface ablation with corneal topography, testing for dry eyes, and regional pachymetry. These tests may need to be expanded after phacoemulsification for those patient who require laser vision enhancement. The process includes preoperative counseling about the potential need for an enhancement (eg, via LASIK or surface treatment, or bioptics for those with high preoperative corneal astigmatism).

For example, a premium-IOL patient anticipating excellent uncorrected distance and near vision was referred to my practice for a postoperative laser vision enhancement. A topographic analysis revealed keratoconus, which had not been diagnosed or discussed before cataract surgery. Preoperative topographic assessments after patients discontinue wearing their contact lenses for an appropriate length of time can enhance the accuracy of keratometry, aid in planning astigmatic treatment, and circumvent the aforementioned unfortunate postoperative surprise.

Undetected dysfunction of the macula or optic nerve can be avoided in many cases through the use of diagnostic devices such as the AMA Optics retinal acuity meter (AMA Optics Inc., Miami Beach, FL) (Figure 2). This device assists with preoperative assessments of macular function and can detect comorbid retinal (eg, diabetic retinopathy or age-related macular degeneration) and/or optic nerve disorders in cataract surgery patients.[2] Depending on the macular disorder's severity or likelihood of progression, an accommodating or aspheric monofocal lens may be a more suitable option than a multifocal IOL, which could further compromise the patient's contrast sensitivity.

IN SUMMARY

Surgeons offering premium-channel IOLs must understand that these patients demand good uncorrected distance vision. If their results are less than satisfactory after IOL surgery, these individuals will require some form of postoperative enhancement, and they should be informed of this possibility preoperatively. ■

This article originally appeared in the August 2007 issue of CRSToday.

1. Pepose JS, Qazi MA, Davies J, et al. Visual performance of patients with bilateral versus combination Crystalens, ReZoom and ReSTOR intraocular lens implants. Available at: http://www.ajo.com/article/PIIS0002939407005193/abstract. Accessed July 24, 2007.
2. Hofeldt AJ, Weiss MJ. Illuminated near card assessment of potential acuity in eyes with cataract. *Ophthalmology.* 1998;105:1531-1536.

CHAPTER 175

Combining the Crystalens and the AcrySof Restor IOLs

J. TREVOR WOODHAMS, MD

The advent of presbyopia-correcting IOLs opened a door for the precataract baby boomers. Theoretically, these individuals have independent lifestyles and a willingness to undergo elective surgical procedures that may enhance their standard of living. Serendipitously, refractive lens exchange is often easier and safer to perform then traditional cataract surgery, because a fully developed lenticular pathology is not yet present. A patient whose visual acuity can be readily refracted to nearly 20/20 prior to surgery, however, is more demanding of his postoperative visual outcome than one whose cataract has long since severely compromised his visual acuity, night vision, and contrast sensitivity. This article discusses my experience with presbyopia-correcting IOLs, with an emphasis on mixing the Crystalens accommodating IOL (Eyeonics, Inc., Aliso Viejo, CA) and the AcrySof Restor lens (Alcon Laboratories, Inc., Fort Worth, TX).

TWO PRESBYOPIA-CORRECTING IOLS

The Crystalens

Currently, there are two distinct categories of presbyopia-correcting IOLs: accommodating and multifocal (both refractive and diffractive). These lenses work in significantly different fashions, and both have strengths and weaknesses.

As the first accommodating IOL on the US market, the Crystalens presented surgeons with a steep learning curve but allowed them to provide patients with quality distance and intermediate vision, albeit with mixed results in terms of consistent reading vision. Although most patients were quite pleased with the Crystalens, many needed supplemental readers postoperatively for sustained near work. A formerly +3.00 D hyperopic presbyope may not mind wearing reading glasses, but a former -3.00 D myope may be dissatisfied.

The AcrySof Restor Lens

The AcrySof Restor lens, introduced shortly after the Crystalens, uses concentric multifocality with apodization to suppress image-related confusion and internal reflectivity in presbyopes. This lens provides +3.50 D of magnification at a typical reading distance of 12 to 14 inches. Undesirable optical side effects include an unsatisfactory intermediate focal point (18 to 35 inches) and what many early recipients of the lens described as *waxy vision*.

The source of this waxiness can be identified by comparing the modulation transfer function of the AcrySof Restor and Crystalens under in vitro conditions (Figure 1). The steep drop-off in the modulation transfer function curve is indicative of a significant loss of contrast across a wide range of frequencies that is perceived as (among other things) a loss of crisp edges and a general difficulty in perceiving objects with less-than-brightly-lit backgrounds with both lenses. This reduction in the area under the curve is roughly equivalent to the Strehl ratio, a measure of the overall quality of any optical device and is also evident in vivo. This drastically decreased area under the modulation transfer function curve reflects a significantly negative impact on overall visual acuity. The modulation transfer function curve's "cutoff," or where that curve drops to the x-axis is also clinically significant. This cutoff corresponds to the best visual acuity achieved by the lens, and often indicates where there has been a loss of best spectacle corrected acuity, especially in the better than 20/20 ranges. The cutoff can also be objectively determined in vivo using the double-pass technique employed by the Optical Quality Assessment System (Visiometrics, SA, Terrassa, Spain).

MIXING IOLs

The rationale for combining the Crystalens and the AcrySof Restor IOL in a single patient is twofold. First, the pairing provides maximum visual acuity at distance because of the higher resolution and better optical performance of the accommodating IOL. Surgical planning typically dictates putting the Crystalens in the patient's dominant eye and the AcrySof Restor in his fellow eye. Second, this strategy in my experience achieves better-quality visual performance at intermediate and close reading distances than bilateral maximally distance-targeted accommodating IOLs.

Assuming that the patient tolerates the different optics of the two IOLs, both of his eyes will perceive equal levels of acuity at distance under bright lighting conditions, based on my experience. His dominant eye's perceived image, however, will have significantly higher levels of contrast sensitivity, which will provide finer levels of visual discrimination that would otherwise be adversely affected

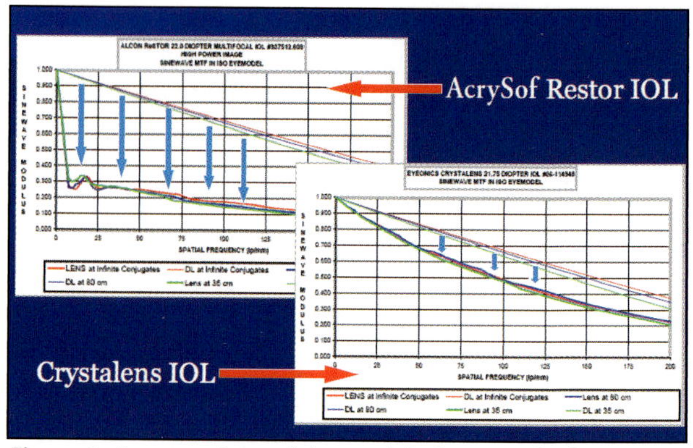

Figure 1. A comparison of the modulation transfer functions of the AcrySof Restor and Crystalens IOLs.

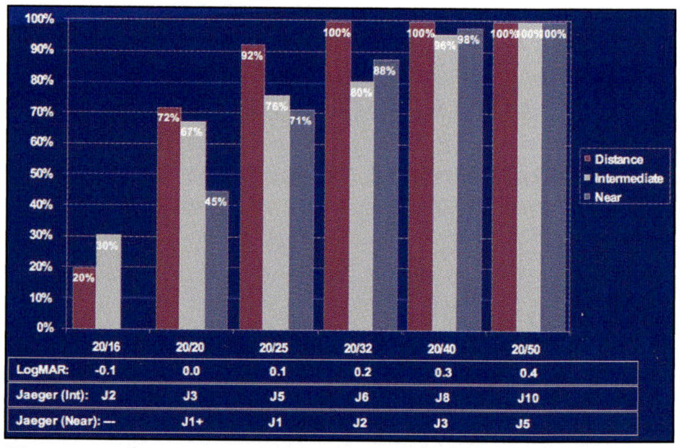

Figure 2. The mixing of the Crystalens with the AcrySof Restor lens demonstrates the degree of acuity at distance, intermediate distance, and near when the patient is allowed to choose his preferred range.

under dim lighting conditions (the depressed modulation transfer function of the multifocal IOL). At close reading distances (11 to 13 inches), however, the AcrySof Restor can relieve the accommodative strain on the ciliary muscle through the high magnification inherent in its design. At intermediate distances, there is typically enough accommodation associated with the Crystalens to comfortably meet my patients' moderate accommodative demand, especially when they use the computer. In my experience, the bilateral AcrySof Restor patients' most frequent complaint is poor intermediate distance vision, and the mixed-IOL strategy relieves this problem.

Does mixing the Crystalens with the AcrySof Restor lens work in the real world? Although it is probably not the best possible solution to every presbyope's need, I find the combination is effective and often works better than bilaterally matched presbyopia-correcting IOLs (Figure 2).

Studies

According to a prospective, nonrandomized cohort of 50 consecutive patients undergoing refractive lens exchange in which the Crystalens was implanted in their dominant eye and the AcrySof Restor in their other eye, 100% saw at least 20/32 binocularly and the equivalent of 20/40 at both near and intermediate distance.[1] These results compare with a series of 13 consecutive bilateral IOL patients who received either two AcrySof Restor lenses or two Crystalens AT45 IOLs (Eyeonics, Inc.).[2] As expected, near vision was better in patients with bilateral AcrySof Restor lenses, and intermediate vision over an impressive depth of field was better in patients with bilateral Crystalens IOLs. This conclusion is based on a recent clinical study we did in which a prospective, matched, nonrandomized set of 15 patients in each of two groups received bilateral presbyopia-correcting IOLs (Crystalens AT45 or AcrySof Restor). We compared these two groups with a previous cohort of mixed patients (Crystalens in the dominant eye, AcrySof Restor in the fellow eye).

Postoperative Vision

What may dissatisfy patients about a mixed-IOL approach? I find it is rarely a perceptual disparity in viewing at distance. The occasional person will spontaneously mention a waxy image through the multifocal IOL. Even when questioned about waxy vision specifically, those who notice a difference will relate it more often to the close reading distance and describe letters as having "ghost image" edges. The high degree of magnification of the AcrySof Restor lens at about 12 inches will often be compared preferably to that of the Crystalens at that same distance.

Intermediate distance vision is rarely, if ever, a source of complaints in those of my patients with mixed IOLs. Most are unaware that their two eyes see differently at 14 to 36 inches . This finding coupled with my patients' extremely high degree of satisfaction with their distance vision (under all conditions: scotopic; mesopic; and photopic) has convinced me that the AcrySof Restor/Crystalens combination works well for refractive lens exchange in most of my patients over age 50 (my rough cutoff age when selecting patients for this surgery).

CONCLUSION

I anticipate combining the Crystalens and AcrySof Restor lens at least until Alcon Laboratories, Inc., releases a ±1.50 D-add model of its multifocal IOL. It will be interesting to see whether the company's forthcoming aspheric version of the lens will significantly improve its modulation transfer function. If so, the current drawbacks of bilaterally implanting the AcrySof Restor lens will decrease dramatically.

As manufacturers improve the degree of dioptric or linear magnification at near with accommodating IOLs like the Crystalens, the relative advantage of the AcrySof Restor lens will disappear. Once accommodating IOLs provide a dependable range of magnification at near without an unreasonable demand on accommodative reserve, I believe that they will completely replace multifocal IOLs because of their superior optical performance, as documented objectively by modulation transfer function and subjectively by patients' satisfaction. ■

This article originally appeared in the August 2007 issue of CRSToday.

1. Woodhams JT, Carpenter H. Mixing presbyopia-correcting IOLs: binocular + contralateral vision in Crystalens/Restor IOL combination. Paper presented at: the AAO/APAO Joint Meeting; November 2006; Las Vegas, NV.
2. Woodhams JT, Carpenter H. Why multifocal IOLs will not prevail in the race for a surgical correction of presbyopic ametropia. Paper presented at: the ASCRS Symposium on Cataract, IOL and Refractive Surgery; May 1, 2007; San Diego, CA.

CHAPTER 176

Why I Do Not Mix IOLs

RICHARD TIPPERMAN, MD

When examining the subject of mixing and matching IOLs, one must first review the proposed benefits and downsides of each approach. This article discusses why I feel mixing multifocal IOLs does not produce a greater percentage of happy patients and, in the long run, is likely to make more patients unhappy. Patients are most pleased following multifocal IOL surgery if they can function normally on a day-to-day basis with minimal dependence on spectacles.

NIGHTTIME VISUAL DISTURBANCES

One of the reasons why I prefer the AcrySof Restor multifocal IOL platform (Alcon Laboratories, Inc., Fort Worth, TX) is that I have found it produces fewer difficulties with nighttime glare and halos than the ReZoom zonal refractive IOL (Advanced Medical Optics, Inc., Santa Ana, CA). In early 2007, I presented a poster at the ASCRS meeting describing the results of an optical bench evaluation of nighttime visual symptoms with various multifocal IOLs.[1] I found the least distortion with the AcrySof Restor platform (Figure 1). Similarly, for a poster presented at the 2007 ESCRS meeting, investigators analyzed visual disturbances in a simulated night-driving environment.[2] They found the fewest visual disturbances with the AcrySof Restor platform (Figure 2). Obviously, in order to justify placing a ReZoom IOL in a fellow eye, the surgeon must feel that the known disadvantage of nighttime dysphotopsia will be offset by a significant improvement for the patient in another parameter of visual function.

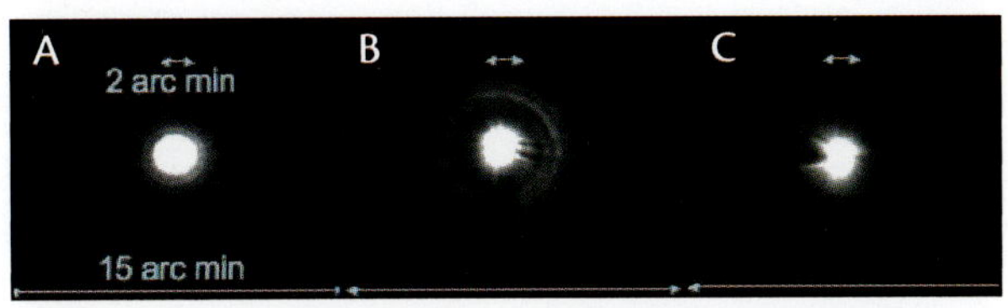

Figure 1. This optical bench simulation shows the visual images that would be seen through the AcrySof Restor lens (A), ReZoom IOL (B), and Tecnis Multifocal lens (not available in the US; Advanced Medical Optics, Inc.) (C) using a white light source. The lowest amount of glare and halos occurs with the AcrySof Restor IOL.

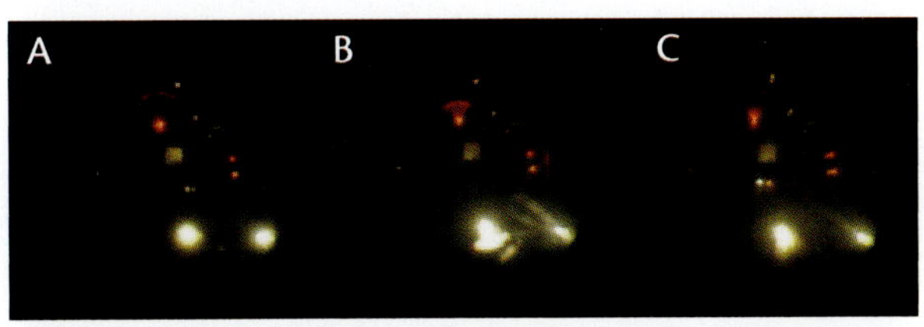

Figure 2. In this simulation of nighttime driving with the AcrySof Restor lens (A), ReZoom IOL (B), and Tecnis Multifocal lens (C), the least dysphotopsia occurs with the AcrySof Restor IOL.

WHEN I MIX PRESBYOPIA-CORRECTING IOLs

I am very comfortable placing an AcrySof Restor IOL (Alcon Laboratories, Inc., Fort Worth, TX) in the second eye of a patient who has received a monofocal IOL. Such individuals have the best personal understanding of the absolute presbyopia that accompanies pseudophakic emmetropia. Many received their monofocal IOL when it was the only available option, and they are very interested in and are excellent candidates for the AcrySof Restor IOL.

The other patients in whom I will mix lens designs have excellent vision after the implantation of an AcrySof Restor IOL in their first eye but are bothered by dysphotopsias. Although most patients will neuroadapt and eventually cease to be bothered by the halos, there is a subgroup of individuals for whom the dysphotopsias do not lessen. If the patient otherwise has excellent vision for distance and near in his eye with an AcrySof Restor IOL, he may desire to keep the lens and try to adapt. In these cases, placing a monofocal IOL in the fellow eye that targets distance vision can often significantly improve these patients' overall clinical function, because the pure distance image from the monofocal IOL can allow them to suppress the distance-vision dysphotopsias in the eye with the multifocal lens. Other surgeons would consider the placement of a Crystalens (Eyeonics, Inc., Aliso Viejo, CA) in the fellow eye. I have avoided this lens platform for the same reasons I have chosen not to implant plate-haptic design lenses in general.

A third group that may require mixed IOLs has extreme midrange concerns (ie, professional musicians, automobile mechanics). If they are pleased with their overall vision following the initial implantation of an AcrySof Restor IOL, I will match their second eye to their first. If they have concerns regarding their midrange vision, then I will adjust their second eye in the manner described by Blaylock et al, which is to target a mildly myopic error (-1.00 D) in their nondominant eye to improve their midrange vision.[1] Others would place a ReZoom IOL (Advanced Medical Optics, Inc., Santa Ana, CA) in the patient's second eye, but I think this approach is likely to induce more nighttime visual disturbances.

1. Blaylock JF, Si Z, Vickers C. Visual and refractive status at different focal distances after implantation of the Restor multifocal intraocular lens. *J Cataract Refract Surg.* 2006;32:1464-1473.

INTERMEDIATE VISION

Proponents of mixing other IOLs with the AcrySof Restor platform propose that doing so improves patients' intermediate vision without any disadvantages, because their brains adjust to improve the image.[3]

My patients rarely report significant midrange visual problems after the bilateral implantation of the AcrySof Restor IOL. Their experience may be explained by several factors. First, preoperative counseling is critical to my success with multifocal IOLs. I inform patients that this lens technology entails a bilateral procedure and that they will see best once they receive their second implant. Second, I explain to patients that their vision will improve with both bilateral summation and neuroadaption, which take time. Third, I show patients where their near visual point will be immediately after surgery. I actually move their hands approximately 12 to 14 inches from their faces and say, "Early on, this is where you will see best up close. Over time, your vision will push outward." It is important for patients to understand this phenomenon preoperatively so they will be comfortable postoperatively. Finally, I address midrange vision by telling patients that the AcrySof Restor lens' design has one peak for reading up close and one for distance and emphasize that the IOL is not quite as strong—but is still functional—in the midrange.

Data from other clinicians also demonstrate that the midrange "difficulties" of the AcrySof Restor lens have been overestimated. In a prospective study of patients who received the AcrySof Restor or ReZoom IOL bilaterally and in a retrospective study of patients who received the Crystalens accommodating IOL (Eyeonics, Inc., Aliso Viejo, CA) bilaterally, David Chang, MD, found that the AcrySof Restor group had the strongest midrange vision when tested through their best distance correction to produce an emmetropic eye.[4]

Another study reviewed the data from a group of ophthalmologists that included Robert Cionni, MD; Stephen Lane, MD; Eric Donnenfeld, MD; Kerry Solomon, MD; James McCulley, MD; and Dr. Chang.[5] This study included more than 150 patients who had received the AcrySof Restor IOL bilaterally at least 6 months earlier. The investigators found that the patients had an extremely high degree of satisfaction with their overall visual function for distance, intermediate, and near vision. When asked specifically about their use of computers, the patients again reported a high degree of satisfaction.

INTERMEDIATE VISION: OBSERVATIONS VERSUS COMPLAINTS

How do I reconcile my positive experiences with those of colleagues who have been concerned about intermediate vision with the AcrySof Restor lens? The issue may be one of observations versus complaints. For ophthalmologists, cataract surgery is routine, but it is a unique experience for patients. They may voice numerous questions or observations out of a desire for reassurance. For example, many of my patients mention that their eyes feel scratchy postoperatively. They are not complaining but are asking if the sensation is normal. Once they hear it is, they are usually relieved.

Similarly, after receiving the AcrySof Restor IOL, those of my patients who make observations regarding their midrange vision have the sharpest overall vision (eg, 20/20, J1). Their vision is so strong at distance and near that they often notice the drop-off at midrange. They will often ask why their midrange vision is less clear. Because I understand that this is usually an observation rather than a complaint, I will answer that the phenomenon is normal. I also remind them of our preoperative discussion, during which I explained that, initially, they would see best at near and distance but that their midrange vision would improve over time. These patients usually confirm remembering this discussion.

STUDIES EVALUATING MIXING

Richard Mackool, MD, performed a prospective study of mixing multifocal IOLs. His series consisted of 15 consecutive patients (13 undergoing cataract surgery and two undergoing refractive lens exchange for hyperopia) who received an AcrySof Restor IOL in one eye and a ReZoom IOL in the other.[6] He asked patients which eye they preferred for distance, intermediate, and near vision and asked them to rate the overall quality of their vision. There was no difference between either lens' objectively measured or subjectively perceived distance acuity postoperatively. Nearly all of the patients preferred their AcrySof Restor eye for near, however, and many favored their ReZoom eye for intermediate vision. One patient requested to have his ReZoom lens removed because of poor distance, near, and intermediate vision, and four patients (including the two refractive lens exchange patients) insisted on having this lens explanted because of poor near vision. Two of these patients listed the symptoms of nocturnal glare and halos as an additional reason for explantation. No patient requested the removal of an AcrySof Restor lens, and all patients who had their ReZoom lens explanted were happy with bilateral AcrySof Restor IOLs.

Dr. Solomon and colleagues also conducted a prospective, randomized study on mixing and matching multifocal IOL platforms.[7] He found that the subjects who received two AcrySof Restor lenses had the best overall reading and near vision, the best visual summation, and the fewest nighttime vision symptoms at 3 and 6 months. Mixing and a Blaylock approach (the bilateral implantation of the AcrySof Restor lens with a planned myopic result of approximately 1.00 D in the nondominant eye)[8] provided a better range of vision but at the expense of near vision and night vision symptoms.

Paul Mann, MD, and colleagues evaluated his personal experience with 205 patients who received presbyopia-correcting IOLs (32 received the Crystalens bilaterally, 82 received the AcrySof Restor lens bilaterally, 49 received the ReZoom IOL bilaterally, and 42 received an AcrySof Restor lens in one eye and a ReZoom IOL in their fellow eye).[9] For more on his results, read Dr. Mann's article on page 69. To summarize, most patients were pleased with their outcomes. Moreover, there were clear data that mixing the AcrySof Restor and ReZoom lenses did not yield higher levels of spectacle independence than the bilateral implantation of either IOL.

Nonetheless, a few physicians have reported better results from mixing the AcrySof Restor and ReZoom IOLs than implanting them bilaterally. I cannot reconcile these clinical findings with either my own clinical experience or that of the physicians I have mentioned. Perhaps these patients and physicians have lower expectations. I have actually seen a number patients with mixed IOLs and have documented for my files their unhappiness with this approach.

SUMMARY

It is possible to make patients happy with any of the presbyopia-correcting IOLs or a combination thereof. Without question, each lens has its strengths and weaknesses, and some of the variance in different investigators' results may represent differences in how they counsel and manage their patients. Each physician needs to evaluate the benefits of these technologies objectively and decide on the most reasonable approach.

I believe, however, that a careful review of the objective data available clearly shows that the bilateral implantation of the AcrySof Restor IOL will produce the greatest percentage of happy patients and, more importantly, the least likelihood of significant clinical problems. With the imminent release of the aspheric AcrySof Restor platform, it is likely that the rationale for implanting this lens bilaterally will be even stronger. ■

This article originally appeared in the August 2007 issue of CRSToday.

1. Tipperman R. Pinhole image comparison with white-light source for 3 multifocal IOL designs. Poster presented at: The ASCRS Symposium on Cataract, IOL and Refractive Surgery; April 27 to May 2, 2007; San Diego, CA.
2. Schwiegerling J, Ye X, Choi J, Ernest P. Night-time visual quality with different multifocal IOLs. Poster presented at: XXIV Congress of the ESCRS; September 10-13, 2006; London, UK.
3. Bucci FA Jr. Mixing multifocal IOLs. *Cataract & Refractive Surgery Today.* March 2007;7:3:76-77.
4. Chang D. Comparing presbyopic IOLs. Paper presented at: The EyeWorld Symposium on Presbyopic IOLs; May 2, 2007; San Diego, CA.
5. Cionni RJ. Bilateral implantation of an apodized diffractive IOL: six-month results. *Ocular Surgery News.* January 15, 2007. Available at: http://www.osnsupersite.com/view.asp?rid=20012. Accessed July 13, 2007.
6. Mackool RJ Sr. Randomized implantation of ReSTOR and ReZoom IOLs in contralateral eyes: results and recommendations. Paper presented at: The ACRS Symposium on Cataract, IOL and Refractive Surgery; April 29, 2007; San Diego, CA.
7. Solomon KD, Fernandez de Castro LE, Vroman DT, Sandoval HP. Mix and match versus bilateral implantation of a diffractive multifocal IOL. Paper presented at: The ACRS Symposium on Cataract, IOL and Refractive Surgery; April 29, 2007; San Diego, CA.
8. Blaylock JF, Si Z, Vickers C. Visual and refractive status at different focal distances after implantation of the Restor multifocal intraocular lens. *J Cataract Refract Surg.* 2006;32:1464-1473.
9. Mann PM II, Brunson PB, O'Neal MR. Patient satisfaction survey with presbyopic IOLs. Paper presented at: The ACRS Symposium on Cataract, IOL and Refractive Surgery; April 28, 2007; San Diego, CA.

CHAPTER 177

European Perspective on Mixing and Matching Multifocal IOLs

MICHAEL C. KNORZ, MD

As with many other technologies in the ophthalmic field, here in Europe, we have a slight advantage over our US colleagues in terms of the variety of multifocal IOLs that we are able to implant. This article outlines some of the multifocals currently available in Europe and discusses my experience and thoughts on mixing and matching these IOLs.

THE MULTIFOCAL LENSES AVAILABLE IN EUROPE

Diffractive

AcrySof Restor IOL

The single-piece, acrylic AcrySof Restor lens (Alcon Laboratories, Inc., Fort Worth, TX) has a 6-mm optic and can be injected through a 2.8-mm incision. Its apodized diffractive design has 12 zones with a total add of +4.00 D. It is available in two models, one that filters blue and ultraviolet light and another that blocks ultraviolet light only. The IOL is available in a power range of +10.00 to +30.00 D.

Acri.LISA 366D and 356D

Manufactured by Acri.Tec GmbH (Berlin, Germany), the single-piece, aberration-correcting, aspheric, hydrophobic acrylic, microincisional Acri.LISA IOL (not available in the US) is actually more a hybrid multifocal. In the acronym *LISA*, *L* stands for a light intensity distribution of 65% (refractive) far and 35% (diffractive) near; *I* represents independent from pupillary size; *S* means smooth refractive/diffractive surface profile; and *A* stands for optimized aspheric surface. The Acri.LISA 366D IOL has a total add power of +3.75 D. It is designed for injection through a sub–2-mm cataract incision using the A2-2000 injector (Acri.Tec GmbH). The lens is available in a power range of 10.00 to 32.00 D in 0.50 D increments. IOLs in 1.00 D increments can be specially made with an 8-week lead time.

The company's Acri.LISA 356D IOL has essentially the same diffractive/refractive multifocal design as the 366D except that the former is designed to go through a larger incision. It is available in 0.50 D increments of 10.00 to 30.00 D, with IOLs of 0 to 9.00 D and 31.00 to 44.00 D available with 8 weeks' lead time.

Tecnis ZM900

The three-piece, diffractive, multifocal, silicone Tecnis ZM900 (not available in the US; Advanced Medical Optics, Inc., Santa Ana, CA) has a 6-mm optic. Its diffractive design on the posterior surface creates two focal points that are 4.00 D apart. As a result, light entering the eye is evenly distributed between near and distance vision and is independent of the pupil's size. Additionally, the Tecnis ZM900 has a modified, prolate anterior surface that is intended to compensate for the spherical aberration of the cornea to create an optical system that is free of spherical aberration. This design should allow patients higher image contrast than with a spherical multifocal lens. The Tecnis ZM900 is available in 0.50 D increments from 5.00 to 34.00 D.

Refractive

ReZoom Multifocal IOL

The ReZoom Multifocal IOL (Advanced Medical Optics, Inc.) is a three-piece acrylic lens with five refractive zones: a low-light/distance-dominant zone; a near-dominant zone; a distance zone; another near-dominant zone; and a bright light/distance-dominant zone (moving from the outer zone inward). Transitions provide intermediate vision. With a design the company calls *balance view optics*, the ReZoom multifocal is intended to have 100% light transmission over all five optical zones. The lens has a total near add of +3.50 D and is available from 5.00 to 30.00 D in 0.50 D increments.

MF4 IOL

From Carl Zeiss Meditec AG (Jena, Germany), the MF4 (not available in the US) is a single-piece, hydrophilic acrylic IOL featuring a four-zone optic with a tripod haptic design. It has a 6-mm optic and a total near add of +4.00 D. The manufacturer describes the IOL as an autofocus multifocal IOL. Although this lens was first introduced approximately 4 years ago by IOLTech Laboratories (La Rochelle, France), there has been little published on its results. The MF4 multifocal IOL is available from 15.00 to 26.00 D in 0.50 D increments.

M-Flex Multifocal IOL

The M-Flex Multifocal IOL (not available in the US; Rayner Intraocular Lenses Ltd., Hove, East Sussex, UK) is the newest multifocal on the European market. This hydrophilic acrylic IOL has a 6.25-mm, multizone aspheric optic. It comes with either four or five zones, depending on the base power. The lens is distance dominant with a +3.00 D near add. The first M-Flex Multifocal IOL was implanted in 2005, although no results have been published to date. The lens is available in powers from 14.00 to 25.00 D in 1.00 D increments and from 18.50 to 23.50 D in 0.50 D increments.

MIXING AND MATCHING

With such a wide range of multifocal IOLs available in Europe, it is interesting to note that the idea of combining different types of multifocals in the same patient is fairly new. The novelty of mixing these lenses is motivated by the inherent limitations of each IOL design. Refractive multifocals such as the ReZoom provide excellent distance and good intermediate vision, but certain patients find their near vision to be insufficient with this type of lens. In contrast, diffractive designs such as the Tecnis Multifocal and AcrySof Restor IOLs provide excellent near and good distance vision, but some patients may find their intermediate vision with these lenses to be unsatisfactory. Combining a diffractive and refractive multifocal IOL is an attempt to compensate for each design's limitations.

I routinely use the ReZoom and the Tecnis Multifocal IOLs and have some experience with the AcrySof Restor lens. I have no experience with the other IOLs mentioned in this article. With its distance-dominant design, the ReZoom lens provides very good distance vision, slightly better than the Tecnis Multifocal or the AcrySof Restor IOL, I find. Intermediate vision with the ReZoom lens is good, also better than with the other two lenses in my experience. My patients' near vision is not as good as with the Tecnis Multifocal or the AcrySof Restor IOL. In contrast, the Tecnis Multifocal lens has provided excellent near vision to all of my patients who have received it, although some have been frustrated by their lack of intermediate or computer vision.

After advocating the bilateral implantation of the same IOL design for years, I recently changed my opinion because of some of my patients' complaints (mentioned earlier) regarding reduced intermediate vision with a diffractive IOL design such as the Tecnis Multifocal IOL and insufficient near vision with a refractive IOL design such as the ReZoom lens. The benefit of a mixed approach is that it enables surgeons to balance the strengths and weaknesses of these multifocals in order to provide cataract surgery and refractive lens exchange patients with the best possible range of vision and the greatest degree of independence from spectacles.

The mixing of multifocal IOLs is becoming my standard of care, particularly when I am operating on a 50-something presbyope who still works at a computer, drives a car, and enjoys an active lifestyle. For refractive lens exchange, I will always operate on the patient's dominant eye first. I usually implant a ReZoom multifocal IOL in these eyes because of its strength in the areas of distance and intermediate vision. If the patient is also happy postoperatively with his near vision, I will implant the same IOL in his second eye. If he is not or is unsure, I will implant a Tecnis Multifocal IOL in his second nondominant, eye. With this approach, I hear no more complaints from patients who cannot see their computer screens. Statistically, approximately 30% of my patients receive a ReZoom IOL in both eyes, and 70% receive a ReZoom lens in their dominant eye and a Tecnis Multifocal IOL in their nondominant eye.

OTHER CONSIDERATIONS

I consider two more issues when implanting multifocal IOLs. The first relates to the typical side effects. All patients will see halos with a multifocal IOL, but I would estimate that the phenomenon is transient in approximately 60% of recipients. It is therefore important to mention this side effect before surgery and to use multifocal IOLs only in those patients who do not want to wear spectacles. They should understand that multifocal lenses are a compromise and are only indicated if independence from spectacles is important.

The second issue is closely linked to the requirement of spectacle independence. Because multifocal IOLs cannot achieve emmetropia in all eyes, a certain number of eyes require a refractive enhancement (approximately 10% to 20% in my practice). I will typically perform LASIK in these eyes about 3 months after implanting the IOL. In eyes with a Tecnis Multifocal IOL, I will perform wavefront-guided LASIK using the Visx Star S4 laser (Advanced Medical Optics, Inc.) with iris registration. In eyes with a refractive multifocal IOL such as the ReZoom, I do not find currently available aberrometers reliable and will therefore perform standard LASIK.

For eyes that have relatively high corneal astigmatism prior to IOL surgery (in my hands, this means astigmatism of 2.00 D or more), I will use the IntraLase FS 60 laser (Advanced Medical Optics, Inc.) to cut a flap (100 μm thick, 9 mm in diameter) immediately prior to performing the refractive lens exchange or cataract surgery. I will not lift the flap at that time, which I find is a significant advantage of using the Intralase FS laser. Approximately 4 weeks later, I will lift the flap and perform the laser enhancement. This technique shortens the time between the lenticular and laser surgeries, which means a faster visual recovery for the patient. ■

This article originally appeared in the August 2007 issue of CRSToday.

CHAPTER 178

South American Perspective on Mixing Multifocal IOLs

LEONARDO AKAISHI, MD

Worldwide experience with multifocal IOLs has demonstrated that overall visual performance and, in particular, quality vision at intermediate distance are important to patients' ability to execute the tasks of daily living. None of the available multifocal and accommodating IOLs can meet everyone's expectations, and refractive lens exchange is not a suitable form of presbyopic correction for all patients. At present, however, I believe that multifocal IOLs are the best means for freeing presbyopes from their dependence on spectacles, but their use should be customized to the patient.[1]

ASSESSING PATIENTS

Pedro Paulo Fabri, MD, an expert on quality of vision from Cascavel, Brazil, maintains that a patient's preoperative modulation transfer function is a reliable indicator of optical quality and a patient's candidacy for refractive lens exchange. The optical quality of a youthful, healthy crystalline lens is better than that of a monofocal IOL, which, in turn, is superior to that of a multifocal IOL. Eyes with a high modulation transfer function, therefore, are not guaranteed a successful outcome with multifocal IOLs.

To satisfy patients' visual needs with multifocal IOLs, surgeons must talk with them about their habits and lifestyle. A thorough preoperative evaluation includes assessing patients' contrast sensitivity, higher-order aberrations, and accommodative miosis. Surgeons must also take into account ocular anatomy, anterior chamber depth, and pupillary size. Finally, they must counsel patients to have realistic expectations for the procedure.

PERSONAL EXPERIENCE

Background

During the last 4 years, my colleagues and I have implanted more than 1,000 AcrySof Restor lenses (Alcon Laboratories, Inc., Fort Worth, TX), 1,200 Tecnis Multifocal IOLs (not available in the US; Advanced Medical Optics, Inc., Santa Ana, CA), and 250 ReZoom IOLs (Advanced Medical Optics, Inc.). Table 1 summarizes my own experience.

Distance Vision

We found that the AcrySof Restor IOL provides the highest-quality vision at distance, probably due to its refractive (monofocal) power in the periphery.[2] Other researchers have achieved similar outcomes in their studies.[3,4]

In our experience, the Tecnis Multifocal IOL is very sensitive to small myopic errors. For example, 0.50 D of myopia produced worse vision at distance with this lens compared with the other two IOLs.

Intermediate Vision

The ReZoom IOL performed the best of the three multifocal lenses at intermediate distance.[5] Provided their pupils were larger than 3.5 mm, most of our patients achieved J3 vision with this lens. When patients who received the Tecnis Multifocal lens had a slightly hyperopic refraction (+0.50 D), their intermediate vision was quite similar to that of subjects in the ReZoom group with little compromise of their distance vision. I now regularly target this result when implanting the Tecnis Multifocal lens.

Near Vision

For near visual acuity, the Tecnis Multifocal IOL proved the best. Our patients found their reading distance to be most comfortable with this lens, and they were easily able to read a restaurant's menu under mesopic conditions.

TABLE 1. THE AUTHOR'S EXPERIENCE WITH THREE MULTIFOCAL IOLs						
	Distance Vision	Intermediate Vision	Near Vision	Halos	Pupillary Size	Lighting Level
AcrySof Restor	++++ +	+	++++	+	+ +	+++
ReZoom*	++++ +	++	++	++	+++	-
Tecnis Multifocal	++++	+	+++++	++	-	-

*The ReZoom IOL has a better modulation transfer function in the author's experience.

In contrast, recipients of the AcrySof Restor lens require bright light for reading.[4] Although patients with the ReZoom IOL are able to read J1 to J2, most of them need reading glasses. Moreover, the clarity of these patients' reading vision and their reading speed are low.[6]

Halos

All multifocal IOLs are associated with halos. We heard the fewest complaints about this phenomenon from patients who had received the AcrySof Restor IOL and the most from those who had received the ReZoom lens.

Pupillary Size

Visual performance with both the ReZoom lens and the AcrySof Restor IOL depends on the pupil's size. We found that patients who received the ReZoom lens and had pupils smaller than 3.5 mm were dissatisfied with their vision at near and at intermediate distance. We also noticed that patients with multifocal IOLs who had pupils larger than 4.5 mm had better intermediate vision than individuals with smaller pupils. Alfonso et al reported similar results.[7]

MIXING IOLS

Basic Approach

Recognizing that each of the multifocal IOLs has limitations, my colleagues and I now approach the implantation of these lenses in the following manner. We select the implant for the patient's first eye according to an assessment of that person's particular needs (eg, occupation, hobbies, reading patterns, computer use, nighttime driving). Seven to 15 days postoperatively, we choose the second IOL based on the patient's level of satisfaction with the first implant. We always advise patients not to compare the vision of their eyes and explain to them how neuroadaptation occurs with time.

If patients are satisfied with the vision in their first eye, we will implant the same IOL in their second eye.

Example No. 1

Patients who read a lot and use computers a fair amount receive a Tecnis Multifocal IOL in their first eye. If they complain about their distance vision postoperatively, we select an AcrySof Restor lens for their fellow eye. If they complain about their intermediate vision, we place a ReZoom lens in their second eye, provided their pupil is larger than 3.5 mm. Another option for improving their intermediate vision is to implant a second Tecnis Multifocal IOL with a targeted refraction of +0.50 D. We choose this option for individuals who desire perfect vision at near as well or who have pupils smaller than 3.5 mm.

Example No. 2

For patients who value distance vision and drive at night, we implant an AcrySof Restor IOL in their first eye. If they feel that their near reading point is too close postoperatively (a particular problem, we have found, with tall patients, who have long arms), we choose either a Tecnis Multifocal or a ReZoom lens for their second eye, as described in the previous example.

Patients who complain about needing bright light to read or not being able to see the menu in a restaurant receive a Tecnis Multifocal lens in their second eye, because it functions independently of pupillary size. Some patients—particularly those with long arms and pupils smaller than 3 mm—will require glasses for activities such as using the computer and should be fully informed of this possibility preoperatively.

Example No. 3

For individuals who rely heavily on their intermediate vision (eg, cooks, pianists, frequent users of a computer), we choose a ReZoom IOL for their first eye. If they complain about poor near vision postoperatively, we select a diffractive multifocal IOL for their second eye.

CONCLUSION

None of the patients in whom we have mixed multifocal IOL designs has required an explantation thus far. We have found that, 3 months postoperatively, some of our patients cannot distinguish which IOL is implanted in their right versus left eye. Currently, we recommend mixing IOLs if the first implant is a diffractive multifocal lens and the outcome is worse than J5. ■

This article originally appeared in the August 2007 issue of CRSToday.

1. Solomon KD. Patient selection for refractive IOLs. *Cataract & Refractive Surgery Today.* July 2006. Available at: http://www.crstoday.com/PDF%20Articles/0706/CRST0706_07.html. Accessed July 12, 2007.
2. Davison JA, Simpson MJ. History and development of the apodized diffractive intraocular lens. *J Cataract Refract Surg.* 2006;32:849-858.
3. Carones F. Pseudoaccomodating ReSTOR IOL to correct defocus and presbyopia in refractive lens exchange: clinical results. Paper presented at: The ASCRS Symposium on Cataract, IOL and Refractive Surgery; April 17, 2005; Washington, DC.
4. Bucci FA Jr. Combining multifocal IOLs. *Cataract & Refractive Surgery Today.* March 2006. Available at: http://www.crstoday.com/PDF%20Articles/0306/CRST0306_F10_Bucci.html. Accessed July 20, 2007.
5. Hutz WW, Eckhardt HB, Rohrig B, Grolmus R. Reading ability with 3 multifocal intraocular lens models. *J Cataract Refract Surg.* 2006;32:2015-2021.
6. Hayashi K, Hayashi H. Pupil size before and after phacoemulsification in nondiabetic and diabetic patients. *J Cataract Refract Surg.* 2004;30:2543-2550.
7. Alfonso JF, Fernandez-Veja L, Begonamonde M, Montes-Mico R. Correlations of pupil size with visual acuity and contrast sensitivity after implantation of an apodized diffractive intraocular lens. *J Cataract Refract Surg.* 2007;33:431-438.

CHAPTER 179

Performing Refractive Lens Exchange on the Refractive Patient

STEPHEN S. LANE, MD

When is a refractive IOL an option for a patient who does not have cataracts and desires correction of his refractive error? Would a 45-year-old emmetropic presbyope who wanted to get rid of his reading glasses be a good candidate for refractive lens exchange? This is a difficult question and one that cannot yet be easily answered because of the IOLs that are currently available. Although the present generation of presbyopia-correcting IOLs is very decent, I am not sure that these lenses are good enough to deliver the results necessary for this type of patient. On the other hand, presbyopic hyperopes represent a much better group of patients for refractive lens exchange. Unlike the former group, the presbyopic hyperope has poor uncorrected vision for both distance and near and is therefore more likely to perceive a significant improvement after refractive lens exchange.

As the safety and effectiveness of refractive IOLs improves, they will be used more frequently as an alternative form of vision correction among patients who are poor candidates for laser refractive surgery.

SELECTING PATIENTS

In my experience, the candidates that achieve the highest rates of success after refractive lens exchange are presbyopes with more than 3.00D of hyperopia. Patients with presbyopia and moderate amounts of myopia (eg, 5.00 D) are also good candidates, because this group like the former is totally dependent on spectacles and/or contact lenses for all tasks. Presbyopia-correcting IOLs free them from this dependence.

The candidates that are most difficult to please for refractive lens exchange are mildly myopic individuals, because they do not use their glasses for reading and may only need distance correction occasionally. Their quality of vision for distance and/or near may be off just enough from what they previous had to cause difficulty. Finally, patients with myopia in excess of 7.00 D have an increased risk for retinal detachment, especially men over the age of 45 years with axial lengths greater than 25 mm. Refractive lens exchange as an elective procedure (eg, no cataracts) may not be justified in this group due to the aforementioned associated risks.

Patients with minimal astigmatism are also ideal candidates for refractive IOLs, because surgeons do not have to correct cylinder as part of the procedure. Individuals with higher levels of astigmatism, however, require its correction through surgical techniques such as peripheral corneal relaxing incisions or laser surgery.

DIFFERENCES IN CATARACT VERSUS REFRACTIVE PROCEDURES

The surgical technique for implanting a refractive IOL in a patient without cataract does not differ from conventional cataract surgery. The optics of the presbyopia-correcting IOLs require accurate centration, which demands a well-centered capsulorhexis and zonular integrity necessary for successful outcomes. If a complication such as a compromised capsular bag occurs during refractive lens exchange, one might want to reconsider implanting a multifocal IOL. An accommodative lens would definitely be contraindicated

Accurate biometry, keratometry, and the use of modern regression formulae are critical for determining IOL power. Achieving emmetropia is absolutely essential for the success of presbyopia-correcting IOLs. With the refractive patient, even more importantly than the cataract patient, surgeons need to be more sensitive to the development of posterior capsular opacification. Meticulous cortical cleanup and posterior capsular polishing are therefore crucial to minimizing this complication.

PHACOEMULSIFICATION

Obviously, surgeons should strive to remove the crystalline lens as atraumatically as possible. Complications during routine cataract surgery are tragic enough, but they are particularly upsetting in purely elective procedures like refractive lens exchange. Fortunately, advances in phaco technology such as power modulations have made the lens' removal safer. Other technological improvements include bimanual methods, torsional phacoemulsification, and the use of water pulses (Aqualase; Alcon Laboratories, Fort Worth, TX)

REALISTIC EXPECTATIONS FOR VISUAL IMPROVEMENT

Refractive IOLs can enable patients to see at both distance and near without glasses. Obviously, postoperative results will vary. For the ophthalmologist, an important part of implanting refractive IOLs is choosing the correct lens for each patient's individual needs. Axial length and keratometric data as well as other ocular characteristics are important, but they may not affect postoperative outcomes as much as a patient's personality. Ophthalmologists need to consider what the patient does for a living, how he uses his eyes (eg, does he read more than perform intermediate tasks or vice versa?), the required sharpness of distance vision for his profession or hobbies, etc. Identifying a patient's true expectations is one of the biggest challenges that surgeons face. Some patients ask for results that we frankly cannot deliver. They are inappropriate candidates for refractive lens exchange.

CONCLUSION

Clearly, the bar for visual rehabilitation with IOLs has been raised. We now can insert accommodative and multifocal IOLs through ultra-small incisions. These lenses permit excellent uncorrected simultaneous distance and near vision for patients, minimize aberrations and block ultraviolet and near ultraviolet light. We can now insert lenses that have been preloaded into an injector. Furthermore, if an error in power determination is made, we may soon be able to adjust or modify of the IOL's power after it is placed in the eye. As we begin to imagine the potential synergies between all these technologies it is obvious that we are at the brink of individualizing IOLs on a patient-by-patient basis depending on the need and makeup of each person.

My recommendation to surgeons who desire to practice current state-of-the-art ophthalmology is to get into the refractive IOL game. Do not stand on the sidelines waiting for the perfect answer. Become knowledgeable and experience firsthand what these lenses offer. An exciting armamentarium of technologies that offer the potential for a better life for our patients is now at our disposal. Without question, these are not yet perfected. Although each technology has potential pitfalls they all have far more attributes. Cataract and refractive surgeons have an obligation to be knowledgeable about the available options and willing to discuss presbyopia-correcting IOLs with every prospective patient. Although there can be a potential "poison" with each choice, we now have the ability to provide appropriate patients with something very special, and, for those interested it can be a true miracle.

But, perhaps more important than what techniques and technology will be used is for whom we will use them. Because the advent of technologies and techniques has made the removal of the crystalline lens safer and more effective, I believe that lensectomy with IOL implantation will be the future of refractive surgery. Like I. Howard Fine, MD, of Eugene, Oregon, who was the first person I heard express this idea, I believe that lens removal will become a procedure most commonly performed on patients younger than 65 years. Surgeons will then be reimbursed more fairly for their work, the government will save money as lens removal occurs before patients reach Medicare age, and manufacturers will be more fairly paid for the technologies they develop, which will allow them to continue the expensive and time-consuming R&D and regulatory measures necessary to continue to advance the field. In the end, patients will undergo a safer and more effective procedure and achieve improved outcomes long before they develop cataracts, and spectacles may become exhibits in a museum that our great grandchildren will ask us about. ■

This article originally appeared in the Novemebr/December 2006 issue of CRSToday.

CHAPTER 180

The Challenges of New IOLs

STEVEN J. DELL, MD

The landscape of refractive surgery is undergoing a radical shift, much of which is demographically driven. The LASIK market in the US is relatively flat with low, single-digit growth. Some ophthalmologists blame fuel prices, the economy, or financial uncertainty, but, in reality, the economy remains quite strong. Others believe that, in addition to seasonal variations, LASIK volumes track with overall consumer confidence. With wavefront-guided treatments and femtosecond flaps, we as refractive surgeons are delivering the best results ever seen with keratorefractive surgery. By all accounts, this should be the golden age of laser vision correction, so where have all the LASIK patients gone?

DWINDLING LASIK PROCEDURES

Age

Perhaps much of the decline in surgical volume lies in the fact that many of the correctable patients have simply gotten older. In 1996, the average baby boomer was 41 years old, which is well within the potential age range of patients for laser vision correction. Now, many of these patients are in their early 50s and opting for lens-based surgery instead. In essence, I believe we are penetrating more deeply into the addressable pool of LASIK patients as technology improves and laser vision correction becomes more acceptable. On the other hand, as baby boomers age, the pool of potential patients shrinks.

More Options

With three presbyopia-correcting IOLs on the market in the US, we now have tools with which to treat this huge population of older individuals. Patients with clinically significant cataracts can upgrade to these technologies, and offlabel refractive lens exchange can simultaneously correct ametropia and presbyopia. According to Shareef Mahdavi, if 20% of the cataract market converts to presbyopia-correcting IOLs, it will be the second largest elective medical market among all specialties.1 What is the number 1 market? LASIK. As ophthalmologists, we are fortunate to have the potential to provide the top two elective procedures in all of medicine.

Positive Financial Model for Elective IOL Surgery

The Centers for Medicare & Medicaid Services have allowed doctors to bill patients for these upgraded IOL technologies, which should stimulate incredible scientific innovation. In fact, I can think of no greater economic stimulus for the development of future IOLs than the financial incentive of charging a premium price for these lenses. Although Alcon Laboratories, Inc. (Fort Worth, TX), and Advanced Medical Optics, Inc. (Santa Ana, CA), both contributed significantly to the development of this financial model, much of the credit belongs to Andy Corley, CEO of Eyeonics, Inc. (Aliso Viejo, CA). For years, he single-handedly pushed for the eventual ruling by the Centers for Medicare & Medicaid Services for these IOLs, despite great skepticism from the ophthalmic industry.

WHO WILL PERFORM PRESBYOPIA CORRECTING IOL SURGERY?

I believe it is likely that presbyopia-correcting IOL surgery will probably segment into "haves" and "have-nots" in that a relatively small minority of surgeons will perform most of the volume. There is certainly a much greater hassle involved in educating and counseling these patients, optimizing biometry, and correcting postoperative ametropia. Many surgeons do not feel comfortable asking patients for thousands of extra dollars to upgrade their IOLs. Other ophthalmologists may serve communities where little disposable income is available for these lenses. Moreover, a number of surgeons lack the ability to perform the keratorefractive enhancements needed in a significant percentage of these cases. Still others will conclude that this added work simply overshadows the potential gain. On the other hand, declining reimbursement will spur some surgeons to embrace this technology.

THE CHALLENGE OF DEALING WITH PRESBYOPIC PATIENTS

Regardless of the IOL used, even perfectly executed surgery may not avoid a very dissatisfied patient. Multifocal IOLs are sometimes associated with unwanted images and a loss of overall visual clarity. These issues are typically not associated with the Crystalens (Eyeonics, Inc.), but some patients may not achieve the degree of accommodation for which they hoped. Since patients pay thousands of dollars for these technologies, the potential for frustration is high with all presbyopia- correcting lenses. The temperament we need in order to deal with these patients is a new concept for many of us.

FRESH APPROACHES TO PROMOTING NEW TECNOLOGY

Marketing presbyopia-correcting IOLs will require different strategies. I suspect that interested senior citizens will more likely respond to word of mouth rather than a slick marketing campaign. In my experience, candidates for presbyopia-correcting IOLs are much more likely to ask their friends about surgeons and their reputations than are LASIK candidates. With new IOLs, the patients' experiences and outcomes drive the market.

THE SIGNIFICANCE OF INTERMEDIATE VISION

The need to provide patients with good intermediate vision postoperatively has grown significantly along with increasing computer usage during the past decade. Treatment strategies that emphasize good near and distance vision while ignoring intermediate vision will dissatisfy many patients.

CONCLUSION

The market has clearly demonstrated that there are ways to achieve successful clinical results with all of the available presbyopia-correcting IOLs. These technologies perform well but will inevitably be surpassed by better lenses in the future. Taking full advantage of these IOLs requires a revision of practice patterns, but with judicious application they can be a rewarding modality. ■

This article originally appeared in the March 2007 issue of CRSToday.

1. Mahdavi S. Traps and truths about the marketing of refractive IOLs. Paper presented at: Advanced Medical Optics, Inc.: Developing the New Lenticular Refractive Business; November 11, 2006; Las Vegas, NV.

CHAPTER 181

The Monofocal Solution for Presbyopic Cataract Surgery

J. E. "JAY" MCDONALD II, MD

Monovision is a familiar technique in cataract surgery that enables patients to view both near and far visual targets in the absence of natural visual accommodation. Implanting monofocal IOLs of different focal distances improves the patient's ability to see objects at close range while maintaining excellent distance visual acuity.[1,2] Once a popular choice of surgeons, monovision has competed in recent years with multifocal and accommodative IOL technologies.

LENS DESIGN AND SPHERICAL ABERRATION

Spherical-aberration changes in an aging eye can benefit from a monofocal, aspheric, aberration-free IOL used in a monovision technique. In a young person, the spherical aberrations of the cornea and lens are of opposite sign. This balance, or "good-coupling," between the lens or internal optics of the eye and the cornea reduces the overall amount of aberrations in the entire eye. In an older person, however, the wavefront of the lens (besides being more aberrated) has a shape that does not match the corneal wavefront. As a result of this "decoupling" between corneal and lenticular aberrations, the entire eye is more aberrated.

Removing the crystalline lens changes the results of all previous couplings between the cornea and the internal optics. Inserting a standard spherical IOL adds to the already positive spherical aberration of the cornea. Implanting an IOL with negative spherical aberration, on the other hand, can offset the positive spherical aberration of the cornea for a net-zero effect of spherical aberration. Research has demonstrated, however, that a small amount of positive spherical aberration is beneficial, because it compensates for higher-order aberrations such as coma and trefoil.[3,4]

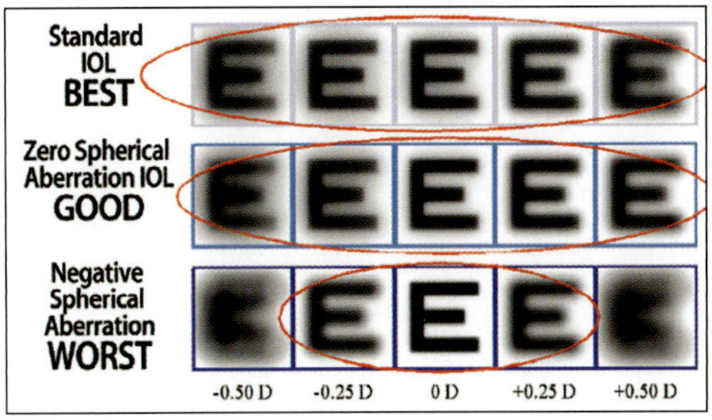

Figure 1. This chart shows the depth of field with three types of monofocal IOLs.

Furthermore, spherical aberration increases an eye's depth of field. When the object distance is infinity, image clarity is sharpest in an eye with no spherical aberration (the IOL with negative spherical aberration produces this). However, as vergence increases, image quality degrades with an IOL that has negative spherical aberration and is better with an aberration-free IOL (Sofport AO

TABLE 1. CURVATURE, POWER, AND INHERENT ABERRATION OF SEVERAL DIFFERENT TYPES OF MONOFOCAL IOLs			
Lens Type	**Curvature**	**Power**	**Spherical Aberration Inherent in Lens**
Standard spherical IOL	Spherical	Increases from center to edge	Positive
Aspheric (Tecnis)	Flattens from center to edge rapidly	Decreases from center to edge	Negative
Aspheric (Sofport AO)	Flattens from center to edge slowly	Constant from center to edge	None

lens; Bausch & Lomb, Rochester, NY) (Table 1 and Figure 1).

An aberration-free lens is forgiving when it is implanted slightly off-center.[5] Eyes that have undergone refractive surgery may have positive or negative spherical aberration, and the optical center of the cornea may be difficult to determine and match with the IOL's optical center. With these unknowns, adding positive or negative spherical aberration to the system could degrade image quality. If other higher-order aberrations are absent or minimal, a centered, negatively aspheric lens can provide image quality equal to or better than the aberration-free IOL in a pseudophakic monovision situation.

STUDY

I achieved great success in my clinic with the Sofport AO aberration-free aspheric IOL for monovision. In a retrospective study with 80 eyes of 40 patients, I implanted a near vision IOL in one eye, with a targeted refraction of -0.75 to -2.00 D, and a distance vision IOL in subjects' other eye, targeted between plano and -0.50 D. Three months postoperatively, all patients had 20/30 binocular vision or better, and 73% had at least 20/20 vision. Near vision was similarly successful, with 88% of patients achieving J2 or better and 48% possessing J1 or better near binocular vision. In a survey on spectacle dependence, only 19% of patients remained dependent on glasses for near vision; in contrast, 11% needed glasses for distance vision, and only 3% needed them for intermediate vision (Figure 2).

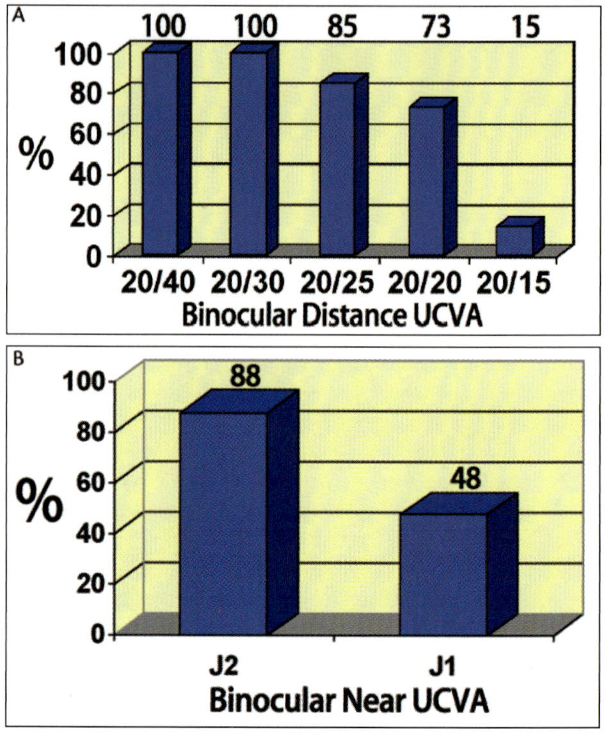

Figure 2. Distance (A) and near (B) visual outcomes in a retrospective evaluation of 80 eyes of 40 patients implanted with the Sofport AO aspheric IOL for monovision are shown.

MONOVISION AND THE HUMAN VISUAL SYSTEM

What attributes of the human visual system facilitate the use of monofocal aspheric implants in overcoming the issues of presbyopia? The monofocal solution is one that cooperates with the brain's natural processes of fusion while maintaining the highest quality of the image.

In developing new ophthalmic technologies, it seems that researchers have not paid enough attention to the naturally structured pathways of the brain. Multifocal IOLs are designed to recapture the phenomenon of accommodation, yet these lenses produce lower contrast sensitivity, are associated with a higher rate of glare and halos, and are highly sensitive to lens decentration.[6-10] According to Claoue and Parmar,[11] patients lose 18% of light energy with multifocal IOLs, which can be attributed to the conflicting and overlapping patterns produced by these lenses. Multifocal IOLs create competing visual images at the outset of the visual pathway that are transferred to the optic nerve and then to the brain, which can cause a significant loss in contrast sensitivity. The degradation in the visual quality that occurs after the implantation of multifocal lenses cannot be reversed with spectacles. A successful monovision procedure, however, allows for visual improvement with glasses.Recent work in neuroscience has paved the way for us to understand the differences between multifocal and monofocal lenses. Multifocal IOLs seem to rely on monoptic suppression. This phenomenon occurs when both eyes are looking at the same target, but, within the target, there are visual cues that promote an alternating focus.[12] For example, in Figure 3, one's eyes are drawn to a number of features; they perceive certain shapes at one moment and focus on others the next. While this occurs, the neural pathway is suppressing pieces of the image as one's focus changes.

Monoptic suppression can be compared to the visual effects caused by multifocal IOLs. With these lenses, near, intermediate, and distance visual information is presented to both eyes simultaneously. Each eye must suppress certain visual information in order to perceive a clear picture. If this suppression stems from the same neural correlates as seen with monoptic suppression, it becomes obvious why multifocal patients are exhibiting significantly lower contrast sensitivity. Humans' visual pathways are not hardwired to distinguish overlapping images and simultaneously produce high-contrast output.[13]

In contrast, utilizing monofocal IOLs for monovision induces binocular fusion when desired clinical outcomes are obtained. Binocular fusion occurs when the eyes perceive two distinct images that are harmonious enough to result in a single visual product. If the images are spatially congruent, fusion can occur

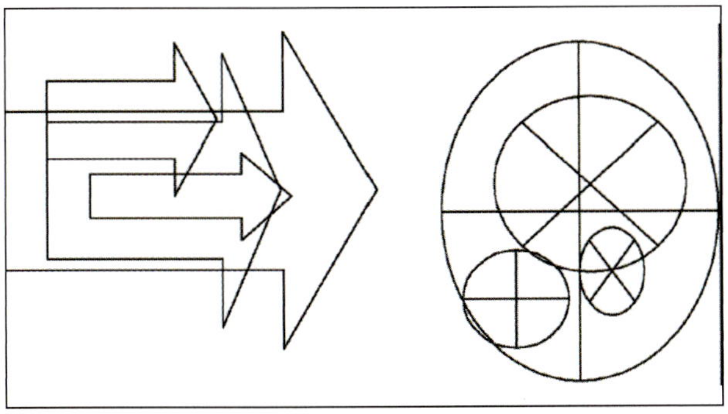

Figure 3. These two images can trigger monoptic suppression.

even if the contrast between the two images varies by a few factors. Images that differ significantly in spatial frequency and orientation prevent binocular fusion.[14-16]

Pseudophakic monovision is a natural choice for cataract replacement or lens exchange surgery, as the contrast difference resulting from monovision permits binocular fusion. The eyes present two images that vary substantially in contrast and clarity, but they are spatially congruent enough to allow fusion to occur. Information from the eyes is transmitted to the visual cortex, where data from the eye producing higher contrast will be accepted as the dominant percept. The visual cortex provides neural feedback to reduce the influence of the lower-contrast eye and thus generate excellent contrast sensitivity and visual acuity at all distances.

CONCLUSION

The theories presented herein help explain the early successes of aspheric IOLs for monovision as well as the visual frustrations and loss of contrast sensitivity that can result from multifocal IOL implants. As research further explains the mechanisms of the brain, I anticipate a more effective solution to the presbyopic problem. ■

This article originally appeared in the March 2007 issue of CRSToday.

1. Boerner CF, Thrasher BH. Results of monovision correction in bilateral pseudophakes. *J Am Intraocul Implant Soc.*1984;10:49-50.
2. Greenbaum S. Monovision pseudophakia. *J Cataract Refract Surg.*2002;28:1439-1443.
3. Artal P, Berrio E, Guirao A, Piers P. Contribution of the cornea and internal surfaces to the change of ocular aberrations with age. *J Opt Soc Am A Opt Image Sci Vis.*2002;19:137-143.
4. Applegate RA, Marsack JD, Ramos R, Sarver EJ. Interaction between aberrations to improve or reduce visual performance. *J Cataract Refract Surg.*2003;29:1487-1495.
5. Altmann GE, Nichamin LD, Lane SS, Pepose JS. Optical performance of 3 intraocular lens designs in the presence of decentration. *J Cataract Refract Surg.* 2005;31:574-585.
6. Chiam PJ, Chan JH, Aggarwal RK, et al. ReSTOR intraocular lens implantation in cataract surgery: quality of vision. *J Cataract Refract Surg.*2006;32:1459-1463.
7. Souza CE, Muccioli C, Soriano ES, et al. Visual performance of AcrySof ReSTOR apodized diffractive IOL: a prospective comparative trial. *Am J Ophthalmol.*2006;141:827-832.
8. Rocha KM, Chalita MR, Souza CE, et al. Postoperative wavefront analysis and contrast sensitivity of a multifocal apodized diffractive IOL (ReSTOR) and three monofocal IOLs. *J Refract Surg.* 2005;21:S808-812.
9. Javitt JC, Steinert RF. Cataract extraction with multifocal intraocular lens implantation: a multinational clinical trial evaluation clinical, functional, and quality-of-life outcomes. *Ophthalmology.* 2000;107:2040-2048.
10. Hayashi K, Hayashi H, Nakao F, Hayashi F. Correlation between pupillary size and intraocular lens decentration and visual acuity of a zonal-progressive multifocal lens and a monofocal lens. *Ophthalmology.* 2001;108:2011-2017.
11. Claoue C, Parmar D. Multifocal intraocular lenses. Dev Ophthalmol. 2002;34:217-237.
12. Sengpiel F, Vorobyov V. Intracortical origins of interocular suppression in the visual cortex. *J Neurosci.*2005;25:6394-6400.
13. Tse PU, Martinez-Conde S, Schlegel AA, Macknik SL. Visibility, visual awareness, and visual masking of simple unattended targets are confined to areas in the occipital cortex beyond human V1/V2. *Proceedings of the National Academy of Sciences of the United States of America.* 2005;102:17178-17183.
14. Schor C, Heckmann T, Tyler CW. Binocular fusion limits are independent of contrast, luminance gradient and component phases. *Vision Res.* 1989;29:821-835.
15. Schor C, Heckmann T. Interocular differences in contrast and spatial frequency: effects on stereopsis and fusion. *Vision Res.* 1989;29:837-847.
16. Liu L, Tyler CW, Schor CM. Failure of rivalry at low contrast: evidence of a suprathreshold binocular summation process. *Vision Res.* 1992;32:1471-1479.

CHAPTER 182

Intentionally Targeting Low Myopia After Cataract Surgery

GARY S. SCHWARTZ, MD

Although presbyopia-correcting IOLs and monovision have the greatest likelihood of providing patients with spectacle independence after cataract surgery, the majority of candidates choose neither of these options. Instead, surgeons typically target a bilateral plano refractive result, thus enabling patients to read the Snellen acuity chart when it is held 20 feet away. Functionally, this allows patients to drive a car without spectacles, but it forces them to wear reading glasses when performing near tasks. I believe that many patients will obtain a higher level of spectacle independence if I target a low myopic result. I therefore recommend that my fellow surgeons consider this option in their surgical planning instead of automatically targeting plano outcomes.

The world of the pseudophake is divided into three distinct zones: distance (eg, driving, television); intermediate (eg, computer, cooking); and near (eg, reading, sewing). When considering a postoperative refractive target, surgeons have the ability to choose in advance which of these activities their patients will most likely be able to perform without spectacles.

ANALYZING WHEN PATIENTS USE SPECTACLES

In addition to treating medical and surgical diseases of the eye, I see a large number of healthy patients whose only ocular problem is ametropia and/or presbyopia. I will often ask patients how often and for what tasks they wear their glasses. I have found that presbyopic and pseudophakic patients who wear glasses the least amount of hours of the day are those who have approximately 1.00 D of myopia.

Pseudophakic emmetropes tend to wear spectacles for near and intermediate tasks only. Individuals who have vocations or avocations that involve reading, computer work, knitting, solving crossword puzzles, etc., may wear their glasses quite frequently. In fact, an emmetropic, pseudophakic attorney or accountant may use his reading glasses 8 to 10 hours a day while working and only take them off to drive to and from work. He may then put his glasses back on at home while he eats dinner, reads the newspaper, and checks e-mail. It may be surprising, but this pseudophakic patient may in fact be wearing glasses the overwhelming majority of his waking hours, despite the emmetropic result.

Pseudophakes with a refractive error of approximately -1.00 D have clear intermediate vision, allowing them to easily use a computer, eat or cook a meal, read the newspaper, see items on shelves while shopping, and play the piano without glasses. Many use reading glasses only to read small print (eg, pill bottles) or in poor lighting conditions (eg, to see menus in dimly lit restaurants). Because pseudophakic patients have a low level of myopia, they can usually drive a car legally without spectacles, often wearing glasses only to drive at night. Instead of buying expensive multifocal glasses, many of these patients are content to use one pair of single-vision prescription glasses for driving and a separate pair of low-plus "dime store" glasses for reading.

OFFERING AN ALTERNATIVE TO EMMETROPIA

We cataract and refractive surgeons have expanded our preoperative consultations to include discussions of phakic, toric, accommodating, and multifocal IOLs. For the sake of completeness, I believe that we can better serve our patients' needs by reviewing the option of targeting a low degree myopia in both eyes after cataract surgery. I have found that the ideal myopic target is around -1.00 D, and I will often target -0.75 D in the dominant eye and -1.25 D in the nondominant eye to increase the depth of focus.

As with any such preoperative discussion, surgeons should emphasize functional vision and try to minimize using terms such as *near-sighted* or *myopia*. I have found it best to concentrate on how many hours patients spend doing specific activities and which ones they would most like to perform without glasses. Often, the discussion is as simple as asking, "Which would you rather be able to do without glasses, drive or use a computer?"

The patients who achieve the most success with targeted low myopia are those who are still working, specifically those who spend a lot of time on a computer. Also, I reserve this option for patients who do not desire either monovision or a presbyopia-correcting IOL.

In summary, presbyopic patients with low myopia are often less dependent upon spectacles than emmetropic ones. Surgeons who successfully incorporate this option into their practices will find patients' satisfaction very high, and they will often offer it to their presbyopic patients undergoing keratorefractive procedures such as LASIK, PRK, and conductive keratoplasty. ■

This article originally appeared in the March 2008 issue of CRSToday.

CHAPTER 183

Pseudophakic Monovision

WILLIAM F. MALONEY, MD

In this month's edition of *Cataract & Refractive Surgery Today,* the cover series' overarching topic—mixing presbyopia-correcting IOLs—highlights ophthalmologists' growing realization that we do not yet have an off-the-shelf, comprehensive presbyopia-correcting IOL. No lens delivers all ranges of vision. Typically, the AcrySof Restor IOL (Alcon Laboratories, Inc., Fort Worth, TX) misses intermediate vision, whereas the ReZoom IOL (Advanced Medical Optics, Inc., Santa Ana, CA) and the Crystalens accommodating IOL (Eyeonics, Inc., Aliso Viejo, CA) fail fully to deliver focus at near.

Mixing IOL technologies between contralateral eyes represents ophthalmologists' attempt to mitigate the effects of these fixed reading-zone deficiencies by pairing lenses that complement one another. I believe that this approach is effective in that regard. These strategic IOL combinations also have solid support in the current theories of the neurophysiology of binocular vision.[1-8]

PHYSIOLOGIC BINOCULAR RIVALRY

Strategically pairing IOLs with different reading capabilities is an effective strategy, because the patient instantly puts the one with better focus for the task at hand to use, while images from the ineffectual lens are readily suppressed and remain unnoticed. The moment the task changes (eg, from computer work to reading the stock charts), the brain shifts to focusing through the other lens. This continual interocular contest for visual awareness is binocular rivalry at work.

Along with fusion and stereopsis, rivalry is a regular aspect of physiologic binocular vision. Binocular vision employs a neural circuitry that evolved to mediate interocular differences. Primates are hardwired to make effective use of just the sort of differences that these IOL pairings present.

PSEUDOPHAKIC MONOVISION

Pseudophakic monovision means mixing conventional IOLs with different focal lengths, each with just the right amount of myopic focus. The resulting anisometropic rivalry becomes the vehicle to ride these neural rails and deliver a made-to-order range of uncorrected focus selected to best meet each patient's particular goals.

A candidate's unique anisometropic "sweet spot" is unambiguously revealed by preoperative assessments, including interocular defocus tolerance, suppression capacity, targeting, and oculomotor dominance. The most important test measures sensory dominance separately for near and distance vision. In my experience, with sensory dominance correctly identified, the vast majority of patients instantly and effortlessly accept 2.00 D or more of anisometropia. Usually, however, no more than 1.50 to 1.75 D of anisometropia is needed because of the additional 1.00 D of accommodative effect derived from pseudoaccommodation—a very useful property of every conventional IOL. Thus, neuroadaptation is not experienced by patients with authentic pseudophakic monovision, who typically report that their results feel "completely natural" within 1 to 2 days. That may not be the case with multifocal patients, as discussed in the next section of this article.

NEUROADAPTATION: THE FOREMOST CONCERN WITH MULTIFOCALITY

Combining complementary multifocal IOLs can effectively address the particular focus-zone deficiency inherent in each lens. This mixture does nothing, however, to address the prolonged neuroadaptive period these lenses typically require.

The concept of multifocality is fundamentally at odds with current theories of the neurophysiology of binocular vision. Again, the structure and function of the visual cortex evolved to mediate interocular image disparity. Multifocality's intraocular disparity has no physiologic precedent. Without a neural template to separate out and convey the needed focus into awareness, a prolonged neuroadaptive period is required to put in place the necessary neural tracks. As the brain adapts, the "smeared" vision emblematic of truncated focal distinction slowly moderates and often, but not always, gradually disappears. It is a testament to the astonishing plasticity of the visual cortex that neuroadaptation occurs at all, let alone within 6 to 12 months. When adaptation falls short and the patient loses faith, bilateral explantation is sometimes the only answer, regardless of a technically perfect procedure. Clearly, ophthalmologists must identify and exclude those patients who are less likely to neuroadapt. The question is how.

MISCONCEPTIONS OF MONOVISION

A large part of the conventional wisdom concerning pseudophakic monovision is either incomplete or simply incorrect. Here are some key misconceptions.

1. Pseudophakic monovision is like permanent contact lens monovision. Despite the paucity of preoperative assessments with and problems related to the contact lenses themselves, contact lens monovision has a relatively high acceptance rate among patients (65% by my estimate). Authentic (surgical) pseudophakic monovision, which includes a comprehensive preoperative assessment, has an acceptance rate of greater than 95% among those of my cataract surgery patients who select presbyopic correction. The difference is due to the larger anisometropic "sweet spot" that results from pseudophakic pseudoaccommodation.

2. Surgeons cannot charge for pseudophakic monovision. Because this approach uses a conventional IOL, there is no uncovered device charge. The charges for the surgeon's services in conjunction with presbyopic correction are for appropriate refractive assessments and procedures. These are uncovered and apply regardless of the IOL employed.

3. Pseudophakic monovision creates troublesome visual compromise. Part of a recent letter to me from a colleague is perhaps the best response here (Figure 1). I was struck by what his account of his experience with pseudophakic monovision did not include: (1) any period of neuroadaptation; (2) any compromise in stereopsis, depth perception, contrast sensitivity, reading of fine print, or intermediate focus; and (3) any need for exercises to strengthen his accommodative ability.

THE RIGHT QUESTION

Pseudophakic monovision is perhaps the most versatile approach to presbyopic correction, because the accommodative effect is not fixed but rather entirely created by the amount of anisometropia. Furthermore, combining multifocal IOLs introduces an important new degree of versatility to the premium IOL category. A comprehensive treatment methodology requires that ophthalmologists shift from a single IOL-centric approach to asking the right question: "Which combination of IOLs is best for this patient?" Surgeons should be fully familiar with each alternative in order to select the one best able to deliver the candidate's unique reading goals. ■

This article originally appeared in the August 2007 issue of CRSToday.

1. Blake R, Logothetis N. Visual competition. *Nat Rev Neurosci.* 2002;3:13-21.
2. Blake R, Overton R. The site of binocular rivalry suppression. *Perception.* 1979;8:143-152.
3. Blake R. A neural theory of binocular rivalry. *Psychol Rev.* 1989;96:145-167.
4. Lehky S, Blake R. Organization of binocular pathways: modeling and data related to rivalry. *Neural Comput.* 1991;3:44-53.
5. Ooi TL, He ZJ. Binocular rivalry and visual awareness: the role of attention. *Perception.* 1999;25:551-574.
6. Polonski A, Blake R, Braun J, Heeger J. Neuronal activity in human primary visual cortex correlates with perception during binocular rivalry. *Nat Rev Neurosci.* 2000;3:1153-1159.
7. Sengpiel F, Blakemore C, Harrad R. Interocular suppression in the primary visual cortex: a possible neural basis of binocular rivalry. *Vision Res.* 1995;35:179-195.
8. Tong F, Nakayama K, Vaughan JT, Kanwisher N. Binocular rivalry and visual awareness in human extra striate cortex. *Neuron.* 1998;21:753-759.

CHAPTER 184

Determining the Mechanism of Pseudophakic Accommodation

ADRIAN GLASSER, PhD

When considering pseudophakic accommodation, one must distinguish between accommodation and pseudoaccommodation. This article seeks to clarify the concepts and apply them to accommodative IOLs.

DEFINING THE TERMS

Accommodation is an active, dynamic dioptric change in the eye's refracting power; it is not simply the ability of a distance-corrected eye to see clearly at near. To establish with certainty whether accommodation is occurring, the optical refracting power of the eye should be measured objectively. The term *pseudoaccommodation* refers to the achievement of functional near vision in distance-corrected presbyopic eyes through nonaccommodative means. These methods include multifocality (by means of IOLs, contact lenses, corneal refractive procedures, or progressive addition lenses), monovision, an increased depth of field due to small pupil diameters, and induced ocular aberrations (eg, astigmatism or spherical aberration). Pseudoaccommodation can provide functional near vision in a distance-corrected eye but without an optical change in the eye's refracting power.

Whether achieved through accommodation or pseudo-accommodation, functional near vision in a distance-corrected presbyope is unquestionably of benefit to the patient. To understand if accommodation can be, or is, restored by an IOL (or any other approach, for that matter), however, it is necessary to demonstrate objectively that the eye undergoes an increase in optical refracting power (a change in refraction) with accommodation. Further, in order to reliably achieve pseudophakic accommodation in all patients, it is necessary to understand the mechanism(s) by which it occurs.

In a normal, young eye, an effort to focus on a near object results in accommodation, a convergence of the eyes, and pupillary constriction. These three physiologic responses are connected in the brain and are referred to as the *accommodative triad.* Presenting a stimulus to induce convergence alone also results in neuronally coupled accommodation and pupillary constriction. The constriction of the pupil aids near vision—although through pseudoaccommodative means—by increasing the eye's depth of field. This effect that pupillary constriction has in aiding accommodation is especially true in older eyes in which accommodation is reduced, pupil sizes are small, and the accommodative pupillary constriction is greater.

In pseudophakic eyes, pseudoaccommodation may also arise from sources other than increased depth of field due to pupillary constriction. Corneal incisions necessary for the insertion of the IOL can induce astigmatism or ocular aberrations, and the IOL itself may cause or increase the amount of ocular spherical aberration or higher-order aberrations.

DIFFERENTIATING BETWEEN ACCOMMODATION AND PSEUDOACCOMMODATION

To distinguish accommodation from pseudoaccommodation, one must use objective methods to measure either an optical change in the eye's refracting power or a physical change in the lens (eg, movement, separation of the optics, or an increase in thickness). Objective methods distinguish the true accommodative optical changes from the pseudoaccommodative effects that contribute to improved near vision without accommodation. Subjective methods that rely on patients' reporting when they first perceive blur and even functional near reading tests do not unequivocally distinguish between accommodation and pseudoaccommodation. Because techniques such as the push-up near reading test[1] and dynamic retinoscopy[2] rely on patients' or clinicians' subjective interpretation, they are not objective methods. Although dynamic retinoscopy may agree well with objective methods in the hands of skilled retinoscopists,[2] the subjective interpretation of the retinoscopic reflex by different clinicians can result in inconsistent results.[3]

MEASURING ACCOMMODATION

The Stimulus

The proximity of a target, among other things, stimulates accommodation by blur and by inducing a convergence of the two eyes. A visual stimulus viewed binocularly that provides blur as well as proximal and convergence cues is therefore a compelling accommodative stimulus. The stimulus should be composed of middle and high spatial frequencies and should be high in contrast. A black Maltese cross or fine black text on a white background is appropriate. Accommodative stimuli are often presented through Badal optical systems. A Badal optical stimulus is a relatively deprived and far less compelling accommodative stimulus relative to a real target, because it can generally only be viewed monocularly, eliminates proximal cues, and stimulates accommodation using blur cues alone. The presentation of the most compelling accommodative stimulus to the subject is most likely to produce an accommodative response.

Subjective Versus Objective Methods

The measurement of accommodative changes in refracting power is important, but so, too, are objective methods that show biometric changes in the eye. Accommodation studies have used A-scan ultrasound,[4,5] continuous ultrasound biometry,[6] ultrasound biomicroscopy,[7] partial coherence interferometry,[8-10] Scheimpflug slit-lamp imaging,[11,12] high-resolution MRI,[13] and optical coherence tomography.[14] Investigators can employ all of these techniques to objectively measure or demonstrate accommodative movements of an IOL in order to elucidate the mechanism whereby the accommodative refractive changes may be occurring. Although all these methods may show movement of an IOL inside the eye, they do not measure the optical refractive change in the power of the eye. This refractive change quantifies the extent of accommodation that the eye actually undergoes. Subjective testing of patients with accommodative IOLs may show functional benefits,[15] but objective methods are necessary to show IOL movement and accommodative optical changes.[16]

Instrumentation

Instruments that objectively measure the optical refracting power of the eye include optometers, autorefractors, and wavefront aberrometers. If they are reliable, accurate, and able to perform measurements through small pupils, these instruments can measure pseudophakic eyes. Several are no longer commercially available, however, such as the Hartinger coincidence refractometer (Carl Zeiss Meditec AG, Jena, Germany)[12,17,18] and PowerRefractor (PlusOptix, Nürnberg, Germany),[19-21] both of which have often been used in accommodation studies and have been shown to be reliable and accurate in phakic eyes.

Although commercially available autorefractors are designed for use on phakic eyes and have been validated for phakic accommodation measurement,[2,22,23] these instruments have not yet been validated on pseudophakic eyes. Special problems exist for the measurement of pseudophakic accommodation. Senile pupillary miosis and strong accommodative pupillary constriction, which are normal in older populations, require that the autorefractors be capable of measuring through small pupils. Clinicians can use phenylephrine to dilate the iris without causing cycloplegia, but dilation increases the amount of optical aberrations present and therefore may decrease the ability of the patients to deliver a normal accommodative response. The high-refractive-index IOL materials result in bright Purkinje images reflected off the IOL's anterior surface. These images can produce optical artifacts that make measurements with an autorefractor inaccurate or impossible. Additionally, the presence of posterior capsular opacification or secondary cataract can degrade the optical quality of the eye and produce inaccuracies or variability in autorefractors' measurements.

Because small accommodative amplitudes are likely to occur with pseudophakic accommodation, objective instruments must have sufficient accuracy and resolution to invoke confidence in the measured amplitudes. Although autorefractors or wavefront aberrometers may well be capable of accurately measuring pseudophakic accommodation, they must be validated as appropriate instruments for accommodation measurement and for accurate measurements of pseudophakic eyes before they can routinely be used to measure pseudophakic accommodation.

CONCLUSION

In summary, subjective testing of distance-corrected near reading ability, objective measurements of dioptric changes in the refracting power of the eye, and objective measurements of biometric changes in the pseudophakic eye are, in conjunction with each other, important for proving the existence of pseudophakic accommodation. The objective tests are necessary for distinguishing between true accommodation and pseudoaccommodation. Many biometric techniques currently exist that are reliable methods for demonstrating and measuring accommodative movements in pseudophakic eyes. The ultimate test and proof of the existence of pseudophakic accommodation, however, depends on (1) the identification of commercially available instruments that can reliably and reproducibly measure small, accommodative, optical refractive changes in pseudophakic eyes and (2) the validation of these instruments for measuring pseudophakic accommodation. ■

This article originally appeared in the July 2004 issue of CRSToday.

1. Duane A. Normal values of the accommodation at all ages. *J Am Med Assoc.* 1912:1010-1013.
2. McClelland JF, Saunders KJ. The repeatability and validity of dynamic retinoscopy in assessing the accommodative response. *Ophthalmic Physiol Opt.* 2003;23:243-250.
3. Whitefoot H, Charman WN. Dynamic retinoscopy and accommodation. *Ophthalmic Physiol Opt.* 1992;12:8-17.
4. Beauchamp R, Mitchell B. Ultrasound measures of vitreous chamber depth during ocular accommodation. *Am J Optom Physiol Opt.* 1985;62:523-532.
5. Vilupuru AS, Glasser A. Dynamic accommodative changes in rhesus monkey eyes assessed with A-scan ultrasound biometry. *Optom Vis Sci.* 2003;80:383-394.
6. Beers APA, Van Der Heijde GL. In vivo determination of the biomechanical properties of the component elements of the accommodative mechanism. *Vision Res.* 1994;34:2897-2905.
7. Bacskulin A, Bergmann U, Horoczi Z, Guthoff R. Continuous ultrasound biomicroscopic imaging of accommodative changes in the human ciliary body. *Klin Monatsbl Augenheilkd.* 1995;207:247-252.
8. Drexler W, Baumgartner A, Findl O, et al. Biometric investigation of changes in the anterior eye segment during accommodation. *Vision Res.* 1997;37:2789-2800.
9. Findl O, Kiss B, Petternel V, et al. Intraocular lens movement caused by ciliary muscle contraction. *J Cataract Refract Surg.* 2003;29:669-676.
10. Petternel V, Koppl CM, Dejaco-Ruhswurm I, et al. Effect of accommodation and pupil size on the movement of a posterior chamber lens in the phakic eye. *Ophthalmology.* 2004;111:325-331.
11. Dubbelman M, Van Der Heijde GL, Weeber HA, Vrensen GFJM. Changes in the internal structure of the human crystalline lens with age and accommodation. *Vision Res.* 2003;43:2363-2375.
12. Koretz JF, Cook CA, Kaufman PL. Accommodation and presbyopia in the human eye. Changes in the anterior segment and crystalline lens with focus. *Invest Ophthalmol Vis Sci.* 1997;38:569-578.
13. Strenk SA, Semmlow JL, Strenk LM, et al. Age-related changes in human ciliary muscle and lens: A magnetic resonance imaging study. *Invest Ophthalmol Vis Sci.* 1999;40:1162-1169.
14. Baikoff G, Lutun E, Wei J, Ferraz C. Anterior chamber optical coherence tomography study of human natural accommodation in a 19-year-old albino. *J Cataract Refract Surg.* 2004;30:696-701.
15. Mastropasqua L, Toto L, Nubile M, et al. Clinical study of the 1CU accommodating intraocular lens. *J Cataract Refract Surg.* 2003;29:1307-1312.
16. Langenbucher A, Huber S, Nguyen NX, et al. Measurement of accommodation after implantation of an accommodating posterior chamber intraocular lens. *J Cataract Refract Surg.* 2003;29:677-685.
17. Vilupuru AS, Glasser A. Dynamic accommodation in rhesus monkeys. *Vision Res.* 2002;42:125-41.
18. Wold JE, Hu A, Chen S, Glasser A. Subjective and objective measurement of human accommodative amplitude. *J Cataract Refract Surg.* 2003;29:1878-1888.
19. Schaeffel F, Wilhelm H, Zrenner E. Inter-individual variability in the dynamics of natural accommodation in humans: relation to age and refractive errors. *J Physiol.* 1993;461:301-320.
20. Seidemann A, Schaeffel F. An evaluation of the lag of accommodation using photorefraction. *Vision Res.* 2003;43:419-430.
21. Kasthurirangan S, Vilupuru AS, Glasser A. Amplitude dependent accommodative dynamics in humans. *Vision Res.* 2003;43:2945-2956.
22. Wolffsohn JS, Gilmartin B, Mallen EA, Tsujimura S. Continuous recording of accommodation and pupil size using the Shin-Nippon SRW-5000 autorefractor. *Ophthalmic Physiol Opt.* 2001;21:108-113.
23. Nakatsuka C, Hasebe S, Nonaka F, Ohtsuki H. Accommodative lag under habitual seeing conditions: comparison between adult myopes and emmetropes. *Jpn J Ophthalmol.* 2004;47:291-298.

CHAPTER 185

Tetraflex Accommodating IOL

PAUL J. DOUGHERTY, MD

The Tetraflex accommodating IOL (Lenstec, Inc., St. Petersburg, FL) is one of the exciting new technologies to which European surgeons, unlike most American surgeons, have access to as part of their surgical refractive armamentarium. Despite the small size of the lens' manufacturer, the Tetraflex accounts for more than 30% of the presbyopic IOL market in Europe (data on file with Market Scope, LLC, Manchester, MO). In addition to implanting the Tetraflex IOL as a principal investigator in the FDA trial, I also implant the Acrysof Restor IOL (Alcon Laboratories, Inc., Fort Worth, TX), Crystalens (Eyeonics, Inc., Aliso Viejo, CA), and Rezoom IOL (Advanced Medical Optics, Inc., Santa Ana, CA) in my practice.

THE TETRAFLEX IOL

Design

The Tetraflex (Figure 1) is an anteriorly vaulted, single-piece, foldable, accommodating IOL that is implanted using a custom-designed injector system through an incision as small as 3mm. The lens' optic is 5.75 mm and is made of a highly biocompatible hydrophilic acrylic material. The IOL's two haptics, each with two footplates, sit posteriorly in the peripheral capsular bag. The surgeon performs his standard capsulorhexis and phacoemulsification technique are performed. Lenstec, Inc. recommends that surgeons create a 5.5- to 6.0-mm circular capsulorhexis. They should not implant the Tetraflex if an anterior capsular radial tear is created during surgery. The lens is used internationally for both cataract and refractive lensectomy surgery.

The Mechanism of Action

The mechanism of action of the Tetraflex is multifactorial. On ultrasound biomicroscopy (UBM) the lens moves forward during accommodative effort (Figures 2 and 3). I think this movement occurs due to the contraction of the ciliary muscle that loosens the zonules as well as increases vitreous pressure. In addition, the anterior surface of the optic curves more than the posterior surface during anterior vaulting of the lens. This higher radius of curvature of the lens' anterior surface increases the net refractive power of the lens as well as induces coma. The later is an important part of the normal accommodative process in the prepresbyopic phakic eye. The accommodative effect of the lens may be seen using three-dimensional ray tracing, which shows increased depth of focus and mean and maximum myopia in eyes implanted with the Tetraflex during the accommodative effort (D. Sanders, MD, oral communication, December 2005) (Figure 4).

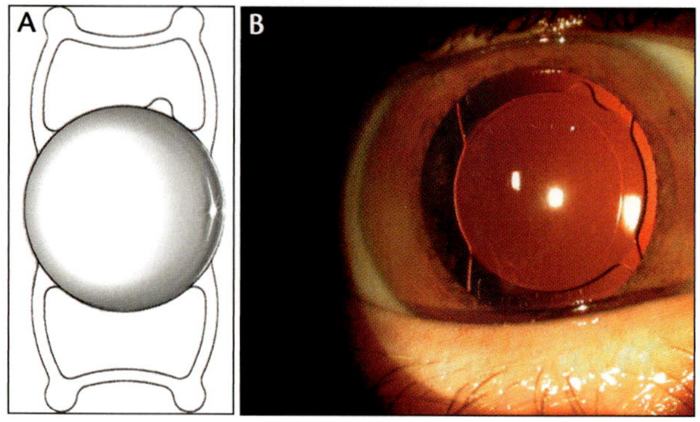

Figure 1. Pictured is a schematic of the Tetraflex accommodating IOL (A). The slit-lamp photograph shows the Tetraflex IOL in an eye (B).

(Courtesy of Michal Janek, MD.)

US Clinical Trial

The Tetraflex IOL is currently in phase 3 FDA clinical trials in seven centers in the US. To date, more than 150 lenses have been implanted in this country, with 53 of eyes having 6 months or more of follow-up (data on file with Lenstec, Inc.). Of those 53 eyes, 60% achieved a distance UCVA of 20/20 or better, and 90% achieved a UCVA of 20/40 or better. In terms of evaluating the near performance of any presbyopic lens, distance-corrected near vision is considered the gold standard. Fifty-five percent of eyes demonstrated a monocular distance-corrected near vision of J5 (print size of stock quotes) or better, and 90% have a distance-corrected near vision of J8 (standard newspaper print) or better. European data of near visual function show that the near performance of Tetraflex is even better when the lens is implanted bilaterally versus monocularly (data on file with Lenstec, Inc.). In terms of accommodative amplitude in the FDA study, 100% of eyes had at least 2.00 D, and 69% had at least 3.00 D of accommodation at 6 months postoperatively using the "Push Down" amplitude of accommodation test. Currently, none of the patients implanted with the Tetraflex, either domestically or internationally, have experienced any capsular issues.

My experience as a principal investigator in the FDA trial of this lens has been excellent. So far, I have implanted 35 of these IOLs. The lens is simple to implant, has none of the visual side effects (such as glare, halo, and loss of contrast sensitivity) of multifocal lenses, and is consistently giving my patients functional near vision without correction. Because there is a single point of focus through all distances, the quality of vision through the lens is excellent. I consider this lens equivalent in distance performance to any monofocal lens that I use with the fringe benefit of improved near vision. Like any accommodative lens, however, I do not promise that all patients will throw away their glasses. Some patients achieve lesser accommodative effect and may require near spectacles part of the time, particularly with low lighting and low-contrast print. I have found that patients with shorter axial lengths tend to have better subjective near vision with the Tetraflex than patients with longer axial lengths.

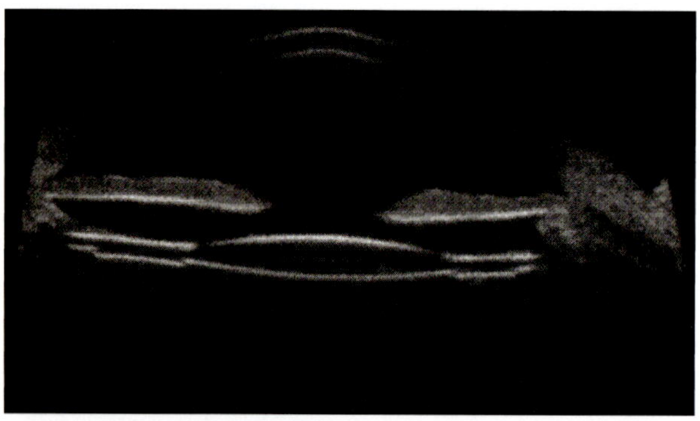

(Courtesy of David Brown, MD and Sonomed, Inc.)

Figure 2. Pictured is a UBM photograph of the Tetraflex IOL in the unaccommodated (distance) position.

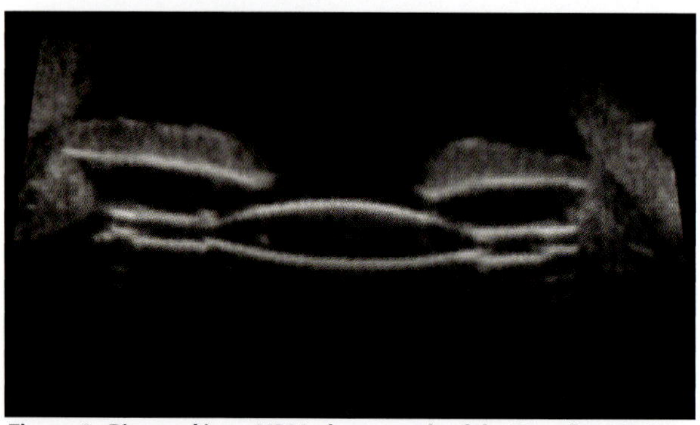

(Courtesy of David Brown, MD and Sonomed, Inc.)

Figure 3. Pictured is an UBM photograph of the Tetraflex IOL in the accommodated (near) position. Note that the anterior portion of the lens has moved closer to the posterior surface of the iris, the anterior chamber depth has diminished by 7%, and the ciliary muscle has thickened compared with the unaccommodated (distance) position.

CONCLUSION

Thus far, I have not noted any complaints of glare or halos at night in my Tetraflex patients, which is likely due to both the monofocal nature of the lens as well as its 5.75-mm optic. Although I have needed to perform a YAG posterior capsulotomy on only a few eyes after the IOL's implantation, the laser does not seem to negatively affect accommodation, and all lenses have remained in perfect position postoperatively.

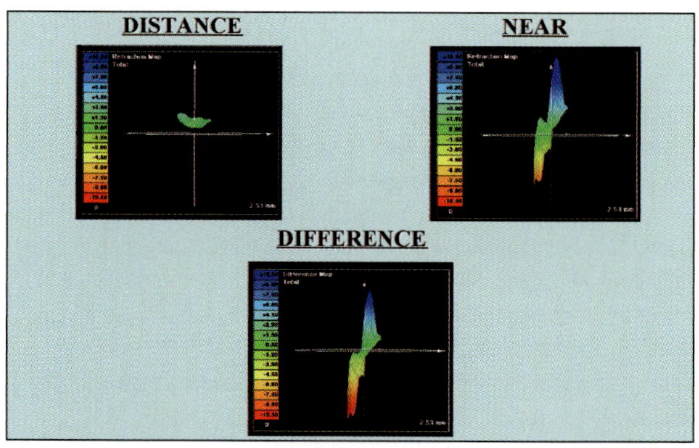

(Courtesy of Don Sanders, MD.)

Figure 4. Three-dimensional ray tracing portrays the refractive power across the pupil in an eye with the Tetraflex IOL. The upper left graph represents the refractive power across the pupil in the unaccommodated (distance) state, the upper right graph shows the power in the accommodated (near) state, and the lower graph displays the difference in power between distance and near states. Noteworthy is the increase in maximum myopia and depth of focus when the patient is fixated on a near target with the Tetraflex IOL.

Many different lenses are available to treat presbyopia in the US, including both monofocal and multifocal IOLs. European surgeons have access to many exciting ophthalmic technologies not currently available here. One of these, the Tetraflex IOL, shows significant promise in helping the surgeon to deal with the presbyopic patient. I believe this lens, when and if approved by the FDA, will be the presbyopic IOL of choice. ■

This article originally appeared in the January 2007 issue of CRSToday.

CHAPTER 186

Functional Vision With a Dual Optic Accommodating IOL

RICARDO ALARCON, MD, AND VICTOR BOHÓRQUEZ, MD

Accommodation allows the eye to change its refractive status to produce a clear image at near. In classic theory, Helmholtz[1] showed that accommodation is achieved when the ciliary muscle contracts. As this muscle contracts, the release of circumferential tension on the zonules leads to a curvature change of the crystalline lens, resulting in a dioptric power change in the eye. Loss of accommodative amplitude (ie, presbyopia) usually occurs after 40 years of age.

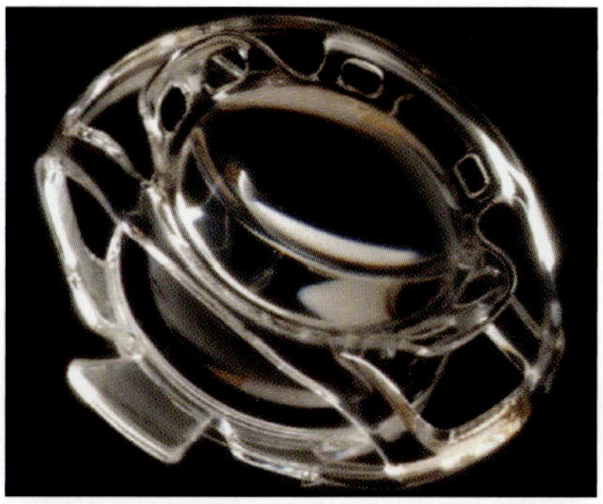

Figure 1. The Synchrony is a single-piece silicone accommodating IOL.

The Synchrony Dual Optic lens (not available in the US; Visiogen, Inc., Irvine, CA) (Figure 1) is a single-piece silicone IOL with a high plus anterior optic—always 32.00 D—coupled with a negative posterior optic. For distance vision, the two optics rest close together. When the patient focuses on a near target, forward movement of the front optic causes an increase in effective IOL power. As the ciliary body relaxes, capsular bag tension brings the front optic back to the resting state, thus restoring emmetropic distance focus. We have proved this with ultrasound biomicroscopy testing (Figure 2). We have also proved that this IOL kept functioning with adequate movement of the optics during accommodation in patients implanted more than 1 year ago.[2]

INCLUSION, EXCLUSION CRITERIA

We have implanted the Synchrony IOL after conventional phacoemulsification in more than 100 patients. Thirtytwo patients were implanted binocularly. Inclusion criteria were (1) aged 40 or more years, (2) the presence of cataracts, (3) fewer than 2.00 D of preoperative astigmatism, and (4) the ability to comply with follow-up visits. Exclusion criteria were (1) a patient having only one eye with potentially good vision, (2) a significant ocular pathology, (3) history of intraocular surgery, (4) diabetes, or (5) use of systemic medications that affect accommodation.

The surgery consisted of conventional clear-cornea phacoemulsification and complete cortical cleanup with anterior capsule polishing. The lens was implanted with Synchrony's preloaded injector, through a 3.6-mm to 3.8-mm incision. The injector delivers the lens into the bag in one easy and controlled step. A standard regimen of antibiotics-steroids was given after surgery. Follow-up visits were scheduled at 1, 3, 6, and 12 months after surgery. Early Treatment of Diabetic Retinopathy Study charts for distance, intermediate (80 cm), and near (40 cm) vision were used for visual acuity testing. Retroillumination photographs were taken at each visit to evaluate IOL centration and capsular bag opacification. Reading speed was also assessed in a subgroup of patients.

RESULTS

From the 32 binocular patients evaluated, 65% were female. Mean follow-up was 10.4 months, and the mean age was 61 years (range, 41 years to 74 years). The mean visual acuities were outstanding: average UCVA was 0.02 logMAR (20/21 Snellen); uncorrected intermediate visual acuity was -0.10 logMAR (20/16 Snellen); and uncorrected near visual acuity was 0.1 logMAR (20/25 Snellen). After correcting these patients for distance, best corrected distance visual acuity was -0.08 logMAR (20/17 Snellen). Distance corrected intermediate visual acuity and distance corrected near visual acuity remained unchanged (Figure 3).

Ninety-one percent of the patients achieved this 20/40 for distance, 97% for intermediate, and 84% for near vision. With distance correction in place, the percentage of patients achieving 20/40 or better improved to 100% for intermediate and 87% for near.

COMPARED WITH THE ACRYSOF

We performed reading speed in a subset of patients (n=25) and compared it with a cohort of 15 patients matched for age, who were binocularly implanted with the Acrysof IOL (Alcon Laboratories, Inc., Fort Worth, TX). This test was performed with full distance correction in place, and without near add power. Reading acuity was better with the Synchrony IOL (logRAD 0.17 [Snellen 20/30]) versus the Acrysof IOL (logRAD 0.51 [Snellen 20/65]), and this difference was statistically significant (P<.001). At newspaper print size (logRAD 0.4), the average reading speed for Synchrony was 160 words/minute versus 23 words/minute for the control (P<.001), with 88% of Synchrony patients reading at least 80 words/minute (ie, the lower reading speed threshold) versus 13% of control patients.

We have worked with this lens for more than 2 years and found

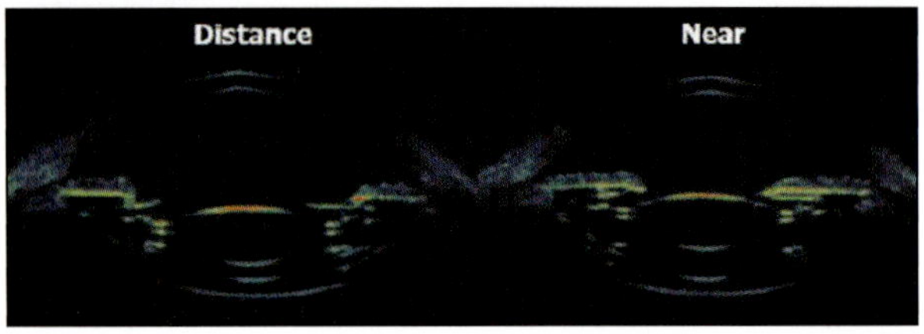

Figure 2. Ultrasound biomicroscopy has shown that emmetropic distance focus is restored when the front optic returns to the resting state.

that it combines the advantages of a monofocal IOL (ie, quality of vision, excellent contrast sensitivity) with improved near and intermediate function, without inducing photopic phenomena (ie, halos and glare). It is worth noting that our first concern with this lens was not its performance but the possibility of interlenticular opacification (ie, Elshnig pearls and fibrosis between the two optics). Our initial cohort of patients have been implanted with this lens for more than 2 years, and we have not seen one case of this disease. The capsular bag remains clean and functional, which we believe is due to continuous aqueous exchange between the bag and the anterior chamber that keeps the lens epithelial cells quiet.

SECOND-GENERATION IOLS

Presbyopic correction has been a challenge for the ophthalmic community for many years. Second-generation accommodative IOLs, including the Synchrony, are a promising alternative for pseudophakic presbyopia. This dual optic accommodating IOL

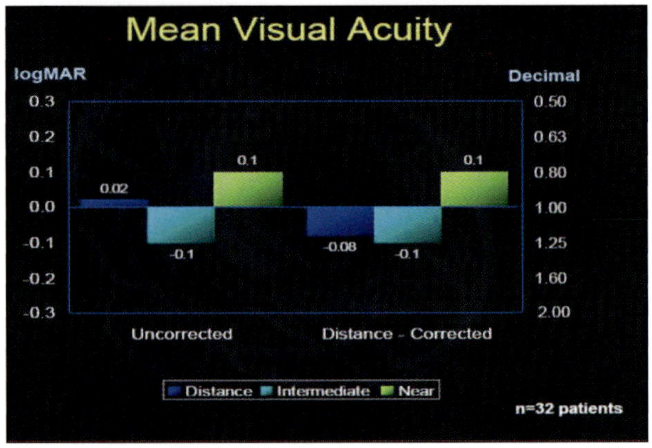

Figure 3. Distance (blue), intermediate (teal), and near (green) mean visual acuities.

provides very good UCVA and, with distance correction in place, maintains or improves near and intermediate vision. The Synchrony also demonstrated good reading performance. It shows potential advantages over multifocal IOLs, because intermediate vision for activities, including computer work, dashboard viewing, cell phone dialing, and grocery shopping, is excellent. ■

This article originally appeared in the March 2007 issue of CRSToday.

1. Southall JPC, ed. Helmholtz's Treatise on Physiological Optics. Translated from the 3rd German edition. New York: Dover Publications; 1962.
2. Bohorquez V, Alarcon R. Accommodative amplitude and Synchrony dual optic IOL. A pilot study. Presented at: The ESCRS 2006 Annual Meeting; September 9-13, 2006; London, UK.

CHAPTER 187

Pseudophakic Wavefront Correction

DANIEL M. SCHWARTZ, MD

Despite advances in both IOL design and biometry, it remains challenging to achieve predictable refractive outcomes.[1-5] In particular, ideal centration and correction of defocus are critical to maximizing the visual function of patients who receive aspheric IOLs. The Light Adjustable Lens (LAL; Calhoun Vision, Inc., Pasadena, CA; not available in the US) is a silicone, three-piece, foldable IOL, the refractive power of which can be precisely adjusted with UV light postoperatively.[6-8] Preclinical and clinical studies of the LAL indicate that it can be adjusted to correct spherical and astigmatic errors as well as spherical aberration.

BACKGROUND

In addition to the silicone polymer and UV blocker contained in conventional silicone IOLs, the LAL has short-chain silicone macromers and a photoinitiator embedded in the lens matrix. Ordinarily, 1 to 4 weeks after cataract surgery, one adjusts the LAL using a Digital Light Delivery (DLD) device manufactured by Carl Zeiss Meditec AG (Jena, Germany). Irradiating the LAL with spatially differentiated UV light causes the selective polymerization of the embedded macromers and the subsequent diffusion of the unexposed macromers into the irradiated zone. For example, if the center of the LAL is irradiated preferentially, then the macromers polymerize centrally, and residual macromers from the unexposed periphery of the LAL diffuse centrally to increase the lens' power (ie, correct hyperopia). Then, 1 to 4 days after the LAL's adjustment, one irradiates the entire lens to polymerize the remaining macromers and lock in the power. Arturo Chayet, MD, of Tijuana, Mexico, and, more recently, José Güell, MD, of Barcelona, Spain, have precisely and reproducibly corrected spherical and astigmatic error in approximately 50 patients based on the spatial-intensity pattern, duration, and intensity of the UV irradiation (unpublished data to be presented by Dr. Chayet at the 2007 AAO Annual Meeting).

The DLD (Figure 1) creates customized spatial-intensity patterns of UV light using a digital mirrored device. Found in the LCD projectors used for Powerpoint presentations (Microsoft Corp., Redmond, WA), the device has approximately 750,000 micromir-

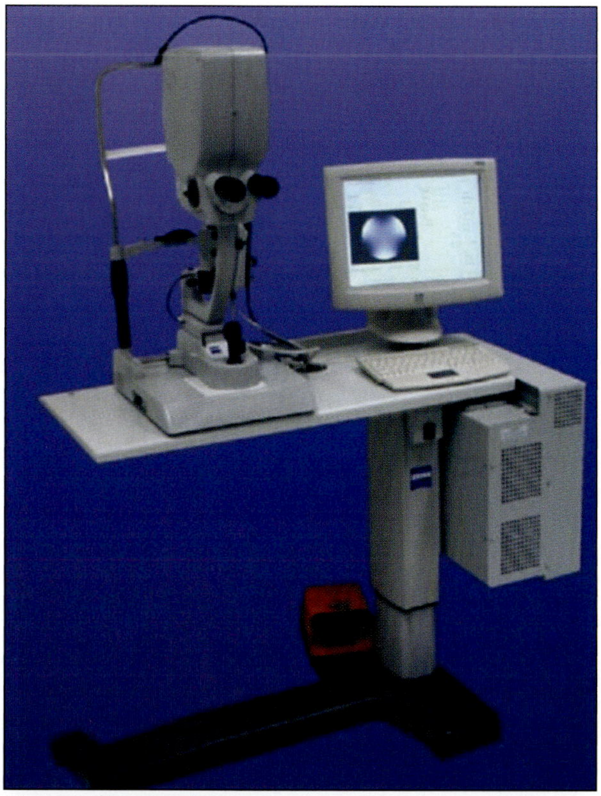

Figure 1. The DLD device.

rors that move extremely rapidly into the "on" or "off" position. The more a single micromirror is on, the brighter the pixel of light it creates; the more it is off, the dimmer the pixel is. Thus, the DLD enables one to define precisely a specific spatial-intensity profile, program it into the digital mirrored device, and then irradiate the LAL. One aligns the DLD's optics with the patient's visual axis by means of a fixation target paracentral to the delivery beam.

The DLD may be capable of writing an aspheric pattern onto the LAL in situ that can be centered on the visual axis. Although an aspheric IOL such as the Tecnis Z9000 (Advanced Medical Optics, Inc., Santa Ana, CA) has a modified prolate anterior surface to increase the patient's visual function by enhancing his contrast sensitivity, this IOL's optical advantage decreases if it is as little as 0.4mm off center.[9] Furthermore, the negative spherical aberration of the Tecnis lens is derived from the mean positive corneal spherical aberration of a study of 71 patients.[10]

Rather than an approach of one size fits all, it would be preferable to correct each individual's spherical aberration following cataract surgery. It may be possible to perform wavefront-driven irradiation of the LAL using the DLD. Moreover, by writing an aspheric correction on an LAL that they adjust to emmetropia and center on the patient's visual axis, surgeons could minimize the untoward optical effects of defocus and decentration on these aspheric IOLs.

To test whether a customized aspheric optic could be written onto a monofocal LAL, scientists at Calhoun Vision, Inc., and Dr. Chayet conducted preliminary in vitro and in vivo studies.

IN VITRO STUDIES

We simultaneously adjusted 32 LALs to correct 1.50 D of hyperopia and remove positive spherical aberration in the lens. We measured the wavefront in the exit pupil of the LAL using a phase-shifting Fizeau Interferometer (Wyko Model 400; Vecco Instruments, Inc., Woodbury, NY) before and after irradiation.

Our analysis of the irradiated LALs showed a mean hyperopic correction of 1.45 D with a standard deviation of less than 0.10 D. In addition, approximately 0.30 D of positive spherical aberration had been removed from the treated lenses. This laboratory study confirmed the possibility of simultaneously correcting refractive error and spherical aberration in the LAL with a specified spatial-intensity pattern programmed into the DLD.

IN VIVO STUDIES

We implanted two New Zealand white rabbits with 20.00 D LALs and then adjusted the lenses for the simultaneous correction of hyperopia and spherical aberration. We irradiated the LALs 1 day after their implantation and then explanted them 1 day after the adjustment. Analysis was interferometrical.

The starting spherical aberration of the LAL was +0.35 D. Our analysis of the irradiated and explanted lenses showed that we had removed approximately 0.50 D of spherical aberration to confer negative spherical aberration on the LALs. As a result, the lenses would neutralize the inherently positive spherical aberration of the human cornea.

Recently, we adjusted, locked in, and then exchanged an LAL from a patient with advanced macular degeneration and visually significant cataract. Optical analysis of the explanted lens showed an approximately 0.30-D reduction in spherical aberration after irradiation. The explanted LAL had excellent resolution and a modulation transfer function of 0.5 at 100 line pairs per millimeter. Chemical analysis of the explanted lens demonstrated consumption of the macromer and a successful lock-in. This result indicates the feasibility of correcting both ametropia and spherical aberration in eyes implanted with an LAL.

Although we are able to establish proof of concept for aspheric corrections, treating more complex wavefront aberrations would require tracking technology on the DLD, not a feature of the current machine. ■

This article originally appeared in the November/December 2006 issue of CRSToday.

1. Brandser JR, Haaskjold E, Dorsum L. Accuracy of IOL calculation in cataract surgery. *Acta Ophthalmol Scan.* 1997;75:162-165.
2. Olsen T, Thim K, Corydon L. Accuracy of the newer generation intraocular-lens power calculation formulas in long and short eyes. *J Cataract Refract Surg.* 1991;17:187-193.
3. Olsen T. Sources of error in intraocular-lens power calculation. *J Cataract Refract Surg.* 1992;18:125-129.
4. Pierro L, Modorati G, Brancato R. Clinical variability in keratometry, ultrasound biometry measurements, and emmetropic intraocular-lens power calculation. *J Cataract Refract Surg.* 1991;17:91-94.
5. Sedgewick JH, Orillac RO, Link C. Array multifocal intraocular lens in a charity hospital training program. *J Cataract Refract Surg.* 2002;28:1205-1210.
6. Schwartz DM. Light-Adjustable Lens. *Trans Am Ophthalmol Soc.* 2003;101:417-436.
7. Schwartz DM, Sandstedt CA, Chang SH, et al. Light-Adjustable Lens: development of in-vitro nomograms. *Trans Am Ophthalmol Soc.* 2004:102:67-72; discussion 72-74.
8. Olson R, Mamalis N, Haugen B. A light adjustable lens with injectable optics. *Ophthalmol Clin North Am.* 2006;19:135-142.
9. Altmann GE, Nichamin LD, Lane SS, Pepose JS. Optical performance of 3 intraocular lens designs in the presence of decentration. *J Cataract Refract Surg.* 2005;31:574-585.
10. Packer M, Fine IH, Hoffman RS. Wavefront technology in cataract surgery. *Curr Opin Ophthalmol.* 2004;15:56-60.

CHAPTER 188

Topography and Premium IOL Surgery

WILLIAM B. TRATTLER, MD

Premium IOLs can achieve visual outcomes that are superior to what traditional IOLs can provide. Ensuring patients' satisfaction with advanced IOL technology, however, can be challenging. Clearly, the most important preliminary step is to educate patients and set realistic expectations. Even so, those who receive superb preoperative counseling may still feel significant disappointment over their visual outcomes or other postoperative matters. By carefully evaluating preoperative tests such as topography, surgeons can identify important issues that they must address and discuss with patients prior to the procedure.

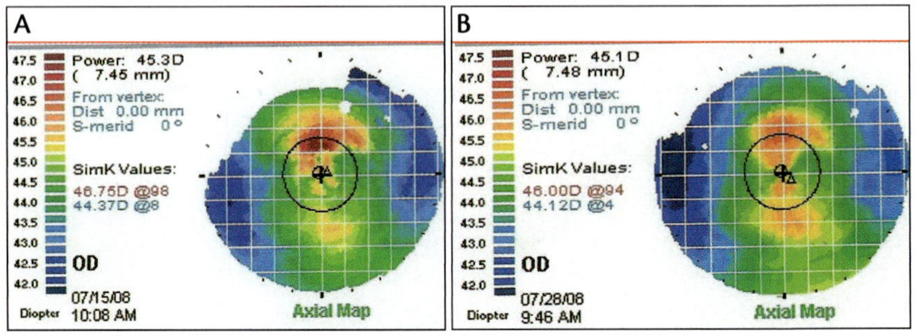

Figure 1. Preoperative topography showed dry eye spots and irregular astigmatism in the right eye of a 62-year-old patient interested in presbyopia-correcting IOLs (A). Two weeks after treatment with a combination of Restasis and AzaSite, the astigmatism was more symmetrical (B).

DRY EYE DISEASE AND MEIBOMIAN GLAND DYSFUNCTION

Preoperative corneal topography provides an extensive amount of useful information about potential candidates for premium IOLs. All of the available corneal topographers can analyze the status of the cornea or the precorneal tear film. The first step in interpreting corneal topography is to determine whether the image obtained is of high quality. In patients with preexisting dry eye disease and/or meibomian gland dysfunction, preoperative topography may be unreliable. These conditions can cause the image to appear asymmetric and/or irregular.

Places on topographic maps where the image appears to drop

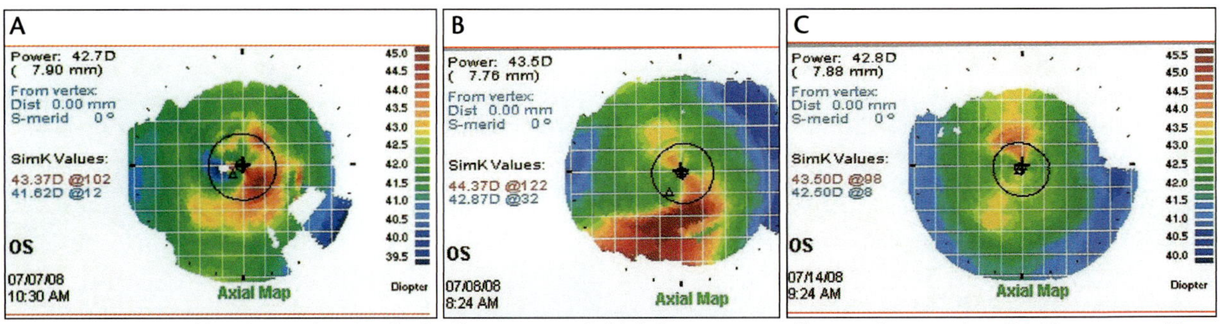

Figure 2. A 58-year-old patient with a visually significant cataract in his left eye expressed interest in a premium IOL. The topographic map dropped out superiorly, and irregular astigmatism was evident (A). One day after beginning treatment with lubricating drops, no dry spots were evident on topography, but the astigmatism appeared to be very irregular (B). One week after beginning treatment with Pred Forte in addition to lubricating drops, the patient had improved results on topography, including less corneal irregularity (C).

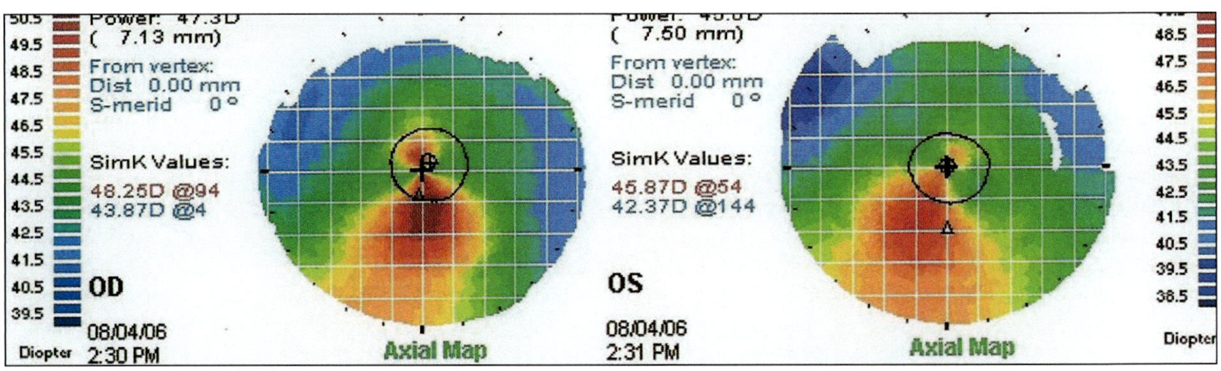

Figure 3. Topography demonstrated keratoconus with inferior steepening in both eyes.

out, often seen as white areas, are a major indicator of dry eye disease. For example, Figure 1A shows a topographic map for a patient interested in presbyopic correction with IOLs. Significant portions of the image drop out, and irregular astigmatism is evident. Based on these topographic findings, it was apparent that the patient had either dry eye disease or meibomian gland dysfunction, which had resulted in a poor tear film. A slit-lamp examination revealed significant meibomian gland dysfunction as well as a low tear film volume. The patient received treatment with topical cyclosporine 0.05% (Restasis; Allergan, Inc., Irvine, CA) b.i.d. as well as AzaSite (Inspire Pharmaceuticals, Inc., Durham, NC) OU q.h.s. Two weeks later, he returned, and the topography was more regular (Figure 1B). Just as importantly, the improvement in the health of the ocular surface resulted in more reliable keratometry readings on the IOLMaster (Carl Zeiss Meditec, Inc., Dublin, CA).

A compromised ocular surface can make topographic images appear suspicious for forme fruste keratoconus. For example, the father of a local optometrist was interested in cataract surgery, but the topographic map of his left eye appeared to be irregular with a number of dry spots (Figure 2A). I instructed the patient to instill artificial tears every 2 hours. Topography from the next day (Figure 2B) provided more information on his ocular state but still looked very suspicious for forme fruste keratoconus. I began treating his underlying dry eye disease with Pred Forte (Allergan, Inc.), and topography performed 6 days later revealed more regular astigmatism (Figure 2C).

CONTRAINDICATIONS

Preoperative topography is critical prior to cataract surgery to determine whether a patient is eligible for a premium IOL. Patients with forme fruste keratoconus, keratoconus, or pellucid marginal degeneration are poor candidates for presbyopia-correcting IOLs, because they have a high chance of reduced BCVA from their corneal condition. For example, topography revealed keratoconus with significant inferior steepening bilaterally, despite a normal slit-lamp examination, in the eyes of a patient who was interested in premium IOLs (Figure 3). Alternatives included a toric or a standard IOL. A presbyopia-correcting IOL was not an ideal option for this patient, because he would not have been eligible for a reduction of his astigmatism with incisional procedures. I also felt that he was a poor candidate for surface ablation. Although some surgeons offer PRK for eyes with forme fruste keratoconus and the medical literature supports this treatment option, the situation is different with eyes that have presbyopia-correcting lens implants. In the United States, I do not believe that current excimer laser technology is able to reduce both astigmatic refractive error and corneal asymmetry adequately to achieve a satisfactory quality of vision for a patient with forme fruste keratoconus and a presbyopia-correcting IOL.

EPITHELIAL BASEMENT MEMBRANE DYSTROPHY

Corneal topography can identify patients with irregular astigmatism due to epithelial basement membrane dystrophy (EBMD). Although this condition is visible at the slit lamp, it can be subtle. In addition, it is difficult to know the degree to which EBMD will affect a patient's vision following cataract surgery. I have found corneal topography useful in these cases. It identifies the irregular astigmatism caused by EBMD and allows me to discuss the potential impact of the disease with patients prior to cataract surgery.

CONCLUSION

I routinely use topography to identify patients with corneal conditions that may affect whether or not they are eligible for premium IOL surgery. Moreover, because I am working with an older population of patients, topography occasionally identifies asymmetric or irregular astigmatism due to dry eye disease or meibomian gland dysfunction. In many cases, improving the ocular surface produces better, more regular corneal topographic images, which may make patients eligible for a premium IOL. Although ophthalmologists may not bill insurance carriers or Medicare for the performance of routine testing prior to cataract surgery, I believe that the information obtained from preoperative corneal topography is worth the expense to my practice. ■

This article originally appeared in the September 2008 issue of CRSToday.

CHAPTER 189

Communicating With Unhappy Refractive Surgery Patients

JOHN POTTER, OD

It is unfortunate when a patient has an unexpected postoperative result from refractive surgery. Sometimes, these patients experience a great sense of visual loss, and they may go through several different stages of grief.

Dealing with disappointed patients is challenging for you and your staff. In this article, I attempt to explain the various phases of unhappiness a patient may endure after a failed refractive procedure and suggest how to help them and your staff cope with the situations, based upon my experiences.[1]

STATE OF SHOCK

Patients' first response is usually shock, which can last for a few days. This reaction protects patients from having to deal with a difficult concept: they have not gotten what they expected from their refractive surgery procedure.

Patients are sometimes accepting of their current situation, because they are numb to its impact. Stay in close contact with patients that achieved a less-than-favorable visual result from refractive surgery. I suggest seeing them weekly for a month or so.

Patient/surgeon contact remains important as patients advance to the second stage of grief.

EXPRESSION OF EMOTION AND ANGER

After their sense of shock passes, patients usually become highly expressive of their emotions—typically, anger and frustration. A natural response is to back away, and it may be prudent to put some space between you and your patient initially. It is important, however, for you to strive to become closer emotionally with the patient.

The next critical step is to say what the patient needs to hear, not necessarily what you want to articulate. At this stage of the grieving process, the patient will remember nearly every word you say. Because inconsistency and a lack of sincerity on your part can damage your relationship with the patient, I suggest creating and following a rubric for these interactions.

When expressing remorse to patients with an error, I suggest you use the five Rs: (1) recognition; (2) regret; (3) responsibility; (4) remedy; and (5) realignment. In my opinion, it is best to recognize that a problem exists first. Next, sincerely express your regret without asking for the patient's forgiveness or attempting to distance yourself emotionally from the patient. Asl for forgiveness can cause a patient to exclaim that you have no idea what he is experiencing and the level of suffering he has to endure. Next, take responsibility, and ask the patient what you can do to help improve the situation. You should then determine a remedy. If you are aware of the next steps for treating the patient, tell him so. The final step is realignment. Errors occur infrequently. It is appropriate to tell your patient so and to ask for him to share with you his progress so that, if an error in treatment occurs again, you will be better prepared to help the patient.

DEPRESSION AND LONELINESS

Patients may feel confused, which can lead to a depressed mood and a sense of loneliness. It is not uncommon for patients to tell their surgeons that they have thoughts of ending their lives. Although I have not encountered any patient who has followed through on these ideas, it is important to recognize these thoughts and address them. Based on my experience, you should see these patients at least monthly. A telephone call is adequate from time to time, and you need not say a lot. Be sure, however, to communicate your concern for the patient's well-being effectively.

PHYSICAL SYMPTOMS

For surgeons, perhaps the most alarming phase of patients' grief occurs next. They may start complaining that their vision is so poor they cannot see to work or perform basic daily duties. Other symptoms may arise that are unrelated to their eyes. Address these emotions and find out if the patient is still working and performing daily activities. Do not challenge patients on their assessments. Show compassion and understanding or risk damaging the doctor/patient relationship.

ANXIETY

Patients may fixate on their poor postoperative vision and become extremely anxious. In my experience, at this stage, surgeons make the most mistakes in judgment. Patients are desperate and will do almost anything to correct their visual defects. Additional surgery is not an option for an anxious patient who is grieving about his current results from refractive surgery. Often, the outcomes of another procedure are not what the patient or surgeon wanted, which further strains their relationship.

GUILT

Although I have found that patients' feelings of guilt seem to last approximately 2 weeks,it is important to recognize these emotions and be prepared for them. Patients may ask if they should have had refractive surgery in the first place. Acknowledge that this is a natural and reasonable concern. If you have had similar encounters with patients before, you might share that with the patient. Finally, support the patient by communicating that these feelings of grief will diminish with time.

ANGER AND RESENTMENT

Anger and resentment over what the surgeon did, or did not do, is the next phase of the grieving process. During this period, the patient may have an overwhelming sense that you have forgotten how much he has suffered.

Patients may express their suffering to you for months, even years. Some will communicate their dissatisfaction on the Internet via anti-refractive surgery Web sites. It is important for your patients to seek advice from you or another physician; the Internet is simply not a very good doctor.

RESISTANCE

A patient may resist further intervention. You may schedule another surgery only to have patients say they do not want the treatment or not show up for appointments. The harder you push the patient for additional treatment and/or appointments, the more resistant he will likely become. I suggest backing off after communicating that an additional procedure is an important decision and telling the patient to take the time to consider if another treatment is right for him.

HOPE

Gradually, hope returns, and your patients will begin to experience their lives differently and for the better. Also, you may find that your patients are now ready to pursue additional surgery to improve their vision.

AFFIRMATION

I have had patients apologize for their past behavior, and countless others have offered to help patients who have had similar experiences. In my opinion, medical malpractice is a rarity when surgeons and patients work together toward a possible resolution of postoperative visual problems. You can preserve your relationships with patients by recognizing and respecting the different phases of their grief. ■

This article was adapted from Potter J. Communicating with the unhappy refractive IOL patient. In: Chang DF, ed. Mastering Refractive IOLs: the Art and Science. *Thorofare, NJ: Slack, Inc.; 2008:807-810.*

This article originally appeared in the June 2008 issue of CRSToday.

CHAPTER 190

Handling Postoperative Issues With Refractive IOLs

D. REX HAMILTON, MD, MS

The 80 million baby boomers in the United States began turning 60 in 2006. By 2011, when this demographic starts becoming eligible for Medicare, there will be an estimated 40 million people over the age of 65 in this country. By 2020, that number will be close to 55 million. This group of individuals differs greatly from previous senior populations. As a whole, the boomers have significant disposable income, they are well educated and computer savvy, and they engage in active lifestyles. With more than 50% of patients over the age of 65 suffering from visually significant cataracts, it is clear that anterior segment surgeons will not only be busy in the coming decade, but they will also have more demanding patients than in years past.

Refractive IOLs are here to stay despite the currently challenging economic times. While keratorefractive surgery was down 11% in the first quarter of 2008 compared with the first quarter of 2007, IOL procedures were up 3.4%, and refractive lens exchange was up 11.0% from the first quarter of 2007.[1] In 10 years, we may not be using the same IOLs we are today, but we will most definitely be dealing with patients' postoperative expectations that are at least equivalent to those of today's refractive cataract surgery patients (see *Preoperative Screening and Setting Expectations*).

This article reviews the main postoperative issues that we anterior segment surgeons can expect to deal with today, as we incorporate refractive IOLs into our practices.

WHY ARE PATIENTS UNHAPPY AFTER RECEIVING REFRACTIVE IOLS?

Spherical Ametropia

Spherical ametropia is the number-one cause of postoperative unhappiness among patients who have received refractive IOLs. Personalized A-constants along with consistent keratometry and biometry (using either immersion A-scan or the IOLMaster [Carl Zeiss Meditec, Inc., Dublin, CA]) are essential to achieving emmetropia with refractive IOLs. When myopia occurs early on in the first eye of a patient receiving the Crystalens (Bausch & Lomb, Rochester, NY), first ensure that your technician or optometrist is not "over-minussing" the patient during the manifest refraction. Verify that the patient's unaided distance and near vision are consistent with the refraction. If the eye is truly myopic, ensure that the lens is well centered with both haptics positioned in the peripheral capsular bag and that there is no significant capsular contraction. Highlight for the patient the exceptional unaided near vision that he has achieved, a result that has far exceeded your expectations. Proceed with the implantation of a Crystalens in the patient's second eye after adjusting the refractive target to account for the unexpected effective lens position that you observed in the first eye. For example, if the first eye ends up with -0.75 D sphere for a goal of plano, target +0.50 to +0.75 D in the second eye. Do not correct the myopia in the patient's first eye with keratorefractive surgical techniques or a lens exchange prior to placing a lens implant in the second eye.

It is less likely that multifocal lens patients will end up with spherical myopia due to a more consistent effective lens position. It is more likely, however, that a keratorefractive or IOL exchange procedure will be required in patients who end up myopic after receiving a multifocal lens, but you should still wait to perform an adjustment until after operating on the second eye, if possible. Hyperopic ametropia can be easily addressed with conductive keratoplasty. This minimally invasive procedure has an advantage over PRK and LASIK: it has essentially no effect on dysfunctional tear syndrome, a disorder that is prevalent in the cataract population, particularly among postmenopausal women. In my experience, the main downside to conductive keratoplasty, regression of refractive effect, occurs to a much lower degree in older patients.

Astigmatic Ametropia

Residual astigmatism will often have a negative impact on patients' acceptance of their unaided near and distance vision. Treat refractive IOL patients like keratorefractive surgery patients; topographic analysis is an essential component of the preoperative evaluation. Patients with less than 1.50 D of regular corneal astigmatism can usually be successfully treated with limbal relaxing incisions or astigmatic keratotomy at the time of the IOL surgery. Those with more than 1.50 D of corneal cylinder are most effectively treated with keratorefractive surgery following IOL implantation. PRK may be performed as soon as 1 month after IOL surgery, whereas LASIK should be delayed for at least 6 weeks following IOL surgery to allow the clear corneal incision time to heal. With the Crystalens, patients usually have good visual function with postoperative astigmatism of 0.75 D or less. Multifocal lenses generally require that there be 0.50 D of astigmatism or less for optimal performance. Ideally, when beginning to implant refractive IOLs, choose patients with less than 0.50 D of preexisting corneal astigmatism. Individuals with topographic keratoconus are not the best candidates for refractive IOLs.

If you are lucky enough to have a patient seeking independence from spectacles who has successfully worn monovision contact lenses for many years, a toric IOL such as the AcrySof Toric (Alcon Laboratories, Inc., Fort Worth, TX) should be your first choice in terms of lenses. With one surgery, you can treat this patient's cataract and astigmatism and provide a high level of spectacle independence.

Suboptimal Scotopic Visual Function

Unwanted nighttime visual disturbances are inherent to multifocal lens designs and should not come as a surprise to patients receiving these IOLs. The halos and glare become less problematic with neuroadaptation. The decreased contrast sensitivity does not improve with neuroadaptation, however, because the loss of contrast relates directly to the amount of light used to form the retinal image. Newer lens designs such as the AcrySof Restor Aspheric (SN6AD3; Alcon Laboratories, Inc.) offer improved contrast sensitivity compared with older designs.

A patient who primarily complains of the halos and glare from lights in the early postoperative period but does not complain about difficulty seeing street signs at night will likely accept the multifocal design as neuroadaptation occurs. Do not be dissuaded from implanting another multifocal lens in this person's second eye. Patients whose primary complaint is of waxy vision at night and difficulty seeing street signs may have a bigger problem. Remind them of their wonderful unaided near vision by having them read through -3.00 D spectacles. After ruling out ametropia as a cause of waxy nighttime vision, consider placing an aspheric monofocal IOL or the Crystalens in his fellow eye, depending on his need for the best possible unaided distance vision versus unaided intermediate vision. A patient who was doing well after the implantation of a multifocal IOL but developed suboptimal scotopic visual function in the late postoperative period merits an evaluation for other ocular comorbidities, with posterior capsular opacification at the top of the list of differential diagnoses.

Suboptimal Unaided Intermediate Vision

There is no question that the Crystalens is the refractive IOL of choice for patients requiring excellent unaided intermediate vision. The latest design, the Crystalens HD, still provides excellent intermediate visual acuity but augments patients' unaided near vision. This lens allows surgeons to reduce the postoperative anisometropia necessary to achieve clear unaided near vision with the current Five-O model.

Phase 4 trials have begun on the AcrySof Restor Aspheric SN6AD1 lens. This model features a lower add (+3.00 D) at the IOL plane, which should improve patients' unaided intermediate vision with this lens. Individuals receiving the current AcrySof Restor Aspheric SN6AD3 should be warned that they may need glasses if they spend many hours at the computer each day. Patients complaining of inadequate unaided intermediate vision with an AcrySof Restor lens in their first eye may benefit from a Crystalens HD in their second eye to improve their computer-range vision.

OTHER OCULAR COMORBIDITIES

Dysfunctional Tear Syndrome

All refractive surgery patients must be evaluated for dysfunctional tear syndrome as a possible contraindication for surgery. Refractive IOL patients are no exception and are more likely to be affected, due to their overall older age demographic. Treat dysfunctional tear syndrome aggressively and early in patients with preexisting symptoms. The mainstay of therapy includes cyclosporine A 0.05% (Restasis ophthalmic emulsion; Allergan, Inc., Irvine, CA), oral omega-3 fatty acid supplements such as BioTears (Biosyntrx, Inc., Lexington, SC), punctal occlusion, and lid hygiene. The role of dysfunctional tear syndrome in suboptimal results with refractive IOLs cannot be over-

PREOPERATIVE SCREENING AND SETTING EXPECTATIONS

The importance of the screening and counseling process cannot be overstated. Surgeons who have experience dealing with keratorefractive surgical patients have an advantage here, because they understand the mindset of patients seeking spectacle independence. An excellent source of multiple opinions and pearls on the screening/counseling process is section VII of *Mastering Refractive IOLs: The Art and Science*, a comprehensive textbook edited by David F. Chang, MD.[1]

1. Chang, DF, ed. *Mastering Refractive IOLs: The Art and Science.* Thorofare, NJ: Slack, Inc.; 2008:332-431.

FACTORS IN THE CHOICE OF IOL DESIGN

As in other forms of refractive surgery, the preoperative evaluation of patients is key to success with refractive IOLs. Certain preexisting conditions and prior surgeries have a bearing on visual outcomes and should influence your selection of lenses.

EPIRETINAL MEMBRANE

Carefully evaluate patients who have a preexisting epiretinal membrane with optical coherence tomography prior to refractive IOL surgery. Even subtle epiretinal membranes may adversely affect the performance of a multifocal IOL. In addition, multifocal optics may make membrane peeling surgery more challenging for the vitreoretinal surgeon. The Crystalens HD (Bausch & Lomb, Rochester, NY) may be a better choice for these patients.

AGE-RELATED MACULAR DEGENERATION AND DIABETIC RETINOPATHY

Macular dysfunction can significantly affect the performance of multifocal IOLs. Patients with preexisting dry macular degeneration or moderate diabetic retinopathy may not be the best candidates for multifocal technology. Even if their macular function is currently adequate, these patients are at somewhat higher risk of decreased macular function in the future, a problem that may be compounded by the multifocal IOL optic. The Crystalens HD may be more forgiving of subtle macular dysfunction and is therefore a somewhat better choice for these patients.

POSTREFRACTIVE SURGERY PATIENTS

Multifocal lenses are likely to produce suboptimal results in eyes that have undergone LASIK or PRK, and they are very likely to perform poorly in post-RK eyes. These corneas have reduced contrast sensitivity due to their oblate shape, which then amplifies the decrease in contrast sensitivity associated with multifocal optics. The top choice for postrefractive surgery patients is aspheric monofocal IOLs, possibly in a monovision configuration if the corneal irregularity is not too severe. Future aspheric versions of refractive IOLs should have better results in these patients than current models of these lenses.

stated and should be foremost in your mind when evaluating these patients.

Posterior Capsular Opacity

Even subtle posterior capsular opacities can be clinically relevant in eyes with refractive IOLs. Particularly with multifocal lenses, even a single capsular fold across the diffractive portion of the IOL can decrease performance. Have a very low threshold for performing an Nd:YAG capsulotomy in these eyes.

Cystoid Macular Edema

Prophylaxis against cystoid macular edema (CME) is essential for all refractive IOL patients. Prior to the introduction of these lenses, ophthalmologists may not have treated angiographic CME, because they considered it to be subclinical. Today, angiographic CME is now optical coherence tomography-positive CME and should be treated in all cases due to patients' high expectations and the sensitive performance characteristics of refractive IOLs, multifocal designs in particular. Patients should begin taking NSAID drops at least 2 days prior to surgery and continue them for at least 4 weeks postoperatively along with topical steroids. Evaluate patients who present with decreased BCVA after refractive IOL surgery with optical coherence tomography and promptly start them on NSAID/prednisolone acetate 1% combination therapy for macular thickening. Patients with persistent CME that is refractory to topical therapy should be referred for a retinal evaluation. ■

This article originally appeared in the September 2008 issue of CRSToday.

1. Harmon D, Freeman W. The Surgeon's Quarterly Survey Report: Q1 2008. St. Louis, MO: Marketscope, LLC; June 30, 2008.

CHAPTER 191

Patients Unhappy With Presbyopia-Correcting IOLs

ERIC D. DONNENFELD, MD

Most patients who receive presbyopia-correcting IOLs are extremely happy. You can take several steps, however, to increase postoperative success dramatically. The first is to set realistic expectations preoperatively. Before surgery, I discuss patients' common concerns, such as glare, halo, their quality of vision, residual refractive error, and the possible need for enhancements. I cannot overemphasize how important it is to have these discussions. When you tell a patient he may have glare and halo after he receives a multifocal IOL, he expects that to happen. I tell him it is going to get better or we can treat it. When you do not tell patients about glare and halos, these visual disturbances become complications. The patient grows defensive, as do you, and they believe you did something wrong. My advice is to tell your patients before surgery about things that they can commonly expect postoperatively.

ADDRESSING THE CAUSES OF UNHAPPINESS

We can effectively correct six different reasons why patients are unhappy with their presbyopia-correcting IOL. Number one is the implantation of a monocular IOL. I do not expect patients to be fully functional until the second IOL is placed in their fellow eye. I warn them about this lack of utility preoperatively. Bilateral implantation is critical to the success of the procedure, as is providing an adequate neuroadaptive period.

Other causes of suboptimal results are minimal refractive error, posterior capsular opacities, ocular surface disease, cystoid macular edema (CME), and an off-center IOL. When I see a patient with a multifocal IOL, I go through the list of possible complications he may be experiencing. When I have exhausted that list, then I know I am out of options. By that point, however, approximately 99% of patients are happy (I have only explanted one of 400 presbyopia-correcting IOLs). In fact, most patients are ecstatic about their results.

REFRACTIVE MYTHS

Small Refractive Errors

A refractive legend regarding presbyopia-correcting IOL patients is that they will tolerate small refractive errors; this could not be more wrong. Presbyopia-correcting IOL patients are incredibly sensitive to small refractive errors, and you have to be willing and able to handle them. My rule for astigmatism is a follows: if a patient has greater than or equal to 0.50 D but less than 1.50 D of cylinder, I perform limbal relaxing incisions (LRIs). Surgeons who choose to implant presbyopia-correcting IOLs need to know how to perform LRIs. For patients who have more than 1.50 D of cylinder, I will also debulk the astigmatism with an LRI and then treat the residual cylinder with PRK or LASIK or refer them for laser refractive surgery. If a cataract surgeon does not perform excimer laser photoablation, then the patient can be referred for laser refractive surgery.

LASIK

Another refractive legend is that surgeons who implant presbyopia-correcting IOLs need to learn to perform LASIK. I disagree. You should learn to perform PRK, which is not too difficult; you can learn the procedure in an afternoon. If you want to learn LASIK later, you can, but start with PRK. Surface ablation is less stressful for you and the patient and often produces better outcomes. The epithelium is less adherent in older, presbyopic patients, so there are fewer problems of epithelial sloughing and basement membrane disease.

Neither must you learn to perform customized ablations. Conventional ablations are probably better for 90% of patients receiving presbyopia-correcting IOLs. I treat 95% of my patients who have LASIK or PRK with customized ablations. I almost always perform conventional correction on patients who received presbyopia-correcting IOLs, however, because the aberrometer will not recognize the multifocal IOL accurately. I mark the cornea, scrape off the a 9-mm–diameter area of epithelium, wipe the bed very gently with a Weck-Cel sponge (Medtronic Xomed Ophthalmics, Inc., Minneapolis, MN), and then perform the ablation. I place a bandage contact lens on the eye and follow the patient until his epithelium heals. His vision should improve in approximately 4 days. In about 2 months, his vision is optimized. A skill necessary for PRK is the postoperative management of patients to ensure the epithelium heals well.

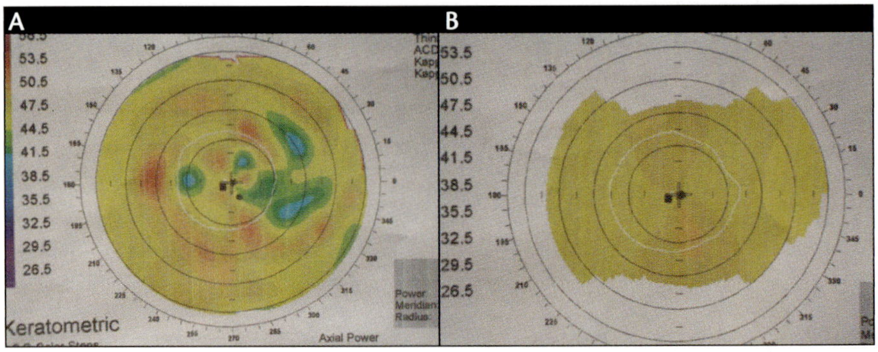

Figure 1. Topography before and after the use of topical cyclosporine 0.05% is shown.

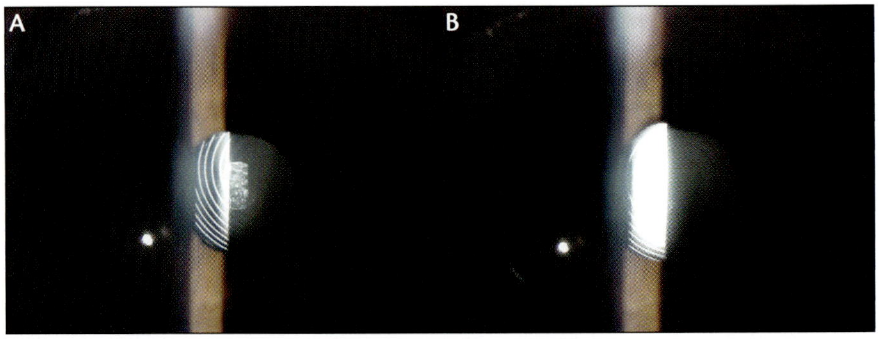

Figure 2. The IOL is not centered under the pupil (A), so the author performed an argon laser iridoplasty. The eye had this appearance after the procedure (B).

Nomograms

You do not have to learn nomograms for PRK after implanting multifocal IOLs, because you are dealing with treatments of 1.00 D or less most of the time. If you are off by 0.10 D, it does not make a difference. I aim for +0.10 D. If I end up with +0.20 D, that is fine. If I get a plano result, that is also OK. Do not attempt any nomogram adjustments for the patient's age or humidity.

Posterior Capsulotomy

I perform many more YAG laser procedures on patients who receive presbyopia-correcting IOLs than I have ever done in the past, because their eyes are incredibly sensitive. The loss of contrast sensitivity and the glare created by a multifocal IOL is made worse by any capsular opacity. I perform a large capsulotomy on these eyes. Once I open the posterior capsule, I perform an IOL exchange. For patients who are very unhappy with a presbyopia-correcting IOL, I explain, "If I open the posterior capsule, I will probably make your vision better, but, if I break it, you buy it." Once the posterior capsule is open, you have exposed the patient to a whole other level of complications, so I will not remove a presbyopia-correcting IOL after a YAG capsulotomy. I inform patients of this policy prior to their capsulotomy.

CME

CME is incredibly important and common. Patients who have conventional cataract surgery with no risk factors and no capsular breakage have up to a 70% chance of developing macular thickening visible on ocular coherence tomography (OCT)[1] and a 12% chance of having visually significant CME if topical NSAIDs are not used perioperatively.[2] I prescribe Acular LS (Allergan, Inc., Irvine, CA) q.i.d. for 3 days preoperatively, and the therapy is continued for 3 to 4 weeks postoperatively. This treatment regimen is becoming the standard. Many studies in the literature state that you must use an NSAID.[2,3]

The loss of contrast sensitivity associated with a multifocal IOL is worsened by CME.[3] Once the normal architecture of the retina is lost, visual quality is degraded for life. Snellen visual acuity will improve, but contrast sensitivity will be permanently reduced.

The best way to look for CME after cataract surgery is with OCT. In addition, OCT is a very effective preoperative screening tool for foveal membranes, which will reduce quality of vision after cataract surgery.

Dry Eye

Dry eye disease is common in older patients. Even a mild breakdown of the corneal epithelium reduces the tear film's ability to smooth out the ocular surface (Figure 1). A study my colleagues and I performing shows that eyes treated with cyclosporine had significantly improved mesopic and scotopic contrast sensitivity compared with eyes that received only an artificial tear. A more regular tear film and ocular surface improve quality of vision.

Centration of the Lens

If all other options have been exhausted, I look for the centration of the IOL beneath the pupil. The pupil and the center of the capsular bag often do not coincide, so the lens will appear to be decentered (Figure 2). In such cases, I perform an argon laser iridoplasty. I place four spots in the iris' midperiphery in the direction I want to pull the pupil. I use a power of 500 mW and a spot size of 500 μm in diameter for a duration of 0.5 seconds. I perform the argon laser iridoplasty when a patient complains of glare and halos and when I am going to perform an excimer laser enhancement. I want to center the IOL on the pupil so my ablation is not off the visual axis or off the center of the lens.

CONCLUSION

There are many ways to improve the vision of patients with multifocal IOLs. Look at organic problems before saying that neuroadaption is going to resolve all of your patient's visual complications. With attention to residual refractive error, the ocular surface, CME, the posterior capsule, and pupillary centration over the IOL, you can satisfy most patients who are unhappy after receiving presbyopia-correcting IOLs. ■

This article originally appeared in the May 2007 issue of CRSToday.

1. Rossetti L, Autelitano A. Cystoid macular edema following cataract surgery. *Curr Opin Ophthalmol.* 2000;11:65-72.
2. Donnenfeld E, Perry HD, Wittpenn J, et al. Preoperative ketorolac tromethamine 0.4% in phacoemulsification outcomes: pharmacokinetic-response curve. *J Cataract Refract Surg.* 2006;32:1474-1482.
3. Donnenfeld E, Solomon K. The effect of a topical NSAID on quality of vision with a multifocal IOL. Paper presented at: The ASCRS/ASOA Symposium and Congress; March 19, 2006; San Francisco, CA.

CHAPTER 192

Managing Patients' Dissatisfaction With Multifocal IOLs

BONNIE AN HENDERSON, MD

Of the three currently available presbyopia-correcting IOLs available in the United States, I use the AcrySof Restor Aspheric IOL (Alcon Laboratories, Inc., Fort Worth, TX) for the majority of my patients for a number of reasons. Most significantly, this IOL almost guarantees spectacle-free near vision combined with very good distance vision. None of the current presbyopia-correcting IOLs, however, is perfect for every patient. One of the most common complaints with the AcrySof Restor IOL (Alcon Laboratories, Inc.) is of sunbursts and glare. Although the incidence of this unwanted visual phenomenon is infrequent,[1] it can be bothersome when it occurs. This article examines the problem and suggests how to address it.

CASE NO. 1

Presentation

A 74-year-old female (Figure 1) with significant bilateral cataracts complained of difficulty driving at night. Her preoperative manifest refraction was +4.50 -0.50 X 90 = 20/50 OD and +6.00 -0.50 X 90 = 20/60 OS. Her keratometry (K) readings were 42.50/42.25 OD and 42.50/42.00 OS. Her preoperative pupils measured 5 mm in dim light and 3 mm in bright light.

The patient underwent uncomplicated phaco surgery with the implantation of the AcrySof Restor lens (the aspheric model was not available at the time of her surgery) in her nondominant right eye. On the first postoperative day, her UCVA was 20/40 distance and J1+ near. The IOL was well centered, and the patient was happy with her outcome.

She returned for her 1-week postoperative visit with complaints of sunbursts and glare that were especially noticeable at nighttime. Her UCVA was 20/30 and J1+. A manifest refraction did not yield any subjective improvement in her vision or symptoms. Corneal topography was normal, and the postoperative K readings were similar to the preoperative values. I started the patient on a trial of brimonidine tartrate 0.5% (Alphagan; Allergan, Inc., Irvine, CA) in hopes that the mild pupillary constriction would improve her symptoms.

On her 3-week postoperative visit, the patient's UCVA remained 20/30 and J1+, and she was still symptomatic and unhappy. Her BCVA was 20/25 with a manifest refraction of +0.25 -0.75 X 107.

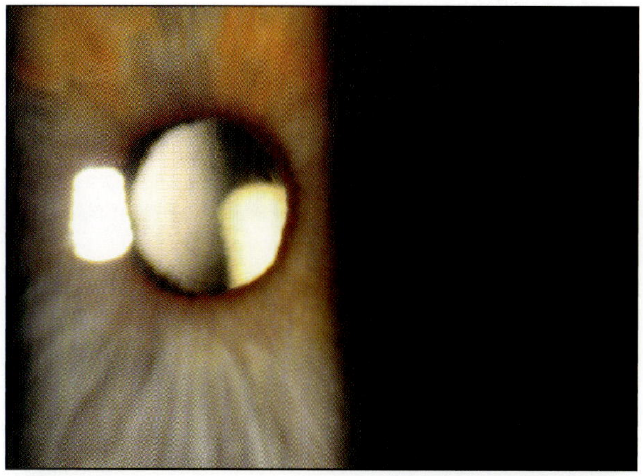

Figure 1. One week postoperatively, the AcrySof Restor lens is centered.

The patient required the removal of the cataract in her fellow eye and was bothered by anisometropia, because she was a +6.00 D hyperope.

Management

Options for this patient included an IOL exchange with either an accommodating or monofocal IOL. Another option was to perform cataract surgery on her second eye with either an accommodating or a monofocal IOL and then, in all likelihood, to perform an IOL exchange on her first eye after her second eye had stabilized.

The patient elected to undergo cataract surgery on her second eye with a monofocal IOL and a distance target. An IOL exchange with a monofocal lens was planned for her first eye in several weeks.

Uncomplicated surgery on the patient's second eye with an aspheric monofocal IOL produced a UCVA of 20/30. Postoperatively, the patient no longer suffered from sunbursts or glare when both of her eyes were open, and she expressed satisfaction with her uncorrected vision at distance and near. The IOL exchange scheduled for her first eye was canceled.

CASE NO. 2

Presentation

A 73-year-old retired engineer with a "type A" personality required cataract removal. He played tennis, sailed, skied, and traveled often. Significant cataracts were interfering with his sporting activities. The patient had pseudoexfoliation (PXF) and strongly desired independence from spectacles. He did not tolerate monovision spectacles and did not wear contact lenses.

The patient's preoperative BCVA was 20/40 OU but dropped to 20/100 on brightness acuity testing due to dense posterior subcapsular cataracts. His preoperative manifest refraction was -2.25 D sphere OD and -2.00 D sphere OS. His K readings were 44.25 D in his right eye and 45.00 D in his left eye.

Although the patient was fully aware that his diagnosis of PXF was a contraindication for accommodating or multifocal IOLs, he decided that the benefits of uncorrected distance and near vision were worth the risk of the IOL's possible decentration. He elected to have the AcrySof Restor Aspheric IOL implanted in both of his eyes.

Cataract surgery on the right eye was uncomplicated. On the first postoperative day, the patient's UCVA was 20/25 and J1. The lens was well centered. He was satisfied with his vision but also anxious and guarded. During his first postoperative week, the patient experienced a drop in his acuity. His UCVA was 20/30 and J1. He noticed glare and a loss of visual clarity, and a manifest refraction did not improve his vision. K readings, corneal topography, and optical coherence tomography were unremarkable. The clinical examination was also unremarkable except for a very slight (0.5 mm) superior decentration of the IOL.

Management

The patient's symptoms and examination remained unchanged for 3 weeks, after which he became so unhappy with his vision that he requested an IOL exchange. The procedure was uncomplicated, and his multifocal lens was replaced by an aspheric monofocal IOL with a target refraction of -0.25 D. His postoperative UCVA was 20/20 and J16 at near. He was happy with his distance vision but dissatisfied with his poor uncorrected near vision.

EFFECTIVE COUNSELING PRACTICES, SATISFACTORY OUTCOMES

I find that the majority of patients who receive presbyopia-correcting IOLs are satisfied with their outcomes, regardless of the lens selected. Each IOL design has limitations, however, that may result in patients' postoperative dissatisfaction. It is important to discuss these limitations in depth when counseling individuals for surgery. The Acrysof Restor is the most commonly used presbyopia-correcting IOL in the United States at this time.[2] I find that this lens achieves excellent outcomes. In my experience, the most common reasons for failure with it are sunbursts and glare.

My tips for minimizing patients' postoperative dissatisfaction with the Acrysof Restor lens are as follows. First, ensure that the IOL is properly centered at the end of surgery by using topical anesthesia and having the patient look directly up at the microscope's light. The light reflex from the microscope can be used as a guide to center the lens optic.

Center the optic more nasally rather than temporally and avoid placing a multifocal or accommodating IOL in patients with PXF.

If a patient has bilateral cataracts, place the AcrySof Restor IOL in the nondominant eye first. If he experiences sunbursts in his first eye, the symptoms may become negligible after cataract surgery in his second eye with a monofocal or accommodating IOL. This mixture of lens types can provide patients with sharp uncorrected near vision and clear distance vision. If the patient is happy with the first AcrySof Restor IOL, then he is quite likely to be happy with this lens' bilateral implantation. Bear in mind that these symptoms of sunbursts and glare generally resolve over time. Most of my patients who experience mild-to-moderate symptoms describe a complete resolution by 3 to 6 months postoperatively. ■

This article originally appeared in the September 2008 issue of CRSToday.

1. Javitt JC, Steinert RF. Cataract extraction with multifocal intraocular lens implantation: a multinational clinical trial evaluating clinical, functional, and quality-of-life outcomes. *Ophthalmology.* 2000;107(11):2040-2048.
2. Market Scope 4th quarter 2007 data. www.market-scope.com.

CHAPTER 193

Diagnosing Dysphotopsia With Multifocal IOLs

AUDREY TALLEY-ROSTOV, MD

Resolving complications associated with multifocal IOLs begins preoperatively by ensuring that patients' expectations are realistic. If patients are dissatisfied with their vision postoperatively despite excellent UCVA or BSCVA, surgeons need to be prepared to acknowledge the concerns and to offer solutions.

Using case examples, this article describes strategies for correcting dysphotopsia after the implantation of multifocal IOLs.

CASE EXAMPLES

No. 1

During a refractive surgery consultation, a 53-year-old white female expressed interest in undergoing refractive lens exchange with presbyopia-correcting IOLs. Her preoperative refraction was -5.00 +0.75 X 78 OD and -4.00 +0.50 X 81 OS. Her central corneal thickness measured 496 µm OD and 490 µm OS.

After uneventful bilateral refractive lens exchange with ReZoom multifocal IOLs (Advanced Medical Optics, Inc., Santa Ana, CA), the patient's BCVA measured -1.00 +0.50 X 90 = 20/20 OD and -0.50 +0.50 X 88 = 20/20 OS. She complained of severe dysphotopsia, night glare, and halos, which were present during the day with fluorescent lights and exacerbated at night, especially when driving. The patient was reassured that her problems would improve with time and neuroadaption, but she was still unhappy with her vision and underwent PRK in her right eye 5 months postoperatively to correct her residual refractive error. It was hoped that this procedure would mitigate her dysphotopsia. Although her spherical error was reduced to -0.25 D OD, she continued to complain of dysphotopsia and subsequently underwent a YAG capsulotomy in her right eye 6 months after PRK. The patient's visual acuity and dysphotopsia remained unchanged after this procedure, and they improved only slightly after the implantation of a piggyback IOL in her right eye 11 months after PRK.

Fourteen months after the initial refractive lens exchange, the surgeon replaced the ReZoom IOL in her left eye with a Tecnis IOL (Advanced Medical Optics, Inc.). She immediately noted a dramatic reduction in her dysphotopsia bilaterally (greater in the left vs the right eye) and stated that she was happy with her vision.

No. 2

A 51-year-old diabetic female who presented with a BCVA of 20/40 OU due to bilateral nuclear sclerotic and posterior subcapsular cataracts underwent uncomplicated phacoemulsification. She received a ReZoom IOL in her dominant left eye and an AcrySof Restor IOL (Alcon Laboratories, Inc., Fort Worth, TX) in her nondominant left eye. Postoperatively, the patient's UCVA was 20/20 OU (-0.25 D OD and plano OS). Her near visual acuity measured J2 OU (J3 OD and J1 OS).

The patient was very happy with the vision in her right eye, but she complained of halos and waxy vision in her left eye when reading. Her symptoms did not improve after a YAG capsulotomy in her left eye 6 months postoperatively. The patient later underwent two argon laser pupilloplasties in her left eye in an attempt to improve the AcrySof Restor IOL's centration and decrease the dysphotopsia. Her symptoms remained unchanged, however, and she was not satisfied with the vision in her left eye until the surgeon replaced the AcrySof Restor IOL with a ReZoom lens approximately 10 months after the initial cataract surgery.

DISCUSSION

Setting Patients' Expectations

Patients who are interested in multifocal IOLs should be counseled preoperatively about the potential for postoperative dysphotopsia. This visual disturbance, which includes nighttime glare, halos, starbursts, waxy vision, and decreased contrast sensitivity, can be replicated preoperatively by means of visual aids, charts, and night-driving simulators. Patients who are extremely phobic about the potential for dysphotopsia or who have professions that could be negatively affected by visual disturbances (ie, engineers, truck/taxi drivers) may be happier with accommodating IOLs, as may individuals who previously had refractive or corneal surgery.

Reassuring Patients

Almost all patients who receive multifocal IOLs experience some visual disturbances during the immediate postoperative period. Instead of dismissing patients' complaints, surgeons should reassure them that some dysphotopsia is normal and will improve over the coming months with neuroadaptation.

Identifying the Problematic Lens

Each multifocal lens design is associated with specific visual disturbances. For example, patients who receive the ReZoom IOL often complain of glare and halos, whereas those with AcrySof Restor IOLs tend to describe waxy vision and decreased contrast sensitivity.[1] As demonstrated in the earlier case examples, however, patients who receive the same type of IOL may experience different complaints. In addition, a symptom that is well tolerated by one patient may be more bothersome to another.

For example, the patient described in case No. 1 experienced disabling glare and halos with the ReZoom IOL. The patient from case No. 2 was very happy with her ReZoom IOL but was bothered by waxy vision and decreased contrast sensitivity in the eye with the AcrySof Restor IOL. Surgeons should try to isolate and differentiate the symptoms that patients may be experiencing in each eye.

Creating a Treatment Plan

It is advisable to wait a minimum of 6 months after the implantation of multifocal IOLs before performing additional procedures such as a YAG capsulotomy, excimer laser ablation, or an IOL exchange. If a patient still complains of severe dysphotopsia 6 months after cataract surgery or refractive lens exchange with a multifocal IOL, the surgeon's first step should be to rule out residual refractive error as the source of the postoperative visual disturbances. If eyeglasses or contact lenses significantly reduce or eliminate the patient's complaints, the surgeon can recommend that the patient either continue to use these corrective devices or undergo more permanent refractive options such as LASIK, PRK, or conductive keratoplasty (CK; Refractec LLC, Irvine, CA).

Surgeons should consider an IOL exchange for patients who continue to complain of dysphotopsia after sufficient time has elapsed for neuroadaptation (at least 3 months). As illustrated in the provided case examples, exchanging IOLs is sometimes the most effective strategy to eliminate postoperative visual disturbances.

It is worth remembering that exchanging IOLs is technically easier in eyes that have intact posterior capsules. Surgeons should therefore consider performing an exchange before a YAG capsulotomy in order to minimize the risk of cystoid macular edema and vitreous loss.

CONCLUSION

Although some dysphotopsia can be resolved by the correction of residual refractive error, the most severely affected patients may require additional surgical intervention such as the explantation and exchange of their multifocal IOLs. Screening patients carefully and setting realistic expectations preoperatively may help improve their visual outcomes with these lenses. Listening to patients and working with them to resolve their postoperative complaints can also improve their satisfaction with these procedures. ■

This article originally appeared in the September 2008 issue of CRSToday.

1. Bucci FA Jr. "Vaseline vision dysphotopsia" and explantation of the ReStor multifocal implant. Poster presented at: The Annual Meeting of the Association for Research in Vision and Ophthalmology; May 8, 2007; Fort Lauderdale, FL.

CHAPTER 194

Solving Multifocal Mysteries

ROBERT J. CIONNI, MD

When faced with patients who are unhappy after receiving multifocal IOLs, surgeons may be tempted to assume immediately that the problem is primarily caused by the lenses themselves. A wide range of factors, however, can affect patients' satisfaction with presbyopia-correcting IOLs.

CASE EXAMPLES

No. 1

A 67-year-old hyperopic female who was diagnosed with clinically significant cataracts desired independence from spectacles for distance and near vision after phacoemulsification. One week after uneventful cataract surgery and the placement of an AcrySof Restor IOL (model SN60D3; Alcon Laboratories, Inc., Fort Worth, TX) in her right eye, the patient stated that she was unhappy with her vision, especially at distance.

Her manifest refraction was significantly myopic with a refractive error of -2.50 + 0.50 X 167 = 20/20. The patient's keratometry readings (obtained manually, topographically, and with the IOLMaster [Carl Zeiss Meditec, Inc., Dublin, CA] and axial length were unchanged from preoperatively. A slit-lamp examination showed a normal anterior segment. Although the posterior capsule was against the back surface of the IOL (ruling out a capsular distension syndrome) and the IOL was completely inside the capsular bag, the optic appeared to be in very close proximity to the posterior surface of the iris. UBM clearly showed that the IOL was displaced anteriorly and demonstrated a nearly complete closure of the angle (Figure 1A). The patient's IOP remained normal, however, and the only symptom of her nearly closed angle was myopia. UBM of the patient's fellow cataractous eye revealed a shallow chamber and angle (Figure 1B).

If the patient had not requested a spectacle-free outcome, my colleagues and I would have recommended that she wear eyeglasses to address her postoperative refractive error. Because she was obviously concerned and unhappy with the result of her cataract surgery, we discussed her symptoms with glaucoma and retina specialists who agreed that her myopia could be caused by mild aqueous misdirection syndrome.

We decided against the implantation of a piggyback IOL, because the ciliary sulcus was too small to accommodate another lens. We also considered performing an IOL exchange but concluded that the outcome would be too uncertain. We instead observed the IOL for 1 month to see if it would spontaneously move posteriorly. When it did not, we performed a pars plana vitrectomy to relieve the suspected aqueous misdirection. One week after the procedure, UBM showed the IOL in a normal axial position (Figure 2). The patient's refraction also improved postoperatively to a spherical equivalent of -0.50 D. She expressed happiness with the vision in her right eye.

Based on the UBM examination of the patient's cataractous left eye and the complications resulting from surgery on her right eye, we decided to perform a primary pars plana vitrectomy at the time of the phacoemulsification and implantation of an AcrySof Restor IOL in her second eye.

After the uncomplicated procedure, the IOL remained in the expected position, and the patient did not experience a refractive surprise.

No. 2

A 48-year-old male with a history of bilateral cortical cataracts presented for evaluation 2 months after undergoing phacoemulsification and the implantation of an AcrySof Restor IOL (model SN60D3) in his right eye by an outside surgeon. Although the patient had good visual acuity postoperatively (20/25 at distance and J1 at near), he complained that his distance vision was hazy. He was also unhappy with his vision for computer use and resistant to the original surgeon's plan to implant the same type of IOL in his left eye.

Upon examination, the visual acuity of the patient's pseudophakic eye was nearly plano with minimal cylinder. His pupils measured 4.5 mm in diameter under normal lighting conditions. After a detailed discussion of his options, the patient underwent phacoemulsification with the implantation of a ReZoom IOL (Advanced Medical Optics, Inc., Santa Ana, CA) in his left eye. By 1 month postoperatively, the patient was happy with the vision

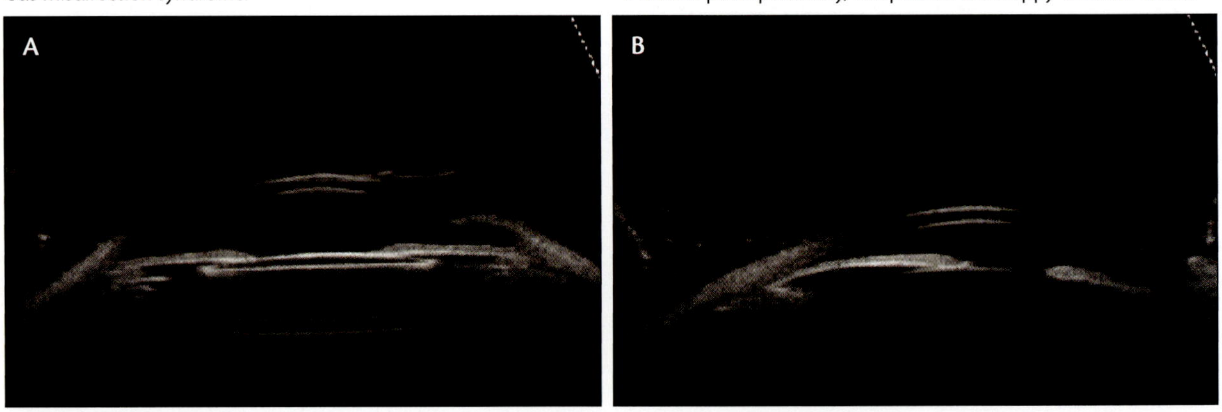

Figure 1. Ultrasound biomicroscopy (UBM) of a patient's right eye showed anterior displacement of the IOL and an almost complete closure of the angle (A). Her cataractous left eye also had a shallow anterior chamber and angle (B).

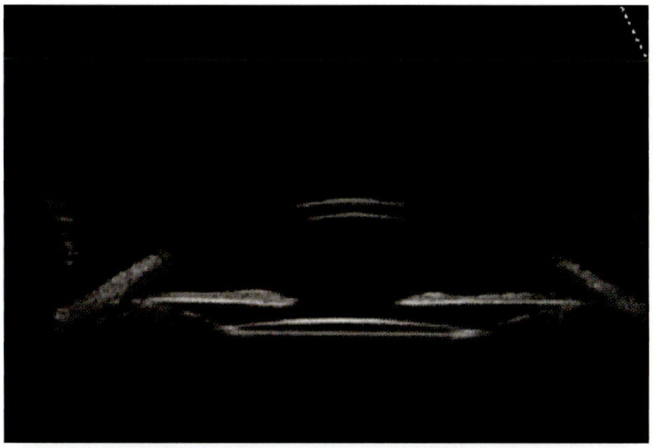

Figure 2. One week after a pars plana vitrectomy, the IOL shown in Figure 1 was in a normal axial position.

in his left eye at distance. He requested that we exchange the AcrySof Restor IOL in his right eye for a ReZoom lens, however, because he preferred the vision provided by the latter.

Despite achieving a nearly plano result and a bilateral UCVA of 20/25 (+2 at distance, 20/25 for intermediate, and J2 at near) after an uncomplicated IOL exchange, the patient stated that the ReZoom lens did not improve the vision in his right eye. The etiology of his visual complaints remains unknown, but it clearly was not due to the design of the diffractive multifocal IOL.

No. 3

A 48-year-old female business consultant who had worn rigid gas permeable contact lenses for 33 years was diagnosed with mild-to-moderate cataracts during an evaluation for LASIK at my colleagues' and my practice. She reported that she had stopped wearing her contact lenses 3 weeks prior to the consultation. At the time of her evaluation, her refraction was -6.00 +1.00 X 140 = 20/20 glare = 20/70 OD and -7.00 + 0.50 X 096 = 20/25 glare = 20/50 OS. Her pupils measured 4 mm in ambient light. Keratomety readings were consistent with the refraction of her right eye but somewhat variable for her left eye.

After discussing presbyopia-correcting IOLs with her surgeon, the patient decided that the AcrySof Restor lens (model SN6OD3) would provide the best near visual acuity and the lowest risk of nighttime glare postoperatively. The AcrySof Restor Aspheric IOL (model SN6AD3; Alcon Laboratories, Inc.) had not yet been cleared for clinical use.

During an uneventful procedure, the surgeon implanted AcrySof Restor IOLs in the patient's right (12.00 D, goal = +0.25 D) and left (11.00 D, goal = +0.29 D) left eyes. He operated on the steep axis of the right eye and placed a small limbal relaxing incision in the left eye.

One month postoperatively, the patient expressed unhappiness with her visual outcome. She had a UCVA of 20/50 and J3 in both eyes. Her manifest refraction was +0.50 +0.75 X 140 = 20/20 OD and +1.25 +0.75 X 65 = 20/20 OS.

A slit-lamp examination showed significant folds and mild haze in the patient's posterior capsules bilaterally. Fundoscopy and optical coherence tomography were normal for both eyes. After a lengthy discussion with the patient, the surgeon performed a YAG capsulotomy bilaterally. The patient did not report any improvement in her vision after this procedure.

She was then referred to a refractive surgeon who treated her residual hyoperopia and astigmatism with bilateral LASIK. The surgeon used a femtosecond laser to create the corneal flaps. By 2 months postoperatively, the patient's manifest refraction measured -0.25 +0.25 X 150 = 20/30- OD and -0.50 +0.50 X 180 = 20/30+ OS. Her bilateral postoperative UCVA was 20/50 and J7 at near. Her BCVA was now diminished without a discoverable etiology, and the patient was becoming more unhappy with her vision.

Wavefront analysis and topographic imaging of the patient's corneas with the Pentacam Comprehensive Eye Scanner (Oculus, Inc., Lynnwood, WA) demonstrated a higher degree of astigmatism in her right eye than was reflected by its refraction (Figure 3). In contrast, the left eye had less than 0.50 D of astigmatism and mild myopia (Figure 4). The surgeon also noted spherical aberration in both of the patient's eyes. With her consent, he decided to lift her flaps and treat her residual refractive error with additional LASIK. The treatment was designed to correct astigmatic myopia and aspheric myopia in the patient's right and left eyes, respectively.

By 2 months postoperatively, the patient's second refractive enhancement had not produced the expected results. Despite having open posterior capsules, pristine corneas, normal maculae, and two LASIK enhancements, the patient had a bilateral UCVA of

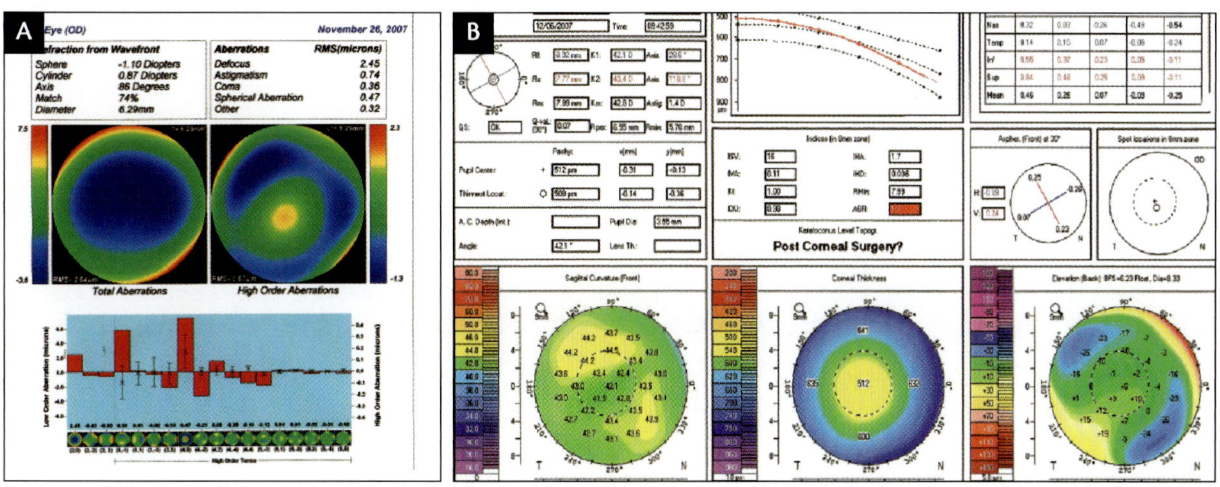

Figure 3. Wavefront (A) and topographic (B) analyses of the patient's right eye showed a higher degree of astigmatism than described by manifest refraction.

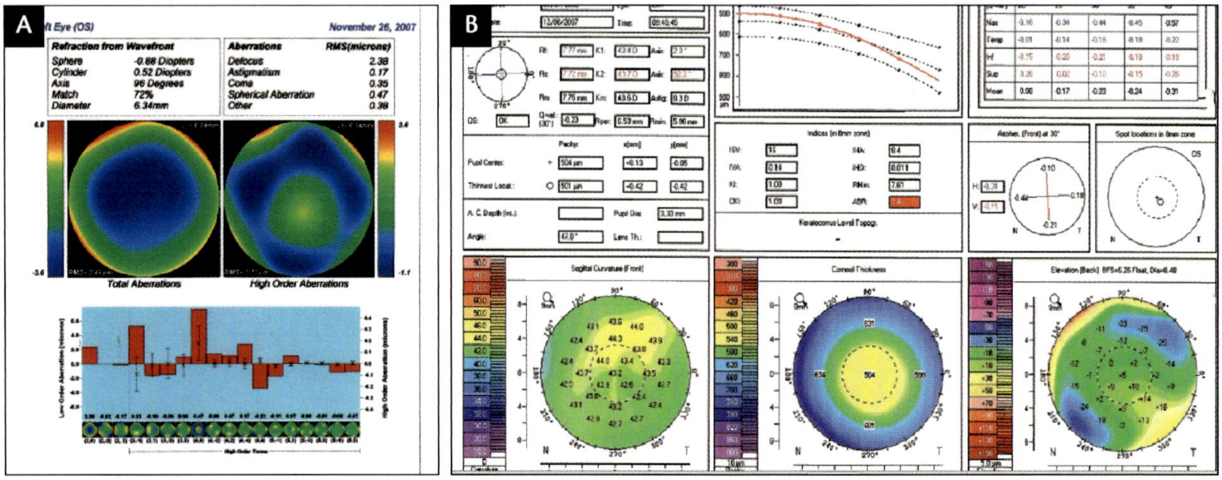

Figure 4. Wavefront (A) and topographic (B) analyses of the left eye of the same patient described in Figure 3 showed mild myopia and less than 0.50 D of astigmatism.

20/50 and J3 at near (+0.25 +0.25 X 180 = 20/40- OD and -0.25 +1.25 X 172 = 20/25- OS). Bitterly disappointed with her refractive outcome, the patient left our practice to seek a second opinion.

DISCUSSION

The case examples presented herein highlight several factors that affect patients' satisfaction with presbyopia-correcting IOLs. Cases No. 1 and 2 show that not all of the problems that patients experience can be attributed to the implanted lenses. In most cases, a careful consideration of the patient's complaint and a thorough investigation into its etiology will lead surgeons to possible solutions that do not require explanting the IOL.

The patient described in case No. 2 probably had some degree of amblyopia in his right eye that was not detected before cataract surgery and that prevented him from achieving his desired vision with the ReZoom IOL.

Case No. 3 illustrates the importance of careful patient selection. My colleagues and I were not able to meet the patient's expectations, and we overlooked several clues that her demanding personality would influence her surgical outcome. The patient's insistence on wearing hard contact lenses up until 3 weeks before her preoperative consultation indicated that she was not prepared to adapt to the visual changes associated with presbyopia-correcting IOLs. Given her 33-year history of wearing contact lenses, it would have been best for her to have discontinued her lenses at least 6 to 7 weeks before presenting for preoperative testing. Had she done so, we might have been able to better determine the IOL power and need for LRIs during the original procedure.

Although we knew that the refusal of the patient in case No. 3 to suspend contact lens wear for longer than 3 weeks could allow for continued corneal changes after cataract surgery, we felt that her vision would be good enough to preclude her need for contact lenses and, if necessary, would allow us to enhance her vision with LASIK. Due to the patient's travel schedule, however, and her stated difficulty of working after her initial surgery, her first enhancement was expedited. I suspect that her first and second enhancements produced disappointing results because they were performed too soon after the initial cataract surgery.

I believe that a very small subset of patients (<1%) has difficulty processing multifocal vision. Unfortunately, I do not have a method that can help me preoperatively identify individuals who are incapable of adapting to presbyopia-correcting IOLs. Instead, I strive to educate patients about the risks associated with these lenses and inform them that I can always exchange their multifocal IOL with a different model if needed. If the patient from case No. 3 had had clear, smooth posterior capsules and a nearly plano refraction without significant visual complaints after her initial cataract surgery, my colleagues and I probably would have replaced her AcrySof Restor IOL with a monofocal lens instead of trying to improve her vision with laser vision correction.

CONCLUSION

We surgeons must realize that not every patient will be thrilled with the refractive outcomes provided by presbyopia-correcting IOLs. The most common reason for patients' dissatisfaction is residual (usually cylindrical) refractive error. Patients who report improvement in their vision with trial lenses are candidates for an enhancement with PRK or LASIK. If their complaints do not appear to be caused by refractive error, surgeons should examine other likely etiologies such as dry eye, retinal edema, and posterior capsular opacification before they conclude the presbyopia-correcting IOL is not working properly. ■

This article originally appeared in the September 2008 issue of CRSToday.

CHAPTER 195

Halos With Multifocal IOLs

DWAYNE K. LOGAN, MD

With the refractive, diffractive, and accommodating lens technologies available, surgeons must be familiar with each type as well as the benefits of mixing and matching these IOLs in order to provide the best care for their patients. A staged implantation strategy allows for customized lens selection that addresses patients' lifestyles and visual needs. This approach provides a postoperative patient-satisfaction safety net by allowing patients to participate in the selection of their lenses.

I primarily use the ReZoom IOL (Advanced Medical Optics, Inc., Santa Ana, CA) for presbyopic correction due to its strengths in the areas of distance vision in daylight and near intermediate vision in dim lighting. I find that this IOL best simulates the natural human crystalline lens the most compared with the AcrySof Restor IOL (Alcon Laboratories, Inc., Fort Worth, TX) and the Crystalens (Bausch & Lomb, Rochester, NY). ReZoom patients with moderately dilated pupils may complain of nighttime visual aberrations, however, in the form of halos and/or starbursts when looking at lights. In my experience, patients seldom describe these symptoms with either the AcrySof Restor IOL or the Crystalens.

I retrospectively reviewed 50 consecutive bilateral ReZoom patients and found that 31% complained of dysphotopsia and fewer than 2% experienced severe halos that prevented them from driving at night during the their initial 90-day postoperative period.

In comparison, out of 25 consecutive bilateral AcrySof Restor IOL patients, fewer than 8% complained of nighttime or daytime halos, and one patient complained of a loss of normal color perception. After implanting more than 700 multifocal IOLs, I have explanted the lens of only one patient who complained of lost color vision.

I have limited experience with the Crystalens 4.5 and Five-O IOLs and have no documented complaints of nighttime visual symptoms. The unpredictability of the refractive outcome and minimal accommodation with the Crystalens, however, have left my patients dissatisfied with their unaided near vision.

My experience with multifocal IOLs began with the bilateral implantation of the ReZoom IOL. Because of patients' complaints about their early postoperative nighttime vision and difficulty when reading small newspaper print in bright light, I switched to implanting the AcrySof Restor IOL bilaterally. Very few of the AcrySof Restor patients complained of nighttime halos, but a significant number of them had poor intermediate vision and decreased distance and near vision in dim light.

Due to my aforementioned experience, I developed a mix-and-match, staged-implantation approach that I described earlier as a patient-satisfaction safety net. After I implant a ReZoom IOL in a patient's dominant eye, I will then address any of his visual issues or concerns. If the patient is happy, I will implant a second ReZoom lens in his fellow eye. If the patient complains of inadequate near vision, I will implant an AcrySof Restor IOL in his fellow eye. If the patient's chief complaint is nighttime halos, I will spend extra chair time explaining my clinical plan to help the patient neuroadapt to his new multifocal IOLs.

TECHNIQUE FOR REDUCING HALOS

Neuroadaptation

Neuroadaptation is a new buzzword for refractive cataract surgeons. Recent data presented as part of an online patient registry involving 20 surgeons showed that, on average, approximately 65% to 67% of the 98 patients included in a 6-month follow-up group achieved an improvement in halos, glare, and ghost images[1] (Figure 1). Although many patients adapt quickly and successfully to multifocal lenses, some adjust more slowly or not at all.

I explain the concept of neuroadaptation to all of my symptomatic patients and tell them that their halos will likely dissipate in time. In my experience, the process of neuroadaptation cannot begin until I have eliminated all postoperative variables, including an inadequate tear film, corneal epithelial and stromal haze, spherocylindrical refractive errors, decentration of the IOL, capsular fibrosis, vitreous opacities, and cystoid macular edema (CME).

Dry Eye

The incidence of dry eye symptoms, such as blurry and fluctuating vision, increases dramatically after cataract surgery and intraoperative limbal and corneal relaxing incisions in patients with preoperative ocular surface disease.[1-3] Tear film insufficiency can result in decreased visual acuity, excessive glare, and halos at night. I instruct my multifocal IOL patients to use artificial tears, Lotemax (Bausch & Lomb), and Restasis (Allergan, Inc., Irvine, CA) for at least 3 to 6 months postoperatively, with the understanding that Restasis takes 3 to 4 weeks to start working. I also place silicone punctal plugs if necessary.

Astigmatism

I recommend treating astigmatism intraoperatively with limbal and/or corneal relaxing incisions based on the patient's corneal topography. More than 0.50 D of sphere and 0.50 D of cylinder increase patients' perception of halos at night. Because I believe cylindrical refractive error plays the more significant role in the severity of halos, I feel that controlling astigmatism at the time of surgery is important. At 12 weeks postoperatively, surgeons can treat stable residual refractive cylinder by repeating limbal relaxing incisions, and surface ablation can remedy remaining spherical refractive errors. If I am only treating cylinder, I prefer a limbal or corneal relaxing incision to correct up to 3.00 D of cylinder. If I am treating mixed astigmatism or greater than 3.00 D of cylinder I will perform LASEK.

The IOL's Centration

It is not uncommon for my patients to complain that they see a comma or crescent secondary to decentration of the pupil on the central optic of the ReZoom lens. I find this problem more irritating than the 360° halo some patients perceive despite a perfectly centered ReZoom IOL.

My first step is to determine if the lens is optically centered. I have the patient look into the center of the two half-moon lights from a microscope, and I adjust the IOL so that the light reflex is

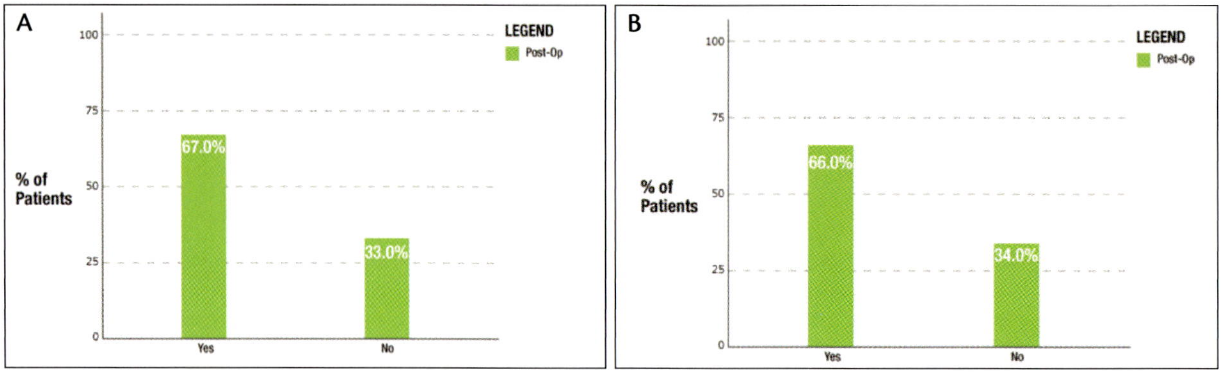

Figure 1. Sixty-seven percent of patients reported an improvement in halos between the 6-week and 6-month follow-up periods (A). More than 65% of patients reported an improvement in glare between the 6-week and 6-month follow-up periods (B).

directly in the center of the ReZoom or AcrySof Restor IOL. If the microscope has only one light source, I instruct the patients to stare at it while I center the central optic on the light reflex.

If the pupil is not symmetrical around the central optic, I often perform an iridoplasty with an argon laser. This procedure not only decreases visual aberrations, but it also improves patients' near vision with either the ReZoom or AcrySof Restor IOL.

Capsular Fibrosis

During the first postoperative month, early capsular fibrotic changes can occur, giving the appearance of an orange peel on the capsule. At night, patients may see starbursts. With monofocal IOLs, I typically wait 3 months before considering an Nd:YAG capsulotomy. With the ReZoom and AcrySof Restor IOLs, however, I have found that performing this procedure 4 to 6 weeks postoperatively effectively reduces patients' visual aberrations and halos and permits neuroadaptation to begin. I consistently confirm that the IOL is properly centered prior to performing an Nd:YAG capsulotomy. I have repositioned eight AcrySof Restor lenses and three Rezoom IOLs; many of these patients were referred to me because they were unhappy with their vision and results after a Nd: YAG capsulotomy results. Repositioning or explanting a multifocal IOL with an open capsule may result in vitreous loss and require an anterior vitrectomy. I have explanted one AcrySof Restor IOL in an eye that had an open capsule following an Nd:YAG laser treatment and required an anterior vitrectomy. I recommend avoiding a Nd:YAG capsulotomy if you are considering explantation.

Vitreous Opacities

Even if they do not cause halos, vitreous opacities can be very annoying to patients. I refer these patients to a retinal specialist for possible surgical intervention.

CME

I have found that patients with decreased visual acuity secondary to CME sense that halos are symptomatic. Several modulators can contribute to the cause of CME, including interleukins and prostaglandin E2 that are released by lens epithelial cells. These and other mediators break down the blood-retina barrier, which leads to CME.[4] I believe that excellent cleanup of residual lens cortex along with the pre- and postoperative use of topical NSAIDs mandatory to prevent CME.

IN SUMMARY

After I have eliminated or stabilized the aforementioned variables and I am happy with the surgical outcome, I can confidently tell patients that they are doing great. I have found that, when I am happy, my patients are, too. The primary concern of my Rezoom IOL patients is the mild halos they see around lights at night during the initial 6-month postoperative period. The mistake I made when I began implanting the ReZoom IOL was expecting patients' halos to disappear quickly. In reality, this dysphotopsia slowly dissipates over 6 to 12 months, as patients' brains adapt to the multifocal zones of the IOL. I now explain to my patients that the ReZoom IOL offers an effective combination of stable distance and near-intermediate vision. I tell them that, in the long run, the neuroadaptive process will enable them to enjoy lifelong benefits. ■

This article originally appeared in the September 2008 issue of CRSToday.

1. Li XM, Hu L, Hu J, Wang W. Investigation of dry eye disease and analysis of the pathogenic factors in patients after cataract surgery. *Cornea*. 2007;26:S16-S20.
2. Beiko, G. Bilateral ReZoom multicentre study; comparison of 6 week and 6 month results. Paper presented at: The ASCRS Symposium on Cataract, IOL and Refractive Surgery. April 2007; San Diego, CA.
3. Roberts, CW, Elie, ER. Dry eye symptoms following cataract surgery. *Insight*. 2007;32:14-21.
4. Nishi O, Nishi K, Imanishi M. Synthesis of interleukin-1 and prostaglandin E2 by lens epithelial cells of human cataracts. *Br J Ophthalmol*. 1992;76:338-341.

CHAPTER 196

Helping Unhappy Premium Lens Patients

JOHNNY L. GAYTON, MD, FSEE

Premium lenses have made a huge impact on both cataract and refractive surgery. Assertively addressing the postoperative concerns of patients unhappy with their presbyopia-correcting lenses is important to a practice's success. The process is challenging, however, because many of these individuals expected to have perfect or nearly perfect vision after surgery. I have many techniques for quieting their discontent.

DRY EYES

Excellent vision starts with a healthy tear film. Any disruption of the ocular surface can negatively affect preoperative measurements and thus surgery and its results. Postoperative dry eye disease decreases contrast sensitivity, blurs vision, and can cause glare and halos.

I prescribe artificial tears postoperatively for all patients undergoing laser eye surgery and/or IOL implantation. At night, I have them use fluorometholone eye ointment, which is a low-potency steroid. I also recommend the use of nutritional supplements, such as omega-3 fatty acids. Finally, I encourage patients to make environmental changes, especially avoiding tobacco smoke and circulating air from cars' air conditioning systems, ceiling fans, etc.

CYSTOID MACULAR EDEMA

With a late onset of 4 to 6 weeks postoperatively, cystoid macular edema (CME) is the most frequent cause of visual decline following uncomplicated cataract surgery.[1] The disease occurs in an estimated 12% of low-risk cataract cases.[2] The complication is due in part to a prostaglandin-mediated breach of the blood-retinal barrier.[3]

Although angiographic CME may not be associated with a significant loss of Snellen visual acuity, it can induce some astigmatism and hyperopia despite a BCVA of 20/20. Patients with clinical CME experience leaking vessels and a visual acuity of 20/40 or worse. Today's definition of clinical CME is becoming stricter (20/25 or worse), however, due to patients' heightened expectations and premium IOLs. Even a small amount of CME results in a decrease in contrast sensitivity. Because multifocal lens technology decreases contrast by dividing light, a small amount of CME can result in a very unhappy patient.

In my opinion, there is no excuse for ophthalmologists not to use NSAIDs prophylactically in patients to prevent CME, especially with all the drugs that are currently available. Dr. Michael Raizman's pioneering study clearly demonstrated the benefits of NSAID prophylaxis in preventing CME.[4] The concurrent use of NSAIDs helps to achieve control of postoperative inflammation faster than steroids alone. The rapid and permanent control of inflammation is critical to decreasing the incidence of postoperative CME. Although all of the NSAIDs are effective, I personally prefer bromfenac. In the phase 3 trials submitted to the FDA, bromfenac controlled inflammation quickly and effectively.[5] Due to the drop's rapid penetration of the cornea and other ocular tissues and strong affinity to the COX-2 enzyme, it only has to be used one to two times per day. The infrequency of dosing improves patients' compliance, especially when you want them to use it for 6 weeks or longer. I use the NSAID for 6 weeks in low-risk patients, but in diabetics and other higher-risk patients, I use the NSAID for at least 8 weeks.

ASTIGMATISM

Limbal Relaxing Incisions

Patients with residual ametropia after surgery with premium IOLs can have a low tolerance for blurry distance vision. Even slight residual astigmatism can markedly decrease the effectiveness of multifocal lenses by further reducing contrast sensitivity.

My colleagues and I conducted a study in which we combined the AcrySof Restor IOL (Alcon Laboratories, Inc., Fort Worth, TX) with limbal relaxing incisions (LRIs) in 14 eyes of 10 patients with refractive cylinder ranging from 0.50 to 2.25 D. After surgery, 10 eyes had slightly less cylinder, two eyes had not changed, and two had experienced an increase of 0.25 D. The two patients that had an increase in cylinder had lenticular cylinder that was neutralizing corneal cylinder. If LRIs had not been used, the astigmatism would have increased even more. I have performed LRIs for many years, and I always tell patients that the procedure is meant to reduce astigmatism but not eliminate it. LRIs are not as potent or as predictable as laser vision correction, but they are a useful tool in managing small-to-moderate amounts of astigmatism.

Surface Ablation

Unless the patient only has a small amount of astigmatism with a nearly plano spherical equivalent, I perform surface laser vision correction. I prefer surface ablation to LASIK, because the latter procedure is more likely to cause dry eye due to the corneal flap, especially immediately postoperatively. Also, with surface ablation, surgeons can perform an enhancement surgery earlier without having to make a preoperative flap, because a suction ring does not have to be applied to the eye.

For surface laser vision correction, I plan for myopia when calculating IOL power (eg, if a patient has 2.00 D of cylinder before phacoemulsification, my desired pre-laser refraction is plano to -1.00 D with 2.00 D of minus cylinder). Of course, if the patient has had previous RK and has a very flat cornea, I then prefer to steepen the cornea with a hyperopic ablation. I make sure that the patient understands that myopia after phacoemulsification is temporary (ie, his uncorrected distance visual acuity is supposed to be blurry in order to maximize his final vision). I offer an inventory of loaner glasses to help patients "survive" the 6-week period before their enhancement procedure. I will consider an Nd:YAG laser treatment prior to performing surface ablation.

In my experience, patients who undergo LASEK after receiving the AcrySof Restor IOL achieve a marked improvement in their astigmatism. For example, I performed laser vision correction on a 42-year-old female who had a history of lensectomy with the AcrySof Restor IOL in both eyes. I targeted myopia because I was going to treat her astigmatism later with surface ablation—1.50 D of cylinder OD and 2.25 D OS. The patient achieved an improvement in her uncorrected distance and near acuity (from uncorrected distance vision of 20/40 OD and 20/60 OS and uncorrected near vision of 20/30 OD and 20/50 OS to 20/20 near and distance in both eyes).

TORIC LENSES

Toric lenses are an excellent method of addressing corneal astigmatism, especially in patients who should not have additional corneal surgery and in those with coexisting cataract and astigmatism. These lenses are not contraindicated in patients with conditions that decrease their contrast sensitivity, because the IOLs improve contrast. These lenses not only accurately correct astigmatism, but they are also very forgiving. Even if they are implanted 15° off axis, patients achieve 50% correction of their astigmatism. In my experience with my first 100 eyes using the AcrySof Toric lens (Alcon Laboratories, Inc.), the patients' average preoperative cylinder was 1.78 D and average postoperative cylinder was 0.26 D. In eyes that have more than 2.00 D of astigmatism, I will combine technologies (eg, toric IOL and LRIs or toric lens and laser vision correction).

Caring for unhappy premium lens patients is not only critical to your success it can be very rewarding. I have cared for patients that others and I have implanted. Converting them to happy patients frequently results in their becoming referral sources for my practice. The two most important things that I can share seem like platitudes, but they are critical to caring for patients. The first is that patients do not care how much you know until they know how much you care. A caring attitude goes a long way in calming an anxious or unhappy patient. The second is a remark from one of my ophthalmic heroes, J. Lawton Smith, MD, who said, "listen to your patient and they will tell you what is wrong." Listening will usually enable you to tell whether the patient has a medical problem, or if he simply needs more education about how to use the lens. It will also demonstrate that you care. Follow these principles, and you should have a very rewarding premium lens practice. ■

This article originally appeared in the August 2008 issue of CRSToday.

1. Samiy N, Foster CS. The role of nonsteroidal anti-inflammatory drugs in ocular inflammation. *Int Ophthalmol Clin.* 1996;36:195-206.
2. McColgin AZ, Raizman MB. Efficacy of topical Voltaren in reducing the incidence of postoperative cystoid macular edema. *Invest Ophthalmol Vis Sci.* 1999;40:S289.
3. Mishima H, Masuda K, Miyake K. The putative role of prostaglandins in cystoid macular edema. *Prog Clin Biol Res.* 1989;312:251-264.
4. Raizman MB. Comparing NSAIDs in aqueous humor. *Eyeworld.* July 9, 2007. http://www.eyeworld.org/ewweeksupplementarticle.php?id=214. Accessed July 9, 2008.
5. Donnenfeld ED, Holland EJ, Stewart RH, et al. Bromfenac ophthalmic solution 0.09% (Xibrom) for postoperative ocular pain and inflammation. *Ophthalmology.* 2007;114:1653-1662.

CHAPTER 197

Dry Eyes and Premium IOLs

ERIC D. DONNENFELD, MD

An evaluation of the ocular surface is one of the most important aspects of my preoperative routine for any patient who is considering a premium IOL. Dry eye can significantly compromise patients' quality of vision, even after routine cataract surgery. With multifocal IOLs, problems related to dry eyes are magnified by the inherent decrease in contrast sensitivity with this lens type. Although we often talk about dry eye in the context of LASIK, in my experience, cataract surgery is even more commonly associated with the condition. According to a recent report, well over half the patients undergoing cataract surgery experienced significant postoperative dry eye.[1]

THE REASONS FOR DRY EYES AFTER CATARACT SURGERY

There are a number of reasons to expect dry eyes after cataract surgery. The cataract surgery patient population is older and has a higher incidence of preoperative dry eye than younger patients. Furthermore, multifocal IOL patients, in my opinion, are generally active and may frequently engage in situations that contribute to ocular dryness (eg, computer use, outdoor activities).

Another reason why a patient may develop dry eye is that their pre- and postoperative topical medications contain preservatives. They may be intrinsically toxic compounds that damage the ocular surface, especially the goblet cells. Also, in addition to the cataract incision, many patients will have limbal relaxing incisions in the periphery of the cornea where the corneal nerves enter the eye. Significant corneal anesthesia and dry eye may ensue. Furthermore, there is a 5% to 10% excimer laser enhancement rate with multifocal IOLs (the risk of dry eye disease increases from multiple surgeries).

PREOPERATIVE EVALUATION

During my preoperative evaluation of patients considering cataract surgery, my first step is to take a thorough ocular history, including contact lens intolerance, foreign body sensation, grittiness, and a record of ocular symptoms that worsen later in the day. The most important indication I look for is fluctuating visual acuity, which almost always suggests ocular surface disease. When I hear a potential patient complain of any of the aforementioned warning signs, I examine him carefully for dry eye syndrome. I observe the tear meniscus and the corneal and conjunctival epithelium (for hyperemia, redundant conjunctiva, etc.) to assist my diagnosis.

Most important in the evaluation of ocular surface disease is vital dye staining of the conjunctiva and/or cornea. Fluorescein staining of the cornea is typical in mild-to-moderate dry eye disease, because epitheliopathy is not yet apparent at this stage. Lissamine green staining (Accutome Inc., Malvern, PA) is probably the most useful test I perform, because it reveals damage to ocular tissue at its earliest stages and will stain the conjunctival epithelium when there is no fluorescein staining. Typically, there is an interpalpebral staining pattern of the conjunctiva. A reduced tear breakup time (≤ 15 seconds) can indicate a lipid deficiency and a less-than-optimal quality to the tear film. Although Schirmer's testing is the standard method by which to measure tear production, it is generally not considered helpful for diagnosing dry eye syndrome at its early stages, because the results are often in the normal range in these patients. I rely on Schirmer's testing most commonly in patients with collagen vascular disease.

PRETREATMENT OF MULTIFOCAL IOL PATIENTS

I begin by prescribing transiently preserved tears such as Blink Contacts Lubricant Eye Drops (Advanced Medical Optics, Inc., Santa Ana, CA), Optive (Allergan, Inc., Irvine, CA), Genteal (Novartis Ophthalmics, Inc., Duluth, GA), and TheraTears (Advanced Vision Research, Inc., Woburn, MA) four times a day. The ideal artificial tear coats the cornea well and smoothes out the ocular surface, thus regularizing the tear film. The most recent generations of artificial tears offer the advantages of high adherence to the ocular surface without blurring patients' vision. Oral nutritional supplementation with flaxseed oil and fish oils also help individuals with dry eye disease, but it is most useful in patients with mixed mechanisms of dry eye and meibomian gland disease. Any patient with even mildly dry eyes who is undergoing cataract surgery, however, deserves immunomodulation.

IMPROVEMENT OF POSTOPERATIVE RESULTS

Cyclosporine has been shown to improve corneal staining at all follow-up visits ($P<.001$). At month 4, the improvement in staining with the help of cyclosporine was significantly greater than with the vehicle ($P\leq.05$). Patients treated with cyclosporine A 0.05% emulsion experienced statistically significant reductions in corneal staining by month 8 ($P=.008$), and they exhibited statistically and clinically significant reductions in blurred vision versus the vehicle at all time points ($P\leq.05$), as measured by the Snellen chart. The mean visual improvement was approximately 24%.[2]

The therapeutic efficacy of cyclosporine is important for patients receiving multifocal IOLs. A recent prospective, randomized, masked, bilateral, multicenter study evaluated 28 eyes of 14 patients without a history of dry eye who were scheduled to undergo bilateral phacoemulsification with the implantation of a multifocal IOL.[3] One eye received topical cyclosporine b.i.d. whereas the other received artificial tears b.i.d. for 1 month prior to and 2 months following cataract surgery. After 3 months of treatment, fluorescein corneal staining was significantly less in the cyclosporine group ($P=.034$). Two months postoperatively, the mean UCVA was significantly better in the eyes treated with cyclosporine as opposed to artificial tears (logMar of 0.11 vs 0.19, $P=.045$). Similarly, BCVA 2 months postoperatively was zero with cyclosporine and 0.1 with tears ($P=.005$). Contrast sensitivity under mesopic and photopic conditions improved with and without glare. The patients who expressed a preference were significantly more likely to favor the cyclosporine-treated eye ($P=.007$).

Cyclosporine can take several weeks or months to have an effect, and 17% of patients who use Restasis (Allergan, Inc.) experience burning upon instillation.[3] The irritation improves over 6 months, but the burning and stinging may cause patients to discontinue using the drug before its therapeutic impact is realized.

Although cyclosporine inhibits inflammatory mediators that are produced by activated T lymphocytes, corticosteroids block several pathways associated with dry eye, including the production of cytokines, chemokines, and metalloproteinases. To control the entire inflammatory process and break the cycle at an earlier stage, clinicians should consider agents such as corticosteroids in combination with cyclosporine therapy. Studies have shown that the concominant use of loteprednol with cyclosporine rapidly treats dry eye disease and reduces the burning and stinging associated with cyclosporine and the pathology.[4]

CONCLUSION

Although the measures I have outlined may sound like a lot of work, they are a worthwhile investment in the postoperative outcome. A healthy ocular surface gives whatever lens technology we use the best chance of success. By addressing dry eye proactively, we help our cataract/IOL patients see better faster with less discomfort after surgery. I have also found it helpful to discuss with patients what I am doing with respect to their dry eyes. This conversation lets patients know that they can help to ensure the best possible surgical outcome. The resulting "wow effect" and patients' high level of satisfaction build referrals for the practice.

Improving visual acuity and quality of vision starts with optimizing the tear film. Because advances in refractive and cataract surgery have raised patients' expectations, it is important to address their ocular surface disease preoperatively in order to improve their visual outcomes after IOL surgery. ■

This article originally appeared in the March 2008 issue of CRSToday.

1. Li XM, Hu L, Hu J, Wang W. Investigation of dry eye disease and analysis of the pathogenic factors in patients after cataract surgery. *Cornea*. 2007;26:S16-S20.
2. Sall K, Stevenson OD, Mundorf TK, Reis BL. Two multicenter, randomized studies of the efficacy and safety of cyclosporine ophthalmic emulsion in moderate to severe dry eye disease. CsA Phase 3 Study Group. *Ophthalmology*. 2000;107:631-639.
3. Donnenfeld E, Roberts C, Perry H, et al. Efficacy of topical cyclosporine versus tears for improving visual outcomes following multifocal IOL implantation. Paper presented at: The ASCRS/ASOA Symposium on Cataract, IOL and Refractive Surgery; April 2006; San Diego, CA.
4. Donnenfeld, E, Sheppard, J, Holland E. Prospective, multi-center, randomized controlled study on the effect of loteprednol etabonate on initiating therapy with cyclosporin A. Poster presented at: The 2007 AAO Annual Meeting; November 2007; New Orleans, LA.

CHAPTER 198

Capsular Complications With an Accommodating Lens

JACK A. SINGER, MD

I believe that the Crystalens Five-O (Bausch & Lomb, Rochester, NY) has a multifactorial mechanism of action. It includes forward movement of the lens during accommodation that is secondary not only to direct anterior tilting of the ciliary muscle, but also to vitreous pressure. Accommodative arching, as described by Kevin Waltz, MD, induces negative spherical aberration and coma, which increase depth of focus.[1] Astigmatism increases in most cases, likely secondary to some tilting of the lens or asymmetric changes in its central anterior shape. The flipside of this accommodative movement and arching can adversely affect vision when the IOL moves, arches, and vaults in unwanted ways due to contraction of the capsular bag. The Crystalens Five-O is much more resistant (but not immune) to capsular contraction syndrome than its smaller predecessor, the AT45SE, particularly in patients under 60 years of age and those with compromised zonular integrity.

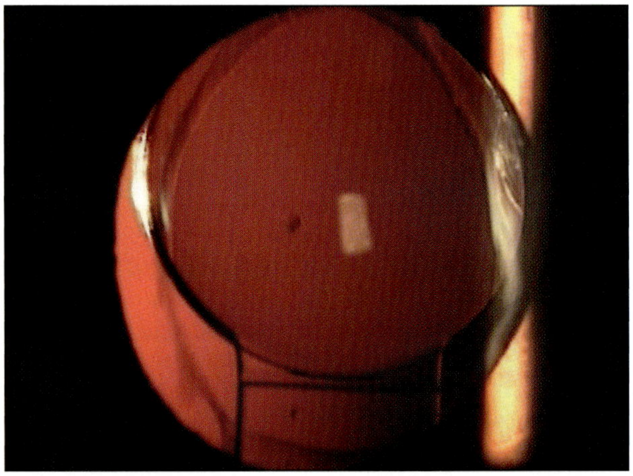

Figure 1. Crystalens Five-O with asymmetric vaulting secondary to contractile fibrosis and ovalization of the capsulorhexis.

ASYMMETRIC VAULTING WITH CONTRACTION OF THE CAPSULORHEXIS

A 36-year-old female with a history of blunt head trauma from an automobile accident developed posterior subcapsular cataracts with mild zonular dehiscence. She underwent phacoemulsification in her left eye with implantation of the Crystalens Five-O. Three weeks postoperatively, she developed symptoms of blurred vision and an inferior crescent, and her surgeon implanted a capsular tension ring (CTR) without rotating the IOL. The patients' symptoms returned 2 hours after the CTR's implantation.

Six weeks postoperatively, the patient presented to me with uncorrected distance vision of 20/30, uncorrected near vision of J8, and a BCVA of 20/20 with a refraction of -0.75 +1.50 X 78. I found asymmetric vaulting of the Crystalens Five-O with contractile fibrosis and ovalization of the capsulorhexis[2] (Figure 1). The superior plate haptic had excessive posterior vaulting (Figure 2A), and the inferior plate haptic had excessive anterior vaulting (Figure 2B).

Early capsular contraction with atypical vaulting of the IOL can usually be treated with a YAG laser posterior and/or anterior capsulotomy, which relieves tension in the capsule and reduces stress on the IOL. In this case, the CTR was insufficient to withstand the force of the contractile anterior capsular fibrosis in the face of zonular dehiscence. The patient wanted to keep her accommodating IOL, if possible, so I attempted a surgical solution.

Viscodissection with Healon GV (Advanced Medical Optics, Inc., Santa Ana, CA) opened the capsular bag, and I used a Sinskey hook to tease out the IOL's four polyimide loops while applying counter traction on the anterior capsule with an iris retractor. I temporarily moved the Crystalens, once freed, into the anterior chamber. I instilled additional Healon GV to inflate the capsular bag and maintain the anterior chamber, while I enlarged the anterior capsulotomy by excising the contractile fibrous band with the Duet intraocular forceps and scissors (MicroSurgical Technology, Redmond, WA) (Figure 3). In order to keep it vaulted posteriorly, the Crystalens was placed underneath the CTR and oriented to give maximal clearance between the sides of the optic and the anterior capsule, which happened to be perpendicular to its original position.

Proper posterior vaulting of the Crystalens was restored, but the refraction turned out to be hyperopic by +1.75 D (20/15), because the lens was located behind the CTR. I implanted a +3.00 D AQ5010V three-piece IOL (STAAR Surgical Company, Monrovia, CA) in a piggyback fashion in the ciliary sulcus (Figure 4). Fourteen months after this procedure, the Crystalens Five-O remains well positioned. The patient has uncorrected distance vision of 20/20, uncorrected intermediate vision of 20/16, uncorrected near vision of J1, and a manifest refraction of -0.50 +0.25 X 57.

ASYMMETRIC VAULTING WITH RETRACTION OF THE CAPSULORHEXIS

A 48-year-old female was referred to me by her surgeon 2 months after she underwent phacoemulsification with implantation of the Crystalens Five-O. She had experienced a myopic shift of -1.50 D sphere, and there was asymmetric vaulting of the IOL. The superior plate haptic had excessive anterior vaulting with the hinge located anterior to the iris plane, and the inferior plate had excessive posterior vaulting (Figure 5). The anterior capsulotomy was retracted superiorly, almost up to the distal end of the plate haptic, and gonioscopy showed the superior loops to be covered with a small amount of fibrotic anterior capsule. Her surgeon reported that the anterior capsule had originally overlapped the plate haptic up to the hinge. The posterior capsule was intact with folds radiating from behind the superior haptic.

After opening the capsular bag via viscodissection with Healon GV, I implanted a CTR through a 1-mm sideport incision. I freed the four polyimide loops, cleaned the capsule with ultra-

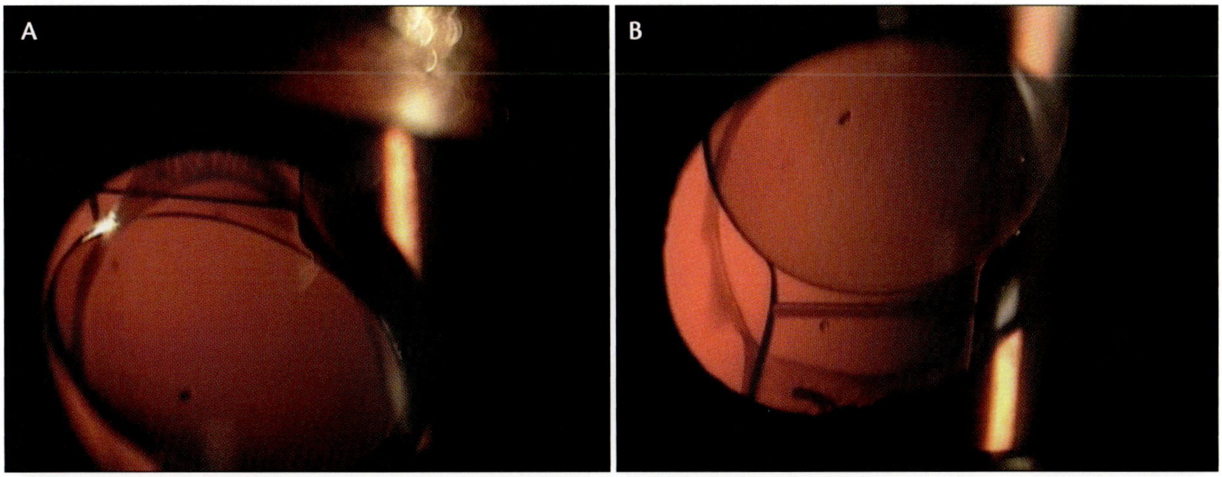

Figure 2. Upgaze showed excessive posterior vaulting of the superior plate haptic (A). Downgaze showed excessive anterior vaulting of the inferior plate haptic (B).

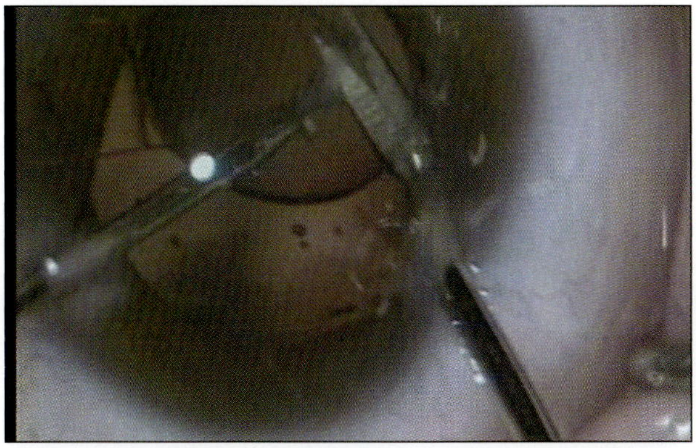

Figure 3. The surgeon enlarged the anterior capsulotomy by excising the contractile fibrous band with Duet intraocular forceps and scissors.

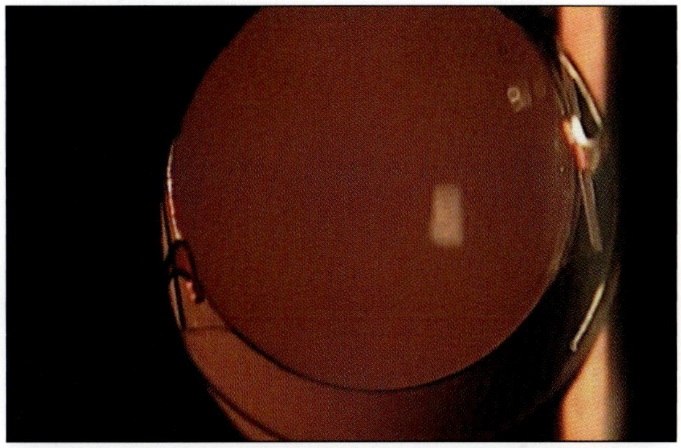

Figure 4. The surgeon piggybacked a model AQ5010V three-piece IOL in the ciliary sulcus over the repositioned Crystalens Five-O and a CTR.

sonic I/A using gravity-powered outflow (Surgical Design Corp., Armonk, NY), rotated the IOL horizontally, and placed it behind the CTR. The lens vaulted symmetrically posteriorly such that there was adequate anterior capsular overlap of the plate haptics and a sufficient gap between the capsulorhexis and the sides of the optic. The patient's UCVA was 20/15 at distance and J6 at near 8 days postoperatively (Figure 6). Her near vision should improve over time.

THE PREVENTION OF CAPSULAR CONTRACTION

Capsular contraction syndrome, reported in 1993 by Davison[3] and by Hanson et al[4] is a complication of the continuous curvilinear capsulorhexis with an exaggerated reduction in the equatorial diameter of the capsular bag. Histologically, lens epithelial cells line the internal surface of the anterior capsule and capsular fornix. Pathologically, these cuboidal epithelial cells can undergo metaplasia with myofibroblastic transformation. The altered cells contain smooth muscle actin, and contraction occurs in the resultant fibrous membrane. Eradicating most of these cells will therefore help to prevent capsular contraction syndrome. This step can be accomplished in two basic ways: (1) removing a greater portion of the anterior capsule by making a large anterior capsulotomy and (2) meticulous cleaning of the anterior capsule and capsular fornix.

In a presentation at the 2008 annual meeting of the ASCRS, I demonstrated the effects of making a 6 X 7-mm capsulorhexis (Figure 7) in combination with the removal of lens epithelial cells using an ultrasonic I/A tip and Shepherd Capsule Polishers (Momentum Medical, Inc., Tampa, FL) (Figure 8). Of 100 eyes, none showed even the slightest contraction of the anterior capsulotomy (based on slit-lamp photographs), and the mean change in refraction between 1 to 3 weeks and 4 to 6 months was only 0.08 D.[5]

In his presentation during the 2008 ASCRS Innovators Award Session, David Apple, MD, showed postmortem specimens of three-piece AcrySof IOLs (Alcon Laboratories, Inc., Fort Worth, TX) with extensive proliferation of lens epithelial cells around the haptics and behind the optic in more than 50% of the eyes.[6] Earlier published reports of the rate of posterior capsular opacification (PCO) with this IOL were as low as 3%.[7] Claiming that "cadavers never lie," Dr. Apple stated, "It is not a matter of if PCO will happen; it is a matter of when PCO will happen. LECs [lens epithelial cells] retained in the capsule bag continue living and proliferate, and will form a Soemmering's ring, which is a precursor to PCO." Dr. Apple showed postmortem specimens in which proliferating lens epithelial cells were displacing the loops and/or optic of the Acrysof IOLs. He concluded, "Stable and long-term fixation of refractive IOLs in the capsular bag will require extensive cleanup or eradication of LECs from the lens capsule. This will be particularly important for accommodating

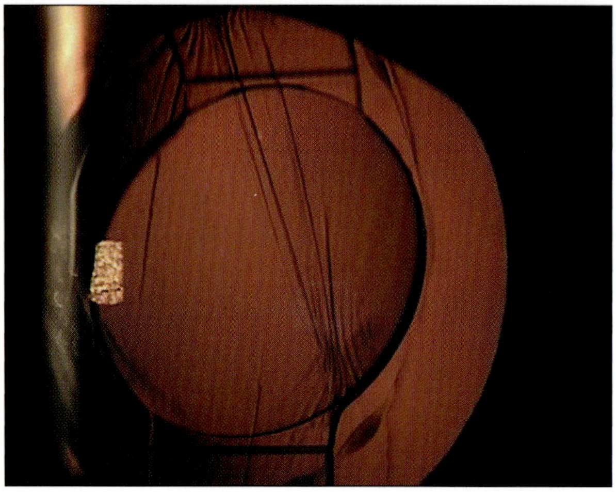

Figure 5. A Crystalens Five-O with asymmetric vaulting and retraction of the capsulorhexis. The superior plate haptic had excessive anterior vaulting with the hinge located anterior to the iris plane. The inferior plate had excessive posterior vaulting.

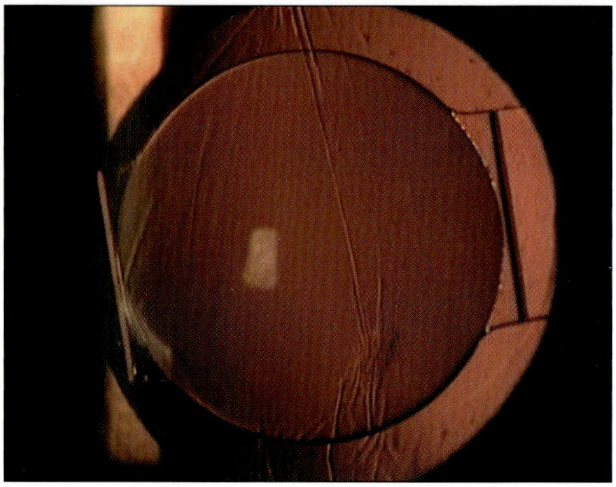

Figure 6. A repositioned Crystalens Five-O with a CTR and posterior capsular folds.

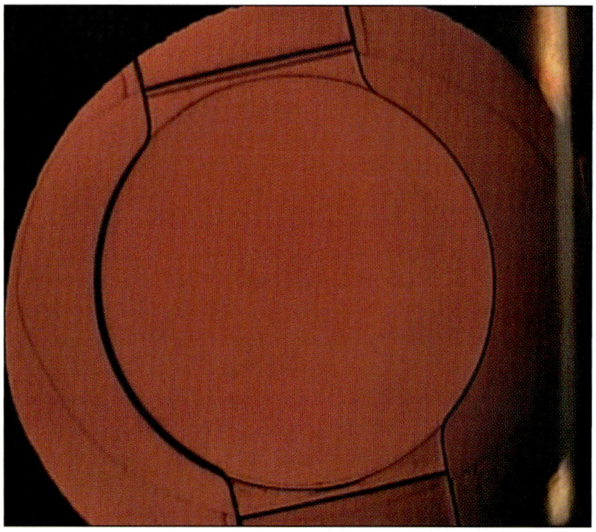

Figure 7. The surgeon created a 6 X 7-mm capsulorhexis through which to implant the Crystalens Five-O.

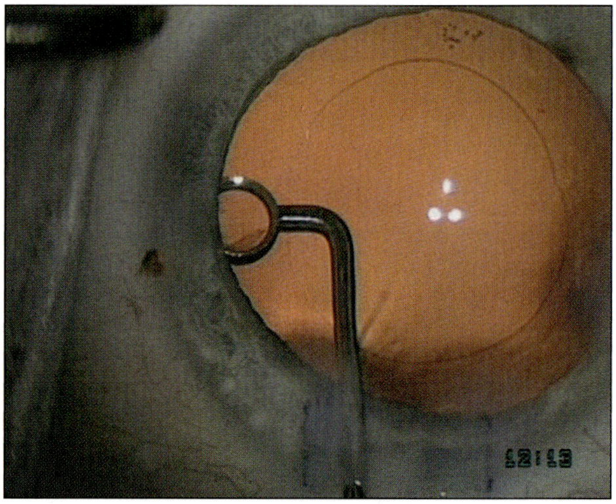

Figure 8. Shepherd Capsule Polishers.

IOLs."[6] My 5.5 years of experience with the Crystalens Five-O and AT-45SE implants along with the removal of lens epithelial cells (using a combination of ultrasonic I/A with gravity-powered outflow and Shepherd Capsule Polishers) has borne out Dr. Apple's prediction. ■

This article originally appeared in the September 2008 issue of CRSToday.

1. Waltz K. Accommodative arching of the natural lens and the Crystalens IOL. Paper presented at: The ASCRS Symposium on Cataract, IOL and Refractive Surgery; March 19, 2006; San Francisco, CA.
2. Singer J. Asymmetric vaulting of Crystalens AT50SE following phaco of traumatic cataract and secondary CTR implantation in a 32-year old. Paper presented at: The ASCRS Symposium on Cataract, IOL and Refractive Surgery; April 7, 2008; Chicago, IL.
3. Davison JA. Capsule contraction syndrome. *J Cataract Refract Surg.* 1993;19:582-589.
4. Hanson S, Crandall A, Olson R. Progressive constriction of the anterior capsular opening following intact capsulorhexis. *J Cataract Refract Surg.* 1993;19:77-82.
5. Singer J. Stability of capsulorhexis size and refraction following Crystalens Five-0 implantation with anterior capsule lens epithelial cell removal. Paper presented at: The ASCRS Symposium on Cataract, IOL and Refractive Surgery; April 6, 2008; Chicago, IL.
6. Apple DJ. Eradication and cleanup of lens substance and LECs: providing stable and long-term fixation of specialized IOLs in the capsular bag. Paper presented at: The ASCRS Symposium on Cataract, IOL and Refractive Surgery; April 7, 2008; Chicago, IL.
7. Prosdocimo G, Tassinari G, Sala M, et al. Posterior capsule opacification after phacoemulsification: silicone CeeOn Edge versus acrylate AcrySof intraocular lens. *J Cataract Refract Surg.* 2003;29(8):1551-1555.

CHAPTER 199

Pearls for IOL Exchanges With Multifocals

STEVEN J. DELL, MD

Some premium IOL patients experience a host of problems in the early postoperative period, rather than a chief complaint. Multiple irritations can compound one another until the patient is so frustrated that he cannot rationally describe what is bothering him. This can result in a flood of complaints that seem insurmountable. The trick to assuaging these patients is to maintain a calm and helpful demeanor and then systematically break each complaint down into a manageable component.

ASK A LOT OF QUESTIONS

I have found that some patients have a difficult time differentiating between problems they *see* and problems they *feel*, and they may assume the two types of complaints are linked. For example, if a patient says, "I feel like there's something in my eye," you must ask him to clarify. Is he seeing something in his field of vision, or is he feeling an irritant in his eye? Is he seeing unwanted images? You must determine whether this is a refractive error, or if it is something like cystoid macular edema or capsular opacification. Is the accommodation insufficient, or is the near visual range in the wrong place? Is he simply unhappy with his intermediate vision? Is the problem something he is feeling; is it an irritation due to the cataract incision, a limbal relaxing incision, dry eye, or blepharitis? These things are obviously important to differentiate, and they often coexist.

REFRACTIVE PROBLEMS

Contact Lens Trial

The next level of possibilities revolve around the IOL power and any remaining astigmatism. With any multifocal or accommodating lens, does the complaint resolve when the eyes are taken to their refractive target (if the original target was not achieved)? Try placing the patient in trial frames, contact lenses, or spectacles that give him the prescription you originally intended. For instance, if you planned -0.75 D OD and -0.25 D OS, and you achieved -2.00 D OD and 0.25 D OS, take the eyes to their target and see if the problem goes away. The best and most precise solution for refractive enhancements in my experience is the excimer laser.

Red Glasses

Sometimes, a patient who has received bilateral diffractive multifocal IOLs appears perfect on paper, but he still dislikes his postoperative vision for nonspecific reasons. After excluding all other remedies, you might want to try this test. Alcon Laboratories, Inc. (Fort Worth, TX), makes a pair of red-framed glasses in -3.00 D. You ask the unhappy patient to try them on, and these glasses will take his near point out to infinity, forcing him to use his near focus for distance. With no near focal point, he will experience the absolute presbyopia of pseudophakia. Explain that that is what his vision would be like with standard monofocal IOLs. Often, these patients instantly decide that the vision they have is not so bad after all, and they quickly become quite satisfied.

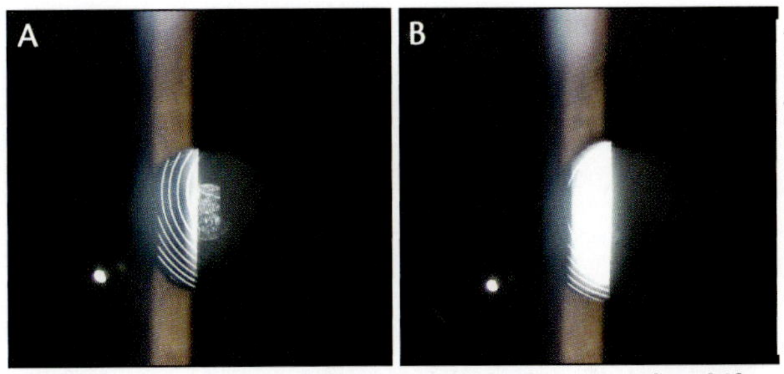

(Courtesy of Eric D. Donnenfeld, MD.)

Figure 1. One approach for correcting a decentered multifocal diffractive IOL is to apply four iridoplasty treatment spots with an argon laser to align the pupil with the IOL. Shown here are the pre- (A) and postoperative (B) images.

EXCHANGING

Setting Expectations

If you have exhausted other forms of visual correction and the patient still wishes to have his IOL(s) exchanged, it is critical that he be willing to accept any possible complications that can occur with the procedure. If I feel I need to get this point across to a patient, I may say something like, "Important parts of your eye might need to be removed along with the IOL." Furthermore, I often suggest that the patient seek a second opinion, because they can be very helpful in such emotional situations.

Does the Lens Always Have to Come Out?

It is possible that an IOL needs only to be repositioned rather than replaced. The ideal placement for multifocal diffractive IOLs is controversial. Some surgeons believe that they should be centered on the entrance pupil, but I tend to center them on the best approximation of the visual axis. One reliable way to do this is to instill a little bit of Miostat (Alcon Laboratories, Inc.) and let the pupil come down to a mid-dilated range, and then nudge the lens slightly nasally from the center of the pupil. For eyes in which these lenses are clearly decentered, Eric D. Donnenfeld, MD, of Rockville Centre, New York, has a slightly different approach. He makes four spots with an argon laser (500 mw for 500 milliseconds to produce a 500-µm spot size) to pull the pupil toward the IOL, instead of moving the IOL to the pupil (Figure 1A and B).

What if a patient has a Crystalens accommodating IOL (Bausch & Lomb, Rochester, NY) with insufficient accommodation? All the data from the patients in the Crystalens FDA clinical trial[1] indicate that their accommodation improved with time. Furthermore, the new Crystalens HD (Bausch & Lomb) offers improved near vision over the original Crystalens AT-45, so perhaps this issue will be less of a problem in the future. In general, I prefer discussing complaints of insufficient accommodation over those relating to distorted vision from a multifocal, because the former discussion usually ends when I tell the patient that the remedy is a weak pair of readers worn occasionally.

CONCLUSION

Multifocal IOLs require a mixed application of art and science. Recall that preoperatively, we practitioners actively solicit complaints from our patients to determine their need for cataract surgery. We prompt them to describe things such as glare and halos in detail, and we document their lifestyle impairments due to these visual problems. We shouldn't be surprised or defensive, therefore, when they continue this pattern of complaint reporting postoperatively. The first steps toward resolving postsurgical dissatisfaction is correctly identifying the problem(s), and then helping the patient understand the available options for solving them together. ■

This article originally appeared in CRSToday's *August 2008 Best of Source supplement.*

1. Data on file with Bausch & Lomb.

CHAPTER 200

Microinstrumentation in IOL Exchange

JENNIFER CALAFATI, MD; DIAMOND Y. TAM, MD; AND IQBAL IKE K. AHMED, MD, FRCSC

Anterior segment surgery has evolved from large-incision intracapsular cataract extraction to bimanual microincisional phacoemulsification. Complications related to the inadvertent intraoperative injury of the capsule or zonules, the bag/sulcus placement of an IOL, postoperative trauma, capsular contraction syndrome, or progressive zonulopathy from pseudoexfoliation syndrome may require the surgical repositioning of the optic. An IOL exchange may become necessary if the lens is sufficiently unstable or dislocated, if the IOL is improperly sized or centered, if lenticular opacification or dysphotopsias occur, or if the IOL causes an ocular comorbidity (eg, corneal edema, anterior chamber inflammation, uveitis-glaucoma-hyphema syndrome, or cystoid macular edema). When manipulating an IOL in such situations, exquisite control of the anterior segment, and at times the posterior segment, is of great utility to the surgeon. Microinstrumentation and small incisions can enhance the stability of the anterior chamber, vitreous management, and the security of the IOL.

MicroSurgical Technology (MST; Redmond, WA) manufactures the microanterior segment set, which consists of a micrograsper, a microtying forceps, microscissors (straight and angled), and an optional IOL cutting scissors (Figure 1). Two different types of handle are available, and the differing functional heads can be interchanged. One of the handles only permits the interchanging of the different heads, whereas the other allows an additional 360° rotation of the instrument's head. In order to close the forceps' or scissors' tip, the surgeon squeezes his thumb and index finger in a pincer grasp around the handle while the shaft of the handle rests on his middle finger.[1] This article reviews the microinstruments from MST and their use.

MICROGRASPER

The micrograsper has a 23-gauge tip, allowing this instrument to access the anterior chamber through a sub–1-mm incision. The

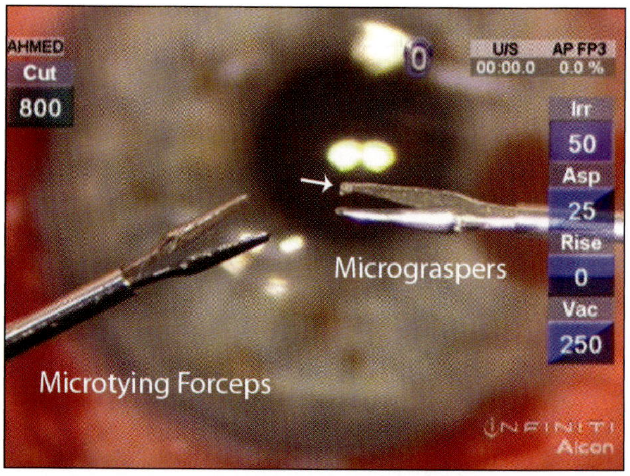

Figure 1. The microtying forceps is shown left. On the right, an arrow indicates the angled tip of the micrograsping forceps.

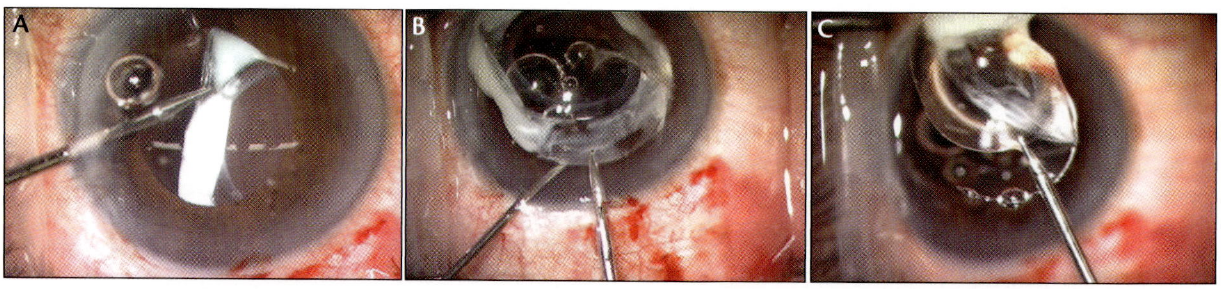

Figure 2. The micrograsper secures the haptic of a subluxated single-piece PMMA IOL at the haptic/optic junction (A). The surgeon has prolapsed a single-piece PMMA IOL into the anterior chamber and has secured the proximal haptic with the micrograsping forceps in preparation for the lens' explantation (B). The forceps holds the explanted IOL/capsular bag complex (C).

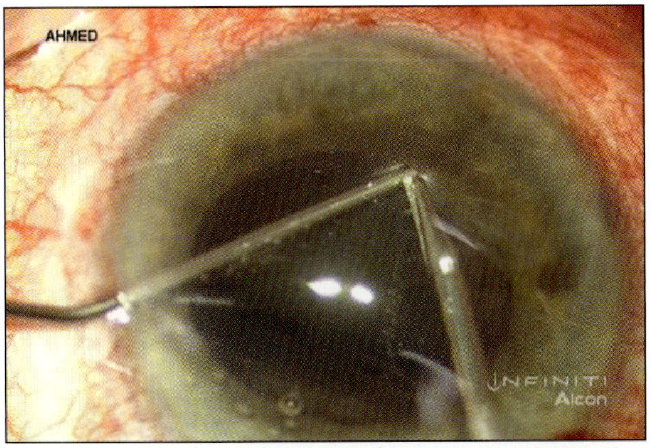

Figure 3. During the explantation of an in-the-bag PCIOL, the surgeon uses the micrograsper to engage the edge of the capsulorhexis and lift the anterior capsule off the IOL's optic to facilitate the injection of viscoelastic into the bag.

forceps' angled, semisharp tip enables the instrument to engage and grasp tissue (eg, iris, capsule) or an IOL easily. The inner surface of the jaws is smooth to avoid traumatizing ocular tissue during maneuvers in the anterior chamber. We prefer the straight design, which allows for easy 360° rotation of the tip.

During IOL exchange, the main use of the micrograsper is for securing the IOL. It is not uncommon for a subluxated IOL in the posterior chamber to be floating freely on the anterior hyaloid face, from where it is dangerously close to falling posteriorly toward the retina. We use the micrograsper to secure the IOL by its haptic, its optic, or the anterior capsule, provided that the adhesion between the IOL and the capsular remnant is sufficient to ensure that grasping the capsule means securing the IOL. After the IOL has been captured and freed of vitreous adhesions, the surgeon may use the micrograsper to bring the IOL forward into the anterior chamber with the assistance of instruments such as a Kuglen or Sinskey hook. The pupil may then be constricted with intracameral acetylcholine and the microforceps, and the IOL may be explanted (Figure 2).

When a PCIOL must be explanted from the capsular bag—with or without an intact posterior capsule—we find the micrograspers useful for lifting the anterior capsule off the optic or the posterior capsule so that we may viscodissect the capsular bag to free the PCIOL (Figure 3). Once the optic and haptics are mobile, we use the micrograsper and a hook to dial the PCIOL out of the bag. If we cannot move a haptic, we use the micrograsper and IOL cutting scissors to amputate it.

We also find the micrograsper useful for handling iris tissue during the implantation of iris-claw–style IOLs. The forceps is an alternative to an enclavation needle. We fixate the IOL with a microtying forceps. We use the micrograsping forceps to engage the iris beneath the claw haptic and bring the iris tissue anteriorly through each side of the claw[2] (Figure 4). We repeat the procedure with the other haptic to fixate the IOL completely.

If profound zonular weakness is destabilizing the IOL but the capsular bag is intact or in the setting of primary cataract extraction, we may use a capsular tension segment (requires an exemption for compassionate use from the FDA) to safely fixate an endocapsular IOL. The capsular tension segment's precise positioning is essential as we pass the needle through the fixation islet, and we have found the micrograsper useful for manipulating the device (Figure 5).

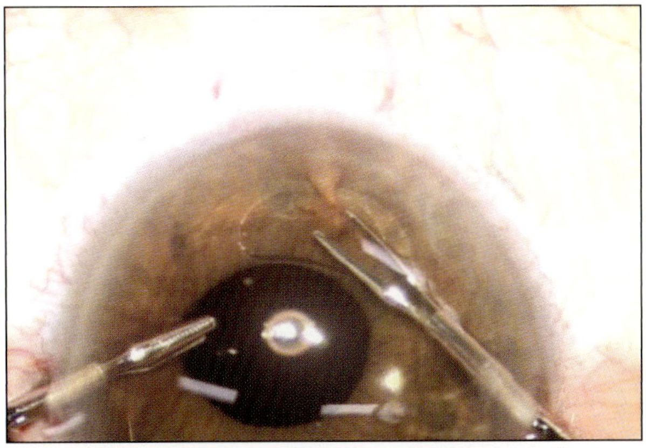

Figure 4. The surgeon uses the microtying forceps to fixate an iris claw IOL (left) and employs the micrograsper to enclavate iris tissue into the claw haptic (right).

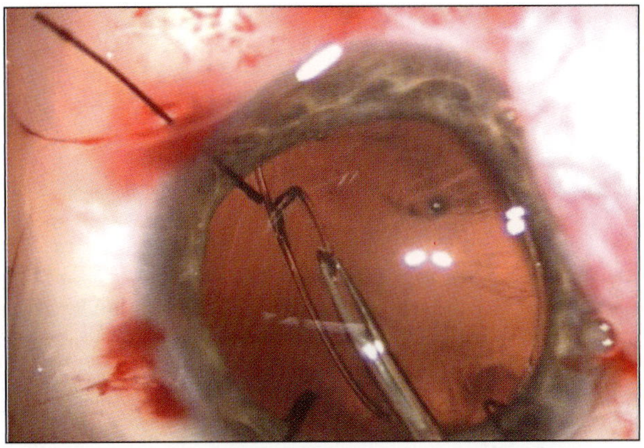

Figure 5. The micrograsper facilitates the positioning of a capsular tension segment in the anterior chamber.

MICROTYING FORCEPS

The microtying forceps has a smooth, rounded, 23-gauge tip and a smooth inner surface to minimize trauma to the suturing material. The instrument is designed to fit through incisions of approximately 1 mm. Iris fixation of IOLs as well as pupillary repair and iris suturing require the ab interno tying of sutures. Although the McCannel suturing technique and the Siepser sliding knot and its variations are the most commonly utilized methods of tying sutures passed through the iris, these techniques require that iris tissue be brought to a corneal incision for tying a secure knot. Tears in the iris, iridodialysis, and/or hyphema may occur, resulting in a haptic's slipping off the suture knot fixating it to the iris. Using two microtying forceps to tie a suture knot in the anterior chamber minimizes manipulation of and trauma to the iris. The use of microincisions helps to maintain anterior chamber stability (Figure 6). We then use a microscissors to cut the ends of the suture (typically 10–0 polypropylene) after tying the knot and positioning the IOL (Figure 7A).

MICROSCISSORS

MST manufactures two types of microscissors: straight, available in 21- and 23-gauge sizes, and angled vertical, available in 21 gauge. In addition to their aforementioned utility when cutting suture knots, we use these scissors to sever thin strands or small sheets of vitreous present in the anterior chamber and attached to corneal incisions. Surgeons may also use microscissors to create

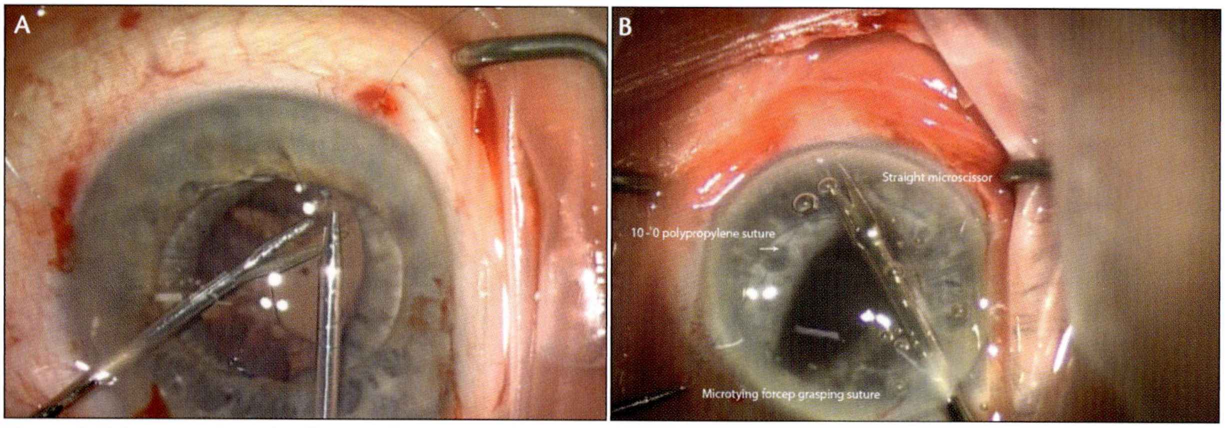

Figure 6. Using two microtying forceps, the surgeon ties a suture knot around the PMMA haptic of a three-piece foldable IOL and iris tissue (A). He then cuts the suture ends with straight microscissors (B).

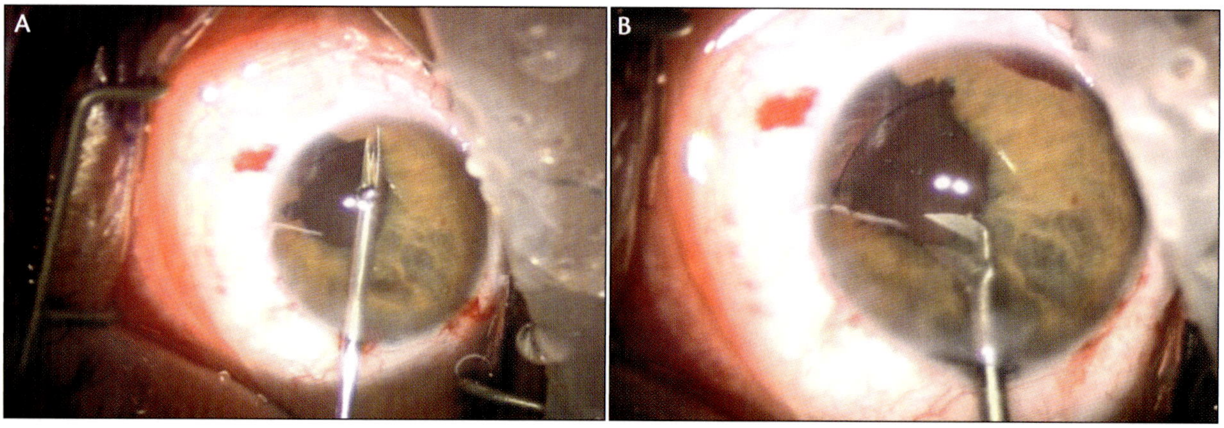

Figure 7. Using a microscissors, the surgeon creates relaxing incisions to facilitate subsequent pupilloplasty in an iris coloboma (A). Angled vertical scissors access iris tissue that is proximal to the incision (B).

small sphincterotomies in the iris at the pupillary margin to enlarge a small pupil, to create relaxing incisions in iris tissue to facilitate pupilloplasty, and to incise the anterior or posterior capsule to facilitate the enlargement or creation of a capsulorhexis (Figure 7B).

IOL CUTTERS

The 19-gauge IOL cutters are slightly heavier duty than MST's microscissors. The IOL cutter fits through a standard 2.5-mm clear corneal coaxial phaco incision. In cases of a malpositioned acrylic or silicone IOL, the surgeon may use the IOL cutter to segment the lens to allow for its removal through an incision smaller than the optic[3] (Figure 8). This instrument may also be used to amputate a haptic from the optic if required.

CONCLUSION

Although the endocapsular implantation of an IOL is usually successful, complications may arise that necessitate an IOL exchange. Microinstrumentation enables anterior segment surgeons to use small incisions and work in a closed system, and it provides exquisite control of anterior chamber stability as well as greater ease of vitreous management. When iris repair or iris-sutured fixation of an IOL becomes necessary, we find that microinstrumentation enables us to handle delicate ocular tissues without further injury or trauma. ■

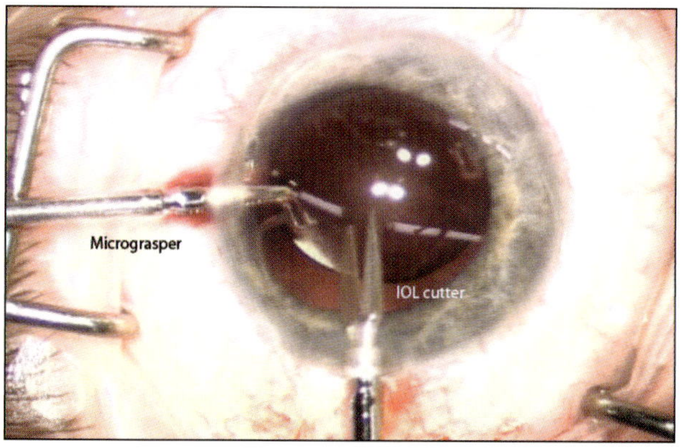

Figure 8. The IOL cutting scissors segment a subluxated IOL that is fixated in the anterior chamber by a micrograsper on the left side.

This article originally appeared in the October 2008 issue of CRSToday.

1. Ahmed I. Micro Instrumentation in the Anterior Segment [video]. http://www.mstsurgical.com/LL/index.php?/weblog/video_tempate_2.0_late_2006/. Accessed July 18, 2008.
2. Teichman J, Ahmed I. Improved technique with the Artisan Aphakic IOL. *Review of Ophthalmology*. 2007;14(10):59-65.
3. Chang D. IOL Exchange in FloMax Patient Using the MST Packer/Chang IOL Cutters [video]. http://www.mst-surgical.com/LL/index.php?/weblog/video_tempate_2.0_late_2006/. Accessed July 18, 2008.

NOTES

NOTES

NOTES

NOTES

NOTES

NOTES

NOTES

NOTES

NOTES

NOTES

NOTES

NOTES